UPDATE

ALTERNATE ITEM FORMAT

The format of the entire NCLEX-RN is not changing. Alternate item format has been introduced as of April 2003. Alternate item format includes: multiple choice items that will require you to choose more than one option, fill-in-the-blank items, identify an area on a picture or graphic image, and numerical entry items.

Here are examples of questions that represent these new types of questions.

Use the 60 test-taking tips and strategies discussed and illustrated in Unit 2 of this book (pp. 47–51) to help you answer these questions, especially tips #9, #14, #23, #24, #32, #34, #37, #39, #43, #44, #45, #48, #50, #51. #55, #56, #60.

Sample Psychosocial Question: Multiple Response Format
How would a nurse caring for a patient with receptive and expressive aphasia communicate with the patient?
 Check all approaches that specifically apply and are most relevant in the care of this patient.

☐ 1. Speak loudly
☐ 2. Use a picture board or flash cards
☐ 3. Use hands to communicate
☐ 4. Speak slowly
☐ 5. Encourage the patient to initiate meaningful communication
☐ 6. Provide support and encouragement

Sample Maternal-Newborn Question: Diagram and Fill-in-the-Blank Format
The client, 39 weeks gestation, gravida 2, para 1, is in active labor and complains of frequent, painful uterine contractions. Which fetal monitor pattern would require <u>immediate</u> nursing intervention?

Fill in the number of the correct pattern: _____ Name the pattern: _____

1.

2.

3.

Sample Pharmacological & Parenteral Therapy Question: Fill-in-the-Blank/Numerical Entry Format
The physician has ordered heparin 900 units/hour IV for a client. The pharmacy sends a solution that has 25,000 units of heparin in 500cc D5W. What would be the flow rate in cc/hour to infuse this order?

Fill in the correct answer: _____

Sample Pediatric Question: Fill-in-the-Blank Format
The nurse is assessing a child with a suspected communicable disease. The child has the following clinical manifestations:

Fever
"Slapped-face" appearance
Symmetrical, maculopapular, red rash on upper and lower extremities
Progression of rash from proximal to distal body surfaces

What communicable disease would the nurse be most concerned about?

Sample Psychosocial Question: Multiple Response Format
Answer/Rationale–correct answers are in **bold**
1. The nurse needs to speak distinctly, <u>not</u> loudly.
2. **A visual mode is helpful when the patient has difficulty hearing (auditory aphasia, receptive) or writing (visual, expressive aphasia).**
3. **Using gestures such as pointing is one way to establish and encourage communication.**
4. **Face the patient and speak slowly, allowing time to respond.**
5. With expressive aphasia, the patient will have difficulty in initiating speech, but may be able to articulate words that have no meaning.
6. Although support and encouragement need to be offered, these are general nursing approaches and not specific to this patient.

<u>Test-Taking Tip</u>
Be aware that the stem asks for specific approaches. Option #1 can be eliminated because hearing is not always impaired. Option #5 can be eliminated because it is theoretically incorrect. Option #6 can be eliminated because it is not specific to this patient.

Codes: Implementation, Psychosocial Adaptation

Sample Maternal-Newborn Question: Diagram and Fill-in-the-Blank Format
Answer/Rationale–correct answer is in **bold**
1. This option is incorrect because the pattern is early decelerations and is caused by compressions of the fetal head descending through the birth canal. No nursing intervention is needed.
2. **This is the correct answer because the pattern is late decelerations and is caused by uteroplacental insufficiency. The fetal heart rate is tachycardic, baseline heart rate of 180 BPM with decreased baseline variability. The nurse must immediately attempt to correct the pattern by turning the client on her side, giving a fluid bolus and oxygen via mask. The physician must also be immediately notified.**
3. This is incorrect because this pattern is variable decelerations, caused by compression of the umbilical cord. The fetus demonstrates good oxygen reserve since the baseline variability is normal and the fetal heart rate rapidly returns to baseline after the deceleration. Immediate intervention in this type of pattern is not required, but continued close observation of the pattern is needed.

<u>Test-Taking Tip</u>
To determine the type of deceleration, draw a line from the lowest part of the deceleration down to the uterine contraction, to establish the relationship as early, variable, or late between the deceleration and the uterine contraction.

Codes: Analysis, Physiological Adaptation

Sample Pharmacological & Parenteral Therapy Question: Fill-in-the-Blank/Numerical Entry Format
Answer
18 cc/hour

Rationale
The solution contains 50 units/cc. It is a simple matter to divide 900 units/hour of heparin by 50 units/cc to obtain the hourly flow rate.

<u>Test-Taking Tip</u>
The first step in completing this calculation is to determine how many units of heparin are in each cc of IV fluid:
25,000 units/500 cc = 50 units/cc.

Because there are 50 units in each cc of IV fluid, how many ccs will it take to deliver 900 units? $\dfrac{900 \text{ units/hour}}{50 \text{ units/cc}} = 18$ cc/hour

Code: Implementation, Pharmacological & Parenteral Therapies

Sample Pediatric Question: Fill-in-the-Blank Format
Answer

_____

(Erythema Infectiosum/Fifth's Disease)

_____

The rash associated with erythema infectiosum/fifth disease appears in three stages:
1. A brief period of erythema on the face and cheeks resulting in a "slapped-face" appearance.
2. Symmetrical, maculopapular, red rash on the upper and lower extremities. Rash progresses from proximal to distal surfaces and usually appears about one day after the facial rash and may last up to a week.
3. Rash gradually disappears but can reappear if the skin is irritated or traumatized. The child is in the early stages of erythema infectiosum/fifth disease. Chickenpox (varicella) is characterized by simultaneous macules, papules, and vesicles and pruritus. Measles (rubeola) is characterized by macules, papules, and Koplik spots. German measles (rubella) is characterized by macules, papules, and malaise. Mumps is characterized by an earache that is aggravated by chewing and parotitis.

<u>Test-Taking Tip</u>
Know all of the types of rashes associated with the most common communicable diseases and the one characteristic associated ONLY with that disease process.

Codes: Analysis, Physiological Adaptation

Davis's
NCLEX-RN Success

Edited by

Sally L. Lagerquist, RN, MS

Written by

Geraldine C. Colombraro, PhD, RN

Assistant Dean for Administration, Leinhard School of Nursing, Pace University, New York

Sally Lambert Lagerquist, RN, MS

Former Instructor of Undergraduate, Graduate, and Continuing Education in Nursing,
University of California, San Francisco, School of Nursing; President,
Review for Nurses, Inc., and RN Tapes Company, San Francisco

Bobbi Morrison, ARNP, MN, PhD Candidate

Women's Health Nurse Practitioner; Instructor, Intercollegiate Center for Nursing Education,
Washington State University College of Nursing, Spokane, Washington

Robyn Marchal Nelson, DNSc, RN

Chair and Professor, Division of Nursing, California State University, Sacramento

Janice Horman Stecchi, RN, EdD

Dean, College of Health Professions, University of Massachusetts Lowell, Lowell, Massachusetts

F. A. DAVIS COMPANY
Philadelphia

F.A. Davis Company
1915 Arch Street
Philadelphia, PA 19103
www.fadavis.com

A modified version of this text was previously published as *Addison-Wesley's Nursing Examination Review* by Addison-Wesley Nursing, A Division of The Benjamin/Cummings Publishing Company, Inc. Copyright © 1991; and *Little, Brown's NCLEX-RN Examination Review* by Little, Brown and Company. Copyright © 1996 by Sally L. Lagerquist.

Printed in the United States of America

Last digit indicates print number: 10 9 8 7 6 5 4 3

Acquisitions Editor: Melanie Freely
Cover Designer: Louis J. Forgione

As new scientific information becomes available through basic and clinical research, recommended treatments and drug therapies undergo changes. The author(s) and publisher have done everything possible to make this book accurate, up to date, and in accord with accepted standards at the time of publication. The authors, editors, and publisher are not responsible for errors or omissions or for consequences from application of the book, and make no warranty, expressed or implied, in regard to the contents of the book. Any practice described in this book should be applied by the reader in accordance with professional standards of care used in regard to the unique circumstances that may apply in each situation. The reader is advised always to check product information (package inserts) for changes and new information regarding dose and contraindications before administering any drug. Caution is especially urged when using new or infrequently ordered drugs.

Library of Congress Cataloging-in-Publication Data

Davis's NCLEX-RN success / edited by Sally L. Lagerquist.
    p.   cm.
Includes bibliographical references and index.
ISBN 0-8036-0816-0
   1. Nursing—Examinations, questions, etc. I. Title: NCLEX-RN success. II. Lagerquist, Sally L.

RT55 .D386 2001
610.73′076—dc21

00-064388

Dedications

I dedicate this book—

To my husband, Tom—you are one-of-a-kind!

I treasure all my days and all the 35 years we spent together—caring and sharing . . . there is no comparing—I am grateful that life presented you.

I am proud of you and your "gifts" of quiet strength, gentleness, and devotion to us.

I can't imagine a husband who is more compassionate nor a father who is more giving than you are. You provide such humor, care, concern, perspective and stability!

What an incredible role model you are!

To our daughter, Elana—

All that is beautiful is encompassed in you!

Your growth into womanhood and progress in academia are wondrous to watch, as your life unfolds—as an educator in theater arts and as a partner with Dan.

You are adventurous and uniquely creative, with your own blend of traditionalism, and special caring family ways.

To Dan—

Welcome to the family! We are proud of you! Here is to sharing all the joys that are yet to be!

To our son, Kalen—

I look at you with love, and great appreciation for all that you have done for us, for "Review for Nurses" all these countless years! You have been our mainstay; we could not have continued without you.

I look to you with hope and pride, as you explore possibilities in what is yet to be in your "trip" to somewhere new and great. You have so many skills!

I will encourage you as you give shape to your dreams and meet the challenges that define your life.

My love is always there.

My heart will gladly share.

To Adair Tench, my dear long-term friend and my very own editorial assistant—

I greatly acknowledge, with immense appreciation, your assistance (each and every moment of it!) as we prepared this book for publication.

I couldn't have done this book without your enthusiasm, your extraordinary support and patience (yes, my handwriting was impossible, and electronic publishing was a challenge that you mastered for this project!)

I will long remember your many "long day journeys into the night" at Woodside, assisting me in putting together contributors' work; your months at the computer with my own chapters; and the hours spent at the copier.

Your caring and warm personality, along with your energy and commitment to this project, is what led us to success in the creation of this book.

In my book, you "passed the test"!

—Sally L. Lagerquist

To my husband of 26 years, Bruce, with all my love and thanks;
I could not have done it without you.
For your support and all the meals you cooked while I typed,
For your smiles and all the faith you always have in me,
For your tenderness and caring,
For your pride in my accomplishments,
For your love throughout the years.
You are *the best* husband and father a woman could be married to.
—*Geraldine C. Colombraro*

This is dedicated to my soul-mate, Ron. I am continually amazed at every stage of our lives how much we are alike. I am forever grateful that throughout our journey we have experienced our "epiphanies" together. Your acknowledgment of who I am has inspired me more than you will ever know. Thank you!

I also dedicate this to my nursing students, who challenge and motivate me to work harder and know more everyday. For you, I lovingly prepare these words to help you succeed in your careers. It will be an amazing journey, I promise!
—*Bobbi Morrison*

I feel a bit like a member of a relay team . . . passing the baton of professional practice to my team members . . . those of you who are taking the licensing examination and entering the profession of nursing in the 21st century. You are racing to the "finish line" of this stage of your educational experience! Grip the baton firmly and never waver in your commitment to nursing. Your trophy will be a lifetime of professional service essential to the health of the community in which you practice and personal rewards that are unmatched by many career choices.

No race would be complete without the "cheers" from the grandstand—thanks to my husband, Dean, daughters, Kelly and Tina, parents, Gordon and Patty Marchal, and to my faculty colleagues who "coach" the new members of the nursing team!

You are all winners!!
—*Robyn M. Nelson*

To Dave, my husband and best friend for over forty years, you have always been the one to encourage me to reach for the prize and never complain when that takes so much of "our time." Thank you. There are very few who have such a generous and understanding mate. To our sons, Dave, Bill, and Joe, all in New England again. It is so nice to share our times together. We are very proud of each of you and love you very much. Stay healthy and happy. Many fond memories of our son Tommy, my parents, Esther and Joe Horman and my father-in-law Dave came to me during the writing of this book. I miss each of you. To my mother-in-law Helen, we love you and wish you good health as you begin a new part of your life.

To all nurses who will read this book. Your patients need more than just your technical skills. They need your knowledge, understanding, and recognition of what they are experiencing. They need you to help them through their problems in this ever-changing health care system, now more than ever before. I hope nursing is as rewarding for you as it has been for me. Your greatest reward will come when *you* know that *you* have made a difference in a patient's life.
—*Janice Horman Stecchi*

About the Editor/Authors

Sally Lambert Lagerquist, RN, MS, is the author and editor of four editions of *Practice Questions and Answers for NCLEX-RN*, published by Review for Nurses Tapes Co.; *How to Pass Nursing Exams*, published by Review Press; four editions of *Addison Wesley's Nursing Examination Reviews* (1977–1992); four books for *NURSENOTES* series: *Psychiatric-Mental Health, Maternal-Newborn, Pediatrics, Medical-Surgical*, published by Lippincott; *Little, Brown's NCLEX-RN Examination Review*, and *Little, Brown's Nursing Q&A: Critical-Thinking Exercises*, published by Little, Brown and Company. She is president and course coordinator of *Review for Nurses, Inc.* She has coordinated RN licensure exam review courses on campuses nationwide since 1976. She is presently a lecturer on test-taking techniques at workshops held nationwide for graduating senior nursing students. She has produced and developed The *NCLEX-RN Board Game* and audio and video tapes on *Nursing Review* and *Successful Test-Taking Techniques for Nurses*. She originated, developed, and has presented *national satellite telecourses* for NCLEX-RN review since June 1989. She is also a marriage, family, and child counselor and a member of Sigma Theta Tau. She has been a faculty member at the University of California at San Francisco School of Nursing for over ten years, where she also received her BS and MS degrees.

Gerrie Colombraro, PhD, RN, has been a nurse for over 25 years and has a broad range of clinical educational, and administrative experiences. After graduation from her baccalaureate program, Gerrie practiced extensively in pediatric and neonatal nursing. She first began teaching national licensure exam reviews in 1981, and has remained active in this area ever since. In addition to teaching review courses, Gerrie has been a contributing author of national and international licensure review books, question-and-answer books, and pediatric study guides; she has also published professional articles about licensure preparation. In addition to her review course experience with *Review for Nurses, Inc.*, Gerrie has worked as an educator in entry-level nursing programs where she taught pediatrics. Gerrie is currently the Assistant Dean for Administration at the Lienhard School of Nursing at Pace University in New York.

Bobbi Morrison, ARNP, MN, PhD candidate, is a Women's Health Nurse Practitioner, and an instructor of nursing at Washington State University College of Nursing in Spokane, Washington. She has been a lecturer for several years for *Review for Nurses, Inc.* She received her BSN from Gonzaga University, her MN from Washington State University, and is currently a doctoral candidate at Gonzaga University. She has practiced maternity and women's health nursing for over 25 years.

Robyn M. Nelson, DNSc, RN, is chairperson and professor in the Division of Nursing at California State University, Sacramento. She currently teaches research and issues and ethics at the graduate level over distance education and the web. She received her BS in Nursing from Loma Linda University, her MS from Boston University, and a Doctor of Nursing Science degree from the University of California, San Francisco. In addition to F.A. Davis's *NCLEX-RN Success*, she is co-author of *Nurse Notes: Medical-Surgical Nursing* (Lippincott), a contributor to *Nursing Q and A* (Lippincott), and has developed a number of audio and visual aids for students preparing for the licensure examination. Dr. Nelson has been a lecturer for *Review for Nurses, Inc.*, for 20 years both at on-site national review courses and as one of the faculty for the "first ever" nationally televised satellite review course that was offered for 7 years. She holds memberships in Sigma Theta Tau International, ANA, ANA/California, and Phi Kappa Phi. Dr. Nelson is a member of the Bioethics Committee of Sutter Community Medical Center, and Vice President of Planning for LearnWell, Inc., a nonprofit education group.

Janice Stecchi, EdD, RN, is presently Dean of the College of Health Professions at the University of Massachusetts Lowell. The College graduates students in nursing, exercise physiology, physical therapy, health services administration, health education, medical technology, and clinical laboratory sciences. Dr. Stecchi is Professor of Nursing and the Director of the Center for Health Promotion. She received her BS in Nursing from Boston College, MEd from Salem State

College, MS in Nursing from Boston University, and Doctorate in Education from Boston University. In addition to F.A. Davis's *NCLEX-RN Success,* she is co-author of *Nurse Notes: Medical Surgical Nursing* (Lippincott), a contributor to *Nursing Q and A* (Lippincott), and author of other professional journal articles. Dr. Stecchi was a lecturer for *Review for Nurses, Inc.,* for 20 years. She has served as a program evaluator for the National League for Nursing for 10 years and served a term on the Board of Review for Baccalaureate and Higher Degree Programs. Dr. Stecchi holds membership in ANA, NLN, Sigma Theta Tau, and Sigma Xi. Dr. Stecchi is the Vice Chair of the Board of Trustees of Saints Memorial Medical Center in Lowell, Massachusetts. Her present scholarly activities are focused on a multidisciplinary project, the Medical Translator, an electronic device that allows the health care provider to obtain vital information from patients who do not speak English. Dr. Stecchi's idea has become a reality with the partnership formed with electrical engineering faculty and students.

Money Back Guarantee

If you are a graduate of a nursing program accredited in the United States, take the NCLEX-RN for the first time, and do not pass after using *Davis's NCLEX-RN Success,* return the book to **F. A. Davis Company, Customer Service, 404-420 N. 2nd Street, Philadelphia, PA 19123**. Enclose your original receipt for purchase of the book and copies of your official test results notification and your certification of graduation. We will refund the price you paid for the book. If you have any questions, please call 800-323-3555.

Preface

We are very pleased that you have selected our book to help you on your path to success on NCLEX-RN.

Our aim is to lead you all the way, to have *PASSING NCLEX-RN MADE EASY* for you—the *first-time test-taker,* the *international* nurse and the *repeat test-taker.*

With a conceptual framework based on the components of the current NCLEX-RN Test Plan (four client needs & their ten subcategories), this book differs significantly from other nursing review books. It is the only nursing review book that thoroughly covers the content in the current NCLEX-RN Test Plan **and has a test tip for each of the 2001 questions!**

Each unit incorporates all the components of the most current test plan. However, **Unit 3** specifically includes content that focuses on **Safe, Effective Care Environment** (with *Management of Care*). **Units 4** and **5** emphasize **Health Promotion and Maintenance** (*Growth and Development, Prevention and Early Detection of Disease,* and *Safety and Infection Control*). **Unit 6** focuses specifically on **Psychosocial Integrity** (*Coping and Adaptation);* **Units 7, 8, 9,** and **10** emphasize **Physiological Integrity** (with **Unit 7** specifically addressing *Basic Care and Comfort, Infection Control, Prevention and Early Detection of Disease, Physiological Adaptation);* **Unit 9** is on *Nutrition and Diet Therapy;* **Unit 10** is devoted to *Pharmacological and Parenteral Therapies;* and **Unit 11** specifically emphasizes *Reduction of Risk Potential.*

In addition, **Unit 2** is a *new* unit that addresses the needs of the **international nurses** and **repeat test-takers;** and the *new* **Unit 8** addresses the needs of the *Older Adult.*

To locate where in the book you will find the *theory* and *practice questions* for each of the above named 10 subcategories of client needs that are tested on the exam, see **Appendices C, D,** and **E.**

Proven Results

This is the only review book for NCLEX-RN that has evolved from and has been tested with over 300,000 NCLEX-RN candidates who have taken our national nursing exam review courses over the last **30 years** and **passed!** These courses emphasize a comprehensive review of *commonalities* in client care throughout the life span and in a variety of clinical settings. The content, the framework, the sequence of topics, the test-taking guidelines, and the practice exam questions and answers in this book have been tested during the past 30 years with *actual examination candidates* who have passed the RN licensure exam with highly successful results. **This gives the material an authenticity and relevance that is difficult to attain in any other way.**

Conceptual Framework

The conceptual framework of this book concentrates on nursing concerns for *client needs* and the essential requirements for safe, effective, competent nursing care. The text emphasizes *practical application* of clinically relevant data. Each unit is organized in terms of the eight areas of human functions (which are subtopics of the four *client needs):* (1) Protective; (2) Sensory-Perceptual; (3) Comfort, Rest, Activity, and Mobility; (4) Nutrition; (5) Growth and Development; (6) Fluid-Gas Transport; (7) Psychosocial-Cultural, and (8) Elimination functions. (See **Appendix H** for definitions of these key terms, and **Appendices I** and **J** for an index to content (theory) in these key categories in the **text** and **test questions.)** Separate units emphasize the content areas of *nutrition; pharmacology; common diagnostic procedures, treatments, and nursing care;* and *management of care* including *ethical and legal aspects in nursing.* A *new* unit on the *older adult* has been added.

Special Features

There are many special features in this *abundantly illustrated* book that make it stand out from all other nursing review books. The most unique features to help you prepare for exams are **test-taking tips for each of the questions,** an *expanded* section on **memory aids (Appendix N),** lists of **common abbreviations and clinical signs (Appendices L** and **M)** that provide quick and interesting ways to review, and 14 detailed examples of *Clinical/Critical Pathways* (also known as *Patient Care Management Plans).* In the **Orientation** section of **Unit 1,** you'll also find **study tips and relaxation exercises,** along with more memorizing ideas.

Other features include:

- A practice **computer test** (CD-ROM) for self-assessment and familiarization with the NCLEX-RN computer testing format now includes **test-taking tips with each answer.**
- Many **easy-to-use and easy-to-find** tables summarize information for *quick* review and emphasize nursing responsibilities in a *visual* way.
- Boxed lab data, diagnostic tests indicated by a ▯, **drug information** indicated by a ⬭, **diets** indicated by a ▮●▮, **position** indicated by a ◪, **standard precautions** indicated by a ⬡, **mnemonic memory aids** indicated by a ♡, and **hands-on nursing care** indicated by a ▶ in the margin for quick reference. Also, **nursing diagnoses, positions, diets,** and **nursing procedures** are *italicized* for visual reinforcement.
- Easy-to-find **content divisions** are marked with black page tabs at the outer margin of each page.
- Unique **indexes to content and test questions** related to **10 specific subcategories of client needs (Appendices C** and **E)** and **4 general** (broad) **client needs (Appendix D),** as well as an index to **test questions** found at the end of each unit that cover specific steps of the **nursing process (Appendix G).** These indexes are based on the

official **NCLEX-RN Test Plan** and especially useful in facilitating review for **repeat exam-takers.**

■ Emphasis on **all five steps of the nursing process,** especially *health teaching* and specific *outcome criteria for evaluation* of the effectiveness of nursing care.

■ Current NANDA-approved *nursing diagnoses* as a structure for presenting nursing interventions.

■ A thorough **question-and-answer review** at the end of *each unit,* in a nursing process format reflecting **diverse cultural** influences.

This review book has been updated and revised to incorporate the latest knowledge and current trends in nursing practice, and to parallel the latest NCLEX-RN Test Plan. All content has been submitted to outstanding educators and nursing practitioners for their review and critique. We would like to express our appreciation to this editorial review panel for their contributions, which make this book the best to use for *complete* nursing review.

In **Unit 1, Orientation and Pre Test,** you will find suggestions on how to use this book and how to plan your study, information about the NCLEX-RN, *study tips and strategies,* help with memorization, and relaxation exercises. At the end of this unit is the **PreTest,** to use as self-assessment before reading the nursing content units that follow.

Unit 2, Guidelines and Tips for International Nurses and Repeat Test-takers is new. *No other book* addresses the special concerns of candidates who have taken the test more than once or are graduates of nursing programs outside of the United States. Unit 2 covers:

■ **risk factors** for not passing the first time.
■ 5 steps for what to do to pass next time.
■ how to know if you are prepared to take the exam again.
■ 60 test-taking tips and guidelines to use in answering questions.

Unit 3 has been greatly expanded and retitled **Management of Care—Cultural Diversity, Ethical and Legal Aspects, and Nursing Trends.** *New* content has been added: 10 aspects of *cultural* diversity relevant to nursing practice, as well as *religious* and *spiritual* influences on health; advance directives, advocacy, organ donation; bioethics and client rights; concepts of *management:* case management, quality assurance, variance reports, resource management, supervision, delegation, disaster planning.

New questions and answers with *test-taking tips* have been added.

An expanded review of patient restraints and nursing responsibilities has also been added.

Unit 4, Nursing Care of the Childbearing Family, is streamlined, visually enhanced, and up-to-date; it contains the most exam-relevant content for both pregnancy and care of the neonate. It is the only nursing review book that features **critical pathways** (intrapartum, postpartum, newborn). The unit includes *detailed* information regarding many important *diagnostic tests,* such as chorionic villi sampling and biophysical profile testing, to identify the woman

and fetus at risk. *New illustrations* have been included: amniocentesis, fetal circulation, and ectopic pregnancy. We include the latest information on *emergency care* in labor and birth, perinatal acquired immune deficiency syndrome, sexually transmitted diseases, and preterm labor. We provide information regarding new drug therapies during the perinatal period recommended for the at-risk infant. *Client teaching* and *nursing interventions* are delineated for each of these areas of practice. The question and answer sections also address these advances in technology and care.

Unit 5, Nursing Care of Children and Families, has *new* content on the role of the Pediatric nurse in *management of care* of infants, children, and adolescents, in *safety and infection control* (two **new tables**), in *prevention* and *early detection of disease* (two **new tables:** *preventive care timeline,* recommended *health screenings*); pediatric *emergencies;* and includes updated information concerning cardiac, respiratory, orthopedic systems, and communicable diseases, that has been synthesized into table format for *easier reading, recall, and application* to client care. Diagrams show genetic transmission of sickle cell anemia and hemophilia. *New illustrations* depict: five cardiac defects, pediatric CPR, TEF and esophageal atresia, developmental hip dysplasia, and scoliosis. Coverage is provided for Reye syndrome; Kawasaki disease; and salicylate, Tylenol, and lead poisoning. Content includes greatly expanded coverage in all areas of physical growth, normal development concerns, and parental counseling, as well as appreciation of cultural diversity in assessment and nursing interventions.

Unit 6, Nursing Care of Behavioral and Emotional Problems Throughout the Life Span, presents psychiatric disorders that have been organized under DSM-IV guidelines. We have included *thorough* coverage of suicide precautions, *midlife* crises, mental health of the *elderly,* substance abuse, panic disorders, posttraumatic disorder, amnestic disorders, personality disorders, sleep and eating disturbances, and affective disorders. Content includes a detailed section on psychiatric *emergencies* and therapeutic communication techniques. *Theoretical model* section has been greatly expanded to include Piaget's age-specific developmental levels, Duvall's Family Development, Kaplan's mental health model.

Also, three *new* developmental sections have been added: a table on development of *body image* (includes disturbances and four phases of crises); *human sexuality* throughout the life cycle (with causes of dysfunction, sexual health counseling, and sexual assessment interview format); and a table on *emotional disturbances in children.*

The *most unique* feature is the inclusion of six **clinical/ critical pathways** (eating disorder, alcohol withdrawal, posttrauma, depression, manic, schizophrenic psychoses).

Nine *new* sections are added: *domestic violence* (battered woman and child, and elder abuse/neglect); *diagnostic tests* (for dementia/cognitive disorders and alcohol abuse); mental status assessment (individual, cultural); interviewing; general principles of health teaching; self-concept; coping mechanisms; treatment modes; and an extensive glossary.

Unit 7, Nursing Care of the Acutely Ill and the Chronically Ill Adult, presents content under appropriate categories of human functions. *Risk factors* have been identified for all conditions, *goals of nursing* are clearly stated, five sample **clinical/critical pathways** have been added (MI, CHF, stroke, spinal fusion, hip arthroplasty), and a brief description of *pathophysiology* has been incorporated with each condition. **New tables** have been added: *Adult Immunizations* and *Preventive Care Timetable*. Other *tables* on fluid and electrolyte imbalances, acid-base disorders, assessment differences with valvular defects, hazards of immobility, complications of diabetes, and malignant disorders supplement the *condensed* and *consolidated content*. **New content** includes: hip fracture, GERDS, latex allergies, and Joint Commission requirements for Pain Assessment. The up-to-date content also includes acquired immune deficiency syndrome, Lyme disease, compartment syndrome, Crohn's disease, ulcers, external fixation devices for fractures, and lithotripsy. **New illustrations** have been added: 12 types of fractures, 8 skin & skeletal tractions, and testicular self-exam. The *many tables, charts,* and *diagrams* include cardiac dysrhythmias, comparison of causes of chest pain, burn care, the Glasgow Coma scale, breast and testicular self-exams, chest drainage, comparison of hepatitis types, postoperative complications, enteric and standard precautions, respiratory isolation, care of the adult patient with medical and surgical emergencies, pain assessment, preventing TPN complications, and TPN dressing changes. *Nursing interventions* are grouped according to the goal of care and identify appropriate treatments and drug therapies. More detailed discussions follow in two special units on *pharmacology* (**Unit 10**) and *diagnostic procedures* and *treatments* (**Unit 11**).

Unit 8, The Older Adult, is a *new* unit. It is concise and highly readable; and the unit synthesizes 12 key problems associated with care of the older adult. There is an expanded section on *assessment of the older adult* that includes material on normal changes of aging. *Five functional rating scales* and a *functional screening* exam are included to make management of care easier:

- social resources rating scale.
- economic resources rating scale.
- mental health rating scale.
- physical health rating scale.
- performance rating scale for activities of daily living.

Unit 9, Review of Nutrition, contains unique information regarding ethnic food patterns, eating problems, nutritional needs of the elderly, religious and ethnic food preferences, and cultural disease treatments involving food. Special and therapeutic diets are featured. Two updated and completely revised tables have been included: *Recommended Dietary Allowances* and *Physiologic Functions and Deficiency Syndromes of Common Vitamins*.

Unit 10, Review of Pharmacology, contains drug classifications and drug treatments with emphasis on **nursing implications.** *New* content has been added: neuroleptic malignant syndrome and selective serotonin reuptake inhibitors (SSRI). Pediatric medication administration, obstetric analgesia, and psychotropic and mindaltering substances are included; **95 new drugs** have been added, as well as **5 new**

tables (e.g., *antipsychotic agents comparison, antianxiety agents, antineoplastic drug classifications, food and fluid considerations with drugs, equianalgesic dosing for opioid analgesics*).

Unit **11, Common Diagnostic Procedures, Intravenous and Oxygen Therapy, Isolation Precautions, and Hands-on Nursing Care,** includes content on commonly used tubes, fluid and electrolyte therapy, oxygen therapy, and colostomy care, as well as many other diagnostic procedures commonly tested on NCLEX-RN. Six *new* tables have been added (e.g., diagnostic tests to evaluate *fetal well-being, newborn screening* procedures, *bladder* and *bowel* training, guidelines for *isolation* precautions, and commonly used *IV fluids*). A *new* **figure** illustrates common patient *positions*. *New* content on *intubation* and *ventilation* has been added.

Appendices in this book include indexes to content and test questions related to **4 general client needs** (**Appendices C and D**) and **10** subcategories of these 4 client needs (**Appendix E**). These indexes, which **are not found in any other book,** provide immediate, easy reference to topics from the NCLEX-RN Test Plan that are covered in this book. Other appendices cover: lab values, common abbreviations and clinical signs, and fun-to-use memory aids.

Four Unique Self-Evaluation Tools—Over 2001 Test Questions and Test-Taking Tips

This book contains four special, *integrated* tests to help you assess your knowledge before taking the NCLEX-RN. The **Pre Test** at the end of **Unit 1** is intended for students to take after reading the **Orientation** section, but *before* reading the rest of this book. It is a pre-assessment tool to let you find your areas of strength and weakness before beginning focused study. The **Practice Test** is intended to be taken *after* reviewing the material in this book to evaluate your progress. The **Final Test,** the third exam tool, will assess your readiness to take NCLEX-RN and identify any last-minute knowledge gaps.

Use the practice **Computer Test** on CD-ROM anytime in your preparation when you need extra practice or want to become familiar with the NCLEX-RN testing format.

In addition to these four tests, there are new and updated **review questions and answers following each unit.** Their purpose is to help students *review each content area separately* before taking the integrated tests. All questions at the *end of units* and in the integrated tests have been field-tested for several years with students—a diverse group of candidates who have successfully passed the exam—from all over the United States. These questions have also been reviewed by an editorial panel for appropriateness. The Answers/Rationale sections in each unit contain detailed explanations about why a particular answer is best and *why* the other options are incorrect, with a **test-taking tip** for **each** question. We expect that these special integrated tests, end-of-unit review questions, and corresponding answer sections will prove to be invaluable review tools for each and every student.

In the answers for each of the end-of-unit review question sections, and for the **Pre Test, Practice Test, Final Test,** and **Computer Test,** you will find a four-part code to help you understand exactly what is being tested by each question. The code refers to the step of the *nursing process,* the *category of human function,* the *client need* and the *subcategory* of client need that applies to that question. See the code legend on the first page of each Answers/Rationale section. The **Computer Test** will track these codes for you, to identify your problem areas. Use these codes as a guide for review when you find you did not select the best answer. **The test-taking tips** and **codes are unique to this book;** they are an added study tool to help you assess your strengths and pinpoint problem areas as you prepare for the NCLEX-RN.

S.L.L.
G.C.C.
B.M.
R.M.N.
J.H.S.

Acknowledgments

Thank you to the editorial, production, and marketing people of FA Davis, for their dedication to publishing excellence. Carol O'Connell, production editor, has shepherded this book through its labor-intensive phases of copy editing, galleys and page proofs. Carol, I deeply appreciate your energy, caring, and willingness to backtrack a number of times with changes as we needed them. Your unique contribution was your upbeat spirit and *always* being available to me. You had the gift of making me feel valued and that this book was important to you also. You struck a responsive cord when you recognized the spirit with which we, the authors, wrote this book . . . we wanted it to be the best possible and most unique resource for nurses preparing successfully for the licensure exam, We feel we did it!!

Sally Lagerquist

Contributing Authors to This Edition

Geraldine C. Colombraro, RN, MA, PhD
Assistant Dean for Administration
Lienhard School of Nursing, Pace University, Pleasantville, New York

Sally L. Lagerquist, RN, MS
Former Instructor of Undergraduate, Graduate, and Continuing Education in Nursing, University of California, San Francisco, School of Nursing; President, Review for Nurses, Inc., and RN Tapes Company, San Francisco

Bobbi Morrison, A.R.N.P., MN, PhD Candidate
Women's Health Nurse Practitioner; Instructor, Intercollegiate Center for Nursing Education, Washington State University College of Nursing, Spokane, Washington

Robyn Marchal Nelson, RN, DNSc
Chair and Professor, Division of Nursing, California State University, Sacramento, California

Janice Horman Stecchi, RN, EdD
Dean, College of Health Professions, University of Massachusetts Lowell, Lowell, Massachusetts

Contributing Author to Previous Editions

Irene M. Bobak, RN, PhD, FAAN
Professor Emerita, Women's Health and Maternity Nursing, San Francisco State University, San Francisco

New Test Item Writers for the Disk

Eileen Hackett, RN, MA
Professor of Nursing and Assistant Director of Nursing, College of the Desert, Palm Desert, California

Rosemary J. Mann, RN, JD, PhD.
Assistant Professor, San Jose State University School of Nursing, San Jose, California

Lynda Schweid, MS, RN
Assistant Dean, Health Sciences, Contra Costa College, San Pablo, California

Kathleen Snider, RN, MSN, CNS
Professor of Nursing, Department of Health Science, Los Angeles Valley College, Valley Glen, California

List of Tables

List of Figures

Contents

UNIT **6**

Nursing Care of Behavioral and Emotional Problems Throughout the Life Span (Client Need: Psychosocial Integrity)   297

Sally L. Lagerquist

UNIT 7

Nursing Care of the Acutely Ill and the Chronically Ill Adult   428

Robyn Nelson and Janice Stecchi

UNIT 1

Orientation and Pre Test

Sally L. Lagerquist, Geraldine Colombraro, Bobbi Morrison, Robyn Nelson, and Janice Stecchi

ORIENTATION

How to Use This Review Book as a Study Guide

Although nursing students may know that they are academically prepared to take the computer adaptive National Council Licensure Examination (NCLEX-RN), many find that reviewing nursing content for the licensure examination itself presents special concerns about *what* and *how* to study.

Some typical concerns about **what to study** are reflected in the following questions:

- Considering that there will be up to 265 questions on the exam, and every candidate gets a different exam, how does one select what is the most important content for review? How does one narrow the focus of study and distinguish the relevant from the irrelevant material?
- What areas should be emphasized?
- How detailed should the review be?
- How does one know what areas to review first?
- Should basic sciences, such as anatomy, physiology, microbiology, and nutrition, be included in the study?

Concerns relating to **how to study** include:

- How does one make the best of limited review time to go over content that may be in lecture and clinical notes compiled during 2 to 4 years of schooling?
- Is it best to review from all the major textbooks used in nursing school?
- Should material be memorized, or should one study from broad principles and concepts?

We have written this nursing review book with the *general* intent of assisting nurses in identifying what they need to study in a format designed to use their study time effectively, productively, and efficiently while preparing for the examination.

The contributing authors have selected content and developed a style of presentation that has been tested by thousands of nursing students attending review courses coordinated by the editor in various cities throughout the United States. This book is the result of this study.

This review book can be used in a variety of ways: (a) as a *starting point* for review of essential content specifically aimed at NCLEX or Canadian exam preparation, (b) as an *end point* of studying for the examinations, (c) as an *anxiety-reduction tool*, (d) as a general guide and *refresher* for nurses not presently in practice, and (e) as a guide for graduates of nursing schools *outside of the United States*, as well as *repeat test-takers* (see **Unit 2**).

As a Starting Point

This text can be used in early review when a longer study period is needed to *fill in gaps* of knowledge. One cannot remember something if one does not know or understand it. A lengthy review before the exam allows students time to rework and organize notes accumulated during 2 to 4 years of basic nursing education. In addition, an early review allows time for *self-evaluation*. We have provided questions and answers to help students identify areas requiring further study and to help them *integrate* unfamiliar material with what they already know.

As an End Point

This text can also be used for a *quick review* (a) to *promote retention and recall* and (b) to aid in determining *nursing actions* appropriate to specific health situations. During the time immediately preceding the examination, the main objective might be to *strengthen previous learning* by refreshing the memory. Or a brief overview may serve to *draw together* the isolated points under key concepts and principles in a way that shows their relationships and relative importance.

As an Anxiety-Reduction Tool

In some students, anxiety related to taking examinations in general may reach such levels that it causes students to be unproductive in study and to function at a lower level during the actual examination. Sections of this text are directed toward this problem and provide simple, *practical approaches to the reduction of general anxiety.* For anxiety specifically related to unknown aspects of the licensure examination itself, the section on the *structure, format, and mechanics of the RN examination* might bring relief through its focus on basic examination information.

For anxiety related to lack of confidence or skill in test-taking "know-how," the special section on *test-taking techniques* may be helpful.

As a General Study Guide and as a Refresher for Nurses Not Presently in Practice

Many nursing students will find this review book useful throughout their education as a general study guide as they prepare patient care plans and study for midterm and final exams. It will help them put information into perspective as they learn it. And nurses who have not been in practice for several years will find it a useful reference tool and review device.

Where To Begin

In using this review book to prepare for the licensure examination, the nurse must:

1. Be prepared mentally.
   a. Know the purpose of the examination.
   b. Know the purpose of reviewing.
   c. Anticipate what is to come.
   d. Decide on a good study method—set a study goal before beginning a particular subject area (number of pages, for example); plan the length of the review period by the amount of material to be covered, not by the clock.
2. Plan the work to be done.
   a. Select one subject at a time for review, and establish and follow a sequence for review of each subject.
      (1) Answer the practice questions following the outline of the selected subject area. (Set a time limit, because pacing is important.)
      (2) Compare your answers with those provided following the questions as a means of evaluating areas of competence.
   b. Identify those subjects that will require additional concentrated study in this review book as well as in basic textbooks.
   c. Study the review text outlines, noting headings, subheadings, and *italics* and **boldface** type for emphasis of relative importance.
   d. Study the content presented in chart format to facilitate memorization, understanding, and application.
   e. Repeat the self-evaluation process by taking the test again.
   f. Look up the answers for the correct response to the multiple choice questions. Do not memorize the answers. Read the rationale explaining *why* it was the correct response. (These explanations serve to correct as well as reinforce. Understanding the underlying

principles also serves as an aid in applying the same principles to questions that may be based on similar rationale, but phrased differently on the actual examination.)
   g. If necessary, refer to basic textbooks to relearn any unclear aspects of anatomy, physiology, nutrition, or basic nursing procedures. Look up unfamiliar terminology in a medical dictionary.

While Reviewing

1. Scan the outline for main ideas and topics.
   a. Do not try to remember verbatim what is on each page.
   b. Paraphrase or explain this material to another person.
2. Refer to basic textbooks for details and illustrations as necessary to recall specific information related to basic sciences.
3. Integrate reading with experience.
   a. Think of examples that illustrate the key concepts and principles.
   b. Make meaningful associations.
   c. Look for implications for nursing actions as concepts are reviewed.
4. Take notes on the review outline—use stars and arrows, underscore, highlight with highlighter pens, and write comments in margins, such as "most important" and "memorize," to reinforce the relative importance of points of information.

After Reviewing

1. Repeat the self-evaluation process as often as necessary to gain mastery of content essential to safe nursing practice.
2. Continue to refer to major textbooks to fill in gaps where greater detail or in-depth comprehension is required.
3. Look for patterns in your selection of responses to the multiple choice practice questions—identify sources of difficulty in choosing the most appropriate answers.
4. Review test-taking strategies (see **Unit 2,** pp. 47–51).

Key Points to Recall for Better Study

1. *Schedule*—study time should be scheduled so that review begins close to the time at which it will be used. Retention is much better following a well-spaced review. It may be helpful to group material into small learning segments. Study goals should be set before beginning each period of study (number of pages, for example).
2. *Organize*—many students have better retention of material after they have reorganized and relearned it.
3. *Rephrase and explain*—try to rephrase material in your own words or explain it to another person. Reinforce learning through repetition and usage.
4. *Decide on order of importance*—organize study time in terms of importance and familiarity.

5. *Use mechanical memory aids*—mnemonic (memory) devices simplify recall. For example, in "On Old Olympus's Towering Top a Finn and German Viewed Some Hops," the first letter of each word identifies the first letter of a cranial nerve. (See **Appendix N.**)
6. *Association*—associate new material with related concepts and principles from past experience.
7. *Original learning*—if an unfamiliar topic is presented, do more than review. Seek out sources of additional information.
8. *Make notes*—look for key words, phrases, and sentences in the outlined review material, and mark them for later reference.
9. *Definitions*—look up unfamiliar terms in a dictionary or the glossary of a basic text, or in **Appendix L.**
10. *Additional study*—refer to other textbook references for more detailed information.
11. *Distractors*—keep a pad of paper on hand to jot down extraneous thoughts; get them out of the mind and onto the paper.

Memorization: Purpose and Strategies

You'll need to memorize some items before you can rapidly assess or apply that knowledge to a particular situation; for example, you need to be able to recall the standard and lethal doses of a drug before deciding to administer it. Items you should memorize include, but are not limited to:

1. Names of common drugs.
2. Lethal and therapeutic doses.
3. Lab norms and values.
4. Growth and development norms.
5. Foods high or low in iron, protein, sodium, potassium, or carbohydrates.
6. Conversion formulas.
7. Anatomical names.
8. List of cranial nerves and their innervations.

To facilitate memorizing these and other essentials, here are some strategies.

1. Before you work on training your mind to remember, you must *want* to remember the material.
2. You cannot memorize something that you do not understand; therefore, *know* your material.
3. Visualize what you want to memorize; picture it; draw a picture.
4. Use the familiar to provide vivid mental pictures, to peg the unfamiliar.
   a. When needing to remember a *sequence*, use your body to turn material into a picture. Draw a person, then list the first item to be memorized on top of the head, the next item on the forehead, and so on for nose, mouth, neck, chest, abdomen, thighs, knees, and feet.

b. Use what you already know to tie in with what you want to remember; make it memorable.
c. Use as pegs the unexpected, the exaggerated. Weird imagery is easiest to recall.
5. Use the blank-paper technique:
   a. Place a large blank sheet on the wall.
   b. After you have studied, draw on the blank paper what you remember.
   c. When you have drawn all that you can recall, check with the book and study what you did correctly and incorrectly.
   d. Take another sheet and do it again. Purpose: to reinforce what you already know and work with what you want to remember.
6. Make up and use mnemonic devices to help you remember the important elements (see **Appendix N**).
7. Repetitively explain to another person the material you want to memorize.
8. Saturate your environment with the material you want to memorize.
   a. Purpose: to overcome the mind's tendency to ignore.
   b. Tape facts, formulas, concepts on walls.
9. Above all, feel confident in your ability to memorize!

The Mechanics of the National Council Licensure Examination for Registered Nurses–Computer Adaptive Test (NCLEX-RN)

Since 1994, the licensure examination for registered nurses has been administered year-round by computer, in an adaptive format: NCLEX-RN. Frequently, candidates for the exam have many questions about the structure and format of the test itself and the rules and regulations concerning the examination procedure.

As an aid to reducing apprehension and time spent on speculation, this section is intended to provide information that candidates need, in outline form; the last segment offers a "question-and-answer" format for specific questions frequently asked by nursing students.

This information was verified as correct at the time that it was compiled from information provided by the National Council of State Boards of Nursing, Inc., and other parties involved in the testing. If you have further questions, contact the board of nursing in your state (see **Appendix O**).

I. **What NCLEX is**
   A. National Council Licensure Examination, developed and administered by the National Council of State Boards of Nursing, Inc., with services provided by VUE (Virtual University Enterprises), an NCS (National Computer Systems) Pearson Company.
   B. Tests for minimum nursing competence according to a national standard.

C. Pass/fail result; must pass to be issued license from state board of registered nursing.
D. National exam. Application procedure and licensing requirements are determined by each state board and may differ from state to state.

II. CAT: How it works

A. Stands for "computer adaptive testing."
B. "Adaptive" because the computer estimates the candidate's ability after each question; the next question is chosen based on the candidate's estimated ability so far. The test is therefore "adapted" to each candidate; everyone takes a different, "customized" test.
C. Estimated ability is recalculated after each question until it is precise enough to determine whether the candidate is above or below minimum competence level, in all areas of the test plan. The test will stop as soon as this is determined.
D. Example: The first question is of a fairly easy level. The candidate answers correctly, so the computer estimates that the candidate's ability level is above the level of this question and selects a harder question; or if the candidate answers incorrectly, it selects an easier question, to pinpoint where the candidate's ability level lies, in each area of the test plan.

III. Some specifics

A. Format
1. Multiple choice questions, each with four or more options.
2. One question at a time appears on screen (Figure 1–1).
3. Each question stands alone (no "scenarios" with several spin-off questions); no question will relate to information given in previous questions.
4. Some items will be fill in, others may have diagrams, charts, numerical entry.
B. Answering
1. As candidate chooses the answer to each question, he or she will be asked to confirm that answer, *or* can change that answer before confirming.

FIGURE 1–1 Computer screen.

```
Question•que          ♦1 Answer option
stion•questi
on•question•          ♦2 Answer option
question•que
stion•questi          ♦3 Answer option
on•question•
                      ♦4 Answer option
```

2. Must answer every question (no penalty for guessing; will simply count as a correct or incorrect answer and adjust difficulty of next question accordingly).
3. Cannot go back to previous questions either to review or change answers (because *subsequent* questions are administered based on *previous* answers).
C. Number of questions
1. 75–265, including about 15 "tryout" questions that are not scored (these are questions being field tested for use on future exams).
2. Depends on number needed to determine whether candidate is definitely above or definitely below minimum competence level.
3. Taking only the minimum can mean **either pass or fail;** it indicates that it took fewer questions to determine whether this candidate is above or below minimum competence, but does not indicate which!
D. Timing
1. No time limit for each question.
2. Maximum time for test is 5 hours.
3. A preprogrammed optional break is given after 2 hours; a second preprogrammed optional break may be taken after another 1½ hours.
E. The test will stop when any *one* of the following occurs:
1. A "pass" or "fail" determination can be made.
2. The maximum number of questions has been taken (265).
3. The test has lasted for 5 hours.
F. The computer
1. Computer experience will not be necessary.
2. After April 1, 2001, a mouse has been used to move down the list of options and select and confirm answer choice; all keys will be "turned off." An on-screen calculator will be available.
3. Candidate receives a brief orientation in the use of the mouse and on-screen calculator with sample questions before beginning the exam.

IV. Administration

A. Application and scheduling
1. Involves three parties: the state board of nursing, VUE, and Pearson Professional Center.
2. Candidate applies to the board of nursing in the state in which licensing is desired; must meet requirements of that state board. (There is a test fee and some state boards may also require an administrative fee.)
3. After state board determines eligibility and fees are received, candidate will be mailed an *Authorization to Test (ATT)* and information on available Pearson Professional Testing Centers, which serve as testing sites (at least one per state; some states have many more).
4. Candidate must schedule an appointment to take the exam by calling NCLEX Candidate Services or going to the NCLEX Candidate

The Mechanics of the National Council Licensure Examination for Registered Nurses–Computer Adaptive Test (NCLEX-RN) **5**

Orientation

Website. (NOTE: These procedures differ in some states, e.g., Massachusetts. Candidates should follow instructions from state board.)

5. Candidate contacts Pearson Professional Testing Center (or other designated test site) to set up testing appointment (5 days/wk, 15 hr/day, in 5 hr time slots). Candidates may test at any test center in any state (they do not have to take the test in the same state to which they have applied for licensure).

6. After testing, results are communicated to state board to which the candidate applied, which mails results to candidate (time frame will differ by state). Candidates who do not pass will receive a Candidate Performance Report, indicating performance in each area of the test plan relative to the passing standard, and information about retesting.

B. Test environment: Pearson Professional Testing Center test sites

1. Up to 30 workstations, each with computer terminal, desk lamp, work surface, and scratch paper.
2. Designed for security, monitored by a proctor and by videotape.
3. Candidate must present *Authorization To Test* and two signed pieces of identification, one with picture; candidate must sign in and be fingerprinted and photographed.
4. Lockers or other secured storage provided; personal items restricted in testing room.

V. **Test plan, development**
A. Test plan*

1. *Client needs* are the bases, or "dimensions," for the test plan. See Table 1–1.
2. Health needs of clients: The test plan primarily emphasizes meeting the clients' physical needs in actual or potentially life-threatening, chronic, or recurring *physiological* conditions and the needs of clients who are at risk for complications or untoward effects of treatment. Subneeds include (1) basic care and comfort (7–13%), (2) pharmacological and parenteral therapies (5–11%), (3) reduction of risk potential (12–18%), and (4) physiological adaptation (12–18%).

The second two highest categories of emphasis are *safe, effective care environment,* which focuses on (1) management of care (7–13%) and (2) safety and infection control (5–11%); and *health promotion and maintenance,* covering (1) growth and development throughout the life span (7–13%) and (2) prevention and early detection of disease (5–11%).

Finally, 10–22% of the test plan concerns *psychosocial adaptation coping* (5–11%) and *adaptation* (5–11%) in stress- and crisis-related situations throughout the life cycle.

3. *Nursing process* (nursing behaviors): The exam integrates steps of the nursing process, as applied to client situations from all stages in the life cycle and to common health problems in all the major health areas and based on current morbidity studies.

4. Levels of cognitive ability: Most items are at the *application* and *analysis* level (application of principles, ideas, theories; and analysis of data to set priorities and see relationships), but include knowledge and comprehension.

5. Categories of nursing knowledge and other concepts that are commonly tested:
   a. Caring ways by which nursing can assist individuals to maintain health and cope with health problems (see *nursing care plan/implementation* sections in *each* unit).
   b. Communication (**see Unit 6).**
   c. Effect of age, sex, culture, ethnicity, and religion on health needs (sociocultural components) are integrated into all units; for special emphasis **see Unit 3** and **Unit 9** (dietary implications).
   d. Documentation; legal and ethical aspects of nursing, accountability (**see Unit 3).**
   e. Self-care.
   f. Teaching-learning (see *health teaching* sections [after the conditions] that are part of **Nursing Care Plan/implementation**).
   g. Nursing fundamentals (**see Unit 11).**
   h. Nutrition and diet therapy (**see Unit 9).**
   i. Pharmacology (**see Unit 10).**
   j. Communicable diseases (**see Unit 5).**
   k. Natural and behavioral sciences (integrated into all units).

---

*Source: National Council of State Boards of Nursing.

TABLE 1–1   Exam Weight Given to Each Category of Health Needs of Clients Based on Current Practice Analysis Study (1999)

Client Health Needs Tested (subneeds)	Total Percentage of Test
Safe, effective care environment (Management of Care, Safety & Infection Control)	12–24
Health promotion and maintenance (Growth & Development, Prevention & Early Detection)	12–24
Psychosocial integrity (Coping & Adaptation, Psychosocial Adaptation)	10–22
Physiological integrity (Basic Care & Comfort, Pharmacological Parenteral Therapies, Reduction of Risk Potential, Physiological Adaptation)	36–60

l. Normal growth and development (**see Units 4, 5, and 6**).

m. Basic human needs (**see Unit 6**).

n. Individual coping mechanisms (**see Unit 6**).

o. Actual or potential health problems (**see Units 4, 5, 7, and 8**).

p. Life cycle (consult the table of **Contents** to see how the conceptual framework for this book is organized by life cycle).

q. Patient environment (there is continual reference throughout this book related to protection from harm against airborne irritants, cold, and heat; identification of environmental discomforts such as noise, odors, dust, and poor ventilation; elimination of potential *safety hazards;* maintenance of environmental order; and *cleanliness*).

B. Development

1. The Examination Committee of the National Council prepares the test plan, which is approved by the delegates representing the state boards of nursing. It is designed to reflect the knowledge and skills needed for *minimum competence by a newly licensed nurse to be a safe and effective practitioner in entry-level nursing,* as determined by studies of nursing practice (performed every 3 years to reflect current nursing practice).

2. State boards take turns nominating item writers (faculty, clinical nurse specialists, or beginning practitioners); the Board of Directors of the National Council then selects from this group those who meet the criteria for item writing based on expertise in a particular area of nursing, type of nursing program, credentials, regional balance, etc. The item writers write questions based on common clinical situations and according to the test plan. Then the questions are researched and reviewed by a panel of experts (nominated by the state boards), by those state boards that choose to review, and by the National Council's Examination Committee.

3. Finally, the questions are field tested to eliminate questions that may be ambiguous, irrelevant, or not equally applicable to all regions of the United States. (Each candidate taking NCLEX will take 15 of these "tryout" questions, mixed in with the regular questions; they will *not* count toward that candidate's performance.) The data gained through field testing are also used to analyze and determine the difficulty level of a question.

C. Passing standard: The passing standard is *criterion referenced;* this means that there is no fixed percentage of candidates that pass or fail. Passing depends solely on performance in relation to the level of minimum competence. The passing standard is reviewed every 3 years.

VI. Frequently asked questions and answers about NCLEX-RN

A. Test questions, test plan

1. *How many questions will there be?* You will take anywhere from 75 to 265 multiple choice questions. (See III. **Some specifics**, p. 4.)

2. *Where do the questions come from?* The state boards of nursing nominate item writers, who must meet various criteria. (See **V. B.** Development, p. 6.)

3. *Will there be questions involving conditions with which I may not have had experience in my nursing program?* Most of the questions are about patients with conditions familiar to you and are representative of common health problems on a national basis. Some questions may relate to nursing problems with which you may not have had prior experience; their purpose is to test your ability to *apply* knowledge of specific principles from the physical, biological, and social sciences to *new* situations.

4. *Can some questions have more than one answer?* Yes. Only *one* of the four options is the *best* answer. You may be asked to choose more than one option as your answer.

5. *Will I get partial credit for selecting the next-to-the-best answer?* No. Your answer will be treated only as correct or incorrect.

6. *If everyone takes a different test, how can it be fair?* Each candidate is tested according to the *same test plan,* and the *same passing standard.* It may simply require more items to reach a stable pass/fail determination for one candidate, while another may require fewer questions to demonstrate competence level.

7. *Do diploma, associate, and baccalaureate graduates all take the same test? What about graduates from schools outside the United States?* All candidates are held to the *same test plan and passing standard,* and take the "same test." (Of course, due to the nature of CAT, each will receive an "individualized" test, without regard to degree, or to state or country of education.)

8. *Does the exam differ by state?* The exam is a national exam; all candidates are held to the *same test plan and passing standard,* and take questions from the same pool. (Again, through CAT, each candidate receives an "individualized" test, but without regard to state.)

9. *How is the exam different from the old "paper-and-pencil" test?* The purpose, test plan, and nursing knowledge and skills tested *did not change* significantly with the advent of CAT (there were minor adjustments to the test plan in October 1995, unrelated to the change to computer testing). The *main differences* lie in the efficiency of the computerized testing (maximum of 5 hours and 265 questions, compared to the old 2-day test with up to 372 questions) and the adaptive nature, which precludes skipping questions and changing answers.

B. Taking the test/after the test

1. *Can I skip questions?* No. You must answer each question in order to move on to the next. You also will not be able to return to previous questions to try them again or change the answer (because *subsequent* questions are administered based on *previous* answers).

2. *What if I just don't know the answer?* Use the tips in **Sixty Strategies in Answering Questions,** pp. 47–51, to make your best guess. You will need to answer the question in order to move on to the next question.

3. *When will I know my results? Will the computer tell me?* You will not learn your pass/fail status at the testing center; the results will be communicated directly to your state board of nursing, who will mail the results to you. The time frame may differ from state to state, but most candidates should receive their results within 2 to 4 weeks after taking the exam. Some states provide a Results-by-Phone Service, where unofficial results are available 3 business days after taking the exam. There is a flat fee for this service. **NOTE:** Taking only the minimum number of questions, or taking the maximum, is not an indication of whether you have passed or failed. It merely indicates that a lesser, or greater, number of items was required to reach a determination.

4. *What percentage must I answer correctly to pass?* Because of the nature of CAT, a percentage rate is *not* used to determine passing or failure. The test determines whether you are above or below standard competence by determining not the *number* of questions you answer correctly, but rather the *difficulty level* you can consistently answer correctly. The process of administering harder or easier questions, as described in **II. CAT: How it works,** p. 4, continues until you reach the level where you answer approximately 50% of the complex questions correctly. **NOTE:** When practicing with questions of mixed difficulty, such as those in this book, you may wish to use 80% correct as a "benchmark" goal for yourself.

5. *If I do not pass, can I retest only those areas of the test plan in which I tested poorly?* No. The whole exam is on a pass/fail basis.

6. *Can I repeat the exam before I get my results?* No.

7. *How many times can the exam be repeated, and when?* The National Council allows you to repeat the exam a maximum of four times per year, but not more than once in any 90-day period; however, each state board may set its own, more restrictive time limits and retake requirements.

8. *Who grants the nursing license?* The license is granted by the state board of nursing to which you applied and for which you took the exam.

C. Testing facilities

1. *Can I bring any materials into the examination room?* There are severe restrictions on personal items allowed in the examination room; you will be provided with a locker or other secure place for your belongings. Do *not* take any study materials (books, notes, calculators, etc.) pens, food, watches, beepers, cell phones, purses, wallets, or cameras into the examination building.

2. *How many people will take the test at the same time?* Up to 30 people may be at computer workstations in your testing room; however, they may not all be taking the NCLEX, because Pearson Professional Test Centers also offer other services.

3. *When and where will I take the test?* After you receive your authorization (ATT), you must contact a Pearson Professional Center facility to set up your own testing appointment (5 days/wk, 15 hr/day, in 5 hr time slots). There is at least one facility per state, although most states have many more.

4. *What accommodations are available for candidates with disabilities?* All test centers are accessible to candidates with disabilities. Other accommodations will be made only with the prior authorization of the board of nursing; contact your state board *before* submitting your application.

How to Prepare for and Score Higher on Exams

The Psychology of Test Taking

Many nursing students know the nursing material on which they are being tested, and can demonstrate their nursing skills in practice, but do not know how to prepare themselves for taking and passing examinations.

It is not just a matter of taking exams but of *knowing how* to take them, taking steps to ensure you can function at full capacity, and using the allotted time in the most productive way. You must learn to use strategy and judgment in answering questions, and to make educated guesses when you are not sure of the right answer.

This section offers practical suggestions to help ensure that you are "at your best" on exam day, and discusses practical strategies for eliminating wrong answers and for increasing your chances of selecting the best ones.

Prepare Physically and Mentally

1. *On the morning of an exam, avoid excessive oral intake of products that act as diuretics for you.* If you know that coffee or cigarettes, for example, increase urgency and frequency, it is best to limit their intake. Undue physiological discomforts can distract your focus from the exam at hand.

2. *Increase your oral intake of foods high in glucose and protein.* These foods reportedly have been helpful to some examinees for keeping up their blood-sugar level. This may enhance your concentration and problem-solving ability at the times when you most need to function at a high level. On the other hand, avoid carbohydrates such as doughnuts, which slow down thinking.

3. *Before examination days, avoid eating exotic or highly seasoned foods to which your system may not be accustomed.* Avoid possible gastrointestinal distress when you least need it!

4. *Use hard candy or something similar* during a test, if it is allowed in the exam room, to help relieve the discomfort of a dry mouth related to a state of anxiety.

5. *Wear comfortable clothes that you have worn before.* The day of an exam is not a good time to wear new clothes or footwear that may prove to be constricting, binding, or uncomfortable, especially at the waistline and shoulder seams.

6. Anxiety states can bring about rapid increases and decreases in body temperature. *Wear clothing that can be shed or added on.* For example, you might bring a sweater that can be put on when you feel chilled or removed when your body temperature fluctuates again.

7. *Women need to be prepared for late, irregular, or unanticipated early onset of menses* on exam day, a time of stress.

8. Exam jitters can elicit anxiety-like reactions, both physiological and emotional. Because anxiety tends to be contagious, *try to limit your contacts with those who are also experiencing exam-related anxiety or who elicit those feelings in you.*

9. *The night before an exam is a good time to engage in a pleasurable activity* as a means of anxiety reduction. You need stamina and endurance for sitting, thinking, and reacting. Give yourself a chance for restful, not energy- or emotion-draining, activities in the days before an exam.

10. *Try a relaxation process* if anxiety reaches an uncomfortable level that cannot be channeled into the service of learning (see **How To Reduce Anxiety,** p. 9).

11. When you arrive home after an exam, *jot down content areas that were unfamiliar to you.* This may serve as a key focus for review.

Tips for NCLEX-RN

1. Get an early start on the day you take the examination, to avoid raising your anxiety level before the actual exam starts. Allow yourself time for delays in traffic and in public transportation or for finding a parking place. Even allow for a dead battery, flooded engine, flat tire, or bus breakdown. If you are unfamiliar with the area in which the test center is located, find it the day before.

2. Remember that *you do not need to get all the answers right to pass.* The exam is designed to test for *minimum* competence; demonstrating a higher level will not earn a special designation on your license, or any other bonus. Moreover, due to the adaptive nature of the test, you will probably reach a level where you are answering only 50% of the questions correctly; this is *normal* for this test and *should not* in itself be taken as an indication of poor performance (you may be answering 50% of the *very difficult* questions correctly)!

3. Because you cannot skip questions and go back to them, or go back to change answers, it is important that you simply *do the best you can* on a particular question, using the **Sixty Strategies in Answering Questions, Unit 2,** pp. 47–51, and *move on.* The adaptive test will give you another chance to show your competence, should you get that question wrong.

4. Remember that although you cannot change answers you have already "confirmed," you *may change your answer during the selection process.* As you make your answer selection, you will *choose* an answer (by pressing the enter key once) and then *confirm* it (by pressing the key a second time); you will be able to change your mind *before confirming* your answer choice.

5. Although the exam uses different levels of difficulty to estimate your competence level, *do not try to figure out the difficulty level* of each question; likewise, do not try to keep track of the number of questions you are answering. You will only distract yourself and raise your anxiety. Again, simply answer each question to the best of your ability and move on.

6. When taking practice questions, it is a good idea to *aim for an average of 1 minute per question,* so that you will be at a speed to finish the exam even if you *do* need to take the maximum number of questions. For the actual exam, however, the 5-hour time limit is not a problem for most candidates, so go ahead and *take the time to work through a difficult problem,* and make use of the scratch paper provided (but *don't* dwell on a question you "just can't get!").

Tips for Other (Pencil-and-Paper) Tests and Exams

1. *Answer the easy questions first.* Too often students focus on 1 question for 10 minutes, for example, instead of going on to answer 20 additional questions during this time. The main goal in this type of exam is to answer correctly as many questions as possible.

2. *Your first hunch is usually a good one.* Pay attention to your intuition, which may indicate which answer "feels" best.

3. *Be wise about the timing.* Divide your time. For example, if you have 90 questions and 1½ hours for the test, aim for an average of 1 question per minute. Keep working! Do not lose time looking back at your answers.

4. *If you cannot decide between two multiple choice answers, make a note of the numbers of the two choices.* This will narrow down your focus when you come back to this question. Leave the question; do not spend much time on those in doubt. When you have completed the test, go back and spend more time on those with which you had trouble.

5. *Exercise care and caution when using electronically scored answer sheets or booklets.* It is essential that you use only the type of pencil or ink specified in the instructions. If erasing is possible, be sure to erase completely; a mere trace might throw out the answer.

6. When using a separate answer sheet or booklet, be especially careful to *mark your answer in the space for the cor-*

rect question number. It might be helpful to say to yourself as you answer each question, "Choice No. 4 to question No. 3," to make sure that the right answer goes with each question number.

7. *Stay the entire time allotted.* If you complete the test early, check your answers. On a second look, after you have completed the test, you may find something that you are *now sure* you marked in error the first time. If you were undecided between two possible answers on any questions, use leftover time to reconsider those answers. (Also, look for and erase stray marks, if using electronically scored answer sheets.)

How To Reduce Anxiety

Most people have untapped inner resources for achieving relaxation and tension-release in stressful situations (such as during an examination) when they need to function at their highest potential. The goal of this discussion is to help you experience a self-guided approach to reducing your anxiety level to one that is compatible with learning and high performance.

In anxiety-producing settings whenever you feel overwhelmed or blocked, a fantasy experience can be of help in mastering the rising anxiety by promoting a feeling of calm, detached awareness, and a sense of deeper personal coping resources. Through the fantasy you can gain access to a zone of *tranquility* in the center of your being. Guided imagery often carries with it feelings of serenity, warmth, and comfort.

Fantasy experiences are, of course, highly individual. Techniques that help one person experience serenity may frustrate another. Try out the self-guided experiences suggested here, make up your own, and select ones that are best for you. There are endless possibilities for fantasy journeys. The best approach is to work with whatever fantasy occurs to you at the moment. The ideas for a journey presented here are meant to be a springboard for variations of your own.

A fantasy will be more effective if you take as comfortable a physical position as possible, with eyes closed and attention focused on the inner experience. Get in touch with physical sensations, your pattern and rate of breathing, your heartbeat, and pressure points of your body as it comes in contact with the chair and floor.

When you take a fantasy journey by yourself, it is important for you to read over the instructions several times so that you will be able to recall the overall structure of the fantasy. *Then*, close your eyes and take your trip without concern for following the instructions in detail.

Progressive Relaxation

Relaxation approaches are used in a variety of anxiety states whenever stress interferes with the ability to function.

Progressive relaxation training was originated in 1929 by Dr. Edmund Jacobson. It is a technique for attaining self-control over skeletal muscles in order to induce low-level tonus in the major muscle groups. The approach involves learning systematically and sequentially to tense and relax various muscle groups throughout the body.

The *objectives* of this approach are to soothe nerves, combat hypertonus in muscles, and substitute relaxing activities for stressful ones in order to feel comfortable in and more alert to the internal and external environments.

The *theory* behind this method takes as its basis the idea that muscular relaxation and anxiety states produce directly opposite physiologic effects and thus cannot coexist. In other words, it is not possible to be tense in any body part that is completely relaxed.

The *physiological changes* during relaxation include decreased oxygen consumption, decreased carbon dioxide elimination, and decreased respiratory rate.

The basic factors vital to eliciting a relaxation response include the following:

1. *Quiet setting*—eliminate unnecessary internal and external stimuli.
2. *Passive, "let-it-happen" attitude*—empty your mind of thoughts and distractions.
3. *Comfortable position*—sit or recline in one position for 20 minutes or so.
4. *Constant stimulus on which to focus*—a repetitive sound, constant gaze on an object or image, or attention to one's own breathing pattern.

Relaxation training is a procedure that can be defined, specified, and memorized until you can go through the exercises mechanically. If you regularly practice relaxation, you will be able to cope more effectively with difficult situations by reaping the physiological and psychological benefits of a balanced and relaxed state.

Instructions

- Sit comfortably in a chair. Shut your eyes and chase your thoughts for a minute; go where your thoughts go.
- Then, let the words go. Become aware of how you *feel,* here and now, not how you would like to feel.
- Shift your awareness to your feet. Do not move them. Become aware of what they are doing.
- Spend 20 to 30 seconds focusing progressively on different parts of your body. Relax each part in turn:

  Relax each of your toes; the tops of your feet; the arch of each foot; the insteps, balls, and heels; and your ankles, calves, knees, thighs, and buttocks. Become aware of how your body is contacting the chair in which you are sitting. Let go of your abdominal and chest muscles; relax your back. Release the tension in your shoulders, arms, elbows, forearms, wrists, hands, and each finger in turn; relax the muscles in your throat, lips, and cheeks. Wrinkle your nose; relax your eyelids and eyebrows (first one and then the other); relax the muscles in your forehead and top and back of your head. Relax your whole body.

  Concentrate on your breathing; become aware of how you breathe. Allow yourself to inhale and exhale in your usual way. Become aware of the depth of your breathing. Are you expanding the lungs all the way? Or is your breathing shallow? Increase your depth of breathing. Now focus on the rate at which you are breathing. See if you can slow the rate down. When you breathe in, can you feel an inflow of energy that fills your entire body?

- Now concentrate on the sounds in the room.
- Focus on how you feel right now.
- Slowly open your eyes.

Suggestions for Additional Experiential Vignettes

- Imagine yourself leaving the room. In your mind's eye go through the city and over the fields. Come to a meadow covered with fresh, new grass and flowers. Look out on the meadow and focus on what you see, hear, smell, and feel. Walk through the meadow. See the length and greenness of the grass; see the brilliance and feel the warmth of the sunlight.
- For a more expansive feeling, visualize a mountain in the distance. Fantasize going to the country and slowly ascending a mountain. Walk through a forest. Climb to the top until at last you reach a height where you can see forever. Experience your awareness.

- Focus on a memory of a beautiful place you have been to, enjoyed, and would like to enjoy again. Be there; experience it.
- Imagine that you are floating on your back down a river. It may help at first to breathe deeply and feel yourself sinking. Visualize that you are coming out on a gentle river that is slowly winding its way through a beautiful forest. The sun is out and the rays feel warm on your skin. You pass trees and meadows of beautiful flowers. Smell the grass and flowers. Hear the birds. Look up in the blue sky; see the lazy tufts of clouds floating by. Leave the river and walk across the meadow. Enjoy the grass around your ankles. Come to a large tree . . .

Fill in the rest of the trip—what do you see now? Where do you want to go from here?

Sally L. Lagerquist

PRE TEST

Introduction

The **Pre Test** is an *initial assessment* tool intended to help you to assess your strengths and weaknesses in your ability to apply the material you have learned in specific clinical areas to any nursing situation. By taking the **Pre Test,** you can focus your subsequent review of content, based on your own analysis of your results.

We suggest that you take the **Pre Test** before you read any of the content units in this book. After taking the **Pre Test,** you should:

1. Score your answers.
2. Take another look at the questions where your answer was wrong.
3. Identify the clinical areas where you need further review (e.g., Childhood and Adolescence, Behavioral and Emotional).
4. Read those specific content units in detail.
5. Then test yourself again on the **Practice Test.**

Questions

1. The nurse can quickly assess volume depletion in a patient with ulcerative colitis by:
   1. Measuring the quantity and specific gravity of the patient's urine output.
   2. Taking the patient's blood pressure first supine, then sitting, noting any changes.
   3. Comparing the patient's present weight with weight on a previous admission.
   4. Administering the oral water test.
2. Physical assessment of a patient admitted for a bronchoscopy revealed a thin, muscular man with wheezes in the left lung and some wheezes in the right lower lobe. Wheezes are due to:
   1. Total obstruction of small bronchioles.
   2. Partial obstruction of bronchi and bronchioles.
   3. Fluid in the alveoli.
   4. Inflammation of the pleura.
3. Which of the following best describes the metabolic functions of the liver?
   1. Detoxification of endogenous and exogenous substances.
   2. Fluid volume control and acid-base balance.
   3. Erythrocyte and leukocyte breakdown.
   4. Concentration and storage of bile.
4. In response to a patient's questions regarding the cause of glomerulonephritis, the nurse explains that acute glomerulonephritis is the result of:
   1. Acute infection of the kidney by gram-negative bacteria.
   2. An immune response of the glomerular membrane to protein of the beta-hemolytic streptococcus.
   3. Destruction of the glomerular membrane by gram-positive streptococci.
   4. Ischemia of glomerular capillary and vasa recta.
5. A patient who is scheduled for repair of bilateral inguinal hernias has a history of obesity, smoker's cough, and heavy lifting following a previous inguinal hernia repair. The *most* likely cause for the herniation is:
   1. Intestinal obstruction.
   2. Failure of resected muscles in previous operations to heal properly.
   3. Chronic cough and vigorous exercise.
   4. Obesity.
6. The nurse knows that the function of the gallbladder is to:
   1. Synthesize and manufacture bile.
   2. Collect, concentrate, and store bile.
   3. Collect and dilute bile.
   4. Regulate bile flow into the duodenum.
7. The most accurate description the nurse could give a colleague about a thyroid scan is that it:
   1. Assists in differentiating between primary and secondary hypothyroidism.
   2. Demonstrates increased uptake of radioactive iodine in areas of possible malignancy.
   3. Demonstrates decreased uptake of radioactive iodine in areas of possible malignancy.
   4. Measures the effect of TSH on thyroid function.
8. A stat cesarean birth is ordered for a woman in labor; her husband is with her. The *primary* priority of the nurse at this time would be to:
   1. Obtain an operation permit.
   2. Attempt to alleviate the couple's anxiety.
   3. Monitor maternal and fetal signs closely.
   4. Provide emotional and physiological support.
9. The nurse knows that a decreased hematocrit occurs in chronic renal failure because:
   1. Secretion of erythropoietin factor by the diseased kidney is decreased.
   2. Chronic hypertension tends to suppress bone marrow centers.
   3. Metabolic alkalosis tends to increase red blood cell fragility.
   4. Excretion of red blood cells in the urine is increased.
10. A routine preoperative assessment for the patient having vein ligation and stripping would include the following laboratory studies:
    1. VDRL, NA, K, Cl.
    2. Prothrombin time, ALT (SGOT), VDRL.
    3. UA, CBC, prothrombin time.
    4. WBC, VDRL, serum glucose.
11. The nurse finds a marijuana joint under an adolescent patient's pillow. After being confronted, the patient promises not to smoke marijuana again if the nurse will not report the incident. The nurse fears that the patient is being manipulative. The *most* therapeutic nursing intervention when working with manipulative patients is to:
    1. Make decisions for them.
    2. Reinforce use of alternative behaviors.
    3. Set rigid limits.
    4. Confront them in front of others.
12. A multiparous woman is admitted to the birth unit for induction of labor. The nurse performing Leopold's maneuvers notes that uterine tonicity is normal and the presenting part (the sacrum) is high, not engaged. The nurse expects that medical management will probably consist of:
    1. Delaying induction until the presenting part is at 0 station.
    2. Piper forceps–assisted vaginal birth.
    3. Spontaneous, vaginal birth.
    4. Cesarean birth.
13. The nurse knows the acetonuria develops in diabetes due to:
    1. Excessive oxidation of fatty acids for energy, which increases ketones in glomerular filtrate.
    2. Osmotic diuresis, accompanying elevation in serum-glucose levels, which decreases exchange of electrolytes in renal tubules.

3. Failure of sodium-hydrogen ion exchange mechanism in the renal tubules to secrete excess hydrogen ions.
4. Increased volatile H^+ ions and decreased nonvolatile H^+ ions in the glomerular filtrate.

14. A woman experienced an incomplete spontaneous abortion. After evacuation of the uterus, an oxytocic agent is ordered to prevent hemorrhage. An ergot product (e.g., ergonovine) is ordered. The nurse knows that ergot products are contraindicated:
1. Until the uterus is emptied.
2. When the woman is normotensive.
3. If her religion proscribes the use of blood products.
4. If she is a candidate for receiving $Rh_0(D)$ immune globulin.

15. A woman who is diabetic gives birth to an 8-pound 11-ounce boy at 38 weeks. On her first postpartum day she is eating a full diet and her insulin has been cut to one-third of the dosage during pregnancy. The night nurse is making rounds and wants to assess the sleeping woman for signs indicating her response to the lowered insulin dosage. Which indicates this woman is hyperglycemic?
1. A flash of light in her face does not elicit a squint or turn of the head.
2. She seems restless, her face is flushed, her pulse is rapid, and her respirations are deep.
3. She is perspiring profusely.
4. She awakens with a headache.

16. The nurse expects hyperkalemia on assessment to occur in chronic renal dysfunction because:
1. As metabolic acidosis increases, the kidneys selectively secrete more H^+ than K^+ in exchange for Na^+.
2. As edema forms, sodium diffuses into the interstitial space and is balanced by increased serum potassium.
3. Respiratory compensation for metabolic acidosis tends to increase K^+ reabsorption by the kidneys.
4. The nausea and vomiting that occur with metabolic acidosis tend to increase serum potassium to compensate for chloride losses.

17. A patient has second-degree burns of the left leg and thigh. The nurse plans to help prevent contractures in the burned leg by:
1. Maintaining abduction of the left leg, extension of the left knee, and flexion of the left ankle.
2. Maintaining abduction of the left leg and extension of the left knee and ankle.
3. Maintaining abduction of the left leg and flexion of the left knee and ankle.
4. Maintaining adduction of the left leg, flexion of the left knee, and extension of the left ankle.

18. A truss is a pad of firm material that is placed over a hernial opening and held in place with a belt. When should the nurse apply a hernia truss on a patient?
1. After the patient gets out of bed but before engaging in strenuous activity.
2. After the hernia has been reduced, with the patient lying down with feet elevated.
3. At any time, whether or not the hernia has been reduced, to prevent further extrusion of the bowel.
4. Not at all, for physicians no longer recommend the use of a truss, because athletic supporters are sufficient in preventing further herniation.

19. To correctly administer a tuberculin skin test, the nurse would inject 5 TU (tuberculin units) of PPD (purified protein derivative) of tuberculin:
1. Intradermally.
2. Subcutaneously.
3. Intramuscularly.
4. Subdermally.

20. If bile flow into the duodenum is obstructed, absorption of fat-soluble vitamins is reduced. Which complication would the nurse therefore observe?
1. Peripheral neuritis.
2. Scurvy.
3. Increased bleeding tendencies.
4. Macrocytic anemia.

21. The preoperative nursing care plan for a patient having cataract surgery includes:
1. Keeping the patient flat in bed.
2. Applying eye patches to both eyes.
3. Orienting the patient to the environment and nursing personnel.
4. Teaching the patient eyedrop instillation.

22. Following a thyroid scan with ^{131}I for a thyroid nodule, the nurse should plan for:
1. No special radiation precautions.
2. Full radiation precautions to be instituted, including segregating the patient in a private room.
3. Radiation precautions that are limited to urine and feces.
4. Full radiation precautions to be instituted for 8 hours (the half-life of ^{131}I).

23. To prevent displacement of radium implants in the cervix, the nurse should position the patient:
1. With the foot of the bed elevated.
2. Flat in bed.
3. With the head elevated 45 degrees (semi-Fowler's).
4. On the side only.

24. A woman in labor is moved into the Cesarean room. Her husband enters the room and appears anxious. The nurse should ask him:
1. "How are you feeling?"
2. "Are you feeling up to this?"
3. "Would you rather wait outside?"
4. "Can I get you anything?"

25. The parents of a newborn who has a unilateral cleft lip and palate are anxious to have surgery performed as soon as possible to repair the deformities. The most appropriate response to the couple's questions about when the surgery may be performed would be to:
1. Reinforce what the physicians have told the parents.
2. Inform the parents that the baby's lip may be repaired during the first few weeks of life and the palate repaired at 12–18 months, before speech develops.
3. Refer the couple to the surgeon.
4. Tell the couple that a complete repair may be performed when their baby weighs at least 10 pounds.

26. A total thyroidectomy is ordered following discovery of a cold nodule. In this case of *hyperthyroidism* versus malignancy, the nurse anticipates that the patient will have:
1. A complete thyroidectomy also.
2. A partial thyroidectomy (approximately one-half of the thyroid is removed).
3. A partial thyroidectomy (approximately five-sixths of the thyroid is removed).
4. Administration of thyroid medication.

27. Besides jaundice of the sclera and skin, what other clinical parameters might indicate biliary obstruction in the patient?
1. Increased systolic and diastolic pressures.
2. Frequent eructation between meals.
3. Darkened urine and clay-colored stools.
4. Longitudinal ridging of the fingernails.

28. A patient who has a long-term history of smoking and a smoker's cough is scheduled for bilateral herniorrhaphy. Which preoperative nursing action will be a priority?
1. Explanation of the surgical procedure.
2. Respiratory hygiene measures and instructions in deep breathing.
3. Discussion of postoperative nursing care measures.

4. Assurance that pain medication will be available whenever needed.

29. A patient has been NPO for the last 12 hours in preparation for an intravenous pyelogram (IVP) and has been complaining of thirst. The specific gravity of the patient's urine has been averaging 1.008. The nurse's explanation for these signs and symptoms is:
    1. The hypothalamus is stimulating increased secretion of ADH.
    2. Extracellular fluid has become hypo-osmolar.
    3. The kidneys are no longer able to concentrate urine, making the extracellular fluid hyperosmolar.
    4. Most patients complain of thirst after fluid restriction.

30. Which contributes to the development of ascites in cirrhosis of the liver?
    1. Portal hypertension, venous dilation, and stasis.
    2. Increased hepatic synthesis of albumin.
    3. Decreased serum levels of aldosterone and ADH.
    4. Increased blood volume causing increased blood hydrostatic pressure in the capillary bed.

31. The nurse explains to a patient that a bronchoscopy is:
    1. An x-ray procedure that allows for multiple views of the lungs.
    2. A procedure utilizing a lighted mirror lens to observe the walls of the trachea, mainstem bronchus, and major bronchial tubes.
    3. A diagnostic test during which a radiopaque substance is inserted into the tracheobronchial tree for clear visualization.
    4. A needle puncture of the lung mass, identified on an x-ray with aspiration of cells for microscopic examination.

32. With severe diarrhea, electrolytes as well as fluids are lost. The nurse would conclude that the patient is experiencing hypokalemia if which of the following were observed?
    1. Spasms, high T waves on ECG, irregular pulse.
    2. Kussmaul breathing, thirst, furrowed tongue.
    3. Apathy, weakness, GI disturbance.
    4. Pitting edema, confusion, bounding pulse.

33. A woman anticipating a stat cesarean birth expresses some concern over feeling the incision and experiencing pain. The most appropriate response would be:
    1. "You will feel nothing at all."
    2. "You may feel some pressure in the area during surgery."
    3. "You may feel slight pain when the incision is made."
    4. "If you feel any pain, it is only your imagination."

34. After discharge following ileostomy surgery, a patient calls the nurse at the hospital to report the sudden onset of abdominal cramps, vomiting, and watery discharge from the ileostomy. What should the nurse advise?
    1. Call the physician if symptoms persist for 24 hours.
    2. Take 30 ml of m.o.m. (milk of magnesia).
    3. NPO until vomiting stops.
    4. Call the physician immediately.

35. To safely transport a patient who has chest tube drainage to the x-ray department to assess the degree of lung reexpansion, the nurse would:
    1. Remove the chest tubes, immediately covering the incision site with a sterile petrolatum gauze to prevent air from entering the chest.
    2. Disconnect the drainage bottles from the chest tubes, covering the catheter tip with a sterile dressing to prevent contamination.
    3. Send the patient to x-ray with the chest tube clamped but still attached to the drainage system to prevent air from entering the chest wall if the bottles are accidentally broken.
    4. Send the patient to x-ray with the chest tube attached to the drainage system, taking precautions to prevent interruption in the system.

36. Which statement would the nurse make to differentiate ketoacidosis from insulin shock?
    1. Deep and rapid respirations are characteristic of ketoacidosis, whereas slow, shallow respirations are characteristic of insulin shock.
    2. Acetone breath characterizes ketoacidosis, whereas the breath of the patient in insulin shock is frequently fetid.
    3. Warm, dry, flushed skin and loss of turgor characterize the patient with ketoacidosis, whereas the skin of the patient with insulin shock is usually pale, cool, and diaphoretic.
    4. Apprehension, irritability, and combative behavior occur with ketoacidosis, whereas the patient in insulin shock is more likely to be confused, lethargic, or comatose.

37. The nurse explains to the patient and family that because of excessive bleeding, an emergency hysterectomy will need to be performed:
    1. Upon completion of the necessary surgical preparation.
    2. Immediately.
    3. Within 24 hours.
    4. At the start of the next surgical day.

38. The nurse can anticipate a marked improvement in the patient's prognosis if a hepatic coma lasts no longer than:
    1. 24 hours.
    2. 36 hours.
    3. 48 hours.
    4. 72 hours.

39. The effectiveness of peritoneal dialysis will be measured by:
    1. Serum potassium less than 3.5 mEq/L and serum sodium greater than 148 mEq/L.
    2. Unchanged quantity and specific gravity of urine.
    3. BUN less than 20 mg/dL, serum creatinine less than 1.2 mg/dL.
    4. Moderately soft abdomen and dullness on percussion.

40. After explaining peritoneal dialysis procedures to a patient and the family and obtaining a signed operative permit, the nurse's next action is to:
    1. Have the patient empty the bladder.
    2. Position the patient in a comfortable supine position.
    3. Weigh the patient and record vital signs.
    4. Cleanse and drape the abdomen.

41. Of the following activities of daily living, which should the nurse recommend that a patient (who has had a bilateral hernia repair) avoid after discharge?
    1. Driving to and from work.
    2. Walking 3 miles a day.
    3. Washing and polishing the car.
    4. Carrying out the garbage cans.

42. A patient has had a spinal anesthetic. In the recovery room, it will be important that the nurse immediately position this patient:
    1. On the side to prevent obstruction of airway by tongue.
    2. Flat on the back.
    3. On the back, with knees flexed 15 degrees.
    4. Flat on the stomach, with head turned to side.

43. After positioning a patient who has had spinal anesthesia, the recovery room nurse initially should make which observation?
    1. Status of reflexes.
    2. Vital signs.
    3. Patient's level of consciousness.
    4. Integrity of airway.

44. While giving diet instructions after a cholecystectomy, the nurse would inform the patient that:
    1. The diet will not include fatty food for at least 1 year.
    2. After approximately 3 months polyunsaturated fats can be added to the diet.
    3. There are no specific dietary restrictions in the postoperative period, but the patient will be more comfortable if large, fatty meals are avoided.
    4. The diet will be limited to 20 g of fat per day.

45. While assisting a patient who has had a thyroidectomy to dangle at the bedside on the first postoperative evening, the most appropriate nursing action would be to:
    1. Support the patient under the axilla while bringing the feet over the bedside.
    2. Bring the patient's feet to the side of the bed and support the back of the neck while assisting the patient to assume a sitting position.
    3. Allow the patient to assume the sitting position at the patient's own pace, unassisted unless necessary.
    4. Bring the patient's feet to the side of the bed, then pull the patient forward.

46. New parents of a baby with a cleft lip and palate are experiencing a reactive depression in response to the birth of their infant, who is in the high-risk newborn nursery. The primary difference between a reactive (situational) depression and major depressive disorder—melancholic type (endogenous depression) is that in a reactive depression:
    1. There is substantial weight loss, usually over 10 pounds.
    2. The individual does not respond to environmental stimuli.
    3. The individual generally feels worse as the day progresses.
    4. The precipitating event is usually difficult to identify.

47. An Apgar score of 4 at 1 and 5 minutes indicates that the neonate's condition is:
    1. Excellent.
    2. Good.
    3. Fair.
    4. Poor.

48. A toddler who fractured the right femur in a car accident is placed in Bryant's traction and admitted to the hospital. During the first night in the hospital, the toddler lies still in the crib, sucks a thumb, and occasionally sobs quietly in a monotone voice. The nurse should interpret these behaviors to mean that the toddler:
    1. Wants his or her mother.
    2. Might prefer to sleep in a bed.
    3. Probably does not sleep through the night at home.
    4. May be experiencing painful muscle spasms due to the fracture.

49. Most accidental pregnancies in couples using "natural" family planning methods have been related to unprotected intercourse *before* ovulation. Which factor explains why pregnancy may be achieved by unprotected intercourse during the preovulatory period?
    1. Spermatozoal viability.
    2. Ovum viability.
    3. Tubal motility.
    4. Secretory endometrium.

50. Parents of an infant with deformities may use which of the following defense mechanisms in attempting to cope with their anxiety?
    1. Fixation.
    2. Displacement.
    3. Conversion.
    4. Sublimation.

51. The parents of an infant born with a cleft lip and palate express concern about caring for their infant. They are especially worried about paying excessive hospital bills because insurance has set limits. The most appropriate nursing action would be to:
    1. Refer the couple to a social worker.
    2. Validate the couple's perceived needs.
    3. Discuss alternatives with the couple.
    4. Implement health teaching regarding the physical care of the infant.

52. The nurse suggests that premenopausal breast self-examinations are best carried out:
    1. During the middle of the menstrual cycle.

2. On the first day of each month.
    3. One week after the onset of menses.
    4. The week before the onset of menses.

53. In preparing a patient for an IV cholangiogram, it is important for the nurse to ascertain:
    1. If the patient has ever had the procedure before.
    2. If the patient has any known allergies, particularly to fish or other iodine-containing substances.
    3. If the patient's epigastric discomfort occurs only with fatty-food ingestion.
    4. If there is a family history of gallstones.

54. The nurse suspects abdominal wound dehiscence, and lifts the edges of the patient's dressings. The nurse notes that the wound edges are entirely separated. What is the *next* nursing action?
    1. Tell the patient to remain quiet and not to cough.
    2. Offer the patient a warm drink to promote relaxation.
    3. Position the patient in a chair with the feet elevated.
    4. Apply a scultetus bandage.

55. Which of the following signs and symptoms are *least* likely to occur during peritoneal dialysis if fluid drainage is inadequate?
    1. A negative balance between the amount drained and the amount instilled.
    2. Confusion, lethargy, and coma.
    3. Moist crackles and rhonchi.
    4. Flattened neck veins in a supine position.

56. Which nursing action is designed to reduce ammonia intoxication in a patient with bleeding esophageal varices who is jaundiced, edematous, and in a hepatic coma?
    1. Active and passive range-of-motion exercises to prevent venous stasis.
    2. Tap-water enemas to remove blood that may still be in the gut from the bleeding esophageal varices.
    3. Administration of insulin and glucagon to reduce serum-potassium levels.
    4. Holding all antibiotic medications so that the action of the intestinal bacteria on protein is enhanced.

57. In analyzing the BBT record of a woman who has a normal 30-day cycle, on which of the following days would the nurse expect to find evidence of ovulation?
    1. Day 5 or 6.
    2. Day 13 or 14.
    3. Day 16 or 17.
    4. Day 28 or 29.

58. The nurse explains to a patient's family that the surgical treatment *most* often implemented for excessive vaginal bleeding due to uterine fibroids is:
    1. Panabdominal hysterectomy.
    2. Vaginal hysterectomy.
    3. Dilation and curettage.
    4. Abdominal hysterectomy.

59. Following surgery, a patient with diabetes complains of nausea and appears lethargic and flushed. BP 108/78, P 100, R 24 and deep. The first nursing action should be:
    1. Call the attending physician.
    2. Check the patient's blood glucose.
    3. Administer an antiemetic.
    4. Decrease the patient's IV infusion rate.

60. Passive arm exercises are instituted on a patient's left arm 4 hours after lobectomy surgery. The nurse assists with these exercises to prevent which dysfunction?
    1. Hyperflexion of the wrist.
    2. Ankylosis of the shoulder.
    3. Flexion of the elbow.
    4. Spasticity of the intercostal muscles.

61. The nurse initiates ileostomy teaching with a patient during the early postoperative period. The primary objective of this procedure is:
    1. To facilitate maintenance of intake and output records.
    2. To control unpleasant odors.

3. To prevent excoriation of the skin around the stoma.

4. To reduce the risk of postoperative wound infection.

62. When teaching families about cleft lip and palate, the nurse would need to be aware that:
    1. Cleft lip occurs most frequently in girls.
    2. Cleft palate occurs most frequently in boys.
    3. Cleft lip and palate almost always occur simultaneously.
    4. Cleft lip and palate are both influenced by hereditary factors.

63. A pregnant woman was instructed to report signs and symptoms of preterm labor. The nurse knows that the woman failed to follow instructions about evaluating her signs and symptoms when she telephoned *before* she:
    1. Waited to see if uterine contractions were occurring every 10 minutes.
    2. Assessed that her contractions continued after she emptied her bladder.
    3. Drank a glass of water for hydration.
    4. Rested in bed on her side for 1 hour.

64. The Trendelenburg test is frequently used to evaluate the competence of venous valves. Prior to administering the test, the nurse tells the patient that this test will consist of:
    1. Walking back and forth so the nurse can observe venous changes during walking.
    2. Injecting a contrast medium into the veins and taking multiple x-rays as the dye flows in the veins.
    3. Stripping a superficial vein, occluding flow, and then releasing the vein and observing the direction of filling.
    4. Elevating the involved leg to empty the veins, applying a tourniquet to the upper thigh while the patient is first lying down and then standing, and then removing the tourniquet to observe the filling of the superficial veins.

65. A woman who is anticipating a stat cesarean birth for a fetus in transverse lie questions the nurse about the type of incision the physician will use in her operation. The nurse should realize that this woman's *primary* concern involves the possibility of:
    1. Infection.
    2. Bleeding.
    3. Scarring.
    4. Rupture.

66. A patient asks the nurse whether marijuana is addictive. The most appropriate response by the nurse would be:
    1. "It is addictive."
    2. "It causes a psychological dependence."
    3. "It is not addictive."
    4. "It is physiologically addictive."

67. Following the insertion of a catheter into the abdominal cavity, warmed dialyzing solution is allowed to run rapidly (10–20 minutes) into the abdominal cavity. The nurse warmed the solution to body temperature to prevent abdominal pain and to:
    1. Expand the molecules and increase the osmotic gradient.
    2. Increase dilation of the peritoneal vessels, thereby increasing urea clearance.
    3. Decrease the likelihood of peritonitis due to constriction of peritoneal vessels.
    4. Expedite the movement of the dialyzing solute into the abdomen.

68. Preoperative teaching measures unique to the patient having a thyroidectomy should encompass:
    1. Active flexion exercise of the neck, special coughing instructions, voice rest, and antithyroid medications postoperatively.
    2. Active flexion and extension neck exercises, deep breathing and coughing, and thyroid replacement when necessary.
    3. Instruction on supporting the back of the neck when repositioning and ambulating, and avoiding hyperextension and flexion of the neck when coughing.

4. Instruction on supporting the back of the neck when ambulating and repositioning and active flexion exercises of the neck.

69. The nurse will plan to read the reaction to an intradermal tuberculin test in:
    1. 6–12 hours.
    2. 12–24 hours.
    3. 24–48 hours.
    4. 48–72 hours.

70. Which are precautionary nursing measures to be used when caring for a patient being treated with internal radioisotopes?
    1. Maintain strict patient isolation, and limit professional contact with patient.
    2. Limit exposure, and maximize distance between patient, professional, and family.
    3. Position the patient in a prone position, and restrict turning to mealtimes only.
    4. Maintain the legs in a flexed position to decrease the likelihood of dislodgement.

71. The nurse explains to a patient who is diagnosed with cirrhosis that the anemia is the result of:
    1. Increased RBC fragility due to folic acid deficiencies from inadequate dietary intake.
    2. Decreased efficiency of Kupffer cells in the liver.
    3. Increased blood-ammonia levels.
    4. Decreased amino acid breakdown and synthesis.

72. Postoperative vital signs for a patient with diabetes are BP 108/78, pulse 100, respirations 24 and deep. IV intake has been 2100 mL and urine output 2000 mL. The nurse recognizes that the patient is experiencing:
    1. Increased ADH release in response to physiological stress of surgery.
    2. Decreased extracellular fluid (ECF) volume due to osmotic diuresis.
    3. A hypo-osmolar fluid imbalance.
    4. Circulatory overload.

73. Following bronchoscopy, what is the nurse's most important observation?
    1. Blood pressure, pulse, and temperature.
    2. Color and consistency of sputum.
    3. Function of the tenth cranial nerve.
    4. Presence of urticaria.

74. The nurse knows that emergency procedures increase the surgical risk to the patient because:
    1. The surgery is performed immediately.
    2. There is little time for psychological/physical preparation.
    3. There is decreased physiological stress.
    4. The anesthesia of choice is different for emergency surgery.

75. Care of the patient on peritoneal dialysis must allow a dwell time, or equilibration period, of the dialyzing fluid, which is normally:
    1. 10–15 minutes.
    2. 20–30 minutes.
    3. 50–60 minutes.
    4. More than 1 hour.

76. The Billings method (or cervical mucus method) of natural family planning incorporates patient examination of cervical mucus. Which characteristics are typical of the cervical mucus during the "fertile" period of the menstrual cycle?
    1. Thick, cloudy.
    2. Thin, clear, good spinnbarkeit.
    3. Yellow, sticky.
    4. Absence of ferning.

77. An elderly patient asks about the type of anesthesia used for cataract surgery. The nurse replies that this surgery is generally performed using a:
    1. Local.
    2. General.

3. Intravenous.
4. Rectal.

78. A patient has frequent stools, with poor oral intake of both fluids and solids. While administering the ordered parenteral hyperalimentation, it is important to remember that hyperalimentation solutions are:
    1. Hypotonic solutions used primarily for hydration when hemoconcentration is present.
    2. Hypertonic solutions used primarily to increase osmotic pressure of blood plasma.
    3. Alkalyzing solutions used to treat metabolic acidosis, thus reducing cellular swelling.
    4. Hyperosmolar solutions used primarily to reverse negative nitrogen balance.

79. A newborn's Apgar score at 1 and 5 minutes is 4. The nurse assisting with the care of this newborn should realize the *primary* goal is to:
    1. Establish an airway.
    2. Maintain an adequate temperature.
    3. Reassure the parents.
    4. Monitor the infant's vital signs.

80. The nurse concludes from a patient's assessment and history of muscle fatigue and ankle swelling that vein-stripping is indicated, because of:
    1. Advancing varicosities and cosmetic reasons.
    2. Stasis ulceration and thrombophlebitis.
    3. Lymphedema and Raynaud's disease.
    4. Advancing varicosities only.

81. Besides omission of food and fluids by mouth, other nursing considerations in the preparation of a patient for IVP would include:
    1. Ingestion of contrast medium the morning of the procedure.
    2. Administration of cathartics or enemas to improve visualization of contrast medium in renal structures.
    3. A low-protein and low-salt diet the evening before to increase hyperosmolarity of ECF.
    4. Institution of an intravenous line to maintain fluid and electrolyte balance.

82. The nurse gives postoperative explanation to a patient with diabetes that regular or crystalline insulin is used as an adjunct to NPH therapy because:
    1. There is increased tissue metabolism with surgery.
    2. Insulin production is decreased even further with the stress of surgery.
    3. Physiological and psychological stress increases serum-glucose levels via sympathetic nervous system stimulation.
    4. An increased insulin load is necessary to prevent hyperkalemia.

83. Three days after successful resuscitation from cardiac arrest after myocardial infarction, the patient states to the nurse, "I'm all washed up. I don't think I'll ever be the same man again." The nurse's best response to this statement would be:
    1. "Most patients who have been as ill as you feel that way."
    2. "How do you feel you have changed from before your illness?"
    3. "Getting depressed won't help you get better."
    4. "Tell me more."

84. The nurse recognizes dyspnea as:
    1. Increased awareness of respiratory effort.
    2. Decreased alveolar ventilation.
    3. Increased rate and depth of respiration.
    4. Decreased oxygen saturation of venous blood.

85. A teenage patient in a substance abuse facility feels very isolated from his peer group because he has been placed in an adult unit. In planning care for this patient, which would be most effective?
    1. Assisting the patient to develop a working relationship with a 51-year-old patient.

2. Encouraging friends to visit frequently.
3. Asking the adolescent what he enjoys doing.
4. Establishing a one-to-one relationship with the patient.

86. A patient asks what type of anesthesia is usually used during vein-stripping. The nurse tells the patient to expect:
    1. Local.
    2. Topical.
    3. Regional.
    4. General.

87. A patient with a history of many years of smoking and a smoker's cough is scheduled for bilateral herniorrhaphy. Which type of surgical anesthesia may be most appropriate for this situation?
    1. General.
    2. Intravenous.
    3. Spinal.
    4. Local infiltration.

88. Pulmonary function testing on a patient with a long history of smoking revealed a vital capacity within normal limits but a reduced forced expiratory volume (FEV_1). The nurse explains to the family that this means that the patient:
    1. Has difficulty moving air in and out of the lungs.
    2. May have some airway obstruction.
    3. Has weakened expiratory muscles of respirations.
    4. May have some areas of atelectasis in the lungs.

89. A patient has a long leg cast due to a fractured right tibia and fibula. Which is an appropriate exercise for this patient to prevent complications of immobility?
    1. Quadriceps setting.
    2. Extension of the right knee.
    3. Passive range of motion of the hip.
    4. Flexion of the right knee.

90. The nurse concludes that an intradermal TB test result is positive if the following is present:
    1. An induration of 10 mm or more.
    2. An induration of 10 cm or more.
    3. An induration of 5–9 mm.
    4. A hivelike vesicle.

91. In providing emotional support for a couple whose infant is unhealthy or has an abnormality, the nurse should realize that at first they will probably:
    1. Wish to talk with other couples who have experienced the same circumstances.
    2. Wish to be left alone, unless they seek out someone to talk to.
    3. Need reassurance and emotional support.
    4. Avoid discussing the situation at this time.

92. In assessing the acid-base status of a patient diagnosed with glomerulonephritis, the nurse would be alert to the following signs of metabolic acidosis:
    1. Hyperreflexia, paresthesias, and tetany.
    2. Giddiness, irregular respiratory pattern, and moist, cool skin.
    3. Muscle weakness, and numbness and tingling in the extremities.
    4. Lethargy, disorientation, and increased rate and depth of respirations.

93. On the second day after a lobectomy, the fluid in the water-seal chamber ceases to fluctuate. The nurse knows that this most likely indicates:
    1. The chest tube is plugged by fibrin or a clot.
    2. There is an air leak in the system.
    3. Pulmonary edema has occurred due to increased blood volume in remaining lung tissue.
    4. The patient's position needs to change to facilitate drainage.

94. What side effects would a patient demonstrate if he or she received hyperalimentation solution at too rapid an infusion rate?

1. Cellular dehydration and potassium depletion.
2. Circulatory overload and hypoglycemia.
3. Hypoglycemia and hypovolemia.
4. Potassium excess and congestive heart failure.

95. Which nursing action is _least_ likely to assist parents to adjust to the psychological trauma of the birth of a deformed child?
    1. Encouraging verbalization of anxiety, fears, and concerns.
    2. Explaining all treatments and prognosis.
    3. Interacting normally with the infant.
    4. Expressing sympathy.

96. Nursing measures that should decrease the incidence of hemorrhage after thyroidectomy are:
    1. Frequent checking of dressing, semi-Fowler's position, and ice packs to neck.
    2. Frequent checking of dressing, supine position, and ice packs to neck.
    3. Frequent checking of dressing, coughing every 2 hours, and moist packs to neck.
    4. Frequent checking of dressings and maintenance of neck flexion.

97. The nurse must assess past medical history and use of medications for any surgical candidate. Which drugs can negatively interfere with anesthesia or contribute to postoperative complications?
    1. Anticoagulants and antihypertensives.
    2. Anticoagulants and insulin.
    3. Digoxin and thiazide diuretics.
    4. Vitamins and mineral replacements.

98. Anticipatory guidance planned for a woman with diabetes who has just given birth includes health teaching regarding self-care health maintenance actions in the postpartum period. She wants to breastfeed her baby. Which should be emphasized as part of her postpartum instructions?
    1. Breastfeeding is contraindicated because it stimulates gluconeogenesis.
    2. Her caloric needs will decrease during the postpartum period, so she must be alert for signs of hyperglycemia.
    3. She should breastfeed the baby before feeding herself so that she can relax; stress inhibits the flow of breast milk.
    4. She must prevent hypoglycemia because it can inhibit the let-down reflex and decrease her milk supply.

99. To assess accurately a patient's functional and vocational rehabilitation potential with myasthenia gravis, the nurse must _first_ ascertain:
    1. The degree of physical and emotional stress in the patient's present occupation.
    2. The activities of daily living that cause the greatest degree of muscle weakness and fatigue.
    3. The patient's understanding of and attitude toward myasthenia gravis, as well as the ability to cope with activity restrictions.
    4. Whether or not the patient's current occupation allows opportunities to sit down and rest when necessary.

100. The nurse tells a patient that NPH insulin reaches its peak action:
    1. 4 hours after injection.
    2. 6–12 hours after injection.
    3. 12–14 hours after injection.
    4. 15–18 hours after injection.

101. A patient has multiple fractures of both legs; treatment includes bed rest with skeletal traction. The nursing intervention that would be _most_ effective in prevention of footdrop would be use of:
    1. A bed cradle.
    2. A footboard.
    3. Passive range of motion every shift.
    4. A trochanter roll.

102. While providing care for a newborn with a cleft lip and palate, the nurse must also be aware of the parents' feelings. Both appear stunned. However, they are still in touch with reality and are asking appropriate questions focused on the newborn's condition. At what level of anxiety is the couple functioning at this time?
    1. Mild.
    2. Moderate.
    3. Severe.
    4. Panic.

103. Which nursing action is inappropriate in the preparation of a patient for _oral_ cholecystography?
    1. Administering a fat-free diet the evening before the test.
    2. Administering Telepaque (iopanoic acid) tablets in 5-minute intervals 1 hour after supper.
    3. Administering at least 6 oz of water with each Telepaque (iopanoic acid) tablet.
    4. Allowing the patient, after ingesting the tablets, to drink water until midnight, then NPO.

104. A preoperative _nursing priority_ for a patient having a tracheostomy is:
    1. Establishing postoperative communication.
    2. Drawing blood for serum-electrolyte and blood gas determinations.
    3. Inserting a Foley catheter and attaching it to dependent drainage.
    4. Doing a surgical prep of the neck and upper chest wall.

105. The nurse explains to a patient that the purpose of intermittent positive-pressure breathing (IPPB) with normal saline is to maintain patent airways and to mobilize secretions. To accomplish this, IPPB exerts:
    1. Positive pressures on inspiration.
    2. Negative pressures on inspiration.
    3. Positive pressures on expiration.
    4. Negative pressures on expiration.

106. A 3-month-old infant brought unconscious to the emergency department (ED) by the parents was pronounced dead. The mother becomes hysterical, crying uncontrollably. The father asks the nurse to "do something." The most appropriate nursing action would be:
    1. Providing the parents with privacy.
    2. Obtaining an order for a tranquilizer.
    3. Sitting quietly with the couple.
    4. Asking the mother to calm down.

107. A pregnant woman tells the nurse that she has a family history of cystic fibrosis and wonders if her unborn child is at risk for this disorder. The nurse's response is based on knowledge that most inborn errors of metabolism are:
    1. Autosomal-dominant inherited disorders.
    2. Autosomal-recessive inherited disorders.
    3. X-linked recessive inheritance disorders.
    4. Multifactorial inheritance disorders.

108. The drainage period during peritoneal dialysis generally takes 20 minutes, though this may vary from patient to patient. If fluid is not draining properly, the nurse can facilitate return by:
    1. Turning the patient to a prone position.
    2. Manipulating the indwelling catheter.
    3. Elevating the head of the bed, thereby increasing intraabdominal pressures.
    4. Elevating the foot of the bed, thereby increasing abdominal pressures and gravity flow.

109. The nurse needs to know that the essential purpose of the water-sealed drainage system for a patient following a lower left lobectomy is to:
    1. Prevent early precipitous reinflation of the lung.
    2. Drain off excess fluid and air, thereby promoting reestablishment of negative intrapleural pressures.

3. Drain off excess fluid and air, thereby promoting reestablishment of positive intrapleural pressures.

4. Decrease atelectasis in unaffected lung tissue and to monitor blood loss.

110. In providing post-operative nursing care for the infant after a cleft lip repair, the nurse should:
   1. Place the infant in a prone position to facilitate drainage.
   2. Avoid moving the infant too much in order to keep from dislodging the Logan bar.
   3. Cleanse the suture area frequently to prevent scarring.
   4. Encourage the infant to cry to promote adequate lung aeration.

111. Muscular twitching and hyperirritability of the nervous system indicate tetany (hypocalcemia). The nurse can assess for this complication by:
   1. Checking the urine calcium.
   2. Palpating the calf muscle, with the ankle hyperflexed.
   3. Tapping the facial nerve just proximal to the ear.
   4. Checking for ankle clonus.

112. Which problem should the nurse expect following uterine isotope insertion?
   1. Bladder atony.
   2. Constipation.
   3. Foul-smelling vaginal discharge.
   4. Loss of sexual libido.

113. Preoperative nursing measures for a patient having a cholecystectomy due to cholelithiasis and cholecystitis include:
   1. Observing for bruising or easy bleeding due to potential prothrombin deficiency.
   2. Informing the patient of the purpose of the postoperative Jackson-Pratt drain.
   3. Providing relief for abdominal discomfort by placing a heating pad on the upper abdomen.
   4. Providing a low-carbohydrate diet to stimulate release of glycogen stores in the liver.

114. Which of the following is the best single nursing measure of fluid volume status in a patient with chronic renal dysfunction?
   1. Skin turgor.
   2. Vital signs.
   3. Daily weights.
   4. Intake and output.

115. The nurse discusses available methods for family planning with the patient. Which method acts by preventing implantation of the zygote if fertilization occurs?
   1. Tubal ligation.
   2. Intrauterine device.
   3. Oral contraceptives.
   4. Diaphragm and spermicidal jelly.

116. Which recreational activity for a hospitalized adolescent would be most appropriate for the nurse to support?
   1. A television to watch in the two-bed hospital room.
   2. Schoolwork that can be brought to the hospital.
   3. A board game such as checkers or Monopoly.
   4. Various novels the adolescent wants to read.

117. Women who tend to delay seeking medical advice after discovering a lump in the breast are displaying what common defense mechanism?
   1. Suppression.
   2. Denial.
   3. Repression.
   4. Intellectualization.

118. When can the nurse expect a patient who is receiving NPH insulin to *most* likely have a hypoglycemic reaction?
   1. Before lunch (10–11 A.M.).
   2. Early afternoon (1–3 P.M.).
   3. Late afternoon (4–7 P.M.).
   4. After supper (8–10 P.M.).

119. The physician has left orders to deflate a patient's Sengstaken-Blakemore tube, used to stop esophageal bleeding, for 5 minutes every 12 hours to prevent esophageal erosion. Two hours following the second reinflation, the patient suddenly becomes severely dyspneic and dusky. The nurse should:
   1. Call a code blue (cardiac arrest).
   2. Deflate the balloons.
   3. Decrease the traction on the tube where it enters the nose.
   4. Irrigate the tube with ice-cold saline to facilitate movement of the balloons into the stomach.

120. The nurse explains that the surgical preparation for a patient scheduled for bilateral herniorrhaphy would include cleansing and shaving:
   1. The entire abdomen from just below the nipple line to the midthigh.
   2. The entire abdomen from the axilla to the pubis.
   3. From the waistline of the abdomen to below both knees.
   4. Lower abdomen, the pubic area, perineum, and inner sides of thighs and buttocks.

121. Postoperative coughing and deep breathing may become a nursing problem following cholecystectomy because:
   1. Patients having abdominal surgery are prone to pulmonary complications.
   2. Patients with biliary surgery tend to breathe shallowly to prevent pain and discomfort.
   3. Many people tend to be thoracic breathers rather than diaphragmatic breathers.
   4. Patients with upper-abdominal surgery usually have a nasogastric tube in place, which inhibits deep breathing.

122. A newborn is admitted to the high-risk neonatal nursery. The father requests permission to see the mother and baby immediately. The most appropriate nursing response would be to:
   1. Take him to see the mother.
   2. Inform him that they both need their rest.
   3. Refer him to the mother's physician.
   4. Allow him to go see the infant.

123. Which statement is correct regarding nursing care of a patient receiving hyperalimentation?
   1. The patient's urine should be tested for glucose acetone every 8–12 hours.
   2. The hyperalimentation subclavian line may be utilized for CVP readings and/or blood withdrawal.
   3. Occlusive dressings at the catheter insertion site are changed every 48 hours using the clean technique.
   4. Records of intake and output and daily weights should be kept.

124. During the procedure to remove the opacified lens, an iridectomy will also be performed. The nurse tells the patient that this procedure is done:
   1. To prevent secondary glaucoma from developing in the postoperative period.
   2. To increase pupillary dilatation postoperatively.
   3. To facilitate circulation and postoperative healing.
   4. To prevent corneal scarring during the procedure.

125. In a closed chest drainage system (Pleur-evac), the nurse knows that:
   1. The first chamber establishes the suction pressure and the second chamber collects the drainage.
   2. The first chamber establishes the suction pressure and the second is attached to motor suction.
   3. The first chamber collects the drainage and the third chamber provides easy access for removing drainage specimens.
   4. The first chamber collects the drainage and the second contains the water seal.

126. Women selecting oral contraceptives as their chosen method of family planning should be instructed to notify the clinic if

they develop symptoms of potential problems. Which symptom requires prompt evaluation?
1. Mild to moderate nausea during the first few days on the medication.
2. Chloasma.
3. Leg cramps or headaches.
4. Breast tenderness and weight gain.

127. In anticipation of emergency complications after thyroidectomy, which nursing measure is essential in the postoperative period?
1. Having calcium gluconate available for possible tetany.
2. Having a thoracentesis tray available to reduce edema.
3. Having a tracheostomy tray available for possible airway obstruction.
4. Having pressure dressings available for possible hemorrhage.

128. A patient's skin test and sputum smear and culture are positive. The chest x-ray demonstrated four small lesions and one of moderate density. Diagnosis: tuberculosis. Respiratory isolation is initiated by the nurse. This means:
1. Both patient and attending nurse must wear masks at all times.
2. Full isolation; that is, caps and gowns are required during the period of contagion.
3. Nurse and visitors must wear masks until chemotherapy is begun. Patient is instructed in cough and tissue techniques.
4. Gloves are worn when handling the patient's tissues, excretions, and linen.

129. The physician recommends an inpatient, short-term drug treatment program for an 11-year-old with a substance abuse problem. The adolescent's father becomes very hostile and states, "My child is no addict and isn't going to be put away in any crazy house." To assess the father's reaction to the physician's recommendation, the nurse should realize that the father is:
1. Expressing anger about the accurate diagnosis.
2. Denying that his child is a drug abuser.
3. Projecting the blame elsewhere.
4. Looking for another, better solution.

130. The preoperative laboratory data of a patient recorded an Hgb of 8.5. What is the nurse's *first* responsibility?
1. To attach the lab report to the chart.
2. To hang a unit of blood.
3. To notify the physician immediately.
4. To chart the report in the nurses' notes.

131. The nurse explains to a patient that methyldopa acts to decrease hypertension by:
1. Dilating peripheral blood vessels and increasing renal flow.
2. Depleting norepinephrine at postganglionic synapses.
3. Inhibiting formation of dopamine, a precursor of norepinephrine.
4. Depressing reticular activating system activity.

132. The mother of a newborn on an apnea monitor tells the nurse that her baby looks so frail and sick. The best response for the nurse to make is:
1. "Your baby does have a life-threatening illness."
2. "Have you seen many newborns?"
3. "Try not to think of your baby like that. Think positive!"
4. "I know how you must feel. It can be very scary to see your baby looking like this."

133. A patient refuses to cough after surgery "because it hurts." The nurse's action would be to:
1. Administer an analgesic and wait a few minutes.
2. Assist the patient to sit up on the side of the bed and splint the incision with a pillow during coughing.
3. Allow the patient to rest this time, but inform the patient that coughing will be expected the next time.

4. Increase fluid intake so as to loosen secretions and ease expectoration.

134. The postoperative nursing care plan following vein-stripping would include which of the following?
1. Administration of anticoagulants to prevent clotting.
2. Elastic stockings/bandages from toe to groin.
3. Sitting in a chair.
4. Bed rest for 48 hours after surgery.

135. On her third postpartum day, a woman with diabetes prepares to return home with her new infant. Which of the following is the priority information to be discussed with this woman before she leaves the hospital?
1. The statistical probability of her infant developing diabetes.
2. The type of medical and obstetric problems that may occur in subsequent pregnancies.
3. Coping strategies with her new baby and diabetes in the immediate postpartum period.
4. Follow-up medical visits for both the infant and herself in the next 6 weeks.

136. The patient returns to the surgical unit following a bilateral hernia repair. The nurse observes that his scrotum is quite swollen. The *first* nursing action is to:
1. Notify the surgeon stat.
2. Elevate the scrotum on a rolled towel and apply ice bags.
3. Administer prn pain medication.
4. Encourage vigorous deep breathing and coughing.

137. A patient with chest tubes returns to the unit. The first nursing measure concerning the closed chest drainage system is:
1. Milking the tubing to prevent accumulation of fibrin and clots.
2. Raising the bottle to bed height to accurately assess the meniscus level.
3. Attaching the chest tubes to the bed linen to ensure that airflow and drainage are unhindered by kinks.
4. Marking the time and the amount of drainage in the collection bottle.

138. For which complication of thyroidectomy would the nurse monitor?
1. Hypercalcemia.
2. Respiratory obstruction.
3. Elevated serum T_4.
4. Paralytic ileus.

139. Which precaution would the nurse implement when caring for a neonate born to a woman who is HIV positive?
1. The nurse should wear gloves until all blood and amniotic fluid have been removed.
2. The woman should be encouraged to breastfeed.
3. The HIV-positive father should have limited contact with the child.
4. The parents should be encouraged to place the infant for adoption since the outlook for the mother is poor.

140. After the birth of an abnormal or unhealthy infant, the nurse should expect the parents' *initial* reactions to include:
1. Depression.
2. Apathy.
3. Withdrawal.
4. Anger.

141. During a postoperative period following a cholecystectomy, the patient has a T-tube connected to gravity drainage. The nurse knows that the purpose of the T-tube is to:
1. Maintain patency of the common bile duct.
2. Reduce the occurrence of postoperative hemorrhage.
3. Prevent infection.
4. Reduce bile flow into the duodenum.

142. A patient being admitted for modified radical mastectomy was restless and had the following vital signs: BP, 186/110 mm Hg; pulse, 90 bpm; respirations, 22; and temperature, 98.4°F. A half-hour later the nurse retakes the patient's vital

signs: BP, 132/86 mm Hg; pulse, 80 bpm; and respirations, 16. The patient's initial elevated BP indicated:

1. She may be an individual who is highly sensitive to sympathetic nervous system stimulation.
2. She is emotionally labile and will need to be assessed closely in the postoperative period.
3. She is psychologically unprepared for surgery and a psych consult is in order.
4. She is denying the possible loss of her breast.

143. A patient diagnosed with cirrhosis has been placed on a moderate-protein, high-carbohydrate, high-calorie, low-salt diet. Which statement would the nurse select as the best rationale for this diet?
    1. Because the liver may not be able to detoxify proteins, carbohydrates are substituted to meet metabolic and nutritional needs.
    2. Proteins are given in sufficient amount to facilitate tissue repair. High-carbohydrate diet prevents further weight loss and spares proteins from energy metabolism. Sodium restriction facilitates management of fluid imbalances.
    3. High-protein foods are harder to digest and also have a high sodium content. Carbohydrates are more palatable and will more quickly correct the patient's weight loss.
    4. High-carbohydrate diets, particularly if they contain adequate fiber, are more likely to decrease dyspepsia and diarrhea. Sodium is always restricted when the patient is edematous.

144. Neomycin is administered by the nurse before ileostomy surgery:
    1. To decrease the incidence of postoperative atelectasis due to decreased depth of respirations.
    2. To increase the effectiveness of the body's immunologic response following surgical trauma.
    3. To reduce the incidence of wound infections by decreasing the number of intestinal organisms.
    4. To prevent postoperative bladder atony due to catheterization.

145. A patient has been diagnosed with cirrhosis and placed on a special diet. One nursing measure that might increase the patient's acceptance of the diet is to:
    1. Sit with the patient until he or she has eaten everything.
    2. Give a family member the responsibility of seeing that the patient eats.
    3. Feed the patient yourself.
    4. Offer frequent, small feedings instead of three large ones.

146. The most important postoperative thoracic surgical activity a patient performs is:
    1. Arm exercises to prevent shoulder ankylosis.
    2. Deep breathing and coughing up of sputum to prevent airway obstruction.
    3. Leg exercises to prevent thrombophlebitis due to prolonged bed rest.
    4. Deep breathing only to prevent undue suture stress while maintaining ventilation.

147. A patient becomes extremely lethargic following administration of meperidine HCl 100 mg IM for pain. What is the most appropriate nursing action?
    1. Give only 50 mg of meperidine next time if pain medication is required.
    2. Administer an oral preparation of meperidine instead of the intramuscular preparation.
    3. Consult with physician about decreasing the amount of pain medication ordered.
    4. Try to prolong the time between medication dosages by employing alternative pain relief strategies.

148. Postoperatively, a patient with a cataract should be positioned:
    1. In a semi-Fowler's position.
    2. In a prone position only.

3. On the back or on the unoperated side.
4. On the operative side.

149. To evaluate a woman's understanding of the use of a diaphragm for family planning, the nurse asks her to explain, in her own words, how she will use the appliance. Which response indicates a need for further health teaching?
    1. "I really need to use the diaphragm and jelly most during the middle of my menstrual cycle."
    2. "The diaphragm must be left in place for at least 6 hours after intercourse."
    3. "I may need a different size diaphragm if I gain or lose more than 20 pounds."
    4. "I should check the diaphragm carefully for holes every time I use it."

150. In observing the drainage from the T-tube during a patient's early postoperative cholecystectomy period, the nurse would notify the physician if:
    1. The drainage contained blood during the first 2–4 hours after surgery.
    2. The drainage was less than 500 mL on the first postoperative day.
    3. The drainage turned greenish brown in color.
    4. The drainage was more than 500 mL on the fourth postoperative day.

151. When a toddler's mother comes to visit, the toddler clings to the aide, who is washing her, and refuses to look at her mother. How should the nurse explain this behavior to the mother?
    1. The toddler is upset because her mother left her at the hospital.
    2. The toddler is spoiled and needs firm, consistent limits set for her.
    3. The toddler has adjusted well to the hospital and is doing fine.
    4. The toddler may be trying to make her mother jealous of the aide.

152. A couple asks to see their baby, who is in a high-risk newborn nursery. The most appropriate nursing action would encompass:
    1. Assessing and analyzing the couple's level of readiness.
    2. Arranging for the couple to see and hold their baby immediately.
    3. Teaching the couple what to expect.
    4. Preparing the couple for what to expect while making the arrangements for visitation.

153. Paracentesis is a minor surgical procedure done at the bedside; its purpose is to remove ascitic fluid. After explaining the procedure to the patient, the *next* nursing action would be to:
    1. Position the patient in a chair or in high Fowler's position.
    2. Instruct the patient to void.
    3. Take vital signs.
    4. Drape the abdomen with sterile towels.

154. Following ileostomy, the nurse would expect the drainage appliance to be applied to the stoma:
    1. 24 hours later, when edema has subsided.
    2. In the operating room.
    3. After the ileostomy begins to function.
    4. When the patient is able to begin self-care procedures.

155. The best explanation the nurse could give for the signs and symptoms (edema, joint pain, oliguria, muscle cramps, and lethargy) a patient with a history of renal disease has on admission would be:
    1. Renal ischemia due to increase in circulating toxins and chronic hypertension.
    2. A decrease in the number of functioning nephrons, which further decreases glomerular filtration.
    3. Increased water and salt loss due to flushing effect in the diseased kidney tubules.

4. Water and salt retention due to insufficient renal blood flow.

156. One potential complication of an abdominal hysterectomy is abdominal distention. Postoperative nursing measures designed to *avoid* abdominal distention are:
    1. Auscultation of the abdomen for bowel sounds.
    2. Abdominal massage and bed rest.
    3. Insertion of nasogastric and rectal tubes and ambulation, as ordered.
    4. Progression of postoperative diet.

157. The most appropriate plan for immediate follow-up care for a family whose baby has died would include:
    1. Referring the family to a psychotherapist.
    2. Arranging for the social worker to visit the family.
    3. Asking the family to identify their needs.
    4. Assessing the family's need for follow-up care.

158. Ten hours after bilateral hernia surgery, a male patient has not been able to void, despite repeated efforts, including standing to void. He states that he feels like he could void but just can't seem to get his stream started. The nurse should:
    1. Try getting him up in a standing position once again.
    2. Insert a Foley catheter stat.
    3. Run water while he attempts to use the urinal.
    4. Consult with his physician to obtain either a medication or catheterization order.

159. Because ascitic fluids are rich in serum proteins, for which complication following a paracentesis would the nurse observe the patient?
    1. Disequilibrium.
    2. Hypotension.
    3. Hypoalbuminuria.
    4. Paralytic ileus.

160. A patient receiving internal radiation therapy for treatment of adenocarcinoma complains of nausea and a general feeling of weakness. The patient's stools are loose. The nurse might suspect:
    1. Extension of the cancer to the abdominal contents.
    2. Radiation syndrome.
    3. Electrolyte imbalances.
    4. Depression.

161. Signs and symptoms of post-thyroidectomy respiratory obstruction vary with the degree of severity. Early warnings observed by the nurse might include:
    1. Hoarseness and weakness of the voice.
    2. Stridor and cyanosis.
    3. Vague feeling of choking, difficulty swallowing, and fullness of the throat.
    4. Pale nailbeds, disorientation, and combative behavior.

162. Objective data seen with hypoglycemic reactions include:
    1. Irritability, confusion, and lethargy.
    2. Increased temperature and flushing of skin.
    3. Muscle tremors and hyperreflexia.
    4. Decreased blood pressure and fatigue.

163. Which of the following activities of daily living must a patient be given instructions to avoid to prevent complications upon returning home following cataract removal?
    1. Self-feeding.
    2. Self-dressing.
    3. Adjusting shoelaces.
    4. Ambulating.

164. A woman who had rheumatic fever at age 8 is admitted in labor 4 days before her EDB. If implemented during labor and birth, which of the following would *increase* the stress on her heart?
    1. Maintaining a semirecumbent position.
    2. Monitoring her pulse more frequently than her other vital signs.
    3. Preparing her for regional anesthesia (epidural).

4. After complete dilation, coaching her to bear down only once per contraction.

165. Which instruction would be *inappropriate* preoperative instruction for a patient regarding thoracic surgery and postoperative care?
    1. Explain that he or she will be surrounded, for example, by chest tubes, oxygen equipment, and IV infusions, and that these are routine.
    2. Tell the patient that he or she will have periods of rest but will be awakened approximately every 2 hours for turning, coughing, and deep breathing.
    3. Assure the patient that he or she will receive medication that will assist in relieving the discomfort.
    4. Assure the patient that anesthesia will not have any untoward effects on respiratory status.

166. Nursing measures to eliminate the cause of joint pain from chronic renal failure would include:
    1. Using Amphogel (aluminum hydroxide) to lower the elevated blood phosphate that occurs with renal failure.
    2. Preparing for dialysis to decrease serum-creatinine levels.
    3. Increasing the patient's activity level.
    4. Implementing a low-purine diet to decrease uric-acid level.

167. The physician orders a magnesium sulfate infusion for a woman with preeclampsia. Which assessment is most important when administering this drug?
    1. Monitoring the serum-magnesium level every 8 hours.
    2. Evaluating the apical heart rate every 4 hours.
    3. Counting the respiratory rate every hour.
    4. Auscultating bowel sounds before meals.

168. A patient is treated with isoniazid (INH) 300 mg PO, and rifampin (RMP). Which vitamin would the nurse expect this patient to receive to prevent the peripheral neuritis that may occur with INH therapy?
    1. Ascorbic acid (vitamin C).
    2. Pyridoxine (vitamin B_6).
    3. Vitamin E.
    4. Vitamin B_{12}.

169. The nurse explains to a patient that urinary retention may be a problem after spinal anesthesia because:
    1. Conduction of autonomic nervous system impulses as well as central nervous system impulses is inhibited.
    2. Sensation and motor responses are decreased.
    3. Patients tend to secrete less ADH with spinal anesthesia than they do with general anesthesia.
    4. Vasomotor depression, which occurs with spinal anesthesia, reduces the glomerular filtration rate.

170. During discharge teaching with a patient following abdominal hysterectomy, the nurse should include the following instruction:
    1. Avoid sitting for long period of time.
    2. Evacuate bowels daily.
    3. Restrict sexual activity for 6 months after hysterectomy.
    4. Avoid all household chores for 2 months.

171. The labor room nurse decides to intervene when the fetal heart rate (FHR) pattern indicates:
    1. A baseline range of 110–160 bpm.
    2. Absence of variability.
    3. Early decelerations.
    4. Mild variable decelerations.

172. The nurse would explain to a patient that elevation of the foot of the bed after vein-stripping surgery is done to:
    1. Decrease pain.
    2. Aid venous return.
    3. Increase blood supply to feet.
    4. Make the patient more comfortable.

173. Which goals would be described as the highest nursing priority to a patient recovering from ileostomy surgery?
    1. Relief of pain to promote rest and relaxation.

2. Assisting the patient with self-care activities.

3. Maintenance of fluid, electrolyte, and nutritional balances.

4. Skin care and control of odors.

174. A woman's initial reaction to seeing her infant in the high-risk neonatal nursery is to cry and tremble slightly. The most appropriate nursing intervention would be to:
1. Remove her from the area immediately.
2. Monitor her for vital signs.
3. Allow her to cry.
4. Ask her what she is feeling.

175. On the fourth postoperative day after a cholecystectomy, the surgeon orders a patient's T-tube clamped for 1 hour before the first solid meal. The nurse explains to this patient that the purpose of clamping the T-tube is to:
1. Inhibit excessive bile drainage during meals.
2. Allow bile to flow into the duodenum and aid digestion.
3. Relieve abdominal distention and promote normal peristalsis.
4. Assess the patency of the common bile duct.

176. When ECG changes would the nurse anticipate a patient who is in chronic renal failure to demonstrate on assessment, given a potassium level of 6.5 mEq/L?
1. Peaked T waves.
2. Flattened T waves.
3. ST-segment depression.
4. ST-segment elevation.

177. In reviewing an infant's admission history, the nurse should know that intussusception most typically presents with which two signs or symptoms?
1. Currant-jelly stools and paroxysmal abdominal pain.
2. Olive-shaped mass in the right upper quadrant and projectile vomiting.
3. Obstinate constipation and increasing abdominal girth.
4. Excessive amounts of mucus and abdominal distention.

178. The nurse can anticipate that the amount of ascitic fluid removed during a paracentesis will generally be:
1. 500 mL.
2. 1000 mL.
3. 2000 mL.
4. 3000 mL.

179. The husband of a woman having a modified radical mastectomy has arrived early to be with his wife before surgery. After his wife leaves for the operating room, the nurse would *initially*:
1. Tell him to go on to work and come back in the early evening, when his wife is likely to be more responsive.
2. Explain that, following surgery, his wife will be taken to the recovery room, but the surgeon will contact him when the procedure is over.
3. Get him a cup of coffee and tell him to make himself comfortable, because it will be some time before his wife returns to her room.
4. Encourage him to express his feelings and concerns so as to plan for postoperative family teaching.

180. One week after surgery, a patient was fitted with cataract glasses. Which nursing statement would best prepare this patient for adjusting to these glasses?
1. "The cataract lenses magnify objects so that they will seem closer to you than they really are."
2. "While your central vision may be somewhat distorted, you will be able to see well peripherally."
3. "These lenses will enable you to see as well as you did before the cataract formed."
4. "The lenses on these glasses are quite narrow, and therefore you may have some double vision."

181. Upon returning from the recovery room after a thyroidectomy, the patient begins to complain of a choking sensation. The immediate nursing action should be to:
1. Elevate the head to high Fowler's.

2. Suggest the patient suck on some ice chips.

3. Assess the wound and dressing for increased swelling, and loosen dressing if necessary.

4. Call the physician.

182. The blood gases of a patient with chronic renal failure reveal the following: pH, 7.36; PO_2, 90; PCO_2, 34; serum bicarbonate, 20 mEq/L. The nurse's interpretation would be:
1. Metabolic acidosis.
2. Compensated metabolic acidosis.
3. Respiratory alkalosis with metabolic compensation.
4. Metabolic acidosis with minimal respiratory compensation.

183. Four days after admission for cirrhosis of the liver, a patient began to bleed from an esophageal varix. The earliest indications of bleeding noted by the nurse would include:
1. Tachycardia, restlessness, and pallor.
2. Tachycardia, lethargy, and flushing.
3. Sudden drop in blood pressure of 10 mm Hg or more.
4. Increasing combativeness and widening pulse pressure.

184. Initially, a new mother is reluctant to touch or hold her son, who is in a high-risk newborn nursery. She says, "I don't know what to do. He's so small, so helpless. He looks so awful." Crying, she turns into her husband's arms. Which nursing diagnosis is the *least* accurate interpretation of her behavior?
1. Altered parenting.
2. Ineffective family coping: compromised.
3. Impaired verbal communication.
4. High risk for altered family processes.

185. Objective assessment data indicating circulatory overload in a patient who has chronic renal failure would include:
1. Neck vein distention, apprehension, soft eyeballs.
2. Periorbital edema, distended neck veins, moist crackles.
3. Increased blood pressure, flattened neck veins, shock.
4. Decreased pulse pressure, cool, dry skin, decreased skin turgor.

186. On the fifth postoperative day, a patient who has had abdominal surgery complains of a "giving" sensation around the wound when walking about. After assisting the patient back in bed, the nurse notes that the dressing covering the incision is saturated with clear, pink drainage. The nurse should suspect:
1. Late hemorrhage.
2. Dehiscence.
3. Infection.
4. Evisceration.

187. The nurse working with a family who experienced SIDS (sudden infant death syndrome) should:
1. Be knowledgeable about various theories of psychotherapy.
2. Have extensive experience working with dying patients.
3. Be able to identify personal feelings about death.
4. Be able to suppress personal feelings about death.

188. The nurse knows that a Sengstaken-Blakemore tube is primarily used to:
1. Prevent bleeding by applying pressure to the esophageal varices.
2. Prevent accumulation of blood in the GI tract, which could precipitate hepatic coma.
3. Stop bleeding by applying pressure to the cardiac portion of the stomach and against the esophageal varices.
4. Reduce transfusion requirements.

189. Which postoperative instruction for a patient who had an abdominal hysterectomy includes *inaccurate* information?
1. Monitor vaginal drainage and report any color changes.
2. Expect that vaginal discharge will diminish and cease gradually.
3. Plan on contraception, considering that her ovaries are still intact.
4. Expect that menses will no longer occur.

190. While the T-tube is clamped, the nurse should observe a patient after a cholecystectomy for signs of:
    1. Abdominal discomfort or pain.
    2. Eructation.
    3. Jaundice.
    4. Increased respiratory rate. \

191. Although chemotherapy for TB renders a patient noninfectious within days to a few weeks, barring side effects, the patient is instructed by the nurse to continue INH therapy for:
    1. 6 months.
    2. 1 year.
    3. 2 years.
    4. The rest of the patient's life.

192. Before lobectomy surgery for squamous cell carcinoma of the left lower lobe, pulmonary function tests are done and blood is drawn for blood gas analysis to establish baseline data on a patient admitted with fever, tachypnea, productive cough, wheezes, and a smoking history that covered 30 years. Given the respiratory symptomatology, which outcome would the nurse expect to find?
    1. Increased vital capacity and respiratory acidosis.
    2. Decreased vital capacity and respiratory alkalosis.
    3. Increased total lung capacity and metabolic acidosis.
    4. Decreased FEV_1 and respiratory acidosis.

193. When teaching the parents about the care of their baby with a cleft lip and palate, the nurse should inform them that:
    1. It is important to use a nipple with large holes to make sucking easier.
    2. The infant will have difficulty feeding because the baby cannot create a vacuum in the mouth.
    3. The infant should be given small amounts of formula while being maintained in a supine position to facilitate feeding.
    4. It is important to isolate the infant from others to prevent possible infection.

194. After presenting a brief class on various methods of family planning to students in a health course, the nurse administers a post test. If teaching has been effective, which statement should the students select as true?
    1. To be effective, rhythm requires avoiding intercourse during the last week of the menstrual cycle.
    2. Couples using coitus interruptus may become pregnant accidentally due to escape of pre-ejaculatory fluid containing spermatozoa.
    3. Spermicidal jellies are highly effective whether used alone or with a diaphragm.
    4. The intrauterine device is the most effective method of contraception.

195. The nurse would recognize signs of hypovolemia, which include:
    1. Dry mucous membranes and soft eyeballs.
    2. Decreased hematocrit and hemoglobin.
    3. Decreased pulse rate and widened pulse pressure.
    4. Dyspnea and crackles.

196. Newborn assessment revealed a scaphoid-shaped abdomen. The nurse knows that this finding suggests a:
    1. Diaphragmatic hernia.
    2. Normal newborn abdomen.
    3. Imperforate anus.
    4. Gastroschisis or omphalocele.

197. During a predischarge teaching session, the nurse tells a patient who has had vein ligation surgery that elastic stockings are best applied:
    1. Before rising in the morning, to prevent pooling of blood in the lower extremities.
    2. After showering and application of skin care to the legs, to prevent undue dermal irritation.
    3. After 15 minutes of vigorous leg exercises designed to increase blood flow.

    4. Only when the patient plans to be standing for an extended period of time because undue constriction of the veins can cause a recurrence of varicosities.

198. Which assessment finding provides data to validate an 8-week gestation?
    1. Fundal height.
    2. Auscultation of fetal heart tones.
    3. Positive radioimmunoassay (RIA) test.
    4. Leopold maneuvers.

199. On the third postoperative day after a mastectomy, the patient voiced concern about her husband's reaction to her surgery. Which approach by the nurse is most likely to help minimize this patient's concern?
    1. Emphasizing the lifesaving aspects of her surgery.
    2. Explaining that depression and anxiety are common behaviors following radical surgery.
    3. Interviewing the husband to learn about his real reaction to his wife's surgery.
    4. Encouraging her to identify the strengths in her relationship with her husband.

200. The nurse must be alert to the development of spontaneous bleeding (ecchymoses) in cirrhosis due to:
    1. Rupture of esophageal varices.
    2. Decreased synthesis of blood-clotting factors by the liver.
    3. Failure of the gut to absorb water-soluble vitamins needed to promote coagulation.
    4. Decreased venous pressures and slow blood flow.

Answers/Rationale

1. (2) Postural blood pressure readings are an excellent mode for assessing volume depletion. If the systolic blood pressure decreases more than 10 mm Hg and there is a concurrent increase in the pulse rate, a volume depletion problem is indicated. Urine output and specific gravity (**Answer 1**) are better measures of the adequacy of fluid volume replacement than of fluid volume depletion. Comparing the prior and present weight of the patient (**Answer 3**) will give the nurse an estimate of the slow catabolism of body stores that occurs with ulcerative colitis. There is no *oral* water test (**Answer 4**).

    Test-taking tip—Key words are "quickly" (something the nurse can do without a great deal of equipment and something that can be done easily) and "volume depletion."
    AS, 8, HPM, Prevention and Early Detection of Disease

2. (2) Wheezes occur when there is partial obstruction of the bronchi or bronchioles. Sounds are due to the increased vibration of air molecules as they pass over these obstructions. **Answer 1** is incorrect because total obstruction would produce *no* sounds. **Answer 3** is incorrect because the sounds produced by fluid in the alveoli are the finer, less harsh sounds generally referred to as crackles. **Answer 4** is incorrect because inflammation of the pleura creates a grating sound referred to as a friction rub.

    Test-taking tip—The question is looking for the reasons why these sounds occur. With a wheeze, think "squeeze"—air through a narrow tube.
    AN, 6, PhI, Physiological Adaptation

Key to codes following rationales *Nursing process:* **AS,** Assessment; **AN,** Analysis; **PL,** Plan; **IMP,** Implementation; **EV,** Evaluation. *Category of human function:* **1,** Protective; **2,** Sensory-perceptual; **3,** Comfort, Rest, Activity, and Mobility; **4,** Nutrition; **5,** Growth and Development; **6,** Fluid-Gas Transport; **7,** Psychosocial-Cultural; **8,** Elimination. **Client need: SECE;** Safe, Effective Care Environment; **PhI,** Physiological Integrity; **PsI,** Psychosocial Integrity; **HPM,** Health Promotion/ Maintenance. See appendices for full explanation.

3. **(1)** Liver functions are many and varied, including detoxification of chemicals (estrogen, adrenocorticoids, aldosterone, drugs, poisons, and heavy metals); synthesis of plasma proteins (albumin, fibrinogen, globulin) and several clotting factors (prothrombin, factor VII); storage of glycogen, iron, and vitamins (A, D, E, K, and B$_{12}$); gluconeogenesis (glucose from amino acids and fats); and deamination of amino acids. Fluid volume control and acid-base balance are functions of the *kidney* (**Answer 2**). Most erythrocyte and leukocyte breakdown occurs in the *spleen* (**Answer 3**). The *gallbladder* concentrates and stores bile (**Answer 4**), and the liver is involved with synthesis and secretion of bile.

   Test-taking tip—The question is focusing on what is the liver supposed to do, what is the normal physiology of the liver. The key words "best describes" are asking for the most accurate and complete answer. Clue—look for a "metabolic" process.

   AN, 4, PhI, Physiological Adaptation

4. **(2)** Acute glomerulonephritis is an autoimmune response to an antigen produced by beta-hemolytic streptococci. Antibodies produced to fight the antigen also react against the glomerular tissue. This causes proliferation and swelling of endothelial cells in the glomerular capillary wall and results in passage of blood cells and protein into the glomerular filtrate. Acute glomerular nephritis is *not* the result of direct infection (**Answers 1 and 3**) or of hypoxia (**Answer 4**).

   Test-taking tip—The key word is "cause" of glomerulonephritis. The question is asking for an explanation of the pathophysiology of the disease. Look for a pattern—three options are *direct* infections.

   IMP, 8, PhI, Physiological Adaptation

5. **(3)** Coughing, vigorous exercise, and straining or lifting increase intra-abdominal pressures, which tend to extrude the intestines through weakened areas of the abdominal wall. This patient's history includes all of the above. Other causes of hernia include combinations of **Answers 1, 2, and 4;** *alone* they are less likely causes.

   Test-taking tip—Patient history identifies several risk factors/behaviors. Select the answer that is most inclusive, the one that lists more than one risk.

   AN, 8, PhI, Physiological Adaptation

6. **(2)** The functions of the gallbladder are to collect, concentrate, and store bile, which is produced by the *liver, not* by the gallbladder (**Answer 1**). Bile reaches the gallbladder via the hepatic duct, which later joins the cystic duct emanating from the gallbladder to form the common bile duct. The common bile duct joins the pancreatic duct, which opens into the duodenum. Bile is not diluted (**Answer 3**). **Answer 4** is incorrect because contraction of the gallbladder and therefore flow of bile are stimulated by the hormone cholecystokinin, which is secreted by the duodenal mucosa when food enters the duodenum.

   Test-taking tip—This question is looking for knowledge of physiology of the gallbladder. What does the gallbladder do under normal circumstances? Be cautious of all statements in the options because some may be correct but are placed with some that are incorrect. Look at each word or phrase and decide right or wrong for each part of the option.

   AN, 4, PhI, Physiological Adaptation

7. **(3)** A thyroid scan utilizes the uptake of ^{131}I by the thyroid gland to determine the size, shape, and function of the gland. Also identified are areas of increased uptake (hot areas), indicating increased metabolic function, as in hyperthyroidism, not malignancy (**Answer 2**), and areas of decreased or no uptake (cold areas), which are associated with malignancy. **Answers 1 and 4** both describe the TSH stimulation test.

   Test-taking tip—The question is asking for the *most accurate* description of a thyroid scan. This test uses iodine uptake to identify normal and abnormal findings.

   IMP, 3, PhI, Reduction of Risk Potential

8. **(4)** This is the most appropriate response because it attempts to provide total intervention for all parties involved. **Answer 1** is essentially the physician's role. It would be almost impossible to alleviate the couple's anxiety at this time (**Answer 2**). The most appropriate intervention is to assist the couple to cope with their anxiety as effectively as possible. **Answer 3** is essential, but it neglects the psychological needs of the woman and her family.

   Test-taking tip—Focus on the nurse's roles/responsibilities in the operating room when caring for patients undergoing cesarean birth, not the MD's (**1**). When two options are good, (**3, 4**) choose the more inclusive option (physiological *plus* psychological).

   PL, 7, PsI, Coping and Adaptation

9. **(1)** The kidneys secrete the erythropoietin factor, which stimulates the bone marrow to produce red blood cells. In chronic kidney disease, secretion of this factor decreases as greater portions of the kidney are destroyed by the disease process. Hypertension does *not* suppress bone marrow centers (**Answer 2**), because local blood flow regulators tend to compensate over the long run by supplying tissue with adequate blood flow for metabolic purposes. Unlike metabolic acidosis, metabolic alkalosis does *not* increase RBC fragility (**Answer 3**). Frank bleeding into the urine is uncommon in chronic renal disease (**Answer 4**).

   Test-taking tip—Take each option by itself and determine if it is correct or incorrect in relation to the normal or abnormal kidney function seen in chronic failure.

   AN, 8, PhI, Physiological Adaptation

10. **(3)** For patients having elective surgery, *routine* preoperative laboratory studies generally include a complete blood count, urinalysis, and prothrombin time. Some institutions also require a VDRL. The urinalysis provides information about specific gravity (indicating the ability of the kidney to concentrate and dilute urine); the presence of albumin or pus, indicating renal infection; and the presence of sugar and acetone. The CBC detects the presence of anemia, infection, allergy, and leukemia. Prothrombin time (increased) may indicate a need for preoperative vitamin K therapy. Electrolytes (**Answer 1**), enzymes such as ALT (SGOT), (**Answer 2**), and serum glucose (**Answer 4**) are ordered *only if* the patient's history or physical condition warrants a more complete workup.

    Test-taking tip—Key word in this question is "routine" for each patient having surgery. The incorrect options all suggest an underlying medical problem, but none is discussed in the stem (e.g., VDRL).

    AS, 6, PhI, Reduction of Risk Potential

11. **(2)** Many times, patients who are manipulative are not aware of any other mechanisms for fulfilling their needs. Teaching them to identify manipulative behaviors may help them to avoid being manipulative and to eventually adopt more appropriate means for meeting their needs. The patients should be *involved* in the decision-making process (**Answer 1**). Limits must be *realistically* established (**Answer 3**). Public confrontation (**Answer 4**) may only exacerbate the power struggle.

    Test-taking tip—Therapeutic nursing process calls for supportive care (e.g., reinforce), *not* a dominant, controlling approach (e.g., rigid, confronting).

    PL, 7, PsI, Psychosocial Adaptation

12. **(4)** For this woman, a cesarean birth may be expected. With the fetus in breech presentation, there is a risk of prolapsed cord if membranes rupture in early labor (the presenting part is not engaged as yet). Induction (**Answer 1**) may not be considered since the presenting part is the sacrum and it is high. Vaginal birth (**Answer 2**) may not be considered; however, if breech birth is vaginal, Piper forceps are used to assist in the birth of the after-coming head. Spontaneous vaginal birth (**Answer 3**) may not be possible for this woman.

Test-taking tip—Note the fetal presentation (high), and eliminate two options that call for *vaginal* delivery (**Answer 1** also implies probable vaginal). Choose the option that is different from the others (i.e., nonvaginal).

PL, 6, SECE, Management of Care

13. (**1**) When excessive quantities of fatty acids are oxidized, blood buffer systems may become exhausted. Ketoacidosis develops and acetone bodies are excreted in the urine. In an emergency room situation, diabetic acidosis can be recognized not only by the increased rate and depth of respirations (Kussmaul's respirations) but also by the odor of acetone on the breath. *Neither* osmotic diuresis (**Answer 2**) *nor* failure in the sodium-hydrogen ion exchange (**Answer 3**) causes acetonuria. In the latter case, failure to excrete excess hydrogen ions would decrease urinary acids. Volatile hydrogen ions (CO_2) are excreted by the lungs; a decrease in nonvolatile hydrogen ions in the glomerular filtrate (**Answer 4**) would move the pH of the urine toward the alkaline side.

Test-taking tip—The word "acetonuria" tells you something is evident in the urine. Improper fat metabolism produces acetonuria.

AN, 6, PhI, Physiological Adaptation

14. (**1**) Ergot products such as ergonovine, which contract the uterus and cervix, are contraindicated until the uterus is emptied to avoid retention of placental fragments or tissue. Retained fragments predispose to uterine relaxation and puerperal infection. **Answer 2** is incorrect because ergot products are not given to women if they are *hypertensive* because of the vasoconstrictive properties of these products. Ergot products are *not* blood products (**Answer 3**). **Answer 4** is incorrect because ergot products are *not contraindicated* if she is also a candidate for $Rh_0(D)$ immune globulin (i.e., she is Rh negative and Coombs negative.)

Test-taking tip—The stem asks for when *not* to administer ergot. Focus on risk factors and eliminate those that do not apply (**2, 4**). Eliminate **Answer 3** because ergot is not related to a *blood* product.

EV, 5, PhI, Pharmacological/Parenteral Therapy

15. (**2**) The woman who seems restless, with flushed face, rapid pulse, and rapid deep respirations, is exhibiting signs of hyperglycemia. **Answer 1** is incorrect because failure to react to a flash of light in the face is associated with an *insulin* reaction (hypoglycemia). **Answer 3** is wrong because diaphoresis during sleep is associated with *insulin* reactions. **Answer 4** is wrong because headaches are associated with *insulin* reactions.

Test-taking tip—Recognize that three of the options describe insulin reaction (hypoglycemia) and therefore do not meet the condition in the stem (hyperglycemia). Review signs and symptoms of hypoglycemia and hyperglycemia. Understand the expected changes in glucose levels and insulin requirements in the immediate postpartum period.

AN, 4, PhI, Physiological Adaptation

16. (**1**) Hyperkalemia tends to develop in renal dysfunction for two reasons: In the kidneys, more hydrogen ions than potassium ions are selectively secreted in exchange for sodium ions, and decreasing glomerular filtration and urine output tends to decrease the excretion of all electrolytes and waste products of metabolism. Potassium does not move out of the cell to balance sodium shifts in edema (**Answer 2**), nor does respiratory alkalosis affect potassium reabsorption in the kidneys (**Answer 3**). Nausea and vomiting (**Answer 4**) cause hypokalemia.

Test-taking tip—Know the role of potassium in the body and the pathophysiology of chronic renal failure.

AN, 8, PhI, Physiological Adaptation

17. (**1**) To prevent contractures, the affected limb is kept straight (knee extension) and slightly abducted (to prevent pressure in hip joint), and the foot is supported (ankle flexion) to prevent footdrop. **Answers 2, 3, and 4** are incorrect because all or part of each response could produce a contracture.

Test-taking tip—Key word is "contractures." Look for anything that is suggested to extend the limb or keep it straight.

PL, 3, PhI, Reduction of Risk Potential

18. (**2**) A truss should be applied *before* the patient gets out of bed or after the hernia has been reduced, by having the patient lie down with the feet elevated in bed or in the bath. If the hernia cannot be reduced, the truss should not be applied (**Answers 1 and 3**). Although the truss is not a cure for a hernia and its use is not as common as it once was, it is far more effective in keeping a hernia reduced than is an athletic supporter (**Answer 4**).

Test-taking tip—A truss keeps the internal organs from protruding through the herniated area. Look for the *best time.*

AN, 3, PhI, Reduction of Risk Potential

19. (**1**) The PPD for the tuberculin skin test is injected intradermally on the polar aspect of the forearm. If the test is correctly administered, a pale elevation similar to a mosquito bite should be apparent. **Answers 2, 3,** and **4** are not used for this test.

Test-taking tip—*Correct* technique is just under the skin. Only *one* option will produce a bubble. You want to be able to see results from the administration of this injection, so you do not want to give deep injections.

IMP, 1, HPM, Prevention and Early Detection of Disease

20. (**3**) Fat-soluble vitamins, particularly vitamin K, are poorly absorbed in the absence of bile. Decreased absorption of vitamin K results in decreased levels of circulating prothrombin, thus reducing normal clotting levels. Peripheral neuritis (**Answer 1**) occurs with vitamin B_6 deficiencies, and scurvy (**Answer 2**) occurs with deficiency in vitamin C; these are *water-soluble* vitamins. Macrocytic anemia (**Answer 4**) is consistent with a vitamin B_{12} deficiency, which may be due to lack of intrinsic factor in the stomach.

Test-taking tip—Need to know fat-soluble vitamins (A, D, E and K). Associate vitamin K with increased bleeding tendencies.

AN, 4, PhI, Physiological Adaptation

21. (**3**) Even though the patient will have only one eye patched after surgery, familiarization with the physical environment and with nursing personnel will decrease the occurrence of disorientation (this is especially important with elderly patients). It is not necessary to keep the patient flat in bed before or after surgery (**Answer 1**). Patches (**Answer 2**) are not generally applied to both eyes. Eye-drop instillations (**Answer 4**) are part of the *postoperative* or predischarge teaching plan.

Test-taking tip—The key word is "preoperative." Orienting the patient to prevent injuries in the post-op period is priority.

PL, 2, PsI, Coping and Adaptation

22. (**1**) Following an injection of the small dose of ^{131}I used in a thyroid scan, no radiation precautions are necessary. Full radiation precautions (**Answer 2**) are utilized for radium implants. **Answer 3** may be employed when ^{131}I therapy is utilized to control and reduce hypersecretion by the thyroid (*hyperthyroidism*). **Answer 4** is not an example of normal radiation therapy policy.

Test-taking tip—There is no identification of *treatment* with radioactive substance, just a scan. Look for a pattern—three of the options are inappropriate precautions.

PL, 3, PhI, Reduction of Risk Potential

23. (**2**) Patients with radioactive implants should be positioned flat in bed to prevent dislodgement of the vaginal packing. The patient may roll to the side for meals, but the upper body should not be raised more than 20 degrees. **Answers 1, 3, and 4** are incorrect because these positions are more likely to change the position of the cobalt seeds.

Test-taking tip—Radium implants are localized treatment for known cancer; therefore it is important that they remain in the correct position. The best option to maintain the implants in the correct position is to have the patient lie flat in bed. Visualize the patient in each position. Which one would have no effect on placement of implant?

IMP, 1, PhI, Physiological Adaptation

24. (1) This is an open-ended question that allows the husband to identify what his needs are at this time. **Answer 2** is too threatening. **Answer 3** assumes he cannot tolerate the situation, which is unfair. **Answer 4** is unrealistic because the nurse has many responsibilities at this time. In addition, the husband would have to leave the room anyway to drink or take anything.

Test-taking tip—Choose an *open*-ended question. Notice that three of the options can be answered with a "yes-no" response that closes communication.

IMP, 7, PsI, Coping and Adaptation

25. (2) This answer provides the parents with accurate information specific to the questions they have asked. **Answer 1** is incorrect because the nurse may or may *not* be fully informed as to what the physicians may have told the parents. **Answer 3** is incorrect because it avoids answering their questions and may actually increase their anxiety. **Answer 4** is incorrect because the palate repair is generally not done until the infant is at least *1 year of age,* when the infant should be well *over* 10 pounds. This delay allows for the growth of the bony structures of the jaw and mouth, but is done before the infant begins to use speech.

Test-taking tip—Use process of elimination; omit the two options referring to MD; select the more complete, precise, factually correct answer.

IMP, 1, PhI, Reduction of Risk Potential

26. (3) Surgical treatment of hyperthyroidism involves a subtotal thyroidectomy in which approximately five-sixths of the thyroid tissue is removed. While this procedure does not cure hyperthyroidism, it reduces the amount of circulating thyroid hormone by reducing the amount of functioning tissue. **Answer 1,** complete or total thyroidectomy, is *rarely* done for hyperthyroidism today but *is* indicated for thyroid malignancy. **Answer 2,** removal of half of the thyroid, would leave enough functioning hyperactive tissue to prevent diminution of symptoms in the patient. **Answer 4** is incorrect because the patient with hyperthyroidism needs no additional thyroid hormone; he or she receives antithyroid medications such as propylthiouracil (PRU) or methimazole (Tapazole) to reduce both circulating and stored thyroid hormone.

Test-taking tip—When you have two good choices, select the one that includes the other.

AN, 3, PhI, Physiological Adaptation

27. (3) Obstruction of the bile duct will cause elevated serum and urine bilirubin (dark urine) as well as a decreased amount of urobilinogen in the feces (clay-colored stools). Bilirubin is an end product of hemoglobin breakdown. Normally it is conjugated in the liver and secreted, in the bile, into the intestines, where it is converted into urobilinogen and excreted in the stools. **Answer 1** is incorrect because biliary obstruction itself does not directly affect blood pressure. However, if the obstruction is acute and accompanied by pain, changes in blood pressure in response to increased sympathetic tone can be expected. **Answer 2** is incorrect because between-meal eructation is a symptom of ulcer disease. Eructation in gallbladder disease occurs after eating, particularly if large amounts of fat have been ingested. **Answer 4** is also incorrect; longitudinal ridging of the fingernails is a sign seen frequently in anemia.

Test-taking tip—The question is focused on what would you see when there is an obstruction of the bile duct. If bile cannot be excreted into the intestines, the bile goes to the serum and urine. The lack of bile in the intestines will cause the stools to be lighter in color. It is bile that gives stool its normal color.

AS, 4, PhI, Physiological Adaptation

28. (2) This patient's smoking history and history of chronic cough necessitate directing preoperative nursing measures toward clearing the respiratory tract of excess secretions that might lead to postoperative complications. Besides oral hygiene, the following may be instituted or ordered before surgery: postural drainage, incentive spirometers, IPPB, and mucolytic agent. Because postoperative coughing is contraindicated with hernia repairs, removal of secretions is a priority, as is instruction in deep-breathing techniques. **Answers 1, 3, and 4,** though *not top priority,* are correct and should also be included in the preoperative teaching plan.

Test-taking tip—This is a *priority* question. The patient is at greater risk for respiratory infection and complications.

AN, 6, PhI, Reduction of Risk Potential

29. (3) This patient's urine specific gravity indicates that the kidneys have lost their ability to concentrate urine. Therefore the patient has a greater water loss than would normally be expected. ADH secretion (**Answer 1**) would produce an elevated specific gravity. **Answer 2** is incorrect because water loss without concomitant electrolyte loss causes the extracellular fluids to become hyperosmolar (that is, the patient is dehydrated). **Answer 4** is incorrect because hyperosmolarity of ECF causes the thirst receptors in the hypothalamus to shrink (which stimulates the thirst mechanism).

Test-taking tip—Know what is normal. It is normal to be thirsty and have a dry mouth after 12 hours, but it is not normal to have a specific gravity of 1.008 (normal is 1.010–1.020). Focus attention on the kidneys.

IMP, 6, PhI, Physiological Adaptation

30. (1) The portal system becomes obstructed, causing a rise in portal venous pressure and portal hypertension, venous dilation, and stasis. In cirrhosis, there is *decreased* hepatic synthesis of albumin, not increased (**Answer 2**), and *increased* levels of aldosterone, not decreased (**Answer 3**). Blood volumes are *decreased,* not increased (**Answer 4**), while total body fluid is increased due to the physiological effects of hypoproteinemia (decreased serum proteins). These factors, plus increasing obstruction of the portal vein, cause fluids, electrolytes, and serum proteins to move out of the vascular compartment and into the intestines. The abdomen provides a large potential space for the accumulation of these fluids.

Test-taking tip—Know where ascites is found and how fluid is able to shift (some type of intravascular problem).

AN, 4, PhI, Physiological Adaptation

31. (2) Bronchoscopy provides direct visualization of the airways by utilizing a long, slender, hollow instrument through which a light is reflected. Bronchoscopy can be utilized for diagnostic purposes, for removal of foreign objects, for removal of mucous plugs, or for obtaining a biopsy or bronchial washings for cytology. **Answer 1** is an example or a fluoroscopic exam. **Answer 3** characterizes a bronchogram, and **Answer 4,** a lung biopsy.

Test-taking tip—Try to take words apart: "bronch" means lungs and "scope" means use an instrument to *look* into a body part or cavity. The other options use x-ray or needle biopsy as the method of making a diagnosis.

IMP, 6, PsI, Coping and Adaptation

32. (3) Potassium deficit leads to decreased muscular function, causing muscle weakness, decreased intestinal motility, and a variety of GI symptoms (vomiting, abdominal distention,

flatulence). There is also decreased neuromuscular irritability, which contributes to apathy, lethargy, and mental confusion. **Answer 1** is partially correct (spasms or tetany and irregular pulse), but high T waves occur in *hyperkalemia;* low flat waves occur in hypokalemia. **Answer 2** is incorrect because the symptoms indicated would likely be seen in metabolic acidosis and dehydration. Hyperkalemia would be expected. Pitting edema and bounding pulse (**Answer 4**) are seen in fluid overload, which would be consistent with hyperkalemia and renal impairment. Confusion does occur in hypokalemia.

> **Test-taking tip**—Know the influences of potassium on tissues and body functioning. Understanding that potassium is lost in severe diarrhea, you would be looking for low potassium levels and symptoms caused by hypokalemia, not hyperkalemia. Look carefully at each option. Often one correct statement is combined with an incorrect statement.

AS, 6, PhI, Physiological Adaptation

33. (2) The effect of the anesthesia will be closely checked prior to making the incision, and the level of anesthesia will be monitored throughout the procedure. Many times the woman *will complain* of tightness or pressure in the area where the physician is working (**Answer 1**). No significant pain should be felt as long as the anesthesia is closely monitored and maintained (**Answer 3**). **Answer 4** is inappropriate because it makes her feel that she should not complain about pain even if she actually does feel it.

> **Test-taking tip**—Look at some key words in the options: "feel *nothing*" (1); "pain when incision" (3); "only your *imagination*"(4). Eliminate: **Answer 4** because it is demeaning; **Answer 3** because there should be no pain *during* surgery/anesthesia; **Answer 1** because pressure sensations *do* exist.

IMP, 7, PsI, Coping and Adaptation

34. (4) Abdominal cramps, vomiting, and watery or no discharge are signs of intestinal obstruction, a complication that requires immediate medical intervention. **Answers 1, 2, and 3** are incorrect, not only because they can delay appropriate medical intervention but also because they increase the risk of severe fluid and electrolyte imbalance. Although obstruction of an ileostomy is a rare problem, a very small stoma or one that is contracted may need to be dilated regularly so that the little finger can be inserted easily.

> **Test-taking tip**—The key word is "*sudden.*" Suspect something serious with onset of multiple symptoms. Look for a pattern—three options delay diagnosis.

IMP, 4, PhI, Physiological Adaptation

35. (4) Normal functioning of chest tubes is maintained, and the drainage system is transported below the level of the chest. Chest tubes are not removed (**Answer 1**) to facilitate transportation of the patient; they are removed only after the physician is satisfied with the degree of reexpansion. Removing the chest tubes from the suction drainage system (**Answer 2**) will result in an equalization of intrapleural pressures with atmospheric pressures, thus also increasing the risk of pneumothorax. Current practice precludes the clamping of the chest tubes (**Answer 3**). It is believed that clamping increases the risk of a tension pneumothorax because air may enter the intrapleural space during inspiration but cannot escape during expiration.

> **Test-taking tip**—The reason why chest tubes are inserted is to re-expand the lung. Avoid any option that would interfere with the purpose of the chest tube. Look for the independent nursing action—nurses do *not* "remove," "disconnect," or "clamp" routinely.

IMP, 6, PhI, Reduction of Risk Potential

36. (3) Hypoglycemic or insulin reactions are the result of decreased circulatory serum glucose to the brain. This stimulates epinephrine release. Early symptoms include cold, clammy skin, nervousness, tremors, numbness of the hands or around the lips, and cardiac palpitations. Later symptoms

may mimic alcoholic intoxication, such as staggering gait, slurring of words, combative behavior, or uncontrolled weeping. As hypoglycemia deepens, the patient may develop convulsions and coma. **Answer 1** is incorrect, in that respirations in insulin shock, though shallow, are increased. **Answer 2** is incorrect because the breath of the patient in insulin shock is noncontributory, not fetid. Fetid breath may occur with liver failure or poor dental hygiene. Behavioral responses in **Answer 4** are switched; that is, confusion and lethargy are common with ketoacidosis, and apprehension and irritability is consistent with insulin shock.

> **Test-taking tip**—Look for the signs and symptoms of insulin shock. Consider each sign or symptom individually; eliminate those options with incorrect signs and symptoms.

AN, 4, PhI, Physiological Adaptation

37. (1) Emergency surgery must be performed to save the life of the patient, save the function of an organ or limb, remove a damaged organ or limb, or stop hemorrhage. Few emergency situations are so urgent as to require immediate response (**Answer 2**), eliminating the necessary laboratory data to evaluate the patient's physiologic response to the situation. Surgical preparation would be completed within 24 hours (**Answer 3**), but this is not the *best* answer. True emergency situations cannot be postponed to the following surgical day (**Answer 4**).

> **Test-taking tip**—*Emergency* means "right away;" *however,* important things need to be done *before* the surgery can begin. There are preliminary measures such as establishing baseline assessment data, establishing IV lines, determining allergies, and having blood on hand for replacement if necessary. Consider what is best for patient.

IMP, 1, SECE, Management of Care

38. (1) Prognosis is generally poor if hepatic coma lasts longer than 24 hours. Other measures that have been utilized to decrease serum ammonia and allow for regeneration of hepatocytes include hemodialysis, exchange blood transfusions, and administration of lactalose, which, when degraded in the large bowel, decreases the pH of the feces, thus preventing formation of ammonia and promoting its excretion. **Answers 2, 3, and 4** all exceed the 24-hour threshold.

> **Test-taking tip**—The longer the patient is in the coma, the more complications will increase in number and effect.

AN, 2, PhI, Physiological Adaptation

39. (3) A BUN of less than 20 mg/dL and serum creatinine less than 1.2 mg/dl would be optimal outcome measures for this patient (that is, within normal range). **Answers 1, 2, and 4** are incorrect because a serum K^+ of less than 3.5 mEq/L would be indicative of hypokalemia and a serum Na^+ above 148 mEq/L indicates hypernatremia (**Answer 1**); quantity of urine output *should increase* to over 500 mL/24 hours (**Answer 2**); and the abdomen should be soft and tympanic to percussion; so dullness to percussion in the abdomen is consistent with *fluid excess* (**Answer 4**).

> **Test-taking tip**—The key word is "effectiveness." How well is the dialysis working? The closer to normal the values are, the more effective the treatment. Know normal lab values.

EV, 8, PhI, Physiological Adaptation

40. (3) Before the dialysis procedure is started, baseline information needs to be collected so that the therapy can be accurately evaluated. Baseline information will include vital signs, body temperature, weight, ECG, and electrolyte levels. If the patient does not have a Foley catheter (often by this time he or she does because of the need to assess hourly outputs), then the patient is asked to void. Following voiding, the patient is positioned in a supine or low Fowler's position and the abdomen is prepared and draped. **Answers 1, 2, and 4** are actions subsequent to **Answer 3**.

Test-taking tip—With renal problems, weight is often the correct answer.

IMP, 8, PhI, Reduction of Risk Potential

41. **(4)** All straining and lifting should be avoided for at least 3 weeks to prevent undue stress on the sutures. Other less strenuous activities, such as **Answers 1, 2, and 3,** are appropriate, though good body mechanics should be reviewed with the patient.

Test-taking tip—Look at all the activities and determine which one would be the most strenuous for the patient.

PL, 3, PhI, Basic Care and Comfort

42. **(2)** To avoid the complication of a painful spinal headache that can last for several days, the patient is kept flat in a supine position for approximately 4–12 hours postoperatively. Headaches are believed to be due to the seepage of cerebral spinal fluid from the puncture site. By keeping the patient flat, cerebral spinal fluid pressures are equalized, which avoids trauma to the neurons. **Answer 1** is the position for patients having general anesthesia. **Answer 3** is incorrect because knees are flexed. **Answer 4** is the position for patients with head traumas.

Test-taking tip—When a question is asked about the recovery room, you know that this is the immediate postoperative period. Select the position that would be used first and would prevent spinal headache.

IMP, 1, PhI, Reduction of Risk Potential

43. **(2)** Patients who have had spinal anesthesia have varying degrees of hypotension due to the vasodepressor effect of the anesthetic agent on the autonomic nervous system. Reflexes **(Answer 1)** will be depressed in the lower extremities because of the anesthetic and should be checked *after* circulatory status. However, sensory impulses remain blocked longer than motor activity, so safety measures should be instituted to prevent injury from bedding, poor positioning, or sources of heat. Because the patient is awake with a spinal anesthetic, level of consciousness **(Answer 3)** and airway integrity **(Answer 4)** are lower priorities than circulatory status.

Test-taking tip—Think *baseline data* in the postoperative period. You need to know what the vitals were and how they progress over time. With spinal anesthetic, circulatory problems are more likely.

AS, 1, PhI, Reduction of Risk Potential

44. **(3)** There are no specific dietary restrictions following cholecystectomy. Patients are advised, however, to avoid foods high in fats. Most patients tend to avoid these foods anyway because they are more comfortable if they do so. Generally, after about 3 months, patients may begin to experiment with certain foods to ascertain their tolerance to them. **Answer 1** is incorrect because some fat *is* allowed in the diet at all times. **Answer 2** is incorrect because fats are not limited to those classified as polyunsaturates. **Answer 4** is incorrect because fats *are* allowed in the postcholecystectomy diet, to tolerance.

Test-taking tip—Understand the purpose of the gallbladder and why it needed to be removed. Bile is stored in the gallbladder and sent out of the gallbladder when fat needs to be digested. Fatty foods are avoided when there is gallbladder disease because of the pain that occurs when there is a demand but the gallbladder is not able to respond. The obstruction or inflammation has been solved with the removal of the gallbladder. Most patients are fearful of the return of severe pain and are hesitant to eat a fatty meal initially.

IMP, 4, PhI, Basic Care and Comfort

45. **(2)** The patient who has had thyroid surgery should be assisted in supporting the head and neck whenever the position is changed during the first 3 postoperative days. Supporting the head is particularly important during early ambulation procedures, when sudden movement may result in hyperextension of the neck. **Answers 1, 3, and 4** are incor-

rect because none of these responses takes into account the need to prevent hyperextension of the neck.

Test-taking tip—Think of where the surgical incision is for this surgery. Support the head to prevent any trauma to the incision.

IMP, 3, PhI, Reduction of Risk Potential

46. **(3)** This diurnal variation is characteristic of a *reactive* (situational) depression. The individuals experiencing a melancholic type depression usually feel worse in the morning but better as the day progresses. In reactive depression there is usually a weight loss of *less* than 10 pounds **(Answer 1)**. The individuals usually do respond to environmental stimuli **(Answer 2)**. The precipitating event is usually an *identifiable* stressor, such as the birth of an unhealthy baby **(Answer 4)**.

Test-taking tip—Knowing the difference between reactive depression (situational) and melancholia will point to the correct answer. You can also eliminate **Answers 2 and 4** because of similarity of terms, such as "reactive" (situational); you would expect a response (reaction) to environment and external stressors (events).

AN, 7, PsI, Coping and Adaptation

47. **(3)** An Apgar score of 4–6 indicates the infant is in fair condition. "Excellent" **(Answer 1)** is not a category in the Apgar score. "Good" **(Answer 2)** is a score of 7–10. "Poor" **(Answer 4)** is a score of 0–3.

Test-taking tip—Review the five areas of assessment and scoring for Apgar. Use this acronym to help remember theory in selecting the answer: **A**—Appearance; **P**—Pulse; **G**—Grimace; **A**—Activity; **R**—Respiratory effort.

EV, 5, HPM, Prevention and Early Detection

48. **(1)** Toddlers will most likely experience separation anxiety when separated from parents. In the "despair" phase, the child appears to be mourning the apparent loss of the parent, as evidenced by nonverbal behavior cues such as monotone crying, regressive behavior (thumb sucking), and sleep disturbances. If this child were experiencing muscle spasms due to her fracture **(Answer 4)**, she would most likely cry out in severe pain intermittently. The other explanations for her behavior **(Answers 2 and 3)** do not take her developmental level into account.

Test-taking tip—Know age-typical (toddler) behavior in relation to the concept of separation anxiety.

AN, 5, PsI, Coping and Adaptation

49. **(1)** Sperm deposited during intercourse may remain viable for about 3 days. If ovulation occurs during this period, conception may result. **Answer 2** is incorrect because the ovum is present only *after* ovulation. **Answer 3** is wrong because tubal motility is important in the union of ovum and sperm (and transport of the zygote) *after ovulation*. **Answer 4** is wrong because the uterine endometrium becomes secretory postovulation.

Test-taking tip—The question asks for when pregnancy might occur *preovulation;* three of the answers focus on *postovulation.*

AN, 5, HPM, Growth and Development

50. **(2)** Both parents will probably attempt to place the blame for their infant's deformities on someone or something else, such as "inadequate prenatal care," "bad counseling," or "God's wish." **Answer 1** involves a state in which personality development is arrested in one or more aspects at a level short of maturity. **Answer 3** involves unconsciously translating emotional problems into physical symptoms. **Answer 4** involves channeling a destructive or instinctual impulse that is socially unacceptable into a socially acceptable behavior, such as coping with anger by participating in sports that require the release of a lot of energy.

Test-taking tip—Know definitions of common defense mechanisms.

AN, 7, PsI, Coping and Adaptation

51. (2) It is important to assess and validate the parents' perceived needs in order to plan care effectively. The parents may need a social worker as well as a public health nurse, speech pathologist, audiologist, etc. Therefore it is essential to first make an accurate and continual assessment of the family's needs before referral (**Answer 1**). Alternatives (**Answer 3**) may be more appropriately identified *after* performing a total assessment. Health teaching (**Answer 4**) is necessary, but it must be based on an assessment and validation of the family's needs as well as of their level of readiness.

> **Test-taking tip**—Assessment ("validate") comes before referral (**1**), discussing alternatives (**3**), or doing health teaching (**4**).

PL, 7, PsI, Coping and Adaptation

52. (3) Breast self-examinations are best done the week *following* onset of menses. The breasts are then the softest, and any lumps not associated with hormonal changes are more evident. **Answer 1** is incorrect because breast changes due to hormonal changes, such as fullness or tenderness, may occur at this time, obscuring possible pathology. **Answer 2** is a good idea (that is, having a *regular* time or pattern for examination), but does *not take into account* the normal breast-tissue changes during the *menstrual cycle*. **Answer 4** is incorrect for the same reason as **Answer 1**.

> **Test-taking tip**—The question asks for the best time period—before, during, or after menses. Key factor is to avoid hormonal influence; therefore, eliminate **Answer 1** (middle), **Answer 2** (first day), **Answer 4** (week before).

IMP, 1, HPM, Prevention and Early Detection of Disease

53. (2) The contrast medium utilized in IV cholangiograms, like that used in intravenous pyelograms, contains iodine. It is important to ascertain before the test whether the patient is aware of any allergy to iodine. Saltwater fish generally leave a high iodine content, so it is helpful to ascertain if the patient has an allergy to fish, and if so, to what kind. **Answer 1** is helpful in planning patient teaching. **Answers 3 and 4** are less specific responses that provide interesting, though not essential, data.

> **Test-taking tip**—Priority for any diagnostic study using a contrast medium is to determine if the patient has an allergy to the substance being used.

AS, 1, PhI, Reduction of Risk Potential

54. (1) The patient should remain quiet in a low Fowler's or horizontal position. He or she should be cautioned not to cough so as not to extrude any intestines by increasing intraabdominal pressures. The physician should be notified next. Remain with the patient, reassuring him or her, monitoring vital signs, and having others bring equipment such as IV setup, nasogastric tube, and suction equipment. The surgeon should also be notified that the patient will be returning to the operating room. The patient should be kept NPO (**Answer 2**) in the above position (**Answer 3**) and the dressing left in place to prevent evisceration (**Answer 4**).

> **Test-taking tip**—This is an emergency situation. Look for the answer that will not add to the damage. Getting the patient out of bed to a chair may cause the entire wound to open and all contents of the cavity to eviscerate. This new wound will need surgical correction, so patient should be kept NPO.

IMP, 1, PhI, Physiological Adaptation

55. (4) Flattened neck veins in a supine position are characteristic of hypovolemia. Inadequate drainage would result in fluid retention and hypervolemia. Indications of fluid retention include inadequate fluid drainage (greater intake than output), increased blood pressure, and signs of congestive heart failure, for example, *distended* neck veins, increased dependent edema, crackles, and decreased mentation (**Answers 1, 2, and 3**).

> **Test-taking tip**—The key word is "least likely"; this could also be rephrased by saying what will *not* happen. Look for fluid volume excess, *not* deficit.

EV, 8, PhI, Reduction of Risk Potential

56. (2) Ammonia is formed in the intestines by the action of intestinal bacteria on proteins. Tap-water enemas may be given to remove protein-rich blood that has resulted from bleeding esophageal varices. Because ammonia is formed during muscle contraction, active range-of-motion exercises are contraindicated (**Answer 1**). To prevent skin breakdown in a patient who is jaundiced and edematous, passive exercises, turning, and frequent skin care are indicated. In an effort to reduce serum-ammonia levels, potassium levels need to be increased, not reduced (**Answer 3**), because potassium is necessary for cerebral metabolism of ammonia. Antibiotics that are poorly absorbed by the intestines, such as neomycin, are given, rather than withheld (**Answer 4**), to decrease the intestinal flora that manufacture ammonia.

> **Test-taking tip**—Only one option includes an intervention for a possible cause for an ammonia increase—blood.

IMP, 4, PhI, Physiological Adaptation

57. (3) Ovulation occurs most commonly 14 days *before* the next menstrual period. In a 30-day cycle, this would be day 16 or 17. **Answers 1 and 2** are incorrect because they describe a time prior to normal ovulation; **Answer 4** is wrong because ovulation occurs *before* the last week of the menstrual cycle.

> **Test-taking tip**—Understand the phases of a woman's menstrual cycle and the fertile period. **Answers 1 and 2** describe a time *prior* to ovulation; **Answer 4** occurs at the *end* of the menstrual cycle. Think *middle* of the month, middle option, a midpoint number (i.e., 16–17) among the options.

AN, 5, HPM, Growth and Development

58. (4) An abdominal hysterectomy is generally the treatment of choice for uterine fibroids with excessive vaginal bleeding. If the ovaries are not pathologic, there is no reason for surgical removal. **Answer 1**, *pan*abdominal hysterectomy, involves the removal of the uterus, fallopian tubes, and ovaries and is usually performed for *extensive endometriosis or carcinoma*. A vaginal hysterectomy (**Answer 2**) is the treatment of choice for a prolapsed *uterus*, and a D&C (**Answer 3**) is primarily a *diagnostic* tool, *not* a measure to *control excessive* uterine bleeding.

> **Test-taking tip**—The key word is "fibroids," which do not require extensive removal of tubes, ovaries and uterus. Thus, eliminate **1**. The difference between **Answer 2** (vaginal) and **Answer 4** (abdominal) is that **Answer 2** is done for a prolapsed uterus, *not* for excessive vaginal bleeding from fibroids.

IMP, 5, SECE, Management of Care

59. (2) Before notifying the physician (**Answer 1**), it is necessary to collect the data, blood sugar and urine sugar and acetone, on which the physician will base the insulin order. The physician should also be notified of the patient's vital signs and intake and output. Generally, urinary output is depressed for about 36 hours after surgery due to increased circulating levels of ADH. Given that the patient has also had insensible water loss (respirations and perspiration), the assessment data strongly indicate dehydration or hypovolemia. An antiemetic (**Answer 3**) may be administered if nausea persists *after* blood sugar and fluid balance are rectified. The physician may order an increase in the amount and rate of intravenous fluids (contrary to **Answer 4**).

> **Test-taking tip**—The key consideration here is that the patient is a diabetic. During surgery the normal routine of the diabetic patient is interrupted. The first thing the nurse should do in this situation is to get baseline information, which includes glucose level for a diabetic patient. Then the nurse has accurate assessment data to report. Choose the first step of the nursing process—*assess*.

AN, 4 ,PhI, Reduction of Risk Potential

60. (2) Arm exercises are initiated to prevent ankylosis of the shoulder. Most patients tend to splint incisional discomfort by limiting movement on the affected side. This protective mechanism may lead to "frozen shoulder," or ankylosis. Therefore, it is important to initiate movement early to maintain muscle tone and joint integrity. **Answer 1** is an example of wristdrop due to poor positioning of wrist joints. **Answer 3** is usually a normal finding, although it may occur with improper positioning with upper motor neuron lesions. Intercostal muscle spasticity (**Answer 4**) is rare and is not due to positioning.

Test-taking tip—Visualize the incision. It is natural to protect an area (to splint) to reduce the pain. The shoulder will lose mobility very quickly if passive range of motion does not begin in the early postoperative phase.
IMP, 1, PhI, Reduction of Risk Potential

61. (3) The primary objective of stoma care is to *prevent* skin irritation and excoriation. The surrounding skin should be washed with mild soap and water, rinsed thoroughly, and patted dry. The ostomy appliance should be fitted *close to the stoma to further prevent skin irritation*. Although fecal material is measured as output (**Answer 1**), this procedure is *secondary* to control of skin damage. A tight-fitting seal on the drainage bag and a well-ventilated room will decrease odor problems (**Answer 2**). Likewise, a tight-fitting appliance will prevent contamination of the abdominal incision (**Answer 4**).

Test-taking tip—The key words are "primary objective." Focus on *prevention* of skin excoriation. The gastric enzymes in the ileostomy drainage are very irritating to the tissue surrounding the stoma.
PL, 8, PhI, Reduction of Risk Potential

62. (4) The exact cause of the failure of the embryonic structures of the face to form a union is unclear. However, there is a significant familial pattern, and a hereditary factor is involved. Cleft palate is seen more frequently in girls, whereas cleft lip is seen more frequently in boys (**Answers 1 and 2**). Although cleft lip and palate sometimes do occur together (**Answer 3**), in many cases they occur independently.

Test-taking tip—Choose the more general "heredity" response than gender-specific responses (**1, 2**); eliminate the option with "always" in the stem.
AN, 5, HPM, Prevention and Early Detection of Disease

63. (3) The woman should have waited to telephone until she had assessed her signs and symptoms *after* drinking three to four 8 oz glasses of water for hydration. She is correct to call when her contractions are every 10 minutes (**Answer 1**), to call after she emptied her bladder (**Answer 2**), and to call after she rested in bed for 1 hour (**Answer 4**).

Test-taking tip—The question asks for the action that the patient *should do first* (but did not do) before calling the health care provider. Hydration will often stop uterine irritability. The other answers *would* be appropriate for her to contact the provider.
EV, 5, HPM, Growth and Development

64. (4) The Trendelenburg test evaluates the competency of the superficial veins. While lying down, the patient is asked to elevate the involved leg to empty the veins. A tourniquet is then applied lightly to occlude the superficial veins. The patient is then asked to stand, the tourniquet is removed, and the direction and degree of vein-filling are observed. **Answer 1** is also a test of venous competence: Ordinarily, distended veins decrease markedly during walking because muscular contractions facilitate venous flow in deeper veins. **Answer 2** describes a phlebography, and **Answer 3** is a test generally used on the jugular vein when pump failure is suspected.

Test-taking tip—The key phrase is "competence of the venous valves." To do such a test, you need to empty the veins as best you can (lying down), obstruct the blood flow (tourniquet), have patient stand to have the impact of gravity on the blood flow (competent valves will prevent blood from flowing backwards). As you visualize each option, look for the one that will empty the vein first.
IMP, 6, PhI, Reduction of Risk Potential

65. (3) Usually with a transverse lie the classic or longitudinal incision is used, and the woman is concerned about her body image. **Answers 1, 2, and 4** may be concerns, but they are not usually primary in the woman's mind.

Test-taking tip—Compare the answers given here, and determine which could cause the patient to be concerned about *body image*. **Answers 1, 2**, and **4** do not relate to body image.
AN, 7, HPM, Growth and Development

66. (2) There is a physical tolerance, but the dependence is purely psychological. **Answers 1 and 3** are imprecise; and **Answer 4** is incorrect because this drug is not physiologically addictive.

Test-taking tip—Know what is the effect of marijuana in relation to dependency/addiction.
IMP, 7, PsI, Psychosocial Adaptation

67. (2) The dialysate is warmed to body temperature before administration to minimize discomfort and optimize clearance of waste products. Warming the fluid tends to dilate the peritoneal vessels, increasing the amount of urea that passes through the membrane. It has little effect on the osmotic gradient (**Answer 1**), does not prevent peritonitis, which is secondary to infection (**Answer 3**), and does not speed infusion time (**Answer 4**), although it does make it more comfortable.

Test-taking tip—The purpose of dialysis is to act as a filtration when the kidneys are unable to function correctly. Know the effect of "warming"—improves blood flow to an area.
PL, 8, PhI, Reduction of Risk Potential

68. (3) To prevent undue stress on the suture line and underlying surgical repair, the patient is taught to support the back of the neck when repositioning and to avoid both hyperextension and flexion of the neck. **Answer 1** is incorrect because active flexion of the neck is avoided and because after a total thyroidectomy the patient will receive thyroid medications to prevent hypothyroidism and to maintain a euthyroid state. **Answer 2** is also incorrect due to the focus on active flexion and extension neck exercises, which would put undue stress on the suture line. **Answer 4** is partially correct; however, again, active flexion exercises are contraindicated.

Test-taking tip—Visualize the incision line. Only one option supports the head in a neutral position.
IMP, 3, PhI, Reduction of Risk Potential

69. (4) The intradermal tuberculin test is read in 48–72 hours. Color is observed, and the injection site is palpated for induration. Reading the test in less than 48 hours may lead to inaccurate interpretation (**Answers 1, 2, and 3**).

Test-taking tip—It takes *time* for a reaction (more than 2 days).
EV, 1, HPM, Prevention and Early Detection of Disease

70. (2) It is not necessary to isolate a patient with radioactive implants (**Answer 1**), but to prevent undue exposure to radiation contacts, contact time should be brief and distance between the patient and others maximized. Specific instructions as to the amount of time permitted with the patient and the safe distance should be posted. **Answers 3 and 4** are incorrect because the best position for the patient is supine.

Test-taking tip—It is important to maintain patient position so that the implant is in the correct position; but *none of these options* describes the correct position (lying flat on back). The *other important consideration* is to protect the staff and family visitor from unnecessary exposure. Patients who have radiation implants have active radiation ongoing for a number of hours. Know the concepts of *time* (as short a time of exposure to others as possible), *distance* (stay as far away as possible from the source of radiation), and *shielding* (protect with a lead barrier such as apron) when dealing with radiation therapy.

IMP, 1, SECE, Safety and Infection Control

71. (1) Anemia occurs in cirrhosis due to (a) erythrocyte destruction in the engorged spleen, (b) gastrointestinal blood losses, and (c) folic acid deficiencies from inadequate dietary intake. Kupffer cells (**Answer 2**) line the venous sinusoids in the liver and are primarily macrophagic. **Answers 3 and 4** are incorrect because decreased amino acid breakdown and synthesis result in increasing serum-ammonia levels, which may further inhibit dietary intake.

Test-taking tip—Use process of elimination and a clue from the stem—anemia; look for low RBCs.

AN, 6, PhI, Physiological Adaptation

72. (2) The patient's vital signs and urine output reflect a decrease in extracellular volume secondary to osmotic diuresis. Increased ADH release *decreases* urinary output (**Answer 1**). A hypo-osmolar fluid imbalance is one in which there is more water than solute in the extracellular fluid compartment (**Answer 3**). Like circulatory overload (**Answer 4**), symptoms of a hypo-osmolar imbalance include widened pulse pressure, increased blood pressure, distended neck veins, and respiratory crackles.

Test-taking tip—Blood pressure is low and pulse is fast in fluid volume deficit.

AN, 6, PhI, Physiological Adaptation

73. (2) After bronchoscopy the patient generally produces a large amount of sputum that must be observed carefully for signs of hemorrhage, particularly if a biopsy specimen has been taken during the procedure. Although the sputum is generally blood streaked, any pronounced bleeding should be reported immediately. Patency of the airway is the *first priority*. **Answers 1 and 3** are also observations made after a bronchoscopy. Vital signs are observed until stable, and food and fluids are withheld until the gag reflex returns. **Answer 4**, urticaria, does not occur following bronchoscopy, though it may after a bronchogram if the patient reacts to the iodine-based dye.

Test-taking tip—Think of the organ just examined and look for any signs and symptoms that identify a problem in that organ or system. Priority—assessment of system affected by procedure (e.g., patency of airway).

AS, 6, PhI, Reduction of Risk Potential

74. (2) Few surgeries warrant immediate treatment (**Answer 1**); however, the urgency of the situation does decrease preparation time. Consequently, the patient's physiologic stress will increase, not decrease (**Answer 3**), placing greater demands on metabolic functions and increasing the risk of complications. Emergency surgery does not compromise the use of general anesthesia (**Answer 4**). It is imperative to ascertain before an emergency surgery the time, type, and amount of the last oral intake, as gastric lavage or suctioning may be necessary to prevent aspiration during the surgery. Generally patients are NPO 12 hours before surgery.

Test-taking tip—When more than one answer looks good look for an answer that is broad and includes another option.

AN, 1, PhI, Physiological Adaptation

75. (2) Generally, the dwell time of the dialysate is 20–30 minutes, occasionally longer. The dwell time as well as the instillation and outflow times are prescribed by the physician according to the patient's needs. Ten to 15 minutes (**Answer 1**) is too short a time to allow for diffusion of waste products. Equilibrium between dialysate and body fluids occurs in 15–30 minutes. Longer times (**Answers 3 and 4**) are not necessary.

Test-taking tip—Think about what is happening in the procedure and determine how long it would take to be effective.

IMP, 1, PhI, Physiological Adaptation

76. (2) Under high estrogen levels, during the period surrounding ovulation, the cervical mucus becomes thin, clear, and elastic (spinnbarkeit), facilitating sperm passage. **Answer 1** is incorrect because cervical mucus becomes thicker and opaque under *progesterone* stimulation *after* ovulation. **Answer 3** is wrong because cervical mucus is essentially colorless, and *postovulation,* under progesterone stimulation, it becomes thick and sticky. **Answer 4** is wrong because ferning is *absent* during the postovulatory period.

Test-taking tip—The question asks for characteristics of the fertile period (i.e., during high estrogen level). Eliminate three of these answers, because they indicate characteristics during *postovulation* (under progesterone simulation). Compare the signs of fertile mucus versus nonfertile periods of a woman's menstrual cycle.

AS, 5, HPM, Growth and Development

77. (1) Local anesthesia is used in cataract surgery, not only because this surgery is a short procedure but also because most patients are elderly, with one chronic disease or more, which may be exacerbated by general anesthesia (**Answer 2**). Intravenous anesthesia (**Answer 3**) with thiopental sodium (Pentothal) is most frequently used when unconsciousness is desirable for short procedures or when an anesthetic induction is desired for general anesthesia. Rectal anesthesia (**Answer 4**), though rarely used today, has been employed to induce short-term anesthesia in children.

Test-taking tip—The procedure is fast, and the eye is easily anesthetized. Most patients are elderly, and are high risk with general anesthesia.

IMP, 2, PsI, Coping and Adaptation

78. (4) Parenteral hyperalimentation solutions are hyperosmolar solutions containing amino acids, 10–25% glucose, multivitamins, and electrolytes. These solutions are administered through large veins such as the subclavian to avoid the inflammation or thrombosis that these hyperosmolar solutions tend to cause in peripheral veins. These solutions are given to patients with disturbances to *ingestion,* digestion, or absorption that are combined with excessive catabolism. Hypotonic solutions (**Answer 1**) have osmolality less than blood plasma osmotic pressures and cause fluids to enter the cells. They are used for fluid replacement when some sodium is also necessary. **Answer 2** is partially correct, in that hyperalimentation solutions are hypertonic; that is, they have an osmolarity greater than that of the plasma. However, the goal of hyperalimentation is not to reduce cellular swelling but to *reverse negative nitrogen balance.* Hypertonic solutions utilized to reduce cellular swelling are indicated in water intoxication and severe sodium depletion. Rapid infusion of hyperalimentation solution, however, will cause cellular dehydration. **Answer 3** is incorrect because it is *not* a hyperosmolar fluid.

Test-taking tip—Look for the clue in the stem—"hyper"; from two choices with the prefix "hyper," choose one that would *improve* poor intake.

IMP, 6, PhI, Pharmacological and Parenteral Therapies

79. (1) Ensuring adequate oxygenation of the infant's system is the number one priority to sustain life. **Answers 2, 3, and 4** are all appropriate *secondary* goals.

Test-taking tip—Choose the *first* action; think priority (airway). Review Apgar scoring and what scores would require immediate resuscitation of the newborn.

PL, 6, PhI, Physiological Adaptation

80. (1) Vein-stripping is done not only for advancing varicosities but also for cosmetic reasons. Vein-stripping is *not* done for

thrombophlebitis (**Answer 2**), though it is done for stasis ulcerations following successful healing of the ulcer. **Answer 3** is incorrect because lymphedema is due to blockage of lymph channels and Raynaud's disease is a syndrome that affects the *arterial* vasculature. **Answer 4** is incomplete.

Test-taking tip—Look at every word in the options because some correct answers may be combined with incorrect; e.g., thrombophlebitis is not a reason for vein stripping, yet stasis ulceration could be. Many people do have vascular surgery for cosmetic reasons, which would make **Answer 4** less complete than **Answer 1**. Look for options that include others (more than one reason).

AN, 6, PhI, Physiological Adaptation

81. (2) The evening before an intravenous pyelogram (IVP), the patient is administered oral cathartics or enemas to clean the bowel of fecal material and flatus, thereby improving visualization of the kidneys and ureters. The radiopaque dye used in this procedure is injected by a physician in the radiology department, not by the nurse before the procedure (**Answer 1**). **Answer 3** is *not* part of IVP preparation. If the patient is having difficulty maintaining fluid volume balance, an intravenous infusion *may* be initiated to prevent dehydration, but it is not standard (**Answer 4**).

Test-taking tip—If the intestine was not empty, would visualization of the kidney be accurate?

PL, 8, PhI, Reduction of Risk Potential

82. (3) Glycogenolysis and therefore serum-glucose levels are increased due to the stresses of surgery. To control blood-glucose levels and prevent ketoacidosis, secondary to increased tissue metabolism (**Answer 1**), regular insulin is given in doses adjusted according to the results of urine tests (rainbow or sliding scale). Regular insulin may be given alone until results of urine tests for glucosuria and ketonuria stabilize or as a supplement along with an intermediate-acting insulin such as NPH. **Answer 2**, decreased insulin production, results from the extent of the patient's dysfunction, not the stress of surgery. Insulin does facilitate the movement of potassium across the cellular membrane, thus preventing hyperkalemia (**Answer 4**) but this is not the *best* answer.

Test-taking tip—Think of the stress reaction and its effects on the body. Increased stress leads to increased glucose level.

AN, 4, PhI, Pharmacological and Parenteral Therapies

83. (2) Life-threatening illnesses, especially those with complications resulting in prolonged recuperative periods, provoke alterations in body image. To assist a patient experiencing altered body image, the nurse needs to ascertain how the patient viewed his or her body previously and how he or she views it now. Doing this may unleash a torrent of feeling from the patient, which may help the nurse discover ways to help the patient cope. **Answers 1 and 3**, while acknowledging this patient's mood, tend to cut off further response from the patient. **Answer 4** is too open-ended.

Test-taking tip—Hear the words in the options as if they were spoken, and many times the correct option will jump out at you.

IMP, 7, PsI, Coping and Adaptation

84. (1) *Dyspnea* is a term that describes the patient's subjective awareness of increased respiratory effort. The increased work of breathing may indeed be *related* to alveolar hypoventilation (**Answer 2**), which *results* in an increased rate and depth of respiration (**Answer 3**). Oxygen saturation (**Answer 4**) shows whether the *circulation* is normal or tissue demands have changed.

Test-taking tip—Look for the option that is broad: Dyspnea is *subjective* data. The other options have components of *objective* data.

AN, 6, PhI, Physiological Adaptation

85. (3) This allows the patient some control over his care and makes the patient feel that the staff is interested in meeting his needs. **Answer 1** is inappropriate unless they have a common interest. Frequent visits should initially be *dis*couraged (**Answer 2**) to avoid the possibility of receiving drugs from the outside. **Answer 4** may be appropriate; however, it is not as important as allowing the patient some control over his own care.

Test-taking tip—Giving a choice is an effective intervention in a milieu setting for patients who are substance abusers.

PL, 7, PsI, Psychosocial Adaptation

86. (4) Vein-stripping is a painful and tiresome procedure and, for the patient's comfort, is almost always done under general anesthesia. **Answer 1** is incorrect because local anesthesia is limited to small areas such as with laceration repair. Topical anesthesia (**Answer 2**) only decreases pain sensation in mucous membranes And, because the incisions for vein-stripping are made in the groin as well as the ankle, regional anesthesia (**Answer 3**) would be impractical. Vein-stripping could also be done using spinal anesthesia.

Test-taking tip—The best option is the one that would provide most comfort for length of the surgical procedure.

IMP, 6, PsI, Coping and Adaptation

87. (3) Because the patient has a history of chronic cough, and because hernias can be repaired with spinal anesthesia, this approach may have the least amount of risk for postoperative complications. General anesthesia (**Answer 1**) has the greatest risk for respiratory complications after surgery. Intravenous (**Answer 2**) and local infiltration (**Answer 4**) would not supply the depth of anesthesia needed to complete the repair.

Test-taking tip—Look for the anesthesia that will be safest for a high-risk patient.

PL, 1, PhI, Reduction of Risk Potential

88. (2) Timed forced expiratory volume measures the functional ability of an individual to remove air from his or her lungs. Reduction in FEV_1 is usually due to airway obstruction from excess mucus. Vital capacity measures the individual's ability to move a volume of air in and out of the lungs (**Answer 1**). Though inadequate innervation of the intercostals (**Answer 3**) would also reduce the FEV_1, there is nothing in this case to indicate that this patient has neuromuscular problems. Atelectasis (**Answer 4**) is determined by x-ray, clinical symptomatology, and blood gases.

Test-taking tip—Distinguish between the normal and the abnormal findings. Normal vital capacity means no difficulty in moving air in and out of the lungs. Reduced forced expiratory volume means something is interfering with expiratory phase of respiration; air is trapped (COPD?).

IMP, 6, PhI, Physiological Adaptation

89. (1) Quadriceps-setting exercise is an appropriate activity to prevent complications of immobility. Range-of-motion exercises for joints not enclosed in the cast are encouraged. The primary purpose of the cast is to immobilize those joints above and below the fracture site; therefore extension (**Answer 2**) and flexion (**Answer 4**) of the knees are inappropriate. **Answer 3** is not correct because passive range of motion is *not as effective as active* range of motion in the prevention of complications of immobility.

Test-taking tip—Visualize the cast; joints above and below the fracture site will be enclosed in the cast. That eliminates any activity for the ankle and knee. Prevention of complications from immobility is best accomplished with active range of motion rather than passive. The best answer would be quadriceps setting. Prevent atrophy while in the cast.

PL, 3, PhI, Reduction of Risk Potential

90. (1) An induration of 10 mm or more (not cm, as in **Answer 2**) is considered a positive reaction. The skin is generally reddened. Indurations of 5–9 mm (**Answer 3**) are considered doubtful reactions. Individuals with doubtful reactions

should be retested, unless they have had a known contact with persons with tuberculosis. Indurations of less than 5 mm are considered negative reactions. The reaction is not hivelike (**Answer 4**).

> **Test-taking tip**—Visualize the size of each of the options given. Watch the unit of measure (mm versus cm).

EV, 1, HPM, Prevention and Early Detection of Disease

91. (3) Initially this couple will be unable to make appropriate decisions regarding their own needs. They first need tender support, empathy, and reassurance to assist them in coping with this stress. **Answer 1** may be appropriate at a *later* time. **Answer 2** is incorrect because this couple is probably incapable of seeking out someone to talk or to listen to. They need guidance. If left alone, they may isolate themselves, withdraw, and become depressed. Avoidance (**Answer 4**) is nontherapeutic; the problems must be faced eventually.

> **Test-taking tip**—Support and reassurance are priority interventions.

EV, 7, PsI, Coping and Adaptation

92. (4) Lethargy, disorientation, and increased rate and depth of respirations are clinical manifestations of metabolic *acidosis*. As hydrogen ion concentration rises, the central nervous system is depressed, causing the patient to become increasingly lethargic and slower in his or her responses. Likewise, the lungs try to compensate for a metabolic acidosis by increasing both the rate and depth of respirations. Serum bicarbonates provide an estimate of metabolic components of acid-base balance. The level of these ions is controlled by the kidney's ability to secrete hydrogen ions and actively reabsorb bicarbonate ions. Decreased levels of bicarbonate indicate metabolic acidosis, and increased levels of serum bicarbonate indicate metabolic alkalosis. **Answers 1, 2, and 3** are symptoms of *alkalosis*.

> **Test-taking tip**—The diagnosis of glomerulonephritis tells you that the kidneys are not functioning as they should; waste products are not being excreted adequately. Look for a respiratory response to the metabolic acidosis.

AS, 6, PhI, Physiological Adaptation

93. (1) Fluid in the water-sealed compartment will cease to fluctuate when the tubing is plugged by fibrin or a clot and/or when negative intrapleural pressures have been reestablished and the lung has re-expanded. The likelihood of lung re-expansion on the second postoperative day is small. Therefore, it is necessary to check the tubing for fibrin, clots, or severe kinking. If the tubing is kinked, it needs to be repositioned. Milking of the tube may be ordered if fibrin or clots are suspected. **Answer 2** is incorrect because an air leak is indicated by bubbling in the water-sealed compartment. Pulmonary edema (**Answer 3**) would be reflected in dyspnea, orthopnea, crackles, and pink, frothy sputum. **Answer 4** is not entirely incorrect because the patient's position may be such that the chest tubes are unnecessarily looped or kinked and repositioning the patient may facilitate flow; however, it is *not* the *best* answer.

> **Test-taking tip**—The key concepts in this question are *timing* and what *fluctuation* means.

EV, 6, PhI, Reduction of Risk Potential

94. (1) The primary effect of rapid infusion of hyperalimentation solutions is cellular dehydration due to osmosis of water from the cell in response to vascular hyperosmolarity. Occasionally circulatory overload (**Answer 2**) does occur, but with hyperglycemia. When infusion rates are rapid, supplementary insulin should be administered to prevent the effects of hyperglycemia. Hypoglycemia (**Answer 3**) may occur if the infusion rate is suddenly decreased because the body generally adapts to hyperosmolar solutions by increasing insulin release from the pancreas. However, *hypervolemia*, not hypovolemia, generally occurs. Potassium *depletion*, not excess (**Answer 4**), also results.

> **Test-taking tip**—Know the concepts of osmosis and diffusion as they relate to a hypertonic solution, *high* in glucose.

EV, 6, PhI, Pharmacological and Parenteral Therapies

95. (4) Expressing sympathy is *least* likely to assist the family to adjust, whereas empathy and understanding *are* effective in providing emotional support to families in crisis. **Answer 1** is wrong because the family *may* need to openly communicate their anxiety, fears, and concerns about the baby in order to begin positive coping. **Answer 2** is wrong because understanding the treatment being given and the potential for a successful surgical repair *may* aid them in coping with their fears. **Answer 3** is wrong because staff attitudes in working with compromised infants *do* affect parental perceptions of the infant.

> **Test-taking tip**—Note the key word in the stem—*least*.

PL, 7, PsI, Coping and Adaptation

96. (1) Nursing measures designed to reduce the occurrence of post-thyroidectomy hemorrhage include frequent checks of the dressings and bedclothes under the patient, semi-Fowler's position to prevent hyperextension of the neck, and ice packs to reduce hematoma formation and edema. **Answer 2** is partially correct; however, the supine position would increase edema because it prevents gravity drainage of the wound site. **Answer 3** is incorrect because coughing will increase stress on the sutures unless the head and neck are well supported, and moist packs tend to increase local blood flow, which in turn tends to increase edema formation in this patient. **Answer 4** is incorrect because flexion-like hyperextension puts increased stress on the suture line.

> **Test-taking tip**—Visualize the incision. For the patient with a thyroidectomy, breathing is sometimes difficult because of the location of the suture line and the dressings. Think patient comfort, safety, and prevention of complications (e.g., edema, hemorrhage).

IMP, 3, PhI, Reduction of Risk Potential

97. (1) Anticoagulants increase bleeding time and tendency to hemorrhage. Antihypertensives such as reserpine, hydralazine, and methyldopa potentiate the hypotensive effects of anesthetic agents, thereby creating problems with maintenance of blood pressure. Thiazide diuretics may induce potassium depletion and lead to respiratory depression during anesthesia. **Answers 2, 3, and 4** are incorrect because neither insulin, digoxin, nor vitamins and minerals potentiate the central nervous system depression due to anesthesia.

> **Test-taking tip**—Review the options as to potential risk in the postoperative phase. If a part of the option is wrong, the option is wrong even if it contains some part that is correct. Once you have eliminated those components that have something wrong in them, there is usually only one correct answer left. Use the process of elimination.

EV, 1, PhI, Reduction of Risk Potential

98. (4) Hypoglycemia does inhibit the let-down reflex and interfere with successful breastfeeding. Further, maintaining a stable serum-glucose concentration is important to maternal health. **Answer 1** is incorrect because breastfeeding exerts a positive effect on diabetes, reducing blood-sugar levels by transferring glucose from serum to the breast for conversion to lactose; energy is expended in milk production. **Answer 2** is wrong because her caloric needs will *increase* with lactation; insulin dosage must be adjusted to maintain optimum serum-glucose levels. **Answer 3** is wrong because hypoglycemia jeopardizes both successful breastfeeding and maternal status.

> **Test-taking tip**—There are two parts to the best answer. First, determine if it is *OK* or *not* OK to breastfeed. Then, focus on the need to maintain stable serum glucose. Choose a *preventive* option (4). Review the physiological mechanisms involved in lactation, and determine how diabetes mellitus might effect a woman's ability to nurse.

IMP, 5, PhI, Physiological Adaptation

99. (3) Before assessing and planning any rehabilitation program, the nurse must *first* assess the patient's and the family's understanding of and attitudes toward myasthenia, as well as their emotional response and coping abilities. *Before* ascertaining any further information about job stresses (**Answers 1 and 4**) or lifestyle (**Answer 2**), any unusual fears, misconceptions, or problems relating to the patient's condition need to be identified and dealt with. It may be necessary to utilize the skills of a psychiatric nurse specialist, health psychologist, or psychiatrist to evaluate the situation and assist in planning interventions.

> **Test-taking tip**—The question is asking for ordering (i.e., *first*).

AS, 3, PsI, Coping and Adaptation

100. (2) NPH is an intermediate-acting insulin with an onset time of 2 hours, peak action in 6–12 hours, and a duration of action of 24 hours. **Answer 1** is the peak action time for regular insulin. **Answers 3 and 4** are within the range for long-acting insulins.

> **Test-taking tip**—Know onset, peak and duration of each of the insulin preparations. NPH is intermediate, meaning it cannot be used for emergency situations (regular is used for that) and it does not have effects for the whole day. Look for a "middle" time.

IMP, 4, PhI, Pharmacological and Parenteral Therapies

101. (2) Keeping the foot in the correct anatomical position is the *best* method of preventing footdrop, and a footboard is best when the patient is in traction. A bed cradle (**Answer 1**) is effective in keeping pressure off the legs and feet. Passive range of motion (**Answer 3**) is most effective in preventing contractures. A trochanter roll (**Answer 4**) is most effective in preventing external rotation of the hip.

> **Test-taking tip**—Visualize the traction; it has ropes and pulleys and weights. This eliminates the bed cradle. A trochanter roll is used to prevent external rotation, not footdrop. The key phrase is "most effective." Something that is continuous rather than three times a day would be best. Look for clues in the stem—*foot*drop . . . *foot* board.

IMP, 3, PhI, Basic Care and Comfort

102. (2) The couple is able to perceive events and communicate their concerns, although there is overt tension present. **Answer 1** is usually indicated by restlessness and increased alertness. **Answer 3** is indicated by an increase in physical symptoms (headaches, nausea, dizziness, etc.) and perceiving only details. **Answer 4** is indicated by an inability to communicate or function.

> **Test-taking tip**—Review theory on levels of anxiety to eliminate severe (3) and panic (4) levels of anxiety, because the parents are able to focus and ask *appropriate* questions.

AN, 7, PsI, Coping and Adaptation

103. (3) Iopanoic acid (Telepaque) tablets are administered 1 hour after eating a fat-free meal (**Answer 1**), one at a time and in 5-minute intervals (**Answer 2**), with a minimal amount of water (usually 8 oz) to swallow *all* the tablets. Water is allowed until bedtime (**Answer 4**), but food is withheld to allow as much dye as possible to concentrate in the gallbladder. The next morning an initial x-ray is taken, after which the patient is given a fatty meal, and several more pictures are taken to observe the functioning of the gallbladder.

> **Test-taking tip**—The key word is "inappropriate" or what would you *not* do for this patient. Look for the wrong answer, not the correct one, when it asks for what is "inappropriate."

PL, 4, PhI, Reduction of Risk Potential

104. (1) Since tracheostomy inhibits the patient from talking, it is essential to establish a mode of postoperative communication so that the patient can express needs. The mode chosen should be communicated to the rest of the staff so that the approach to the patient is consistent. Blood work (**Answer 2**) may or may not be ordered before tracheostomy, though

blood gas analysis is frequently ordered to establish baseline data in order to evaluate the effectiveness of the intervention. Inserting a Foley catheter (**Answer 3**) is not a priority *unless* urinary output has decreased. A standard surgical prep (**Answer 4**), cleansing and shaving the operative area, is not done before tracheostomy. However, the physician does cleanse the area with an antiseptic before performing the tracheostomy.

> **Test-taking tip**—Do something for the patient directly, then take care of procedures.

AN,7,PsI, Coping and Adaptation

105. (1) IPPB facilitates the flow of air deep into the lungs by exerting pressures greater than atmospheric pressure (positive pressure) on inspiration. The patient needs to learn to take slow, controlled inspirations to prevent hyperventilation. **Answers 2, 3, and 4** are incorrect because negative inspiratory pressures are consistent with CPAP or PEEP ventilatory systems, and pressures normally become more negative as the patient exhales.

> **Test-taking tip**—Key term in this question is "positive pressure." This eliminates two options immediately. To improve respiratory hygiene, you attempt to get more air in on inspiration.

AN, 6, PhI, Physiological Adaptation

106. (3) It is essential that the nurse be readily available to provide physiological, sociological, and psychological support when needed. The father has requested assistance; therefore, although privacy (**Answer 1**) is important, remaining with the couple to provide support and guidance is paramount. **Answer 2** may be appropriate if sitting with the couple does not decrease the mother's anxiety. **Answer 4** will probably be ineffective. Furthermore, she may need to feel that it is OK to express her feelings, and the nurse should encourage her to be as open as possible.

> **Test-taking tip**—In crisis intervention, *support* (sitting quietly) is a first priority.

PL, 7, PsI, Psychosocial Adaptation

107. (2) Usually inborn errors of metabolism are autosomal-recessive inherited disorders; that is, if a woman with the disorder has a child with a man who carries the recessive gene, there is a chance for her child to exhibit the disorder. **Answers 1, 3, and 4** are incorrect, because this disorder is autosomal-*recessive* (individuals carrying the gene are not aware of it until two people with the gene have a child who exhibits the disorder), *not* a *sex*-linked disorder, and not a multifactorial inheritance disorder.

> **Test-taking tip**—Focus on the two "recessive" options and eliminate the sex-linked (X) recessive.

AN, 5, HPM, Prevention and Early Detection of Disease

108. (3) The cumulative inflow and outflow records should show an outflow equal to or in excess of the amount instilled. The amount of excess outflow allowed is also determined by the physician; this rarely exceeds 200 mL per cycle. Occasionally, drainage is less then expected. Nursing measures to enhance outflow include turning the patient from side to side, elevating the head of the bed (increases intraabdominal pressures), and/or gently massaging the abdomen. If the problem continues, notify the physician before initiating another cycle; she or he may attempt to clear the catheter by rotation or by probing it for fibrin clots (**Answer 2**). **Answers 1 and 4** will not improve flow.

> **Test-taking tip**—Visualize where the catheter is placed and what would facilitate the return of fluid. By elevating the head of the bed, intra-abdominal pressure is increased; this in turn helps to force the fluid out through the catheter.

IMP, 3, PhI, Reduction of Risk Potential

109. (2) The primary purpose of the water-sealed drainage system is to remove excess fluid and air from the pleural space, thereby speeding reinflation of the lung, reestablishing normal negative intrapleural pressure, and preventing the devel-

opment of pneumothorax in the unaffected lung. Secondarily, water-sealed drainage enables the nurse to monitor blood loss. **Answers 1 and 3** are incorrect because both effects are the opposite of those intended. **Answer 4** is incorrect because atelectasis is caused by insufficient removal of secretions from the bronchial tree.

> **Test-taking tip**—Chest tubes are inserted to assist in re-expansion of the lung from the surgical intervention. Remember that it is negative pressure in the pleural space. This is the reason that the end of the tube is inserted in water, so air can escape but no air can get back into the tube or pleural cavity. Know normal physiology; only one option explains the purpose.

AN, 6, PhI, Reduction of Risk Potential

110. **(3)** The prevention of scarring is essential. All crusts should be cleaned away as gently as possible, and the area should be cleansed frequently to prevent infection. The infant should be placed on the back or side and minimally restrained to prevent him or her from turning onto the face. The side position is preferred in order to prevent the aspiration of mucus or the regurgitation of milk (**Answer 1**). The infant needs to be repositioned frequently to lessen the danger of hypostatic pneumonia (**Answer 2**). Crying should be minimized as much as possible to avoid unnecessary strain on the suture line (**Answer 4**).

> **Test-taking tip**—Visualize the surgical site anatomically and eliminate **Answer 1** (needs to be face up) and **Answer 4** (what happens to suture line when crying?). Choose the option that *prevents* (3).

PL, 1, PhI, Reduction of Risk Potential

111. **(3)** Tetany caused by hypocalcemia can be assessed for by briskly tapping the facial nerve, which is located near the middle of the masseter muscle just proximal to the ear lobe (Chvostek's sign). A positive reaction occurs when there is facial-muscle contraction, which includes a twitch of the upper lip on that side. Checking urine-calcium levels (**Answer 1**) is not helpful in assessing for early signs of hypocalcemia because urine-calcium levels are dependent not only on parathormone excretion but also on oral intake. **Answer 2** describes Homans' sign, which is used to determine the presence of deep-vein thrombosis. **Answer 4** is a late sign of hypocalcemia.

> **Test-taking tip**—Look for an early sign of tetany. Know the tests for tetany (e.g., Chvostek).

AS, 2, HPM, Prevention and Early Detection of Disease

112. **(3)** During treatment (total insertion time varies from 48–144 hours), vaginal discharge may become foul-smelling due to tissue destruction; however, perineal care is generally not allowed due to the danger of dislodging the needles. Frequently, patients find this quite distressing. A douche given under low pressure following removal of the applicator helps to reduce this side effect of therapy. Bladder atony (**Answer 1**) is a rare complication; diarrhea, rather than constipation (**Answer 2**), is more likely to occur. Sexual libido (**Answer 4**) following this therapy seems more dependent on the relationship of the partners before therapy than on the therapy itself.

> **Test-taking tip**—Look for consistency between stem and option; only one option addresses a problem with the immediate area (vagina, uterus).

AS, 8, PhI, Physiological Adaptation

113. **(1)** Fat-soluble vitamins, particularly vitamin K, are poorly absorbed in the absence of bile. This leads to decreased levels of circulating prothrombin, thus reducing normal clotting and increasing the tendency to bleed. Patients will have a T-tube postoperatively, not a Jackson-Pratt drain (**Answer 2**). Heating pads (**Answer 3**) are not used to relieve the abdominal discomfort of cholelithiasis and cholecystitis since they have little effect on reducing spasms of deeper organs. Instead, antispasmodics are used. A high-carbohydrate diet, rather than a low-carbohydrate one (**Answer 4**), would be given to build up glycogen stores in the liver.

> **Test-taking tip**—Eliminate the wrong answers: Jackson Pratt is not used (T-tube is used), heat is not used (medications are used) to decrease spasms, and low carbohydrate is incorrect. (need *high* carbohydrate to build glycogen stores).

AS, 6, PhI, Reduction of Risk Potential

114. **(3)** The single best measure for assessing fluid volume status is daily weights. Significant water loss must occur before there are changes in skin turgor (**Answer 1**). Similarly, blood pressure (**Answer 2**) may not reflect changes in fluid volume status if the fluid is sequestered in the interstitial spaces (edema formation). Finally, intake and output measures are important (**Answer 4**) but generally do not reflect insensible water losses (water lost per respiration and diaphoresis) and are not always as sensitive to decreases in urine output in chronic renal dysfunction as they are in more acute illnesses.

> **Test-taking tip**—Key word is "best." Other factors influence status of skin, vital signs, and intake and output besides fluid.

AS, 6, PhI, Physiological Adaptation

115. **(2)** Intrauterine devices (IUDs) are believed to prevent conception. The copper-bearing IUD damages sperm in transit to fallopian tubes. The progesterone-bearing IUD causes progestin-related effects on cervical mucus and endometrial maturation. **Answer 1** is incorrect because tubal ligation *prevents union* of sperm and egg by closing the passage. **Answer 3** is wrong because oral contraceptives *prevent maturation* of the graafian follicle and expulsion of the egg. **Answer 4** is wrong because the diaphragm and spermicidal jelly serve as mechanical and chemical *barriers* to prevent viable sperm from gaining access to the egg.

> **Test-taking tip**—Key words are "prevent implantation." Only one method does that. The other methods prevent *union* of sperm/egg; prevent *maturation* of follicle; or provide a mechanical *barrier* to the egg.

AN, 5, HPM, Growth and Development

116. **(4)** Provide activities the patient enjoys. **Answer 1** does not promote intellectual stimulation and may disturb the roommate. Furthermore, the nurse has not validated whether the patient enjoys watching television. **Answer 2** is not a recreational activity. The nurse does not yet know whether the patient enjoys board games (**Answer 3**), and they also require a suitable partner.

> **Test-taking tip**—Note the words *most (age) appropriate* and *recreational activity.* Eliminate the one choice that is *not* a recreational activity and two other options that *assume* the patient's likes.

PL, 5, PsI, Coping and Adaptation

117. **(2)** Denial is a very strong defense mechanism used to allay the emotional effects of discovering a potential threat. Although denial has been found to be an effective mechanism for survival in some instances, such as during natural disasters, it may result in greater pathology in a woman with potential breast carcinoma. Suppression (**Answer 1**) occurs when the individual recognizes the threat but consciously refuses to think about it. Repression (**Answer 3**) is an unconscious mechanism that keeps the knowledge of the threat from coming to one's conscious awareness. Intellectualization (**Answer 4**) occurs when the individual attempts to consciously allay anxiety by attributing symptoms to other possible causes, such as cystic breast disease. However, the patient who intellectualizes does not attempt to deny the possibility that a more serious pathology may be present.

> **Test-taking tip**—Application of definitions of coping mechanism will help select the only correct answer. Denial is also the *most* common.

AN, 7, PsI, Coping and Adaptation

118. **(3)** The patient receiving NPH insulin is most likely to experience a hypoglycemic reaction in the late afternoon. Several factors may be involved, such as increased physical activity or inadequate dietary intake. Patients should be instructed

to carry gumdrops or hard candy as a source of quickly absorbed carbohydrates should symptoms occur. **Answers 1, 2, and 4** are not as likely.

> **Test-taking tip**—Know that intermediate-acting insulin lasts 8–12 hours.

AN, 4, PhI, Pharmacological and Parenteral Therapies

119. **(2)** Symptoms of severe respiratory distress indicate that the tube has dislodged and is obstructing the airway. Re-establishing an airway is the first priority: Deflate the balloons using a syringe. Following deflation, the doctor should be notified to assess the patient's condition and determine ongoing medical therapy. A code blue (**Answer 1**) would be called only *after* establishing the airway. Traction on the Sengstaken-Blakemore tube should be increased or decreased (**Answer 3**) *only by* the attending *physician*. Iced saline (**Answer 4**) is no longer used for irrigation during active bleeding, and this problem is respiratory, *not* hemorrhagic.

> **Test-taking tip**—Think of the common, yet most serious, thing that could happen to this special tube. When it was deflated, the position changed. Dyspnea and skin color change represent airway obstruction. Deflate the balloon and assess again.

IMP, 6, PhI, Physiological Adaptation

120. **(1)** The skin preparation area for hernia repair includes the entire abdomen from just below the nipple line to the mid-thigh. It includes all pubic hair visible when the legs are together, and should extend to the bedline on each side. **Answer 2** is an example of an abdominal prep when the incision is above the umbilicus. **Answer 3** is a lower-extremities prep for surgeries such as a femoral arterial graft. **Answer 4** is a perineal prep used for vaginal or rectal surgeries.

> **Test-taking tip**—Visualize where the incision will be and extend the field in all directions.

IMP, 1, PhI, Reduction of Risk Potential

121. **(2)** Patients having upper-abdominal surgery tend to breathe shallowly after surgery in order to splint incisional discomfort. Consequently, these patients need both assistance and encouragement to breathe deeply and cough. Splinting of the incisional area by the nurse helps, as well as planning deep breathing and particularly coughing times to follow the administration of a pain reliever. **Answers 1 and 3** are correct statements but not the best answers. Patients having abdominal surgery tend to guard against coughing because it increases intra-abdominal pressures and incisional discomfort. Many people do tend to be thoracic breathers and need to be taught abdominal or diaphragmatic breathing in the preoperative period. **Answer 4** is incorrect, because NG tubes do not inhibit deep breathing; rather, they tend to increase oral respirations, which causes drying of the oral mucous membranes.

> **Test-taking tip**—Think of where the incision is and consider what organs/function will be most affected due to pain and splinting. Upper abdominal incisions have a significant impact on respiratory function. Look for an answer that explains *why* deep breathing is a problem.

AN, 6, PhI, Physiological Adaptation

122. **(1)** It is important for the couple to be able to rely on each other at this time. They need time to communicate and to begin to cope with their feelings. As long as the mother's vital signs are stable, it may be most therapeutic to allow the father into the recovery room. **Answer 2** isolates the father from all significant others. **Answer 3** evades the problem and does not alleviate any anxiety. **Answer 4** is a physician's decision, and the infant is probably still being worked up and treated at his time.

> **Test-taking tip**—Priority response by the nurse is to reinforce *couple* interaction.

IMP, 7, PsI, Coping and Adaptation

123. **(4)** Intake and output records, as well as daily weights, provide important measures of the effectiveness of the treat-

ment and are good monitors of fluid balance. Urine testing (**Answer 1**) is done to detect glycosuria every 4–6 hours. In the event glycosuria occurs, the physician should be notified. The physician may order insulin coverage or a decrease in the flow rate. Blood withdrawal and CVP readings (**Answer 2**) are contraindicated because infusion rates must be kept constant to avoid the formation of clots in the catheter. If the catheter insertion site remains dry, dressings are changed every 48 hours utilizing strict aseptic technique, not just clean technique (**Answer 3**). Gloves and masks are used during the dressing change and while the IV tubing and filter are changed.

> **Test-taking tip**—Hyperalimentation is administered through a central line, which is kept open exclusively for this purpose (*no* CVP readings as in **2**). Because the solution is nutrient rich and contains a high content of glucose and other nutrients and additives, frequent monitoring is necessary, not 8–12 hours (**1**). Sterile technique, *not* clean technique, is used (**3**). The stem asks for "correct" action. Only one will be right.

IMP, 6, PhI, Pharmacological and Parenteral Therapies

124. **(1)** An iridectomy, or removal of a wedge from the iris, is performed with cataract removal to prevent the forward push of the aqueous humor from blocking the canal of Schlemm, which would produce a secondary glaucoma. Iridectomy does not affect pupillary dilation (**Answer 2**), facilitate retinal circulation (**Answer 3**), or prevent corneal scarring (**Answer 4**).

> **Test-taking tip**—Think about the normal eye structure. What would removing a wedge of iris do?

IMP, 2, PhI, Reduction of Risk Potential

125. **(4)** In a closed chest drainage system (Pleur-evac), the first chamber collects the drainage from the patient's chest, the second chamber provides the water seal to reestablish negative pressure, and the third chamber is attached to the suction. **Answer 1** is incorrect because the third chamber establishes the suction and the first chamber collects the drainage. **Answer 2** is incorrect because it is the third chamber that is associated with the suction, not the first and second. **Answer 3** is incorrect because the self-sealing diaphragm for drainage sampling is in the first chamber.

> **Test-taking tip**—Picture the device: drainage is collected in the first chamber, which is closest to the patient. The second chamber is the water-seal chamber and the third is the suction. Patient drainage "first"; suction control last.

AN, 1, PhI, Physiological Adaptation

126. **(3)** Women should be instructed to contact the clinic doctor or nurse if they have leg cramps or headaches (signs of possible thrombophlebitis caused by the hypercoagulability that occurs under estrogen/progesterone stimulation). **Answer 1** is incorrect because mild to moderate nonpathological nausea may occur during the first few days on oral contraceptives as the body adjusts to the elevated hormone levels. **Answer 2** is wrong because chloasma, the "mask of pregnancy," is merely hyperpigmentation related to the high hormone levels. **Answer 4** is wrong because breast tenderness and weight gain are nonpathologic and are associated with an increased tendency to retain fluid in the interstitial spaces.

> **Test-taking tip**—Prioritize which signs/symptoms might be life threatening and must be evaluated immediately. Think vascular, think neuro. Eliminate three options that are signs and symptoms associated with physiological adaptation in pregnancy.

AS, 1, PhI, Pharmacological and Parenteral Therapies

127. **(3)** Maintenance of an adequate airway is always the primary goal of nursing care. Respiratory obstruction is a very serious complication; therefore it is wise to have both an emergency tracheostomy set and suctioning apparatus available at the bedside of the patient who has had a thyroidectomy. **An-**

swer 1 is also correct, but it is not the best answer because the onset of this complication is *more gradual.* With adequate nursing observation, it can be handled before it becomes life threatening. **Answer 2** is incorrect because thoracentesis is utilized to remove excess fluid from the *pleural* space. The correct nursing strategy for postoperative bleeding (**Answer 4**) is to notify the *physician immediately.*

> **Test-taking tip**—Visualize the area of the incision. The greatest threat to patient safety is respiratory obstruction. This could be due to damage to the parathyroid gland during surgery. Select the greatest risk to the patient.

PL, 6, PhI, Reduction of Risk Potential

128. (3) Proper handling of sputum is essential to allay droplet transference of bacilli in the air. Patients need to be taught to cover their nose and mouth with tissues when sneezing or coughing. Chemotherapy generally renders the patient non-infectious within days to a few weeks, usually before cultures for tubercle bacilli are negative. Until chemical isolation is established, many institutions require the patient to wear a mask when visitors are in the room or when the nurse is in attendance. Patients should be in a well-ventilated room, without air recirculation, to prevent air contamination. **Answer 1, 2, and 4** are unnecessary precautions.

> **Test-taking tip**—Think of the mode of transmission of this disease (droplets). Selection of the correct answer will need to focus on whatever protects the nurse and others to avoid direct contamination. Select the best choice to *prevent* spread.

IMP, 1, SECE, Safety and Infection Control

129. (2) He is attempting to cope with his anxiety by denying reality. He may also be angry (**Answer 1**), but his behavior and verbalization indicate denial. It is through the use of denial that he is displacing the blame (**Answer 3**), so denial is the more appropriate answer. He is unable to think clearly enough to seek any type of intervention (**Answer 4**); he is reacting rather than problem solving.

> **Test-taking tip**—Denial is the most common coping mechanism. One manifestation of denial can be anger, but denial is the more *inclusive* answer. Eliminate **Answers 3** and **4** because they are not related to the stem.

AN, 7, PsI, Coping and Adaptation

130. (3) The initial response would be to notify the physician of the critical hemoglobin (oxygen-carrying protein) level. A hemoglobin of 10 is desirable for the patient, decreasing the deleterious risks of general anesthetic and hypovolemic shock. The lab slip is then attached to the chart (**Answer 1**). Most likely a blood transfusion will be ordered before surgery (**Answer 2**), but there is no order yet. The nurse's actions will be charted on the nurse's notes (**Answer 4**), but charting is *not* the *first* priority.

> **Test-taking tip**—Know normal values. If no answer involves patient comfort or safety, call MD.

AN, 6, PhI, Reduction of Risk Control

131. (3) Methyldopa acts to decrease blood pressure by inhibiting the formation of dopamine, thus decreasing the amount of norepinephrine that is secreted in adrenergic synapses. Decreased adrenergic stimulation results in decreased vasoconstriction, which causes peripheral vascular resistance. **Answer 1** is an example of the effects of hydralazine; **Answer 2**, of guanethidine SO_4; and **Answer 4**, of diazepam.

> **Test-taking tip**—Read each choice—look for clues, such as "dopamine" for *dopa.*

IMP, 6, PhI, Pharmacological and Parenteral Therapies

132. (2) New parents, especially parents of infants with health problems, may need help focusing on what is normal and healthy in their infant. Discussing how their baby compares with other infants and focusing on the baby's strengths will help parents to focus on these important aspects of development. To tell this mother that her baby has a "life-threaten-

ing illness" (**Answer 1**) could be very frightening and not at all helpful to her at this time. False reassurance (**Answer 3**) and stating you "know how she feels" (**Answer 4**) are also not therapeutic responses.

> **Test-taking tip**—Eliminate two responses that are trite clichés (**Answers 3** and **4**). Choose **Answer 2** because it is at least an attempt to *assess* for mother's knowledge deficit regarding what is normal.

IMP, 7, PsI, Coping and Adaptation

133. (2) Sitting the patient up allows for deeper ventilation, and splinting of the incisional area reduces incisional discomfort. **Answer 1** is also correct but not specific enough. Generally 20–30 minutes should elapse before instituting coughing techniques following administration of an analgesic, to allow for the full effects of the drug. **Answer 3** is incorrect unless the patient is in a good deal of pain; if so, the patient should be medicated, then coughed. **Answer 4** is incorrect because oral intake is withheld until bowel activity is re-established. Secretions can be kept mobilized by frequent turning and deep breathing.

> **Test-taking tip**—Look for the option that has the nurse performing an independent nursing action.

IMP, 6, PhI, Basic Care and Comfort

134. (2) The legs of the patient undergoing vein-stripping are wrapped from foot to groin with elastic bandages. Anticoagulants (**Answer 1**) are not routinely ordered following surgery, although analgesics will be ordered for pain. Sitting in a chair (**Answer 3**) is contraindicated because the pressure this position exerts behind the knees and at the hips impedes venous return and increases dependent venous pressures. **Answer 4** is incorrect because the patient is usually ambulated the day of vein-stripping surgery to enhance venous return by way of muscle contraction.

> **Test-taking tip**—Picture the extent of the surgical wounds and the best action to prevent complications.

PL, 1, PhI, Reduction of Risk Potential

135. (3) The primary goal is to prepare the new mother with diabetes to care for her infant while effectively managing her disease. **Answer 1** is incorrect because it will not ensure adequate home health maintenance of mother and infant. **Answer 2** is incorrect because potential problems will vary, depending on many factors such as maternal age, and it does not address the primary health maintenance goal. **Answer 4** is incorrect because, although follow-up care is an important aspects of discharge teaching, it is subsumed under the broader goal of discussing coping strategies for managing diabetes.

> **Test-taking tip**—Prioritize the most important goals for *both* mother and infant during the immediate postpartum period for a woman with diabetes. The question asks for *early* considerations; **Answers 1, 2,** and **4** are *later* considerations.

PL, 1, SECE, Management of Care

136. (2) Postoperative inflammation and edema underlie the frequent occurrence of scrotal swelling after indirect hernia repair. This complication is very painful, and any movement by the patient results in discomfort. Elevating the scrotum on rolled towels or providing support with a suspensory helps to reduce edema. Ice bags facilitate pain relief. **Answer 1** is inappropriate because this is not an emergency side effect of surgery. Pain medication (**Answer 3**) may also be administered, but vigorous coughing (**Answer 4**) is contraindicated following herniorrhaphy.

> **Test-taking tip**—Look for what the nurse can do to assist with the identified problem. Think of the basic intervention: ice and elevation.

IMP, 3, PhI, Reduction of Risk Potential

137. (4) The first nursing measure should be to mark the time and the amount of drainage in the collection bottle to ensure a baseline measurement for further observations. The milking of chest tubes (**Answer 1**) is a matter of debate at

this time. Although the process of stripping or milking does assist in the removal of fibrin and clots from the chest tubes, compression of the tubes also increases intrapleural pressures by preventing the movement of air and fluid. Whether the chest tubes are milked or not will depend on institutional or individual physician's policies. **Answer 2** is incorrect because the drainage system is always kept in a dependent position to maintain gravity flow of air and fluids. The nurse's next measure is to secure the tubes to the bed linen (**Answer 3**) to prevent kinking or unnecessary looping of the drainage tubes, which would hinder the flow of air and fluid.

Test-taking tip—Think baseline data. Complete assessment first.

IMP, 6, PhI, Reduction of Risk Potential

138. (2) Respiratory obstruction, hemorrhage, tetany, and laryngeal nerve injury are the major complications following thyroid surgery. *Hypocalcemia,* not hypercalcemia (**Answer 1**), is a complication resulting from damage to the parathyroid glands during surgery. Serum T_4 will be *decreased* or absent, not elevated (**Answer 3**), and the patient will need replacement therapy because no thyroid hormone is secreted once the total thyroid gland is removed. **Answer 4** is not a good answer. Because the integrity of the gastrointestinal tract is not interrupted during thyroid surgery, paralytic ileus is a *rare* complication.

Test-taking tip—Think of where this incision is and the first priority—airway.

AN, 3, PhI, Reduction of Risk Potential

139. (1) Standard precautions specify that all health care providers should wear gloves until all blood and amniotic fluid have been removed. Because transmission of the virus may occur via breast milk, breastfeeding is *discouraged* (**Answer 2**). **Answers 3 and 4** are incorrect because the parents are *encouraged to bond* with the child and the nurse needs to support all positive parental feelings.

Test-taking tip—The priority is *infection control,* that is, standard precautions (gloves when in contact with body fluids). See the word "precaution" in the stem and an example of standard precautions in **Answer 1.**

IMP, 1, SECE, Safety and Infection Control

140. (4) This couple is experiencing an actual loss and will probably exhibit many of the same symptoms as a person who has lost someone to death. **Answers 1, 2, and 3** will most likely occur at some *later* time.

Test-taking tip—Note the key word "initial."

EV, 7, PsI, Coping and Adaptation

141. (1) The purpose of the T-tube is to maintain the patency of the bile duct after surgery. Localized edema in the surgery area tends to obstruct the outflow of bile, which is continuously being synthesized by the liver. The T-tube does not directly prevent postoperative hemorrhage (**Answer 2**) or postoperative wound infection (**Answer 3**). A secondary effect of this procedure is that bile flow is directed away from the duodenum (**Answer 4**).

Test-taking tip—Visualize the T-tube. The horizontal part of the T is inserted into the common bile duct to maintain patency. Drainage comes into the tube from both sides of the horizontal portion of the tube into the vertical part of the T, which is connected to a collection apparatus. The T-tube remains in the duct until the edema subsides, because exploration causes swelling.

AN, 4, PhI, Reduction of Risk Potential

142. (1) Anxiety, like pain, glucose imbalance, or changes in blood pressure, stimulates discharge of the sympathetic nervous system. In some patients this increased adrenergic discharge results in moderate to severe increases in systolic and diastolic pressures that decrease to normal levels when emotional equilibrium is restored. The patient may be emotionally labile (**Answer 2**), but at this time there are insufficient data to make this judgment. She is fearful, but that does not

mean she is unprepared for this surgery (**Answer 3**). Should her anxiety remain high, however, the attending physician should be notified. Though the patient may be attempting to employ denial (**Answer 4**), her emotional response (restlessness and increased blood pressure) indicates this defense mechanism is ineffective in allaying her present anxieties (**Answer 4**).

Test-taking tip—When in doubt as to the answer, look for a pattern in the options—three are psychological explanations; choose the one that is different.

EV, 7, PsI, Coping and Adaptation

143. (2) The diet of a patient with cirrhosis should provide ample protein for tissue repair, at least 0.5 g/lb. Some modification occurs *if* serum-ammonia levels are elevated (**Answer 1**). Sufficient carbohydrate intake is needed to sustain weight and prevent proteins from being utilized for energy, *not for the reason* stated in **Answer 3**. **Answer 4** is partially correct. Salt is restricted to assist in decreasing edema formation. However, the reason for high-carbohydrate foods is as discussed above. Fluids may also be restricted to 1000–1500 mL/day. Vitamin supplements, particularly fat-soluble vitamins (A, D, and K), are usually prescribed because of decreased bile production for their absorption and because of the inability of the liver to store them successfully. Initially, if the patient has a very poor appetite, liquid protein supplements such as Sustagen may be given. Frequent, small feedings may also increase intake.

Test-taking tip—How would each dietary restriction or specific allowance relate to the pathophysiology of the disease identified? Patients with cirrhosis often need adequate protein intake. Fluid accumulation is another significant problem to be considered.

PL, 4, PhI, Basic Care and Comfort

144. (3) Neomycin is administered preoperatively because it is a poorly absorbed antibiotic and therefore is effective in reducing the number of intestinal organisms that may cause infection of the suture line. Neomycin is not effective in reducing postoperative atelectasis (**Answer 1**). Prevention of atelectasis is dependent on adequate pulmonary hygiene (deep breathing and coughing up of secretions) in the postoperative period. **Answer 2** is correct, but it is not the *best* answer, because the ability of the body to ward off infection is a result of the decrease in intestinal organisms. **Answer 4** is incorrect because bladder atony is generally due to decreased parasympathetic outflow and bladder tone secondary to anesthesia.

Test-taking tip—Look for an option relating to the *drug action* (i.e., decreased intestinal organisms).

AN, 8, PhI, Pharmacological and Parenteral Therapies

145. (4) Frequent, small meals do not visually overwhelm the patient and they require less energy for ingestion. Because patients with cirrhosis frequently have very poor appetites, the nurse may have to be very creative in approaches to ensure adequate nutritional intake. **Answers 1, 2, and 3** take the responsibility away from the patient and increase his or her dependency.

Test-taking tip—Look for a pattern—three options take away patient control or independence. Choose the one that does not.

IMP, 4, PhI, Basic Care and Comfort

146. (2) Postoperatively, deep breathing and particularly coughing up of sputum are the most important activities engaged in by the patient after chest surgery. These activities reduce bronchotracheal secretions, prevent atelectasis, and promote adequate ventilation. Although **Answers 1 and 3** are also important in preventing postoperative complication, airway integrity is always the *first* priority. **Answer 4** is employed for patients having herniorrhaphies.

Test-taking tip—The question is asking for "most important postoperative activity." Priority should focus on prevention of airway complication if appropriate for the location.

IMP, 6, PhI, Reduction of Risk Potential

147. **(3)** Although most patients are able to rest more comfortably and even sleep after administration of a narcotic, extreme or prolonged lethargy indicates that the medication dose may be too large. The physician should be consulted for both a change of dose and route of administration (**Answers 1 and 2**). Alternative modes of pain relief can and should be instituted if the patients' discomfort is not severe, but not as a delaying tactic (**Answer 4**) when the issue is the appropriateness of a specific medication dose.

> **Test-taking tip**—Three options are *not* nursing decisions, once an adverse effect is noted.

IMP, 2, PhI, Pharmacological and Parenteral Therapies

148. **(3)** Postoperatively the patient with a cataract may be placed in a flat or low Fowler's position on the back or turned to the unoperated side. Turning the patient to the operated side (**Answer 4**) or raising the head of the bed (**Answer 1**) increases the stress on the sutures and may lead to hemorrhage. The patient may assume a prone position with the head turned to the unoperated side (**Answer 2**), though most patients find a side-lying position more comfortable.

> **Test-taking tip**—Visualize which position will lower pressure in the head.

PL, 2, PhI, Reduction of Risk Potential

149. **(1)** The woman must understand that, although the "fertile" period is approximately midcycle, hormonal variations do occur and can result in early or late ovulations. To be effective, the diaphragm should be inserted before every intercourse. **Answer 2** is incorrect because the diaphragm must be left in place for a minimum of 6 hours after intercourse. Premature removal may permit passage of viable sperm. **Answer 3** is incorrect because marked variations in weight may result in the need for a larger or smaller appliance. **Answer 4** is wrong because pin holes in the diaphragm may permit viable sperm to pass the barrier.

> **Test-taking tip**—The question asks for an answer that would require further teaching. Reword the question when it asks for this. The *best* answer will have an incorrect statement.

EV, 5, HPM, Growth and Development

150. **(4)** Normally drainage from the T-tube averages 300–500 mL during the first few days after surgery and then gradually decreases; the tube is generally removed in 7–10 days. By the fourth postoperative day, flow has usually begun to decrease. Excessive drainage at this time should be reported as it indicates possible reobstruction of the duct. **Answers 1, 2, and 3** are normal postoperative findings.

> **Test-taking tip**—Think of timing. Know normal postop course. Would you expect more than 500 mL of drainage on day 4? Usually the patient is ambulatory, discharged home, and healing well. 500 mL is a great deal of T-tube drainage. Nurse should notify the MD for an abnormal finding, *not expected* findings such as in **Answers 1, 2, and 3**.

AN, 6, PhI, Reduction of Risk Potential

151. **(1)** After a settling-in period, the toddler experiencing separation anxiety may enter the phase of "denial," covering up painful feelings toward parents and seeming to turn instead to others, such as the aide. Although it may seem like the toddler is doing fine (**Answer 3**), she is actually denying feelings that are too painful to deal with just now. At her age, she is not trying to make her mother jealous (**Answer 4**); neither does she need discipline (**Answer 2**).

> **Test-taking tip**—Know age-appropriate manifestations of separation anxiety.

AN, 5, PsI, Coping and Adaptation

152. **(4)** It is essential that the couple be prepared for what they will see. However, it is equally as important for them to be able to see, touch, and hold their infant as soon as possible, to begin the attachment process. **Answer 1** merely delays the couple in seeing their infant. The nurse continually assesses the parents' readiness while caring for the infant. Parents *do* need some preparation before seeing their infant (**Answer 2**). Teaching without immediate parent-child contact can increase the parents' anxiety (**Answer 3**).

> **Test-taking tip**—The underlying concept for the best answer is facilitating early bonding and attachment, when complications with the newborn might affect the bonding.

PL, 7, PsI, Coping and Adaptation

153. **(2)** After explaining the procedure to the patient, the nurse should first instruct the patient to void. This prevents accidental nicking or perforation of the bladder during the procedure. The patient is positioned in a chair or in high Fowler's position in bed (**Answer 1**), after the vital signs have been taken to establish baseline information (**Answer 3**) and the abdomen is prepared (**Answer 4**).

> **Test-taking tip**—This question is establishing a priority order. Assume all actions are correct. Instructing the patient to void would be the second thing the nurse would do.

IMP, 6, PhI, Reduction of Risk Potential

154. **(2)** The stoma drainage bag is applied in the operating room. Drainage from the ileostomy contains secretions that are rich in digestive enzymes and highly irritating to the skin. Protection of the skin from the effects of these enzymes is begun at once. Skin exposed to these enzymes even for a short time becomes reddened, painful, and excoriated. **Answers 1, 3, and 4** are incorrect because they would result in skin irritation.

> **Test-taking tip**—Think of the consistency (liquid green, not formed) of the contents and irritability in that portion of the intestine.

IMP, 8, PhI, Basic Care and Comfort

155. **(2)** Chronic renal failure symptomatology is due to a decrease in the number of functioning nephrons, with resultant decrease in glomerular filtration due to the extension of the disease process. **Answer 1** is incorrect because the cause of the renal failure was likely related to intrarenal damage from acute glomerulonephritis. **Answers 3 and 4** are incorrect because the patient has moved from the second stage of chronic kidney disease (renal insufficiency, characterized by water diuresis and mild azotemia) to renal failure, which is characterized by acidosis, marked electrolyte imbalances, fluid retention, anemia, and increases in serum urea, uric acid, and creatinine.

> **Test-taking tip**—The problem is *within* the kidney (the nephrons), not *to* or *from* the kidney.

AN, 8, PhI, Physiological Adaptation

156. **(3)** Manipulation of abdominal contents during surgery produces inhibition of peristalsis for 24–48 hours. Measures to avoid potential distention could include insertion of a nasogastric tube before surgery and continuous postsurgical suction until peristalsis returns; rectal tubes can be inserted to remove excess air in the lower colon; and early ambulation promotes return of gastrointestinal functioning. Auscultation of the abdomen for return of bowel sounds (**Answer 1**) will be necessary in assessing the return and degree of peristalsis. Abdominal massage is *not* recommended (**Answer 2**). *When* bowel sounds return, oral intake (**Answer 4**) may be started.

> **Test-taking tip**—The key word is "avoid."

PL, 1, PhI, Reduction of Risk Potential

157. **(4)** Immediately following a death, the nurse must assess and validate the family's needs for follow-up care. It is important to look at their past ability to cope with stress, how effective these coping mechanisms were, and so forth. However, initially the family will be unable to communicate their feelings and perceptions due to their high level of anxiety. **Answer 1** may be necessary if the family is unable to cope effectively with their anxiety. **Answer 2** would depend on the individual family's needs. **Answer 3** may be appropriate once the family is able to communicate their feelings and needs.

PL,7,PsI, Coping and Adaptation

158. **(4)** If all the secondary measures have been tried and the patient's bladder is distended, the physician should be notified if he or she has not left a catheterization order. Occasionally, drugs such as neostigmine bromide (Prostigmin) are ordered to stimulate bladder contractions before resorting to catheterization. **Answer 1** will only tire the patient more. Catheters should not be inserted without an order (**Answer 2**), nor should the patient be unduly fatigued by continuing to try other measures (**Answer 3**) that most likely were unsuccessful prior to this point in time. The bladder should not be allowed to become overdistended.

Test-taking tip—All usual activities have been tried. It is time to call the physician.

IMP, 8, PhI, Physiological Adaptation

159. **(2)** Hypotension and shock can occur during or after paracentesis. Fluid from the vascular compartment shifts into the abdomen to replace fluids that are withdrawn. This complication can be minimized if withdrawal of ascitic fluid is limited to 1000 ml or if lost fluid is replaced by administration of salt-poor albumin. To assess for this complication, vital signs are taken every 15 minutes during the procedure and afterward until stable, then every hour for 4 hours. Disequilibrium (**Answer 1**) occurs with rapid removal of wastes during renal dialysis. Hypoalbuminuria (no protein in urine) is a normal physical finding; therefore **Answer 3** is incorrect. Paralytic ileus (**Answer 4**) is rarely a complication of this procedure.

Test-taking tip—Look for a pattern—only one option would be an *immediate* response.

AN, 6, PhI, Reduction of Risk Potential

160. **(2)** Local radiation is generally used under four conditions: the tumor is relatively well defined, a larger dose of radiation can be delivered than by an external source, there is a critical need to reduce involvement of other tissue, and the site is accessible for introduction of seeds or implants. As a result of cobalt implantation, diarrhea may occur due to radiation-induced toxicosis of the mucous membranes of the large bowel. Diarrhea may be painful as well as profuse and bloody. **Answer 1** is incorrect because the rationale for doing an implant is that the tumor is generally well defined. The effects of severe diarrhea may indeed be electrolyte imbalance (**Answer 3**), but this is not the cause in this situation. **Answer 4** may indeed be occurring, but is not the basis for the patient's present symptoms.

Test-taking tip—The problem is caused by the treatment, not additional disease. Think of the proximity of the radiation to nearby structures.

AN, 3, PhI, Physiological Adaptation

161. **(3)** In early respiratory obstruction, the patient generally complains of a feeling of fullness or a choking sensation. Swallowing difficulties are fairly common due to tracheal irritation; however, difficulty in swallowing in conjunction with a choking sensation is indicative of airway obstruction. **Answer 1**, hoarseness and weakness of the voice, is common and is secondary to edema of the larynx. **Answer 2**, stridor and cyanosis, is a late sign of airway obstruction. **Answer 4**, disorientation and combative behaviors, is indicative of severe anoxia.

Test-taking tip—Rule out what is *expected* in the postoperative period from what is an *early* sign and what is a *late* sign.

AS, 6, PhI, Physiological Adaptation

162. **(3)** Hypoglycemic or insulin reactions are the result of decreased circulatory serum glucose to the brain. This stimulates epinephrine release. Early symptoms include cold, clammy skin, nervousness, tremors, numbness of the hands or around the lips, and cardiac palpitations. Later symptoms may mimic alcoholic intoxication, such as staggering gait, slurring of words, combative behavior, or uncontrolled weeping. As hypoglycemia deepens, the patient may develop convulsions and coma. **Answers 1, 2, and 4** are symptoms of ketoacidosis, which acts to depress the central nervous system.

Test-taking tip—The key word is "objective" data; decide between hypoglycemia and ketoacidosis.

AS, 4, PhI, Reduction of Risk Potential

163. **(3)** Bending to adjust shoelaces would increase intraocular pressures and should therefore be *avoided* during the early postoperative period; the patient who is ambulatory should wear slip-on shoes or slippers to avoid bending or stooping. Other activities to avoid include coughing, brushing the teeth, shaving, and vomiting. Self-feeding (**Answer 1**) *is* encouraged, to help reduce the patient's perception of helplessness, though food may need to be cut up for the patient to reduce exertion. Self-dressing (**Answer 2**) and ambulation (**Answer 4**) *are* permitted.

Test-taking tip—Look for an option that increases pressure on the operative site as the activity to avoid.

IMP, 2, PhI, Reduction of Risk Potential

164. **(4)** Bearing down is too strenuous for the pregnant cardiac patient. **Answer 1** is incorrect because relaxation in a semi-recumbent position reduces the workload on the heart. **Answer 2** is wrong because frequent monitoring may help identify increased pulse rate as an early sign of cardiac decompensation. **Answer 3** is wrong because regional anesthesia *reduces* pain and the physiological response to pain, which may cause cardiac decompensation. It also pools blood in the lower extremities, thereby preventing the rapid increase in cardiac output that immediately follows birth.

Test-taking tip—Identify the action that would *increase* the stress on the heart and therefore is to be avoided.

AN, 6, PhI, Reduction of Risk Potential

165. **(4)** The rationale for turning, coughing, and deep breathing every 1–2 hours is to rid the lungs of the side effects of anesthesia. Inhalant anesthetics, like cigarette smoke, irritate the mucous membranes lining the bronchi, increasing mucous production. It is exceedingly important that the patient understand that these activities are important in mobilizing and removing these excess secretions. Failure to remove them may lead to atelectasis or hypostatic pneumonias. **Answers 1, 2, and 3** are all appropriate interventions.

Test-taking tip—The key word is "inappropriate." Look for a *wrong* answer, something the nurse should *not* do.

PL, 6, PhI, Reduction of Risk Potential

166. **(4)** Increased circulating levels of uric acid, an end product of purine metabolism, are responsible for the patient's gout-like joint discomfort. Thus the diet will exclude foods high in purines (e.g., high-protein foods, organ meats). Hyperphosphatemia does occur in the third stage of chronic kidney disease. Normally this would stimulate the parathyroid gland to increase parathormone, thus raising calcium levels and lowering phosphate. However, in chronic renal failure the kidney fails to produce a metabolite of vitamin D, which effectively reduces parathormone activity, lowering serum-calcium levels. Amphogel (an aluminum hydroxide preparation) is given to bind the phosphate excreted in the *bowel* (**Answer 1**). Dialysis is used to decrease the serum-creatinine level, which causes central nervous system *depression* (**Answer 2**), not joint pain. Joint pain is usually related to inflammation or trauma rather than decreased activity level. Increasing activity (**Answer 3**) might *aggravate* the pain.

Test-taking tip—Look for a *known* cause of joint pain in answers—increased uric acid, as with gout.

AN, 4, PhI, Basic Care and Comfort

167. (3) Respiratory depression is a cardinal sign of magnesium toxicity. **Answer 1** is incorrect because individual variations in respiratory depression are observed at the same serum-magnesium level. **Answer 2** is incorrect because respiratory compromise normally *precedes* depressed cardiac function and is a *late* sign of magnesium toxicity. **Answer 4** is incorrect because, although decreased peristalsis can occur with a magnesium infusion, it is *not the most important* assessment to make.

> **Test-taking tip**—Assess respirations first, before cardiac status, because respirations are *earlier* signs of toxicity.

AS, 1, PhI, Pharmacological and Parenteral Therapies

168. (2) Pyridoxine (vitamin B$_6$) 25–50 mg a day is ordered prophylactically to prevent symptoms of peripheral neuritis. Serious side effects of INH therapy are rare. **Answers 1, 3, and 4** have no effect on peripheral neuritis.

> **Test-taking tip**—Know the effects of vitamin supplements on the body (C is used to increase healing, prevent infections, and help other substances achieve their goals; E protects red blood cells from hemolysis; B$_{12}$ is essential for red blood cell formation; and B$_6$ is used to prevent peripheral neuritis).

IMP, 4, PhI, Pharmacological and Parenteral Therapies

169. (1) Urinary retention following spinal anesthesia is due to blockage of autonomic nervous system fibers, which innervate the bladder and sensory perception. **Answer 2,** though correct, is not as complete as **Answer 1.** All patients secrete ADH postoperatively because of the surgical insult. However, ADH reduces the volume of urine (**Answer 3**), as does lowered blood pressure (**Answer 4**), but neither causes urinary retention.

> **Test-taking tip**—Think of the action of spinal anesthesia. The medication used during this type of anesthesia inhibits the conduction of autonomic nervous system impulses and central nervous system impulses. When trying to figure out what happens, try to think of *why* it should happen.

AN, 8, PhI, Physiological Adaptation

170. (1) Sitting for long periods of time and wearing constrictive clothing tend to increase pelvic congestion. Daily bowel movements (**Answer 2**) are not necessary as long as a normal pattern is achieved. It is important to reinforce the physician's instructions that sexual activity *may be resumed* within a specific period of time, usually 6–8 weeks. Six months (**Answer 3**) is *too long.* Paced and gradual ambulation aids in increasing venous return and general strength. Complete avoidance of chores for 2 months (**Answer 4**) is *not* necessary. Lifting of heavy objects, however, may injure the incision site and promote bleeding.

> **Test-taking tip**—Look for options that will prevent stasis and pooling of blood to prevent complications. Select the option that is not as restrictive as the other three (i.e., "daily" is not necessary; 6 months is too long; "*all* household chores" is too inclusive). Select the more general answer ("long periods").

IMP, 1, HPM, Prevention and Early Detection

171. (2) Absence of variability (a smooth baseline) is an ominous sign of potential fetal distress. It can result from fetal hypoxia and acidosis and certain drugs that depress the central nervous system. A baseline range of 110–160 bpm is within normal limits (**Answer 1**). Early decelerations (from head compression) are of no clinical significance (**Answer 3**). Mild variable decelerations are usually remedied by changing the woman's position (**Answer 4**).

> **Test-taking tip**—Look at the key words: "baseline," "absence," "early," "mild." An intervention goes with "absence." Understand basic electronic fetal monitoring (EFM) patterns. Compare early, late, and variable decelerations.

EV, 6, PhI, Physiological Adaptation

172. (2) Elevation of the foot of the bed enhances venous return and reduces edema by utilizing the force of gravity. Pain is decreased (**Answer 1**) as the edema is reduced. **Answer 3** is incorrect because raising the foot of the bed should not greatly affect arterial blood flow. Reducing edema is what makes the patient more comfortable (**Answer 4**).

> **Test-taking tip**—Visualize the body positions. Would venous stasis be prevented?

IMP, 6, PhI, Reduction of Risk Potential

173. (3) Postoperatively the potential for severe fluid and electrolyte imbalances exists for several reasons: (a) the ileostomy drainage contains large amounts of sodium and water, (b) postsurgical diuresis increases both water and potassium excretion, and (c) nasogastric suction further decreases fluid and electrolytes by preventing their normal reabsorption. **Answers 1, 2, and 4** are also important measures in this patient's postoperative care; however, maintenance of fluid and electrolyte balance is most critical.

> **Test-taking tip**—Look for the *most* life-threatening option (a priority question).

PL, 8, PhI, Physiological Adaptation

174. (3) Crying is an appropriate, expected, and natural response. **Answers 1, 2, and 4** all invade the woman's need for privacy at this time.

> **Test-taking tip**—Choose "allow" rather than "remove" or "ask." Omit the physical aspects of care (vital signs) when a psychosocial response is the priority here because it is a psychological shock.

IMP, 7, PsI, Coping and Adaptation

175. (2) The T-tube is clamped before eating to increase bile flow into the duodenum and assist in the digestion of fats. **Answer 1** is incorrect because the act of eating normally stimulates bile secretion, and clamping of the T-tube will not inhibit its flow except to the dependent drainage bag. **Answer 3** is incorrect because bile does not affect peristalsis, although inadequate bile flow can result in abdominal distention. **Answer 4** is also correct, though it is not the best answer. If the patient is able to tolerate clamping of the T-tube, bile is flowing normally into the duodenum and the duct is patent.

> **Test-taking tip**—It is a test to see if the body is ready for the tube to be removed. Look for a choice that allows bile to do its job.

IMP, 4, PhI, Reduction of Risk Potential

176. (1) Increased serum potassium (hyperkalemia) causes the T waves to lose their normal, rounded configuration and become more pointy or peaked (the difference in shape between a mountain and a mound); therefore **Answer 2** is incorrect. ST segments are not significantly affected by this electrolyte imbalance (**Answers 3 and 4**).

> **Test-taking tip**—Think "mountains" for high K$^+$ and "mounds" for low K$^+$—T-wave changes.

AS, 6, PhI, Reduction of Risk Potential

177. (1) Severe, crampy, intermittent pain accompanies the progressive telescoping of the bowel wall found in intussusception; as this progresses, the stools become bloody and full of mucus ("currant jelly"). An olive-shaped mass in the right upper quadrant and projectile vomiting (**Answer 2**) are found in pyloric stenosis. Obstinate constipation and increasing abdominal girth (**Answer 3**) are found in Hirschsprung's disease. Excess mucus and abdominal distention (**Answer 4**) are found in tracheoesophageal fistula.

> **Test-taking tip**—Know distinguishing classic symptoms between TEF, Hirschsprung's disease, pyloric stenosis, and intussusception.

AS, 8, PhI, Physiological Adaptation

178. (2) Hypotension and shock can occur during or after paracentesis. Fluid from the vascular compartment shifts into the abdomen to replace fluids that are withdrawn. This complication can be minimized if withdrawal of ascitic fluid is limited to 1000 mL or if lost fluid is replaced by administration of salt-poor albumin. To assess for this complication, vital

signs are taken every 15 minutes during the procedure and afterward until stable, then every hour for 4 hours. **Answers 1, 3, and 4** are incorrect amounts.

Test-taking tip—The general rule of thumb is to not remove more than 1000 mL of fluid from anywhere at one time without observation of the patient's vital signs.

AN, 6, PhI, Physiological Adaptation

179. **(2)** After the patient has left for surgery, family members should be told the approximate time the patient will be in surgery and that from there the patient will go to the recovery room until awake and all vital signs are stable. Clarify that delays may occur and that the induction of, as well as the emergence from, anesthesia takes time. **Answers 1 and 3** are incorrect because family members should be allowed to decide whether they will stay or go and come back later. If family members decide to wait, direct them to a waiting area where they can be comfortable. Assure them that you will direct the surgeon to them after the surgery is finished. **Answer 4** is not an initial action. The nurse does answer any questions and concerns the family members may have, being as supportive as possible.

Test-taking tip—Look at the action words carefully: "*tell* him," "*explain* that," "*get* him," or "*encourage* him." Best answer is to *encourage* him.

IMP, 7, PsI, Coping and Adaptation

180. **(1)** Patients should be informed that the cataract glasses will magnify objects; this not only causes distortions in the shape of an object but also may result in color distortions. The spatial changes that result from these lenses may cause the patient to underreach for an object or have difficulty walking and climbing stairs. Peripheral vision is decreased (**Answer 2**), so the patient needs to be taught to turn the head and utilize the central vision provided by the lenses. **Answers 3 and 4** are incorrect because the magnification created by these lenses (up to 35%) is not similar to the size perception before the cataract formed, nor do they cause double vision.

Test-taking tip—Think of the *purpose* of the glasses—magnification.

IMP, 2, SECE, Safety and Infection Control

181. **(3)** An immediate response to the choking sensation is assessment of the surgical site by examining under the dressing. If the area appears edematous, loosen the dressing and have someone remain with the patient. Elevating the head to a high Fowler's position (**Answer 1**), though the preferred position for improving ventilation of the lung, will not reduce upper-airway obstruction. **Answer 2** is inappropriate for this situation and may actually increase the patient's distress. Notify the physician (**Answer 4**), who might order the sutures or clips to be removed, *after* assessing the surgical site.

Test-taking tip—Choose the first step of the nursing process—assess, before implementation.

IMP, 6, PhI, Physiological Adaptation

182. **(2)** This patient's blood gases indicate mild acidosis. pH is still within normal limits. **Answer 1** is incorrect because the remaining functional nephrons and the lungs have been able to compensate for the increase in circulating hydrogen ions. If respiratory alkalosis (**Answer 3**) were the underlying pathology, the pH would demonstrate alkalosis (pH above 7.40). **Answer 4** is incorrect because the patient does have respiratory alkalosis, but it represents respiratory compensation rather than the primary pathologic mechanism.

Test-taking tip—Know the normal values. The pH is normal—only one option says "compensated."

AN, 6, PhI, Reduction of Risk Potential

183. **(1)** The earliest clinical signs of bleeding include restlessness, pallor, tachycardia, and cooling of the skin. These symptoms occur as the result of vasoconstriction (increased sympathetic stimulation) in order to maintain venous return and cardiac output. **Answer 2** represents symptoms of ketoacidosis. When the vasoconstrictive mechanisms discussed above are no longer effective, the blood pressure begins to fall (**Answer 3**). It is essential to identify bleeding early because liver cells are very susceptible to ischemia. **Answer 4** may occur with increases in intracranial pressure.

Test-taking tip—The key word is "earliest." Look for *restlessness.*

AS, 6, PhI, Physiological Adaptation

184. **(3)** The mother *is* communicating her feelings of distress at seeing her physiologically compromised son. **Answer 1** is wrong because interference with the bonding process may affect later parenting. **Answer 2** is wrong because the mother is demonstrating her inability to cope with the situation at present. **Answer 4** is wrong because the family system is unable to meet the neonate's emotional needs at present due to being overwhelmed by their own reactions to the baby.

Test-taking tip—Note key phrase in the stem: "least accurate."

AN, 7, PsI, Coping and Adaptation

185. **(2)** Symptoms of circulatory overload result from varying degrees of cardiac decompensation, with blood backing up into the pulmonary (moist crackles) and systemic circuits (neck vein distention, dependent edema, periorbital edema, and hepatomegaly). Symptoms of circulatory *failure* or hypovolemia include apprehension, soft eyeballs, flattened neck veins, shock, decreased pulse pressure, and poor skin turgor (**Answers 1, 3, and 4**).

Test-taking tip—Because the question is asking for objective data, eliminate subjective information (apprehension). What would you *see* with fluid volume deficit and fluid volume overload? Renal failure means fluids are held in, unable to be excreted.

AS, 6, PhI, Physiological Adaptation

186. **(2)** Given the patient's complaint and evidence of pink drainage, the nurse should suspect dehiscence. Dehiscence is characterized by a gush of pink serous drainage and a parting of the wound edges. Dehiscence generally occurs in the fifth to seventh day following surgery, due to increased intra-abdominal pressures from flatus, coughing, retching, or inadequate tissue support. Late hemorrhage (**Answer 1**) would be accompanied by signs of shock such as decreased blood pressure, rapid pulse, and diaphoresis. Wound infection (**Answer 3**) would be characterized by pain, redness, and fever. Evisceration (**Answer 4**) occurs after dehiscence when loops of intestine escape through the opened incision.

Test-taking tip—Sound out and visualize what the patient said about a "giving" sensation, similar to a "splitting" or "moving away" feeling. Considering that the patient has an abdominal incision, the nurse should be alerted that the problem could be dehiscence (separation of the wound). Evisceration is when the internal contents protrude through the opened wound. Know the risks of abdominal surgery. Dehiscence comes before evisceration, just as a "d" comes before "e" in the alphabet.

AN, 1, PhI, Physiological Adaptation

187. **(3)** It is important for all health team members to be in touch with their feelings about death and dying in order to help the family work through *their* feelings. **Answers 1 and 2** may help the nurse teach the family to express their feelings, but **Answer 3** is still primary. **Answer 4** is inappropriate because suppression may lead to avoidance and to the ineffective resolution of feelings.

Test-taking tip—Ask yourself, Is it knowledge and experience that is primary? Or is it "feelings"? "Feelings" are primary. Then ask, Is it suppression or identification of feelings? Being in touch with your own feelings is a primary nursing concept.

PL, 7, PsI, Coping and Adaptation

188. **(3)** The Sengstaken-Blakemore tube is a triple-lumen tube composed of a catheter that goes to the stomach for suctioning, a lumen that ends in a gastric balloon, and a lumen that ends in an esophageal balloon. The *primary* purpose of this tube is to stop bleeding by applying pressure to the cardiac portion of the stomach and against the esophageal varices. Thus, **Answer 1** is only partially correct. The *secondary* purposes of the tube are (a) to prevent accumulation of blood in the gastrointestinal tract (**Answer 2**), which could precipitate hepatic coma, and (b) to reduce blood transfusion requirements (**Answer 4**).

Test-taking tip—With two good choices, pick the most comprehensive answer that covers them both. (**Answer 1** is correct but not as complete as **Answer 3**.)

PL, 6, PhI, Reduction of Risk Potential

189. **(3)** Once the uterus is removed, the woman is infertile and contraception is *not* necessary. **Answers 1, 2, and 4** *should* be included in the teaching plan. Following a hysterectomy, the vaginal flow is usually brownish in nature and will gradually diminish and cease. If the flow continues and is obviously red in nature, the physician must be notified. These signs could indicate a bleeding vessel. Menses will be absent following removal of the uterus.

Test-taking tip—When a question asks for *inaccurate* information, choose the one that is wrong.

IMP, 5, HPM, Growth and Development

190. **(1)** Following clamping of the T-tube, observe the patient for signs of abdominal distress, pain, nausea, chills, or fever. These symptoms may be due to a localized reaction to the bile, edema, or obstructed flow. Severe abdominal pain may indicate leakage of bile into the peritoneal cavity. Eructation (**Answer 2**) or burping may occur after eating if bile flow was insufficient. Jaundice (**Answer 3**) is a late symptom of biliary obstruction. An increased respiratory rate (**Answer 4**) may occur if the patient has abdominal discomfort, pain, or nausea.

Test-taking tip—Know the purpose of the T-tube—allow for bile to flow into the intestine. Bile in the abdominal cavity causes pain and discomfort.

AS, 3, PhI, Reduction of Risk Potential

191. **(3)** Because tubercle bacilli multiply very slowly, and because antitubercular drugs are bacteriostatic, not bactericidal, the patient must continue therapy for at least 2 years to allow time for the body's defenses to contain the organisms. Six months (**Answer 1**) would be insufficient treatment. Individuals who have been inspected for tuberculosis but who do not have evidence of active disease are treated prophylactically with INH for a 1-year period (**Answer 2**). **Answer 4** is an excessive length of time.

Test-taking tip—The difference between *noninfectious* and *effectively treated* is significant.

IMP, 1, PhI, Pharmacological and Parenteral Therapies

192. **(2)** Space-occupying lesions and pneumonia tend to decrease vital capacity by reducing inspiratory capacity. In order to maintain arterial oxygen levels, the respiratory rate is increased, which results in excess CO_2 excretion by the lungs (respiratory alkalosis). It is important to remember that patients can be hypoxic ($\downarrow PO_2$) but not hypercapnic ($\uparrow CO_2$—respiratory acidosis) because of the facility with which carbon dioxide passes through the respiratory membrane. **Answer 1** is incorrect because the patient's pathology tends to decrease, *not* increase, vital capacity. The total lung capacity (**Answer 3**) is usually increased with the hyperinflation of obstructive airway disease. Even though the patient has an extensive smoking history, neither the health history nor the physical assessment findings indicate hyperinflation (chronic cough, barrel chest). **Answer 4** is partially correct and partially incorrect. With extensive wheezes, the nurse would expect a slight to moderate decrease in the forced expiratory volume in 1 second (FEV_1); however, the respiratory rate and lack of other symptoms (lethargy, easy fatigue) tend to contradict the occurrence of respiratory acidosis.

Test-taking tip—Something is filling the normal capacity (tumor). What effect will signs and symptoms have on acid-base balance? Remember that the patient is getting rid of CO_2 (alkalosis) rather than retaining it (acidosis).

EV, 6, PhI, Physiological Adaptation

193. **(2)** The nurse must meet the parents at their level of readiness while at the same time providing them with enough information to allow them to care adequately for the infant. Sucking needs to be *avoided* in an infant with a cleft palate because of the possibility of aspiration and because the infant will not be allowed to suck postoperatively (**Answer 1**). A special nipple or feeder is helpful, such as Lamb's nipple or Brecht feeder. The infant should be fed in an *upright* position to decrease the likelihood of aspiration (**Answer 3**). The infant needs to be isolated *only* from those individuals with *infectious* diseases such as colds or chickenpox (**Answer 4**). The infant should be treated as normally as possible to stimulate growth and development.

Test-taking tip—Eliminate three of the options (too specific *and* incorrect); instead, select the most *general* response ("difficulty feeding").

IMP, 4, PhI, Reduction of Risk Potential

194. **(2)** Withdrawal of the penis before orgasm is not reliable as a method of birth control because fluid containing semen, stored in the prostate or Cowper's glands, may release viable sperm around or into the vaginal canal before ejaculation. **Answer 1** is incorrect because the rhythm method of birth control requires avoiding intercourse around the time of ovulation (approximately 14 days *before* next menses). **Answer 3** is incorrect because spermicidal jellies are most effective when used in *conjunction* with the barrier diaphragm. **Answer 4** is wrong because long-acting *Progestin implants* provide the most effective modern method of contraception when used appropriately.

Test-taking tip—Three of the answers indicate that the students need further teaching. Choose the one that would indicate that the students understand.

EV, 5, HPM, Growth and Development

195. **(1)** Decreases in body fluids lead to dryness of mucous membranes and softness of eyeballs. Weight loss and decreased urinary output would also be present. **Answer 2** is incorrect because hemoglobin and hematocrit are elevated due to hemoconcentration. **Answer 3** is incorrect because the pulse *elevates* to increase blood flow to vital organs; and crackles and dyspnea (**Answer 4**) would be present in fluid *overload*.

Test-taking tip—Look for data that indicate not enough fluid.

AS, 6, PhI, Physiological Adaptation

196. **(1)** A scaphoid-shaped abdomen suggests a diaphragmatic hernia. The newborn abdomen should have a symmetric, slightly rounded contour. Diaphragmatic hernia is the most urgent of the neonatal emergencies. The abdominal viscera are in the thoracic cavity. If extensive, the viscera in the thoracic cavity during embryonic life prevent the normal development of pulmonary tissue. **Answer 2** is incorrect because a normal newborn abdomen should have a symmetric, slightly rounded contour. Imperforate anus does not manifest with a scaphoid-shaped abdomen (**Answer 3**). **Answer 4** is incorrect because gastroschisis is an abdominal wall defect at the base of the umbilical stalk, and omphalocele is a congenital defect resulting from failure of the abdominal wall or muscles to close and leads to herniation of abdominal contents through the navel.

Test-taking tip—First decision is whether this is normal or *not*. Then recall the assessment findings for diaphragmatic hernia versus imperforate anus versus omphalocele.

AN, 5, PhI, Physiological Adaptation

197. **(1)** Elastic stockings are applied before standing up in order to prevent stagnation of blood in the lower extremities. If the patient has been standing or exercising (**Answer 3**), he or she should sit in a chair, with legs elevated, for at least 15 minutes before applying the stockings. Elastic stockings should be removed *regularly,* both to inspect the skin and to provide skin care (**Answer 2**). The patient should be cautioned not to sit or stand in any one position for a prolonged period of time (**Answer 4**). Stockings should fit properly and be kept wrinkle free because when improperly used they can cause venous stasis, the condition they are designed to prevent.

Test-taking tip—Look for a pattern—in three options the patient is standing. Choose the one that is different.

IMP, 3, PhI, Basic Care and Comfort

198. **(3)** Serum radioimmunoassay (RIA) is accurate within 7 days of conception. This test is specific for HCG, and accuracy is not compromised by confusion with LH levels. **Answer 1** is incorrect because the pregnant uterus is not palpable at or above the pubic symphysis before 12-week gestation. **Answer 2** is incorrect because fetal heart tones are not audible by present methods before 9–12 weeks (Doppler) or 20 weeks (fetoscope). **Answer 4** is wrong because Leopold maneuvers are neither possible nor applicable until much later in pregnancy.

Test-taking tip—Note the *time* element in the stem: 8-week gestation. Three of the options are possible *later* than 8 weeks. Choose the option that is different (does not involve hands-on assessment)—a blood test.

AS, 5, PhI, Reduction of Risk Potential

199. **(4)** Initial intervention when patients are reacting to the loss of a significant body part is to encourage verbalization of their fears and to assist them in identifying how they see the change in their body image as well as how it may affect their relationships. One of the most important factors in the patient's response to mastectomy surgery is the reaction of her husband or the person with whom she is intimately involved. **Answers 1 and 2** tend to cut off communication in this instance. Many partners are very supportive; others are not. It is therefore also important to assist the partners to talk with each other, not just to the nurse, to acknowledge feelings and concerns (**Answer 3**). The patient needs the reassurance of the partner's love and support to work through her own emotional reaction and begin the work of recovery.

Test-taking tip—Focus on the patient, *not* the husband (**3**); focus on feelings, *not* cognitive explanations (**1 and 2**).

IMP, 7, PsI, Psychosocial Adaptation

200. **(2)** Ecchymoses occur in cirrhosis due to decreased synthesis of clotting factors as well as decreased vitamin K storage. Dilation and slow blood flow in veins cause the formation of spider angiomas (particularly on the upper chest), palmar redness, and varicosities (esophageal and rectal are common). Esophageal hemorrhage (**Answer 1**) results in the *vomiting* of bright red blood. Vitamin K is fat soluble, *not* water soluble (**Answer 3**). Venous pressures will increase, *not* decrease (**Answer 4**), due to mechanical obstruction in the liver, which results in increased capillary fragility.

Test-taking tip—Recall the normal physiology of the organ and trace what functions will be interfered with during the disease. Vitamin K and synthesis of clotting factor take place in the normal liver; and in disease, these functions are decreased or absent. Visualize where "ecchymoses" would be seen—on the skin (spider angiomas) due to slow blood flow (↓ vitamin K).

AN, 6, PhI, Physiological Adaptation

Guidelines and Tips for International Nurses and Repeat Test-Takers

Sally L. Lagerquist

This unit addresses the special concerns of candidates who have taken the test more than once, as well as international nurses who are graduates of nursing programs outside of the United States.

Since 1977, the authors of this book have had a long history of highest passing results in helping repeat test-takers and international nurses to pass, because we have developed *an approach that works!* We give you guidelines, strategies, and tips that give *you* the skills and confidence to PASS.

This unit will help put you in the frame of mind of an exam question writer and an entry-level nurse (which is what is tested on the exam), so that logic, practice, and a systematic approach can lead you to the best answer.

Tips for NCLEX-RN Candidates Who Must Repeat the Exam

Purpose of This Section

Repeat test-takers have somewhat different needs, different starting points, and a different time frame from those who are first-time NCLEX-RN candidates: that is, figuring out *why* they did not pass, what the diagnostic profile *means* that they received, and what to do *next*.

Also refer to **Unit 1—Orientation** in **How to Use This Book as a Study Guide: Where to Begin, While Reviewing, After Reviewing; Key Points to Recall; Memorization Strategies;** information about the structure and format of the computer-adaptive NCLEX-RN; and **How to Prepare Physically and Mentally.**

What Is the Difference Between Taking This Exam for the First Time and Repeating It?

You are "ahead of the game"! You have already received feedback about your exam-related strengths and weaknesses. You know what the exam is really like and what areas to emphasize. You also know what study methods did *not* work for you. Look at the experience you had in taking the exam as a "dry-run" for helping you to *pass next time.*

What Are Some Risk Factors for Not Passing the First Time?

1. It can readily be *what* you used to study. Often, it is a matter of *what* review materials you used that were not as helpful as other resources could be. Remember, some study aids are better than others. For next time, get a *fresh* start. Use *different* review materials.
2. Using *too many study aids,* from *too many different resources.* You wind up finding that theory and questions in books contradict each other; and there is no one to "referee" as to which books have the right information when books disagree.
3. Reviewing *only with questions and answers in books* will not help you to systematically cover *all* the theory that you need to review.
4. Reviewing *primarily with computer tests* is too time-consuming. You can cover more questions in less time by using a book. In addition, when you get through the thousands of questions, you still cannot be sure that you have reviewed all that you need to know in each subject area, because the material is fragmented (i.e., it is not by concepts or systems). Also, picture the dimensions of the computer screen—it limits how much can be presented. Compare this with a book that has *detailed* explanations for wrong and correct answers, where so much *more* helpful information can be seen at a glance on each page.
5. Taking the exam when you are *not ready, just because* you set an exam date.
6. Going into the exam with little or no review because of life circumstances (e.g., illness, moving, vacations, marriage, baby, job).

It Is Not a Matter of How Much You Study for the Test, but *How* You Use the Review Material

At this point in your exam prep, do not start with page 1 and go through page 800+. This is usually overwhelming and not confidence building. *You* need a *focused* review, starting with your *weakest* area and leaving what you feel most comfortable with toward the end of your reviewing. Discern if you mostly need a review of theory, test-taking strategies, or both. This will determine where you start.

How Do You Know What You Need to Review?

This is based on knowing what the NCLEX-RN Diagnostic Profile means. Look at the four "General Client Needs" and their 10 subcategories listed in the Diagnostic Profile that came with your NCLEX results. Look at the areas where the **boldface** print states that you need **very large, large,** or **moderate** improvement. This means that these are the areas (#1 through #10) that should be the major focus of your content review to **PASS NEXT TIME** (e.g., *Management of Care, Safety and Infection Control, etc.*).

If the computer stopped when you took only 75–100 questions, this probably means that you have significant deficiencies and gaps in certain areas of *nursing content.*

If the computer stopped when you took more than 100 but less than 200 questions, this usually means that you have *some* identifiable areas where you need to review certain content, as well as to improve your test-taking skills. **Appendix C** will show you where to go in this book to *read* in your areas where **very large, large,** or **moderate** improvement is needed.

If the computer stopped between 200 and 265 (the maximum number) questions, you were close to passing. Your problem area may very well be a difficulty with or an inconsistency in *answering the questions* when more than one answer could be correct. In this case, help is on the way! Go right to the **Sixty Guidelines and Test-taking Tips** section in this unit. These test-taking strategies are designed to help you to pull the question apart to show you:

1. How to choose the best answer when all four options could be right.
2. How to narrow your choices down to two possible answers.
3. How to decide between two options.
4. What to do when you haven't a clue!

You *can learn* our *proven* test-taking techniques for success on NCLEX-RN. By following our guidelines before you repeat the exam, you can get quick feedback on your exam-related problem areas in order to better predict your next NCLEX results *before* you take it (i.e., whether you are at risk for not passing).

What to Do to Pass Next Time

STEP ONE: ASSESS yourself. In this book, take the **Pre Test, Practice Test,** and **Final Test** all at once (a total of 500 questions).

STEP TWO: Score yourself at the end. Determine what percent correct you had in each of these three integrated tests.

STEP THREE: In any of the tests where you got less than 80% correct, tally the **client need subcategories** that your wrong answers represented. Each question is coded by various categories; *you* need to focus primarily on the *last* category (i.e., the 10 subcategories that are written out). The codes are found after the rationale paragraphs for each question in the answer section of each test. For example, if most of the questions that you missed in the **Pre Test, Practice Test,** and **Final Test** were represented by the code *Management of Care,* **Appendix C** will list the pages in this book where this content is covered.

STEP FOUR: Go to **Appendix C** and look up where to find *content* in your most problematic area(s). *Read* these pages carefully.

STEP FIVE: Go to **Appendix E** and look up *where* there are all the *questions* in the book that focus on your *most problematic* area(s). Let's say it is *Management of Care; take* each of those questions that are listed, unit by unit, in your problem area(s). *Score* yourself. Go for 80% correct on these *difficult* questions.

How Will You Know That You Are Well Prepared and Ready to Retake the Exam?

When you are getting 80% correct in all of the 2000 questions in this book and on the accompanying disk, you are ready!

Most of all, you are ready when you change the "tape recorder" in your mind that keeps saying "I have failed" to "I haven't **PASSED** yet"; from "I hope I pass" to **"I WILL PASS!"**

A Guide for Graduates of Nursing Schools Outside the United States

International nurses who are educated outside the United States can use this book to serve their special needs.

1. To check their experiences, skills, and knowledge for *equivalency* to those of nursing candidates from U.S. programs, in terms of their ability to deliver effective and safe health care as determined by U.S. standards of practice.
2. To identify cultural differences in perception of patient needs and nursing responses and actions (see **Unit 3: Management of Care, Legal and Ethical Aspects in Nursing** and **Cultural Diversity**).
3. To obtain state board of nursing addresses, to find out requirements and procedures to apply to take the RN licensure exam in their state (see **Appendix O**).
4. To learn about the structure and format of the exam (see **Unit 1**).
5. To learn how to prepare for the exam (see **Unit 1**).
6. To practice taking tests made up of multiple choice questions (see questions and test-taking tips in **Units 1, 3, 4, 5, 6, 7, 8, 9, 10, 11, 12,** and **13**).
7. To assess the level of language difficulty in reading the exam.
8. To become skilled in test-taking techniques (see following section).

If you are an international nurse and wish to compare your preparation with that of U.S.-educated nurses, you will find that the practice questions with detailed answers with test-taking tips for each question that are included at the end of each major content unit can serve as an effective **self-assessment** guide. If you find that you need further in-depth study after taking the practice tests and reviewing the essential content presented in outline format throughout the book, you may wish to seek assistance from review courses or self-paced review on videocassette or audiocassette tapes. In addition, **Unit 10** may help you review **drugs** used in the United States that may be called by other names outside the United States.

Cultural differences may be one cause of incorrect answers stemming from your different perception of patients' needs or nursing action. In addition, **Unit 3** contains the code of ethics and standards of nursing practice and legal aspects that pertain to nursing *in the United States*. We suggest that the international nurse become familiar with these sections to determine what is *emphasized* in this country. **Appendix B** addresses important client needs.

To assist the nurse in making contact with Boards of Registered Nursing, **Appendix O** contains a directory of addresses to write for information about each state's specific requirements for application to take the RN licensing exam.

The **Orientation** unit (see **Unit 1**) is designed to help the international nurse know **what to expect during the exam**, what the **exam structure and format** will be like, **what content will be covered,** and how it will be **scored.** It will also help him or her learn **how to study** for the test, **how to take a multiple choice test,** and **how to reduce test-taking anxiety.**

If you are concerned about your ability to read and comprehend English as it might be used in the exam, first check yourself by looking at the exam questions in this book. The terms used here are those used in the health care field and are considered to be those a nurse needs to know and use. If the vocabulary is different from yours or is difficult, look at the list of common terms in **Appendix L.** You may also want to consult local colleges for courses in *English as a second language (ESL courses).*

If you are not familiar with or proficient in taking exams with multiple choice questions when more than one answer looks good, the approximately 2000 sample test questions in this book and the accompanying disk will provide you with sufficient practice for taking such a test. The following section on test-taking tips was specifically included to help you choose the best answer by *narrowing* your choices to *increase* your chances of selecting the best answer.

Test-Taking Tips and Guidelines: Sixty Strategies to Use in Answering Questions

If you can systematically eliminate false answers, you can reduce a four-answer question to a two-answer one and thereby make your chances as good as those in the true-false type of question; that is, odds will favor your guessing half of the answers correctly.

We think that the following ⌐ narrow down your choices systema⌐

1. *Always, all, everyone, never, none,* ⌐ clude *global* words such as these sho⌐ tion because they imply that there ar⌐ are very few instances in which a cor⌐ solute. Any suggested answer, such as i⌐

   Nurses should exercise caution in interv⌐ ⌐coholics because:
   1. Alcoholics *always* exaggerate.
   2. Alcoholics are *never* consistent.

   should be looked at with care because any exception will make that a false response. A more reasonable answer to the preceding might be "Alcoholics may not be reliable historians."

2. *Broadest, most comprehensive answers.* Choose the answer that includes all the others, which is referred to here as the *"umbrella effect."* For example, in answering the question:

   A main nursing function in group therapy is to:
   1. Help patients give and receive feedback in the group.
   2. Encourage patients to bring up their concerns.
   3. Facilitate group interaction among the members.
   4. Remind patients to address their comments to the group.

   Number 3 is the best choice because all the other choices fall under it.

3. Test how *reasonable* the answer is by posing a specific situation to yourself. For example, the question might read, "The best approach when interviewing children who have irrational fears is to: (1) Help them analyze why they feel this way." Ask yourself if it is reasonable to use Freudian analysis with 2-year-old children.

4. *Focus on the patient.* Usually the reason for doing something with a patient is *not* to preserve the good reputation of the *doctor, hospital,* or *nurse* or to enforce *rules.* Wrong choices would focus on enlisting the patient's cooperation for the purpose of fulfilling orders or because it is the rule. On seeing a patient out of bed against orders, instead of just saying, "It's against doctor's orders for you to get up," you might better respond by focusing on how the patient is reacting to the restriction on his mobility, by saying, for example, "I can see that you want to get up and that it is upsetting to you to be in bed now. Let me help you get back to bed safely and see what I can do for you."

5. *Eliminate any answer that takes for granted that anyone is unworthy or ignorant.* For example, in the question, "The patient should not be told the full extent of her condition because . . .," a poor response would be, ". . . she would not understand." Choose an answer that focuses on the patient as a worthy human being.

6. When you do *not* know the best answer, and need to guess, *look for the answer that may be different from the others.* For example, if all choices but one are stated in milligrams and the exception reads "1 g," that choice may be a *distractor* or the *best choice.*

7. Read the question carefully to see if a *negative* modifier is used. If the question asks, "Which of the following is least helpful," be sure to gear your thinking accordingly. Emphasize a key word such as *least* as you read the questions.

Guidelines

not look for a pattern in the correct answers. If you have already selected option 3 for several questions in a row, do not be reluctant to choose option 3 again, if you think that it is the correct response.

9. *Look for the choices that you **know are** either correct or may be incorrect.* You can save time and narrow your selection by using this strategy.

10. In eliminating potentially wrong psychosocial answers, remember to look for examples of what has been included in the *nontherapeutic response* list in **Unit 6.**

11. Wrong choices tend to be either *very brief* or *very long and involved.*

12. Better psychosocial nursing responses to select are those responses that (a) focus on *feelings* (unless safety is at stake!): "How did that make you feel?" (b) *reflect* the patient's comments: "You say that made you angry"; (c) communicate *acceptance* of the patient by the nurse rather than criticism or a value judgment; (d) *acknowledge* the patient: "I see that you are wincing"; and (e) stay in the *here-and-now:* "What will help now?" Examples of better choices can be found in the *therapeutic responses* list in **Unit 6.**

13. Look for the *average, acceptable, safe, common, typical,* "*garden variety*" responses, not the "exception to the rule," esoteric, or controversial responses.

14. Eliminate the response that may be the best for a *physician* to make. Look for an *RN role-appropriate psychosocial response;* for example, *psychiatrists* analyze the *past,* and *nurses* in general focus on *present* feelings and situations.

15. *Look for similarities and groupings* in responses and the one-of-a-kind key idea in multiple choice responses.

> Example: *At which activity would it be important to protect the patient who is on phenothiazines from the side effects of this drug?*
> 1. *Sunday church services.*
> 2. *A twilight concert.*
> 3. *A midday movie in the theater.*
> 4. *A luncheon picnic on the hospital grounds.*

Choices 1, 2, and 3 all involve indoor activities. Choice 4 involves outdoor exposure during the height of the sun's rays. Patients need to be protected against photosensitivity and burns when on phenothiazines.

16. Be sure to note whether the question asks for what is the *first* or *initial* response to be made or action to be taken by the nurse. The choices listed may all be correct, but in this situation selecting the response with the *highest priority* is important. If the question asks for an *immediate* action, probably all answers are correct and you need to choose the *priority* answer.

17. When you do not know the specific facts called for in a question, use your *skills of reasoning;* for example, when an answer involves amounts or time (mainly *numbers*) and you do not know the answer and cannot find any basis for reasoning (all else being equal), *avoid the extreme* responses (the highest or lowest numerical values).

18. *Give special attention to questions in which each word counts.* The purpose of this type of question may be not only to test your knowledge but also to see if you can read accurately and find the main point. In such questions, each answer may be a profusion of words, but there may be one or two words that make the critical difference. If the option has several aspects, *all* the parts must be correct for that answer to be correct. If you can eliminate one aspect in an answer, you can eliminate the other options with that aspect.

19. All else being equal, select the response that you best *understand.* Long-winded statements are likely to be included as distractors and may be a lot of words signifying little or nothing, such as "criteria involved in implementing conceptual referents for standardizing protocol." You may want to eliminate *unusual* or *highly technical* language. Relate the situation to something that is *familiar* to you.

20. *Apply skim-reading techniques.* Read the practice questions in this book quickly. Pick out *key* words (write them down, if that is helpful to you). Translate, into *your own* words, the gist of what is asked in the question. You might close your eyes at this point and see if the answer "pops" into mind. *Then,* skim the answer choices, looking for the response that corresponds to what first came into your mind. Key ideas or themes to look for in psychosocial responses have been covered in this section—look for a "feeling" response, acceptance, acknowledgment of the patient, and reflection, for example.

21. Look for the *best* answer; not the right answer; for example, *incorrect* action may be the *best* answer *if* the stem asks for an action that is *not appropriate* (e.g., "Which of the following is an inappropriate action?" can be rephrased to say "Which action is wrong?").

22. To narrow down the choices, first find two *contradictory* options; for example, hypo—hyper, flex—extend, give—withhold, dilate—constrict; then focus on which one may be the correct or best choice.

23. Focus on the *age-appropriate* answer (e.g., "When caring for a *toddler,* with what safety issue should the nurse be concerned?").

24. *Time* sequence points to the best choice; e.g., ask yourself *when* is this taking place (e.g., prenatal or postpartum; preoperative or postoperative; before, during, or after; early or late; immediately?).

25. In medication administration questions, apply the *5 rights:*

> Right Medication, Right Route, Right Patient, Right Dosage, Right Time

26. When more than one answer looks right, choose the *first step* of the nursing process (*assess* before "implement"). Assessment words and phrases indicate priority:

> Ascertain
> Assess
> Check
> Collect
> Detect
> Determine
> Find out
> Identify
> Look
> Monitor
> Observe
> Obtain information
> Recognize

27. Isolate the *verbs* from the rest of the question (e.g., *ask* is better than tell, give, or ignore).
28. Do not overlook the obvious answer: **KIS** (**K**eep **I**t **S**imple); for example, the best answer for what to do when there is a malodor in the room of a patient with a colostomy is to "check the stoma for fecal leakage." If it smells like feces, check for feces.
29. As you read what is given for assessment findings (e.g., signs and symptoms) ask yourself: Is this *OK*? Or is it *not OK*?
30. When two options are correct, choose the one that covers them *both* (i.e., *incorporates* the other, like a telescope).

    Example: *Two hours after a liver biopsy, the nurse finds the patient lying on the left side. What is the best nursing action at this time?*
    1. *Check for bleeding.*
    2. *Turn the patient onto the right side.*

    Both options are correct, but choose option 2 because it incorporates option 1; it is possible to *check for bleeding* while *turning* the patient over onto the right side (where the liver is), to put pressure on the site (as a *preventive* measure when postbiopsy bleeding is possible).
31. Look at *root* words to give you a clue: for example, hemi = one half (hemianopsia = "half without vision"). Break down unfamiliar words in the stem.
32. Remember *Maslow*—"soma before psyche"—physiological needs are *before* psychosocial (i.e., physical needs first). Use Maslow's hierarchy to establish *priorities* when more than one answer looks correct.

    Example: *What is the priority nursing care for a patient after ECT?*
    1. *Reorient to time and place.*
    2. *Put the side rails up.*
    3. *Explain that memory loss is an expected outcome.*

    When all three options are good (as in this case), select the *physical* aspect of care first (option 2) rather than either of the two psychosocial options.
33. Think *safety* as the best choice when more than one answer could be right. Safety is a *priority*. See the preceding example, where putting side rails up is a "safety" action.
34. *Visualize the condition, behavior, situation,* and the options to help you choose the best answer. Form a *mental image* (e.g., what *flexion* looks like versus *extension*); *visualize and sound out the answers* (e.g., to eliminate trite clichés or "authoritarian"-sounding responses such as "That's not allowed here").
35. "Would that you could that the *ideal* be possible." Choose an answer for the "ideal," not real, world. Do not use real world experiences to answer NCLEX questions (i.e., on the exam, answer as if you *have* all the time, all the staff, and all the equipment).
36. When in doubt as to which answer is best, use the *process of elimination* first (e.g., eliminate what you know is incorrect) to narrow your choice to two options. The best choice will provide an answer to what the question is *asking*.

37. Apply the *ABCS* when the question calls for priorities:

    - **Airway**
    - **Breathing**
    - **Circulation**
    - **Safety**

38. An important goal is to *maximize* patient actions. For example, choose options that have indicator words for "encourage":

    Reinforce
    Support
    Facilitate
    Assist
    Help
    Aid
    Foster

39. Try to turn options into *true-or-false responses* if possible in order to narrow down to two possible options; for example, when a question asks about adjusting insulin dosage, ask yourself, "What is true about adjusting the dose?" "Is it true or false that dosage is increased when the patient has an infection?" (True.) "Is it true or false that dosage is decreased when blood glucose level increases?" (False.) If you find no "true" answers, look at the choices for a "maybe" answer.
40. Use *acronyms* and memory aids to help remember theory in selecting an answer (see **Appendix N**).

    SWISS—management of Cushing's:
    - **S**ugar (hyperglycemia)
    - **W**ater (fluid retention)
    - **I**nfection (prone to . . .)
    - **S**odium (retention)
    - **S**ex changes (no menses)

    5 P's of fracture:
    Pain
    Pallor
    Pulselessness
    Paresthesia
    Paralysis

    WOUND healing—affected by:
    - **W**ound dimensions
    - **O**verweight
    - **U**ndiagnosed infections
    - **N**utritional deficiencies
    - **D**iabetes, **D**isabilities (e.g., immunosuppressed)

41. *Reword* the question if the stem says "further teaching is necessary" (e.g., the *best* answer will have an *incorrect* statement).
42. Recognize what is *normal*, for example, the data presented is normal. Or is the sign/symptom presented an "*Oh! Oh!*" (meaning that a problem exists)?
43. Do *not delegate* functions of assessment, evaluation, and nursing judgment to an LVN/LPN or CNA (Certified Nursing Assistant) (e.g., do *not* delegate admitting a patient from the OR to the unit, nor establish a plan of care, nor teach or give telephone advice; do *not* handle invasive lines).

44. *Do delegate* activities to LVN/LPN or CNA for *stable* patients with *predictable* outcomes (e.g., help ambulate a patient who is 2 days postsurgery). *Do delegate* to LVN/LPN or CNA activities that involve *standard*, unchanging procedures (e.g., take vital signs after ambulation, *do* clean catheterizations, simple dressing changes, suction chronic tracheostomies using clean technique).

45. In *positioning* a patient, decide what you are trying to *prevent* (e.g., contractures) or *promote* (e.g., venous return).

46. To help decide in which position to place a patient, form a mental image of each position in the options (e.g., picture supine, high Fowler, semi-Fowler, Sims, prone, Trendelenburg, lithotomy, dorsal recumbent).

47. When none of the options looks good, identify the nursing *concept* implied in the *options* given (e.g., risk factors for infection).

48. When in doubt, reread *answer choices* to obtain clues, rather than rereading the question. When you come across a question that is about unfamiliar nursing content (e.g., paracentesis), ask yourself, "What is the topic of the question?" "What do the *answer choices mean?*" Then reword the question using the clues from the *options*.

> Example: *What is most important for the nurse to ask a patient immediately after a paracentesis?*
> 1. *"Are you in pain?"*
> 2. *"Do you feel dizzy?"*
> 3. *"Does your underwear fit better around the belt line?"*
> 4. *"Do you need to urinate?"*

Based on rereading the options, you can reword the question to, "What is an untoward reaction (complication) after this procedure?" The answer choices relate to *expected* outcomes (1, 3), a question that is not relevant to ask *after* the procedure (4), and a *complication* (2), which is the correct option.

49. Recognize *expected* outcomes of drugs and treatments/procedures.

> Example: *What will indicate improvement in the condition of the patient who has anorexia nervosa?*
> 1. *The patient has gained weight.*
> 2. *The patient weighs herself every day.*
> 3. *The patient eats all the foods served to her.*
> 4. *The patient asks the parents to bring her favorite foods.*

Choose the option that shows progress toward the goal (in this condition, it is weight gain that is expected).

50. When you do *not* know the answer, choose what will cause the *least harm.*

> Example: *The nurse suspects abdominal wound dehiscence when lifting the edges of the patient's dressings. What should the nurse do next?*
> 1. *Tell the patient to remain quiet and not cough.*
> 2. *Offer a warm drink to help relax the patient.*
> 3. *Place the patient with feet elevated.*
> 4. *Change the dressing.*

Option 1 is the best answer, because it will not *add* damage that could happen with changing the position or the dressing.

51. Take care of the *patient first,* not the equipment or the family (unless a family member is the focus of the question).

52. If one option has *generally, usually, tends to* but other options do not have these qualifiers, use the one option that does have the qualifier as the best answer.

53. Look for a *similar* word or phrase used in the question and in one of the options. For example, if the question states that the patient is on an *intermediate*-acting insulin (NPH), and the stem asks for its peak action, look for a *middle* time—between a choice of: 4 hours after the injection, 6–12, 12–14, or 15–18. Choose 6–12 hours (as the midpoint).

54. If two options say the same thing, *neither* can be the answer because both are distractors.

> Example: *What might the nurse expect to see when a patient with cirrhosis is hospitalized with ascites?*
> 1. *Patient is likely to be anorexic.*
> 2. *Patient's intake will be poor, especially if served large portions.*

You can eliminate both of these options because they are saying the same thing in different words: the patient is likely to be uninterested in eating.

55. Don't "pass the buck"—think what is a *nursing action* that an RN can do *before* calling the MD.

> Example: *After surgery, a patient with diabetes complains of nausea, appears lethargic and flushed, with BP 108/78, P 100, R 24 and deep. What is the next action?*
> 1. *Call the MD.*
> 2. *Check the patient's glucose.*
> 3. *Give an antiemetic.*
> 4. *Change the IV infusion rate.*

The nurse should *assess* (option 2) *before* calling the MD (who may *then* order an antiemetic, option 3, and alter the IV infusion rate, option 4).

56. Focus on key words in the *stem* of the question as your clue:

Best
Essential
Highest
Immediate
Least likely
Most
Most appropriate
Most likely
Vital

57. "Action" does not always mean choose an "implementation" type of answer. The question may ask: "What is the best nursing action?" However, the answer may be an "assessment" option.

> Example: *What is the best action for the nurse to take when a mother at the clinic reports that her diabetic child is hyperglycemic in the morning (215 mg/dL), although the child has been well controlled with NPH and regular insulin before breakfast and dinner?*
> 1. *Suggest that the mother give the bedtime snack earlier.*
> 2. *Suggest that the insulin be given later in the evening.*
> 3. *Suggest that they continue with the same regimen.*

4. *Check the blood sugar now, and suggest that the mother check it during the night.*

Choose "check," which is an "assessment" response (option 4), although the question (the stem) is phrased as an implementation ("best action" is an implementation).

58. Remember the *nursing hierarchy.* Go to the next line of *nursing* authority (e.g., staff → charge nurse; LPN/LVN → staff nurse) when the question asks to whom to report a situation; for example, if the question is about an LVN/LPN, the best answer is to report to the staff nurse.

59. When the question includes lab values, ask yourself whether the given value is "Oh! Oh!" (meaning too high or too low); or "Eh" (meaning not a particular problem). For example, a serum K^+ of 8.5 is "Oh! Oh!" (too high).

60. *Prevention* is a key concept (e.g., when the question deals with infection control, and in health teaching).

> Example: *The primary objective in ileostomy teaching with a patient during early postoperative period is to:*
> 1. *Facilitate maintenance of intake and output records.*
> 2. *Control unpleasant odors.*
> 3. *Prevent skin excoriation around the stoma.*
> 4. *Reduce the risk of postoperative wound infection.*

Choose "prevention" (option 3), which in turn may prevent contamination of abdominal incision (option 4). Options 1 and 2 are *secondary* objectives.

Confidence, Performance, Pass!

This **Unit 2** is aimed at helping you to take NCLEX-RN with more and improved test-taking skills.

THINK: ↑ confidence
THINK: ↑ performance
THINK: PASS NCLEX-RN

UNIT **3**

Management of Care—Cultural Diversity, Ethical and Legal Aspects, and Nursing Trends

Sally L. Lagerquist

CULTURAL DIVERSITY IN NURSING PRACTICE

With increasing ethnocultural diversity among health care clients and staff, health care providers must increase their sensitivity to and knowledge of cultural concepts, be aware of both similarities and differences in values and beliefs that exist across cultures, and know how this may affect health care delivery. Important objectives are to increase respect and sensitivity for diversity in order to minimize potential for transgressing cultural norms, and to provide culturally conscious health care and working relationships among clients and staff from dissimilar cultures.

The purpose of this section is to provide a framework/structure for assessing, planning, and implementing culturally conscious interventions.

We have selected 10 essential areas as guidelines for assessing cultural characteristics that have implications for health and health care: **communication, family roles, biocultural ecology, high-risk health behaviors, nutrition, pregnancy and childbearing practices, death rituals, spirituality, health care practices,** and **health care practitioners.**

I. **Communication**
   A. *Language*
      1. What is the usual *volume* and *tone* of speech?
         a. *Guidelines:* use interpreters (to provide meaning behind words) rather than translators (who just restate words); *avoid* use of relatives and children; use interpreters of same age and gender when possible. Select the words you use carefully, avoiding buzz

words and jargon. Speak clearly, pacing yourself to be neither too fast nor too slow. Words that are slurred, have many syllables in them, or are too technical make communication more difficult. Speaking too fast may overload the client and make it difficult for the client to follow. Speaking too slowly may lose the client's attention.
         (1) Select the gestures you use with care, using your nonverbal behavior to underscore your words and your actions. The proper use of gestures can clarify a message, and drawings can sometimes be helpful. Be careful, however; not all gestures mean the same thing in all cultures.
   B. *Cultural communication patterns*
      1. Willingness to share their *thoughts and feelings.*
      2. Use and meaning of *touch* between family, friends, same sex, opposite sex, with healthcare provider.
      3. *Personal space:* meaning of distance and physical proximity.
      4. *Eye contact:* special meaning for staring (rude, "evil eye"); for avoidance of eye contact (e.g., not caring, not listening, not trustworthy); variation of eye contact among family, friends, strangers, and socioeconomic groups.
      5. *Facial* expression: how emotions are shown (or not) in facial expressions; use and meaning of smiles.
      6. *Standing, greeting* strangers: what is acceptable.
   C. *Concept of time:* past, present or future oriented; social time vs. clock time.
   D. *Names:* expected greetings by health-care providers.

Source: © Sally Lagerquist (was in *Addison-Wesley's Nursing Examination Review*, ed. 2, Addison-Wesley, Menlo Park, CA, 1982, p. 693, Unit 7).

II. Family roles

A. *Gender roles:* patriarchal or egalitarian; change in perceived head of household during different life stages; male/female norms (e.g., stoic, modest)

B. *Prescriptive (should do), restrictive (should not do), taboo* behaviors for children and adolescents
1. *Prescriptive:* e.g., "Fat children are healthy."
2. *Restrictive* practices: e.g., silence, not anger, at parents.
3. *Taboo:* e.g., discussion of sexuality.

C. *Family roles and priorities*
1. Family goals and priorities (family needs may have priority over individual health needs).
2. Developmental tasks.
3. Aged: status and role.
4. Extended family (biologic and nonbiologic): role and importance.
5. How social status is gained: through heritage? Educational accomplishments?

D. *Alternative lifestyles*
1. Nontraditional families: single parents, blended families, communal families, same-sex families.

III. Biocultural ecology

A. *Variations in color of skin* and *biologic variations*
1. *Skin color:* special problems/concerns: assessment of jaundice, mongolian spots, and blood/oxygenation levels in dark skin. *Considerations for health care:*
   a. Assessment of anemia: examine oral mucosa and nail bed capillary refill.
   b. Assessment of jaundice (e.g., in Asian people): look at sclera.
   c. Get a baseline of skin color from family.
   d. Use direct sunlight.
   e. Look at areas with least amount of pigmentation.
   f. Rashes: palpate.
   g. Compare skin in corresponding areas.
2. *Biologic* variations in *body, size, shape, and structure:* long bones, width of hips and shoulders, flat nose bridges (relevance for fitting eyeglasses), shorter builds (at variance with normative growth curves); mandibular and palatine dimensions (relevance for fitting dentures); teeth (peg, extra, natal, large size); ears (free, floppy, attached); eyelids (epicanthic folds).
3. *Diseases and health conditions:*
   a. Specific risk factors related to climate, topography (e.g., air pollution, mosquito-infested tropical areas).
   b. *At-risk groups for endemic* diseases (those that occur continuously in a specific ethnic group): e.g., malaria, liver and renal impairment, infectious blindness and scleral infections, otitis media, respiratory diseases (e.g., tuberculosis, coccidiomycosis).
   c. Increased genetic *susceptibility* for diseases and health conditions (e.g., diabetes, dwarfism, muscular dystrophy, cystic fibrosis, myopia, keloid formation, gout, cancer of stomach is more prevalent in blood type O, sickle cell anemia, Tay-Sachs).
4. Variations in *drug metabolism:* e.g., cardiovascular effects of propranolol in Chinese; peripheral neuropathy in Native Americans in isoniazid.
5. Variations in *blood groups,* e.g., Native Americans usually are type O and no type B; Rh negative nonexistent in Eskimos, more often in Whites; twinning (dizygote) is highest among African-Americans.

IV. High-risk behaviors

A. Use of alcohol, tobacco, recreational drugs
B. Level of physical activity; increased calorie consumption
C. Use of safety measures (e.g., seat belts and helmets and safe driving practices)
D. Self-care using folk and magicoreligious practices before seeking professional care

V. Nutrition

See also **Unit 9, Cultural Food Patterns**.

A. *Meaning* of food: symbolic, socialization role; denotes caring and closeness and kinship, and expression of love and anger
B. Common foods and rituals
1. Major ingredients commonly used (high sodium, fat, spices).
2. Preparation practices, e.g., Kosher does not mix meat with dairy (cooking, eating, serving).
3. Afternoon tea (British), morning coffee (American).
4. Fasting (e.g., Muslims, Catholics, Jews).
5. Foods not allowed (e.g., no shell fish or pork in kosher diet).
C. Nutritional deficiencies and food limitations
1. Enzyme deficiencies (e.g., in glucose-6-phosphate dehydrogenase deficiency, fava bean can cause hemolysis and acute anemic crisis).
2. Food intolerances (e.g., lactose deficiency).
3. Significant nutritional deficiencies, such as calcium (Southeast Asian immigrants).
4. Native food limitations that may cause special health difficulties, such as poor intake of lysine and other amino acids (Hindu).
D. Use of food for health promotion, to treat illness, and in disease prevention
1. "Hot and cold" theories.

VI. Pregnancy and childbearing practices

A. *Fertility* and views toward pregnancy, contraception, and abortion
B. *Prescriptive, restrictive, and taboo* practices related to *pregnancy, birthing* practices, and *postpartum period*
1. *Pregnancy:* foods, exercise, intercourse, and avoiding weather-related conditions.

Cultural Diversity

2. *Birthing process:* reactions during labor, presence of men, position for delivery, preferred types of health-care practitioners, place for delivery.
3. *Postpartum* period: bathing, cord care, exercise, foods, role of men.

VII. Death rituals
A. Death rituals and expectations
  1. Cultural expectations of response to death and grief.
  2. Meaning of death, dying, and afterlife.
    a. Euthanasia.
    b. Autopsies.
B. Purpose of death rituals and mourning practices
C. Specific burial practices (e.g., cremation)

VIII. Spirituality
A. Use of prayer, meditation or symbols
B. Meaning of life and individual sources of strength
C. Relationship between spiritual beliefs and health practices

IX. Health care practices
A. *Health-seeking beliefs and behaviors*
  1. Beliefs that influence health-care practices.
    a. Perception of illness (e.g., punishment for sin, work of malevolent persons).
  2. Health promotion and prevention practices.
    a. Acupuncture.
    b. Yin and yang.
      (1) Increased yin results in nervous, digestive disorders.
      (2) Increased yang results in dehydration, fever, irritability.
B. *Responsibility* for health care
  1. Acute care: curative or fatalistic.
  2. Who assumes responsibility for health care?
  3. Role of health insurance.
  4. Use of over-the-counter medications.
C. *Folklore practices*
  1. Combination of folklore, magicoreligious beliefs, and traditional beliefs that influence health-care behaviors.
D. *Barriers to health care* (e.g., language, economics, geography)
E. *Cultural responses to health and illness*
  1. Beliefs and responses *to pain* that influence interventions.
    a. Special meaning of pain.
  2. Beliefs and views about *mental illness/mental health care.*

a. Therapies must include *extended* families as opposed to individuals or nuclear families.
b. Cultural and racial as well as individual components must be considered when assessing precipitating or predisposing causes of illness (e.g., need to atone for sins).
c. Values may conflict: for example, individualism versus concern for family or social interactions; self-actualization versus survival needs.
d. Some ethnic groups *do not value or possess* qualities required for some psychiatric therapies, such as verbal skills, introspection, ability to delay gratification, ability to discuss personal problems with strangers.
e. Therapy resources *may not be accessible or considered useful or relevant* for members of some ethnic groups.
f. Common feelings and behavior patterns may be shared by many "minority" groups:
  (1) Feelings of *inferiority and inadequacy,* often a result of prejudice and racism.
  (2) *Incompetent* behavior as an outcome of feeling inferior and inadequate.
  (3) *Suppressed anger,* resulting in displaced hostility and paranoid ideas.
  (4) *Withholding and withdrawal;* not comfortable with sharing feelings or experiences.
  (5) *Selective inattention;* may block out or deny frustration or insults.
  (6) *Overcompensation* in some areas to make up for denied opportunities in other areas.
  3. Different perception of *mentally and physically* handicapped.
  4. Beliefs and practices related to *chronic* illness and *rehabilitation.*
  5. Cultural perceptions of the *sick role.*
F. *Acceptance of blood transfusions and organ donation*

X. Health care practitioners
A. Traditional vs. biomedical care
  1. Does the *age* of practitioner matter?
  2. Does the *gender* of practitioner matter?
B. Status of health-care provider
  1. How different members of health-care practice see each other.

RELIGIOUS AND SPIRITUAL INFLUENCES ON HEALTH

Religious and spiritual beliefs can have a major impact on health and illness. Each religion has its own rituals and traditions that must be observed, with the belief that if these are not followed, the outcomes may negatively affect the patient's well-being or their family.

I. Definition:
  A. *Religion*—an organized belief system in God or supernatural, using prayer, meditation, or symbols
  B. *Spirituality*—encompasses more than religious beliefs; includes values, meaning, and purpose in life; can provide inspiration and sustain a person or group during crisis
  C. *Values clarification*—aligns values and beliefs so that they are consistent with goals

◆ **II. Assessment** *of religious and spiritual beliefs*
  A. Beliefs about birth and what follows death
  B. Code of ethics about right and wrong
  C. View of health, causes of illness, or what may be the cure for the problem
  D. Dietary laws
  E. Relationship of mind, body, and spirit
  F. Importance of work and money as they relate to religion
  G. Pain: purpose of, response to, treatment for
  H. Importance of family
  I. Meaning of life, individual sources of hope and strength
  J. Religious practices that conflict with health practices and use of health services

◆ **III. Analysis/nursing diagnosis**
  A. *Risk for spiritual distress* related to prolonged pain; health-care choices that are in conflict with religious practices; anxiety and guilt due to violating religious beliefs; lashing out against the religion

◆ **IV. Nursing care plan/implementation**
  A. Acknowledge patient's beliefs
    1. Provide contact with clergy of choice.
    2. Provide opportunity to carry out practices not detrimental to patient's health.
  B. Do *not* impose beliefs and values of health-care system

◆ **V. Evaluation/outcome criteria**
  A. Increased satisfaction related to medical care decision
  B. Decrease in feelings of stress, guilt, depression, anger

Cultural Diversity

NURSING ETHICS

Nursing ethics involves rules and principles to guide right conduct in terms of moral duties and obligations to protect the rights of human beings. In nursing, ethical codes provide professional standards and formal guidelines for nursing activities to protect both the nurse and the patient.

I. **Code of ethics**—serves as a frame of reference when judging priorities or possible courses of action. *Purposes:*
   A. To provide a basis for regulating relationships between nurse, patient, co-workers, society, and profession.
   B. To provide a standard for excluding unscrupulous nursing practitioners and for defending nurses unjustly accused.
   C. To serve as a basis for nursing curricula.
   D. To orient new nurses and the public to ethical professional conduct.

II. **ANA Code of Ethics for Nurses** incorporates the following key elements of what the nurse needs to do*:
   A. Demonstrate respect for *human dignity* and *uniqueness* of individual regardless of health problem or socioeconomic level
   B. Maintain patient's *right to privacy* and *confidentiality*
   C. Protect the patient from *incompetent, unethical,* or *illegal* behavior of others
   D. Accept *responsibility* for informed individual nursing judgment and behavior
   E. Maintain *competence* through ongoing professional development and *consultation*
   F. Maintain responsibility when *delegating* nursing care, based on competence/qualification criteria
   G. Work on maintaining/improving standards of care in employment setting
   H. Protect consumer from misinformation/misrepresentation

III. **Bioethics**—a philosophical field that applies ethical reasoning process for achieving clear and convincing reasons to issues and dilemmas (conflicts between two obligations) in health care.†
   A. Purpose of applying ethical reflection to nursing concerns:
      1. Improve quality of professional nursing decisions.
      2. Increase sensitivity to others.
      3. Offer a sense of moral clarity and enlightenment.

   B. Framework for analyzing an ethical issue:
      1. Who are the relevant participants in the situation?
      2. What is the required action?
      3. What are the probable and possible benefits and consequences of the action?
      4. What is the range of alternative actions or choices?
      5. What is the intent or purpose of the action?
      6. What is the context of the action?
   C. Principles of bioethics:
      1. *Autonomy*—the right to make one's own decisions.
      2. *Nonmalfeasance*—the intention to do no wrong.
      3. *Beneficence*—the principle of attempting to do things that benefit others.
      4. *Justice*—the distribution, as fairly as possible, of benefits, resources, and burdens.
      5. *Veracity*—the intention to tell the truth.
      6. *Confidentiality*—the social contract guaranteeing another's privacy.

IV. **Patient bill of rights†**
   A. Right to appropriate treatment that is most supportive and least restrictive to personal freedom.
   B. Right to individualized treatment plan, subject to review and reassessment.
   C. Right to active participation in treatment, with the risk, side effects, and benefits of all medication and treatment (and alternatives) to be discussed.
   D. Right to give and withhold consent (exceptions: emergencies and when under conservatorship).
      1. *Advance directives:* legal, written, or oral statements made by a mentally competent person about treatment preferences. In the event the person is unable to make these determinations, a designated surrogate decision-maker can do so. Each state has own specific laws with restrictions.
         a. **Living will:** legal document stating person does not wish to have extraordinary lifesaving measures when not able to make decisions about own care.
         b. **Durable power of attorney:** legal document giving designated person authority to make health-care decisions on client's behalf when client is unable to do so.
   E. Right to be free of experimentation unless following recommendations of the National Commission on Protection of Human Subjects (with informed, voluntary, written consent.)
   F. Right to be free of restraints and seclusion except in an emergency.
   G. Right to humane environment with reasonable protection from harm and appropriate privacy.
   H. Right to confidentiality of medical records.
   I. Right of access to personal treatment record.

---

*Source: Adapted from ANA Code for Nurses, Kansas City, MO.
†Source: Adapted from recording at JONA and Nurse Educator's Joint Leadership Conference, 1981, A.J. Davis, "Ethical Dilemmas in Nursing."

J. Right to as much freedom as possible to exercise constitutional rights of association (e.g., use of telephone, personal mail, having visitors) and expression.

K. Right to information about these rights in both written and oral form, presented in an understandable manner at outset and periodically thereafter.

L. Right to assert grievances through a grievance mechanism that includes the power to go to court.

M. Right to obtain advocacy assistance.
   1. *Definition:* an *advocate* is a person who pleads for a cause or who acts on a client's behalf.
   2. *Goals:* help client gain greater self-determination and encourage freedom of choices; increase sensitivity and responsiveness of the health-care, social, political systems to the needs of the client.
   3. *Characteristics:* assertiveness; willingness to speak out for or in support of client; ability to negotiate and obtain resources for positive outcomes; willingness to take risks, and take necessary measures in instances of incompetent, unethical, or illegal practice by others that may jeopardize client's rights.

N. Right to criticize or complain about conditions or services without fear of retaliatory punishment or other reprisals.

O. Right to referral to complement the discharge plan.

V. Conflicts and problems—Ethical dilemmas

A. *Personal values versus professional duty*—nurses have the right to refuse to participate in those areas of nursing practice that are against their personal values, as long as a patient's welfare is not jeopardized. *Example:* therapeutic abortions.

B. *Nurse versus agency*—conflict may arise regarding whether or not to give out needed information to a patient or to follow agency policy, which does not allow it. *Example:* an emotionally upset teenager asks a nurse about how to get an abortion, a discussion that is against agency policy.

C. *Nurse versus colleagues*—conflict may arise when determining whether to ignore or report others' behavior. *Examples:* you see another nurse steal medications; you know that a peer is giving a false reason when requesting time off; or you observe an intoxicated colleague.

D. *Nurse versus patient/family*—conflict may stem from knowledge of confidential information. Should you tell? *Example:* patient or family member relates a vital secret to the nurse.

E. *Conflicting responsibilities*—to whom is the nurse primarily responsible when needs of the agency and the patient differ? *Example:* an MD asks a nurse not to list all supplies used for patient care, because the patient cannot afford to pay the bill.

F. *Ethical dilemmas*—stigma of diagnostic label (e.g., AIDS, schizophrenic, addict); involuntary psychiatric confinement; right to control individual freedom; right to suicide; right to privacy and confidentiality.

VI. Trends in nursing practice

A. Overall characteristics
   1. Some trends are subtle and slow to emerge; others are obvious and quickly emerge.
   2. Trends may conflict; some will prevail, others get modified by social forces.

B. General trends
   1. *Broadened focus of care*—from care of ill to care of sick and healthy, from care of individual to care of family. Focus on prevention of illness, promotion of optimum level of health, holism.
   2. *Increasing scientific base*—in bio-social-physical sciences, not mere reliance on intuition, experience, and observation.
   3. *Increasingly complex technical skills* and use of *technologically advanced equipment,* such as monitors and computers.
   4. *Increased independence* in use of judgment, such as teaching nutrition in pregnancy and providing primary prenatal care.
   5. *New roles,* such as *nurse-clinician,* require advanced skills in a particular area of practice. *Examples:* psychiatric nurse consults with staff about problems; *primary care* nurse takes medical histories and does physical assessment; one nurse coordinates 24-hour care during hospital stay; *independent nurse practitioner* has her or his own office in community where patients come for care; case management.
   6. *Community nursing services* rather than hospital based; needs of the healthy are served as well as those of the ill.
   7. *Development of nursing standards* to reflect specific nursing functions and activities.
      a. Ensure *safe* standard of care to patients and families.
      b. Provide criteria to measure *excellence* and *effectiveness* of care.

C. Trends in care of childbearing family
   1. *Consumerism:*
      a. Consumer push for humanization and individualization of health care during the childbearing cycle to reflect patient's role in decision making, preferences, and cultural diversity.
      b. Emphasis on family-centered care (including father, siblings, grandparents).
      c. Increase in options available for conduct of birth experience and setting for birth: birthing homes, alternative birth center (ABC) in hospitals; birthing chairs; side-

lying position for birth; family-centered cesarean birth; health-care provider (MD, RN, lay midwife); length of postpartum stay.

    d. Increased consumer awareness of legal issues, patient's rights.

    e. Major nursing role: patient advocate.

  2. *Social trends:*

    a. Alternative lifestyles of families—single parenthood, communal living, surrogate motherhood, marriages without children.

    b. Earlier sexual experimentation—availability of assistance to emancipated minors.

    c. Increase in number of older (>38 yr) primiparas.

    d. Legalization of abortion; availability to emancipated minors.

    e. Smaller families.

    f. Rising divorce rates.

  3. *Technologies:*

    a. Development of genetic and bioengineering techniques.

    b. Development of prenatal diagnostic techniques, with options for management of each pregnancy.

    c. In vitro fertilization and embryo transplantation.

D. Trends in community mental health (1960s–1990s)

  1. Shift from institutional to community-based care.

  2. Preventive services.

  3. Consumer participation in planning and delivery of services.

  4. Original 12 essential services (1975) reduced to 5 (indicated by asterisk [*]) (1981).

    *a. 24-hour inpatient care.

    *b. Outpatient care.

    *c. Partial hospitalization (day or night).

    d. Emergency care.

    *e. Consultation and education.

    f. Follow-up care.

    g. Transitional services.

    h. Services for children and adolescents.

    i. Services for elderly.

    *j. Screening services (courts).

    k. Alcohol abuse services.

    l. Drug abuse services.

  5. Protecting human rights of persons in need of mental health care.

  6. Developing an advocacy program for chronically mentally ill.

  7. Improving delivery of services to underserved and high-risk populations (e.g., minorities).

E. ANA Standards of Clinical Nursing Practice*

  1. Use of *nursing process:* assessment, nursing diagnosis, planning, implementation, evaluation, outcome identification.

  2. Performance appraisal review.

  3. Continuing education.

  4. Collegiality; *peer review.*

  5. Ethics.

  6. Interdisciplinary collaboration.

  7. Research.

  8. Resource utilization—utilization of community health systems.

F. *Four levels* of nursing practice

  1. *Promotion of health* to increase level of wellness. *Example:* provide dietary information to reduce risks of coronary artery diseases.

  2. *Prevention of illness or injury. Example:* immunizations.

  3. *Restoration of health. Example:* teach how to change dressing, care for wound.

  4. *Consolation of dying*—assist person to attain peaceful death.

G. *Five components* of nursing care

  1. *Nursing care activities*—assist with basic needs, give medications and treatments; observe response and adaptation to illness and treatments; teach self-care; guide rehabilitation activities for daily living.

  2. *Case management—a process that includes coordination of total patient care*—all health team members should work together toward common goals.

  3. *Continuity of care*—process of ensuring that ongoing physical, medical, and emotional health-care needs are assessed, planned for, and coordinated with all providers, for desired outcomes, without interruption of service when the location of care is transferred.

  4. *Evaluation of care*—flexibility and responsiveness to changing needs: patients' reactions and perceptions of their needs.

  5. *Delegate responsibility and direct nursing care provided by others*—based on particular patient/family needs and on job description, roles, functions, and skills of other nursing personnel: client's condition (stable or medically fragile), *complexity* of required care, *potential risks for harm* to client, degree of needed *problem-solving* expertise, *predictability* of outcome, type and *level of client interaction* required. *Important:* The person who delegated the task has the responsibility and final accountability for effective completion of task.

H. *Three main nursing roles* in relation to care of patients and their families (emphasis of each role varies with the situation, with adaptation of skills and modes of care as necessary)

---

*Source: Adapted from the complete description in American Nurses' Association: *1998 Standards of Clinical Nursing Practice.* American Nurses' Association, Washington, DC, 1998. Reprinted with permission. (Rationale and assessment factors for the Standards of Clinical Nursing Practice are available from the American Nurses' Association.)

1. *Therapeutic role* (instrumental). Function: work toward "cure" in acute setting.
2. *Caring role* (expressive). Function: provide support through human relations, show concern, demonstrate acceptance of differences.
3. *Socializing role.* Function: offer distractions and respite from focus on illness.

VII. Concepts of Management
A. *Definitions*
1. *Case management*—process that involves comprehensive coordination of activities and services provided to the client throughout the continuum of care or episode. *Activities* include case finding, screening, intake, assessment, problem identification, prioritization of client's problems and needs, planning, reassessment, evaluation, documentation, designing and monitoring critical pathways, and identification of variances.
2. *Continuous quality improvement*—process used to make improvements in client care; indicators of excellence are identified and process involves actively including input from and collaboration with the client (whose needs are at the center of the process), the family, and all health-care team members.
3. *Incidents/variance reports*—part of quality improvement, where occurrences take place in a health-care agency that are not typical according to medical orders, may be an accident, or may be a violation of policy and procedures (e.g., wrong medication dose, a client or visitor falls, needle stick by nurse). These are considered unexpected incidents, exceptions that happen during client care.
4. *Quality assurance*—activities that evaluate the quality of care provided to clients to ensure that it meets predetermined standards of excellence.
5. *Resource management*—providing appropriate number and type of resources needed by clients to achieve desired outcomes.
6. *Supervision*—process of guiding, encouraging, and assessing the work of others to whom tasks were delegated.

B. *Management theories*
1. *Microlevel* theories: clarify and predict behavior (e.g., motivation) of the individual, with input on the group/organization (e.g., group dynamics).
2. *Macrolevel* theories: focus on best ways to make changes within an organization, organizing projects, obtaining resources, attaining goals.
3. *Intrapersonal/interpersonal* theories:
   a. *Cognitive:* belief—a person's motivation is based on expectations about what will happen as a result of own behavior; involves goal setting, with regular feedback to increase motivation to achieve.
   b. *Scientific management:* belief—repetition of task will result in expertise.
   c. *Neoclassical management:* based on Maslow (i.e., person continuously strives to meet higher level needs); **ERG** (**E**xistence, **R**elatedness, **G**rowth); job redesign (i.e., ensures that task has validity, significance, autonomy, and feedback).
   d. *Social/reinforcement:* belief—motivation comes from learning from those with whom a person identifies; conditioned by reinforcement.

C. *Management behaviors*
1. *Decision maker*
   a. Initiator of new projects.
   b. Crisis handler (e.g., interpersonal conflicts among staff).
   c. Resource allocator (people, physical, financial).
   d. Negotiator.
2. *Communicator*
   a. Monitor of data collection and processing.
   b. Dissemination of collected information.
   c. Speaker on behalf of agency.
3. *Representative*
   a. Institutional figurehead.
   b. Group leader.
   c. Liaison between agency and community.

VIII. Disaster Planning
A. *Definition:* any man-made (e.g., toxic material spill, riot, explosion, structural collapse) or naturally occurring (e.g., communicable disease epidemic, flood, hurricane, earthquake) event that results in destruction or devastation that causes suffering, creates human needs, and cannot be alleviated without support
B. *Goal:* reduce vulnerability to prevent recurrence
C. *Benefits* of a disaster plan
1. Decrease in costs of damage control.
2. Decreased extent and duration of injury.
3. Decreased loss of life.
4. Increased ability to respond to unforeseen disasters.
D. *Health-care components*
1. Early warning signals, with *realistic* expectations.
2. Brief and succinct assessment of those at risk.
3. Simple, flexible rescue chains that unfold in organized stages/steps.
E. *Nursing responsibilities*
1. *Nurses at the scene:* assisting with rescue, evacuation, and first aid.
2. *Nurses at the hospital:* triaging victims and providing acute care.
3. *Nurses at community shelters or health clinics:* assessing, planning, implementing, and evaluating ongoing health care needs of victims.
F. *Level of prevention*

Disaster Planning

1. *Primary prevention:* prevention of disaster and limiting consequences when cannot be prevented.
   a. *Nursing activities:* identification of factors that pose actual or potential problem.
2. *Secondary prevention:* responding to the disaster, halting it, and resolving problems caused by it.
   a. *Nursing activities:* assessment of extent of injuries; tagging victims for treatments and evaluation; providing first aid; identi-fying complications; coordinating activities of shelter workers.
3. *Tertiary prevention:* recovery and prevention of recurrence.
   a. *Nursing activities:* implementing community's disaster plan; providing continuous assessment, planning, implementation, and evaluation; providing counseling as needed to victims and co-workers; educating the public about disaster preparedness.

NURSING ORGANIZATIONS

I. **International Council of Nurses (ICN)**
   A. *Purpose:* to provide a medium through which national nursing associations can work together and share common interests; formed in 1899
   B. *Functions*
      1. Serves as representatives of and spokespersons for nurses at international level.
      2. Promotes organization of national nurses' associations.
      3. Assists national organizations to develop and improve services for public health practice of nursing and social/economic welfare of nurses.

II. **World Health Organization (WHO)**—special intergovernmental agency of the United Nations, formed in 1948
   A. *Purpose:* to bring all people to the highest possible level of health
   B. *Functions:* provides assistance in the form of education, training, improving health standards, fighting disease, and reducing water pollution in member countries

III. **American Nurses' Association (ANA)**—national professional association in the United States, composed of the nurses' associations of the 50 states, Guam, Virgin Islands, Puerto Rico, and Washington, DC
   A. *Purpose:* to foster high standards of nursing practice and promote the education and welfare of nurses
   B. *Functions:* officially represents professional nurses in the United States and internationally; defines practice of nursing; lobbies and promotes legislation affecting nurses' welfare and practice

IV. **National League for Nursing (NLN)**—composed of both individuals and agencies
   A. *Purpose:* to foster the development and improvement of all nursing services and nursing education
   B. *Functions*
      1. Provides educational workshops.
      2. Assists in recruitment for nursing programs.
      3. Provides testing services for both RN and LPN (LVN) nursing programs.

Nursing Organizations

LEGAL ASPECTS OF NURSING

I. Definition of terms

A. *Common law:* accumulation of law as a result of judicial court decisions.

B. *Civil law* (private law): law that derives from legislative codes and deals with relations between private parties.

C. *Public law:* concerns relationships between an individual and the state. The thrust of public law is to attain what are deemed valid public goals, such as reporting child abuse.

D. *Criminal law:* concerns actions against the safety and welfare of the public, such as robbery. It is part of the public law.

E. *Informed consent:* implies that significant benefits and risks of any procedure, as well as alternative methods of treatment, have been *explained;* person has had *time* to ask questions and have these answered; person has agreed to the treatment *voluntarily* and is legally competent to give consent; and communication is in a *language known to the patient.*

F. *Reasonably prudent nurse:* nurse must react as a reasonably prudent nurse trained in that specialty area would react. For example, if a nurse works with fetal monitors, she must know how to use the monitors, know how to read the strips, and know what actions to take based on the findings.

II. Nursing licensure—mandatory licensure required in order to practice nursing.

A. *Nurse Practice Act:* each state has one to protect nurses' professional capacity to set educational requirements, to distinguish between nursing and medical practice, to define scope of nursing practice, to legally control nursing through licensing, and to define standards of professional nursing.

B. *American Nurses' Association* (1980): "The practice of nursing means the performance for compensation of professional services requiring substantial specialized knowledge of the biological, physical, behavioral, psychological, and sociological sciences and of nursing theory as the basis for assessment, diagnosis, planning, intervention, and evaluation in the promotion and maintenance of health; the casefinding and management of illness, injury, or infirmity; the restoration of optimum function; or the achievement of a dignified death. Nursing practice includes but is not limited to administration, teaching, counseling, supervision, delegation, and evaluation of practice and execution of the medical regimen, including the administration of medications and treatments prescribed by any person authorized by state law to prescribe. Each registered nurse is directly accountable and responsible to the consumer for the quality of nursing care rendered" (American Nurses' Association: *The Nursing Practice Act; Suggested State Legislation.* American Nurses' Association, Kansas City, MO, 1980, p 6. Reprinted with permission).

C. *Revoking a license:* Board of Examiners in each state in the United States and each province in Canada has the power to revoke licenses for just cause, such as incompetence in nursing practice, conviction of crime, drug addiction, obtaining license through fraud, or hiding criminal history (see pp. 65–66, section **X A, B, C**).

III. Crimes and torts

A. *Crime:* an act committed in violation of societal law and punishable by fine or imprisonment. A crime does not have to be intended (as in giving a patient an accidental overdose that proves to be lethal).

1. *Felonies:* crimes of a serious nature (such as murder) punishable by imprisonment of longer than 6 months.

2. *Misdemeanors:* crimes of a less serious nature (such as shoplifting), usually punishable by fines or short prison term or both.

B. *Tort:* a wrong committed by one individual against another or another's property. Fraud, negligence, and malpractice are torts (such as losing a patient's hearing aid or bathing the patient in water that burns her or him).

1. *Fraud:* misrepresentation of fact with intentions for it to be acted on by another person (such as falsifying college transcripts when applying for a graduate nursing program).

2. *Negligence:* "Omission to do something that a reasonable person, guided by those *ordinary* considerations which ordinarily regulate human affairs would *do,* or doing something which a reasonable and prudent person would *not* do" (Creighton H: *Law Every Nurse Should Know.* Saunders, Philadelphia, 1986). Types of negligent acts related to:

   a. Sponge counts: incorrect counts or failure to count.

   b. Burns: heating pads, solutions, steam vaporizers.

   c. Falls: side rails left down, baby left unattended.

   d. Failure to observe and take appropriate action—forgetting to take vital signs and check dressing in a newly postoperative patient.

   e. Wrong medicine, wrong dose and concentration, wrong route, wrong patient.

   f. Mistaken identity—wrong patient for surgery.

   g. Failure to communicate—ignore, forget, fail to report complaints of patient or family.

h. Loss of or damage to patient's property—dentures, jewelry, money.

3. *Malpractice:* part of the law of negligence as applied to the *professional* person; any professional misconduct, unreasonable lack of skill, or lack of fidelity in professional duties, such as accidentally giving wrong medication or forgetting to give correct medication or instilling wrong strength of eyedrops into the patient's eyes. Proof of intent to do harm is not required in acts of commission or omission.

IV. **Invasion of privacy**—compromising a person's right to withhold self and own life from public scrutiny. *Implications for nursing*—avoid unnecessary discussion of patient's medical condition; patient has a right to refuse to participate in clinical teaching; obtain consent before teaching conference.

V. **Libel and slander**—wrongful action of communication that damages person's reputation by print, writing, or pictures (libel), or by spoken word using false words (slander). *Implications for nursing*—make comments about patient only to another health team member caring for that patient.

VI. **Privileged communications**—information relating to condition and treatment of patient requires confidentiality and protection against invasion of privacy. This applies only to court proceedings. Selected person does not have to reveal in court a patient's communication to him or her. The purpose of privileged communication is to encourage the patient to communicate honestly with the treating practitioner. It is the patient's privilege at any time to permit the professional to release information.

Therefore, if the patient asks the nurse to testify, the nurse must truthfully give all information. However, if the nurse is a witness against the patient, without the patient's permission to release information, the nurse must keep the information confidential by invoking the privileged communication rule if the state law recognizes it and if it applies to the nurse.

VII. **Assault and battery**—violating a person's right to refuse physical contact with another.
   A. Definitions
      1. *Assault*—the attempt to touch another or the threat to do so and person fears and believes harm will result.
      2. *Battery*—physical harm through willful touching of person or clothing, without consent.
   B. Implications for nursing—need to obtain consent to treat, with special provisions when patients are underage, unconscious, or mentally ill.

VIII. **Good Samaritan Act**—protects health practitioners against malpractice claims resulting from assistance provided at scene of an emergency (unless there was willful wrongdoing) as long as the level of care provided is the same as any other reasonably prudent person would give under similar circumstances. Also see section VI on p. 65.

IX. **Nurses' responsibilities to the law**
   A. A nurse is liable for nursing acts, even if directed to do something by an MD.
   B. A nurse is not responsible for the negligence of the employer (hospital).
   C. A nurse is responsible for refusing to carry out an order for an activity believed to be injurious to the patient.
   D. A nurse cannot legally diagnose illness or prescribe treatment for a patient. (This is the MD's responsibility.)
   E. A nurse is legally responsible when participating in a criminal act (such as assisting with criminal abortions or taking medications from patient's supply for own use).
   F. A nurse should reveal patient's confidential information only to appropriate health care team members.
   G. A nurse is responsible for explaining nursing activities but not for commenting on medical activities in a way that may distress the patient or the MD.
   H. A nurse is responsible for recognizing and protecting the rights of patients to refuse treatment or medication, and for reporting their concerns and refusals to the MD or appropriate agency people.
   I. A nurse must respect the dignity of each patient and family.

X. **Organ donation**
   A. Legal aspects to protect potential donors and to expedite acquisition
      1. Prohibits selling of organs (National Organ Transplant Act).
      2. Guidelines regarding who can donate, how donations are to be made, and who can receive donated organs (Uniform Anatomical Gift Act).
      3. Legal definition of brain death (Uniform Determination Death Act): *absence of breathing movement, cranial nerve reflex, response to any level of painful stimuli, and cerebral blood flow; and flat EEG.*
   B. Donor criteria
      1. Contraindications for being organ donor: *HIV-positive* status and *metastatic cancer.*
      2. Prospective donors of both organs and tissues: those with no neurological functions, but have cardiopulmonary functions.
      3. Prospective donors of only tissues: those with no cardiopulmonary function (e.g., can donate corneas, eyes, saphenous veins, cartilage, bones, skin, heart valves).

C. Management of donor
> 1. Maintain body temperature at greater than 96.8°F with room temperature at 70°–80°F, warming blankets, warmer for intravenous fluids.
> 2. Maintain greater than 100% PaO_2 and suction/turn and use positive end-expiratory pressure (PEEP) to prevent *hypoxemia* caused by airway obstruction, pulmonary edema.
> 3. Maintain central venous pressure at 8 to 10 mm Hg and systolic blood pressure at greater than 90 mm Hg to prevent *hypotension* caused by complete dilation of systemic vasculature due to destruction of brain's vasomotor center, cessation of antidiuretic hormone production, and decreased cardiac output. Give fluid bolus and vasopressors, and monitor sodium levels.
> 4. Maintain fluid and electrolyte balance due to volume depletion. Monitor for hyponatremia, hyperkalemia and hypokalemia, and intake and output.
>   5. Prevent infections due to invasive procedures (e.g., tubes, catheters) by using *aseptic* technique.

Questions Most Frequently Asked by Nurses About Nursing and the Law

I. Taking orders
A. *Should I accept verbal phone orders from an MD?* Generally, no. Specifically, follow your hospital's by-laws, regulations, and policies regarding this. Failure to follow the hospital's rules could be considered negligence.
B. *Should I follow an MD's orders if (a) I know it is wrong, or (b) I disagree with his or her judgment?* Regarding (a)—no, if you think a reasonable, prudent nurse would not follow it; but first inform the MD and record your decision. Report it to your supervisor. Regarding (b)—yes, because the law does not allow you to substitute your nursing judgment for a doctor's medical judgment. Do record that you questioned the order and that the doctor confirmed it before you carried it out.
C. *What can I do if the MD delegates a task to me for which I am not prepared?* Inform the MD of your lack of education and experience in performing the task. Refuse to do it. If you inform him or her and still carry out the task, both you and the MD could be considered negligent if the patient is harmed by it. If you do not tell the MD and carry out the task, you are solely liable.

II. Obtaining patient's consent for medical and surgical procedures: *Is a nurse responsible for getting a consent for medical/surgical treatment?* Obtaining consent requires explaining the procedure and risks involved, which is the MD's responsibility. A nurse may accept responsibility for *witnessing* a consent. This carries with it little legal liability other than obtaining the correct signature and describing the patient's condition at time of signing.

III. Patient's records (documentation)
A. *What should be written in the nurse's notes?* All facts and information regarding a person's condition, treatment, care, progress, and response to illness and treatment. Document consent or refusal of treatment. Purpose of record: factual documentation of care given to meet legal standards; used to refute unwarranted claims of negligence or malpractice.
B. *How should data be recorded?* Entries should:
  1. State date and time given.
  2. Be written, signed, and titled by caregiver or supervisor who observed action.
  3. Follow chronological sequence.
  4. Be accurate, factual, objective, complete, precise, and clear.
  5. Be legible; use black pen.
  6. Use universal abbreviations.
  7. Have all spaces filled in on documentation forms; leave no blank spaces.

IV. Confidential information
A. *If called on the witness stand in court, do I have to reveal confidential information?* It depends on your state, because each state has its own laws pertaining to this. Consult a lawyer. Inform the judge and ask for specific directions before relating in court information that was given to you within a confidential, professional relationship.
B. *Am I justified in refusing (on the basis of "invasion of privacy") to give information about the patient to another health agency to which a patient is being transferred?* No. You are responsible for providing continuity of care when the patient is moved from one facility to another. Necessary and adequate information should be transferred between professional health care workers. The patient's consent for this exchange of information should be obtained. Circumstances under which confidential information can be released include:
  1. By authorization and consent of the patient.
  2. By order of the court.
  3. By statutory mandate, as in reporting cases of child abuse or communicable diseases.

V. Liability for mistakes—yours and others.
A. *Is the hospital or the nurse liable for mistakes made by the nurse while following orders?* Both the hospital and the nurse can be sued for dam-

age if a mistake made by the nurse injures the patient. The nurse is responsible for his or her own actions. The hospital would be liable, based on the doctrine of *respondeat superior*.

B. *Who is responsible if a nursing student or another staff nurse makes a mistake? The supervisor? The instructor?* Ordinarily the instructor and/or supervisor would not be responsible unless the court thought the instructor and/or supervisor was negligent in supervising or in assigning a task beyond the capability of the person in question. No one is responsible for another's negligence unless he or she contributed to or participated in that negligence. Each person is personally liable for his or her own negligent actions and failure to act as a reasonably prudent nurse.

C. *Am I responsible for injury to a patient by a staff member who was observed (but not reported) by me to be intoxicated while giving care?* Yes, you may be responsible. You have a duty to take reasonable action to prevent a patient's injury.

VI. Good Samaritan Act: *For what would I be liable if I voluntarily stopped to give care at the scene of an accident?* You would be protected under the Good Samaritan Act and required to live up to reasonable and prudent nursing standards in those specific circumstances. You would not be treated by the law as if you were performing under professional standards of properly sterile conditions, with proper technical equipment. Also see section VIII on p. 63.

VII. Leaving against medical advice (AMA): *Would I or the hospital be liable if a client left "AMA," refusing to sign the appropriate hospital forms?* None of the involved parties would ordinarily be liable in this case as long as (a) the medical risks were explained, recorded, and witnessed, and (b) the patient is a competent adult. The law permits patients to make decisions that may not be in their own best health interest. You cannot interfere with the right and exercise of the decision to accept or reject treatment.

VIII. Restraints: *Can I put restraints on a patient who is combative even if there is no order for this?* Only in an emergency, for a limited time (not longer than 24 hours), for the limited purpose of protecting the patient from injury—*not* for convenience of personnel. Notify attending MD immediately. Consult with another staff member, obtain patient's consent if possible, and get co-worker to witness the record. Check frequently to ensure restraints do not impair circulation, cause pressure sores, or other injury. Remove restraints at the first opportunity, and use them only as a last resort after other reasonable means have not been effective. Restraints of any degree may constitute *false imprisonment*. Freedom from unlawful restraint is a basic human right protected by law. In July 1992 the Food and Drug Ad-

ministration (FDA) issued a warning that use of restraints "no longer represents responsible, primary management of a client's behavioral problem." It is necessary to advise the patient and family of decision to restrain, explain risks and benefits, and obtain informed consent.

In July 1996, the Joint Commission on Accreditation of Healthcare Organizations (JCAHO) recommended standards to minimize injury and complications from the use of restraints:

- Use *alternatives* to physical restraints whenever possible (e.g., offer explanations; ask someone to stay with patient; use clocks, calendars, TV, and radio).
- Use only under supervision of *licensed* healthcare provider.
- Use according to manufacturer's direction to avoid strangulation or circulation impairment.
- Documentation must include time applied and removed; type; medical reason (description of dangerous behavior) and alternatives tried before application of restraints; response.

▶ **A.** *Nursing responsibilities*
1. Provide padding to protect skin, bony prominences, and intravenous lines.
2. Secure restraints to parts of bed or chair that will move with the patient and not constrict movement. *Never* secure restraints to bed rails or mattress.
3. Use knots with hitches for easy removal, as required.
4. Maintain proper body alignment when securing restraints.
5. Remove restraints at least every 2 hours to allow for activities of daily living.

IX. Wills: *What do I do when a patient asks me to be a witness to her or his will?* There is no legal obligation to participate as a witness, but there is a moral and ethical obligation to do so. You should not, however, help draw up a will because this could be considered practicing law without a license. You would be witnessing that (a) the patient is signing the document as her or his last will and testament; (b) at that time, to the best of your knowledge, the patient (testator) was of sound mind, was lucid, and understood what she or he was doing (i.e., she or he must not be under the influence of drugs or alcohol or otherwise unable to know what she or he is doing); and (c) the testator was under no overt coercion, as far as you could tell, but was acting freely, willingly, and under her or his own impetus.

X. Disciplinary action
A. *For what reasons may the RN license be suspended or revoked?*
1. Obtaining license by fraud (omission of information, false information).
2. Negligence and incompetence; assuming duties without adequate preparation.

3. Substance abuse.
4. Conviction of crime (state or federal).
5. Practicing medicine without a license.
6. Practicing nursing without a license (expired, suspended).
7. Allowing unlicensed person to practice nursing or medicine that places the patient at risk.
8. Giving patient care while under the influence of alcohol or other drugs.
9. Habitually using drugs.
10. Discriminatory and prejudicial practices in giving patient care (pertaining to race, skin color, sex, age, or ethnic origin).
11. Falsifying a patient's record; failure to maintain a record for each patient.
12. Breach in patient confidentiality.
13. Physically or verbally abusing a patient.
14. Abandoning a patient.

B. *What could happen to me if I am proven guilty of professional misconduct?*
1. License may be revoked.
2. License may be suspended.
3. Behavior may be censured and reprimanded.
4. You may be placed on probation.

C. *Who has the authority to carry out any of the aforementioned penalties?* The State Board of Registered Nursing that granted your license.

D. *I am the head nurse. One of my nursing aides has a history of failing to appear to work and not giving notice of or reason for absence. How should I handle this?* An employee has the right to know hospital policies, what is expected of an employee, and what will happen if an employee does not meet the expectations stated in his or her job description or in hospital policies and procedures. As a head nurse, you must document behavior factually, clearly, and concisely, as well as any discussion and decision about future course of action. The employee must have the chance to read and sign this documentation. The head nurse then sends a copy to her or his supervisor.

XI. **Floating:** *Is a nurse hired to work in psychiatry obligated to cover in the intensive care unit (ICU) when the latter is understaffed?* The issue is the hiring contract (implied or expressed). The contract is a composite of the mutual understanding by involved parties of rights and responsibilities, any written documents, and hospital policies. If the nurse was hired as a psychiatric nurse, he or she could legally refuse to go to the ICU. If the hospital intends to float personnel, such a policy should be clearly stated during the hiring process. Also at this time the employer should determine the employee's education, skills, and experience. On the other hand, if emergency staffing problems exist, a nurse should go to the ICU regardless of personal preference, but should request ori-

entation and not assume responsibility beyond level of experience or education.

XII. **Dispensing medication:** *Can a nurse legally remove a drug from a pharmacy when the pharmacy is closed (during the night) if the MD insists that the nurse go to the pharmacy to get the specifically prescribed medication immediately?* Within the legal boundaries of the Pharmacy Act, a nurse may remove one dose of a particular drug from the pharmacy for a particular patient during an unanticipated emergency within a limited time and availability of resources. However, the hospital should have a written policy for the nurse to follow and should authorize a specific person to use the services of the pharmacy under certain circumstances.

XIII. **Illegible orders:** *What should I do if I cannot decipher the MD's handwriting when she or he persists in leaving illegible orders?* Talk to the MD regarding the dangers of your giving the wrong amount of the wrong medication via the wrong route at the wrong time. If that does not help, follow appropriate channels. Do not follow an order you cannot read. You will be liable for following orders you thought were written.

XIV. **Heroic measures:** *The wife of a terminally ill patient approaches me with the request that heroic measures not be used on her husband. She has not discussed this with him but knows that he feels the same way. Can I act on this request?* No. The patient is the only one who can legally make the decision as long as he or she is mentally competent.

XV. **Medication:** *An MD orders pain medication prn for a patient. The patient asks for the medication, but when I question her she says the pain "isn't so bad." If in my judgment the patient's pain is not severe, am I legally covered if I give half of the pain medication dosage ordered by the MD?* A nurse cannot substitute his or her judgment for the MD's. If you alter the amount of medication prescribed by the MD without a specific order to do so, you may be liable for practicing medicine without a license.

XVI. **Malfunctioning equipment:** *At the end-of-shift report the nurse going off duty tells me that the tracheal suctioning machine is malfunctioning and describes how she got it to work. Should I plan to use the machine in the evening shift and follow her suggestions about how to make it work?* Do not plan to use equipment that you know is not functioning properly. You could be held liable because you could reasonably foresee that proper functioning of equipment would be needed for your patient. You have been put on notice that there are defects. Report this to the supervisor or person responsible for maintaining equipment in proper working order.

Ethical and Legal Considerations in Intensive Care of the *Acutely Ill* Neonate

I. Responsibilities of the health agency

  A. Provide a neonatal intensive care unit (NICU) or transfer to another hospital.

  B. *Personnel—adequate number trained in neonate diseases, special treatment, and equipment.*

  C. Equipment—adequate supply on hand, functioning properly (especially temperature regulator in incubator, oxygen analyzer, blood-gas machine).

II. Dying infants

  A. Decision regarding resuscitation in cardiac arrest, with brain damage from cerebral anoxia. It is difficult to predict the effect of anoxia in infancy on the child's later life.

  B. Decision to continue supportive measures.

  C. Issue of euthanasia, such as in severe myelomeningocele at birth.

   1. Active euthanasia (giving overdose).

   2. Passive euthanasia (not placing on respirator).

III. Extended role of nurse in NICU—may raise issues of nursing practice versus medical practice, as when a nurse draws blood samples for blood gas determinations without prior order. To be legally covered:

  A. The nurse must be trained to perform specialized functions.

  B. The functions must be written into the nurse's job description.

IV. Issue of negligence—such as cross-contamination in nursery.

V. Issue of malpractice—such as assigning care of critically ill infant on respirator to untrained student or aide.

  A. May be liable for inaccurate bilirubin studies for neonatal jaundice; may be legally responsible if brain damage occurs in absence of accurate laboratory tests.

  B. May be liable for brain damage in infant due to respiratory or cardiac distress. Nurse must make sure that there are frequent blood gas determinations to ensure adequate oxygen to prevent brain damage. Nurse also must make sure that the infant is not receiving too high a concentration of oxygen, which may lead to retrolental fibroplasia.

Legal Aspects of Psychiatric Care

I. Four sets of criteria to determine criminal responsibility at time of alleged offense

  A. *M'Naghten Rule* (1832)—a person is not guilty if:

   1. Person did not know the *nature and quality* of the act.

   2. Person could not distinguish right from wrong—if person did not know what he or she was doing, person did not know it was wrong.

  B. *The Irresistible Impulse Test* (used together with M'Naghten Rule)—person knows right from wrong, but:

   1. Driven by *impulse* to commit criminal acts regardless of consequences.

   2. Lacked premeditation in sudden violent behavior.

  C. *American Law Institute's Model Penal Code (1955) Test*

   1. Not responsible for criminal act if person lacks capacity to "appreciate" the wrongfulness of it or to "conform" conduct to requirements of law.

   2. Excludes "an abnormality manifested only by repeated criminal or antisocial conduct"—namely, psychopathology.

   3. Includes "knowledge" and "control" criteria.

  D. *Durham Test* (Product Rule—1954): accused not criminally responsible if act was a "product of mental disease." Discarded in 1972.

II. Types of admissions

  A. *Voluntary:* person, parent, or legal guardian applies for admission; person agrees to receive treatment and to follow hospital rules; civil rights are retained.

  B. *Involuntary:* process and criteria vary among states (Figure 3–1).

FIGURE 3–1 Typical procedure for involuntary commitment.

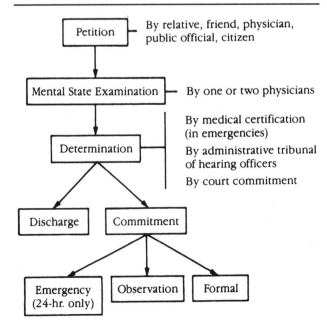

III. **Legal and civil rights of hospitalized patients**—the right to:
  A. Wear own clothes, keep and use personal possessions and reasonable sum of money for small purchases.
  B. Have individual storage space for private use.
  C. See visitors daily.
  D. Have reasonable access to confidential phone conversations.
  E. Receive unopened correspondence and have access to stationery, stamps, and a mailbox.
  F. Refuse: shock treatments, lobotomy.

IV. **Concepts central to community mental health** (Community Mental Health Act, 1980)
  A. *Systems* perspective: scope of care moves beyond the individual to the community, with influences from biological, psychological, and sociocultural forces.
  B. Emphasis on *prevention: primary* (reduce incidents by preventing harmful social conditions); *secondary* (early identification and treatment of disorders to reduce duration); *tertiary* (early rehabilitation to reduce impairment from disorders).
  C. *Interdisciplinary collaboration:* flexible roles based on unique areas of expertise.
  D. *Consumer participation and control.*
  E. *Comprehensive services:* outpatient care, partial hospitalization, 24-hour hospitalization and emergency care; consultation and education; screening services.
  F. *Continuity of care.*

Legal Aspects of Preparing a Patient for Surgery

I. No surgical procedure, however minor, can proceed without the voluntary, informed, and written consent of the patient.
  A. Surgical permits are witnessed by the physician, nurse, or other authorized person.
  B. Surgical permits protect the patient against unsanctioned surgery and also protect the surgeon and hospital staff against claims of unauthorized operations.
  C. *Informed consent* means that the operation has been fully explained to the patient, including possible complications and disfigurements, as well as whether any organ or parts of the body are to be removed.
  D. Adults and emancipated minors may sign their own operative permits if they are mentally competent; permission for surgery of minor children and incompetent or unconscious adults must be obtained from a responsible family member or guardian.

E. The signed operative permit is placed in a prominent place on the patient's chart and accompanies the patient to the operating room.
F. *Legal issues in the emergency room: record keeping* plays an essential role in both the prevention and defense of malpractice suits. Detailed documentation not only provides for continuity of care but also perpetuates evidence that care was appropriately given. Records should:
  1. Be written legibly.
  2. Clearly note events and time of occurrence.
  3. Contain all lab slips and results of other tests.
  4. Describe events and patients objectively.
  5. Clearly note physician's parting instructions to the patient.
  6. Be signed where appropriate, such as with doctor's orders.
  7. Contain descriptions of every event that might lead to a lawsuit, such as fights, injuries, equipment failures.

G. *Consent*—although there is no law requiring written consent before performing medical treatment, all elective procedures can only be performed if the patient has been fully informed and voluntarily consents to the procedure.
  1. If informed consent cannot be obtained because of the patient's condition and immediate treatment is necessary to save life or safeguard health, the emergency rule can be applied. This rule implies consent. However, if time allows, it is advisable to obtain either oral or written informed consent from someone who has authority to act for the patient.
  2. Verbal consents should be recorded in detail, witnessed and signed by *two* individuals.
  3. Written or verbal consent can be given by alert, coherent, or otherwise competent adults, by parents, legal guardian, or person in *loco parentis* (one standing in for the parent with the parent's rights, duties, and responsibilities) of minors or incompetent adults.
  4. If the minor is 14 yr old or older, consent must be acquired from the minor as well as from the parent or legal guardian. *Emancipated minors* can consent for themselves.

Questions

Select the one best answer for each question.

1. A physician orders the elixir form of a medication. The nurse, familiar only with the injectable form of the medication, believes the order is incorrect. The nurse should:
  1. Ask the two physicians who are currently on the unit whether the medication should be given as the nurse understood the order.
  2. Ask the head nurse if the order is correct.
  3. Call the physician who ordered the medication.
  4. Contact the nursing supervisor about the problem.

2. A patient had been receiving a drug by injection over a number of weeks. As the clinical symptoms changed, the physician wrote an order on the patient's order sheet changing the mode of administration from injection to oral. When the nurse on the unit, who had been off duty for several days, was preparing to give the medication by injection, the patient objected and referred the nurse to the physician's new orders. The nurse should:
   1. Go back to the order sheet and check for the order.
   2. Talk with the nurse who had taken care of this particular patient while he or she had been off duty.
   3. Talk with the head nurse about the advisability of using oral rather than injectable medications.
   4. Check the order sheet for the changed order and then speak with the attending physician concerning the changed order.

3. A nurse had been caring for a patient whose vital signs had previously been unstable. The nurse had not had a coffee break or a lunch break all day. By 2 P.M. the patient had been stable for a number of hours. The physician in charge had seen the patient and had told the nurse that the patient appeared "much improved." The nurse should:
   1. Leave for lunch break.
   2. Forego lunch break because of the patient's previous unstable condition.
   3. Arrange to eat lunch in the patient's room.
   4. Discuss the situation with the nurse in charge of the unit and determine who should cover the patient while the staff nurse is at lunch.

4. In a certain hospital, whenever there are patients in the recovery room, two nurses are usually present. The hospital policy expects the nurses to take their breaks before patients arrive from surgery. On this particular day, there are two nurses on duty and two patients in the recovery room who have had minor surgeries performed that morning. One nurse had not had a coffee break that morning. That nurse should:
   1. Stay because hospital policy expects there to be two nurses in attendance while there are patients in the recovery room.
   2. Leave for coffee break because there are only two patients in the recovery room and one nurse can handle two patients quite easily.
   3. Talk with the nursing supervisor and secure permission from him or her.
   4. Leave to get coffee and come right back.

5. While driving down a freeway, a nurse spots an overturned car with the driver lying next to the car. The nurse:
   1. May drive on without stopping, or stop and render emergency first aid, without liability.
   2. May stop, start to render aid, and then leave, without liability.
   3. Must stop at the scene of an accident and render first aid.
   4. May stop and render aid, but if he or she performs a medical act, he or she may be charged with illegal practice of medicine.

6. A patient is terminally ill and has asked the nurse to witness a will. Which statement is true?
   1. The nurse has a legal obligation to act as a witness to a will.
   2. The nurse should help the patient draw up a will.
   3. The nurse should make sure that the patient is of sound mind, is lucid (not under the influence of drugs or alcohol), and understands what he or she is doing.
   4. Only lawyers or family members can act as a witness to a will. If the nurse acts as a witness, the will may automatically be declared invalid.

7. A patient, just returned from the recovery room, complains of pain that is "not too severe" and requests pain medication. The nurse notes that the patient has been given pain medication in the recovery room. Which statement indicates the best action to take?
   1. Administer the dosage the physician had ordered on a prn basis.
   2. Consult the physician and let him or her know that the patient is requesting medication for pain that is "not too severe."
   3. Give half of the pain medication dosage ordered as prn by the physician.
   4. Chart that the patient was complaining of pain but that it was "not too severe."

8. When a nurse is being sued for malpractice, what will occur?
   1. The nurse's license will be revoked or suspended *automatically.*
   2. The nurse will automatically be put on probation until the matter is cleared up.
   3. The nurse will automatically be charged with a crime.
   4. The State Board of Registered Nurses will be notified of the suit, and, depending on the offense and outcome of the suit, it might hold a hearing to determine the status of the license.

9. A nurse's license will be revoked or she or he will be put on probation for which reason?
   1. The nurse lost a malpractice suit.
   2. The nurse was found guilty of practicing while under the influence of drugs or alcohol.
   3. The nurse was accused of negligence.
   4. The nurse gave a wrong medication.

10. A nurse who applies restraints on a patient *may* be held liable by the patient for restraint of freedom of movement (false imprisonment) if the nurse:
   1. Does not immediately obtain an order from the physician.
   2. Does so after other means to subdue the patient have failed.
   3. Tries but fails to obtain the patient's consent.
   4. Applies restraints for the convenience of the personnel.

11. The nurse has been working with a terminally ill male patient for weeks. The patient is lucid. His wife pleads with the nurse not to use heroic measures on her husband but to let him die "with dignity." The nurse should:
   1. Tell the wife that she needs to talk with the attending physician, patient (if possible), and other significant people about her concerns.
   2. Act on the wife's request.
   3. Ignore the wife's request and proceed with the patient's care.
   4. Tell the wife that to do as she requested would be equivalent to murdering the patient.

12. A physician calls the unit, wishing to leave an important order. A new nurse answers the phone so that the senior nurses may continue their conversation. The new nurse does not know the physician nor the patient to whom the order pertains. The nurse should:
   1. Take the telephone order.
   2. Refuse to take the telephone order.
   3. Ask the charge nurse or one of the other senior staff nurses to take the telephone order.
   4. Ask the physician to call back after the nurse has read the hospital policy manual.

13. Which statement concerning consent is *false*?
   1. If an informed consent is not obtained from the patient, the nurse, doctor, and/or hospital may be liable for assault.
   2. One need only obtain a general consent to treatment.
   3. In an emergency a nurse may do what she or he can do to save life and limb, even in cases in which she or he has no consent.
   4. Consent may be given by conduct as well as expressed words.

14. A nurse gave a patient the wrong medication. The patient was seriously injured. The patient sued. Who will most likely be held liable?
    1. The nurse.
    2. No one, because it was just an accident.
    3. The hospital.
    4. The nurse and the hospital.

15. The supervisor of a cardiovascular unit, responsible for checking staffing patterns, assigned a particular staff nurse to work on the unit because that nurse had many years of experience on that unit. That evening, this staff nurse made a treatment error and a patient was injured. Who is liable?
    1. The staff nurse.
    2. The staff nurse and the supervisor.
    3. The staff nurse and the hospital.
    4. The staff nurse, the supervisor, and the hospital.

16. Nurse A noticed that Nurse B was intoxicated while giving care. However, Nurse A did not report this fact to the supervisor. That same day, Nurse B made a medication error and a patient was injured. Who *may* be held responsible?
    1. Nurse B (the one intoxicated).
    2. Nurse A, Nurse B, and the hospital.
    3. Nurse A (the one who did not report Nurse B).
    4. Nurse B (the one intoxicated) and the hospital.

17. A graduate nurse who was new to a unit was caring for an elderly patient. The physician on call ordered a treatment that the nurse had not heard of. The nurse should:
    1. Inform the physician of the nurse's lack of education and experience and refuse to do the treatment without supervision.
    2. Inform the physician of the nurse's lack of education and experience and then proceed to perform the treatment.
    3. Refuse to perform the treatment.
    4. Carry out the treatment to the best of the nurse's ability.

18. Which is *not* true about informed consent?
    1. Obtaining consent is the responsibility of the physician.
    2. A nurse may accept responsibility for witnessing a consent form.
    3. A physician subjects himself or herself to liability if he or she withholds any facts that are necessary to form the basis of an intelligent consent.
    4. If a nurse witnesses a consent for surgery, the nurse is, in effect, indicating that the patient is "informed."

19. The day nurse tells the night nurse that the suction equipment in a patient's room is not working properly. The night nurse, who will be working with this patient, should:
    1. Follow the day nurse's suggestions on how to get the malfunctioning equipment to work.
    2. Continue to use the malfunctioning machine, hoping that it will function for the night shift.
    3. Ask the supervisor how to work with the malfunctioning equipment.
    4. Replace the equipment or report it to whomever is responsible for maintaining equipment in proper working condition.

20. A competent adult patient has refused treatment and wishes to leave AMA (against medical advice). The patient has also refused to sign any of the appropriate AMA forms. Which statement is inaccurate?
    1. The physician and/or hospital is always liable for any injury that might occur as a result of the patient's decision to leave AMA.
    2. The law usually permits competent adult patients to make decisions that may not be in their own best health interest.
    3. Even if the patient is a competent adult, the law may interfere with the patient's decision to refuse medical treatment if the patient has small children that need care.

    4. The physician might be held liable if it can be proved that the patient did not receive sufficient information about risks involved with leaving AMA.

21. The only Spanish-speaking nurse in the emergency department admitted a 6-year-old child. The child's mother explained in Spanish that she had removed two ticks from the child the previous day. The child was now running a very high temperature and had a rash on the abdomen. The nurse reported the information to the emergency department physician, who did not speak Spanish. The nurse failed to tell the doctor about the ticks. The physician diagnosed the child as having measles. Over the course of the day, the child's health deteriorated until the child died. Who is liable?
    1. The nurse.
    2. The nurse and the physician.
    3. The nurse and the hospital.
    4. The physician.

22. A nurse was on weekend call for the operating room. Late Saturday night, the nursing supervisor called the nurse to say that they were expecting an emergency appendectomy within the hour. While gowning the surgeon, the nurse smelled alcohol on the doctor's breath. The nurse mentioned this to the anesthesiologist, who also admitted smelling alcohol on the surgeon. Both the nurse and the anesthesiologist felt the surgeon was somewhat unstable on his feet. However, neither the nurse nor the other doctor said anything. If the patient had been injured during the surgery, who would have been liable?
    1. Nurse, anesthesiologist, surgeon, and hospital.
    2. Nurse and surgeon.
    3. Surgeon and hospital.
    4. Hospital, surgeon, and anesthesiologist.

23. A child about 11 months old was brought by the mother to a hospital for examination, diagnosis, and treatment. The child was seen by a nurse and physician. At the time, the child was suffering from a comminuted spiral fracture of the right tibia and fibula that gave the appearance of having been caused by twisting. The child also had numerous bruises and burns on the body. In addition, there was a nondepressed linear fracture of the skull in the process of healing. When approached, the child demonstrated fear and apprehension. The mother had no explanation for the child's wounds. No further x-rays were taken, and the child was released to the mother without report to concerned agencies. One month later the child was brought in again by the mother and was seen by a different physician. The second physician correctly diagnosed the battered-child syndrome and filed the proper reports. The child was placed in a foster home, and the foster home filed suit. Who may be liable?
    1. First nurse, first doctor, and hospital.
    2. First doctor.
    3. No one.
    4. First nurse.

24. While getting a patient ready for surgery, the nurse removed the patient's dentures. The nurse wrapped the dentures in a towel so as not to break them and left them on the bedside stand. While the nurse was out of the room, two nursing aides stripped the bed and threw all the linen, including the towel, in the laundry hamper. Upon returning from surgery, the patient requested the dentures. However, the nurse and nursing aides were unable to find them. Who is liable?
    1. The nurse.
    2. The nurse and the hospital.
    3. The nurse and nursing aides.
    4. The nurse, nursing aides, and hospital.

25. A teenage girl who had complained of dizziness the previous day wanted to take a shower. The physician gave permission for the patient to shower with assistance. The nurse started to get the girl out of bed and over to the shower. The nurse questioned the patient about her dizziness. The girl replied

that she was not dizzy. The mother then said that she would watch her daughter in the shower and help her back to bed. The nurse then left the room. While the nurse was out, the patient fainted getting back into bed. The patient injured her head. Who is liable?

1. The nurse.
2. The doctor, nurse, and hospital.
3. The nurse and the hospital.
4. No one.

26. What does the Durham Test state about the accused?
    1. The same thing as the M'Naghten Rule.
    2. Accused is not criminally responsible if the act was the product of mental disease.
    3. Accused is not criminally responsible if the act was a result of impulsiveness.
    4. Accused is not criminally responsible if he or she does not appreciate the wrongfulness of the act.

27. What does voluntary admission require of the individual?
    1. The individual must ask to be admitted to a psychiatric hospital and must agree to abide by its rules.
    2. The request for hospitalization must originate with the individual to be admitted.
    3. The individual must make written application to a hospital, agree to treatment, and agree to abide by the rules.
    4. The individual is responsible for the hospital bill.

28. Standards of practice for psychiatric mental health nursing have been developed by:
    1. A joint commission of psychiatric nurses and psychiatrists.
    2. Psychiatric nurses who are members of the American Nurses' Association.
    3. A panel of representative psychiatric nurses in the United States.
    4. The Division on Psychiatric and Mental Health Nursing Practice of the American Nurses' Association.

29. The standards of practice for psychiatric mental health nursing are organized around:
    1. Different models of treatment.
    2. Rights of the clients.
    3. The nursing process.
    4. Legal aspects of treatment.

30. The Community Mental Health Centers Amendments of 1975, Title III of Public Law 94-63:
    1. Cut the flow of funds to community mental health centers and set forth general guidelines for service.
    2. Extended the flow of funds to community mental health centers and set forth specific guidelines for service.
    3. Cut the flow of funds to community mental health centers and set forth specific guidelines for service.
    4. Extended the flow of funds to community mental health centers and set forth general guidelines for service.

31. Congress, in the Mental Health Centers Act of 1974, also stated that it wanted to:
    1. Increase federal operation funds to centers and have centers under federal support.
    2. Provide funding on a declining basis at the federal level and encourage the goal of independence from federal support.
    3. Provide funding on a declining basis at the federal level but maintain federal control.
    4. Get out of the community mental health business.

32. The principal recommendation of the Report of the President's Commission on Mental Health, 1978, was:
    1. The federal government should get out of mental health.
    2. The government should upgrade the old federal grant program for community mental health to encourage the creation of necessary services where they are inadequate and to increase the flexibility of communities planning a comprehensive network of services.
    3. Community mental health programs should strictly adhere to the provision of specific services to all communities.
    4. A new federal grant program should be established for community mental health to encourage the creation of necessary services where they are inadequate and to increase the flexibility of communities planning a comprehensive network of services.

33. For nurses to control their own profession, they must demonstrate:
    1. Expertise in implementing patient care levels already determined by law.
    2. The ability to participate in the drafting of health care laws that directly reflect patient care levels.
    3. The ability to participate in the drafting of laws at all levels and in all areas of health care.
    4. Neutrality by ignoring political power, thus being free from political influence in giving health care.

34. The ICN's Code for Nurses, "Ethical Concepts Applied to Nursing," approved by the Council of Nurse Representatives in 1973, states that:
    1. The professional body of nurses of a particular country carries the responsibility for nursing practice and for maintaining competence.
    2. The hospital employing the nurse carries the responsibility for nursing practice and for maintaining competence.
    3. The laws of the country in which the nurse works carry the responsibility for nursing practice and for maintaining competence.
    4. The individual nurse carries personal responsibility for nursing practice and for maintaining competence by continual learning.

35. The National Health Planning and Resource Development Act of 1974 allows:
    1. Physicians the largest representation on local and state health care boards that make decisions about health care.
    2. Hospital administrators the largest representation on local and state health care boards that make decisions about health care.
    3. The consumer the largest representation on local and state health care boards that make health care decisions.
    4. Health professionals as a group the largest representation on local and state health care boards that make health care decisions.

36. In which situation should the nurse submit a report as a legally mandated reporter?
    1. A pregnant patient states that her boyfriend hit her once when he was drunk.
    2. A patient in the Family Planning Clinic has a positive HIV screening test result.
    3. An elder who is disoriented states that the nurses are yelling at her and calling her names at night.
    4. The neighbors of an elder complain that her son is verbally abusive to her. She denies it.

37. The nurse is reviewing medications on the MD's order sheet and notes a medication with a dose that is two times greater than the customary dose. The nurse should:
    1. Understand that there may be special circumstances in which additional medication is needed and give the medication as ordered.
    2. Ask the patient if the patient has been receiving the dose of medications as ordered.
    3. Check with the nurse from the previous shift to see if the medication was given as ordered.
    4. Discuss the question about the drug with the physician who ordered it and record the results of the discussion.

38. The nurse is supervising the actions of a certified nursing assistant in providing care to three newborns. The nursing assistant erroneously gives a formula feeding to a newborn

who is on water feedings only. The nurse is liable for the mistake of the nursing assistant:
1. Always, because nurses who supervise less-trained individuals are responsible for their mistakes.
2. If the nurse failed to determine whether the nursing assistant was competent to take care of the patient.
3. Only if the nurse agreed that the newborn could be fed formula.
4. Always, as a representative of the institution.

39. The nurse is in charge of the newborn nursery. A postpartum mother notifies the nursery that the wrong baby was brought to her hospital room. The nurse determines that two babies were placed in the wrong cribs. The most appropriate action by the nurse would be to:
1. Record the event in an incident/variance report and notify the nursing supervisor.
2. Reassure both mothers, report to the charge nurse, and do not record.
3. Determine who is responsible for the mistake and terminate his or her employment.
4. Record detailed notes of the event on the mother's medical record.

40. One of the ethical obligations for nursing is accountability. Accountability means that the staff nurse is responsible for:
1. The behavior of patients who are noncompliant.
2. The consequences of his or her actions, even mistakes in judgment.
3. The behavior of other staff members who are negligent in their nursing care.
4. The consequences of an administration decision to decrease nursing staff.

41. The nurse in the labor and delivery unit administered a dose of terbutaline to a patient without checking the patient's pulse. The standard that would be used to determine if the nurse was negligent is:
1. The actions of a reasonably prudent nurse with similar education and experience.
2. The statements in the drug literature about administration of terbutaline.
3. The actions of a clinical nurse specialist who is a recognized expert in the field.
4. The orders of the patient's physician.

42. A nurse is regularly assigned to the newborn nursery. On a particular shift, two of the regularly assigned staff members are on sick time and no new staff is available for assistance. The nurse should:
1. Provide nursing care only to those patients regularly assigned.
2. Prioritize care so that all patients receive reasonably safe care.
3. Refuse the nursing assignment because the increased number of patients makes it unsafe.
4. Take all of the babies out to their mothers to take care of them.

43. The nurse on the labor and delivery unit is assigned to a primigravida in transition complicated by hypertension. A new patient, also in active labor, is admitted to the unit, and the nurse manager informs the nurse that the nurse will be assigned to the new patient as well. The nurse feels that the first patient requires one-to-one care. The nurse should first:
1. Accept the new assignment and provide the best care possible.
2. Accept the new assignment and complete an incident report describing a shortage of nursing staff.
3. Report the incident to the nursing supervisor and request to be floated.
4. Report the nursing assessment of the patient in transitional labor to the nurse manager and discuss misgivings about the new assignment.

44. During a home visit to a new mother with a 1-week-old baby, the nurse observes that the baby appears anxious and distressed and is difficult to console when crying. The fontanels are slightly sunken. The baby has one to two wet diapers per day. The urine is yellow in the diaper. The mother states that the baby has a hard time latching on to the breast nipple but she has not offered supplements because she is determined to breastfeed. The most appropriate case management decision by the nurse would be to:
1. Refer the baby in for a medical evaluation today.
2. Refer the mother to Women, Infants, and Children (WIC) for formula supplements.
3. Refer the mother to Nursing Mother's Council for breastfeeding support.
4. Schedule a repeat home visit in 1 week.

45. The nurse on the postpartum unit is giving medications at 10:00 A.M. The nurse enters the room of a patient, calls the patient by name, checks the name band for accuracy, and administers an oral vitamin. After the patient swallows the pill, she states that another nurse has also given her this same pill 1 hour ago. The nurse checks the medication record and finds that another nurse has signed off the drug entry. The most appropriate action by the nurse is to:
1. Report the first nurse to the nurse manager for not informing the medication nurse that a drug had been given.
2. Submit an incident report describing the circumstances of the medication error.
3. Do nothing because the patient was not harmed by the second vitamin.
4. Notify the patient's physician and ask for advice.

46. What should be included in the nurse's response when the patient asks for factual information about becoming an organ donor?
1. A donor can be any age.
2. Verbal consent would be sufficient.
3. Family members must also give their consent.
4. There are some contraindications for being an organ donor.

47. A terminally ill patient tells the nurse during a home health care visit that he does not want CPR when the time comes. What should be the nurse's next action?
1. Document the request in the health care plan.
2. Talk to the family about this request.
3. Obtain an order from the MD.
4. Share this information with other members of the home health care team.

48. Which is an accurate statement regarding the role of a nurse as a patient advocate?
1. A nurse helps patients gain greater independence and self-determination.
2. A nurse measures the risk and benefits of various health situations while factoring in cost.
3. A nurse has the moral obligation to prevent harm and do good for patients.
4. A nurse may override patients' wishes for their own good.

49. Which assignment would the RN give to a nursing assistant?
1. Assisting a recently admitted post–cerebrovascular accident patient to eat.
2. Admitting a patient to the unit who is being transferred from ICU.
3. Taking vital signs on a postoperative patient whose blood transfusion is about to end.
4. Irrigating a Foley catheter that is not draining well.

50. In providing an orientation for the new graduate nurse on case management, which characteristic should be included in the discussion about what is case management?
1. Main focus is comprehensive coordination of patient care, avoid unnecessary duplication of services, improve resource utilization, and decrease cost.

2. Primary goal is to understand why predicted outcomes have not been met and the correction of identified problems.

3. Main purpose is to identify expected patient, family, and staff performance against the timeline for patients with the same diagnosis.

4. Main objective is a written plan that combines discipline-specific processes used to measure outcomes of care.

51. What level of prevention is the nurse's goal in the community following an earthquake?
    1. Primary level of prevention.
    2. Secondary level of prevention.
    3. Tertiary level of prevention.
    4. Quaternary level of prevention.

52. Which situation would be an example of professional malpractice by a nurse?
    1. An infant is injured as a result of incorrect information provided to the parents by the nurse on the use of a child safety restraint in the car.
    2. The nurse inadvertently throws away the container holding the patient's dentures.
    3. A patient is ambulating in the hall and slips on a recently mopped floor, causing injury to his leg.
    4. A visitor who is sitting by the patient's bed is hit by a falling IV pole while the nurse is changing the IV tubing, and requires stitches for a laceration.

53. The nurse manager has requested a social worker see the following patients. Which one requires assistance first?
    1. A 30-year-old woman who is homeless, newly diagnosed with diabetes.
    2. A 70-year-old man with heart failure and no insurance coverage.
    3. A 55-year-old man, with a history of a recent myocardial infarction, who is in the midst of a divorce.
    4. A 60-year-old woman, post–cerebrovascular accident, who has been living alone.

54. In which one of the following patient situations would it be inappropriate for the RN to delegate the care to the nursing assistant?
    1. A postoperative patient who is stable needs to ambulate.
    2. Routine temperature check that must be done for a patient at end of shift.
    3. A confused elderly woman who needs assistance with eating.
    4. Patient in soft restraints who is very agitated and crying.

55. When checking the IV solution at the beginning of the shift, it was discovered that an incorrect solution was running. After changing the solution to the correct order, an appropriate nursing action would be to:
    1. Report the discovery of the error to the supervisor.
    2. Document the error and correction in the medical record.
    3. Fill out an incident report according to hospital policy.
    4. Assure the patient that the error had no adverse effects.

Answers/Rationale

1. **(3)** The nurse would be negligent for any untoward effects of the drug if she or he failed to contact the physician who

Key to codes following rationales *Nursing process:* **AS,** Assessment; **AN,** Analysis; **PL,** Plan; **IMP,** Implementation; **EV,** Evaluation. *Category of human function:* **1,** Protective; **2,** Sensory-perceptual; **3,** Comfort, Rest, Activity, and Mobility; **4,** Nutrition; **5,** Growth and Development; **6,** Fluid-Gas Transport; **7,** Psychosocial-Cultural; **8,** Elimination. **Client need: SECE;** Safe, Effective Care Environment; **PhI,** Physiological Integrity; **PsI,** Psychosocial Integrity; **HPM,** Health Promotion/ Maintenance. See appendices for full explanation.

ordered the drug before the nurse administered it. In *Norton v. Argonaut Insurance Co.* [144 So. 2nd 249 (La. Ct. App. 1962)], the court stated that it was the responsibility of the nurse to clarify the order with the physician *involved,* not with other nurses (**Answers 2 and 4**). **Answer 1** is incorrect because the doctors on the unit are not the ones who wrote the order.

> **Test-taking tip**—Apply the concept of negligence: omission to do something that a *reasonable* person guided by *ordinary* considerations would *do;* and go directly to the source for clarification.

IMP, 1, SECE, Safety and Infection Control.

2. **(4)** Although **Answer 1** is a correct answer, **Answer 4** is the *best* answer because the nurse would validate the changed order and learn the physician's rationale for the change. In *Larrimore v. Homeopathic Hospital Association* [54 Del. 449, 181 A. 2d 573 (1962)], the court found that the nurse who went ahead and gave the medication was negligent. The courts went on to say that the jury could find the nurse negligent by applying ordinary common sense to establish the applicable standard of care. **Answers 2 and 3** are incorrect because talking with nurses is not the direct way to clarify and validate an order.

> **Test-taking tip**—Eliminate two options related to talking to other nurses. Although the two other choices are good, select the more inclusive option.

IMP, 1, SECE, Safety and Infection Control.

3. **(4)** The nurse would come back to the patient revitalized after having a lunch break, and the patient would be covered the whole time the nurse is away. In deciding that the nurse would not be negligent to leave such a patient, the court would emphasize that the question of liability should be determined in light of the circumstances as they existed at the time. When the nurse left the patient, it was not foreseeable that an increased risk to the patient would result. On the contrary, the patient would be looked after, and the nurse's needs would also be met. *Child v. Vancouver General Hospital* [71 W.W.R. 656 (1979)]. **Answer 1** does not provide for patient's care. **Answers 2 and 3** are not necessary actions, for the patient's condition at the time did not warrant the nurse's foregoing lunch or eating in the patient's room.

> **Test-taking tip**—Patient's condition (stable) allows for continuity of care (by delegation) while the nurse is at lunch. Choose the option that is different (taking a lunch break).

IMP, 7, SECE, Management of Care.

4. **(1)** In a court of law, hospital policy may be used to set the standard of care by which the nurses' actions are judged. Because the hospital policy states that two nurses must be in attendance while patients are in the recovery room, both the nurse who left (**Answers 2 and 4**) and the supervisor who authorized the nurse's absence (**Answer 3**) would be held liable for any untoward effect on the patient. *Laidlaw v. Lions Gate Hospital* [70 W.W.R. 727 (1969)].

> **Test-taking tip**—In following hospital policy, standards of care are met.

IMP, 1, SECE, Management of Care.

5. **(1)** The court has stated that no one is obliged by law to assist a stranger, even if he or she can do so by a word and without the slightest danger to himself or herself. Hence, **Answer 3** is incorrect. But once one has undertaken to give assistance, the law imposes on him or her a duty of care toward the person assisted. Hence **Answer 2** is incorrect. The court also states that under emergency circumstances, a nurse, like any other person, may perform a medical act to preserve life and limb. Either law or custom exempts such actions from coming within the medical practice acts. This, then, would rule out **Answer 4**.

> **Test-taking tip**—Apply the *Good Samaritan Act.*

PL, 7, SECE, Management of Care.

6. **(3)** Anyone can act as a witness. **Answer 1** is incorrect because a nurse has no legal obligation to participate as a witness, only a moral and ethical obligation. **Answer 2** is incorrect because only a lawyer or the patient can draw up a will. If the nurse draws up the will, she or he could be charged with practicing law without a license. If a nurse does act as a witness, he or she should determine that the patient is of sound mind or the will could be declared invalid—not because the nurse acted as a witness (**Answer 4**) but because the patient was not of sound mind.
   Test-taking tip—Eliminate the three *false* statements.
   EV, 7, SECE, Management of Care.

7. **(2)** The physician should be notified of the patient's complaints, and the new orders should be established. This is what the courts would consider prudent under the circumstances and what a reasonable nurse should do. **Answer 1** would not be the best choice because the patient had already been given pain medication in the recovery room, and another full dose might be too much. Without further information, this is a very dangerous choice, and the nurse would be held liable for any untoward effects. **Answer 3** would also be incorrect because a nurse cannot substitute his or her judgment for the physician's without consulting the physician first. If a nurse alters the amount prescribed without an order from the physician, the nurse could be charged with practicing medicine without a license. **Answer 4** is incomplete. A nurse must chart the patient's complaints but must also indicate what was done about them.
   Test-taking tip—Consultation with physician is necessary.
   IMP, 1, PhI, Pharmacological and Parenteral Therapy.

8. **(4)** Only the State Board of Registered Nurses has the authority to revoke or suspend a license. This can occur only after the nurse has been given a fair hearing before an impartial hearing body. Hence, **Answers 1, 2, and 3** are incorrect because they assume a penalty should be applied before the State Board is notified.
   Test-taking tip—For an educated guess, choose the option that is different (three options state "automatically," one does not).
   EV, 7, SECE, Management of Care.

9. **(2)** *All State Practice Acts* list "guilty of practicing while under the influence of drugs or alcohol" as a reason for revocation of a license or for putting a nurse on probation. **Answers 1, 3, and 4** *may* cause revocation of a license; however, *other* circumstances would have to be considered first, such as the frequency with which these had occurred.
   Test-taking tip—Refer to the *State Practice Acts* for reasons for license revocation.
   EV, 7, SECE, Management of Care.

10. **(4)** Freedom from unlawful restraint is a basic human right. Restraints of any type may constitute false imprisonment. False imprisonment is an actionable tort for which a nurse may be held liable by a patient. The patient may have an actionable case of false imprisonment if the restraints were applied for staff convenience only. Most likely the nurse would not be held liable for false imprisonment even if the nurse does not immediately obtain an order from the physician for the restraints. However, **Answer 1** is not the *best* choice. Restraints should be used only in emergency situations, for a limited time, for the limited purpose of protecting the patient, and not for the convenience of the staff. Even though the patient's consent (**Answer 3**) is not usually obtainable under the circumstances, the nurse should try in order to avoid being held liable for false imprisonment. However, these restraints should only be applied as a last resort (**Answer 2**).
   Test-taking tip—Select the option that violates patient's rights.
   EV, 7, SECE, Safety and Infection Control.

11. **(1)** This type of case is an example of the most difficult medical ethical and legal questions today. The answers are ambiguous at best. However, in this case **Answer 1** would be best because neither the nurse (**Answer 3**), the wife (**Answer 2**), nor the doctor can make that decision as long as the patient is a competent adult. **Answer 4** is incorrect because the nurse's values should not supersede the wife's concerns for her husband's welfare.
   Test-taking tip—The best answer includes the patient; the decision is *not* the nurse's to make, and the nurse should not ignore the wife's request.
   IMP, 7, SECE, Management of Care.

12. **(3)** Get a senior nurse who knows the policies, the patient, and the doctor. Generally speaking, a nurse should not accept telephone orders. However, if it is necessary to take one, follow the hospital's policy regarding telephone orders. Failure to follow hospital policy could be considered negligence. In this case, the nurse was new and did not know the hospital's policy concerning telephone orders. The nurse was also unfamiliar with the doctor and the patient. Therefore the nurse should not take the order unless (a) no one else is available and (b) it is an emergency situation. **Answers 1 and 2** are both incomplete, because they do not take into account the mitigating circumstances. The doctor has said that the order is important; therefore the nurse should not delay the doctor while she or he reads the manual. Hence, **Answer 4** is incorrect.
   Test-taking tip—Look for an option calling for supervision of a new nurse.
   IMP, 7, SECE, Management of Care.

13. **(2)** *Assault* is the unjustifiable attempt to touch another person or the threat to do so in such circumstances as to cause the other reasonably to believe that it will be carried out. The lack of informed consent is an important part of the meaning of assault. Consent is a defense to an action for assault. However, if the treatment or procedure goes beyond the patient's consent (as it probably would if consent was only to "general" treatment, as in **Answer 2**), the nurse, the doctor, and/or the hospital may be liable. Hence, **Answer 1** is a *true* statement. In an emergency situation in which the nurse is trying to save the patient's life, if the patient does not or cannot consent to treatment, the nurse usually will not be held to have assaulted the patient. Hence, **Answer 3** is also a *true* statement. Consent may be given by conduct as well as by expressed words, as in **Answer 4**. For example, in a case in which a person held up his arm to be vaccinated, the court said he had consented. However, it is best to get the consent in writing, specifically outlining the treatment or procedure to be performed. The consent will most likely be deemed invalid, however, if the patient is a child, is mentally incompetent, or is intoxicated.
   Test-taking tip—Eliminate the three *true* statements.
   EV, 7, SECE, Management of Care.

14. **(4)** *Both* the nurse and the hospital can be sued for damages if a mistake the nurse makes injures the patient. The nurse is always responsible for his or her own actions. The hospital, as the employer, will be vicariously liable under the *respondeat superior doctrine*—the employer is liable for the negligent conduct of its nurses when the act was committed within the scope of employment. **Answers 1 and 3** are incomplete; **Answer 2** is incorrect.
   Test-taking tip—The best answer is based on the *respondeat superior doctrine*, under which the hospital is also liable.
   EV, 7, SECE, Management of Care.

15. **(3)** The hospital is *always* initially held liable under the theory of *respondeat superior*—vicarious liability of the employer. **Answers 2 and 4** are incorrect because the supervisor would *not* be responsible unless the court thought that the supervisor was negligent in supervising or assigning a task beyond

the capabilities of another. In this case, the staff nurse had had numerous years of experience on the cardiovascular unit. Without further data, the supervisor would not be considered negligent for assigning this nurse to the cardiovascular unit. **Answer 1** is incomplete.

Test-taking tip—The best answer is based on *respondeat superior,* under which the hospital is also liable.

AN, 7, SECE, Management of Care.

16. (2) This answer includes all parties: the hospital, Nurse A, and Nurse B. The hospital, as the employer, might be held liable under the theory of *respondeat superior*—vicarious liability. Nurse B would be held responsible because each nurse is personally liable for his or her own negligent actions. Nurse A might also be held responsible because every nurse is obligated to act so that patients are safe from injury. In this case, Nurse A knew of B's intoxicated state. Nurse A did not act as a *reasonably prudent nurse* in failing to inform a supervisor. **Answers 1, 3,** and **4** are incomplete.

Test-taking tip—The best answer is based on both the doctrine of *respondeat superior* and *reasonably* prudent behavior.

AN, 7, SECE, Management of Care.

17. (1) If the nurse informs the physician and still carries out the treatment (**Answer 2**), both the nurse and the physician could be held liable if the patient is negligently harmed. The nurse would be liable for not acting as a reasonably prudent nurse, and the physician would be liable because he or she knew of the nurse's lack of knowledge and did not step in to protect the patient. If the nurse does not tell the physician and still carries out the treatment (**Answer 4**), the nurse would be solely liable. The nurse should not refuse to perform the treatment (**Answer 3**) unless she or he has no supervision.

Test-taking tip—For an educated guess, first eliminate the two options in which the nurse performs the treatment (**Answers 2 and 4**). Then eliminate **Answer 3** because to refuse without notifying the MD is not enough.

IMP, 7, SECE, Management of Care.

18. (4) The nurse who witnesses a consent for surgery or other procedure is witnessing only that the signature is that of the purported person and that the person's condition is as indicated at the time of signing. The nurse is not witnessing that the patient is "informed." **Answers 1, 2,** and **3** are all true statements.

Test-taking tip—Look for the *false* option; eliminate the three true options that pertain to informed consent.

AN, 7, SECE, Management of Care.

19. (4) As a nurse, you should *not* plan to use equipment that you know is malfunctioning. You could be held liable because you were on notice and could reasonably foresee that properly functioning equipment would be needed by your patient. Hence, **Answers 1, 2,** and **3** are incorrect.

Test-taking tip—Eliminate the three options that involve working *with* malfunctioning equipment.

IMP, 1, SECE, Safety and Infection Control.

20. (1) This is the *only clearly false* option. Neither the physician nor the hospital would ordinarily be liable if (a) the medical risk is explained and a full report concerning the incident is documented and (b) the patient is a competent adult. The court does not usually interfere with one's right to refuse treatment, as in **Answer 2**. However, the court will closely scrutinize a situation in which the patient's refusal to accept treatment results in death or in the patient's inability to care for children. If the children might be left as wards of the court, the court may force the patient to accept treatment, as in **Answer 3**. Hence, **Answers 2, 3,** and **4** do not apply, because they are true.

Test-taking tip—Eliminate the three true/correct options pertaining to AMA.

EV, 7, SECE, Management of Care.

21. (3) The court in *John Ramsey, Jr. et al. v. Physicians Memorial Hospital, Inc. et al.* stated that "evidence supported finding that the failure of nurse to notify physician of client history involving removal of ticks from one of the children constituted a violation of her duties as a nurse, and failure to relate the information to the physician was the contributing proximate cause of death of the child." The hospital is *also* held liable under the doctrine of *respondeat superior* for the negligent conduct of its nurses when committed within the scope of their employment. Hence, **Answer 1** is incomplete because it does not include the hospital. The physician would most likely *not* be held liable because of the language barrier and the nurse's clear failure to communicate. Hence, **Answers 2 and 4** are incorrect.

Test-taking tip—Choose the option that involves the hospital under *respondeat superior doctrine.*

EV, 1, SECE, Management of Care.

22. (1) Both nurses and doctors are under a duty to protect the safety of their patients. In this case, the patient's safety was potentially jeopardized, yet neither the anesthesiologist nor the nurse reported the situation. Therefore, if something had happened to the patient during surgery, the court could have made a good argument that all were negligent. Hence, **Answers 2, 3,** and **4** are incomplete. What can a nurse do in a situation as described here? First, for the nurse's own safety, he or she should prepare a summary of the incidents. The nurse might also consult with nurse colleagues who have worked with the physician, because they could confirm or deny the problem and possibly offer support. Second, the nurse should report the incident to the supervisor and director of nursing, who have a liaison with the surgical/medical staff. If the action is not pursued successfully, the nurse can bring the problem to the attention of the hospital administrator. Again, if no action is forthcoming, the nurse may seek out a board member who might be sensitive to the situation. In any case, these are difficult situations that may arise. There is no easy solution.

Test-taking tip—The best answer is the *most inclusive;* failure to report by *both* nurse and doctor can be seen as negligence, and the hospital will also be liable.

AN, 1, SECE, Management of Care.

23. (1) Most state statutes provide that every hospital to which any person is brought who is suffering from any injuries inflicted by another must report the fact immediately to the local law enforcement authorities. Most state statutes also impose the same duty on other health care professionals, school officials and teachers, child care supervisors, and social workers. Hence **Answers 2 and 4** are incomplete; **Answer 3** is incorrect. From *Landeros v. Flood* as well as other cases, it seems clear that the responsibility of professional people—doctors, nurses, and others who must deal with injured children—includes the duty to report suspicious evidence to the proper authorities.

Test-taking tip—Choose the *most inclusive* answer, involving *all* concerned as mandated by state laws regarding reporting suspected abuse.

AN, 7, SECE, Management of Care.

24. (2) However, it could be argued that **Answer 1** is correct. The nurse's liability for the negligent loss of or damage to a patient's property is based on the nurse's duty as a person, trained or untrained, to act as a reasonable and ordinary, prudent person. In this case, the nurse put the dentures in a towel without a label. The nurse might reasonably expect that aides would be stripping the linen after the patient left for surgery. Therefore, this act was not that of an ordinary prudent person. The nurse would be liable. Because the nurse is liable, the hospital, as employer, *might* also be held liable. This would be for court determination. Because the aides had no knowledge of the dentures, and they were acting reasonably, they would not be liable for the lost dentures. Hence, **Answers 3 and 4** are incorrect.

Test-taking tip—Remember, the hospital may also be liable under *respondeat superior.* Eliminate the two options that include the aides, who were acting as an ordinary prudent person would act.
AN, 7, SECE, Management of Care.

25. **(4)** Although **Answer 4** is best, this is a very close case. When family members help with a hospitalized patient, liability becomes complicated. Where members of the nursing team offer to assist patients in bathing, feeding, and so on, and an apparently capable family member prefers to assist the patient, this is usually acceptable and neither the hospital nor the health care team is liable. Thus, **Answers 1, 2, and 3** can be eliminated as correct choices. However, the nurse should never assume that the presence of a family member obviates the nurse helping the patient.
Test-taking tip—Eliminate options **1, 2, and 3** that include the nurse and the hospital, because they are not liable when family members prefer to assist.
AN, 1, SECE, Safety and Infection Control.

26. **(2)** The Durham Test says that a person is not criminally responsible if the act was a product of mental disease. **Answer 1** is incorrect because the M'Naghten Rule states that a person is insane if he or she cannot determine right from wrong. **Answer 3** is wrong because it is *not* what the Durham Test states. **Answer 4** is wrong because it is an interpretation of the M'Naghten Rule.
Test-taking tip—Know the difference between the Durham Test and M'Naghten Rule, to eliminate **1 and 4**.
*, 7, SECE, Management of Care.

27. **(3)** The request must be in writing. **Answers 1 and 2** are true but incomplete. **Answer 4** has nothing to do with voluntary admission.
Test-taking tip—Choose the *complete* response (**Answer 3**) and eliminate **Answers 1 and 2** as incomplete. Eliminate **Answer 4** as irrelevant to the question.
EV, 7, SECE, Management of Care.

28. **(4)** This division of the ANA sets the standards; therefore, **Answer 1** cannot be correct. **Answers 2 and 3** are also incorrect, although they may be part of **Answer 4**.
Test-taking tip—When two or more options are correct (**Answers 2 and 3**), choose the one that encompasses them (**Answer 4**). Eliminate **Answer 1** because it includes an MD.
*, 7, SECE, Management of Care.

29. **(3)** **Answers 1, 2, and 4** may be referred to in the standards, but the standards were organized around the nursing process.
Test-taking tip—When all four options are right, choose the umbrella option that includes them all.
*, 7, SECE, Management of Care.

30. **(2)** The Amendments extended the flow of funds and set forth specific guidelines for service. **Answer 1** is incorrect because it did not cut funds or set general guidelines. **Answer 3** is incorrect because it did not cut funds. **Answer 4** is incorrect because it did not set general guidelines.
Test-taking tip—Eliminate two options that cut the funding; select the option regarding *specific* guidelines, rather than general.
*, 7, SECE, Management of Care.

31. **(2)** Congress intended to provide funding on a declining basis and to encourage independence from federal support. **Answer 1** is incorrect because Congress does not want centers under continual federal support. **Answer 3** is incorrect because it did not want to maintain federal control. **Answer 4** is incorrect because although Congress wanted declining funding and control, it remains interested in community mental health centers.
Test-taking tip—Eliminate two options that maintain federal control (**Answers 1 and 3**); choose the option that is the opposite of "control," that is, independence from federal control.
*, 7, SECE, Management of Care.

32. **(4)** This was the principal recommendation. **Answer 1** is incorrect. **Answer 3** is incorrect because the commission wanted flexibility in services. **Answer 2** is incorrect because the commission did not want to upgrade the old grant; it wanted to provide a new one.
Test-taking tip—Eliminate **Answer 1** as totally wrong; eliminate **Answer 2** because flexibility is desirable; narrow the choice to upgrade old or provide new grant; choose "new."
*, 7, SECE, Management of Care.

33. **(3)** Nurses, for control and better health care, should be active at all levels and in all areas of health care. **Answer 1** passively carries out others' ideas. **Answer 2** is too limited in scope. **Answer 4** is also passive, with an additional loss of control.
Test-taking tip—Choose the *broadest* scope of involvement ("all areas of health care").
EV, 7, SECE, Management of Care.

34. **(4)** This is what the document states. *Other* choices (**1, 2, 3**) do not give the individual nurse primary responsibility.
Test-taking tip—Eliminate the three options ("body of nurses," "hospital," "laws") that do not focus on the *individual* nurse (**Answer 4**).
*, 7, SECE, Management of Care.

35. **(3)** The Act states that the boards must be composed of 60% *consumers* who are not affiliated with any health professional group; hence, **Answers 1, 2, and 4** are incorrect.
Test-taking tip—Choose the option that focuses on the *consumer.*
*, 7, SECE, Management of Care.

36. **(4)** Emotional abuse of an elder is reportable, and the complaint of neighbors is a reasonable suspicion even if the elder denies it. **Answer 1** is incorrect because, between adults, actual observation of the abuse or of trauma from the abuse is necessary for a report. **Answer 2** is incorrect because HIV results are strictly confidential and may not be disclosed without the patient's permission under any circumstances. **Answer 3** is incorrect because, without corroborating reports, confusion may be causing the elder to misinterpret the situation. It is not enough for a reasonable suspicion.
Test-taking tip—The abused person does not have to admit to the abuse, may deny it, and may even beg to have it go unreported. The nurse is still obligated to file the report.
IMP, 7, SECE, Safety.

37. **(4)** The nurse is ethically and legally obligated to question orders that appear incorrect in order to protect the patient from harm. **Answer 1** is incorrect because, although the ordered dose may be appropriate, the nurse may not assume so without questioning the order first. **Answer 2** is incorrect because the patient is not an appropriate source to validate a medication order. **Answer 3** is incorrect because the actions of nurses on previous shifts do not remove the obligation to question the order, unless there is a clear note that the order has been questioned and the doctor, using medical judgment, has validated the dose.
Test-taking tip—As a patient advocate, the nurse is obligated to protect the patient from harm even if the nurse is exposed to anger or frustration on the part of other health care practitioners. Always select the choice that minimizes the harm to the patient.
IMP, 7, SECE, Safety.

38. **(2)** The nurse who is supervising others has a legal obligation to determine that they are competent to perform the assignment, as well as a legal obligation to provide adequate supervision. **Answer 1** is incorrect because competent individuals are responsible for the consequences of their own behavior. The nurse would not be liable unless the nurse contributed to the mistake or negligence. **Answer 3** is incorrect because the nurse could be liable if the nurse failed to provide adequate supervision or failed to determine that the nursing assistant was competent to perform the assignment. **Answer 4** is incorrect

because the nurse is *not* the employer of the nursing assistant. It is the employer who is liable for the actions of employees.

Test-taking tip—Eliminate options that impose absolutes such as "always" or "never."

AN, 7, SECE, Management of Care.

39. **(1)** Every incident that exposes a patient to harm should be recorded in an incident report, as well as reported to the appropriate supervisors in order to resolve the current problem and permit the institution to prevent the problem from happening again. **Answer 2** is incorrect because the harm to future patients is not prevented, as would be the case if an incident report was filed. **Answer 3** is incorrect because it is usually not the role of the nurse alone to terminate employment, and termination of employment may not be indicated by this incident. **Answer 4** is incorrect because recording the event on the medical record does not adequately put the hospital on notice of potential harm to patients.

Test-taking tip—The duty to protect the patient from harm (to act as patient advocate) almost always involves extensive and appropriate reporting.

IMP, 7, SECE, Safety.

40. **(2)** Accountability means responsibility for nursing actions and the consequences of those actions even if an honest mistake in judgment is made. **Answer 1** is incorrect because the patient has the right to consent to or refuse treatment and the nurse is not responsible for making the patient compliant. **Answer 3** is incorrect because the nurse would *only* be accountable for the actions of other staff members *if* the behavior of the nurse *contributed* to the negligence and negative consequences. **Answer 4** is incorrect because, although the nurse may be responsible for providing correct assessments of the need for nurses, the administrative decision is not within the role of the staff nurse.

Test-taking tip—Nurses are always responsible for the positive and negative consequences of their own behavior. Responsibility for the actions of other staff is a function of the position of the nurse, as well as the potential for harm to the patient.

AN, 7, SECE, Management of Care.

41. **(1)** The standard of care is determined by the average degree of skill, care, and diligence exercised by nurses in similar circumstances. **Answer 2** is incorrect because the drug literature, although informative, cannot recognize all of the circumstances that might be involved in a particular patient situation. **Answer 3** is incorrect because the clinical specialist/ expert may not be a nurse with similar education and experience and would be held to a *higher* standard of care. **Answer 4** is incorrect because the nurse's role is not limited to the direction or order of a physician.

Test-taking tip—Liability/accountability/responsibility is determined by a nursing standard; and levels of education and experience influence the standard of behavior expected of individual nurses.

AS, 7, SECE, Safety.

42. **(2)** In the case of unusual circumstances, a test of reasonableness is applied. The nurse is expected to be flexible enough to prioritize care, and the minimal level of acceptable care is patient safety. **Answer 1** is incorrect because providing customary or ideal care to some patients and leaving others without care would not meet the test of reasonableness. **Answer 3** is incorrect because refusing the assignment would expose the patients to harm from abandonment. **Answer 4** is incorrect because care by family members does not obviate the need for nursing care or attendance by the nurse.

Test-taking tip—The option that includes patient safety without abandonment is usually correct. Options including abandonment are rarely correct. Note that the key word in **Answer 2** is "prioritize," which is a key concept.

PL, 7, SECE, Management of Care.

43. **(4)** The nurse is obligated to inform the nurse manager about changes in the condition of the patient, which may change the decision made by the nurse manager. **Answer 1** is incorrect because the nurse has an obligation to protect the patient from harm, which requires the nurse to inform the nurse manager about the changing status of the patient. **Answer 2** is incorrect because an incident report does not protect the first patient from harm, although an incident report may be indicated to prevent future harm. **Answer 3** is incorrect because, by abandoning the first patient, the nurse exposes the patient to harm and does not protect the patient from harm. Being floated may protect the nurse from harm, but it does not assist the patient.

Test-taking tip—Note the key word "first" in the stem. Answers that involve a reasonable and flexible approach to care with adequate reporting are often correct.

PL, 7, SECE, Safety.

44. **(1)** The infant shows significant signs of dehydration, which requires immediate care. **Answer 2** is incorrect because it fails to deal with the immediate life-threatening situation. **Answer 3** is incorrect because it fails to deal with the immediate life-threatening situation. **Answer 4** is incorrect because it fails to deal with the immediate life-threatening situation.

Test-taking tip—When all the options appear correct, check the question again to determine if there is some key word or phrase that must be interpreted. In this case, all of the options make sense, but, to find the right one, it is necessary to recognize that the baby might have a life-threatening problem.

IMP, 7, SECE, Management of Care.

45. **(2)** It is the legal and ethical obligation of the nurse to report incidents such as medication errors that expose a patient to harm. Failing to check the medication record to see if a drug had been given is a form of medication error. **Answer 1** is incorrect because it fails to discharge the legal and ethical obligation of the nurse to report a medication error. **Answer 3** is incorrect because actual harm to the patient is not a prerequisite for filing an incident report, and failure to report the incident does nothing to prevent future incidents. **Answer 4** is incorrect because it is not the legal and ethical obligation of the physician to inform the nurse about the need to report a medication error.

Test-taking tip—Incidents involving harm to the patient involve a strong obligation to report them adequately, even if it puts the nurse in the position of experiencing negative consequences, and even if the patient is unharmed. It is only necessary to have the potential for harm.

IMP, 7, SECE, Safety.

46. **(4)** The only factually correct answer would include information about contraindications (e.g., HIV-positive status and a person with metastatic cancer). **Answers 1, 2, and 3** have incorrect information: **(1)** a donor must be at least *18 years of age;* **(2)** *written* consent is required; and **(3)** a family member or legal guardian *may* authorize organ donation in the *absence* of written documentation by donor.

Test-taking tip—Knowledge about the Uniform Anatomical Gift Act will identify the only correct option and eliminate the other three options.

IMP, 7, SECE, Management of Care.

47. **(3)** A *Do Not Resuscitate* (DNR) order is required. **Answers 1, 2, and 4** are also appropriate, but not as great a priority as notifying the MD, who must provide a written order.

Test-taking tip—Prioritization is required. Note the key words "next action."

IMP, 7, SECE, Management of Care.

48. **(1)** An advocate *role* encourages freedom of choice, includes speaking out for the patient, and supports the patient's best interests. **Answer 2** is the definition of *cost-benefit analysis.* **Answer 3** is an *ethical principle.* **Answer 4** is a *liberty-limiting*

principle, called *paternalism,* that does not allow patients' preferences.

> **Test-taking tip**—Key word is *role,* not ethical principle (**3, 4**). Cost-benefit analysis is a *course of action,* not a role.

PL, 7, SECE, Management of Care.

49. (**3**) This is a routine function, when the danger of a transfusion reaction is not likely to occur at the conclusion of this treatment. **Answer 1** requires the assessment by a licensed professional for potential for aspiration in a *newly* admitted patient who has had a stroke. **Answer 2** requires assessment of status at admission and is the role of the RN. **Answer 4** may be assigned to an LVN/LPN, *not* a nursing assistant.

> **Test-taking tip**—The key concept is "assessment." Any activity that requires assessment is carried out by an RN, with knowledge, ability, and skills, *not* a nursing assistant.

IMP, 7, SECE, Management of Care.

50. (**1**) There are several models of case management, but the commonality is comprehensive coordination of care to better predict needs of high-risk clients, decrease exacerbations, and continually monitor progress over time. **Answer 2** describes *variance analysis.* **Answer 3** states the purpose of a *care map.* **Answer 4** is the description of a case management tool, the *critical path.*

> **Test-taking tip**—The other options define different *tools* of case management, not the concept itself.

PL, 7, SECE, Management of Care.

51. (**3**) The nurse's goal is to reduce the extent of injury, death, and damage after this crisis (e.g., by providing housing for survivors, obtaining physical care, providing counseling and support for families). **Answer 1** would involve prevention of the crisis from happening (which is not realistic in a natural disaster). **Answer 2** involves reduction of intensity and duration (which is also unrealistic). **Answer 4** is nonexistent as a level of prevention.

> **Test-taking tip**—Picture the aftermath of an earthquake and apply knowledge of levels of prevention used by nurses in disasters.

AN, 1, SECE, Safety and Infection Control.

52. (**1**) The definition of *malpractice* is the "incorrect or negligent treatment of a patient." Included would be incorrect instructions that resulted in injury. **Answers 2 and 3** are careless and would likely require the *hospital* to compensate the patient for the loss or injury. **Answer 4** is an *accident,* not malpractice or negligence.

> **Test-taking tip**—Think of the meaning of the word *malpractice*—"bad practice." Which situation puts the patient at risk because of the nurse's action?

EV, 7, SECE, Management of Care.

53. (**1**) Although all of the patients need social service and discharge assistance, the newly diagnosed diabetic is at greatest risk for complications from the condition and the potential for poor management. Proper diet and safe medication administration would be difficult for a person who is homeless. **Answers 2, 3, and 4** do not pose the most immediate risk to the patient.

> **Test-taking tip**—Note the pattern in the responses: three options are concerned with cardiovascular conditions, one with diabetes. Choose the one that is different (**1**). Two of the conditions are past history; the best option states "newly diagnosed."

PL, 4, SECE, Management of Care.

54. (**4**) The RN cannot delegate the responsibility for assessment and evaluation of patients. The status of the patient in restraints requires further assessment to determine if there are additional causes for the behavior. **Answers 1, 2, and 3** are implementation of the nursing care plan, not assessment.

> **Test-taking tip**—The first step in the nursing process, *assessment,* cannot be delegated by the RN.

IMP, 3, SECE, Management of Care.

55. (**3**) A quality assurance report or incident report should be completed and submitted according to hospital policy. The report would indicate that the MD was notified, the status of the patient, and any orders as a result of the error. The supervisor (**Answer 1**) should be notified, but *not before* completing the incident report. It is also most important to notify the MD before completing the report. Incidents are not usually documented in the patient (medical) record (**Answer 2**). If unsure of hospital policy, hospital risk management should be consulted. Open communication with patients is important (**Answer 4**); however, *unless* there was an adverse effect that required additional treatment or a change in treatment, it is unlikely that the physician will inform the patient.

> **Test-taking tip**—When two options are correct, select the one that encompasses the other. The incident report (**Answer 3**) also serves to inform the supervisor (**Answer 1**).

IMP, 7, SECE, Management of Care.

Nursing Care of the Childbearing Family

Bobbi Morrison

GROWTH AND DEVELOPMENT

Biologic Foundations of Reproduction

General overview: This review of the structures, functions, and important assessment characteristics of the reproductive system provides essential components of the database required for accurate nursing judgments. Comparing normal characteristics and established patterns with nursing assessment findings assists in identifying patient needs and in planning, implementing, and evaluating appropriate goal-directed nursing interventions.

Female Reproductive Anatomy and Physiology

I. **Structure of pelvis** (Figure 4–1)
 A. Two hip bones (right and left innominate: sacrum, coccyx).
 B. False pelvis—upper portion above brim, supportive structure for uterus during last half of pregnancy.
 C. True pelvis—below brim; pelvic inlet, midcavity, pelvic outlet comprise this structure. Fetus passes through during birth.

II. **Pelvic measurements**
 A. Diagonal conjugate—12.5 cm or greater is adequate size; measured by examiner.

 B. Conjugate vera—11 cm is adequate size; measured by x-ray.
 C. Obstetric conjugate—measured by x-ray.
 D. Tuber-ischial diameter—9 to 11 cm indicates adequate size; measured by examiner.

III. **Female external organs**
 A. Mons veneris—protects symphysis.
 B. Labia majora—covers, protects labia minora.

FIGURE 4–1 **The female pelvis.**

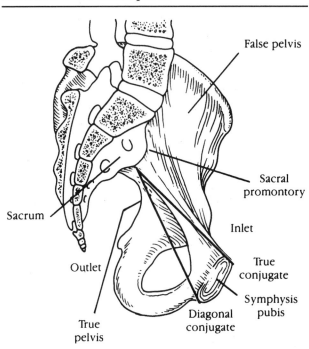

FIGURE 4–2 Female internal reproductive organs.

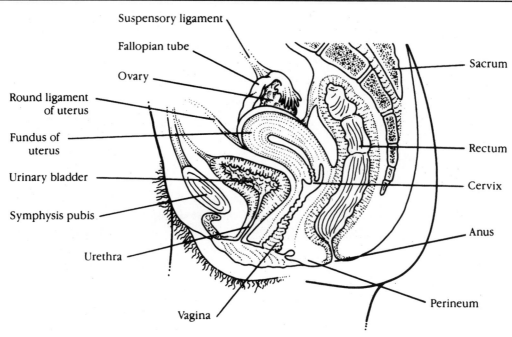

C. Labia minora—two located within labia majora.
D. Clitoris—small erectile tissue.
E. Hymen—thin membrane at opening of vagina.
F. Urinary meatus—opening of urethra.
G. Bartholin glands—producer of alkaline secretions that enhance sperm motility, viability.

IV. **Internal structures** (Figure 4–2)
  A. Vagina—outlet for menstrual flow, depository of semen, lower birth canal.
  B. Cervix—uterine outlet.
  C. Uterus—muscular organ that houses fetus during gestation.
  D. Fallopian tubes—two tubes stretching from cornua of uterus to ovaries; transport ovum.
  E. Ovaries—two oval-shaped structures that produce ovum and hormones (estrogen and progesterone).
  F. Breasts—two mammary glands capable of secreting milk for infant nourishment.

V. **Menstrual cycle** (Figure 4–3)
  A. **Reproductive hormones**
    1. *Follicle-stimulating hormone (FSH)*—secreted during the first half of cycle; stimulates development of graafian follicle; secreted by anterior pituitary.
    2. *Interstitial cell-stimulating hormone, luteinizing hormone (ICSH, LH)*—stimulates ovulation and development of corpus luteum; secreted by pituitary.
    3. *Estrogen*—assists in ovarian follicle maturation; stimulates endometrial thickening; re-

sponsible for development of secondary sex characteristics; maintains endometrium during pregnancy. Secreted by ovaries and adrenal cortex during cycle and by placenta during pregnancy.
    4. *Progesterone*—aids in endometrial thickening; facilitates secretory changes; maintains uterine lining for implantation and early pregnancy; relaxes smooth muscle. Secreted by corpus luteum and placenta.
    5. *Prostaglandins*—substances produced by various body organs that act hormonally on the endometrium to influence the onset and continuation of labor. A medication that may be used to facilitate onset of second trimester abortion; also used to efface the cervix before induction of labor in term pregnancies.
  B. **Ovulation**—maturation and release of egg from ovary; generally occurs 14 days *before* beginning of next menses.
  C. **Menstruation**—vaginal discharge of blood and fragments of the endometrium; cyclic; occurs in response to dropping levels of estrogen and progesterone.
  D. **Fertilization**—impregnation of ovum by sperm.
  E. **Implantation**—fertilized ovum attaches to uterine wall for growth.
  F. **Menopause**—normally occurring cessation of menses with gradual decrease in amount of flow and increase in the time between periods at end of fertility cycle; average age, 51. Early menopause rare but may be influenced by hypothyroidism, surgical ovarian removal, overexposure to radia-

FIGURE 4–3 The menstrual cycle. (From Thomas, CL [ed]: Taber's Cyclopedic Medical Dictionary, ed. 18. FA Davis, Philadelphia, 1997.)

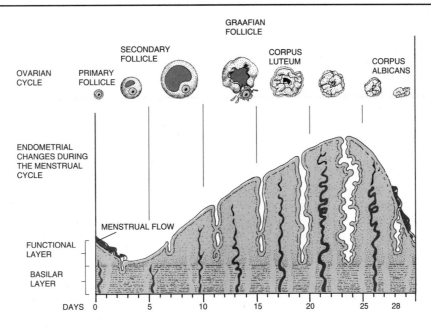

tion. *Treatments* during menopause for symptom relief: hormonal replacement therapy, vitamins B and E for hot flashes, vaginal creams for dyspareunia (painful intercourse), and calcium for osteoporosis.

G. Spinnbarkheit—stretchable, thin cervical mucus present at ovulation.

◆ **VI. Assessment of reproductive tract/reproductive health:**
A. Health history
1. Menarche: onset and duration.
2. Menstrual problems.
3. Contraceptive use.
4. Pregnancy history.
5. Fertility problems.
6. Lifestyle choices that may have an impact on health and reproductive decision making.
B. Physical examination
1. External, internal reproductive organs.
2. Breast examination.
3. *Mammography*—every 1–2 years for women beginning age 40; annually beginning age 50; more frequently if have **risk factors for breast cancer:**
   a. Mother, daughter, or sister had breast cancer.
   b. Menses before age 11, or menopause before age 45 or after age 55.
   c. Previous benign needle biopsies.
   d. Birth of first child > 30 years old.
   e. High-fat diet, obesity.
   f. Nulliparous.
   g. Excessive alcohol consumption.
   h. Personal history of cancer.
   i. Defects in certain genes (BRCA1 and BRCA2).
4. Pap smear—First Papanicolaou (Pap) smear at age 18 or earlier if sexually active; then annually until 3 consecutive normal Paps. After 3 consecutive normal Paps, physician discretion is recommended.
5. Tests for sexually transmitted diseases (STDs).

◆ **VII. Analysis/nursing diagnosis:**
A. *Health-seeking behaviors* related to health promotion.
B. *Health-seeking behaviors* related to menopause.

◆ **VIII. Nursing care plan/implementation:**
A. Discuss anatomy and physiology of reproductive tract.
B. Review menstruation, ovulation, fertilization.
C. Explain need for periodic Pap smears, annual gynecologic exams, including mammography.
D. Discuss lifestyle choices and sexuality issues that might affect health.

◆ **IX. Evaluation/outcome criteria:**
A. Woman displays basic understanding of anatomy and physiology.
B. Woman understands cycle and contraception.
C. Woman regularly seeks preventive care and performs monthly breast self-examination (BSE).

Decision Making Regarding Reproduction

General overview: During the reproductive years, the sexually active woman often faces the decision to postpone, prevent, or terminate a pregnancy. The nursing role focuses on assisting her to make an informed decision consistent with individual needs.

I. Family planning

◆ **A. Assessment:**
   1. Determine interest in and present knowledge of methods of family planning.
   2. Identify factors affecting choice of method: cultural and religious objections, contraindications for individual methods, motivation/ability to follow chosen method successfully, financial considerations, and sexual orientations.

◆ **B. Analysis/nursing diagnosis:** *knowledge deficit* regarding family planning methods/options.

◆ **C. Nursing care plan/implementation**—Goal: *health teaching*—to facilitate informed decision making, selection of option appropriate to individual needs, desires.
   1. Describe, explain, discuss options available and appropriate to the woman. Include information on advantages and disadvantages of each option (Tables 4–1 and 4–2).
   2. Demonstrate, as necessary, method selected.
   3. Quick health teaching reminders for missed oral hormone preparations:
      a. Woman should take one pill at the same time every day for 21 (or 28) days.
      b. If woman misses one pill, she should take it as soon as she remembers it; she should then take the next one at the usual time.
      c. If woman misses two or more pills in a row in the first 2 wk of her cycle, she should take 2 pills for 2 days and use a backup method of contraception for the next 7 days.
      d. If woman misses two pills in the third week, or three or more pills anytime:
         (1) A *Sunday starter* should keep taking pills until the next Sunday, then start a new pack that Sunday. She should use a backup method of contraception for the next 7 days.
         (2) A *day 1 starter* should throw out the rest of the pack and start a new pack that day. She should use a backup method of contraception for the next 7 days.
      e. *28-day pill pack:* If woman misses any of the seven pills that do not have any hormones, she should throw out the pills missed and keep taking one pill a day un-

til the pack is empty. She does not need a backup method of contraception.
   4. Alert woman to discontinue use of *oral hormone contraceptive* preparations and report any of the following symptoms to the physician **stat.** Signs of potential problems: "ACHES"*
      A—Abdominal pain: possible problem with the liver or gallbladder.
      C—Chest pain or shortness of breath: possible clot within lungs or heart.
      H—Headaches (sudden or persistent): possibly caused by cardiovascular accident or hypertension.
      E—Eye problems: possible vascular accident or hypertension.
      S—Severe leg pain: possible thromboembolic process.
   5. Signs of *potential problems* related to IUD use: "PAINS"*
      P—Period (menstrual) late, abnormal spotting or bleeding.
      A—Abdominal pain, pain during coitus (dyspareunia).
      I—Infection, abnormal vaginal discharge.
      N—Not feeling well; fever or chills.
      S—String missing (nonpalpable on vaginal self-examination, or not seen on speculum examination).
   6. **Toxic Shock Syndrome** (TSS)
      a. *Signs/symptoms*
         (1) Fever of sudden onset—over 102°F (38.9°C).
         (2) Hypotension—systolic pressure < 90 mm Hg; orthostatic dizziness; disorientation.
         (3) Rash—diffuse, macular erythroderma (resembling sunburn).
         (4) Sore throat; severe nausea, vomiting.
         (5) Copious vaginal discharge.
      b. *Instructions for prevention*
         (1) General
            (a) *Avoid* use of tampons, cervical caps, and diaphragms during the postpartum period (6 wk).
            (b) Do *not* use any of the above if you have a history of TSS.
            (c) Call physician if you experience sudden onset of a high fever, vomiting, diarrhea, or skin rash.
            (d) Insert clean tampons and contraceptive devices with clean hands.
            (e) Remove within prescribed time limits.
         (2) Tampons
            (a) Change tampons every 3 to 6 hr.

---

*Source: Hatcher, R, et al: Contraceptive Technology, ed. 16. Irving, New York, 1994.

TABLE 4–1   Contraception

Method	Action/Effectiveness	Advantages	Disadvantages and Side Effects
Hormonal Contraceptives Combination of estrogen and progesterone	Suppresses ovulation by suppressing production of FSH and LH *Most efficient* form of contraception (99.7%) if used consistently	▪ Convenient; easy to take ▪ Withdrawal bleeding cycles are predictable ▪ Not related to sex act ▪ Safe for older nonsmoking women until menopause ▪ Many noncontraceptive health benefits	▪ *Absolute contraindications,* e.g., thromboembolic or coronary artery disease, some cancers or liver disease ▪ *Relative contraindications,* e.g., migraines, hypertension, immobility 4 wk or more, abnormal genital bleeding ▪ Some decrease in glucose tolerance ▪ Effectiveness decreased if taken during use of barbiturates, phenytoin, antibiotics ▪ **No protection against STDs**

Progestin only
  Minipill (0) qd
  Depo-Provera (IM) q3mo
	Impairs fertility
	Thickens cervical mucus; decreases sperm penetration
	Alters endometrial maturation
	Effectiveness: Undetermined; can reach 100% reliability if used exactly as prescribed
		▪ (Oral) convenient, easy to take
		▪ (IM) 4 times a yr; lactation OK during this time
			▪ Ovulation may occur
			▪ Irregular bleeding, mood changes, weight gain
			▪ May change glucose and insulin values
			▪ **No protection against STDs**

Emergency Postcoital Contraception Estradiol (100 µg) and Norgestrol (1.0 mg)	Antifertility; taken within 72 h of unprotected coitus Take 2 pills as soon as possible; take 2 pills 12 h later *Effectiveness:* 75–85%	▪ Available, prn	▪ Nausea, headache, dizziness
Intrauterine Devices (IUDs) Small T-shaped device inserted into uterine cavity Medicated: ▪ Copper	Prevents fertility Recommended for women who have had at least one child Damages sperm in transit to fallopian tube	▪ Can be used by women who cannot use hormonal contraception; no disruption of ovulation pattern ▪ Can be used effectively for 10 yr (Copper)	▪ *Contraindications:* history of PID, pregnancy, undiagnosed genital bleeding, genital malignancy, abnormal uterine cavity ▪ *Risks:* uterine perforation, infection (may be followed by PID) in the first 3 mo of insertion; unnoticed expulsion
▪ Progesterone	Alters cervical mucus and endometrial maturation *Effectiveness* rate: 90–99%	▪ Change every yr (Progesterone) ▪ Less blood loss during menses and decreases primary dysmenorrhea	▪ *Side effects* (especially with copper-T): heavy flow, spotting between periods, and cramping within first few months of insertion ▪ Must check for string after each menses and before intercourse ▪ **No protection against STDs**
Mechanical Barriers Diaphragm: shallow rubber device that fits over cervix	Barrier preventing sperm from entering cervix (if it is correct size, undamaged, correctly placed, and is used with spermicide) *Effectiveness:* 83–90%; 99% in highly motivated women	▪ Does not interrupt sex act, except to add spermicide just before act* ▪ Insert up to 6 hr before intercourse and leave in place for 6 hr after last intercourse, but not longer than 24 hr† ▪ Safe: no side effects from well-fitted device if woman is not allergic to diaphragm or spermicide ▪ Decreased incidence of vaginitis, cervicitis, PID	▪ Requires careful cleansing with warm water and mild soap; powder with cornstarch, and store away from heat. Size/fit must be checked after term birth, second/third trimester abortion, weight gain or loss of 15–20 lb or more, or every 2 yr ▪ Spermicide must be reinserted for additional acts that may follow after initial intercourse

Continued

Maternal-Infant

TABLE 4–1 Contraception—cont'd

Method	Action/Effectiveness	Advantages	Disadvantages and Side Effects
Mechanical Barriers (continued)			
Cervical cap: 1¼" to 1½" soft natural rubber dome with a firm but pliable rim	Physical barrier to sperm Spermicide inside cap adds a chemical barrier *Effectiveness* similar to that of diaphragm	■ Worn for 8 hr but not longer than 48 hr ■ No need to add spermicide for repeated acts of intercourse	■ Need a Pap smear every yr: higher rate of conversion from class I to class III‡ ■ If in place over 48 h, it produces an odor and might be associated with TSS† ■ Cannot be worn during menstrual flow (menses) or up to at least 6 wk postpartum ■ *Contraindications:* abnormal Pap smear, hard to fit, history of TSS or genital infection, allergy ■ Change after genital surgery or birth, major change in weight ■ Must be checked each yr ■ **Does not protect against STDs**
Female condom: vaginal sheath of natural latex rubber with flexible rings at both the closed and the open ends	Barrier preventing sperm from entering vagina *Effectiveness* similar to other mechanical methods used with spermicide *Note:* Male and female condoms should not be used at the same time	■ Apply well in advance of intercourse; spermicide added just before intercourse ■ Heightens sensation for man ■ About as satisfying for both woman and man as intercourse without it ■ **Provides protection from STDs**	■ Cost ■ A new one must be used for every act of intercourse
Condom: thin, stretchable latex sheath to cover penis	Barrier preventing sperm from entering vagina, applied over erect penis before loss of preejaculatory drops and is held in place as penis is withdrawn ⬤ Spermicidal foam, jelly, or cream is also used* *Effectiveness* rate: 64–98% when used with spermicide	■ Safety—no side effects ■ **Provides protection from spread of STDs** With spermicide (0.5 g of ⬤ nonoxynol-9) added to interior or exterior surface, provides protection from STDs, including HIV	■ Check expiration date ■ Requires high motivation to use correctly/constantly ■ Must be properly applied and removed ■ Sheath may tear during intercourse
Chemical Barriers			
⬤ Spermicide: aerosol foams, foaming tablets, suppositories, creams, and films (V-Film)	Physical barrier to sperm penetration Chemical action on sperm (kills sperm) ⬤ Nonoxynol-9 has a bacteriostatic action *Effectiveness* rate: 70–98% when used with diaphragm or condoms	■ Increases effectiveness of mechanical barriers ■ Ease of application. Aids lubrication of vagina* ■ Requires no medical examination or prescription ■ May be used during lactation ■ Backup for missed oral contraceptive pills	■ Messy ■ Some people are allergic to preparations ■ Tabs or suppositories take 10–15 min to dissolve ■ If it is only method being used, each intercourse should be preceded (by 30 min) by a fresh application; may be allergenic
Other Methods			
Natural family planning: BBT each morning before any physical activity Symptothermal variation: BBT plus cervical mucus changes Calendar method Predictor test for ovulation	Requires sexual abstinence during woman's fertile period (4 d before ovulation), and for 3 or 4 days after ovulation *Effectiveness:* about 80%	Physically safe to use—no drugs or appliances are used; meets requirements of most religions	■ Effectiveness depends on high level of motivation and diligence ■ Requires fairly predictable menstrual cycle

*Spermicide provides lubrication, but if additional lubrication is needed, use water-based products only, e.g., K-Y jelly.

†TSS: toxic shock syndrome. Although there is no direct link between TSS and use of the diaphragm or cervical cap, a possible association remains (see p. 82).

‡Class I Pap smear: no abnormal cells; Class III Pap smear: suspicious abnormal cells present.

TABLE 4-2   Sterilization

Method	Advantages	Disadvantages and Side Effects
Male Vas deferens is occluded (ligated and severed; bands; clips) to prevent passage of sperm	■ Relatively simple surgical procedure ■ Does not affect endocrine function, production of testosterone ■ Does not alter volume of ejaculate ■ Tubal reconstruction possible (90%)	■ Sterility is not immediate; sperm are cleared from vas after about 15 ejaculations ■ Some men become impotent due to psychological response to procedure ■ Fertility after tubal reconstruction (30–85%)
Female Both fallopian tubes are ligated and severed, or occluded with bands or clips to prevent passage of eggs; fulguration of the tubes at the cornu is most effective	■ Abdominal surgery utilizing 1-inch incision and laparoscopy ■ Greater than 99.5% effective	■ Major surgery (if done by laparotomy) with possible complications of anesthesia, infection, hemorrhage, and trauma to other organs; psychological trauma in some ■ Success rate for pregnancy after tubal reversal using microsurgical techniques: 40–75%
Hysterectomy or oophorectomy or both	■ Abdominal or vaginal surgery ■ Absolute sterility	

Maternal-Infant

(b) Do *not* use superabsorbent tampons.
(c) For overnight protection, substitute other products such as sanitary napkins or minipads.
(3) Diaphragm or cervical cap
(a) *Avoid* use during your menstrual period.
(b) Remove within 8 hr after intercourse (diaphragm must be removed no later than 24 hr; the cap, no later than 48 hr).

◆ **D. Evaluation/outcome criteria:**
1. Woman avoids or achieves a pregnancy as desired.
2. Woman expresses comfort and satisfaction with method selected.

II. Infertility
A. Definition: inability to conceive after 1 yr of unprotected intercourse.
B. Pathophysiology: contributing factors—hormonal deficiencies, reproductive system disorders, congenital anomalies, male impotence, sexual knowledge deficit, debilitating disease.
◆ **C. Assessment:**
1. History—general health, reproduction, social history.
2. *Maternal diagnosis*
   a. Basal body temperature (BBT) (Figure 4–4).
   b. Endocrine studies.
   c. Huhner (postcoital).
   d. Rubins (tubal patency).
   e. Hysterosalpingogram (tubal patency).

3. *Male diagnosis*—history, physical examination, laboratory studies, e.g., semen analysis.
◆ **D. Analysis/nursing diagnosis:** *altered sexuality* related to infertility.
◆ **E. Nursing care plan/implementation:**
1. Provide emotional support.
2. Explain testing procedures for diagnosis.
3. Assist with referral process.
◆ **F. Evaluation/outcome criteria:**
1. The couple conceives, or,
2. If the couple does not conceive, they accept referral for help with adoption, other reproductive alternatives, or childlessness.

III. Interruption of Pregnancy—also known as elective, voluntary, or therapeutic abortion. Once the diagnosis of pregnancy and the length of gestation are established, the woman faces the decision to interrupt or to maintain the pregnancy (Table 4–3, p. 87).
A. Decision-making stage:
◆ 1. **Assessment:**
   a. Health history:
      (1) Determine woman's feelings about the pregnancy, reasons for considering abortion, level of maturity; if decision was already made before she came to clinic, how was decision made? Does she have a support system?
      (2) Identify factors influencing/complicating her decisions (religious beliefs, cultural mores, peer and family pressures).
      (3) Information needs.
   b. Physical examination.
   c. Laboratory tests: blood type, Rh, hemoglobin, hematocrit, urinalysis, pregnancy

Maternal-Infant

FIGURE 4–4 Basal body temperature chart. (From Thomas, CL [ed]: Taber's Cyclopedic Medical Dictionary, ed. 18. FA Davis, Philadelphia, 1997.)

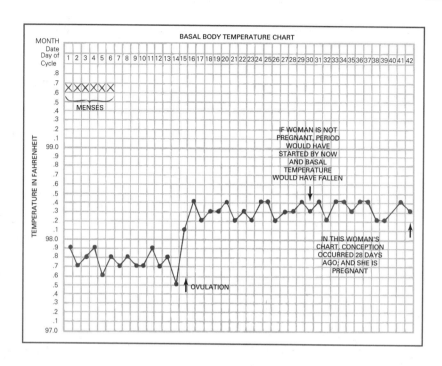

test, antibody titer, other tests dependent on her health status.

◆ 2. **Analysis/nursing diagnosis:**

a. *Ineffective coping* related to emotional conflicts associated with need for decision to continue/terminate pregnancy.

b. *Altered family process* related to intrafamily conflict associated with need for/decision to continue/terminate pregnancy.

c. *Anticipatory grieving* related to loss of pregnancy/child.

d. *Altered self-concept, self-esteem disturbance* related to possible guilt feelings related to pregnancy/termination.

e. *Knowledge deficit* related to available options.

◆ 3. **Nursing care plan/implementation:**

a. Goal: *emotional support* to minimize impact on self-image and self-esteem.

   (1) Maintain accepting, nonjudgmental attitude.

   (2) Encourage verbalization of feelings, perceptions, and values.

   (3) Support woman's decision.

b. Goal: *health teaching* to facilitate informed decision making.

   (1) Explain and discuss available options as applicable (see Table 4–3).

   (2) Describe procedure selected and what to expect after procedure.

c. Goal: *minimize impact on intrafamily relations, family process.* Where applicable,

encourage open communication between deciding partners.

◆ 4. **Evaluation/outcome criteria:**

a. Woman states she understands all information necessary to give consent.

b. Woman expresses comfort and satisfaction with the decision.

B. Preoperative period

◆ 1. **Assessment:**

a. Reassess woman's emotional and physical status and current feelings regarding decision.

b. Determine woman's current knowledge/ understanding of authorization form, anticipated procedure, and consequences (informed consent).

c. Monitor woman's physiological and (if awake) psychological response to procedure.

◆ 2. **Analysis/nursing diagnosis:**

a. *Anxiety/fear* related to procedure, potential complications

b. *Knowledge deficit* related to ongoing procedure, sights, sounds, and sensations experienced.

◆ 3. **Nursing care plan/implementation:**

a. Goal: *provide opportunity to reconsider decision regarding termination of pregnancy.*

   (1) Check to ensure all required permission (informed consent) forms have been signed/filed.

TABLE 4–3 Interruption of Pregnancy (Elective/Voluntary Abortion)

Method	Advantages	Disadvantages and Side Effects
First-Trimester Procedures		
Menstrual extraction—aspiration of endometrium through undilated cervix	Performed for women who have not yet missed a menstrual period 100% effective if implantation site is not missed	Cervical trauma may occur and may lead to incompetent cervix Hemorrhage
RU 486 (mifepristone)—a progesterone antagonist; taken up to 7 wk gestation (56 days LMP); taken orally	Prevents implantation of fertilized egg Most effective in early gestation, during luteal phase, within 10 days of first missed period	Slight nausea and fatigue during period of bleeding Uterine aspiration may be needed if RU 486 does not work
Misoprostol—initiates uterine contractions; given intravaginally	Softens cervix and aids in expelling products of conception	
Uterine aspiration (vacuum or suction curettage)—cannula suction under local anesthesia, following cervical dilatation, usually with laminaria tent	Relatively few complications—minimal bleeding, minimal discomfort Outpatient basis	Performed after one or two missed menstrual periods Cervical or endometrial trauma possible
Surgical dilation and curettage (D & C)—cervix dilated with laminaria tents; endometrium scraped with metal curette or flexible aspiration tip, under local anesthesia (paracervical block)	After cervix is dilated, procedure takes about 15 min Outpatient basis Relatively few complications ($\leq 1\%$)—bleeding like a heavy period, some cramping	Performed after one or two missed periods Possible but rare: cervical trauma, uterine perforation, infection, hemorrhage
Second-Trimester Procedures		
Intraamniotic infusion between weeks 14 and 16; transabdominal extraction of 200 mL amniotic fluid and replacement with equal amount of hypertonic NaCl (20%); or 30% urea in D_5W	Does not require laparotomy Woman may ambulate until labor starts and during early labor Abortion completed within 36–40 hr; $\frac{2}{3}$ of fetuses are aborted in 24 hr With urea: abortion usually occurs within 12 hr; complications less common or serious than with NaCl	Complications increase proportionally with weeks of gestation Risks—*hypernatremia:* tinnitus, tachycardia, and headache *Water intoxication:* edema, oliguria (≤ 200 mL/8 hr), dyspnea, thirst, and restlessness Hemorrhage and possible disseminated intravascular coagulation (DIC); fever with sepsis Woman experiences labor May require D & C
Instillation of 40–45 mg prostaglandin F_2, E_2	Labor is usually shorter than with hypertonic NaCl Avoids complications of water intoxication and hypernatremia	May cause vomiting, diarrhea, nausea Fetus may be born alive
D & E (dilation and evacuation)—extends D & C and vacuum curettage up to 20 wk gestation	Woman does not experience labor Hospitalization is shortened With a skilled operator, complication rate is lower than with intraamniotic injection methods	Requires 3 d to dilate cervix; procedure done on third day
Second- and Third-Trimester Procedures		
Hysterotomy—cesarean delivery	Available for gestations more than 14–16 wk Preferred method if woman wishes a tubal ligation or hysterectomy to follow	*After:* major surgery complications—hemorrhage and infection possible Fetus may be born alive, causing ethical, moral, religious, and legal problems

(2) Refer to physician if woman is ambivalent or insecure in decision.
b. Goal: *reduce anxiety/fear related to procedure.*
  (1) Explain all anticipated preoperative, operative, and postoperative care.
  (2) Assist with procedure; if woman is awake, explain what is happening and what she may be experiencing.
c. Goal: *emotional support* to facilitate effective coping.

(1) Encourage verbalization of feelings, fears, concerns.
(2) Support woman's decision.
◆ 4. **Evaluation/outcome criteria:** woman does not experience physiological or psychological problems during procedure.
C. **Postoperative period**
◆ 1. **Assessment:**
a. Monitor *physiological* response to procedure (vital signs, blood loss, uterine cramping).

b. Determine *psychological* response (happy, relieved; guilt feelings, lowered self-esteem).

c. Determine desire for family planning information.

d. Determine need for Rho(D)immune globulin, *Rubella* vaccination

◆ 2. **Analysis/nursing diagnosis:**

a. *Pain* related to procedure.

b. *High risk for infection* related to lack of knowledge of postabortal self-care.

◆ 3. **Nursing care plan/implementation:**

a. Goal: *provide and explain postoperative care.*

(1) Administer intravenous (IV) fluids.

(2) Administer medications prn for discomfort.

(3) Administer oxytocic meds for uterine atony, prn.

(4) If *Rh-negative* mother, 8 or more weeks of gestation, and laboratory tests indicate no current sensitization (i.e., she is Coombs negative):

(a) Explain rationale for postabortion administration of Rho (D antigen) immune globulin (RhoGAM).

(b) Administer RhoGAM, as ordered.

(5) Provide and explain perineal care

b. Goal: *health teaching* to facilitate active participation in own health maintenance,

informed decision making, provide pre-discharge anticipatory guidance (also provide in written form with attention to woman's level of reading skill and understanding, and in her native language whenever possible):

(1) Immediately report any cramping, excessive bleeding, signs of infection.

(2) Provide name and telephone number of person to call if she has questions.

(3) Schedule a postabortal checkup.

(4) Discuss contraception, if woman indicates interest; or give her place and name to call for information later.

(5) Discuss resumption of tampon use (3 days to 3 wk as ordered) and sexual intercourse (1 wk to 3 wk as ordered).

(6) Discuss need to avoid douching.

◆ 4. **Evaluation/outcome criteria:**

a. Woman returns for postabortal appointment.

b. Woman suffers no adverse physical sequelae to the procedure.

c. Woman suffers no adverse psychological sequelae to the procedure.

d. Woman is successful in achieving her goal of either contraception or conception at the time she desires.

5. Postabortion psychological impact:

a. Majority—relieved and happy.

b. Small number (5–10%)—negative feelings, such as guilt or low self-esteem.

CHILDBEARING: PREGNANCY BY TRIMESTER

General overview: This review of the normal physiological and psychosocial changes occurring during each trimester of pregnancy provides essential components of the database for accurate nursing judgments and anticipatory guidance during the prenatal period. Complications of pregnancy are correlated with the trimester of common occurrence; relationships with other NCLEX categories of human function are described.

I. General aspects of nursing care

◆ **A. Assessment**—based on nursing knowledge of the following:
1. Biophysical and psychosocial aspects of conception and gestation.
2. Parameters of normal pregnancy.
3. Risk factors, signs, symptoms, and implications of deviations from normal patterns of maternal and fetal health.

◆ **B. Analysis/nursing diagnosis:**
1. *Knowledge deficit* related to normal pregnancy-related alterations (physiological and emotional alterations/trimester).
2. *Pain* related to normal physiological alterations in pregnancy.
3. *Altered elimination* related to normal physiological changes during pregnancy (polyuria, constipation).
4. *Altered nutrition* related to increased metabolic needs due to pregnancy.
5. *Impaired adjustment* related to altered self-image; anticipated role change; resurgence of old, unresolved conflicts.

◆ **C. Nursing care plan/implementation:**
1. Goal: *emotional support.*
   a. Encourage verbalization of feelings, fears, concerns.
   b. Validate normalcy of behavioral response to pregnancy.
2. Goal: *anticipatory guidance.*
   a. Facilitate achievement of developmental tasks.
   b. Strengthen coping techniques for pregnancy, labor, birth. Suggest appropriate resources (preparation for childbirth classes).
3. Goal: *health teaching.* Describe, explain, discuss:
   a. Normal physiological alterations during pregnancy.
   b. Common discomforts of pregnancy, management.

◆ **D. Evaluation/outcome criteria:**
1. Woman takes an active, informed part in her pregnancy-related care.

2. Woman copes effectively with common alterations associated with pregnancy (physiological, psychological, role change).
3. Woman successfully carries an uneventful pregnancy to term.

II. Biologic foundations of pregnancy

A. Conception
1. *Egg*—life span, approximately 24 hr after ovulation.
2. *Sperm*—life span, approximately 72 hr after ejaculation into female reproductive tract.
3. *Conception* (fertilization)—usually occurs 12–24 hr after ovulation, within fallopian tube.
4. *Implantation* (nidation)—usually occurs within 7–9 days of conception, or about day 21–23 of a 28-day menstrual cycle.
5. *Ovum*—period of conception until primary villi have appeared; usually about 12–14 days.
6. *Embryo*—period from end of ovum stage until measurement reaches approximately 3 cm; 54–56 days.
7. *Fetus*—period from end of embryo stage until birth.

First Trimester
Susceptible to teratogens
Heart functions at 3–4 wk
Eye formation at 4–5 wk
Arm and leg buds at 4–5 wk
Recognizable face at 8 wk
Brain: rapid growth
External genitalia at 8 wk
Placenta formed at 12 wk
Bone ossification at 12 wk
Second Trimester
Less danger from teratogens after 12 wk
Facial features formed at 16 wk
Fetal heartbeat heard by 18 to 20 wk with a fetoscope/doppler
Quickening at 18–20 wk
Length: 10 inches, weight: 8–10 oz
Vernix: present
Third Trimester
Iron stored
Surfactant production begins in increasing amounts
Size: 15 inches, 2–3 lb
Calcium stored at 28–32 wk
Reflexes present at 28–32 wk
Subcutaneous fat deposits at 36 wk
Lanugo shedding at 38–40 wk
Average size: 18–22 inches, 7.5–8.5 lb at 38–40 wk

B. Anatomical and physiological modifications
1. *Bases of functional alterations*
   a. *Hormonal*—Table 4–4 discusses the effects of estrogen and progesterone during

TABLE 4–4 **Hormones of Pregnancy**

Primary Effects	Clinical Implications for Nursing Actions
Estrogen	
Level rises in serum and urine	Basis of test for maternal/placental/fetal well-being
Uterine enlargement	Probable sign of pregnancy
Breast enlargement	Probable sign of pregnancy; increased tingling, tenderness
Genital enlargement: increased vascularization, hyperplasia	Vaginal growth facilitates vaginal birth
Softens connective tissue	Results in backache and leg ache; relaxes joints to increase size of birth canal and rib cage
Alters nutrient metabolism:	*Gastrointestinal and metabolic changes:*
Decreases HCl and pepsin	Digestive upsets
Antagonist to insulin—makes glucose available to fetus	Anti-insulin effect challenges maternal pancreas to produce more insulin; failure of β-cells to respond leads to "gestational" diabetes. For the insulin-dependent woman, insulin requirements increase by an average of 67% during the second half of pregnancy
Supports fat deposition	Protect source of energy for fetus
Sodium and water retention; edema of lower extremities (nonpitting)	Meet increased plasma volume needs and maintain fluid reserve
Hematological changes:	
Increased coagulability	Increased tendency to thrombosis
Increased sedimentation rate (SR)	SR loses diagnostic value for heart disease
Vasodilation: spider nevi; palmar erythema	Resolves spontaneously after birth
Increased production of melanin-stimulating hormone	Resolves spontaneously after birth; causes chloasma and linea negra
Progesterone	
Development of decidua	High levels result in tiredness, listlessness, and sleepiness
Reduces uterine excitability	Protection against abortion/early birth
Development of mammary glands	Prepares breasts for lactation
Alters nutrient metabolism:	*Nutritional significance:*
Antagonist to insulin	Diabetogenic
Favors fat deposition	Energy reserve
Decreases gastric motility and relaxes sphincters	Favors heartburn and constipation
Increased sensitivity of respiratory center to CO_2	Increased depth, some dyspnea, increased sighing
Decreased smooth-muscle tone:	*Decreased tone can lead to:*
Colon	Constipation
Bladder, ureters	Stasis of urine with ↑ chance of infection
Veins	Dependent edema; varicosities
Gallbladder	Gallbladder disease
Increased basal body temperature (BBT) by 0.5°C	Discomfort from hot flashes and perspiration
Human Chorionic Gonadotropin	
Maintains corpus luteum during early pregnancy	Placenta must "take over" after a few weeks
Stimulates male testes	Increased testosterone in male fetuses
May suppress immune response	May inhibit response to foreign protein, for example, fetal portion of placenta
	Diagnostic value:
	Basis for pregnancy test
	Hydatidiform mole ↑
	Decreased level with threatened abortion
	Increased level with multiple pregnancy
Human Placental Lactogen	
Antagonizes insulin	Diabetogenic; may → gestational diabetes or complicate management of existing diabetes
Mobilizes maternal free fatty acids	Increased tendency to ketoacidosis in pregnant diabetic
Prolactin	
Suppressed by estrogen and progesterone	No milk produced before birth
Increased level after placenta is delivered	Milk production 2–3 days after birth

TABLE 4–4   Hormones of Pregnancy—cont'd

Primary Effects	Clinical Implications for Nursing Actions
Follicle Stimulating Hormone	
Production suppressed during pregnancy; level returns to prepregnant levels within 3 wk after birth	No ovulation during pregnancy; ovulation usually returns within 6 wk for 15%, within 12 wk for 30%
Oxytocin	
Causes uterus to contract when the oxytocin levels exceed those of estrogen and progesterone	Labor induction or augmentation; treatment for postpartum uterine atony

TABLE 4–5   Blood Values

Component	Prepregnant	Pregnant	Postpartum*
WBC	4,000–11,000	9,000–16,000 (25,000—labor)	20,000–25,000 within 10–12 days of birth, then returns to normal
RBC volume	1600 ml	1900 ml	Prepregnant level of 1600 ml
Plasma volume	2400 ml	3700 ml	Prepregnant level of 2400 ml
Hct (PCV)	37–47%	32–42%	At 72°, returns to prepregnant level of 37–47%
Hgb (at sea level)	12–16 g/dl	10–14 g/dl	At 72°, returns to prepregnant level of 12–16 g/dl
Fibrinogen	250 mg/dl	400 mg/dl	At 72°, returns to prepregnant level of 250 mg/dl

*Postpartum values depend on factors of amount of blood loss, mobilization, and physiological edema (excretion of extravascular water). Normal blood loss for vaginal birth is 300–400 mL.

pregnancy. Nursing implications provide the knowledge base for the following:
   (1) Anticipatory guidance regarding normal maternal adaptations.
   (2) Early identification of deviations from normal patterns.
   b. *Mechanical*—enlarging uterus → displacement and pressure; increased weight of uterus and breasts → changes in posture and pressure.
2. *Breasts*—enlarged darkened areola; secrete colostrum.
3. *Reproductive organs*
   a. *Uterus*
      (1) Amenorrhea. Occasional spotting common, especially at time of first missed menstrual period.
      (2) Increased vascularity adds to increase in size and softening of the lower uterine segment (*Hegar's sign*).
      (3) Growth is due to hypertrophy and hyperplasia of existing muscle cells and connective tissue.
      (4) Fundal height measurement landmarks:

Uterus	Nonpregnant	Pregnant (At Term)
Length	6.5 cm	32 cm
Width	4 cm	24 cm
Depth	2.5 cm	22 cm
Weight	50 g	1000 g

   b. *Cervix*
      (1) Increased vascularity → softening (*Goodell's sign*) and deepened blue-purple coloration (*Chadwick's sign*).
      (2) Edema, hyperplasia, thickening of mucous lining, and increased mucus production; formation of mucus plug by end of second month.
      (3) Becomes shorter, thicker, and more elastic.
   c. *Vagina*
      (1) Hyperemia deepens color (*Chadwick's sign*).
      (2) Hypertrophy and hyperplasia thicken vaginal mucosa.
      (3) Relaxation of connective tissue.
      (4) pH acidic (4.0–6.0).
      (5) Leukorrhea—nonirritating.
   d. *Perineum*
      (1) Increases in size—hypertrophy of muscle cells, edema, and relaxation of elastic tissue.
      (2) Deepened color—increased vascularization/hyperemia.
   e. *Ovaries*
      (1) Ovum production ceases.
      (2) Corpus luteum persists; produces hormones to wk 10–12 until placenta "takes over."
C. **Alterations affecting fluid-gas transport**
   1. *Cardiovascular system* (Table 4–5)

a. **Physiological changes**
   (1) Heart displaced upward and to the left.
   (2) Circulation:
      (a) Cardiac volume increases by 20–30%.
      (b) Labor—cardiac output increases by 20–30%.
      (3) Hemoglobin and hematocrit values remain between 10–14 g and 35–42%, normal drop is 10% during second trimester.
      (4) Hypercoagulability—increased levels of blood factors VII, VIII, IX, and X.
      (5) Nonpathologic increased sedimentation rate—due to 50% increase in fibrinogen level.
      (6) Blood pressure should remain stable with drop in second trimester.
      (7) Heart rate often increases 10–15 beats/min at term.
      (8) Compression of pelvic veins → stasis of blood in lower extremities.
      (9) Compression of inferior vena cava when supine → bradycardia → reduced cardiac output, faintness, sweating, nausea *(supine hypotension). Fetal response:* marked bradycardia due to hypoxia secondary to decreased placental perfusion.

◆ b. **Assessment:**
   (1) Apical systolic murmur.
   (2) Exaggerated splitting of first heart sound.
   (3) Physiologic anemia.
   (4) Dependent edema in third trimester (Table 4–6).
   (5) *Vena cava syndrome* (supine hypotension)—drop in systolic blood pressure may occur due to compression of descending aorta and inferior vena cava when supine.
   (6) Varicosities (vulvar, anal, leg).

◆ c. **Nursing care plan/implementation:**
   Goal: *health teaching*
   (1) *Elevate* lower extremities frequently.
   (2) Apply support hose.
   (3) *Avoid* excess intake of sodium.
   (4) Assume *side-lying* position at rest.
   (5) Learn signs and symptoms of pregnancy-induced hypertension.

2. *Respiratory system*
   a. **Physiological changes:**
      (1) Increased tidal volume, vital capacity, respiratory reserve, oxygen consumption, production of CO_2.
      (2) Diaphragm elevated, increased substernal angle → flaring of rib cage.
      (3) Uterine enlargement prevents maximum lung expansion in third trimester.

   ◆ b. **Assessment:**
      (1) Shortness of breath or dyspnea on exertion and when lying flat in third trimester.
      (2) Nasal stuffiness due to estrogen-induced edema (see Table 4–6).
      (3) Deeper respiratory excursion.

   ◆ c. **Nursing care plan/implementation:**
      Goal: *health teaching*
      (1) Sit and stand with good posture.
      (2) When resting assume *semi-Fowler's position*.
      (3) *Avoid* overdistention of stomach.

D. **Alterations affecting elimination**
   1. *Urinary system*
      a. **Physiological changes:**
         (1) Relaxation of smooth muscle results in conditions that can persist 4–6 wk after birth:
            (a) Dilatation of ureters.
            (b) *Decreased* bladder tone.
            (c) Increased potential for urinary stasis and *infection* (UTI).
         (2) *Increased* glomerular filtration rate (50%) during last two trimesters.
         (3) *Increased* renal plasma flow (25–50%) during first two trimesters; returns to near normal levels by end of last trimester.
         (4) *Increased* renal-tubular reabsorption rate—compensates for increased glomerular activity.
         (5) Glycosuria—reflects kidney's inability to reabsorb all glucose filtered by glomeruli (may be normal or may indicate gestational diabetes; glycosuria always warrants further testing).
         (6) *Increased* renal clearance of urea and creatinine (creatinine clearance used as test of renal function during pregnancy).
         (7) Hormone-induced turgescence of bladder and pressure on bladder from gravid uterus (see Table 4–6).

      ◆ b. **Assessment:**
         (1) Urinary frequency, first and third trimesters (see Table 4–6).
         (2) Nocturia.
         (3) Stress incontinence in third trimester.

      ◆ c. **Nursing care plan/implementation:**
         Goal: *health teaching*
         (1) Void with urge, to prevent bladder distention.
         (2) Learn signs and symptoms of UTI.
         (3) Decrease fluid intake in late evening.
         (4) Perform *Kegel* exercises to reduce incontinence.

TABLE 4–6   Common Discomforts During Pregnancy

Discomfort and Cause	Health Teaching
Morning sickness—first 3 mo; nausea and vomiting; may occur anytime, day or night; *cause:* hormonal, psychological, and empty stomach	Alternate dry carbohydrate and fluids hourly; take dry carbohydrate before rising, stay in bed 15 more minutes; *avoid* empty stomach, offending odors, and food difficult to digest (e.g., food high in fat); *avoid* acidic foods
Fatigue (sleep hunger)—first 3 mo; *cause:* possibly hormones; often returns in late pregnancy when physical load is great	Iron supplement if anemic—foods high in *iron, folic acid,* and *protein;* adequate rest
Fainting (syncope)—early pregnancy; due to slightly decreased arterial blood pressure; late pregnancy, due to venous stasis in lower extremities	*Elevate feet;* sit down when necessary; when standing, do not lock knees; *avoid* prolonged standing, fasting
Urinary frequency—enlarging uterus presses on bladder, turgescence of structures from hormone stimulation; relieved somewhat as uterus rises from pelvis; recurs with lightening	*Kegel exercises; limit fluids* just before bedtime to ensure rest; rule out urinary tract infection
Vaginal discharge—mo 2–9; mucus less acidic, and increases in amount (leukorrhea)	Cleanliness important; treat only if infection sets in; douche contraindicated in pregnancy
Hot flashes—heat intolerance, due to increased metabolism → diaphoresis	Alter clothing, bathing, and environmental temperature prn
Headache—cause unknown; possibly blood pressure change, nutritional, tension (unless associated with preeclampsia)	If pain relief needed, consult physician (*avoid* over-the-counter drugs without prescription); reduce tension
Nasal stuffiness—due to increased vascularization; allergic rhinitis of pregnancy	Antihistamines and nasal sprays by *prescription only*
Heartburn—enlarging uterus and hormones slow digestion; progesterone → reverse peristaltic waves → reflux of stomach contents into esophagus	Physician may prescribe an antacid; *"flying exercise"; avoid* use of antacids containing sodium; instead of leaning over, bend at the knees, keeping torso straight; sit on firm chairs; *limit fatty and fried* foods; small, frequent meals
Flatulence—altered digestion from enlarging uterus and hormones	Maintain regular bowel habits, *avoid* gas-forming foods; antiflatulent may be prescribed
Insomnia—fetal movements, fears or concerns, and general body discomfort from heavy uterus	Medication by prescription only; exercise; side-lying *positions* with pillow supports; change position often; back rubs, ventilate feelings
Shortness of breath—enlarging uterus limits expansion of diaphragm	Good posture; cut down/stop smoking; *position*—supine and upright
Backache—increased elasticity of connective tissue, increased weight of uterus, and increased lumbar curvature	Correct posture, low-heeled, wide-base shoes, and abdominal support; do pelvic rock often; *avoid* fatigue
Pelvic joint pain—hormones relax connective tissue and joints and allow movement within joints	Rest; good posture; will go away after giving birth, in 6-8 wk; *avoid* prolonged standing/walking
Leg cramps—pressure of enlarging uterus on nerve supplying legs; possible causes: lack of calcium, fatigue, chilling, and tension	Stretch affected muscle and hold until it subsides; *do not rub* (may release a blood clot, if present); ↑ calcium intake
Constipation—decreased motility (hormones, enlarging uterus) and increased reabsorption of water; iron therapy (oral)	*Diet*—prunes, fruits, vegetables, roughage, and fluids; regular habits; exercise; sit on toilet with knees up; *avoid* enemas, mineral oil, laxatives
Hemorrhoids—varicosities around anus; aggravated by pushing with stool and by uterus pressing on blood vessels supplying lower body	As above, *avoid* constipation; pure Vaseline or Desitin is mild and sometimes soothing; use any other preparation with prescription only
Ankle edema—normal and nonpitting; gravity	Rest legs often during day with legs and hips raised
Varicose veins—lower legs, vulva, pelvis; pressure of heavy uterus; relaxation of connective tissue in vein walls; hereditary	Progressively worse with subsequent pregnancies and obesity; elevate legs above level of heart; support hose may help
Cramp in side or groin—round ligament pain; stretching of round ligament with cramping	To get out of bed, turn to side, use arm and upper body and push up to sitting position

2. *Gastrointestinal system* (see Table 4–6)
   a. **Physiological changes:**
      (1) General decrease in smooth-muscle tone and motility due to actions of progesterone.
      (2) *Intestines:* slowed peristalsis, increased water reabsorption in bowel.
      (3) *Stomach*
         (a) Gastric emptying time is delayed (e.g., 3 hr vs. 1½ hr).
         (b) Gastric secretion of HCl and pepsin decreases.
         (c) Decreased motility delays emptying; increased acidity.
      (4) *Cardiac sphincter* relaxes.
      (5) Increasing size of *uterus* and displacement of *intraabdominal organs.*
      (6) *Gallbladder:* decreased emptying.
   ◆ b. **Assessment:**
      (1) Nausea and vomiting in first trimester.
      (2) Constipation and flatulence.
      (3) Hemorrhoids.
      (4) Heartburn, reflux esophagitis, indigestion.
      (5) Hiatal hernia.
      (6) Epulis—edema and bleeding of gums.
      (7) Ptyalism—excessive salivation.
      (8) Jaundice.
      (9) Gallstones.
      (10) Pruritus due to increased retention of bile salts.
   ◆ c. **Nursing care plan/implementation:**
      Goal: *health teaching*
      (1) Nausea and vomiting
         (a) *Avoid* fatty food; increase carbohydrates.
         (b) Eat small, frequent meals.
         (c) Eat dry crackers in morning.
         (d) *Decrease* liquids with meals.
         (e) *Avoid* odors that predispose to nausea.
      (2) Constipation and flatulence
         (a) *Increase* fluids (6–8 glasses/day).
         (b) Maintain exercise regimen.
         (c) Add *fiber* to diet.
         (d) *Avoid* mineral oil laxatives.
         (e) *Avoid* gas-producing foods (e.g., beans, cabbage).
      (3) Heartburn and indigestion
         (a) *Eliminate* fatty or spicy foods.
         (b) Eat small, frequent meals (6/day).
         (c) Eat slowly.
         (d) *Avoid* gastric irritants (e.g., alcohol, coffee).
         (e) Perform "flying exercises."
         (f) *Avoid* lying flat.
         (g) Take antacids without sodium or phosphorus.
      (h) Sip milk or eat yogurt if heartburn occurs.
      (i) *Avoid* sodium bicarbonate.
   (4) Hemorrhoids
      (a) Increase *fluid and fiber* intake.
      (b) Maintain exercise regimen.
      (c) *Avoid* constipation and straining to defecate.
      (d) Take warm sitz baths.
      (e) Apply witch hazel pads.
      (f) *Elevate* hips and legs frequently.
      (g) Use hemorrhoidal ointments only with advice of health care provider.

E. **Alterations affecting nutrition**
   1. **Physiological changes:**
      a. *Gastrointestinal system*
         (1) Gingivae soften and enlarge due to increased vascularity.
         (2) Increased saliva production.
      b. *Endocrine system*
         (1) *Increased* size and activity of pituitary, parathyroids, adrenals.
         (2) *Increased* vascularity and hyperplasia of thyroid.
         (3) Pancreas—*increased* insulin production during second half of pregnancy, needed to meet rising maternal needs; human placental lactogen (HPL) and insulinase deactivate maternal insulin; may precipitate *gestational diabetes* in susceptible women.
      c. *Metabolism*
         (1) Basal metabolic rate (BMR)—*increases* 25% as pregnancy progresses, due to increasing oxygen consumption; protein-bound iodine (PBI) *increases* to 7–10 μg/dl; metabolism returns to normal by sixth postpartal week.
         (2) Protein—need *increased* for fetal and uterine growth, maternal blood formation.
         (3) Water retention—*increased.*
         (4) Carbohydrates—need *increases* to spare protein stores.
            (a) *First half of pregnancy*—glucose rapidly and continuously siphoned across placenta to meet fetal growth needs; may lead to hypoglycemia and faintness.
            (b) *Second half of pregnancy*—placental production of antiinsulin hormones; normal maternal hyperglycemia; affects coexisting diabetes.
         (5) Fat—*increased* plasma-lipid levels.
         (6) Iron—supplements recommended to meet *increased* need for red blood

cells (RBCs) by maternal/placental/fetal unit.

◆ 2. **Assessment:**
   a. Weight gain: 20–35 lb (11.5–16 kg); depends on Body Mass Index and prepregnant nutritional status.
   b. Normal pattern: first trimester, 2–5 lb (1–2.3 kg); remainder of gestation, approximately 1 lb/wk (0.4–0.5 kg/wk).

◆ 3. **Nursing care plan/implementation:**
   Goal: *health teaching*
   a. Evaluate diet for adequacy of nutrient and caloric intake.
   b. Evaluate cultural, religious, and economic influences on diet.
   c. Review dietary recommendation for pregnancy with woman.
   d. *Avoid* dieting in pregnancy (even if obese).
   e. Supplement diet with *vitamins, iron,* or *folic acid* on advice of health provider.
   f. *Ptyalism:*
      (1) Suck hard candies.
      (2) Perform frequent oral hygiene.
      (3) Maintain adequate oral intake (6-8 glasses/day).
      (4) Use lip balm to prevent chapping.
   g. *Epulis:*
      (1) Frequent oral hygiene.
      (2) Use soft toothbrush.
      (3) Floss gently.
      (4) See dentist regularly.

F. **Alterations affecting protective functions**—*integumentary system*
   1. **Physiological changes**—estrogen-induced vascular and pigment changes.
   ◆ 2. **Assessment:**
      a. Increased pigmentation.
      b. Striae gravidarum (stretch marks).
      c. Increased sebaceous and sweat gland activity.
      d. Palmar erythema.
      e. Angiomas—vascular "spiders."
   ◆ 3. **Nursing care plan/implementation:**
      Goal: *health teaching*
      a. Bathe or shower daily.
      b. Reassure woman that skin changes decrease after pregnancy.

G. **Alterations affecting comfort, rest, mobility**—*musculoskeletal system*
   1. **Physiological changes**
      a. Progesterone, estrogen, and relaxin-induced relaxation of joints, cartilage, and ligaments.
      b. Function in childbearing—increases anteroposterior diameter of rib cage and enlarges birth canal.
   ◆ 2. **Assessment:**
      a. Complaint of pelvic "looseness."
      b. Duck-waddle walk.

   c. Tenderness of symphysis pubis.
   d. Lordosis (exaggerated lumbar curve)—*increased* weight of pelvis tilts pelvis forward; to compensate, woman throws head and shoulders backward; complaint of leg and back strain and fatigue (see Table 4–6)

◆ 3. **Nursing care plan/implementation:**
   Goal: *health teaching*
   a. Good body alignment—tuck pelvis under; tighten abdominal muscles.
   b. Pelvic-rock exercises.
   c. Squat; bend at knees, *not* at waist.
   d. Wear low-heeled, sturdy shoes.
   e. *Avoid* tight-fitting clothing that interferes with circulatory return in legs.

III. **Psychosocial-cultural alterations**
   A. *Emotional changes*—affected by age, maturity, support system, amount of current stresses, coping abilities, physical and mental health status. *Developmental tasks of pregnancy:*
      1. Accept the pregnancy as real: "I am pregnant"; progress from symbiotic relationship with the fetus to perceiving the child as an individual.
      2. Seek and ensure acceptance of child by others.
      3. Seek protection for self and fetus through pregnancy and labor ("safe passage").
      4. Prepare realistically for the coming child and for necessary role change: "I am going to be a parent."
   B. *Physical bases of changes*
      1. *Increased* metabolic demands may result in anemia and fatigue.
      2. *Increased* hormone levels (steroids, estrogen, progesterone)—affect mood as well as physiology.
   C. *Characteristic behaviors*—Table 4–7 describes behaviors commonly exhibited in each trimester.
   D. *Sexuality and sexual expression*—feelings and expressions of sexuality may vary during pregnancy due to maternal adaptations.
   E. *Intrafamily relationships*
      1. Pregnancy is a maturational crisis for the family.
      2. Requires changes in lifestyle and interactions:
         a. Increased financial demands.
         b. Changing family and social relationships.
         c. Adapting communication patterns.
         d. Adapting sexual patterns.
         e. Anticipating new responsibilities and needs.
         f. Responding to reactions of others.

TABLE 4–7   Behavioral Changes in Pregnancy

◆ Assessment/Characteristics	◆ Nursing Care Plan/Implementation
First Trimester	
Emotional lability (mood swings)	Encourage verbalization of feelings, concerns
Displeasure with subjective symptoms of early pregnancy (nausea, fatigue, etc.)	*Health teaching:* diet, rest, relaxation, diversion
Feelings of ambivalence	Validate normalcy of feelings, behaviors
Second Trimester	
Accepts pregnancy (usually coincides with awareness of fetal movement, i.e., "quickening")	Encourage exploration of feelings of dependency, introspection, mood swings
Becomes introspective: resolves old conflicts (feelings toward mother, sexual intimacy, masturbation)	Discuss childbirth preparation and preparation-for-parenthood classes; refer, as necessary
Reevaluates self, lifestyle, marriage	
Daydreams, fantasizes self as "mother"	
Seeks out other pregnant women and new mothers	
Third Trimester	
Altered body image	Encourage verbalization of concerns, discomforts of late pregnancy
Fears body mutilation (stretching of body tissues, episiotomy, cesarean birth)	Help meet dependency needs; offer reassurance, as possible
Distress over loss of control over body functions (ptyalism, colostrum leakage, leukorrhea, urinary frequency, constipation, stress incontinence)	*Health teaching:* Kegel exercises; preparation for labor. Anticipatory guidance and planning for needs of self, baby, and family in early postpartum
Anxiety for baby (deformity, death)	
Fears pain, loss of control in labor	
Acceptance of impending labor during last 2 wk (ready to "move on")	

Prenatal Management

◆ **I. Initial assessment:** Goal: *establish baseline for health supervision, teaching, emotional support, or referral.*

II. Objectives:
   A. Determine woman's present health status and validate pregnancy.
   B. Identify factors affecting or affected by pregnancy.
   C. Determine current gravidity and parity.
   D. Identify present length of gestation.
   E. Establish an estimated date of birth (EDB). Nägele's determination of EDB—subtract 3 mo, add 7 days to last menstrual period (LMP).
   F. Determine relevant knowledge deficit.

◆ **III. Assessment:** *history*
   A. *Family*—inheritable diseases, reproductive problems.
   B. *Personal*—medical, surgical, gynecological, past obstetric, average nonpregnant weight.
     1. *Gravida*—a pregnant woman.
        a. *Nulligravida*—woman who has *never* been pregnant.
        b. *Primigravida*—woman with a *first* pregnancy.
        c. *Multigravida*—woman with a *second or later* pregnancy.
     2. *Para*—refers to *past pregnancies* (not number of babies) that reached viability (20-22 wk) (whether or not born alive).
        a. *Nullipara*—woman who has *not* carried a pregnancy to viability; e.g., may have had one or more abortions.
        b. *Primipara*—woman who has carried *one* pregnancy to viability.
        c. *Multipara*—woman who had *two or more* pregnancies that reached viability.
        d. *Grandmultipara*—woman who has had *six or more* viable pregnancies.
     3. *Examples of gravidity/parity.* Several methods of describing gravidity and parity are in common use. One method (**GTPAL**) describes number of "Gravida" (pregnancies), **T**erm (or full-term infants), **P**reterm infants, **A**bortions, and number of **L**iving children.
        a. A woman who is pregnant for the *first* time and is currently *undelivered* is designated as 1-0-0-0-0. *After* giving birth to

a full-term living neonate, she becomes 1-1-0-0-1.

b. If a woman's second pregnancy ends in abortion and she has a living child from a previous pregnancy, born at term, she is designated as 2-1-0-1-1.

c. A woman who is pregnant for the fourth time and whose previous pregnancies yielded one full-term neonate, premature twins, and one abortion (spontaneous or induced), and who now has three living children, may be designated as 4-1-1-1-3.

d. Others record as follows: number gravida/number para. Applying this system to the examples given above, those mothers would be designated as follows: a—G1P1; b—G2P1; c—G4P2.

e. Others include recording of abortions:
G1P1 Ab0
G2P1 Ab1
G4P2 Ab1

◆ **IV. Assessment: *initial physical aspects:***
  A. Height and weight.
  B. Vital signs.
  C. Blood work—hematocrit and hemoglobin for anemia; type and Rh factor; tests for sickle cell trait, syphilis, rubella antibody titer, and hepatitis B screen (see also Table 4–5).
  D. Urinalysis—glucose, protein, ketones, signs of infection, and pregnancy test (HCG).
  E. Breast examination.
  F. Pelvic examination.
    1. Signs of pregnancy.
    2. Adequacy of pelvis and pelvic structures.
    3. Size and position of uterus.
    4. Papanicolau smear.
    5. Smears for monilial and trichomonal infections.
    6. Signs of pelvic inflammatory disease.
    7. Tests for STD: Gonorrhea (Gonococcus-GC), chlamydia.
  G. *Validation of pregnancy*—physician or midwife makes differential diagnosis between presumptive/probable signs/symptoms of early pregnancy and other signs.
    1. *Presumptive symptoms*—subjective experiences.
      a. Amenorrhea—more than 10 days past missed menstrual period.
      b. Breast tenderness, enlargement.
      c. Nausea and vomiting.
      d. Quickening (wk 16–18).
      e. Urinary frequency.
      f. Fatigue.
      g. Constipation (50% of women).
    2. *Presumptive signs*
      a. Striae gravidarum, linea nigra, chloasma (after wk 16).
      b. Increased basal body temperature (BBT)

3. *Probable signs*—examiner's objective findings.
  a. Positive pregnancy test.
  b. Enlargement of abdomen/uterus.
  c. Reproductive organ changes (after sixth week):
    (1) *Goodell's sign*—cervical softening.
    (2) *Hegar's sign*—softening of lower uterine segment.
    (3) Vaginal changes (*Chadwick's sign*): purple hue in vulvar/vaginal area.
  d. Ballottement (after 16–20 wk).
  e. *Braxton-Hicks* contractions.
4. *Positive signs of pregnancy:*
  ▶ a. Fetal heart tones.
    (1) Doptone: wk 10–12.
    (2) Fetoscope: wk 20.
  b. Examiner visualizes and feels fetal movements (usually after wk 24).
  c. Sonographic examination (after wk 14) when fetal head is sufficiently developed for accurate determination of gestational age. Pregnancy may be detected as early as fifth or sixth week after LMP.

◆ **V. Assessment: *nutritional status:***
  A. Physical findings suggesting poor nutritional status:
    1. Skin: rough, dry, scaly.
    2. Lips: lesions in corners.
    3. Hair: dull, brittle.
    4. Mucous membranes: pale.
    5. Dental caries.
  B. Height, weight, age—average weight gain approximately 24 lb. Range from 24 to 32 lb is best for mother and neonate.
  C. Laboratory values—Hemoglobin: < 10.5/100 mg. Hct: < 32% indicates anemia.
  D. Nutrition history.
◆ **E. Analysis/nursing diagnosis:**
    1. *Altered nutrition: less than body requirements* related to anemia, vitamin/mineral deficit.
    2. *Altered nutrition: more than body requirements* related to obesity.
◆ **F. Nursing care plan/implementation:**
    Goal: *health teaching.* Nutritional counseling for diet in pregnancy and/or lactation.
◆ **G. Evaluation/outcome criteria:**
    1. If *underweight* at conception: should gain 28–42 lb (12.5–18 kg).
    2. If *overweight* at conception: 15–25 lb (7–11.5 kg).
    3. If *obese* at conception: 15 lb (7 kg) or more.

◆ **VI. Assessment: *psychosocial aspects:***
  A. Pregnancy: planned or not; desired or not.
  B. Present plans:
    1. Carry pregnancy, keep baby.
    2. Carry pregnancy, adoption.

Maternal-Infant

3. Abortion.
C. Cultural, ethnic influences on decisions: will influence range of activities, types of safeguarding actions, diet, and health-promotion behaviors.
D. Parenting potential: actively seeking medical care and information about pregnancy, childbirth, parenthood.
E. Family readiness for childbearing and child rearing:
   1. Physical maintenance.
   2. Allocation of resources: identify support system.
   3. Division of labor.
   4. Socialization of family members.
   5. Reproduction, recruitment, launching of family members into society.
   6. Maintenance of order (relationships within family).
F. Perceptions of present and projected family relationships.
G. Review lifestyle for smoking, drugs, alcohol (ETOH), attitudes to pregnancy, health care practices, and risks for hepatitis and human immunodeficiency virus (HIV).

VII. Analysis/nursing diagnosis:
A. *Altered role performance* related to stress imposed by developmental tasks.
B. *Ineffective coping: individual, family* related to stress caused by developmental tasks/crises.
C. *Altered family process* related to developmental tasks. First baby may precipitate individual or family developmental crisis.

VIII. Nursing care plan/implementation:
A. Goal: *anticipatory guidance/support.*
   1. Discuss mood swings, ambivalent feelings, negative feelings.
   2. Reinforce "normalcy" of such feelings.
B. Goal: *increase individual/family coping skills, reduce intrafamily stress.*
   1. Reinforce family strengths (both partners), sense of family identity.
      a. Encourage open communication between partners; share feelings and concerns.
      b. Increase understanding of mutual needs, encourage mutuality of support.
      c. Increase tendency of mother to turn to partner as most significant person (as opposed to physician).
      d. Enhance bond, success of childbirth preparation classes.
   2. Promote understanding/acceptance of role change.
      a. Facilitate/support achievement of developmental tasks.
      b. Reduce probability of postpartal psychological problems.
      c. Promote family bonding.
C. Goal: *health teaching.*

1. *Siblings:*
   a. Alert parents to sibling needs for security, love.
   b. Include sibling in pregnancy experience.
   c. Provide clear, simple explanations of happenings.
   d. Continue demonstrations of love.
   e. Describe increased status ("big sister/brother").
   f. Discuss possible misbehavior to gain attention.
2. *Relatives:* alert parents to possible negative feelings of in-laws.
3. Referral to childbirth preparation/parenting classes.
4. Appropriate community referrals for financial relief to decrease stress and provide aid.

◆ **IX. Evaluation/outcome criteria:**
A. Actively participates in pregnancy-related decision making.
B. Expresses satisfaction with decisions made.
C. Demonstrates growth and development in parenting role.
D. Prepared for the birth and for early parenthood.

Antepartum

I. **Nursing care and obstetric support**
A. **General aspects of prenatal management**
   1. *Scheduled visits:*
      a. Once monthly—until wk 28.
      b. Every 2 wk—wk 28–36.
      c. Weekly—wk 36 until labor.
   ◆ 2. **Assessment:**
      a. General well-being, signs of deviations, concerns, questions.
      b. Weight gain pattern.
      c. Blood pressure (sitting).
   ▶ d. Abdominal palpation:
      (1) Fundal height; tenderness, masses, hernia.
      (2) Fetal heart rate (FHR).
   ▶ (3) Leopold's maneuvers for presentation (after wk 32).
      e. Laboratory tests:
      (1) Urinalysis—for protein, sugar, signs of asymptomatic infection.
      (2) Venous blood—for Hgb, Hct; done initially: VDRL, anti-body titer, sickle cell. HIV recommended for high-risk groups, and hepatitis for high-risk groups.
      (3) Cultures (vaginal discharge; cervical scrapings, for *Chlamydia trachomatis*) prn.
      (4) Tuberculosis (TB) screening in high-risk areas.

(5) Maternal alpha-fetoprotein screen, 16–18 wk optimum time.
(6) Serum-glucose screen, 24–28 wk.

    f. Follow-up on medications (vitamins, iron) and nutrition.

    g. If TB positive during pregnancy, isoniazid (INH) and rifampin given daily. INH is associated with increase in fetal malformations, particularly neurotoxicity. Pyridoxine administered simultaneously to prevent their development.

B. Common minor discomforts during pregnancy (for Assessment, see Table 4–6).

1. **Etiology:** normal maternal physiologic/psychological alterations in pregnancy.

2. **Nursing care plan/implementation:**
   a. Goal: *anticipatory guidance.* Discuss the importance of adequate rest, exercise, diet, and hydration in minimizing symptoms.
   b. Goal: *health teaching* (see Table 4–6).

3. **Evaluation/outcome criteria:** woman avoids, minimizes, or copes effectively with minor usual discomforts of pregnancy.

C. Danger signs:

1. **Etiology:** Specific disease processes are discussed under **Complications.**

2. **Nursing care plan/implementation:**
   Goal: *health teaching*—to safeguard status. Signs to report *immediately:*

> a. Persistent vomiting beyond first trimester or severe vomiting at any time. *Possible cause:* Hyperemesis gravidarum.
> b. Fluid discharge from vagina—bleeding or amniotic fluid (anything other than leukorrhea). *Possible causes:* Placental problem, rupture of membranes (ROM).
> c. Severe or unusual pain: abdominal. *Possible cause:* Abruptio placentae.
> d. Chills or fever. *Possible cause:* Infection.
> e. Burning on urination. *Possible cause:* UTI.
> f. Absence of fetal movements after quickening. *Possible cause:* Intrauterine fetal death.
> g. Visual disturbances—blurring, double vision, "spots before eyes." *Possible cause:* Preeclampsia.
> h. Swelling of fingers or face. *Possible cause:* Preeclampsia.
> i. Severe, frequent, or continual headache. *Possible cause:* Preeclampsia.
> j. Muscle irritability or convulsions. *Possible cause:* Preeclampsia.

3. **Evaluation/outcome criteria:**
   a. Actively participates in own health maintenance/pregnancy management.
   b. Identifies early signs of potentially serious complications during the antepartal period.

    c. Promptly reports and seeks medical attention.

II. Complications during the antepartum
A. General aspects:

1. **Etiology:**
   a. Normal alterations and increasing physiologic stress of pregnancy affect status of coexisting medical disorders.
   b. Conditions affecting mother's general health also affect ability to adapt successfully to normal physiological stress of pregnancy.
   c. Aberrations of normal pregnancy.

2. Goal: *reduce incidence of health problems affecting maternal/fetal health and pregnancy outcome.*
   a. Identify presence of risk factors and signs and symptoms of complications early.
   b. Treat emerging complications promptly and effectively.
   c. Minimize effects of complications on pregnancy outcome.

3. **Assessment:** risk factors:
   a. Age:
      (1) Adolescent.
      (2) Primigravida, age 35 or older.
      (3) Multigravida, age 40 or older.
   b. Socioeconomic level: lower.
   c. Ethnic group
   d. Previous pregnancy history:
      (1) Habitual abortion.
      (2) Multiparity greater than 5.
      (3) Previous stillbirths.
      (4) Previous cesarean birth.
      (5) Preterm labor.
   e. Multifetal pregnancy.
   f. Prenatal care:
      (1) Enters health care system late in pregnancy.
      (2) Irregular/episodic prenatal care visits.
      (3) Noncompliance with medical/nursing recommendations.
   g. Preexisting or coexisting medical disorders:
      (1) Cardiovascular: hypertension, heart disease.
      (2) Diabetes.
      (3) Other: renal, respiratory, infections, acquired immunodeficiency syndrome (AIDS).
   h. Substance abuse.

4. **Nursing care plan/implementation:**
   a. Goal: *health teaching* (discussed under specific health problem).
   b. Goal: *early identification/treatment of emerging health problems* (if any).
      (1) Monitor status and progress of pregnancy.

(2) Refer for medical management, as necessary.

c. Goal: *emotional support.*

◆ 5. **Evaluation/outcome criteria:**

a. Understands present health status, interactions of coexisting disorder and pregnancy.

b. Accepts responsibility for own health maintenance.

c. Makes informed decisions regarding pregnancy.

d. Minimizes potential for complications of coexisting disorder/pregnancy.

(1) Avoids factors predisposing to health problems.

(2) Understands and implements therapeutic management of coexisting disorder/pregnancy.

(3) Increases compliance with medical/nursing recommendations.

e. Carries uneventful pregnancy to successful termination.

B. **Disorders affecting fluid-gas transport: cardiac disease**

1. **Pathophysiology:** cardiac overload → cardiac decompensation → right-sided failure → pulmonary edema.

2. **Etiology:**

a. Congenital heart defects.

b. Valvular damage—due to rheumatic fever (most common lesion is mitral stenosis, which can lead to pulmonary edema and emboli).

c. Increased circulating-blood volume and cardiac output—exceeds cardiac reserve. Greatest risk: *after 28 weeks of gestation*—reaches maximum (30–50%) volume increase; *postpartum*—due to diuresis.

d. Secondary to treatment (tx) (e.g., tocolysis and B methasone)

e. Pregnancy after valve replacement.

3. Normal physiological alterations during pregnancy that *mimic cardiac disorders:*

a. Systolic murmurs, palpitations, tachycardia, and hyperventilation with some dyspnea on normal moderate exertion.

b. Edema of lower extremities.

c. Cardiac enlargement.

d. Elevated sedimentation rate near term.

◆ 4. **Assessment:**

a. Medical evaluation of cardiac status. Classification of severity of cardiac involvement.

(1) *Class I*—least affected; asymptomatic with ordinary activity.

(2) *Class II*—activities somewhat limited; ordinary activities cause fatigue, dyspnea, angina.

(3) *Class III*—moderate/marked limitation of activity; common activities

result in severe symptoms of fatigue, etc.

(4) *Class IV*—most affected; symptomatic (dyspnea, angina) at rest; should avoid pregnancy.

b. **Cardiac decompensation:**

(1) *Subjective symptoms*

Palpitations; feeling that the heart is "racing"

Increasing fatigue or difficulty breathing, or both, with the usual activities

Feeling of smothering and/or frequent cough

Periorbital edema; edema of face, fingers (e.g., rings do not fit anymore), feet, legs

(2) *Objective signs*

Irregular weak, rapid pulse ($\geq$ 100 beats/min)

Rapid respirations ($\geq$ 25 breaths/min)

Progressive, generalized edema

Crackles (rales) at base of lungs, after two inspirations and exhalations

Orthopnea; increasing dyspnea on minimal physical activity

Moist, frequent cough

Cyanosis of lips and nailbeds

◆ 5. **Analysis/nursing diagnosis:**

a. *Fluid volume excess* related to inability of compromised heart to handle increased workload (decreased cardiac reserve → congestive heart failure).

b. *Impaired gas exchange* related to pulmonary edema secondary to congestive heart failure.

◆ 6. **Nursing care plan/implementation:**

a. *Medical management:*

(1) Diuretics, electrolyte supplements.

(2) Digitalis (dose may need to be higher because of dilution in the increased blood volume of pregnancy).

(3) Antibiotics—prophylaxis against rheumatic fever; treatment of bacterial infections during pregnancy.

(4) Anticoagulants. Heparin is preferred because its large molecule cannot easily cross placenta. Occasionally, sequelae may include maternal hemorrhage, preterm birth, stillbirth.

(5) Oxygen, as needed.

(6) Mitral valvotomy for mitral stenosis often brings dramatic relief.

b. Goal: *health teaching.*

(1) Need for compliance with therapeutic regimen, medical/nursing recommendations.

(2) Drug actions, dosage, necessary actions (how to take own pulse, reportable signs/symptoms).

(3) Methods for *decreasing work of heart:*

(a) Adequate *rest*—minimum 10 hr sleep each night; 30 min nap after each meal.

(b) *Avoid* heavy physical *activity* (including housework), fatigue, excessive weight gain, emotional stress, infection.

(c) *Avoid situations* of reduced ambient O_2, such as smoking, exposure to pollutants, flight in unpressurized small planes.

c. Goal: *nutritional counseling.*

(1) Well-balanced *diet;* adequate protein, fresh fruits and vegetables, water.

(2) *Avoid* "junk food," stimulants (caffeine), excessive salt intake.

d. Goal: *anticipatory planning:* management of **labor.**

(1) Goal: *minimize physiological and psychological stress.*

(2) Medical management:

(a) Reevaluation of cardiac status before EDB and labor.

(b) Regional anesthesia for labor/birth.

(c) Low-outlet forceps birth; episiotomy.

◆ (3) **Assessment:** continuous.

(a) Physiological response to labor stimuli—*frequent vital signs* (pulse rate most sensitive and reliable indicator of impending congestive heart failure).

(b) Color, respiratory effort, diaphoresis.

(c) Contractions, etc.—same as for any laboring mother.

◆ (4) **Nursing care plan/implementation:** *labor.*

(a) Goal: *safeguard status.*

(1) Report *promptly:* pulse rate over 100; respirations more than 24 between contractions.

(2) Oxygen at 6 liters, as needed.

(b) Goal: *emotional support*—to reduce anxiety, facilitate cooperation.

(1) Encourage verbalization of feelings, fears, concerns.

(2) Explain all procedures.

(c) Goal: *promote cardiac function.*

Position—semirecumbent; support arms and legs.

(d) Goal: *promote relaxation/control over labor discomfort.* Encourage

Lamaze (or other) breathing/relaxation techniques.

(e) Goal: *reduce stress on cardiopulmonary system.* Discourage bearing-down efforts.

(f) Goal: *relieve stress of pain, eliminate bearing-down.* Prepare for regional anesthesia.

(g) Goal: *maintain effective cardiac function.* Administer medications, as ordered (e.g., digitalis, diuretics, antibiotics).

e. Goal: *anticipatory planning:* **postpartal** management.

(1) Factors increasing risk of cardiac decompensation:

(a) Delivery → rapid, decreased intraabdominal pressure → vasocongestion and rapid rise in cardiac output.

(b) Loss of placental circulation.

(c) Normal diuresis increases circulating blood volume.

◆ (2) **Assessment:**

(a) Observe for tachycardia or respiratory distress.

(b) Monitor blood loss, I&O—potential hypovolemic shock, cardiac overload due to diuresis.

(c) Pain level—potential neurogenic shock.

(d) Same as for any postpartum mother (fundus, signs of infection, etc.).

◆ (3) **Nursing care plan/implementation:** *postpartum.*

(a) Goal: *minimize stress on cardiopulmonary system.*

(i) Rest, dangle, ambulate with aid.

(ii) Gradual increase in activity—as tolerated without symptoms.

(iii) *Position:* semi-Fowler's if needed.

(iv) Extra help with newborn care.

◆ 7. **Evaluation/outcome criteria:**

a. Successfully carries uneventful pregnancy to term.

b. Experiences no cardiopulmonary decompensation during labor, birth, or postpartum.

C. **Disorders affecting fluid-gas transport in fetus: Rh incompatibility**

1. **Pathophysiology**—in an Rh-negative mother: Rh-positive fetal red blood cells enter the maternal circulation → maternal antibody formation → antibodies cross placenta and enter fetal bloodstream → attack fetal red

blood cells → hemolysis → anemia, hypoxia.

a. The pregnant Rh-positive mother carries her infant (Rh negative *or* positive) without incident.

b. The pregnant Rh-negative mother carries an Rh-negative infant without incident.

c. The pregnant Rh-negative mother *usually* carries her first Rh-positive child without problems *unless* she has been sensitized by inadvertent transfusion with Rh-positive blood. *Note:* Fetal cells do not usually enter the maternal bloodstream until placental separation (at abortion, abruptio placentae, amniocentesis, or birth).

2. **Etiology:**

a. The Rh factor is an antigen on the red blood cells of some people (these people are Rh positive); the Rh factor is dominant; a person may be homozygous or heterozygous for Rh factor.

b. An Rh-negative person is homozygous for this recessive trait—does *not* carry the antigen; develops antibodies when exposed to Rh-positive red blood cells (isoimmunization) through transplacental (or other) transfusion.

c. Following birth of an Rh-positive infant, if fetal cells enter the mother's bloodstream, maternal antibody formation begins; antibodies remain in the maternal circulation.

d. At time of next pregnancy with Rh-positive fetus, antibodies cross placenta → hemolysis. *Note: Degree* of hemolysis depends on amount (titer) of maternal antibodies present.

3. Possible serious complication (fetal)—rare today. Hydrops fetalis—most severe hemolytic reaction: severe anemia, cardiac decompensation, hypoxia, edema, ascites, hydrothorax; may be stillborn.

◆ 4. **Assessment:**

a. *Prenatal*—diagnostic procedures:
   (1) Maternal blood type and Rh factor.
   (2) Indirect Coombs test—to determine presence of Rh sensitization (titer indicates amount of maternal antibodies).
   (3) Amniocentesis—as early as 26 weeks of gestation—amount of bilirubin by-products indicates severity of hemolytic activity.
   (4) RhoGAM between 28–32 wk to prevent antibody formation.

b. *Intrapartal* observation of amniotic fluid (after membrane rupture).
   (1) Straw-colored fluid—mild disease.
   (2) Golden fluid—severe fetal disease.

c. *Postnatal*—see III. A. Rh Incompatibility, p. 184.

◆ 5. **Nursing care plan/implementation:**

a. Goal: *prevent isoimmunization in Coombs-negative women*
   (1) *Postabortion*—if no evidence of Rh sensitization (antibody formation) in the Rh-negative mother, administer RhoGAM.
   (2) *Prenatal*—if no evidence of sensitization, administer RhoGAM at 28 weeks of gestation, as ordered, to all Rh-negative women.
   (3) *Postpartum*—if no evidence of sensitization, administer RhoGAM within 72 hr of birth to Rh-negative women who gave birth to Rh-positive baby.

> **Give RhoGAM to:**
> 1. Rh-negative mother who gives birth to Rh-positive neonate.
> 2. Rh-negative mother after spontaneous or induced abortion (>8 wk).
> 3. Rh-negative mother after amniocentesis or chorionic villus sampling (CVS).
> 4. Rh-negative mother between 28 and 32 weeks of gestation.

b. Goal: *health teaching.*
   (1) Explain, discuss that RhoGAM suppresses antibody formation in susceptible Rh-negative women carrying Rh-positive fetus. *Note:* Cannot reverse sensitization if already present.
   (2) Required during and after each pregnancy with Rh-positive fetus.

◆ 6. **Evaluation/outcome criteria:**
   a. Successfully carries pregnancy to term.
   b. No evidence of Rh isoimmunization.
   c. Birth of viable infant.

D. **Disorders affecting nutrition: diabetes mellitus**

1. **Pathophysiology**—increased demand for insulin exceeds pancreatic reserve → inadequate insulin production; enzyme (insulinase) activity breaks down circulating insulin → further reduction in available insulin; increased tissue resistance to insulin; glycogenolysis/gluconeogenesis → ketosis.

2. **Etiology**—increased metabolic rate; action of placental hormones (see below), enzyme (insulinase) activity.

3. *Normal physiologic* alterations during pregnancy that may *affect* management of the *diabetic* woman, or *precipitate gestational diabetes* in susceptible women:
   a. Hormone production:
      (1) Human placental lactogen (HPL)
      (2) Progesterone.
      (3) Estrogen.
      (4) Cortisol.

b. *Effects of hormones:*
   (1) Decreased glucose tolerance.
   (2) Increased metabolic rate.
   (3) Increased production of adrenocortical and pituitary hormones.
   (4) Decreased effectiveness of insulin (increased resistance to insulin by peripheral tissues).
   (5) Increased gluconeogenesis.
   (6) Increased size and number of islets of Langerhans to meet increased maternal needs.
   (7) Increased mobilization of free fatty acids.
   (8) Decreased renal threshold, increased glomerular filtration rate; glycosuria common.
   (9) Decreased CO_2-combining power of blood; higher metabolic rate increases tendency to acidosis.

c. *Effect of pregnancy on diabetes:*
   (1) Nausea and vomiting—predispose to ketoacidosis.
   (2) Insulin requirements—relatively stable or may decrease in first trimester; rapid *increase* during second and third trimesters; rapid *decrease* after birth to prepregnant level.
   (3) Pathophysiological progression (nephropathy, retinopathy, and arteriosclerotic changes) may appear; existing pathology may worsen.

4. *Effect of poorly controlled diabetes on pregnancy*—increased incidence of:
   a. Infertility.
   b. UTI.
   c. Vaginal infections (moniliasis).
   d. Spontaneous abortion.
   e. Congenital anomalies (three times as prevalent).
   f. Preeclampsia/eclampsia.
   g. Polyhydramnios.
   h. Preterm labor and birth.
   i. Fetal macrosomia—cephalopelvic disproportion (CPD).
   j. Stillbirth.

◆ 5. **Assessment:** *gestational diabetes (mellitus)*
   a. History:
      (1) Family history.
      (2) Previous infant 9 lb or more.
      (3) Unexplained fetal wastage—abortion, stillbirth, or early neonatal death.
      (4) Obesity with very rapid weight gain.
      (5) Polyhydramnios (excessive amniotic fluid).
      (6) Previous infant with congenital anomalies.
      (7) Increased tendency for intense vaginal or urinary tract infections.
      (8) Previous history of gestational diabetes

b. Symptoms: **3 "Ps"**—*polydipsia, polyphagia, polyuria*—and weight loss.
c. *Abdominal assessment:*
   (1) Fetal heart rate.
   (2) Excessive fundal height.
      (a) Hydramnios.
      (b) Large-for-gestational-age (LGA) fetus. *Note:* With vascular pathology, small-for-gestational-age (SGA) fetus.
d. *Medical diagnosis*—procedures:
   (1) 50 g oral glucose tolerance test (GTT): woman ingests 50 g oral glucose solution; 1 hr later plasma glucose obtained. If > 140 mg/dl, 3 hr oral GTT ordered.
   (2) Abnormal GTT: two or more of the following findings are diagnostic of gestational diabetes.

   > (a) Fasting blood sugar (FBS) ≥ 105 mg/dl.
   > (b) One hour ≥ 190 mg/dl.
   > (c) Two hours ≥ 165 mg/dl.
   > (d) Three hours ≥ 145 mg/dl.

   (3) *Diabetic classification criteria*
      (a) Class A—gestational or chemical diabetes (abnormal GTT).
      (b) Class B—overt diabetes, onset after age 20, duration less than 10 yr, no vascular involvement.
      (c) Class C—overt diabetes, onset before age 20, duration 10–20 yr, no vascular involvement.
      (d) Class D—overt diabetes, onset before age 10, duration longer than 20 yr, vascular involvement, benign retinopathy, leg calcification.
      (e) Class F—renal impairment.
e. Woman with known diabetes—all classes.
   (1) Knowledge and acceptance of disease and its management:
      (a) Signs and symptoms of hyperglycemia/hypoglycemia (Table 7–27, p. 528).
      (b) Appropriate behaviors (e.g., skim milk for symptoms of hypoglycemia).
   (2) Skill and accuracy in monitoring serum glucose (dextrometer use).
   (3) Skill and accuracy in preparing and administering insulin dosage; site rotation; subcutaneous injection.
   (4) Close monitoring—prenatal status assessment every 2 wk until 30 wk, then weekly until birth. Alert to signs of emerging problems (need for insulin adjustment, polyhydramnios, macrosomia).
   (5) Other—as for any pregnant woman.

Maternal-Infant

◆ 6. **Analysis/nursing diagnosis:**
   a. *Knowledge deficit* related to pathophysiology, interactions with pregnancy, management (e.g., insulin administration).
   b. *Altered nutrition, more or less than body requirements,* related to weight gain.
   c. High-risk pregnancy: high risk for infection, ketosis, perinatal wastage, fetal macrosomia, cephalopelvic disproportion, polyhydramnios, preterm labor and birth, congenital anomalies.

◆ 7. **Nursing care plan/implementation:**
   a. Goal: *health teaching.*
      (1) Pathophysiology of diabetes, as necessary; effect of pregnancy on management.
      (2) Signs and symptoms of hyperglycemia, hypoglycemia; appropriate management of symptoms.
      (3) Hygiene—to reduce probability of infection.
      (4) Exercise—needed to control serum-glucose levels, to regulate weight gain, and for feeling of well-being.
      (5) Need for close monitoring during pregnancy.
      (6) Insulin regulation:
         (a) Requirements vary through pregnancy: *first trimester*—may decrease with some periods of hypoglycemia due to fetal drain; *second trimester*—increased need for insulin; *third trimester*—needs may be triple prepregnant dose; acidosis more common in late pregnancy (precipitated by emotional stress, infection).
         (b) Serum-glucose testing—dextrometer, Acucheck, or other.
         (c) Preparation and self-administration of insulin injection, as necessary.
         (d) Prompt reporting of fluctuating serum-glucose levels.
      (7) Diagnostic testing/hospitalization:
         (a) Nonstress test.
         (b) Sonography.
         (c) Amniocentesis.
   b. Goal: *dietary counseling.*
      (1) Optimal weight gain—about 24 lb.
      (2) Needs 35 calories/kg of ideal body weight.
      (3) Protein—20% (2 g/kg, or about 70 g daily).
      (4) Carbohydrates: 30–45% in complex form (milk, bread).
      (5) Fats—unsaturated.
      (6) Appropriate exchanges.
   c. *Medical management:* hospitalize woman for:

      (1) Regulation of insulin (oral hypoglycemics **contraindicated** in pregnancy, due to teratogenicity; crosses placental barrier).
      (2) Control of infection.
      (3) Determination of fetal jeopardy or indications for early termination of pregnancy.

◆ 8. **Evaluation/outcome criteria:**
   a. Understands and accepts diagnosis of diabetes.
   b. Actively participates in effective management of diabetes and pregnancy.
   c. Maintains serum-glucose levels within acceptable parameters (e.g., 70–120 mg/dl).
      (1) Monitors serum-glucose levels accurately (dextrometer, Acucheck, urine testing).
      (2) Prepares and self-administers insulin appropriately.
      (3) Complies with dietary regimen.

9. **Antepartal** *hospitalization*
◆ a. **Assessment:**
      (1) *Medical evaluation*—procedures:
         (a) Serum-glucose levels (↓120 mg).
         (b) Sonography for fetal growth: biophysical profile (BPP) evaluates fetal physical well-being and volume of amniotic fluid.
         (c) Nonstress testing/contraction stress testing.
         (d) Amniocentesis for fetal maturity (*Note:* L/S ratio may be elevated in diabetic women; *phosphatidylglycerol [PG]* more accurate for diabetic women.)
      (2) **Nursing assessment:**
         (a) Daily weight, vital signs, FHR q4h, I&O.
         ▶ (b) Fundal height and Leopold's maneuvers on admission.
◆ b. **Nursing care plan/implementation.**
      Goal: *emotional support*—to reduce anxiety and tension, which contribute to insulin imbalance.
      (1) Explain all procedures.
      (2) Assist with tests for fetal status.
      (3) Prepare for possibility of preterm or cesarean birth.

10. *Anticipatory planning*—management of **labor**
◆ a. **Assessment:** continuous.
      (1) Signs and symptoms of hyperglycemia, hypoglycemia (Table 7–27, p. 528).
      (2) Electronic fetal monitoring—to identify signs of fetal distress.
      (3) Other—as for any laboring woman.
◆ b. **Nursing care plan/implementation:**
      Goal: *safeguard maternal/fetal status.*

Position: lateral Sims'—to reduce compression of inferior vena cava and aorta due to polyhydramnios or LGA baby. (Supine hypotensive syndrome results from compression; reduced placental perfusion increases incidence of fetal hypoxia/anoxia.)

c. *Medical management*—varies widely.

   (1) Timing—amniocentesis to determine PG and *phosphatidylinositol* levels (estimate fetal pulmonary surfactant).

   (2) Insulin added to intravenous infusion of 0.9 NaCl and titrated to maintain serum glucose approximately 100 mg/dl. 5–10% D/W I.V. needed to prevent hypoglycemia that may lead to maternal ketoacidosis; hyperglycemia may result in newborn hypoglycemia.

   (3) Ultrasound or x-ray pelvimetry to identify CPD.

11. *Anticipatory planning*—management of **postpartum**

  a. Factors influencing serum-glucose levels:

    (1) Loss of placental hormones that degrade insulin.

    (2) Lower metabolic rate. Woman requiring large doses of insulin may need to triple caloric intake and decrease insulin by one-half.

◆ b. **Assessment:**

    (1) Observe for:

      (a) Hypoglycemia.

      (b) Infection.

      (c) Preeclampsia/eclampsia (higher incidence in diabetic women).

      (d) Hemorrhage (associated with polyhydramnios, macrosomia, induction of labor, forceps birth, or cesarean birth).

    (2) Monitor healing of episiotomy/abdominal incision.

◆ c. **Nursing care plan/implementation:**

    (1) *Medical management:* insulin calibration—requirement may drop to one-half or two-thirds pregnant dosage on first postpartum day if woman is on full diet (due to loss of human placental lactogen and conversion of serum glucose to lactose).

    (2) *Nursing management*

      (a) Goal: *euglycemia.* Acucheck, insulin as ordered.

      (b) Goal: *avoid trauma, reduce risk of UTI. Avoid* catheterization, where possible.

      (c) Goal: *health teaching.* Nipple care—to prevent fissures and possible mastitis.

    (d) Goal: *reduce serum-glucose and insulin needs.* Encourage/support breastfeeding → antidiabetogenic effect. *Note:* If *acetonuria* occurs, stop breastfeeding while physician readjusts diet/insulin balance; may pump breasts to maintain lactation. If *hypoglycemic,* adrenalin level rises → decreased milk supply and letdown reflex.

12. *Anticipatory guidance*—**discharge plan/implementation**

  a. Goal: *counseling.* Reinforce recommendations of physicians/genetic counselors.

    (1) Risk of infant inheriting gene for diabetes is greater if mother has early-onset, non-insulin-dependent disease.

    (2) Increased risk of congenital disorders.

  b. Goal: *family planning*

    (1) Oral contraceptives are controversial because they decrease carbohydrate tolerance; may be cautiously prescribed for women with no vascular disease and who are nonsmokers. IUD **contraindicated** because of impaired response to infection. Barrier contraceptives (diaphragm or condoms with spermicides) recommended.

    (2) Tubal ligation: if mother has vascular involvement, i.e., retinopathy or nephropathy, increased risk with later pregnancies (see Table 4–2).

  c. Goal: *health teaching.*

    (1) Self-care measures.

    (2) Importance of eating on time, even if infant must wait to breastfeed or bottle feed.

    (3) Importance of adequate rest and exercise to maintain insulin/glucose balance.

    (4) Organize schedule to care for infant, other children, and her diabetes. Allow time for self.

◆ d. **Evaluation/outcome criteria:**

    (1) Successfully completes an uneventful pregnancy, labor, and birth of a normal, healthy newborn.

    (2) Makes informed judgments regarding parenting, family planning, management of her diabetes.

E. Disorders affecting psychosocio-cultural behaviors: substance abuse

◆ 1. **Assessment:** pregnant substance abuser

  a. *Medical history*

    (1) Infections: HIV-positive status, AIDS, STDs, hepatitis, cirrhosis, cellulitis, en-

docarditis, pancreatitis, pneumonia.
(2) Psychiatric illness: depression, paranoia, irritability.
(3) Trauma related to violence.
  b. *Obstetric history*
(1) Spontaneous abortions.
(2) History of abruptio placentae.
(3) Preterm labor.
(4) Preterm rupture of membranes.
(5) Fetal death.
(6) Low-birth-weight (LBW) infants.
(7) Tremors/seizures.
  c. *Current pregnancy*
(1) Preterm labor contractions.
(2) Hypoactivity or hyperactivity in fetus.
(3) Poor or decreased weight gain.
(4) STD.
(5) Undiagnosed vaginal bleeding.
(6) Drugs being used and methods of self-administration.
  d. *Psychosocial history*
(1) Attitudes re: pregnancy.
(2) Current support system: lacking.
(3) Current living arrangements; lifestyle.
(4) History of psychiatric illness.
(5) History of physical, sexual abuse.
(6) Involvement with legal system.
  e. *Physical examination*
  f. *Commonly abused substances*
(1) Nicotine.
(2) Alcohol (fetal alcohol syndrome [FAS] or fetal alcohol effects [FAE]).
(3) Marijuana.
(4) Stimulants—cocaine, crack, ice, methamphetamine
(5) Opiates—heroin, methadone, Darvon, codeine, Vicodin, Oxycontin.
(6) Sedatives, hypnotics.
(7) Caffeine.
(8) Ecstasy.
  g. *Neonatal outcomes*
(1) LBW, small heads.
(2) Irritable, difficult to console.
(3) Disorganized suck-swallow reflex.
(4) Impaired motor development.
(5) Congenital anomalies: genitourinary, gastrointestinal, limb anomalies.
(6) Cerebral infarctions.
(7) Breastfeeding contraindicated unless mother is drugfree for 3 months.
(8) Poor, slow weight gain; failure to thrive.
◆ 2. **Analysis/nursing diagnosis:**
  a. *Altered nutrition: less than body requirements*—poor weight gain related to poor nutrition.
  b. *Altered nutrition: less than body requirements*—slow fetal growth related to slow gain in weight.
  c. *Altered placental function* related to high risk for abruptio placentae.

  d. *Noncompliance* with health care protocols related to persistent drug use.
  e. *Altered parenting* related to psychological illness (substance dependence).
◆ 3. **Nursing care plan/implementation:**
  a. Early identification of substance abuser.
  b. Stabilize physiological status.
  c. Fetal surveillance.
  d. Urge consistent obstetric care.
  e. Refer for social services.
◆ 4. **Evaluation/outcome criteria:**
  a. Seeks out and uses social services and drug treatment program.
  b. Abstains from illicit substances during pregnancy.
  c. Successfully completes an uneventful pregnancy, labor, and birth of normal healthy infant.

III. Other high-risk women
  A. Pregnant adolescent
    1. **General aspects:**
      a. Pregnancy in female between 12 and 17 years old.
      b. Incidence has started to ↓; approximately one-third of all births are to adolescents.
      c. *Predisposing factors:* early menarche, early experimentation with sex, poor family relationships, poverty, late or no prenatal care, cultural influence.
      d. *Associated health problems:* pregnancy-induced hypertension (PIH), preterm labor, SGA infants, anemia, bleeding disorders, infections, CPD.
      e. *Social problems:* poorly educated mothers, child abuse, single-parent families, mothers who are unemployed or working at minimum wage or who lack support system.
◆ 2. **Assessment:**
      a. Present physical/health status.
      b. Feelings toward pregnancy.
      c. Plans for the future.
      d. Factors influencing decisions related to self, pregnancy, baby.
      e. Signs and symptoms of complications of pregnancy (see A.1.d *Associated health problems*).
      f. Need/desire for health maintenance information (family planning).
◆ 3. **Analysis/nursing diagnosis:**
      a. *Ineffective coping, individual/family,* related to need to alter lifestyle, plans, expectations.
      b. *Altered family processes,* related to unexpected/unwanted pregnancy.
      c. *Altered parenting* related to intrafamily stress secondary to unexpected pregnancy, developmental tasks.
      d. *Self-esteem disturbance* related to altered self-concept, body image, role performance, personal identity.

e. *Knowledge deficit* related to family planning, health maintenance, risk factors, pregnancy options.

f. *Altered nutrition* related to lifestyle

◆ 4. **Nursing care plan/implementation:**

a. Goal: *emotional support.*

   (1) Ensure confidentiality.

   (2) Establish acceptant, supportive environment.

   (3) Encourage verbalization of feelings, concerns, fears, desires, etc.

   (4) Maintain continuity of care—consistency of nursing approach, to establish trust, confidentiality.

b. Goal: *facilitate informed decision making.* Discuss available options; aid in exploring implications of possible decisions.

c. Goal: *nutritional counseling* (anemia).

   (1) Needs for own growth and that of fetus.

   (2) High-quality diet—value for character of skin, return to prepregnant figure.

   (3) Include pizza, hamburgers, milkshakes as acceptable—to minimize anger at being "different."

d. Goal: *health teaching.*

   (1) Rest, exercise, hygiene—as for other women.

   (2) Prevention of infection—STD, UTI, etc.

   (3) Breast self-exam; Pap smear.

   (4) Future family planning options (see Table 4–1).

e. Goal: *assist in achievement of normal developmental tasks.* Encourage exploration of new role and responsibilities.

f. Goal: *referral to appropriate resources.*

   (1) Abortion.

   (2) Preparation for childbirth and parenting classes.

   (3) Family counseling.

   (4) Social services.

g. Goal: *assist in facilitating/continuing/completing basic education.*

   (1) Communicate with school nurse.

   (2) Explore other options available in community.

◆ 5. **Evaluation/outcome criteria:**

a. Makes informed decisions appropriate to individual and family needs, desires.

b. Actively participates in own health maintenance.

   (1) Complies with medical/nursing recommendations.

   (2) Minimizes potential for complications of pregnancy.

c. Copes effectively with normal physiological and psychosocial alterations of pregnancy.

d. Both woman and baby's father express satisfaction with decision and management of this pregnancy. If parenthood is chosen and pregnancy is successful, accepts parenting role.

B. Older mother: primigravida over age 35

1. *General aspects*—higher incidence of congenital anomalies (e.g., Down syndrome), increased possibility of complications of pregnancy. However, generally it is a conscious decision to have postponed childbearing. Individuals are usually used to making own decisions regarding career and health care.

◆ 2. **Assessment:**

a. Same as for other pregnant women.

b. Reaction to reality of pregnancy.

c. Family response to pregnancy.

◆ 3. **Analysis/nursing diagnosis:**

a. *Fear* related to threat to pregnancy.

b. *Knowledge deficit* related to aspects of pregnancy care.

◆ 4. **Nursing care plan/implementation:**

a. Goal: *anticipatory guidance.* Preparation for parenthood, altered lifestyle, potential change of career. Assist with realistic expectations. Refer to "over 30" parents' support group.

b. Goal: *health teaching.* Explain, discuss special diagnostic procedures. See xx Amniocentesis, Figure 4–6, p. 121.

c. Other—same as for other pregnant women.

◆ 5. **Evaluation/outcome criteria:**

a. Experiences normal, uncomplicated pregnancy, labor, and birth of normal, healthy newborn.

b. Expresses satisfaction with decision and outcome of this pregnancy.

C. Older mother: multipara over age 40

1. *General aspects*

a. Increased incidence of preexisting and coexisting medical disorders (hypertension, diabetes, arthritis).

b. Increased incidence of complications of pregnancy (preeclampsia/eclampsia, hemorrhage).

c. Smoking is major risk factor.

◆ 2. **Assessment:**

a. Same as for other pregnant women.

b. Reaction to pregnancy (varies from pleasure at still being "young enough," to despair, if facing decision to abort).

c. History, signs and symptoms of coexisting disorders.

d. Indications of reduced physical ability to cope with normal physiological alterations of pregnancy.

e. Family constellation: stage of family developmental cycle, responses to this

pregnancy (especially adolescents' reaction to parents' pregnancy).
◆ 3. **Analysis/nursing diagnosis:** same as for over-35 age group.
◆ 4. **Nursing care plan/implementation:**
   a. Goal: *emotional support.* Encourage verbalization of feelings, fears, concerns.
   b. Goal: *referral to appropriate resource.*
      (1) Genetic counseling.
      (2) Abortion/support groups.
      (3) Preparation for childbirth and parenthood classes.
   c. Goal: *facilitate/support effective family process.* Involve family in preparation for birth and integration of newborn into family unit.
   d. Other—same as for other pregnant women.
◆ 5. **Evaluation/outcome criteria:**
   a. Makes informed decisions related to pregnancy.
   b. Expresses satisfaction with decision and outcome of this pregnancy.
   c. Experiences uncomplicated pregnancy, labor, and birth of normal, healthy newborn.

D. AIDS
   1. **General aspects**—AIDS is a serious condition affecting the immune system. Heterosexual females are considered at risk if they or their sexual partners:
      a. Are HIV positive.
      b. Are IV drug users (50%).
      c. Received blood between 1977 and 1985 (9%).
      d. Are homosexual or bisexual males (39%).
      e. Are hemophiliacs.
◆ 2. **Assessment**—general symptoms:
   a. Malaise.
   b. Chronic cough; possible tuberculosis.
   c. Chronic diarrhea.
   d. HIV positive.
   e. Weight loss: 10 lb in 2 mo.
   f. Night sweats; lymphadenopathy.
   g. Skin lesions; thrush.
   h. PID; STDs; vulvovaginitis (usually, yeast [*Candidiasis*]), often refractory and severe.
   i. Cervical cytologic abnormalities; often infected with human papillomavirus (HPV).
◆ 3. **Analysis/nursing diagnosis:**
   a. *Altered nutrition, less than body requirements,* related to general malaise.
   b. *Fatigue,* related to altered health status, weight loss.
   c. *Fear* related to progressively debilitating disease.
   d. *Knowledge deficit* related to disease progression, treatment, life expectancy.

   e. *Ineffective individual coping* related to disease progression.
◆ 4. **Nursing care plan/implementation:**
   a. Identify women at risk.
   b. Protect confidentiality.
   c. Implement standard precautions.
   d. Use proper gloves, gown, hand washing.
   e. Use protective eyewear and mask in labor, birth.
◆ 5. **Evaluation/outcome criteria:**
   a. No further transmission of virus.
   b. Woman's confidentiality maintained.
   c. Standard precautions implemented.
   d. Emotional support implemented.
   e. Supportive groups contacted.
   6. **HIV-positive women**—pregnancy management:
      a. *Antepartum*
         (1) Increased incidence of other STD (gonorrhea, syphilis, herpes, HPV).
         (2) Increased incidence of cytomegalovirus (CMV).
         (3) Differential diagnosis for all pregnancy-induced complaints.
         (4) Counsel regarding nutrition.
         (5) Advise about risk to infant.
         (6) Counsel regarding safer sex.
      b. *Intrapartum*
         (1) Focus on prevention of transmission.
         ▶ (2) External electronic fetal monitoring (EFM) preferred.
         (3) Mode of birth not based on disease.
         (4) *Avoid* use of fetal scalp electrodes or sampling.
      c. *Postpartum*
         (1) No remarkable alteration in disease progression.
         (2) Breastfeeding **contraindicated.**
         (3) Implement standard precautions for mother and infant.
         (4) Refer to specialists in AIDS care and treatment.
   7. **Newborn or neonate:**
      a. **General aspects:** Neonatal AIDS—transmission may be transplacental, contact with maternal blood at birth, or postnatal exposure to infected parent (i.e., breastfeeding). Classic signs evident in adult often not present. Common signs: lymphadenopathy, hepatosplenomegaly, oral candidiasis, bacterial infections, failure to thrive.
      b. Implement standard precautions for all invasive procedures. Wear gloves for all contact before first bath.
      c. Provide supportive nursing care (thermoregulation, respiratory).
      d. Encourage parent-infant contact.
      e. Provide opportunities for sensory stimuli and touch.

f. Monitor intake and weight gain.

g. Observe for signs of infection.

h. Initiate social service consultation.

i. Counsel family about vaccinations (should receive all *except* oral polio).

Emergency Conditions by Trimester

See Table 4–8.

Common Complications of Pregnancy

First Trimester Complications

I. **Complications affecting fluid-gas transport: hemorrhagic disorders**

   A. **General aspects** (review Table 4–8)

   ◆ 1. **Assessment:**

   a. Vital signs, output, general status.

   b. Evidence of internal/external bleeding (pad count).

   c. Pain.

   d. Emotional response.

   e. Perineal pads saturated and number.

   f. Speculum examination.

   ◆ 2. **Analysis/nursing diagnosis:**

   a. *Knowledge deficit* related to diagnosis, prognosis, treatment, sequelae.

   b. *Anxiety/fear* related to loss of pregnancy, surgery.

   c. *Fluid volume deficit, potential/actual,* related to excessive blood loss.

   d. *Pain.*

   e. *Ineffective coping, individual/family,* related to knowledge deficit and fear.

   f. *Anticipatory/dysfunctional grieving,* related to loss of pregnancy.

   g. *Disturbance in self-esteem, body image, role performance,* related to threat to self-image as woman and childbearer.

   ◆ 3. **Nursing care plan/implementation:**

   a. Goal: *minimize blood loss, stabilize physiological status.*

   (1) Facilitate prompt medical management.

   ▶ (2) Administer IV fluids, blood, as ordered.

   (3) Administer analgesics, as needed.

   b. Goal: *prevent infection.* Strict aseptic technique.

   c. Goal: *emotional support.*

   (1) Encourage verbalization of anxiety, fears, concerns.

   (2) Supportive care for grief reaction (p. 316).

   ◆ 4. **Evaluation/outcome criteria:**

   a. Blood loss minimized; physiological status stable.

   b. Copes effectively with loss of pregnancy.

   B. **Spontaneous abortion:** *before viable age of 20–22 wk*

   1. **Etiology:**

   a. Defective products of conception.

   b. Insufficient production of progesterone.

   c. Acute infections.

   d. Reproductive system abnormalities, e.g., incompetent cervical os.

   e. Trauma (physical or emotional).

   f. Rh incompatibility.

   ▶ 2. **Assessment:** types

   a. *Threatened*—mild bleeding, spotting, cramping; cervix closed.

   b. *Inevitable*—moderate bleeding, painful cramping; cervix dilated, positive Nitrazine test (membranes ruptured).

   c. *Imminent*—profuse bleeding, severe cramping, urge to bear down.

   d. *Incomplete*—fetal parts or fetus expelled; placenta and membranes retained.

   e. *Complete*—all products of conception expelled; minimal vaginal bleeding.

   f. *Habitual/recurrent*—history of spontaneous loss of three or more successive pregnancies.

   g. *Missed*—fetal death with no spontaneous expulsion within 4 weeks.

   (1) Anorexia, malaise, headache.

   (2) Fundal height—inconsistent with gestational estimate.

   (3) Laboratory—prolonged clotting time, due to resultant concurrent hypofibrinogenemia (disseminated intravascular coagulation [DIC], a major threat to mother).

   h. *Elective abortions* (intentionally introduced loss of pregnancy).

   ◆ 3. **Analysis/nursing diagnosis:**

   a. *Altered family processes* related to pregnancy, circumstances surrounding abortion.

   b. *Sexual dysfunction* related to compromised self-image, altered interpersonal relationship, guilt feelings.

   ◆ 4. **Nursing care plan/implementation:**

   a. *Threatened*—Goal: *health teaching.* Suggest: *avoid* coitus and orgasm, especially around normal time for menstrual period.

   b. *Incomplete, inevitable, imminent.*

   (1) Goal: *safeguard status.*

   (a) Save all pads, clots, tissue for expert diagnosis.

TABLE 4–8 **Emergency Conditions**

First Trimester

◆ Assessment/Observations	Possible Problem	◆ Nursing Care Plan/Implementation
Fluid-Gas Transport		
a. *Cramping*—with or without bleeding or passage of tissue	Abortion (before 24 wk) Threatened Imminent, incomplete, septic	Bed rest, sedation, *avoid* coitus—if threatened; bed rest, start IV fluids and draw blood for laboratory work: CBC, type/crossmatch, electrolytes, platelets, HCG levels
b. *Passage of tissue* (products of conception; grapelike vesicles) or *brown spotting;* fundus too high for gestational age; *blood pressure* elevated. Often associated with hyperemesis gravidarum and preeclampsia	Hydatidiform mole (trophoblastic disease)	Vital signs q5–15 min, prn
c. Severe *pain, shock* out of proportion to amount of overt blood; shoulder-strap pain (*Kehr's sign*), a "referred pain" that indicates intraabdominal bleeding (or rupture of ovarian cyst); amenorrhea of 6–12 wk	Ectopic pregnancy	Save all pads or tissue passed through vagina for physician evaluation **No** rectal or vaginal examination until physician is present
d. Malodorous *discharge; hyperthermia and chills;* tender abdomen	Septic abortion (self-induced or "criminal")	Take complete history, if possible Convulsion precautions if hypertensive
e. *Ecchymosis or bleeding*—with a history that includes any or all of the following: had symptoms of pregnancy, but they subsided; pregnancy test negative; uterine size diminishing; no FHR	Missed abortion with possible DIC (retained dead fetus syndrome)	Emotional support for loss of pregnancy (through nurse's manner, tone of voice, touch, use of woman's name, keep her informed of what is happening); oxygen, prn

Second Trimester

◆ Assessment/Observations	Possible Problem	◆ Nursing Care Plan/Implementation
Fluid-Gas Transport		
a. Cramping; passage of products of conception	Late abortion	Same as for first trimester
b. Labor—cervical changes, "show"	Incompetent cervical os	See physician immediately for possible cerclage
c. *Prolonged* nausea and vomiting; unexplained *hypertension* or *preeclampsia;* passage of dark blood or grapelike vesicles; *absent FHRs;* excessive fundal height for gestation	Hydatidiform mole	Maintain hydration; assess for dehydration; refer to physician
Sensory-Perceptual		
a. *Preeclampsia/eclampsia* *Assessment:* hypertension first noted after 24 wk; followed by increased proteinuria *Symptoms:* blurred or double vision; pain: headache, epigastric (late sign) *Signs:* BP 160/110; 3+ proteinuria Edema: facial, digital; pulmonary Oliguria Hyperreflexia	With increased severity: renal failure, circulatory collapse, CVA, coagulation defects (DIC); abruptio placentae; convulsions	Pharmacological management of hypertension (see Unit 7) **Convulsion precautions:** 1. Emergency tray at bedside 2. Oxygen/suction 3. Start IV 4. Padded siderails 5. Limit environmental stimulation 6. Constant observation 7. Deep-tendon reflexes 8. Daily weight 9. I&O—strict 10. Note any complaints and changes 11. Prepare for lab work (type and crossmatch, CBC, platelets, BUN, and creatinine, uric acid, SGOT, SGPT)

b. *Convulsions* in absence of hypertension, proteinuria, or facial edema	CVA, epilepsy, drug toxicity; intracranial injury; diabetic complications; encephalopathy	**Convulsion care:**
		1. Oxygen/mask; drugs (Valium, magnesium sulfate IV)
		2. Observe:
		  a. Uterine tone, FHR, fetal activity
		  b. Signs of labor
		3. Emotional support for woman and family

TABLE 4–8 Emergency Conditions—cont'd

Third Trimester		
◆ Assessment/Observations	Possible Problem	◆ Nursing Care Plan/Implementation
Fluid-Gas Transport		
a. *Bleeding:* painless, bright red, vaginal Contractions or uterine tone normal	Placenta previa	**No vaginal exam** Apply fetal monitor; assess for labor; *position:* ▨ semi- to high Fowler's; ultrasound to verify placental location
b. *Pain:* abdomen rigid and tender to touch Increased uterine tone; signs of shock disproportionate to visible blood loss; may have loss of FHTs; associated with: preeclampsia, multiparity, precipitous labor, oxytocin induction trauma, cocaine use	Abruptio placentae	▨ As for placenta previa; *position:* Sims' Prepare for possible emergency Cesarean delivery

        (b) Report immediately any change in status, excessive bleeding, signs of infection, shock.

        (c) Prepare for surgery.

    (2) Goal: *comfort measures.*

        (a) Administer analgesics, as necessary.

        (b) Bed rest, quiet diversional activities.

    (3) Goal: *emotional support.*

        (a) Encourage verbalization of fear, concerns.

        (b) Reduce anxiety, as possible.

        (c) If pregnancy terminates, facilitate grieving process; assist in working through guilt feelings (p. 144).

        (d) Supportive care for grief reaction (p. 144).

    (4) Goal: *prevent isoimmunization.* See II. C. 5 Rh incompatibility, p. 102.

    (5) *Medical management:*

        (a) Laboratory—blood type and Rh factor, indirect Coombs, platelets, serum fibrinogen, clotting time.

      ▶ (b) Replace blood loss; maintain fluid levels with IV.

        (c) Dilation and curettage or dilation and evacuation.

        (d) *Habitual*—determine etiology.

◆ 5. **Evaluation/outcome criteria:**

    a. *Threatened*—responds to medical/nursing regimen; abortion avoided, successfully carries pregnancy to term.

    b. *Spontaneous abortion*—after uterus emptied.

        (1) Her bleeding is controlled.

        (2) Her vital signs are stable.

        (3) Copes effectively with loss of pregnancy.

        (4) Expresses satisfaction with care.

    c. *Habitual abortion*—cause identified and corrected; carries subsequent pregnancy to successful termination.

C. **Hydatidiform mole** (complete)

    1. **Pathophysiology**—chorionic villi degenerate into grapelike cluster of vesicles; may be antecedent to choriocarcinoma.

    2. **Etiology**—genetic base of complete mole (sperm enters empty egg and its chromosomes replicate; 23 pairs of chromosomes are all paternal); rare complication; more common in women over 45 yr of age and Asian women.

◆ 3. **Assessment:**

    a. Uterus—rapid enlargement; fundal height inconsistent with gestational estimate.

    b. Brownish discharge—beginning about wk 12; may contain vesicles.

    c. Signs and symptoms of preeclampsia/eclampsia (before third trimester), increased incidence of hyperemesis gravidarum.

    d. *Medical evaluation*—procedures:

        (1) Sonography, x-ray, amniography—no fetal parts present; "snowstorm."

        (2) Laboratory test—for elevated human chorionic gonadotropin (HCG) levels.

        (3) Follow-up surveillance of HCG levels for at least 1 yr; persistent HCG level is consistent with choriocarcinoma; x-ray.

◆ 4. **Analysis/nursing diagnosis:**

    a. *Anxiety/fear* related to treatment, possible sequelae of hydatidiform mole (choriocarcinoma).

    b. *Potential for injury* related to hemorrhage, perforation of uterine wall, preeclampsia/eclampsia.

    c. *Fluid volume deficit* related to hemorrhage.

◆ 5. **Nursing care plan/implementation:**

    a. *Medical management*

        (1) Monitor for pregnancy-induced hypertension (PIH).

        (2) Evacuate the uterus—hysterectomy may be necessary.

(3) Strict contraception for at least 1 yr to enable accurate assessment of status.

● (4) Choriocarcinoma—chemotherapy (methotrexate plus Dactinomycin) or radiation therapy, or both.

b. *Nursing management*

  (1) Goal: *safeguard status.* Observe for hemorrhage, passage of retained vesicles and abdominal pain, or signs of infection (because woman is at risk for perforation of uterine wall).

  (2) Goal: *health teaching.*

    (a) Explain, discuss diagnostic tests; prepare for tests.

    (b) Discuss contraceptive options.

    (c) Importance of follow-up.

  (3) Goal: *preoperative and postoperative care.*

  (4) Goal: *emotional support.* Facilitate grieving (p. 144).

◆ 6. **Evaluation/outcome criteria:**

a. Verbalizes understanding of diagnosis, tests, and treatment.

b. Complies with medical/nursing recommendations.

c. Tolerates surgical procedure well.

  (1) Bleeding controlled.

  (2) Vital signs stable.

  (3) Urinary output adequate.

d. Copes effectively with loss of pregnancy.

e. Returns for follow-up care/surveillance.

f. Selects and effectively implements method of contraception; avoids pregnancy for 1 yr or more.

g. Tests for HCG remain negative for 1 yr; no evidence of malignancy.

h. Achieves a pregnancy when desired.

i. Successfully carries pregnancy to term; normal, uncomplicated birth of viable infant.

D. Ectopic pregnancy (Figure 4–5)

1. **Pathology**—implantation outside of uterine cavity.

2. Types:

  a. Tubal (most common).

  b. Cervical.

  c. Abdominal.

  d. Ovarian.

3. **Etiology:**

  a. PID—pelvic salpingitis and endometritis.

  b. 43% caused by STD-related factors: 25%, chlamydial; 20%, previous STD.

  c. Tubal or uterine anomalies, tubal spasm.

  d. Adhesions from PID or past surgeries.

  e. Presence of IUD.

◆ 4. **Assessment:** dependent on implantation site.

  a. *Early signs*—abnormal menstrual period (usually following a missed menstrual period), spotting, some symptoms of pregnancy; possible dull pain on affected side.

  b. *Impending or posttubal rupture*—sudden, acute, lower abdominal pain; nausea and

FIGURE 4–5 Ectopic pregnancy. (From Thomas, CL [ed]: Taber's Cyclopedic Medical Dictionary, ed. 18. FA Davis, Philadelphia, 1997.)

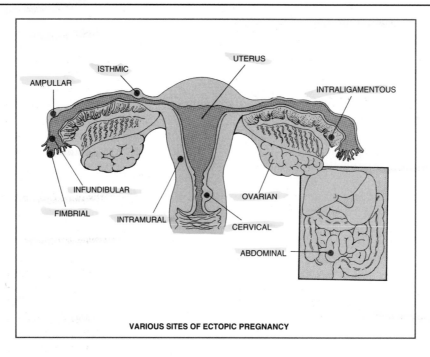

VARIOUS SITES OF ECTOPIC PREGNANCY

vomiting; signs of shock; referred shoulder pain (*Kehr's sign*) or neck pain—due to blood in peritoneal cavity; blood in cul-de-sac may → rectal pressure.

  c. Sharp, localized pain when cervix is touched during vaginal exam; shock and circulatory collapse in some, usually following vaginal examination.

  d. Positive pregnancy test in many women.

◆ 5. **Analysis/nursing diagnosis:**
  a. *Fear* related to abdominal pain and pregnancy status.
  b. *Grief* related to pregnancy loss.

◆ 6. **Nursing care plan/implementation:**
  a. *Medical management:* Surgical removal/repair. Methotrexate, a folic acid antagonist, which acts by inhibiting cell division (may be used in early ectopic pregnancy).
  b. *Nursing management:*
   (1) Goal: *preoperative and postoperative care, health teaching.*
   (2) Goal: *supportive care for grief reaction;* encourage verbalization of anxiety and concerns of further pregnancies.

◆ 7. **Evaluation/outcome criteria:**
  a. Woman experiences uncomplicated postoperative course.
  b. Woman copes effectively with loss of pregnancy.

II. Complications affecting nutrition/elimination: hyperemesis gravidarum

 A. **Pathophysiology**—pernicious vomiting during first 14–16 wk (peak incidence around 10 weeks of gestation); excessive vomiting at any time during pregnancy. Potential hazards include the following:
  1. Dehydration with fluid and electrolyte imbalance.
  2. Starvation, with loss of 5% or more of body weight; protein and vitamin deficiencies.
  3. Metabolic acidosis—due to breakdown of fat stores to meet metabolic needs.
  4. Hypovolemia and hemoconcentration; *increased* blood urea nitrogen (BUN); *decreased urinary output.*
  5. Embryonic or fetal death may result, and the woman may suffer irreversible metabolic changes or death.

 B. **Etiology:**
  1. Physiological—secretion of HCG, decrease in free gastric HCl, decreased gastrointestinal motility. Increased incidence in hydatidiform mole and multifetal pregnancy (due to high levels of HCG).
  2. Psychological—thought to be related to rejection of pregnancy or sexual relations.

◆ C. **Assessment:**
  1. Intractable vomiting.

  2. Abdominal pain.
  3. Hiccups.
  4. Marked weight loss.
  5. Dehydration—thirst, tachycardia, skin turgor.
  6. Increased respiratory rate (metabolic acidosis).
  7. Laboratory—elevated BUN.
  8. *Medical evaluation:* rule out other causes (infection, tumors).

◆ D. **Analysis/nursing diagnosis:**
  1. *Altered nutrition, less than body requirements,* related to inability to retain oral feedings.
  2. *Fluid volume deficit* related to dehydration.
  3. *Ineffective individual coping* related to symptoms, insecurity in role, psychological stress of unwanted pregnancy.
  4. *Personal identity disturbance* related to symptoms or perception of self as inadequate in role, sick, socially unpresentable.

◆ E. **Nursing care plan/implementation:**
  1. Goal: *physiological stability*
   a. Rest GI tract (keep NPO), e.g., maintain IV fluids, parenteral nutrition.
   b. Progress diet, as ordered; present small feedings attractively; ↑CHO, ↓ fat, ↓ acid.
   c. Weigh daily, assess hydration; note weight gain.
   d. Antiemetics (IV, suppository).
  2. Goal: *minimize environmental stimuli.*
   a. Limit visitors and phone calls.
   b. Bed rest with bathroom privileges.
  3. Goal: *emotional support.*
   a. Establish accepting, supportive environment.
   b. Encourage verbalization of anxiety, fears, concerns.
   c. Support positive self-image.

◆ F. **Evaluation/outcome criteria:**
  1. Woman's signs and symptoms subside; she takes oral nourishment and gains weight.
  2. Woman's pregnancy continues to term without recurrence of hyperemesis.

III. Complications affecting protective function: STDs.
This NCLEX category measures applications of knowledge about conditions related to patient's capacity to maintain defenses and prevent physical and chemical trauma, injury, *infection,* and threats to health status.

 A. **Vaginitis**—inflammation of vagina.
  1. **Pathophysiology**—local inflammatory reaction (redness, heat, irritation/tenderness, pain). May cause preterm labor in pregnancy.
  2. **Etiology:**
   a. Common causative organisms:
    (1) Bacteria—streptococci, *Escherichia coli,* gonococci, chlamydia, bacterial vaginosis.
    (2) *Viruses*—herpes type II, CMV, HPV
    (3) Protozoa—*Trichomonas vaginalis.*
    (4) Fungi—*Candida albicans.*

b. Atrophic changes—due to declining hormone level (postmenopausal women).

◆ 3. **Assessment:** differentiate among common vaginal infections:
   a. Vulvovaginal erythema.
   b. Pruritus, dysuria, dyspareunia.
   c. Vaginal discharge.

◆ 4. **Analysis/nursing diagnosis:** *pain* related to inflammation, discharge.

◆ 5. **Nursing care plan/implementation:**
   a. Goal: *emotional support.*
   b. Goal: *health teaching.* Instruct woman in self-care measures to promote comfort and healing:
      (1) Perineal care.
      (2) Sitz baths.
      (3) Douching (as ordered). *Not* recommended during pregnancy.
      (4) Exposing vulva to air.
      (5) Cotton briefs.
      (6) Proper insertion of vaginal suppository.
      (7) Instruct patient on antibiotic use, as ordered.
   c. Goal: *prevent reinfection.*
      (1) Suggest sexual partner use condom until infection is eliminated—or abstain from intercourse.
      (2) Recommend sexual partner seek examination and treatment.
   d. Goal: *medical consultation/treatment.* Refer for diagnosis and treatment.

◆ 6. **Evaluation/outcome criteria:**
   a. Woman is asymptomatic; unable to recover organism from body fluids or tissue.
   b. Woman avoids reinfection.
   c. Woman carries pregnancy to term without complications.

B. Gonorrhea
   1. **Pathophysiology:**
      a. Male—early infection usually confined to urethra, vestibular glands, anus, or pharynx. Untreated: ascending infection may involve testes, causing sterility.
      b. Female—early infection usually confined to vestibular glands, endocervix, urethra, anus (vagina is resistant). May ascend to involve pelvic structures, e.g., PID: fallopian tubes, ovaries; scarring may cause sterility.
      c. Pregnant female—may result in preterm rupture of membranes, amnionitis, preterm labor, postpartum salpingitis.
      d. Sequelae (untreated):
         (1) May develop carrier state (asymptomatic; organism resident in vestibular glands).
         (2) Systemic spread may result in gonococcal:
            (a) Arthritis.
            (b) Endocarditis.
            (c) Meningitis.
            (d) Septicemia.
      e. Newborn—ophthalmia neonatorum (gonococcal conjunctivitis). Untreated sequela: blindness.
   2. **Etiology:** gram-negative diplococcus (*Neisseria gonorrhoeae*).
   3. **Epidemiology:**
      a. Portal of entry—oral or genitourinary mucous membranes.
      b. Mode of transmission—usually sexual contact.
      c. Incubation period: 2–5 days; may be asymptomatic.
      d. Communicable period—as long as organisms are present; to 4 days after antibiotic therapy begun.

◆ 4. **Assessment:**
   a. History of known (or suspected) contact.
   b. *Male:*
      (1) Complaint of mucoid or mucopurulent discharge.
      (2) Medical diagnosis—procedure: urethral discharge gram stain.
   c. *Female:*
      (1) Often asymptomatic; acute infection: severe vulvovaginal inflammation, venereal warts, greenish-yellow vaginal discharge.
      (2) Medical diagnosis—procedure: endocervical culture.
   d. Gonococcal urethritis (male and female)—sudden severe dysuria, frequency, burning, edema.
   e. Salpingitis/oophoritis—severe, sudden abdominal pain, fever (with or without vaginal discharge).

◆ 5. **Analysis/nursing diagnosis:** *impaired tissue integrity* related to tissue inflammation.

◆ 6. **Nursing care plan/implementation:**
   a. Goal: *emotional support.*
   b. Goal: *health teaching* to prevent transmission, sequelae, reinfection.
      (1) Need for accurate diagnosis and effective treatment, follow-up examination in 7–14 days, and culture.
      (2) All sexual partners need examination, treatment.
      (3) Possible sequelae/complications (sterility, carrier state).
   c. Goal: *medical consultation/treatment.*
      (1) Determine allergy to antibiotics.
      (2) Refer for diagnosis and treatment.
         (a) Diagnosis: culture.
         (b) Treatment—ceftriaxone IM, plus doxycycline PO. May use erythromycin or spectinomycin in pregnancy.
         (c) Follow-up culture before birth.
         (d) Notification of sexual partners.

◆ 7. **Evaluation/outcome criteria:**
   a. Verbalizes understanding of mode of transmission, prevention, importance of examination, treatment of sexual contacts.
   b. Informs sexual contacts of need for examination.
   c. Returns for follow-up examinations.
   d. Successfully treated; weekly follow-up cultures: negative on two successive visits.
   e. Avoids reinfection.

C. **Chlamydia trachomatis**
   1. **Pathophysiology:**
      a. Most common sexually transmitted disease in United States.
      b. Initial infection mild in females; inflammation of cervix with discharge.
      c. If untreated, may lead to urethritis, dysuria, PID, tubal occlusion, infertility.
   2. **Etiology:**
      a. *Chlamydia trachomatis* has maternal-fetal effects.
      b. Bacteria can exist only within living cells.
      c. Transmission is by direct contact from one person to another.
   ◆ 3. **Assessment—maternal:**
      a. Inflamed cervix (may be asymptomatic).
      b. Cervical congestion, edema.
      c. Mucopurulent discharge.
   ◆ 4. **Assessment—fetal-neonatal:**
      a. Increased incidence of stillbirth.
      b. Preterm birth may result.
      c. Contact with infected mucus occurs during birth.
      d. Newborn may be asymptomatic.
      e. Conjunctivitis; may lead to scarring.
      f. *Chlamydial* pneumonia.
   ◆ 5. **Analysis/nursing diagnosis:**
      a. *Pain* related to inflamed reproductive organs.
      b. *Fatigue* related to inflammation.
      c. *Knowledge deficit* related to mode of treatment, disease transmission.
   ◆ 6. **Nursing care plan/implementation:**
      a. Treatment with antibiotics, generally doxycycline or azithromycin. Erythromycin in pregnancy.
      b. Provide pain relief, analgesics.
      c. Counsel regarding use of condoms, spermicidal agents (containing nonoxynol-9) to prevent reinfection.
   ◆ 7. **Evaluation/outcome criteria:**
      a. Woman understands treatment and shows compliance.
      b. Woman understands portal of entry and risk for reinfection.

D. **Herpes genitalis**
   1. **Pathophysiology**—initial infection: varies in severity of symptoms, may be local or systemic; duration: prolonged; morbidity: severe.

   2. **Etiology**—Herpes virus type II.
   3. **Epidemiology:**
      a. Portal of entry—skin, mucous membranes.
      b. Mode of transmission—usually sexual.
      c. Incubation: 3–14 days.
      d. Communicable period—while organisms are present.
   ◆ 4. **Assessment:**
      a. Lesions—painful, red papules; pustular vesicles that break and form wet ulcers that later crust; self-limiting (3 wk).
      b. Severe itching or tingling or pain.
      c. Discharge—copious; foul smelling.
      d. Dysuria.
      e. Lymph nodes—enlarged, inflammatory, inguinal.
      f. Pregnant female—vaginal bleeding, spontaneous abortion, fetal death.
      g. May shed virus for 7 wk.
      h. Medical diagnosis: multinucleated giant cells in microscopic examination of lesion exudate; culture for herpes simplex virus (HSV).
   ◆ 5. **Analysis/nursing diagnosis:**
      a. *Pain* related to inflammation process.
      b. *Fear* related to longevity of disease.
      c. *Fear* related to no cure for disease.
      d. *Knowledge deficit* related to transmission to future partners.
   ◆ 6. **Nursing care plan/implementation:**
      a. Goal: *emotional support.*
      b. Goal: *health teaching.*
         (1) Virus remains in body for life (dormant, noninfectious) in 25–30% of population; small percentage have symptoms.
         (2) Recurrence probable; usually shorter and milder.
         (3) Need for close surveillance during pregnancy; cesarean birth may be indicated if woman has active genital lesions or positive culture.
      c. Goal: *promote comfort.*
      d. Goal: *accurate definitive treatment.* Refer for diagnosis and treatment.
         (1) Diagnosis—cervical smears, labial and vaginal smears.
         (2) Treatment—acyclovir (Zovirax, but not in pregnancy), used for suppressive treatment only.
   ◆ 7. **Evaluation/outcome criteria:**
      a. Woman remains asymptomatic.
      b. Pregnancy continues to term with no newborn effects.

E. **Syphilis**
   1. **Pathophysiology:**
      a. *Primary stage:* nonreactive VDRL.
         (1) *Male:* 3–4 wk after contact, painless, localized penile/anal ulcer (chancre); lymph nodes—enlarged, regional.

(2) *Female:* often asymptomatic; labial, vaginal, or cervical chancre.
(3) Medical diagnosis—procedure: dark-field microscopic examination of lesion exudate.
b. *Secondary stage:* reactive VDRL.
(1) 6–8 wk after infection.
(2) Rash—macular, papular; on trunk, palms, soles.
(3) Malaise, headache, sore throat, weight loss, low-grade temperature.
c. *Latent stage:* reactive serologic test for syphilis (STS). Asymptomatic; noninfectious.
d. *Tertiary stage:*
(1) Gumma formation in skin, cardiovascular system, or central nervous system.
(2) Psychosis.
2. **Etiology:** *Treponema pallidum* (spirochete).
3. **Epidemiology:**
a. Portal of entry—skin, mucous membranes.
b. Mode of transmission—usually sexual.
c. Incubation period—9 d–3 mo.
d. Communicable period—primary and secondary stages.
◆ 4. **Assessment:**
a. *Primary*—chancre, when detectable.
Medical diagnosis—procedure: dark-field examination of lesion exudate.
b. *Secondary:*
(1) Malaise, lymphadenopathy, headache, elevated temperature.
(2) Macular, papular rash on palms and soles; may be disseminated.
(3) Medical diagnosis—see d., below.
c. *Tertiary:*
(1) Subcutaneous nodules (gumma).
(2) *Note:* Gumma formation may affect any body system; symptoms associated with area of involvement.
d. Medical diagnosis—procedures: stages other than primary—STS: VDRL, rapid plasma reagin (RPR), *T. pallidum* immobilization (TPI), fluorescent treponemal antibody absorption (FTA). *False-positive STS* in: collagen diseases, infectious mononucleosis, malaria, systemic tuberculosis.
◆ 5. **Analysis/nursing diagnosis:**
a. *Pain* related to inflammation process.
b. *Knowledge deficit* related to treatment and transmission of the disease.
◆ 6. **Nursing care plan/implementation:**
a. Goal: *emotional support*
(1) Nonjudgmental.
(2) Caring, supportive manner.
b. Goal: *health teaching.*
(1) Need for accurate diagnosis and treatment, follow-up examinations.

(2) All sexual partners need examination and treatment.
c. Goal: *medical consultation/treatment.*
(1) Refer for diagnosis and treatment. *Note:* In pregnancy—treatment by 18th gestational week prevents congenital syphilis in neonate; however, treat at time of diagnosis.
(2) Treatment:
(a) Primary, secondary—benzathine penicillin G, 2.4 million U.
(b) Other stages—7.2 million U over 3 wk period.
(c) Erythromycin or doxycycline for penicillin-allergic clients.
◆ 7. **Evaluation/outcome criteria:**
a. If treated by 18th wk of pregnancy, congenital syphilis is prevented.
b. Appropriate treatment after 18th wk cures both mother and fetus; however, any fetal damage occurring before treatment is irreversible.
c. Follow-up VDRL: nonreactive at 1, 3, 6, 9, and 12 mo.
d. *Tertiary*—cerebrospinal fluid examination negative at 6 mo and 1 yr following treatment.
e. Verbalizes understanding of mode of transmission, potential sequelae without treatment, importance of examination/ treatment of sexual contacts, preventive techniques.
f. Informs contacts of need for examination.
g. Returns for follow-up visit.
h. Avoids reinfection.

F. PID
1. **Pathophysiology**—ascending pelvic infection; may involve fallopian tubes (salpingitis), ovaries (oophoritis); may develop pelvic abscess (most common complication), pelvic cellulitis, pelvic thrombophlebitis, peritonitis.
2. **Etiology:**
a. *C. trachomatis.*
b. Gonococci.
c. Streptococci.
d. Staphylococci.
◆ 3. **Assessment:**
a. Pain: acute, abdominal.
b. Vaginal discharge: foul smelling.
c. Fever, chills, malaise.
d. Elevated white blood cell (WBC) count.
◆ 4. **Analysis/nursing diagnosis:**
a. *Pain* related to occluded tubules.
b. *Infertility* related to permanent block of tubes.
c. *Knowledge deficit* related to transmission of disease.
d. *Altered urinary elimination* related to dysuria.

◆ 5. **Nursing care plan/implementation**—for **hospitalized woman:**
  a. Goal: *emotional support.*
  b. Goal: limit extension of infection.
    ◪ (1) Bed rest—*position:* semi-Fowler's, to promote drainage.
    (2) *Force fluids* to 3000 mL/days.
    ⬭ (3) Administer antibiotics, as ordered.
  c. Goal: *prevent autoinocculation/transmission.*
    ▶ (1) Strict aseptic technique (hand washing, perineal care).
    ▶ (2) Contact-item isolation.
    (3) *Health teaching:* if untreated: high risk of tubal scarring, sterility, or ectopic pregnancy; pelvic adhesions; transmission of disease.
  d. Goal: *promote comfort.*
    ⬭ (1) Analgesics, as ordered.
    (2) External heat, as ordered.

◆ 6. **Evaluation/outcome criteria:**
  a. Woman responds to therapy; uneventful recovery.
  b. Woman avoids reinfection.

Second Trimester Complications

See Table 4–8, p. 110.

I. **Complications affecting comfort, rest, mobility: Incompetent cervix**
  A. **Pathophysiology**—inability of cervix to support growing weight of pregnancy; associated with repeated spontaneous second trimester abortion.
  B. **Etiology:**
    1. Unknown; exposure to DES.
    2. Congenital defect in cervical musculature.
    3. Cervical trauma during previous birth, abortion; aggressive, deep, or repeated dilation and curettage.
  ◆ C. **Assessment:**
    1. History of habitual, second trimester abortions.
    2. Painless, progressive cervical effacement and dilation during second trimester.
    3. Signs of threatened abortion or (early third trimester) preterm labor.
  ◆ D. **Analysis/nursing diagnosis:**
    1. *Pain* related to early dilation.
    2. *Fear* related to possible pregnancy loss.
  ◆ E. **Nursing care plan/implementation:**
    1. *Medical management*
      a. Cerclage surgical procedure (*Shirodkar, McDonald*).
    2. *Preoperative nursing management*
      a. Goal: *reduce physical stress on incompetent cervix.* Bed rest, supportive care.
      b. Goal: *emotional support.* Encourage verbalization of anxiety, fear, concerns.

  c. Goal: *health (preoperative) teaching.* Explain procedure—purse-string suture encircles cervix and reinforces musculature.
  d. Goal: *preparation for surgery.*
    3. *Postoperative nursing management*
      a. Goal: *maximize surgical result.* Bed rest, supportive care.
      b. Goal: *health teaching.*
        (1) *Avoid:* strenuous physical activity; straining.
        (2) Report promptly: signs of labor (vaginal bleeding, cramping).
        (3) Need for continued, close health surveillance.
  ◆ 4. **Evaluation/outcome criterion:** woman carries pregnancy to successful termination.

II. **Complications affecting sensory/perceptual functions: pregnancy-induced hypertension (PIH); preeclampsia/eclampsia**
  A. **Pathophysiology**
    1. Generalized arteriospasm → increased peripheral resistance, decreased tissue perfusion, and hypertension.
    2. *Kidney:*
      a. Reduced renal perfusion and vasospasm → glomerular lesions.
      b. Damage to membrane → loss of serum protein (albuminuria). *Note:* Reduced serum albumin/globulin (A/G) ratio alters blood osmolarity → edema.
      c. Increased tubular reabsorption of sodium → increased water retention (edema).
      d. Release of angiotensin contributes to vasospasm and hypertension.
    3. *Brain:* decreased oxygenation, cerebral edema, and vasospasm → visual disturbances and hyperirritability, convulsions, and coma.
    4. *Uterus:* decreased placental perfusion → increased risk of SGA baby, abruptio placentae, oligohydramnios.
  B. **Etiology:** unknown. *Risk factors:*
    1. Pregnancy—occurs only when a functioning trophoblast is present; more common in *first* pregnancies; develops after wk 20 of gestation.
    2. Coexisting conditions—diabetes, multifetal gestation, polyhydramnios, renal disease.
    3. Angiotensin gene T235.
  ◆ C. **Assessment**—types:
    1. *Preeclampsia—mild*
      a. Hypertension—systolic increase of 30 mm Hg or more over baseline; diastolic rise of 15 mm Hg or more.
      b. Proteinuria—1 g/day.
      c. Edema—digital and periorbital; weight gain over 0.45 kg (1 lb)/wk.
    2. *Preeclampsia—severe*
      a. Increasing hypertension—systolic at or above 160 mm Hg or more than 50 mm Hg over baseline; diastolic, 110 mm Hg or

Maternal-Infant

more.

b. Urine: proteinuria (5 g or more in 24 h); oliguria (400 mL or less in 24 h).

c. Hemoconcentration, hypoproteinemia, hypernatremia, hypovolemic condition.

d. Nausea and vomiting.

e. Epigastric pain—due to edema of liver capsule.

f. Cerebral or visual disturbances (before convulsive state):
  (1) Disorientation and somnolence.
  (2) Severe frontal headache.
  (3) Increased irritability; hyperreflexia.
  (4) Blurred vision, halo vision, dimness, blind spots.

g. **HELLP** Syndrome (**H**emolysis, **E**levated **L**iver enzymes, and **L**ow **P**latelets).

3. *Eclampsia*
  a. Tonic and clonic convulsions; coma.
  b. Renal shutdown—oliguria, anuria.

◆ **D. Assessment—hospitalized woman:**

1. Vital signs (blood pressure in side-lying position, pulse, respirations)—q2-4h, while awake (if mild to moderate preeclampsia) or as necessary. *Note:* Record, report persistent hypertension.

▶ 2. Fetal heart tones at time of vital signs.

▶ 3. Deep-tendon reflexes (DTR) and clonus—to identify/monitor CNS hyperirritability.

4. I&O—to identify diuresis. (*Note:* oliguria indicates pathologic progression.)

5. Urinalysis (clean-catch) for protein, daily or after each voiding, as necessary.

6. Signs of pathologic progression (see **C. Assessment**—types, p. 117).

7. Signs of labor, abruptio placentae (*Note:* high blood pressure, or a rapid drop, may initiate abruptio), DIC.

8. Emotional status.

9. Daily weight, amount/distribution of edema (pitting; pedal, digital, periorbital)—to identify signs of mobilization of tissue fluid, diuresis.

◆ **E. Analysis/nursing diagnosis:**

1. *Fluid volume excess:* hemoconcentration, edema related to altered blood osmolarity and sodium/water retention.

2. *Altered nutrition, less than body requirements:* protein deficiency related to loss through damaged renal membrane.

3. *Altered tissue perfusion* related to increased peripheral resistance and vasospasm in renal, cardiovascular system.

4. *Altered urinary elimination:* oliguria, anuria related to hypovolemia, vasospasm.

5. *Sensory/perceptual alterations:* visual disturbances, hyperirritability related to cerebral edema, decreased oxygenation to brain.

6. *Anxiety* related to symptoms, implications of pathophysiology.

7. *Diversional activity deficit* related to need for reduced environmental stimuli, bed rest.

8. *Risk for injury* related to seizure.

F. Prognosis:

1. *Good*—symptoms mild, respond to treatment.

2. *Poor*—convulsions (number and duration); persistent coma; hyperthermia, tachycardia (120 beats/min); cyanosis, and liver damage.

3. *Terminal*—pulmonary edema, congestive heart failure, acute renal failure, cerebral hemorrhage. The earlier the symptoms appear, the poorer the outcome for the pregnancy.

◆ **G. Nursing care plan/implementation:** Goal: *health teaching.*

1. *Rest*—frequent naps in *lateral Sims' position.*

2. Immediate report of **danger signs:**
  a. Digital and periorbital edema.
  b. Severe headache, irritability.
  c. Visual disturbances.
  d. Epigastric pain.

▶ 3. *Do roll-over* test (blood pressure while on back and lateral positions).

4. Importance of regular prenatal visits.

5. Monitoring own blood pressure between prenatal visits.

◆ **H. Nursing care plan/implementation—hospitalized woman:**

1. Goal: *reduce environmental stimuli,* to minimize stimulation of hyperirritable CNS. Limit visitors and phone calls.

2. Goal: *emotional support.*
  a. Encourage verbalization of anxiety, fears, concerns.
  b. Explain all procedures, seizure precautions.

3. Goal: *supportive care.*
  a. Encourage bed rest—to increase tissue perfusion, promote diuresis.
  b. *Position:* lateral Sims'—to reduce risk of supine hypotensive syndrome.

4. Goal: *health teaching.* Rest with reduced stimuli.

5. Goal: *monitor and administer drugs as ordered.*
  a. Anticonvulsants (especially magnesium sulfate).
  b. Antihypertensives.
  c. Diuretics (used rarely, and only in presence of congestive heart failure [CHF]).
  d. Blood volume expanders.

6. Goal: *seizure precautions.* To safeguard maternal/fetal status:
  a. Observe for signs and symptoms of *impending* convulsion:
    (1) Frontal headache.

(2) Epigastric pain.

(3) Sharp cry.

(4) Eyes fixed; unresponsive.

(5) Facial twitching.

b. Emergency items (suction equipment, airway, drugs, IV fluids) immediately available.

▶ 7. *Goal: convulsion care* (woman with eclampsia).

> a. Maintain patent *airway;* administer oxygen.
> b. *Safety*—padded bed rails.
> c. Reduce environmental stimuli: dim lights, quiet.
> d. Observe, report, and record:
>   (1) Onset and progression of convulsion.
>   (2) If followed by coma or incontinence.
> e. Prepare for immediate cesarean delivery; check FHR. Close observation for 48 hr postpartum, even if no further convulsions (or no convulsions to date).

◆ I. Evaluation/outcome criteria:

1. Woman complies with medical/nursing plan of care.
2. Woman's symptoms respond to treatment; progression halted.
3. Woman carries uneventful pregnancy to successful termination.

Third Trimester Complications

See Table 4–8.

I. **Complications affecting fluid-gas transport**

A. **Placenta previa**—abnormal implantation; near or over internal cervical os. Increased incidence with multiparas, multiple gestation, previous uterine surgery.

◆ 1. **Assessment:**

a. Painless vaginal bleeding (may be intermittent); absence of contractions, abdomen soft.

b. If in labor, contractions usually normal.

c. Boggy lower uterine segment—palpated on vaginal exam. (*Note:* If placenta previa is suspected, internal examinations are **contraindicated.**)

d. *Medical diagnosis—procedure:* sonography—to determine placental site.

◆ 2. **Analysis/nursing diagnosis:**

a. *Anxiety* related to bleeding, outcome.

b. *Fluid volume deficit* related to excessive blood loss.

c. *Altered tissue perfusion* related to blood loss.

d. *Altered urinary elimination* related to hypovolemia.

e. *Fear* related to fetal injury or loss.

◆ 3. **Nursing care plan/implementation:**

a. *Medical management*

(1) Sterile vaginal examination under double setup.

(2) Vaginal birth possible if bleeding minimal, marginal implantation; if fetal vertex is presenting so that presenting part acts as tamponade.

(3) Cesarean birth for complete previa.

b. *Nursing management.* Goal: *safeguard status.*

◆ 4. **Evaluation/outcome criteria:** see following section on abruptio placentae and Table 4–9.

TABLE 4–9   Comparison of Placenta Previa and Abruptio Placentae

Pathology	Etiology	◆ Assessment	◆ Nursing Care Plan/Implementation
Placenta Previa Types: *Marginal*—low-lying *Partial*—partly covers internal os *Complete*—covers internal os	More common with multiparity, advanced maternal age Fibroid tumors Endometriosis Old uterine scars Multiple gestation	Painless vaginal bleeding Usually manifests in 8th mo *Postpartum:* signs of hemorrhage, infection	*No* vaginal or rectal examinations or enemas Bed rest (*high Fowler's* if marginal previa) ■ Continuous fetal monitor ■ Maternal vital signs q4h, or prn ■ Note character and amount of bleeding Emotional support
Abruptio Placentae Types: *Partial*—small part separates *Complete*—total placenta separates *Retroplacental*—bleeding (concealed) *Marginal*—occurs at edges; external bleeding	Preeclampsia/eclampsia Before birth of second twin Traction on cord Rupture of membranes High parity Chronic renal hypertension Oxytocin induction/ augmentation of labor Cocaine use Trauma	Pain: sudden, severe Abdomen: rigid Uterus: very tender to touch Fetal hyperactivity; bradycardia, death Shock: rapid, profound Port-wine amniotic fluid Signs of DIC *Postpartum:* signs of atony, infection, pulmonary emboli	*Position:* supine; elevate (right) hip ■ Monitor: vital signs, blood loss, fetus ■ I&O (anuria, oliguria; hematuria) Prepare for surgery Emotional support ■ Fluid, blood replacement

B. Abruptio placentae—premature separation of normally implanted placenta.

◆ 1. **Assessment:**
   a. Sudden onset, severe abdominal pain.
   b. Increased uterine tone—may contract unevenly, fails to relax between contractions; very tender.
   c. Shock usually more profound than expected on basis of external bleeding or internal bleeding.
   d. *Medical evaluation—procedures:* DIC screening (bleeding time, platelet count, prothrombin time, activated partial thromboplastin time, fibrinogen); sonogram to see placental hemoseparation.

◆ 2. **Analysis/nursing diagnosis:**
   a. *Fluid volume deficit* related to bleeding.
   b. *Potential for fetal injury* related to uteroplacental insufficiency.
   c. *Fear* related to unknown outcome.

3. **Potential complications:**
   a. Afibrinogenemia and DIC.
   b. Couvelaire uterus—bleeding into uterine muscle.
   c. Amniotic fluid embolus.
   d. Hypovolemic shock.
   e. Renal failure.
   f. Uterine atony, hemorrhage, infection in postpartum.

◆ 4. **Nursing care plan/implementation:**
   a. *Medical management*
      (1) Control: hemorrhage, hypovolemic shock, replace blood loss.
      (2) Cesarean birth.
      (3) Fibrinogen, crystalloids, blood replacement.
      (4) IV heparin—by infusion pump—to reduce coagulation and fibrinolysis.
   b. *Nursing management.* Goal: *safeguard status.*

◆ 5. **Evaluation/outcome criteria:**
   a. Experiences successful termination of pregnancy.
      (1) Woman gives birth to viable newborn (by vaginal or cesarean method).
      (2) Woman has minimal blood loss.
      (3) Woman's assessment findings within normal limits.
      (4) Woman retains capacity for further childbearing.
   b. No evidence of complications (anemia, hypotonia, DIC) during postpartal period.

II. **Complications affecting comfort, rest, mobility**
   A. **Polyhydramnios**—amniotic fluid over 2000 mL (normal volume: 500–1200 mL).
      1. **Etiology:** unknown. *Risk factors:*
         a. Maternal diabetes.
         b. Multifetal gestation.
         c. Erythroblastosis fetalis.
         d. Preeclampsia/eclampsia.

   e. Congenital anomalies (e.g., anencephaly, upper-GI anomalies, such as esophageal atresia).

◆ 2. **Assessment:**
   a. Fundal height: excessive for gestational estimate.
   b. Fetal parts: difficult to palpate, small in proportion to uterine size.
   c. Increased discomfort—due to large, heavy uterus.
   d. Increased edema in vulva and legs.
   e. Shortness of breath.
   f. GI discomfort—heartburn, constipation.
   g. Susceptibility to *supine hypotensive syndrome*—due to compression of inferior vena cava and descending aorta while in supine position.
   h. *Medical diagnosis—procedures:*
      (1) Sonography—to diagnose multifetal pregnancy, gross fetal anomaly, locate placental site.
      (2) Amniocentesis—to diagnose anomalies, erythroblastosis.

3. **Potential complications:**
   a. Maternal respiratory impairment.
   b. Premature rupture of membranes (PROM) with prolapsed cord or amnionitis.
   c. Preterm labor.
   d. Postpartum hemorrhage—due to overdistention and uterine atony.

◆ 4. **Analysis/nursing diagnosis:**
   a. *Pain* related to excessive size of uterus impinging on diaphragm, stomach, bladder.
   b. *Impaired physical mobility* related to increased lordotic curvature of back, increased weight on legs.
   c. *Altered tissue perfusion* related to decreased venous return from lower extremities, compression of body structures by overdistended uterus.
   d. *Potential fluid volume deficit* related to potential uterine atony in immediate postpartum, secondary to loss of contractility due to overdistention.
   e. *Sleep pattern disturbance* related to respiratory impairment and discomfort in side-lying position.
   f. *Anxiety* related to discomfort, potential for complications, associated with congenital anomalies.
   g. *Altered urinary elimination* (frequency) related to pressure of overdistended uterus on bladder.

◆ 5. **Nursing care plan/implementation:**
   a. *Medical management*
      (1) Amniocentesis—remove excess fluid very slowly, to prevent abruptio placentae.
      (2) Termination of pregnancy—if fetal abnormality present *and* woman desires.

b. *Nursing management*
   (1) Goal: *health teaching.*
       ◼ (a) Need for *lateral Sims' position* during resting; semi-Fowler's may alleviate respiratory embarrassment.
       (b) Explain diagnostic or treatment procedures.
       (c) Signs and symptoms to be *reported immediately:* bleeding, loss of fluid through vagina, cramping.
   (2) Goal: *prepare for diagnostic and/or treatment procedures.*
       (a) Permit for amniocentesis.
   (3) Goal: *emotional support for loss of pregnancy* (if applicable).
       (a) Encourage verbalization of feelings.
       (b) Facilitate grieving: permit parents to see, hold infant; if desired, take photograph, footprints for them.

◆ 6. **Evaluation/outcome criteria:**
   a. Woman complies with medical/nursing management.
   b. Woman's symptoms of respiratory impairment, etc., reduced; comfort promoted.
   c. Woman experiences normal, uncomplicated pregnancy, labor, birth, and postpartum.

III. **Diagnostic tests to evaluate fetal growth and well-being**
   A. **Daily fetal movement count (DFMC)**
      1. Assesses fetal activity.
      2. Noninvasive test done by pregnant woman.
      3. Three movements per hour: normal activity.
      4. Two movements or less per hour may indicate fetal jeopardy or sudden change in movement pattern.
      5. Assess for fetal sleep patterns.
   B. **Nonstress test (NST)**
      1. Correlates fetal movement with FHR. Requires electronic monitoring.
      2. *Reactive test*—three accelerations of FHR 15 beats/min above baseline FHR, lasting for 15 sec or more, over 20 min time period.
      3. *Nonreactive test*—no accelerations or acceleration less than 15 beats/min above baseline FHR. May indicate fetal jeopardy. V/S to differentiate hypoxia from fetal sleep.
      4. Unsatisfactory test—data that cannot be interpreted or inadequate fetal activity; repeat.
   C. **Contraction stress test (CST); oxytocin challenge test (OCT)**
      1. Correlates fetal heart rate response to spontaneous or induced uterine contractions.
      2. Requires electronic monitoring.

3. Indicator of uteroplacental sufficiency.
4. Identifies pregnancies at risk for fetal compromise from uteroplacental insufficiency.
5. Increasing doses of oxytocin are administered to stimulate uterine contractions until 3 in 10-minute period.
6. Interpretation: *negative* results indicate absence of late decelerations with all contractions.
7. *Positive* results indicate late FHR decelerations with contractions.
8. Nipple stimulation (breast self-stimulation test) may also release enough systemic oxytocin to contract uterus to obtain CST.

D. **Biophysical profile (BPP)**
   1. Observation by ultrasound of four variables for 30 min and results of nonstress testing:
      a. Fetal body movements.
      b. Fetal tone.
      c. Amniotic fluid volume.
      d. Fetal breathing movements.
   2. Variables are scored at 2 for each variable if present; score of 0 if not present; score of less than 6 is associated with perinatal mortality.

E. **Ultrasound**
   1. Noninvasive procedure involving passage of high-frequency sound waves through uterus to obtain data regarding fetal growth, placental positioning, and the uterine cavity.
   2. Purpose may include:
      a. Pregnancy confirmation.
      b. Fetal viability.
      c. Estimation of fetal age.
      d. BPD measurement (biparietal diameter).
      e. Placenta location.
      f. Detect fetal abnormalities.
      g. Confirm fetal death.
      h. Identify multifetal gestations.
      i. Amniotic fluid index.
   3. No risk to mother with infrequent use. Fetal risk not determined on long-term basis.

F. **Amniocentesis** (Figure 4–6)
   1. Invasive procedure for amniotic fluid analysis to assess fetal lung maturity or disease; done after 14 weeks of gestation.
   2. Needle placed through abdominal-uterine wall; designated amount of fluid is withdrawn for examination.
   3. Empty bladder if gestation greater than 20 wk.
   4. Risk of complications less than 1%. Ultrasound *always* precedes this procedure.
   5. *Possible complications:* onset of contractions; infections (probably amnionitis); placental punctures; cord puncture; bladder or fetal puncture.
   6. Advise women to observe and report the following to physician: fetal hypoactivity or hyperactivity, vaginal bleeding, vaginal discharge (clear or colored), signs of labor, signs of infection.

FIGURE 4–6 Amniocentesis. (From Thomas, CL [ed]: Taber's Cyclopedic Medical Dictionary, ed. 18. FA Davis, Philadelphia, 1997.)

AMNIOCENTESIS

SYRINGE

(GREATLY ENLARGED) CELLS IN AMNIOTIC CAVITY

INTRAUTERINE CAVITY

UMBILICAL CORD

PLACENTA

FETUS

CHORIONIC VILLI

WALL OF UTERUS

CERVICAL CANAL

CERVIX

SAMPLE OF AMNIOTIC FLUID IS REMOVED, THEN THE NEEDLE IS REMOVED

UTERUS

G. Analysis of amniotic fluid

1. Chromosomal studies to detect genetic aberrations.
2. Biochemical analysis of fetal cells to detect inborn errors of metabolism.
3. Determination of fetal lung maturity by assessing *lecithin-sphingomyelin* ratios.
4. Evaluation of *phospholipids* (PG and PI); aids in determining lung maturity.
5. Determination of *creatinine* levels, aids in determining fetal age. (*Greater than 1.8* mg/dl indicates fetal maturity and the fetal age.)
6. Assesses isoimmune disease.
7. Assesses *alpha-fetoprotein (AFP)* HCG, and estriol (UE₃)levels for determination of neural tube defects and Down syndrome.
8. Presence of meconium may indicate fetal hypoxia.

H. Chorionic villus sampling (CVS)
1. Cervically invasive procedure.
2. Advantage—results can be obtained after 10 weeks of gestation due to fast-growing fetal cells.
3. Procedure—removal of small piece of tissue (chorionic villus) from fetal portion of placenta. Tissue reflects genetic makeup of fetus.
4. Determines some genetic aberrations and allows for earlier decision for induced abortion (if desired) from abnormal results. Does not diagnose neural tube defects; CVS patients need further diagnoses with ultrasound and serum AFP levels.
5. Protects "pregnancy privacy" because results can be obtained before the pregnancy is apparent and decisions can be made regarding abortion or continuation of gestation.
6. Risks involve spontaneous abortion, infection, hematoma, intrauterine death, Rh isoimmunization, and fetal limb defects, if done before 9 weeks of gestation.

THE INTRAPARTAL EXPERIENCE

General overview: This review of the anatomical and physiological determinants of successful labor provides baseline data against which the nurse compares findings of an ongoing assessment of the woman in labor. Nursing actions are planned and implemented to meet the present and emerging needs of the woman in labor.

I. Biologic foundations of labor

A. Premonitory signs

1. *Lightening*—process in which the fetus "drops" into the pelvic inlet.
   a. *Characteristics*
      (1) Nullipara—usually occurs 2-3 wk before onset of labor.
      (2) Multipara—commonly occurs with onset of labor.
   b. *Effects*
      (1) Relieves pressure on diaphragm—breathing is easier.
      (2) Increases pelvic pressure.
         (a) Urinary frequency returns.
         (b) Increased pressure on thighs.
         (c) Increased tendency to vulvar, vaginal, perianal, and leg varicosities.
2. *Braxton-Hicks contractions*—may become more uncomfortable.

B. Etiology: unknown. *Theories* include:

1. Uterine overdistention.
2. Placental aging—declining estrogen/progesterone levels.
3. Rising prostaglandin level.
4. Fetal cortisol secretion.
5. Maternal/fetal oxytocin secretion.

C. Overview of labor process—forces of labor (involuntary uterine contractions) overcome cervical resistance; cervix thins *(effacement)* and opens (0-10 cm *dilation*) (Table 4–10). Voluntary contraction of secondary abdominal muscles during the second stage (e.g., pushing, bearing-down) forces fetal descent. Changing pelvic dimensions force fetal head to accommodate to the birth canal by molding (cranial bones overlap to decrease head size).

Stages of labor:
1. *First*—begins with establishment of regular, rhythmic contractions; ends with complete effacement and dilation (10 cm); divided into three phases:
   a. Latent and early active.
   b. Active.
   c. Transitional.
2. *Second*—begins with complete dilation and ends with birth of infant.
3. *Third*—begins with birth of infant and ends with expulsion of placenta.
4. *Fourth*—begins with expulsion of placenta; ends when maternal status is stable (usually 1–2 hr postpartum).

D. Anatomical/physiological determinants

1. **Maternal**
   a. *Uterine contractions*—involuntary; birth; begin process of involution.
      (1) *Characteristics:* rhythmic; increasing tone *(increment)*, peak *(acme)*, relaxation *(decrement)*.
      (2) *Effects:*
         (a) Decreases blood flow to uterus and placenta.
         (b) Dilates cervix during first stage of labor.
         (c) Raises maternal blood pressure during contractions.
         (d) With voluntary bearing-down efforts (abdominal muscles), expels fetus (second stage) and placenta (third stage).
         (e) Begins involution.
      ◆ (3) **Assessment:**
         (a) Frequency—time from beginning of one contraction to beginning of the next.
         (b) Duration—time from beginning of contraction to its relaxation
         (c) Strength (intensity)—resistance to indentation.
         (d) False/true labor—differentiation (Table 4–11)
         (e) Signs of dystocia (dysfunctional labor). See pp. 141, 145
   b. *Pelvic structures and configuration:*
      (1) *False positive*—above linea terminalis (line travels across top of symphysis pubis around to sacral promontory); supports gravid uterus during pregnancy.
      (2) *True pelvis*—below linea terminalis; divided into:
         (a) Inlet—"brim," demarcated by linea terminalis.
            (i) Widest diameter: transverse.
            (ii) Narrowest diameter: anterior-posterior (true conjugate).
         (b) Midplane—pelvic cavity.
         (c) Outlet.
            (i) Widest diameter: anterior-posterior (requires internal rotation of fetal head for entry).
            (ii) Narrowest diameter: transverse (intertuberous); facilitates birth in occiput anterior (OA) position.

TABLE 4–10 First Stage of Labor

Phases of First Stage	◆ Assessment: Expected Maternal Behaviors	◆ Nursing Care Plan/Implementation
0 to 4 cm: Latent Phase and Early Active Phase		
1. *Time:* multipara 5–6 hr; nullipara 8–10 hr, average	1. Usually comfortable, euphoric, excited, talkative, and energetic, but may be fearful and withdrawn	1. Provide encouragement, feedback for relaxation, companionship
2. *Contractions:* regular, mild, 5–10 min apart, 20–30 seconds duration	2. Relieved or apprehensive that labor has begun	2. Coach during contractions: signal beginning of contraction, mark the seconds, signal end of contraction; "Follow my breathing," "Watch my lips," etc.
3. Low-back pain and abdominal discomfort with contractions	3. Alert, usually receptive to teaching, coaching, diversion, and anticipatory guidance	3. Comfort measures: position for comfort; praise; keep aware of progress
4. Cervix thins: some bloody show		
5. *Station:* Multipara −2 to +1; nullipara 0.		
4 to 8 cm: Midactive Phase, Phase of Most Rapid Dilation		
1. Average *time:* nullipara 1–2 hr; multipara 1½–2 hr	1. Tired, less talkative, and less energetic	1. Coach during contractions; husband (coach) may need some relief
2. *Contractions:* 2–5 min apart, 30–40 seconds' duration, intensity increasing	2. More serious, malar flush between 5 and 6 cm, tendency to hyperventilate, may need analgesia, needs constant coaching	2. *Comfort measures* (to husband too—as needed): position for comfort while preventing hypotensive syndrome; encourage relaxation, focusing her on areas of tension; provide counterpressure to sacrococcygeal area, prn; praise; keep aware of progress; minimize distractions from surrounding environment (loud talking, other noises); offer analgesics and anesthetics, as appropriate; provide hygiene: mouth care, ice chips, clean perineum; warmth, as needed
3. Membranes may rupture now		3. Monitor progress of labor and maternal/fetal response
4. Increased bloody show		4. If monitors are in use, attention on mother; periodically check accuracy of monitor readouts
5. *Station:* −1 to 0		
8 to 10 cm: Transition, Deceleration Period of Active Phase		
1. Average *time:* nullipara 40 min–1 hr; multipara 20 min	1. If not under regional anesthesia, more introverted; may be amnesic between contractions	1. Stay with woman (couple) and provide constant support
2. *Contractions:* 1½–2 min apart, 60–90 seconds duration, strong intensity	2. Feeling she cannot make it; increased irritability, crying, nausea, vomiting, and belching; increased perspiration over upper lip and between breasts; leg tremors; and shaking	2. Continue to coach with contractions: may need to remind, reassure, and encourage her to reestablish breathing techniques and concentration with each contraction; coach panting or "he-he" respirations to prevent pushing
3. Increased vaginal show; rectal pressure with beginning urge to bear down	3. May have uncontrollable urge to push at this time	3. Comfort measures; remind her and husband her behavior is normal and "OK"; coach breathing to quell nausea
4. *Station:* +3 to +4		4. Assist with countertension techniques woman requested: effleurage
		5. Monitor contractions, FHR (after each contraction), vaginal discharge, perineal bulging, maternal vital signs; record every 15 min
		6. Assess for bladder filling
		7. Keep mother (couple) aware of progress
		8. Prepare husband for birth (scrub, gown, etc.)

TABLE 4–11   Assessment: Differentiation of False/True Labor

False Labor	True Labor
Contractions: Braxton-Hicks intensify (more noticeable at night); short, irregular, little change	*Contractions:* begin in lower back, radiate to abdomen ("girdling"), become regular, rhythmic; frequency, duration, intensity increase
Relieved by change of position or activity (e.g., walking)	*Unaffected* by change of position, activity, drinking two glasses of water, or moderate analgesia
Cervical changes—none; *no* effacement or dilation progress	*Cervical changes*—*progressive* effacement and dilation

(3) *Classifications*
   (a) *Gynecoid*—normal female pelvis; rounded oval.
   (b) *Android*—normal male pelvis; funnel shaped.
   (c) *Anthropoid*—oval.
   (d) *Platypelloid*—flattened, transverse oval.

2. **Fetal**
  a. *Fetal head* (Figure 4–7).
   (1) *Bones*—one occipital, two frontal, two parietals, two temporals.
   (2) *Suture*—line of junction or closure between bones; sagittal (longitudinal), coronal (anterior), and lambdoidal (posterior, frontal); permit molding to accommodate head to birth canal.
   (3) *Fontanels*—membranous space between cranial bones during fetal life and infancy.
    (a) *Anterior* "soft spot"—diamond shaped; junction of coronal and sagittal sutures; closes (ossifies) by *18 mo.*
    (b) *Posterior*—triangular; junction of sagittal and lambdoidal sutures; closes by *4 mo of age.*
  b. *Fetal lie*—relationship of fetal long axis to maternal long axis (spine).
   (1) *Transverse*—shoulder presents.
   (2) *Longitudinal*—vertex or breech presents.
  c. *Presentation*—fetal part entering inlet first (Figure 4–8).
   (1) *Cephalic*—vertex (most common); face, brow.
   (2) *Breech*
    (a) *Complete*—feet and legs flexed on thighs; buttocks and feet presenting
    (b) *Frank*—legs extended on torso, feet up by shoulders; buttocks presenting.
    (c) *Footling*—single (one foot), double (both feet) presenting.

  d. *Attitude*—relationship of fetal parts to one another (e.g., head flexed on chest).
  e. *Position*—relationship of presenting fetal part to quadrants of maternal pelvis; vertex most common, occiput anterior on maternal left side (LOA). See Figure 4–8.
◆ 3. **Assessment:** determine presentation and position.
  ▶ a. *Leopold's maneuvers*—abdominal palpation.
   (1) *First*—palms over fundus, breech feels softer, not as round as head would be.
   (2) *Second*—palms on either side of abdomen, locates fetal back and small parts.
   (3) *Third*—fingers just above pubic symphysis, grasp lower abdomen; if unengaged, presenting part is mobile.
   (4) *Fourth*—facing mother's feet, run palms down sides of abdomen to symphysis; check for cephalic prominence (usually on right side), and if head is floating or engaged.
  ▶ b. *Location of fetal heart tones*—heard best through fetal back or chest.
   (1) *Breech* presentation—usually most audible *above* maternal umbilicus.
   (2) *Vertex* presentation—usually most audible *below* maternal umbilicus.
   (3) Changing location of most audible FHTs (fetal heart tones)—useful indicator of fetal descent.
   (4) Factors affecting audibility:
    (a) Obesity.
    (b) Maternal position.
    (c) Polyhydramnios.
    (d) Maternal gastrointestinal activity.
    (e) Loud uterine bruit—origin: hissing of blood through maternal uterine arteries; synchronous with maternal pulse
    (f) Loud funic souffle—origin: hissing of blood through umbilical arteries; synchronous with fetal heart rate (FHR).

FIGURE 4–7 The fetal head. *Bones:* two frontal, two temporal, one occipital. *Sutures:* sagittal, frontal, coronal, lambdoid. *Fontanels:* anterior, posterior. (Used with permission of Ross Products Division, Abbott Laboratories, Inc., Columbus, OH 43216, Clinical Education Aid No. 13.)

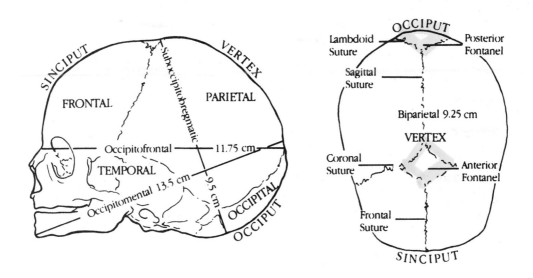

FIGURE 4–8 Categories of fetal presentation. (a) LOA: fetal occiput is in left anterior quadrant of maternal pelvis. (b) LOP: fetal occiput is in left posterior quadrant of maternal pelvis. (c) ROA: fetal occiput is in right anterior quadrant of maternal pelvis. (d) ROP: fetal occiput is in right posterior quadrant of maternal pelvis. (e) LSP: fetal sacrum is in left posterior quadrant of maternal pelvis. (f) Shoulder presentation with fetus in transverse lie. (g) Prolapse of umbilical cord with fetus in LOA position. (Used with permission of Ross Products Division, Abbott Laboratories, Inc., Columbus, OH 43216, Clinical Education Aid No. 18.)

(g) External noise, faulty equipment.

c. *Vaginal examination:* palpable sutures, fontanels (triangular-shaped superior, diamond-shaped inferior=vertex presentation, OA position).

4. *Cardinal movements of the* **mechanisms of normal labor**—vertex presentation, positional changes of fetal head accommodate to changing diameters of maternal pelvis (Figure 4–9).

a. *Descent*—head engages and proceeds down birth canal.

b. *Flexion*—head bent to chest; presents smallest diameter of vertex (suboccipital-bregmatic).

c. *Internal rotation*—during second stage of labor, transverse diameter of fetal head enters pelvis; occiput rotates 90 degrees to bring back of neck under symphysis (e.g., LOT to LOA to OA); presents smallest diameter (biparietal) to smallest diameter of outlet (intertuberous).

d. *Extension*—back of neck pivots under symphysis, allows head to be born by extension.

e. *Restitution*—head returns to normal alignment with shoulders (with LOA, results in head facing right thigh), presents smallest diameter of shoulders to outlet.

f. *Delivery of head*—shoulders in anterior-posterior position.

g. *Expulsion*—birth of neonate completed.

◆ 5. **Assessment:** relationship of fetal head to ischial spines (**degree of descent**).

FIGURE 4–9 Cardinal movements in the mechanism of labor with the fetus in vertex presentation. (a) Engagement, descent, flexion. (b) Internal rotation. (c) Extension beginning (rotation complete). (d) Extension complete. (e) External rotation (restitution). (f) External rotation (shoulder rotation). (g) Expulsion. (Used with permission of Ross Products Division, Abbott Laboratories, Inc., Columbus, OH 43216, Clinical Education Aid No. 13.)

a. *Engagement*—widest diameter of presenting part has passed through pelvic inlet (e.g., biparietal diameter of fetal head).

b. *Station*—relationship of presenting part to ischial spines (IS).

　(1) *Floating*—presenting part above inlet, in false pelvis.

　(2) Station—−5 is at inlet (presenting part well above IS).

　(3) Station 0—presenting part at IS (engaged).

　(4) Station +4—presenting part at the outlet.

E. Warning signs during labor

1. *Contraction*—hypertonic, poor relaxation, or tetanic (greater than 90 sec long and ≤2 min apart).

2. *Abdominal pain*—sharp, rigid abdomen

3. *Vaginal bleeding*—profuse.

4. *FHR*—late decelerations, prolonged variable decelerations, bradycardia, tachycardia (Figure 4–10), decreased variability.

5. *Maternal hypertension.*

6. *Meconium-stained amniotic fluid (MSAF).*

7. *Prolonged ROM.*

II. Participatory childbirth techniques

A. Psychoprophylaxis—Lamaze method

1. Premise—conditioned responses to stimuli occupy nerve pathways, reducing perception of pain. Emphasis is on childbirth as a natural event, with an informed woman as the active participant. The ability to relax effectively reduces the perception of pain, and the involvement of the coach fosters the family concept.

2. Childbirth partners are taught:

　a. Anatomy and physiology of labor.

　b. Psychology of man and woman.

　c. What to expect in the birthing setting.

　d. Conditioned responses to labor stimuli.

　　(1) Concentration on focal point.

　　(2) Breathing techniques.

　　(3) Need for active coaching to enable woman to:

　　　(a) Use techniques appropriate to present stage of labor.

　　　(b) Avoid hyperventilation.

　e. Specific stage—appropriate techniques:

　　(1) *First stage of labor—early:* slow, deep chest breathing; *active:* patterned breathing.

　　(2) *Transition* (8–10 cm)—rapid, shallow breathing pattern, to prevent pushing prematurely.

　　　(a) Panting.

　　　(b) Pant-blow.

　　　(c) "He-he" pattern.

　　(3) *Second stage of labor*

　　　(a) Pushing (or bearing-down) — aids fetal descent through birth canal.

　　　(b) Panting—aids relaxation between contractions; prevents explosive birth of head.

　f. Effects on labor behaviors/coping:

　　(1) Help mother cope with and assist contractions.

　　(2) Prevent premature bearing-down efforts; reduce possibility of cervical lacerations, edema due to pushing on incompletely dilated cervix.

　　(3) When appropriate, improve efficiency of bearing-down efforts.

B. Other methods—include parent classes, classes for siblings, multiparas, and those who plan cesarean birth.

III. Nursing actions during first stage of labor

◆ **A. Assessment:** careful evaluation of:

1. *Antepartal history*

　a. EDB

　b. Genetic and familial problems.

　c. Preexisting and coexisting medical disorders, allergies.

　d. Pregnancy-related health problems (hyperemesis, bleeding, etc.).

　e. Infectious diseases (past and present herpes, etc.).

　f. Past obstetric history, if any.

　g. Pelvic size estimation.

　h. Height.

　i. Weight gain.

　j. Laboratory results:

　　(1) Blood type and Rh factor.

　　(2) Serology.

　　(3) Urinalysis.

　　(4) Hepatitis.

　　(5) Rubella.

　k. Prenatal care history.

　l. Use of medications.

2. *Admission findings*

　a. Emotional status.

　b. Vital signs.

　c. Present weight.

　d. Fundal height.

　e. Estimated fetal weight.

　f. Edema.

　g. Urinalysis (for protein and glucose).

▶ 3. *FHR*—normal, 110–160 beats/min (see Figure 4–10).

　a. Check and record every 15–30 min—monitor fetal response to physiological stress of labor.

　b. *Bradycardia* (mild, 100–110 beats/min, or 30 beats/min lower than baseline reading).

　c. *Tachycardia* (moderate, 160–179 beats/min, or 30 beats/min above baseline reading lasting 5+ minutes).

▶ 4. *Contractions*—every 15–30 min.

　a. Place fingertips over fundus, use gentle pressure; contraction felt as hardening or tensing.

FIGURE 4–10 Fetal heart rate (FHR) decelerations and nursing interventions.

Pattern	Description	Nursing Intervention
Head compression **(HC)**	**Early Decelerations** Early deceleration (HC) 1. FHR begins to slow with the onset of the uterine contraction (UC) and returns to baseline when contraction is over. 2. Fetal head compression occurs. 3. Vagal nerve stimulation. 4. Transient slowing of FHR.	No intervention required. Continue observation.
Compression of vessels Uteroplacental insufficiency **(UPI)**	**Late Decelerations** Late deceleration (UPI) 1. FHR begins to fall at height of the UC and returns to baseline after contraction has ceased. 2. FHR usually remains within normal range. 3. Indicates some degree of uteroplacental insufficiency.	Change maternal position. Turn off Pitocin; increase rate of maintenance IV. Begin oxygen by face mask Notify physician. Check blood pressure and pulse rate. Possible candidate for cesarean birth.
Umbilical cord **Umbilical cord compression (CC)**	**Variable Decelerations** Variable deceleration (CC) 1. Slowing of FHR either with a contraction or in between contractions. Unrelated pattern of FHR and uterine contraction. 2. Pattern may be U shaped or V shaped. Transitory acceleration precedes or follows the deceleration. 3. FHR may fall below 100 beats/min; then returns immediately to baseline. 4. Usually indicates cord compression.	Change maternal position to alleviate cord pressure. Turn off Pitocin; increase rate of maintenance IV. Begin oxygen by face mask. Notify physician. Check blood pressure and pulse rate. Possible candidate for cesarean birth. Possible candidate for amnio infusion.

b. Time: frequency and duration.

c. Intensity/strength at acme:

(1) Weak—easily indent fundus with fingers.

(2) Moderate—some tension felt, fundus indents slightly with finger pressure.

(3) Strong—unable to indent fundus.

5. *Maternal response to labor*—assess for effective coping, cooperation, and using effective breathing techniques.

6. *Maternal vital signs*—between contractions.

a. Response to pain or use of special breathing techniques alters pulse and respirations.

b. B/P, P, RR—if normotensive: on admission, and then every hour and prn; after regional anesthesia: every 30 min (every 5 min first 20 min).

c. Temp—if within normal range: on admission, and then every 4 hr and prn. Every 2 hr after rupture of membranes.

d. Before and after analgesia/anesthesia.

e. After rupture of membranes (see **Amniotic fluid embolism,** p. 147).

7. Character and amount of *bloody show.*

8. *Bladder* status: encourage voiding every 1–2 hr, monitor output.

a. Determine bladder distention—palpate just above symphysis (full bladder may impede labor progress or result in trauma to bladder).

b. Admission urinalysis—check for protein and glucose.

9. Signs of deviations from normal patterns.

10. *Status of membranes:*

a. Intact.

b. Ruptured (nitrazine paper turns blue on contact with alkaline amniotic fluid). Fluid may be placed on a glass slide to dry; a fernlike crystallization of sodium chloride will appear. Note, record, and report:

(1) Time—danger of infection if ruptured more than 24 hr.

(2) FHR stat and 10 min later—to check for prolapsed cord.

(3) Character and color of fluid (see 11.b. and c.).

11. Amniotic fluid.

a. Amount—polyhydramnios (>2000 mL)—associated with congenital anomalies/poorly controlled diabetes.

b. Character—thick consistency or odor associated with infection.

c. Color—normally clear with white specks.

(1) Yellow—presence of bilirubin; Rh or ABO incompatibility.

(2) Green or meconium stained; if fetus in vertex position, indicates recent fetal hypoxia secondary to respiratory distress in fetus.

(3) Port wine—may indicate abruptio placentae.

12. *Labor progress:*

a. Effacement.

b. Dilatation.

c. Station.

d. Bulging membranes.

e. Molding of fetal head.

13. *Perineum*—observe for bulging.

◆ **B. Analysis/nursing diagnosis:**

1. *Anxiety, fear* related to uncertain outcome, pain.

2. *Ineffective individual coping* related to lack of preparation for childbirth or poor support from coach.

3. *Altered nutrition: less than body requirements* related to physiological stress of labor.

4. *Altered urinary elimination* related to pressure of presenting part.

5. *Altered thought processes* related to sleep deprivation, transition, analgesia.

6. *Fluid volume deficit* related to anemia, excessive blood loss.

7. *Impaired (fetal) gas exchange* related to impaired placental perfusion.

◆ **C. Nursing care plan/implementation:**

1. Goal: *comfort measures.*

a. Maintain hydration of oral mucosa. Encourage sucking on cool washcloth, ice chips, lollipops, clear liquids.

b. Reduce dryness of lips. Apply lip balm.

c. Relieve backache. Apply sacral counterpressure (particularly with occiput posterior [OP] presentation).

d. Encourage significant other to participate.

e. Encourage ambulation when presenting part engaged.

2. Goal: *management of physical needs.*

a. Encourage frequent voiding to prevent full bladder from impeding oncoming head.

b. Encourage ambulation throughout labor; *lateral Sims' position with head elevated to:*

(1) Encourage relaxation.

(2) Allow gravity to assist in anterior rotation of fetal head.

(3) Prevent compression of inferior vena cava and descending aorta (*supine hypotensive syndrome*).

(4) Promote placental perfusion.

c. Perineal prep, if ordered to promote cleanliness.

d. Fleet's enema, if ordered—to stimulate peristalsis, evacuate lower bowel. *Note:* **contraindicated** if:

(1) Cervical dilation (4 cm or more) with unengaged head—due to possibility of cord prolapse.

(2) Fetal malpresentation/malposition—due to possible fetal distress.

(3) Preterm labor—may stimulate contractions.

(4) Painless vaginal bleeding—due to possible placenta previa.

3. Goal: *management of psychosocial needs. Emotional support:*

a. Encourage verbalization of feelings, fears, concerns.

b. Explain all procedures.

c. Reinforce self-concept ("You're doing well!").

4. Goal: *management of discomfort.*

a. Analgesia or anesthesia—may be required or desired—to facilitate safe, comfortable birth.

b. Support/enhance/teach childbirth techniques.

▶ (1) Reinforce appropriate *breathing techniques* for current labor status.

(a) If woman is **hyperventilating,** to increase PaCO$_2$, minimize fetal acidosis, and relieve symptoms of vertigo and syncope, suggest:

(i) Breathe into paper bag.

(ii) Breathe into cupped hands.

(b) Demonstrate appropriate breathing for several contractions—to reestablish rate and rhythm.

5. Goal: *sustain motivation.*

a. Offer support, encouragement, and praise, as appropriate.

b. Keep informed of status and progress.

c. Reassure that irritability is normal.

d. Serve as surrogate coach when necessary (if no partner, before partner arrives, while partner changes clothes, during needed breaks); assist with effleurage, breathing, focusing.

e. Discourage bearing-down efforts by pant-blow until complete (10 cm) dilation to avoid cervical edema/laceration.

f. Facilitate informed decision making regarding medication for relaxation or pain relief.

g. Minimize distractions: quiet, relaxed environment; privacy.

◆ **D. Evaluation/outcome criteria:**

1. Woman manages own labor discomfort effectively.

2. Woman maintains control over own behavior.

3. Woman successfully completes first stage of labor without incident.

IV. Nursing actions during second stage of labor

◆ **A. Assessment:**

1. Maternal (or couple's) response to labor.

▶ 2. FHR—continuous electronic monitoring, or after each contraction with fetoscope, Doppler.

3. Vital signs.

4. Time elapsed—average: 2 min to 1 hr; prolonged second stage increases risk of fetal distress, maternal exhaustion, psychological stress, intrauterine infection.

5. Contraction pattern—average every 1½-3 min, lasting 60-90 sec.

6. Vaginal discharge—increases.

7. Nausea, vomiting, disorientation, tremors, amnesia between contractions, panic.

8. Response to regional anesthesia, if administered.

a. Signs of hypotension—reduces placental perfusion, increases risk of fetal hypoxia.

b. Effect on contractions—note and report any slowing of labor.

9. Efforts to bear down—increase expulsive effects of uterine contractions.

10. Perineal bulging with contractions—fetal head distends perineum, crowns; head born by extension.

◆ **B. Analysis/nursing diagnosis:**

1. *Pain* related to strong uterine contractions, pressure of fetal descent, stretching of perineum.

2. *High risk for injury:*

a. Infection related to ruptured membranes, repeated vaginal examinations.

b. Laceration related to pressure of fetal head exceeding perineal elasticity.

3. *Impaired skin integrity* related to laceration, episiotomy.

4. *Fluid volume deficit* related to hypotension secondary to regional anesthesia.

5. *Anxiety* related to imminent birth of fetus.

6. *Ineffective individual coping* related to prolonged sensory stimulation (contractions) and anxiety.

7. *Altered urinary elimination* related to anesthesia and contractions, descent of fetal head.

8. *Sleep pattern disturbance.*

◆ **C. Nursing care plan/implementation:**

1. Goal: *emotional support.*

a. To sustain motivation/control:

(1) Never leave mother and significant other alone during 2nd stage.

(2) Keep informed of progress.

▶ (3) Direct bearing-down efforts (pushing) without holding breath* while pushing. Encourage pushing "out through vagina" and encourage mother to touch crowning head; po-

---

*The woman must be discouraged from using the **Valsalva maneuver** (holding one's breath and tightening abdominal muscles) for pushing during the second stage. This activity increases intrathoracic pressure, reduces venous return, and increases venous pressure. Cardiac output and blood pressure increase, and pulse slows temporarily. During the Valsalva maneuver, fetal hypoxia may occur. The process is reversed when the woman takes a breath.

sition mirror so woman can see perineal bulging with effective efforts; minimize distractions.

b. To allay significant other's anxiety: reassure regarding mother's behavior if she is not anesthetized.

c. Support family choices.

2. Goal: *safeguard status.*

a. Precautions when putting legs in stirrups:

(1) If varicosities, **do not put legs in stirrups.**

(2) *Avoid* pressure to popliteal veins; pad stirrups.

(3) Ensure proper, even alignment by adjusting stirrups.

(4) Move legs simultaneously into or out of stirrups—to *avoid* nerve, ligament, and muscle strain.

(5) Provide proper support to woman not using stirrups. Do **not** hold legs (can cause back injury).

b. Support woman in whatever position selected for birth (e.g., side-lying position).

c. Cleanse perineum, thighs as ordered.

3. Goal: *maintain a comfortable environment.*

a. Free of unnecessary noise, light.

b. Comfortable temperature (warm).

4. *Medical management:*

a. Episiotomy may be performed to facilitate birth.

b. Forceps may be applied to exert traction and expedite birth.

c. Vacuum extraction also used to assist birth.

5. Birthing room birth with alternative positions (squat).

◆ **D. Evaluation/outcome criteria:**

1. Cooperative, actively participates in birth; maintains control over own behavior.

2. Successful, uncomplicated birth of viable infant.

3. All assessment findings within normal limits (vital signs, emotional status, response to birth).

4. Presence of significant other.

V. Nursing actions during third stage of labor

◆ **A. Assessment:**

1. Time elapsed—average: 5 min; prolonged third stage (greater than 25 min) may indicate complications (placenta accreta).

2. Signs of *placental separation:*

a. Increase in bleeding from the vagina.

b. Cord lengthens.

c. Uterus rises in abdomen, assumes globular shape.

3. Assess mother's level of consciousness.

4. Examine placenta for intactness and number of vessels in umbilical cord (normal: three. *Note:* two vessels only—associated with increased incidence of congenital anomalies); condition of placenta for calcification, infarcts, etc.

◆ **B. Analysis/nursing diagnosis:**

1. *Family coping: potential for growth* related to bonding, beginning achievement of developmental tasks.

2. *Fluid volume deficit* related to blood loss during third stage.

◆ **C. Nursing care plan/implementation:**

1. Goal: *prevent uterine atony.* Administer oxytocin, as ordered.

2. Goal: *facilitate parent-child bonding.*

a. While protecting neonate from cold stress, encourage parents to see, hold, touch neonate.

b. Comment about neonate's individuality, characteristics, and behaviors.

c. After neonate is assessed for congenital anomalies (e.g., cleft palate, esophageal atresia), encourage breastfeeding, if desired.

3. Goal: *health teaching.*

a. Describe, discuss common neonatal behavior in transitional period (periods of reactivity, sleep, hyperactivity).

b. Demonstrate removal of mucus by aspiration with bulb syringe.

c. Demonstrate ways of facilitating breastfeeding.

◆ **D. Evaluation/outcome criteria:**

1. Woman has a successful, uneventful completion of labor.

a. Minimal blood loss.

b. Vital signs within normal limits.

c. Fundus well contracted at level of umbilicus.

2. Parents express satisfaction with outcome, demonstrate infant attachment.

VI. Nursing actions during the fourth stage of labor—1–2 hr postpartum.

◆ **A. Assessment**—every 15 min four times; then, every 30 min two times—or until stable—to monitor response to physiological stress of labor/birth.

▶ 1. Vital signs:

a. *Temperature* taken once; if elevated, requires follow-up—may indicate infection, dehydration, excessive blood loss. Note, record, report temperature of 100.4°F (38°C).

b. *Blood pressure*—every 15 min × 4.

(1) Returns to prelabor level—due to loss of placental circulation and increased circulating blood volume.

(2) Elevation may be in response to use of oxytocic drugs or preeclampsia (first 48 hr).

(3) Lowered blood pressure—may reflect significant blood loss during labor/birth, or occult bleeding.

   c. Pulse—every 15 min × 4.
     (1) Physiological bradycardia—due to normal vagal response.
     (2) Tachycardia—may indicate excessive blood loss during labor/birth, dehydration, exhaustion, or occult bleeding.

▶ 2. Location and tone of fundus—every 15 min × 4 to ensure continuing contraction; prevent blood loss due to uterine relaxation.
   a. Fundus—firm; at or slightly lower than the umbilicus; in midline.
   b. May be displaced by distended bladder—due to normal diuresis; common cause of bleeding in immediate postpartum, uterine atony.

3. Character and amount of vaginal flow.
   a. Moderate lochia rubra.
   b. If perineal pad saturated in 15 min, or blood pools under buttocks, excessive loss.
   c. Bright red bleeding may indicate cervical or vaginal laceration.

4. Perineum.
   a. Edema.
   b. Bruising—due to trauma.
   c. Distention/hematoma, rectal pain.

5. Bladder fullness/voiding—to prevent distention.

6. Rate of IV, if present; response to added medication, if any.

7. Intake and output—to evaluate hydration.

8. Recovery from analgesia/anesthesia.

9. Energy level.

10. Verbal, nonverbal interaction between woman and significant other.
   a. Dialogue.
   b. Posture.
   c. Facial expressions.
   d. Touching.

11. Interactions between parent(s) and newborn; signs of bonding.
   a. Eye contact with newborn.
   b. Calls by name.
   c. Explores with fingertips, strokes, cuddles.

12. Signs of postpartal emergencies:
   a. Uterine atony, hemorrhage.
   b. Vaginal hematoma.

◆ **B. Analysis/nursing diagnosis:**
1. *Fluid volume deficit* related to excessive intrapartal blood loss, dehydration.
2. *Altered urinary elimination* related to intrapartal bladder trauma, dehydration, blood loss.
3. *Impaired skin integrity* related to episiotomy, lacerations, cesarean birth.

4. *Altered family processes* related to role change.
5. *Altered parenting* related to interruption in bonding secondary to:
   a. Compromised maternal status.
   b. Compromised neonatal status.
6. *Knowledge deficit* related to self-care procedures.
7. *Fatigue* related to sleep disturbances and anxiety.
8. *Anxiety* regarding status of self and infant.
9. *Altered nutrition, less than body requirements,* related to decreased food and fluid intake during labor.

◆ **C. Nursing care plan/implementation:**
1. Goal: *comfort measures.*
   a. Position, pad change.
  ▶ b. Perineal care—to promote healing; to reduce possibility of infection.
   c. Ice pack to perineum; as ordered—to reduce edema, discomfort, and pain related to hemorrhoids.
2. Goal: *nutrition/hydration.* Offer fluids, foods as tolerated.
3. Goal: *urinary elimination.*
   a. Encourage voiding—to avoid bladder distention.
   b. Record: time, amount, character.
   c. Anticipatory guidance related to nocturnal diuresis and increased output.
4. Goal: *promote bonding.*
   a. Provide privacy, quiet; encourage sustained contact with newborn.
   b. Encourage: touching, holding baby; breastfeeding (also promotes involution).
5. Goal: *health teaching.*
   a. Perineal care—front to back, labia closed (after *each* void/bowel movement).
   b. Hand washing—before and after each pad change; after voiding, defecating; before and after baby care.
   c. Signs to report:
     (1) Uterine cramping.
     (2) Increased vaginal bleeding, passage of large clots.
     (3) Nausea, dizziness.

◆ **D. Evaluation/outcome criteria:**
1. Expresses comfort, satisfaction in fourth stage.
2. Vital signs stable, fundus contracted, moderate lochia rubra, perineum undistended.
3. Tolerates food and fluids well.
4. Voids in adequate amount.
5. Demonstrates eye contact with infant, cuddles.
6. Verbalizes abnormal signs to report to physician.
7. Returns demonstration of appropriate perineal care.
8. Ambulates without pain, dizziness, numbness of legs.

Maternal-Infant

VII. Nursing management of the newborn immediately after birth

◆ **A. Assessment:**

1. Mucus in nasophyarynx, oropharynx.
2. *Apgar score:* note and record—at 1 and 5 min of age (Table 4–12).

> a. Score of 7-10: *good* condition.
> b. Score of 4-6: *fair* condition; assess for CNS depression.
> c. Score of 0-3: *poor* condition; requires immediate intervention. *Asphyxia neonatorum*—fails to breathe spontaneously within 30-60 sec after birth; HR<100.

3. Number of vessels in umbilical stump.
4. Passage of meconium stool, urine.
5. General physical appearance/status.
   a. Signs of respiratory distress (nasal flaring, grunting, sternal retraction, cyanosis, tachypnea).
   b. Skin condition (meconium-stained, cyanosis, jaundice, lesions).
   c. Cry—presence, pitch, quality.
   d. Signs of birth trauma (lacerations, dislocations, fractures).
   e. Symmetry (absent parts, extra digits, gross malformations, ears, palm creases, sacral dimples).
   f. Molding, caput succedaneum, cephalhematoma.
   g. Assess gestational age.
6. Identify high-risk infant.

◆ **B. Analysis/nursing diagnosis:**

1. *Ineffective airway clearance* related to excessive nasopharyngeal mucus.
2. *Ineffective breathing pattern* related to CNS depression secondary to intrauterine hypoxia narcosis, prematurity, and lack of pulmonary surfactant.
3. *Impaired gas exchange* related to respiratory distress.
4. *Fluid volume deficit* related to birth trauma; hemolytic jaundice.
5. *Impaired skin integrity* related to cord stump.
6. *High risk for injury* (biochemical, metabolic) related to impaired thermoregulation.
7. *Ineffective thermoregulation* related to environmental conditions/prematurity.

◆ **C. Nursing care plan/implementation:**

1. Goal: *ensure patent airway.*
   ▶ a. Suction mouth first, then nose; when stimulated, sensitive receptors around entrance to nares initiate gasp, causing aspiration of mucus present in mouth.
   ▶ b. Suction with bulb syringe.
      (1) If deeper suctioning necessary, use DeLee mucus trap attached to suction. Oral use of DeLee is contraindicated due to risk of contact with baby's secretions (new Delee now available that has no such risk).
      (2) *Avoid* prolonged, vigorous suctioning.
         (a) Reduces oxygenation.
         (b) May traumatize tissue, cause edema, bleeding, laryngospasm, and cardiac arrhythmia.
   c. Assist gravity drainage of fluids. *Position:* head dependent (Trendelenburg) and side-lying position.
2. Goal: *maintain body temperature*—to conserve energy, preserve store of brown fat, decrease oxygen needs; prevent acidosis. Prevent chilling:
   a. Minimize exposure; dry quickly.
   b. Warm; apply hat.
   c. Take temperature hourly until stable.
3. Goal: *identify infant:*
   a. Apply Identiband or name beads.
   b. Take infant's footprints and maternal fingerprints.
4. Goal: *prevent eye infection* (gonorrheal and chlamydial ophthalmia neonatorum). Within 1 hr of birth apply antibiotic ointment in each eye.
5. Goal: *facilitate prompt identification/vigilance for potential neonatal complications.*
   a. Record significant data from mother's chart:
      (1) History of pregnancy, diabetes, hypertension, current drug abuse, excessive caffeine, medications, alcohol, malnutrition.
      (2) Course of labor, evidence of fetal distress, medications received in labor.

TABLE 4–12   Apgar Score

Sign	0	1	2
Heart rate	Absent	<100	>100
Respiratory effort	Absent	Slow and irregular	Good and crying
Muscle tone	Flaccid	Some flexion of extremities	Active motions, general flexion
Reflex irritability	No response	Weak cry or grimace	Cry
Color	Blue, pale	Body pink, extremities blue	Completely pink

(3) Birth history of anesthesia.

(4) Apgar; resuscitative efforts.

6. Goal: *facilitate prompt identification/intervention in hemolytic problems of the newborn.*

  a. Collect and send cord blood for appropriate tests:

    (a) Blood type and Rh factor.

    (b) Coombs test.

  b. Give vitamin K to facilitate clotting.

D. Evaluation/outcome criteria: successful transition to extrauterine life.

1. Status satisfactory; all assessment findings within normal limits.

2. Responsive in bonding process with parents.

VIII. Nurse-attended emergency birth (precipitate birth). When woman presents without prenatal care to emergency department, may represent drug abuse.

IMMINENT BIRTH

◆ **A. Assessment:** identify signs of *imminent birth:*

1. Strong contractions.

2. Bearing-down efforts.

3. Perineal bulging; crowning.

4. Mother states, "It's coming."

◆ **B. Analysis/nursing diagnosis:**

1. *Pain* related to:

  a. Strong, sustained contractions.

  b. Descent of fetal head.

  c. Stretching of perineum.

2. *Anxiety/fear* related to imminent birth.

3. *Ineffective individual coping* related to circumstances surrounding birth; anxiety, fear for self and infant.

4. *Injury* (mother) related to lacerations (vaginal, perineal).

5. *Fluid volume deficit* related to:

  a. Lacerations.

  b. Uterine atony.

  c. Retained placental fragments.

6. *Impaired gas exchange* (infant) related to intact membranes after birth.

7. *Risk for injury* (infant) related to:

  a. Precipitate birth.

  b. Trauma.

  c. Hypoxia.

◆ **C. Nursing care plan/implementation:**

1. Goal: *reduce anxiety/fear*—reassure mother.

2. Goal: *delay birth,* as possible.

  a. Discourage bearing-down efforts.

  b. Encourage panting.

  c. *Side-lying position* to slow descent and allow for more controlled birth.

▶ 3. Goal: *prevent infection.*

  a. Provide clean field for birth.

  b. *Avoid* touching birth canal without gloved hands.

  c. Support perineum (and advancing head) with sterile (or clean) towel.

▶ 4. Goal: *prevent, or minimize, infant hypoxia* and perineal lacerations.

  a. If membranes intact as head emerges, tear at neck to facilitate first breath.

  b. Feel for cord around neck (if present, and if possible, slip cord over head; if tight, *and* sterile equipment at hand, clamp cord in two places, cut between clamps, unwrap cord). If unsterile environment, keep fetus and placenta attached—do not cut cord.

▶ 5. Goal: *facilitate/assist birth.*

  a. Hold head in both hands.

  b. Apply gentle downward pressure to bring anterior shoulder under pubic symphysis.

  c. Gently lift head to ease birth of posterior shoulder.

  d. Support infant as body slips free of mother's body.

▶ 6. Goal: *facilitate drainage of mucus and fluid →* patent airway.

  a. Hold infant in head-dependent *position.*

  b. Clear mucus with bulb syringe (if available), or use fingertip, wipe with towel.

▶ 7. Goal: *prevent placental transfusion*—hold infant level with placenta until cord stops pulsating, clamp and cut.

▶ 8. Goal: *prevent chilling.*

  a. Wrap infant in towel or other clean material.

  b. Place infant on side, head dependent, on mother's abdomen.

  c. Dry head, cover with cap or material.

9. Goal: *stimulate respiration.* If neonate *fails to breathe* spontaneously:

  a. Maintain body temperature—dry and cover.

  b. Clear airway

    (1) *Position:* head down.

    (2) Turn head to side.

  c. Stimulate.

    (1) Rub back gently.

    (2) Flick soles of feet.

  d. If no response to stimulation:

    (1) Slightly extend neck to "sniffing" *position* (head tilt–chin lift method).

    (2) Place mouth over newborn's nose and mouth and exhale air in cheeks, saying "ho" (prevents excessive pressure).

▶ 10. Goal: begin *cardiopulmonary resuscitation (CPR)* if no heart rate.

  a. Place infant on firm, flat surface.

  b. With two fingers on sternum depress ½-¾ inch 100 times/min.

  c. Assist ventilation on upstroke of every fifth compression (5:1 ratio).

  d. Go immediately to emergency department.

11. Goal: *maintain infant's body temperature.*

  a. Wrap placenta with baby, if cord intact.

  b. Place infant in mother's arms.

PLACENTAL SEPARATION

◆ **A. Assessment**—*third stage:* identify signs of *placental separation.*

◆ **B. Nursing care plan/implementation:**

1. Goal: *avoid/minimize potential for complications* (everted uterus, tearing of placenta with fragments remaining, separation of cord from placenta).
   a. *Avoid* traction (pulling) on cord.
   b. *Avoid* vigorous fundal massage.
   c. Discourage maternal bearing-down efforts unless placenta visible at introitus.
   d. With fundus well contracted, and placenta visible at introitus, encourage mother to bear down to expel placenta.

2. Goal: *prevent maternal hemorrhage* (uterine atony).
   a. Encourage breastfeeding, or stimulate nipple.
   b. Gently massage fundus, support lower part of uterus, and express clots when uterus is contracted.
   c. Encourage voiding if bladder is full.
   d. Get to a medical facility.

3. Goal: *encourage bonding/stimulate uterine contractions.* Encourage breastfeeding.

4. Goal: *legal accountability* as birth attendant. Record date, time, birth events, maternal and fetal status.

◆ **C. Evaluation/outcome criteria:**

1. Experiences normal spontaneous birth of viable infant over intact perineum.
2. Uncomplicated fourth stage—status satisfactory for both mother and infant.
3. Expresses satisfaction in management and result.

IX. Alterations affecting protective function

A. Induction of labor—deliberate initiation of uterine contractions.

1. Indications for:
   a. History of rapid or silent labors, precipitate birth.
   b. Woman resides some distance from hospital (controversial).
   c. Coexisting medical disorders:
      (1) Uncontrolled diabetes.
      (2) Progressive preeclampsia.
      (3) Severe renal disease.
      (4) Cardiac disease.
   d. PROM—spontaneous rupture of membranes before onset of labor and less than 37 wk from last menstrual period.
      Hazards:
      (1) Maternal—intrauterine infection (chorioamnionitis, endometritis).
      (2) Fetal—sepsis; prolapsed cord.
   e. Rh or ABO incompatibility, fetal hemolytic disease.
   f. Congenital anomaly (e.g., anencephaly).

g. Postterm pregnancy with nonreactive nonstress test (NST), or oligohydramnios.
h. Intrauterine fetal demise.

2. *Criteria for induction:*
   a. Absence of CPD, malpresentation, or malposition.
   b. Engaged vertex of single gestation.
   c. Nearing, or at term.
   d. Fetal lung maturity.
      (1) Survival rate—better at 32 wk or more.
      (2) *Lecithin/sphingomyelin* ratio greater than 2:1.
      (3) Diabetic mother—PG is present in amniotic fluid.
   e. "Ripe" cervix—softening, partially effaced, or ready for effacement/dilation (if not already present). *Note:* Intravaginal or paracervical application of prostaglandin gel, or misoprostol may be used to prepare cervix for labor.

3. *Methods:*
   a. Amniotomy—artificial rupture of membranes with fetal head engaged and dilation of cervix.
   b. Intravenous oxytocin infusion.

4. *Potential complications:*
   a. *Amniotomy*—irrevocably committed to birth. Hazards:
      (1) Prolapsed cord.
      (2) Infection.
   b. *IV oxytocin infusion:*
      (1) Overstimulation of uterus.
      (2) Decreased placental perfusion/fetal distress (neonatal jaundice).
      (3) Precipitate labor and birth.
      (4) Cervical/perineal lacerations.
      (5) Uterine rupture.
      (6) Postpartum hemorrhage.
      (7) Water intoxication—if large doses given in D/W over prolonged period (antidiuretic effect increases water reabsorption).
      (8) Hypertensive crisis.

BEFORE INDUCTION

◆ **5. Assessment**—*before induction:*
   a. Estimate of gestation (EDB, fundal height, cervical status).
   b. *Bishop score:* evaluation of cervical inducibility
   c. General health status:
      (1) Weight, vital signs, FHR, edema.
      (2) Status of membranes.
      (3) Vaginal bleeding.
      (4) Coexisting disorders.
   d. History of previous labors, if any.
   e. Emotional status.
   f. Knowledge/understanding of anticipated procedures:
      (1) Amniotomy (artificial rupture of membranes).

Maternal-Infant

(2) IV oxytocin infusion.

(3) Fetal monitoring

g. Preparation for childbirth (Lamaze, etc.); coping strategies. Identify support person.

◆ **6. Analysis/nursing diagnosis:**

a. *Knowledge deficit* related to process of induction.

b. *Anxiety/fear* related to need for induction of labor.

c. *Ineffective individual coping* related to psychological stress.

d. *Pain* related to uterine contractions.

◆ **7. Nursing care plan/implementation:**

a. Goal: *health teaching.*

(1) Explain rationale for procedures:

(a) *Amniotomy.*

(i) Induces labor.

(ii) Relieves uterine overdistention.

(iii) Increases efficiency of contractions, shortening labor.

(b) *Oxytocin infusion.*

(i) Induces labor.

(ii) Stimulates uterine contractions.

(c) *Internal fetal monitor.*

(i) Provides continuous assessment of uterine response to oxytocin stimulation.

(ii) Provides continuous assessment of fetal response to physiological stress of labor.

(2) *Describe procedure*—to reduce anxiety and increase cooperation.

(3) *Explain advantages/disadvantages*—to ensure "informed consent."

b. Goal: *emotional support*—encourage verbalization of concerns, reassure, as possible.

◆ **8. Evaluation/outcome criterion:** woman verbalizes understanding of process, rationale, procedures, and alternatives.

DURING INDUCTION AND LABOR

◆ **9. Assessment**—*during induction and labor:*

a. *Amniotomy*—same as for spontaneous rupture of membranes:

(1) Observe fluid—note color, amount.

(2) Monitor FHR; assess for fetal distress.

(3) Observe for signs of prolapsed cord.

(4) Assess fetal activity.

(a) Excessive activity may indicate distress.

(b) Absence of activity may indicate distress or demise.

b. *IV oxytocin infusion:*

(1) Continually assess response to oxytocin stimulation/flow rate; always given by controlled infusion.

(a) Uterine contractions.

(b) Maternal vital signs, FHR.

(2) Identify signs of:

(a) *Deviation* from normal patterns:

(i) Lack of response to increasing flow rate.

(ii) Uterine hyperirritability (contractions—less than 2 min apart).

(iii) Lack of adequate uterine relaxation between contractions.

(b) *Side effects* of oxytocin: diminished output—potential water intoxication.

(c) **Hazards** to mother or fetus:

(i) Sustained (over 90 sec) or tetanic (strong, spasmlike) contractions—potential abruptio placentae, uterine rupture, fetal hypoxia/anoxia/death.

(ii) *Fetal* arrhythmias, decelerations.

(iii) *Maternal* hypertension—potential for hypertensive crisis, cerebral hemorrhage.

◆ **10. Nursing care plan/implementation:**

a. Same as for other women in labor.

b. If indications of deviations from normal patterns:

(1) Change maternal position (see Figure 4–6).

(2) Stop oxytocin infusion, maintain IV with Ringer's lactate, etc.

▶ (3) Begin oxygen per mask; up to 8-10 L/min.

(4) Notify physician promptly.

(5) Check maternal blood pressure and pulse rate.

c. Anticipatory guidance: may have strong contractions soon after induction starts.

◆ **11. Evaluation/outcome criteria:**

a. Demonstrates response to oxytocin stimulation.

(1) Establishes desired contraction pattern, not hyperstimulated.

(2) Progresses through labor—within normal limits:

(a) Normotensive.

(b) Voids in adequate amounts.

(c) No evidence of deviation from normal contraction patterns.

b. No evidence of fetal distress.

c. Experiences normal vaginal birth of viable infant.

B. **Operative obstetrics**—procedures used to prevent trauma/reduce hazard to mother or infant during the birth process.

1. **Episiotomy**—incision of perineum to facilitate infant's birth.
   a. Rationale:
      (1) Surgical incision reduces possibility of laceration.
      (2) Protects infant's head from pressure exerted by resistant perineum.
      (3) Shortens second stage of labor.
   b. Types:
      (1) Midline—chance of extension into anal sphincter greater than with mediolateral.
      (2) Mediolateral—healing is more painful than midline.
   ◆ c. **Assessment:**
      (1) **REEDA:**
         (a) *R*edness
         (b) *E*dema
         (c) *E*cchymosis
         (d) *D*ischarge
         (e) *A*pproximation (suture line intact, separated)
      (2) Healing.
      (3) Bruised; hematoma.
      (4) Tenderness; pain. *Note:* Evaluate complaints of pain carefully. If intense, and unrelieved by usual measures, report promptly. May indicate vulvar, paravaginal, or ischiorectal abscess or hematoma.
   ◆ d. **Analysis/nursing diagnosis:**
      (1) *Pain* related to labor process.
      (2) *Impaired skin integrity* related to surgical incision.
      (3) *Fluid volume deficit* related to hematoma.
      (4) *Sexual dysfunction* related to discomfort.
   ◆ e. **Nursing care plan/implementation:**
      (1) Goal: *prevent/reduce edema, promote comfort and healing.*
         (a) Place covered ice pack during immediate postpartum
         (b) Administer analgesics, topical sprays, ointments, witch hazel pads, hydrocortisone.
         (c) Encourage use of sitz bath or rubber ring.
         (d) Encourage Kegel exercises.
         (e) Do *health teaching:*
            (i) Instruct in tightening gluteal muscles before sitting.
            (ii) Instruct to *avoid* sitting on one hip.
      (2) Goal: *minimize potential for infection.*
         (a) Teach/provide perineal care during fourth stage of labor.
         (b) *Health teaching:* instruct in self-perineal care after voiding, defecation, and with each pad change.

   ◆ f. **Evaluation/outcome criteria:**
      (1) Woman's incision heals by primary intention.
      (2) Woman demonstrates appropriate self-perineal care.
      (3) Woman evidences no signs of hematoma, infection, or separation of suture line.
      (4) Woman experiences minimal discomfort.

2. **Forceps-assisted birth**—use of instruments to assist birth of infant.
   a. Indications:
      (1) Fetal distress.
      (2) Maternal need:
         (a) Exhaustion.
         (b) Coexisting disease, such as cardiac disorder.
         (c) Poor progress in second stage.
         (d) Persistent fetal OT or OP position.
   b. *Criteria* for forceps application:
      (1) Engaged fetal head.
      (2) Ruptured membranes.
      (3) Full dilatation.
      (4) Absence of CPD.
      (5) Some anesthesia has been given; usually, episiotomy has been performed.
      (6) Empty bladder.
   c. *Types:*
      (1) Low—outlet forceps.
      (2) Mid—applied after head is engaged (rarely used).
      (3) Pipers—applied to after-coming head in selected breech births.
   d. *Potential complications:*
      (1) *Maternal:*
         (a) Lacerations of birth canal, rectum, bladder.
         (b) Uterine rupture/hemorrhage.
      (2) *Neonatal:*
         (a) Cephalhematoma.
         (b) Skull fracture.
         (c) Intracranial hemorrhage, brain damage.
         (d) Facial paralysis.
         (e) Direct tissue trauma (abrasions, ecchymosis).
         (f) Umbilical cord compression.
   ◆ e. **Assessment:**
      ▶ (1) FHR immediately before—and after—forceps application (forceps blade may compress umbilical cord).
      (2) Observe mother/newborn for injury or signs of complications.
   ◆ f. **Analysis/nursing diagnosis:**
      (1) *Self-esteem disturbance* related to inability to give birth without surgical assistance.

Maternal-Infant

(2) *Anxiety/fear* related to infant's appearance (forceps marks) or awareness of potential complications.

◆ g. **Nursing care plan/implementation:**
   (1) Goal: *minimize feelings of failure due to inability to give birth "naturally."*
      (a) Explain, discuss reasons/indications for forceps-assisted birth.
      (b) Emphasize no maternal control over circumstances.
   (2) Goal: *reduce parental anxiety, maternal guilt over infant bruising/forceps marks.* Explain condition is temporary and has no lasting effects on child's appearance.

◆ h. **Evaluation/outcome criteria:**
   (1) Woman verbalizes understanding of reasons for forceps-assisted birth.
   (2) Woman evidences no interruption in bonding with infant.
   (3) Woman experiences uncomplicated recovery.

3. Vacuum extraction (soft plastic cup with vacuum from a suction pump). Used to assist in rotation or delivery of the fetal head.
   a. Risks may include caput succedaneum and cephelhematoma.
   b. Causes neonatal jaundice, IVH → death.

4. **Cesarean birth**—incision through abdominal wall and uterus to give birth.
   a. Indications for elective cesarean birth:
      (1) Known CPD.
      (2) Previous uterine surgery (e.g., myomectomy), repeated cesarean births (depends on type of incision done).
      (3) Active maternal genital herpes II infection; human papilloma virus (HPV).
      (4) Breech presentation. (*Note:* To reduce infant morbidity/mortality, elective cesarean birth is common method of choice.)
      (5) Neoplasms of cervix, uterus, or birth canal.
      (6) Maternal diabetes with placental aging; fetal macrosomia (CPD); >425 g.
   b. *Criteria* for elective cesarean birth:
      L/S ratio greater than 2:1 —indicates presence of pulmonary surfactant; less risk of respiratory distress syndrome.
   c. *Indications for emergency cesarean birth:*
      (1) **Fetal:**
         (a) *Fetal distress:* prolapsed cord, repetitive late deceleration, prolonged bradycardia.
         (b) *Fetal jeopardy:* Rh or ABO incompatibility.
         (c) *Fetal malposition/malpresentation.*

      (2) **Maternal:**
         (a) Uterine dysfunction; rupture.
         (b) Placental disorders:
            (i) Placenta previa.
            (ii) Abruptio placentae, with Couvelaire uterus.
         (c) Severe maternal PIH/eclampsia.
         (d) Fetopelvic disproportion.
         (e) Sudden maternal death.
         (f) Carcinoma.
         (g) Failed induction.
   d. *Types:*
      (1) Low segment—method of choice:
         (a) Transverse incision through abdominal wall and lower uterine segment.
         (b) Transverse incision through abdominal wall, with vertical incision of lower uterine segment.
         (c) Advantages—fewer complications:
            (i) Less blood loss.
            (ii) More comfortable convalescence.
            (iii) Less adhesion formation.
            (iv) Lower risk of uterine rupture in subsequent pregnancy/labor and birth.
            (v) Cosmetically more acceptable.
      (2) Classic—vertical incision through abdominal wall and uterus. Necessary for anterior placenta previa and transverse lie, <28 weeks prematurity.
      (3) Porro's—hysterotomy followed by hysterectomy. Necessary in presence of:
         (a) Hemorrhage from uterine atony.
         (b) Placenta accreta/percreta.
         (c) Large uterine myomas.
         (d) Ruptured uterus.
         (e) Cancer of uterus or ovary.

◆ e. **Assessment:**
   (1) Maternal physical status.
      (a) Vital signs.
      (b) Labor status, if any.
      (c) Contractions (if any).
      (d) Membranes (intact; ruptured).
      (e) Bleeding.
   (2) Fetal status.
      (a) FHR pattern.
      (b) Color and amount of amniotic fluid.
      (c) Biophysical profile (BPP)
   (3) Maternal emotional status.
   (4) Understanding of procedure, indications for, implications.
   (5) Other—as for any abdominal surgery (see **Unit 7**).

◆ f. **Analysis/nursing diagnosis:**
  (1) *Self-esteem disturbance* related to perceived failure to give birth vaginally.
  (2) *Anxiety/fear* related to impending surgery and/or reasons for cesarean birth.
  (3) *Ineffective individual coping* related to anxiety and fear for self, infant.
  (4) *Fluid volume deficit* related to abdominal surgery or reason for cesarean birth.
  (5) *Pain* related to abdominal surgery.
  (6) *Constipation* related to decreased bowel activity.
  (7) *Altered urinary elimination* related to fluid volume deficit.

◆ g. **Nursing care plan/implementation:**
  (1) *Preoperative:*
    (a) Goal: *safeguard fetal status.*
      (i) Monitor fetal heart rate continually.
      (ii) Notify neonatology and neonatal intensive care unit (NICU) of scheduled surgical birth.
    (b) Goal: *health teaching.*
      (i) Describe, discuss anticipated anesthesia.
      (ii) Explain rationale for preoperative antacids to minimize effects of aspiration: cimetidine, Bicitra, histamine blocker to decrease production of gastric acid. Reglan (metoclopramide), to hasten gastric emptying.
      (iii) Describe, explain anticipated procedures—abdominal shave, indwelling catheter, intravenous fluids—to woman and support person.
    (c) Other—as for any abdominal surgery.
    (d) Prepare for cesarean birth.
  (2) *Postoperative:*
    (a) Same as for other abdominal surgical patients (see **Unit 7**).
    (b) Same as for other postpartum women.

◆ h. **Evaluation/outcome criteria:**
  (1) Verbalizes understanding of reasons for cesarean birth.
  (2) Successful birth of viable infant.
  (3) Evidences no surgical/birth complications.
  (4) Evidences no interference with bonding.
  (5) Expresses satisfaction with procedure and result.

5. **Trial of labor after cesarean (TOLAC)**

  a. Candidates for TOLAC.
    (1) Previous low transverse cesarean birth.
    (2) Head well-engaged in pelvis (vertex presentation).
    (3) Soft anterior cervix.
    (4) Preexisting reason for repeated cesarean birth not apparent.

◆ b. **Assessment:**
    (1) Monitor FHR carefully during trial of labor.
    (2) Monitor contractions carefully for adequate progress of labor.
    (3) Observe mother for signs of complications/uterine rupture.

◆ c. **Analysis/nursing diagnosis:**
    (1) *Knowledge deficit* related to trial of labor.
    (2) *Fear* related to outcome for fetus.
    (3) *Ineffective individual coping* related to labor progress and outcome.

Complications During the Intrapartal Period

I. **General aspects**
  A. **Pathophysiology**—interference with normal processes and patterns of labor/birth result in maternal or fetal jeopardy (e.g., **preterm** labor, **dysfunctional** labor patterns; **prolonged** [over 24] labor; **hemorrhage: uterine rupture**/inversion, **amniotic-fluid embolus**).
  B. **Etiology:**
    1. **Preterm labor**—unknown.
    2. **Dysfunctional labor (dystocia:** see p. 145):
      a. Physiological response to anxiety/fear/pain—results in release of catecholamines, increasing physical/psychological stress → myometrial dysfunction; painful and ineffectual labor.
      b. Iatrogenic factors: premature or excessive analgesia, particularly during latent phase.
      c. *Maternal factors:*
        (1) Pelvic contractures.
        (2) Uterine tumors (e.g., myomas, carcinoma).
        (3) Congenital uterine anomalies (e.g., bicornate uterus).
        (4) Pathological contraction ring (*Bandl's* ring).
        (5) Rigid cervix, cervical stenosis/stricture.
        (6) Hypertonic/hypotonic contractions.
        (7) Prolonged rupture of membranes. *Note:* Intrauterine infection may have caused rupture of membranes or may follow rupture.

(8) Prolonged first or second stage.

(9) Medical conditions: diabetes, hypertension.

d. *Fetal factors:*

(1) Macrosomia (LGA).

(2) Malposition/malpresentation.

(3) Congenital anomaly (e.g., hydrocephalus, anencephaly).

(4) Multifetal gestation (e.g., interlocking twins).

(5) Prolapsed cord.

(6) Postterm.

e. *Placental factors:*

(1) Placenta previa.

(2) Inadequate placental function with contractions.

(3) Abruptio placentae.

(4) Placenta accreta.

f. Physical restrictions: when confined to bed, *flat position,* etc.

◆ **C. Assessment:**

1. Antepartal history.

2. Emotional status.

3. Vital signs, FHR.

4. Contraction pattern (frequency, duration, intensity).

5. Vaginal discharge.

◆ **D. Analysis/nursing diagnosis:**

1. *Anxiety/fear* for self and infant related to implications of prolonged or complicated labor/birth.

2. *Pain* related to hypertonic contractions/dysfunctional labor.

3. *Ineffective individual coping* related to physical/psychological stress of complicated labor/birth, lowered pain threshold secondary to fatigue.

4. *High risk for injury* related to prolonged rupture of membranes, infection.

5. *Fluid volume deficit* related to excessive blood loss secondary to placenta previa, abruptio placentae, Couvelaire uterus, DIC.

◆ **E. Nursing care plan/implementation:**

1. Goal: *minimize physical/psychological stress during labor/birth.* Assist woman in coping effectively:

a. Reinforce relaxation techniques.

b. Support couple's effective coping techniques/mechanisms.

2. Goal: *emotional support.*

a. Encourage verbalization of anxiety/fear/concerns.

b. Explain all procedures—to minimize anxiety/fear, encourage cooperation/participation in care.

c. Provide quiet environment conducive to rest.

3. Goal: *continuous monitoring of maternal/fetal status and progress through labor*—to identify early signs of dysfunctional labor, fetal dis-

tress; facilitate prompt, effective treatment of emerging complications.

4. Goal: *minimize effects of complicated labor on mother, fetus.*

▰ a. *Position* change: lateral Sims'—to reduce compression of inferior vena cava.

b. Oxygen per mask, as indicated.

c. Institute interventions appropriate to emerging problems (see specific disorder).

◆ **F. Evaluation/outcome criteria:**

1. Woman has successful birth of viable infant.

2. Maternal/infant status stable, satisfactory.

II. Disorders affecting protective functions. Preterm labor—occurs after 20 weeks of gestation and before beginning of wk 38.

A. Pathophysiology—physiological events of labor (i.e., contractions, spontaneous rupture of membranes, cervical effacement/dilation) occur before completion of normal, term gestation.

B. Etiology—causes may be from maternal, fetal, or placental factors.

C. *Coexisting disorders:*

1. Infections that may cause PROM.

2. PROM of unknown etiology.

3. PIH (preeclampsia/eclampsia).

4. Uterine overdistention.

a. Polyhydramnios.

b. Multifetal gestation.

5. Maternal diabetes, renal or cardiovascular disorder, UTI.

6. Severe maternal illness (e.g., pneumonia, acute pyelonephritis).

7. Abnormal placentation.

a. Placenta previa.

b. Abruptio placentae.

8. Iatrogenic: miscalculated EDB for repeat cesarean birth (rare).

9. Fetal death.

10. Incompetent cervical os (small percentage).

11. Uterine anomalies (rare).

a. Intrauterine septum.

b. Bicornate uterus.

12. Uterine fibroids.

13. Positive fetal fibronectin assay (protein found in fetal tissue, membranes, amniotic fluid, and the decidua) found in cervical/vaginal fluid first half of pregnancy and normally absent through mid to late pregnancy (↑ risk of PTL by 20%).

D. *Prevention:*

1. *Primary*—close obstetric supervision; education in signs/symptoms of labor.

2. *Secondary*—prompt, effective treatment of associated disorders (see II. C., p. 142).

3. *Tertiary*—suppression of preterm labor.

a. Bedrest.

▰ b. *Position:* side-lying—to promote placental perfusion.

c. Hydration.

d. Pharmacological (may require "informed consent"; follow hospital protocol). Beta-adrenergic agents, MgSO$_4$ (take ECG first) to reduce sensitivity of uterine myometrium to oxytocic and prostaglandin stimulation; increase blood flow to uterus.

e. May be maintained at home with adequate follow-up and health teaching.

E. Contraindications for suppression: Labor is not suppressed in presence of:

1. Placenta previa or abruptio placentae with hemorrhage.
2. Chorioamnionitis.
3. Erythroblastosis fetalis.
4. Severe preeclampsia.
5. Severe diabetes (e.g., "brittle").
6. Increasing placental insufficiency.
7. Progressive cervical dilatation of 4 cm or more.
8. Ruptured membranes (with maternal fever).

◆ **F. Assessment:**

1. Maternal vital signs. Response to medication:
   a. Hypotension.
   b. Tachycardia, arrhythmia.
   c. Dyspnea, chest pain.
   d. Nausea and vomiting.
2. Signs of infection:
   a. Increased temperature.
   b. Tachycardia.
   c. Diaphoresis.
   d. Malaise.
   e. Increased baseline fetal heart rate; ↓ variability
3. Contractions: frequency, duration, strength.
4. Emotional status—signs of denial, guilt, anxiety, exhaustion.
5. Signs of continuing and progressing labor. *Note:* Vaginal examination *only* if indicated by other signs of continuing labor progress.
   a. Effacement.
   b. Dilation.
   c. Station.
6. Status of membranes.
7. Fetal heart rate, activity (continuous monitoring).

◆ **G. Analysis/nursing diagnosis:**

1. *Anxiety/fear* related to possible outcome.
2. *Self-esteem disturbance* related to feelings of guilt, failure.
3. *Impaired physical mobility* related to imposed bed rest.
4. *Knowledge deficit* related to medication side effects.
5. *Ineffective individual coping* related to possible outcome.
6. *Impaired gas exchange* related to side effects of medication (circulatory overload; pulmonary edema).
7. *Diversional activity deficit* related to imposed bed rest, decreased environmental stimuli.
8. *Altered urinary elimination* related to bed rest.
9. *Constipation* related to bed rest.

◆ **H. Nursing care plan/implementation:**

1. Goal: *inhibit uterine activity.* Administer medications as ordered—terbutaline, magnesium sulfate, Procardia, Indocin.
2. Goal: *safeguard status.*
   a. Continuous maternal/fetal monitoring.
   b. I&O—to identify early signs of possible circulatory overload.
   c. *Position:* side-lying—to increase placental perfusion, prevent supine hypotension.
   d. Report **promptly** to physician:

   > (1) Maternal pulse of 110 or more.
   > (2) Diastolic pressure of 60 mm Hg or less.
   > (3) Respirations of 24 or more; crackles (rales).
   > (4) Complaint of dyspnea.
   > (5) Contractions: increasing frequency, strength, duration, or cessation of contractions.
   > (6) Intermittent back and thigh pain.
   > (7) Rupture of membranes.
   > (8) Vaginal bleeding.
   > (9) Fetal distress.

3. Goal: *comfort measures.*
   a. Basic hygienic care—bath, mouth care, cold washcloth to face, perineal care.
   b. Back rub, linen change—to promote relaxation.
4. Goal: *emotional support.*
   a. Encourage verbalization of guilt feelings, anxiety, fear, concerns; provide factual information.
   b. Support positive self-concept.
   c. Keep informed of progress.
5. Goal: *provide quiet diversion.* Television, reading materials, handcrafts.
6. Goal: *health teaching*
   a. Explain, discuss proposed management to suppress preterm labor.
   b. Describe, discuss side effects of medication.
   c. Explain rationale for bed rest, position.

I. If labor continues to progress:

1. Goal: *facilitate infant survival.*
   a. Administer betamethasone, as ordered, 24–48 hr before birth—to increase/stimulate production of pulmonary surfactant.
   b. Give antibiotic to mother to ↓ chance of neonatal sepsis.
   c. Notify neonatal ICU (NICU)—to increase chances for fetal survival, ensure prompt, expert management of neonate, and provide information and support to parents.
   d. Monitor progress of labor to identify signs of impending birth. *Note:* May give birth before complete (10 cm) dilation.
   e. Consider transfer to high-risk facility.
   f. Prepare for birth, or cesarean birth if infant less than 34–36 weeks of gestation.
2. Goal: *emotional support.*

a. Do *not* leave woman (or couple) alone.

b. Encourage verbalization of anxiety, fear, concern.

c. Explain all procedures.

3. Goal: *comfort measures. Note:* Analgesics used conservatively—to prevent depression of fetus/neonate.

4. Goal: *support effective coping techniques.* Encourage support Lamaze (or other) techniques—coach, as necessary; discourage hyperventilation.

5. Goal: *health teaching*—for severe preterm birth.

a. Discuss need for episiotomy, possibility of outlet forceps-assisted birth—to reduce stress on fetal head, or

b. Prepare for cesarean birth—to reduce possibility of fetal intraventricular hemorrhage.

c. Rationale for avoiding use of medications to reduce contraction pain.

J. Immediate care of neonate:

1. Goal: *safeguard status.*

a. Stabilize environmental temperature—to prevent chilling (isolette or other controlled-temperature bed).

▶ b. Suction, oxygen, as needed; may need intubation.

◗ c. Parenteral fluids, as ordered—to support normal acid-base balance, pH; administer antibiotics, as necessary.

d. Arrange transport to high-risk facility, as necessary.

2. Goal: *continuous monitoring of status.*

a. Electronic monitors—to observe respiratory and cardiac functions.

▍ b. Blood samples—to monitor blood gases, pH, hypoglycemia.

K. Postpartum care: Goal: *emotional support.*

1. Facilitate attachment—photos if baby transferred or mother unable to visit.

2. If couple, foster sense of mutual experience and closeness.

3. Help her/them maintain a positive self-image.

4. Encourage touching of infant before transport to nursery or high-risk facility; father/partner may accompany infant and report back to mother.

5. Encourage early contact—to facilitate mother's need to ventilate her feelings.

6. Assist parent(s) with grieving process, if necessary.

7. Refer to support group if necessary.

L. *Other*—as for any postpartum woman.

◆ **M. Evaluation/outcome criteria:**

1. Woman verbalizes understanding of medical/nursing recommendations and treatments.

2. Woman complies with medical/nursing regimen.

3. Woman experiences no discomfort from side effects of therapy.

4. Woman experiences successful outcome—labor inhibited.

5. Woman carries pregnancy to successful termination.

6. If preterm birth occurs, woman copes effectively with outcome (physiologically compromised neonate, neonatal death).

III. Grief and childbearing experience. The loss of a pregnancy or a newborn, or the birth of a physiologically compromised child (preterm, congenital disorder) is a crisis situation. The unexpected outcome can cause the parent(s) to suffer a sense of loss of self-esteem, self-concept, positive body image, feelings of worth (see p. 163).

◆ **A. Assessment:**

1. Response to loss of the "fantasy child"/real child.

a. Behavioral—anger, hostility, depression, disinterest in activities of daily living, withdrawal.

b. Biophysical—somatic complaints (stomach pain, malaise, anorexia, nausea).

c. Cognitive—feelings of guilt.

2. Knowledge/understanding/perception of situation.

3. Coping abilities, mechanisms.

4. Support system.

◆ **B. Analysis/nursing diagnosis:**

1. *Ineffective family coping: compromised* related to psychological stress related to fear for infant, guilt feelings, impact on self-image.

2. *Ineffective individual coping* related to anxiety, stress.

3. *Ineffective family coping: disabling* related to disturbance in intrafamily relations secondary to individual coping deficits, recriminations.

4. *Altered parenting* related to lack of effective bonding secondary to emotional separation from infant, feelings of guilt.

5. *Dysfunctional grieving* related to guilt feelings, impact of loss on self-concept.

6. *Disturbance in body image, self-esteem, role performance* related to perceived failure to complete gestational task, produce perfect, healthy infant; associated with sleep deprivation.

7. *Social isolation* related to severe coping deficit, dysfunctional grieving, disturbance in self-esteem.

◆ **C. Nursing care plan/implementation:**

1. Goal: *emotional support.*

a. Provide privacy; encourage open expression/verbalization of feelings, fears, concerns, perceptions.

b. Crisis intervention techniques.

2. Goal: *facilitate bonding, effective coping, or anticipatory grieving processes.*

a. Encourage contact and participation in care of premature or compromised infant.

b. Keep informed of infant's status.

c. Provide realistic data.

3. Goal: *health teaching.*

   a. Clarify misperceptions, as appropriate.

   b. Discuss, demonstrate infant care techniques (e.g., feeding infant who has cleft lip or palate).

   c. Refer to appropriate community resources.

◆ **D. Evaluation/outcome criteria:**

1. Woman verbalizes recognition and acceptance of diagnosis.

2. Woman verbalizes understanding of relevant information regarding treatment, prognosis.

3. Woman makes informed decision regarding infant care.

4. Woman demonstrates comfort and increasing participation in care of neonate.

5. Woman shows evidence of bonding (eye contact, cuddles, calls infant by name).

IV. Disorders affecting comfort, rest, mobility: dystocia

A. Definition—difficult labor.

💡 **B.** *General aspects (MOTHER, "3 Ps": Psych, Placenta, Position):*

1. **Pathophysiology**—see specific disorders.

💡 2. **Etiology**—due to effects of factors that affect the FETUS (also "3 Ps"):

   a. *POWER:* forces of labor (uterine contractions, use of abdominal muscles).

      (1) Premature analgesia/anesthesia.

      (2) Uterine overdistention (multifetal pregnancy, fetal macrosomia).

      (3) Uterine myomas.

   b. *PASSAGEWAY:* resistance of cervix, pelvic structures.

      (1) Rigid cervix.

      (2) Distended bladder.

      (3) Distended rectum

      (4) Dimensions of the bony pelvis: pelvic contractures.

   c. *PASSENGER:* accommodation of the presenting part to pelvic diameters.

      (1) Fetal malposition/malpresentation.

         (a) Transverse lie.

         (b) Face, brow presentation.

         (c) Breech presentation.

         (d) CPD.

      (2) Fetal anomalies.

         (a) Hydrocephalus.

         (b) Conjoined ("Siamese") twins.

         (c) Meningomyelocele

      (3) Fetal size.

3. **Hazards:**

   a. *Maternal:*

      (1) Fatigue, exhaustion, dehydration—due to prolonged labor.

      (2) Lowered pain threshold, loss of control—due to prolonged labor, contin-

ued uterine contractions, anxiety, fatigue, lack of sleep.

      (3) Intrauterine infection—due to prolonged rupture of membranes and frequent vaginal examinations.

      (4) Uterine rupture—due to obstructed labor.

      (5) Cervical, vaginal, perineal lacerations—due to obstetric interventions.

      (6) Postpartum hemorrhage—due to uterine atony or trauma.

   b. *Fetal:*

      (1) Hypoxia, anoxia, demise—due to decreased O_2 concentration in cord blood.

      (2) Intracranial hemorrhage—due to changing intracranial pressure.

C. Hypertonic dysfunction

1. **Pathophysiology**—increased resting tone of uterine myometrium; diminished refractory period; prolonged latent phase:

   a. *Nullipara*—more than 20 hr.

   b. *Multipara*—more than 14 hr.

2. **Etiology**—unknown. Theory—ectopic initiation of incoordinate uterine contractions.

◆ 3. **Assessment:**

   a. Onset—early labor (latent phase).

   b. Contractions:

      (1) Continuous fundal tension, incomplete relaxation.

      (2) Painful.

      (3) Ineffectual—no effacement or dilation.

   c. Signs of fetal distress

      (1) Meconium-stained amniotic fluid.

      (2) FHR irregularities.

   d. Maternal vital signs.

   e. Emotional status.

   f. Medical evaluation: vaginal examination, x-ray pelvimetry, ultrasonography—to rule out CPD.

◆ 4. **Analysis/nursing diagnosis:**

   a. *Pain* related to hypertonic contractions, incomplete uterine relaxation.

   b. *Anxiety/fear* for self and infant related to strong, painful contractions without evidence of progress.

   c. *Ineffective individual coping* related to fatigue, exhaustion, anxiety, tension, fear.

   d. *Impaired gas exchange (fetal)* related to incomplete relaxation of uterus.

   e. *Sleep pattern disturbance* related to prolonged ineffectual labor.

◆ 5. **Nursing care plan/implementation:**

   a. Medical management:

      (1) Short-acting barbiturates (see **Unit 10**)—to encourage rest, relaxation.

      (2) Intravenous fluids—to restore/maintain hydration and fluid-electrolyte balance.

(3) If CPD, cesarean birth.
b. Nursing management:
(1) Goal: *emotional support*—assist coping with fear, pain, discouragement.
(a) Encourage verbalization of anxiety, fear, concerns.
(b) Explain all procedures.
(c) Reassure. Keep couple informed of progress.
(2) Goal: *comfort measures.*
◪ (a) *Position:* side-lying—to promote relaxation and placental perfusion.
(b) Bath, back rub, linen change, clean environment.
(c) Environment: quiet, darkened room—to minimize stimuli and encourage relaxation, warmth.
(d) Encourage voiding—to relieve bladder distention; to test urine for ketones.
(3) Goal: *prevent infection.* Strict aseptic technique.
(4) Goal: *prepare for cesarean birth* if necessary.
◆ 6. **Evaluation/outcome criteria:**
a. Relaxes, sleeps, establishes normal labor pattern.
b. Demonstrates no signs of fetal distress.
c. Successfully completes uneventful labor.
D. **Hypotonic dysfunction during labor**
1. **Pathophysiology**—after normal labor at onset, contractions diminish in frequency, duration and strength; lowered uterine resting tone; cervical effacement and dilation slow/cease.
2. **Etiology:**
a. Premature or excessive analgesia/anesthesia (epidural block or spinal block).
b. CPD.
c. Overdistention (hydramnios, fetal macrosomia, multifetal pregnancy).
d. Fetal malposition/malpresentation.
e. Maternal fear/anxiety.
◆ 3. **Assessment:**
a. Onset—may occur in latent phase; most common during active phase.
b. Contractions: normal previously, demonstrate:
(1) Decreased frequency.
(2) Shorter duration.
(3) Diminished intensity (mild to moderate).
(4) Less uncomfortable.
c. Cervical changes—slow or cease.
d. Signs of fetal distress—rare.
(1) Usually occur late in labor due to infection secondary to prolonged rupture of membranes.
(2) Tachycardia.

e. Maternal vital signs may indicate infection (↑temperature).
▯ f. Medical diagnosis—procedures: vaginal examination, x-ray pelvimetry, ultrasonography—to rule out CPD (most common cause).
◆ 4. **Analysis/nursing diagnosis:**
a. *Knowledge deficit* related to limited exposure to information.
b. *Anxiety/fear* related to failure to progress as anticipated; fear for fetus.
c. *High risk for injury* (infection) related to prolonged labor or ruptured membranes.
◆ 5. **Nursing care plan/implementation:**
a. Medical management:
(1) Amniotomy—artificial rupture of membranes.
◖▢ (2) Oxytocin augmentation of labor—intravenous infusion of oxytocin to increase frequency, duration, strength, and efficiency of uterine contractions (see Induction of labor, p. 137).
(3) If CPD, cesarean birth.
b. Nursing management:
(1) Goals: *emotional support, comfort measures, prevent infection*—as for Hypertonic dysfunction, see p. 145.
(2) Other—see Induction of labor, p. 137.
◆ 6. **Evaluation/outcome criteria:**
a. Reestablishes normal labor pattern.
b. Experiences successful birth of viable infant.

V. **Disorders affecting fluid-gas transport:** *maternal*
A. **Uterine rupture**
1. **Pathophysiology**—stress on uterine muscle exceeds its ability to stretch.
2. **Etiology:**
a. Overdistention—due to large baby, multifetal gestation.
b. Old scars—due to previous cesarean births or uterine surgery.
c. Contractions against CPD, fetal malpresentation, pathological retraction ring (*Bandl's*).
d. Injudicious obstetrics-malapplication of forceps (or application without full effacement/dilation).
e. Tetanic contraction—due to hypersensitivity to oxytocin (or excessive dosage) during induction/augmentation of labor.
◆ 3. **Assessment:**
a. Identify predisposing factors early.
b. *Complete rupture*
(1) Pain: sudden, sharp, abdominal; followed by cessation of contractions; tender abdomen.
(2) Signs of shock; vaginal bleeding.
(3) Fetal heart tones—absent.

(4) Presenting part—not palpable on vaginal examination.
c. *Incomplete rupture*
(1) Contractions: continue, accompanied by abdominal pain and failure to dilate; may become dystonic.
(2) Signs of shock.
(3) May demonstrate vaginal bleeding.
(4) Fetal heart tones—absent/bradycardia.

4. **Prognosis**
a. Maternal—guarded.
b. Fetal—grave.

◆ 5. **Analysis/nursing diagnosis:**
a. *Pain* related to rupture of uterine muscle.
b. *Fluid volume deficit* related to massive blood loss secondary to uterine rupture.
c. *Anxiety/fear* related to concern for self, fetus.
d. *Altered tissue perfusion* related to blood loss secondary to uterine rupture.
e. *Altered urinary elimination* related to necessary conservation of intravascular fluid secondary to blood loss.
f. *Anticipatory grieving* related to expected loss of fetus; inability to have more children.

◆ 6. **Nursing care plan/implementation:**
a. Medical management:
(1) Surgical—laparotomy, hysterectomy.
(2) Replace blood loss—transfusion, packed cells.
(3) Reduce possibility of infection—antibiotics.
b. Nursing management:
(1) Goal: *safeguard status.*
(a) Report *immediately;* mobilize staff.
(b) Prepare for immediate laparotomy.
▶ (c) Oxygen per mask—to increase circulating oxygen level.
(d) Order stat type and crossmatch for blood—to replace blood loss.
▶ (e) Establish IV line—to infuse fluids, blood, medications.
▶ (f) Insert indwelling catheter—to deflate bladder.
(g) Abdominal prep—to remove hair, bacteria.
(h) Surgical permit (informed consent) for hysterectomy.
(2) Goal: *emotional support*—to allay anxiety (woman and family).
(a) Encourage verbalization of fears, anxiety, concerns.
(b) Explain all procedures.
(c) Keep family informed of progress.

◆ 7. **Evaluation/outcome criteria:**
a. Experiences successful termination of emergency; minimal blood loss.

b. Postoperative status stable.
B. **Amniotic fluid embolus (Anaphylactoid Syndrome)**
1. **Pathophysiology:** acute cor pulmonale—due to embolus blocking vessels in pulmonary circulation; massive hemorrhage—due to DIC resulting from entrance of thromboplastin-like material into bloodstream.
2. **Etiology**—amniotic fluid (with any meconium, lanugo, or vernix) enters maternal circulation through open venous sinuses at placental site; travels to pulmonary arterioles. Triggers cardiogenic shock and anaphylactoid reaction.
a. Rare.
b. Associated with: tumultuous labor, abruptio placentae, AROM, placement of intrauterine catheter.
3. **Prognosis**—poor; often fatal to mother.

◆ 4. **Assessment:**
a. May occur during labor, at time of rupture of membranes, or immediately postpartum.
b. Sudden dyspnea and cyanosis.
c. Chest pain.
d. Hypotension, tachycardia.
e. Frothy sputum.
f. **Signs of DIC:**
(1) Purpura—local hemorrhage.
(2) Increased vaginal bleeding—massive.
(3) Rapid onset of shock.

◆ 5. **Analysis/nursing diagnosis:**
a. *Impaired gas exchange* related to pulmonary edema.
b. *Risk for fluid volume deficit* related to DIC.
c. *Anxiety/fear* for self and fetus related to severity of symptoms, perception of jeopardy.

◆ 6. **Nursing care plan/implementation:**
a. Medical management:
(1) IV heparin, whole blood.
(2) Birth: immediate, by forceps, if possible; or cesarean birth.
(3) Digitalize, as necessary.
b. Nursing management:
(1) Goal: *assist ventilation.*
(a) *Position:* semi-Fowler's.
▶ (b) Oxygen under positive pressure.
▶ (c) Suction prn.
(2) Goal: *facilitate/expedite administration of fluids, medications, blood.*
▶ (a) Establish intravenous line with large-bore needle.
(b) Administer heparin, fluids, as ordered.
(3) Goal: *restore cardiopulmonary functions, if needed.* Cardiopulmonary re
▶ suscitation techniques.
(4) Goal: *emotional support* of woman, family.

(a) Allay anxiety, as possible.

(b) Explain all procedures.

(c) Keep informed of status.

◆ 7. **Evaluation/outcome criteria:**

a. Dyspnea relieved.

b. Bleeding controlled.

c. Successful birth of viable infant.

d. Uneventful postpartum course.

VI. **Disorders affecting fluid-gas transport:** *fetal*

A. **Fetus in jeopardy**—general aspects:

1. **Pathophysiology**—maternal hypoxemia, anemia, ketoacidosis, Rh isoimmunization, or decreased uteroplacental perfusion.

2. **Etiology**—*maternal:*

a. Preeclampsia/eclampsia.

b. Heart disease.

c. Diabetes.

d. Rh or ABO incompatibility.

e. Insufficient uteroplacental/cord circulation due to:

(1) Maternal hypotension/hypertension.

(2) Cord compression:

(a) Prolapsed.

(b) Knotted.

(c) Nuchal.

(3) Hemorrhage; anemia.

(4) Placental problem:

(a) Malformation of the placenta/cord.

(b) Premature "aging" of placenta.

(c) Placental infarcts.

(d) Abruptio placentae.

(e) Placenta previa.

(5) Postterm gestation.

(6) Maternal infection.

(7) Hydramnios.

(8) Hypertonic uterine contractions.

f. Premature rupture of membranes (PROM) with chorioamnionitis.

g. Dystocia (e.g., from CPD).

◆ 3. **Assessment**—intrapartal:

a. Amniotic fluid examination—at or after rupture of membranes. *Signs of fetal distress:* meconium stained, vertex presentation—due to relaxation of fetal anal sphincter secondary to hypoxia/anoxia. *Note:* Fetus "gasps" in utero—may aspirate meconium and amniotic fluid.

b. Fetal activity:

(1) Hyperactivity—due to hypoxemia, elevated CO_2.

(2) Cessation—possible fetal death.

▶ c. Methods of monitoring FHR:

(1) Fetoscope.

(2) Phonocardiography with microphone application.

(3) Internal fetal electrode—attached directly to fetus through dilated cervix after membranes ruptured.

(4) Doppler probe using ultrasound flow.

(5) Cardiotocograph—transducer on maternal abdomen transmits sound.

d. Abnormal FHR patterns (see p. 130, Figure 4–10).

(1) Persistent arrhythmia.

(2) Persistent tachycardia of 160 or more beats/min.

(3) Persistent bradycardia of 100 or fewer beats/min.

(4) *Early deceleration*—due to vagal response to head compression.

(5) *Late deceleration*—due to uteroplacental insufficiency.

(6) *Variable deceleration*—due to cord compression.

(7) Decreased or loss of variability in FHR pattern.

e. Medical evaluation—procedures: fetal blood gases, pH.

(1) Purpose—to identify fetal acid-base status.

(2) Requirements for:

(a) Ruptured membranes.

(b) Cervical dilation.

(c) Engaged head.

(3) Procedure—under sterile condition, sample of fetal scalp blood obtained for analysis.

(4) Signs of fetal distress:

(a) pH <7.20 (normal range is 7.3–7.4).

(b) Increased CO_2.

(c) Decreased PO_2

◆ 4. **Analysis/nursing diagnosis:**

a. *Impaired gas exchange, fetal,* related to decreased placental perfusion/insufficient cord circulation.

b. *Altered tissue perfusion* related to hemolytic anemia.

c. *High risk for fetal injury* related to hypoxia.

B. **Prolapsed umbilical cord**

1. **Pathophysiology**—cord descent in advance of presenting part; compression interrupts blood flow, exchange of fetal/maternal gases → fetal hypoxia, anoxia, death (if unrelieved).

2. **Etiology:**

a. Spontaneous or artificial rupture of membranes before presenting part is engaged.

b. Excessive force of escaping fluid, as in hydramnios.

c. Malposition—breech, compound presentation, transverse lie.

d. Preterm or SGA fetus—allows space for cord descent.

◆ 3. **Assessment:**
   a. Visualization of cord outside (or inside) vagina.
   b. Palpation of pulsating mass on vaginal examination.
   c. Fetal distress—variable deceleration and persistent bradycardia.

◆ 4. **Analysis/nursing diagnosis:**
   a. *Impaired gas exchange, fetal,* related to interruption of blood flow from placenta/fetus.
   b. *Anxiety/fear, maternal,* related to knowledge of fetal jeopardy.

◆ 5. **Nursing care plan/implementation:**
   a. Goal: *reduce pressure on cord.*
      ▰ (1) *Position:* knee to chest; lateral modified Sims' with hips elevated; modified Trendelenburg.
      (2) With gloved hand, support fetal presenting part.
   ▶ b. Goal: *increase maternal/fetal oxygenation:* oxygen per mask (8–10 L/min).
   ▶ c. Goal: *protect exposed cord:* continuous pressure on the presenting part to keep pressure off cord.
   d. Goal: *identify fetal response* to above measures, reduce threat to fetal survival: monitor FHR continuously.
   e. Goal: *expedite termination of threat to fetus:* prepare for immediate cesarean birth.
   f. Goal: *support mother and significant other* by staying with them and explaining.

◆ 6. **Evaluation/outcome criteria:**
   a. FHR returns to normal rate and pattern.
   b. Uncomplicated birth of viable infant.

VII. Summary of danger signs during labor

A. Contractions—strong, every 2 min or less, lasting 90 sec or more; poor relaxation between contractions.
B. Sudden sharp abdominal pain followed by boardlike abdomen and shock—abruptio placentae or uterine rupture.
C. Marked vaginal bleeding.
D. **FHR** periodic pattern decelerations—late; variable; absent (see Figure 4–10).
E. Baseline.
   1. Bradycardia (<100 beats/min).
   2. Tachycardia (>160 beats/min).
F. Amniotic fluid.
   1. Amount: excessive; diminished
   2. Odor.
   3. Color: meconium stained; port-wine; yellow.
   4. 24 hr or more since rupture of membranes.
G. Maternal hypotension, or hypertension.

Maternal-Infant

Maternal-Infant

CRITICAL PATHWAY for Intrapartal Stages

Category	First Stage	Second and Third Stage	Fourth Stage Birth to 1 Hour Past Birth
Referral	Review prenatal record Advise CNM/physician of admission	Labor record for first stage	Report to recovery room nurse
Assessments ◆	**Admission assessments:** Ask about problems since last prenatal visit; labor status (contraction frequency and duration), membrane status (intact or ruptured); coping level; support; woman's desires during labor and birth; ability to verbalize needs; laboratory testing (blood and UA) **Intrapartal assessments:** Cervical assessment: from 1 to 10 cm dilation; nullipara (1.2 cm/hr), multipara (1.5 cm/hr) Cervical effacement: from 0% to 100% Fetal descent: progressive descent from −4 to +4 Membrane assessment: intact or ruptured; when ruptured, Nitrazine and Fern positive, fluid clear, no foul odor Comfort level: woman states is able to cope with contractions Behavioral characteristics: facial expressions, tone of voice and verbal expressions are consistent with comfort level and ability to cope **Latent Phase:** • BP, P, R q1h if in normal range (BP 90–140/60–90 or not >30 mm Hg systolic or 15 mm Hg diastolic over baseline; pulse 60–90; respirations 12–20/min, quiet, easy) • Temp q4h unless >37.6°C (99.6°F) or membranes ruptured >q2h • Uterine contractions q30min (contractions q5–10min, 15–40sec, mild intensity) • FHR q60min (for low-risk women) and q30min (for high-risk women) if reassuring (reassuring FHR has baseline 110–160, LTV average, accelerations with fetal movement, no late or variable decelerations); if nonreassuring, position on side, start O₂, assess for hypotension, monitor continuously, notify CNM/physician **Active Phase:** • BP, P, R q1h if WNL • Temp as above • Uterine contractions q30min: contractions q2–3min, 60 sec, moderate to strong • FHR q30min (for low-risk women) and q15min (for high-risk women) if reassuring; if nonreassuring, institute interventions **Transition:** • BP, P, R, q30min	**Second stage assessments:** • BP, P, R q5–15min • Uterine contraction palpated continuously • FHR q15min (for low-risk women) and q5min (for high-risk women) if reassuring; if nonreassuring, monitor continuously Fetal descent: descent continues to birth Comfort level: woman states is able to cope with contractions and pushing Behavioral characteristics: response to pushing, facial expressions, verbalization **Third Stage Assessments:** • BP, P, R q5min • Uterine contractions, palpate occasionally until placenta is delivered, fundus maintains tone and contraction pattern continues to birth of placenta **Newborn Assessments:** • Assess *Apgar* score of newborn • Respirations 30–60, irregular • Apical pulse: 120–160 and somewhat irregular • Temperature: skin temp above 36.5°C (97.8°F) • Umbilical cord: two arteries, one vein (if one artery, assess for anomalies and urine output) • Gestational age: 38–42 wk	**Expected Outcomes:** Appropriate resources identified and used **Immediate postbirth assessments of mother q15min for 1 hr:** • *BP:* 90–140/60–90; should return to pre-labor level • *Pulse:* slightly lower than in labor; range is 60–90 • *Respirations:* 12–20/min; easy; quiet • *Temperature:* 36.2–37.6°C (98–99.6°F) • *Fundus:* firm, in midline, at the umbilicus • *Lochia:* rubra; moderate amount; <1 pad/hr; no free flow or passage of clots with massage • *Perineum:* sutures intact; no bulging or marked swelling; minimal bruising may be present; no c/o severe pain or rectal pain • *Bladder:* nondistended; spontaneous void of >100 ml clear, straw-colored urine; bladder nondistended following voiding • If hemorrhoids present, no tenseness or marked engorgement; <2 cm diameter Comfort level: <3 on scale of 1 to 10 Energy level: awake and able to hold newborn **Newborn assessments if newborn remains with parents:** • *Respirations:* 30–60; irregular • *Apical pulse:* 120–160 and somewhat irregular • *Temperature:* skin temp above 36.5°C (97.8°F); skin feels warm to touch • *Skin color:* noncyanotic • *Mucus:* small amount, clear, easily suctioned with bulb syringe without skin color change • *Behavioral:* newborn opens eyes widely if room is slightly darkened • *Movements:* rhythmic; no hand tremors present **Expected Outcomes:** Findings indicate normal progression with absence of complications

CRITICAL PATHWAY for Intrapartal Stages—cont'd

Category	First Stage	Second and Third Stage	Fourth Stage Birth to 1 Hour Past Birth
Assessments —cont'd	• Uterine contractions q15–30min: contractions q2min, 60–75 sec, strong • FHR q30min (for low-risk women) and q15min (for high-risk women) if reassuring; if nonreassuring, see above		
Teaching/ psychosocial	Establish rapport Orient to environment, expected assessments, and procedures Answer questions and provide information Orient to EFM if used Teach relaxation, visualization, and breathing pattern if needed Explain comfort measures available Assume advocacy role for woman/ family during labor and birth	Orient to expected assessments and procedures Answer questions and provide information Explain comfort measures available Continue advocacy role	Explain immediate assessments and care after this first hour Teach self-massage of fundus and expected findings Instruct to call for assistance if mother desires to get OOB Begin newborn teaching; bulb syringe, positioning; maintaining warmth Assist parents in exploring their newborn Assist with first breastfeeding experience **Expected Outcomes:** Client and partner verbalize/demonstrate understanding of teaching
Nursing care management and report ▶	Straight cath prn if bladder distended If regional block administered monitor BP, FHR, sensation per protocol Provide continuing status reports to CNM/physician Perineal clip per woman's request Small enema per woman's request Perform sterile vaginal examination as indicated	Straight cath prn if bladder distended Continue monitoring VS, FHR and sensation if regional block has been given	Straight cath if bladder distended Monitor return of motor ability and sensation if regional block has been given Weigh perineal pads if lochia flow >1 saturated pad in 15 min, presence of boggy uterus and clots; ↓BP, ↑P **Expected Outcomes:** • Maternal/fetal well-being maintained and supported • Mother and newborn experience safe labor and birth • Family participates in process as desired
Activity	Encourage ambulation unless contraindicated Maintain bed rest immediately after administration of IV pain medication, or following regional block Woman rests comfortably between contractions	Position comfortably for birth Woman rests comfortably between pushing efforts and while awaiting birth of placenta	Position of comfort **Expected Outcomes:** • Activity maintained as desired unless contraindicated • Comfort enhanced by positioning/ movement
Comfort ▶	Institute comfort measures: ambulation, frequent position change, effleurage, focal point, patterned paced breathing, visualization, therapeutic touch, back rub, moist cloths to face, holding hand, words of encouragement, changing underpad, shower, whirlpool, staying with the woman/family, warmed blanket at back, sacral pressure Offer pain medication or administer if requested Assist with administration of regional block	Institute comfort measures • *Second stage:* cool cloth to forehead, encouragement, coaching, help support legs while pushing, position of comfort for pushing and birth • *Third stage:* cool cloth to forehead, assist parents to see newborn, position mother to hold newborn, provide encouragement	Institute comfort measures: • *Perineal* discomfort: gently cleanse and apply ice pack; position to decrease pressure on perineum • *Uterine* discomfort: palpate fundus gently • *Hemorrhoids:* ice pack • *General fatigue:* position of comfort, encourage rest • Administer pain medication **Expected Outcomes:** • Optimal comfort level maintained • Active reduction of pain/discomfort achieved

Maternal-Infant

Continued

CRITICAL PATHWAY **for Intrapartal Stages—cont'd**

Category	First Stage	Second and Third Stage	Fourth Stage Birth to 1 Hour Past Birth
Nutrition	Ice chips and clear fluids Evaluate for signs of dehydration	Ice chips and clear fluids	Regular diet if assessments are WNL Encourage fluids **Expected Outcomes:** Nutritional needs met
Elimination	Voids at least q2h; urine clear, straw-colored, negative for protein Bladder nondistended May have bowel movement Monitor I & O with IVs	May void spontaneously with pushing May pass stool with pushing	Voids spontaneously **Expected Outcomes:** Urinary bladder and bowel function unimpaired
Medications	Administer pain medication per woman's request	Local infiltration of anesthetic agent for birth by CNM/physician Pitocin 10 units IM, IVP per IV tubing, or added to IV fluids	Continue Pitocin infusion Administer pain medication **Expected Outcomes:** Comfort enhanced by pain relieving techniques, administration of analgesia agent or an analgesic or anesthetic block
Discharge planning	Evaluate knowledge of labor and birth process Evaluate support system and need for referral after birth		Provide information if mother to be moved from LDR room Provide opportunity for parents to ask questions regarding newborn Evaluate knowledge of normal postpartum, newborn care **Expected Outcomes:** Mother and newborn transferred to low-risk postpartal and newborn care
Family involvement	Identify available support person(s) Recognize possible impact of culture on responses Observe interaction between woman and partner Create moment alone with woman to identify possible abuse Assess current parenting skills	Provide opportunities for woman and support person(s) to watch newborn assessments Perform newborn assessment on mother's abdomen/chest if possible	Provide opportunity for parents to be with baby Encourage skin-to-skin contact Darken room to encourage eye-to-eye contact Provide quiet time for new family Parenting: demonstrates early culturally expected parenting behaviors **Expected Outcomes:** ■ Incorporation of newborn into family ■ Family verbalizes comfort with newborn care

Source: Maternal-Newborn Nursing (6th ed), by Olds, London, Ladewig © 2000. Pp. 548-550. Reprinted by permission of Prentice-Hall, Inc., Upper Saddle River, NJ.

Maternal-Infant

THE POSTPARTAL PERIOD

General overview: This review of the normal physiological and psychological changes occurring during the post-partal period (birth to 6 weeks after) provides the database necessary for assessing the woman's progress through involution, planning and implementing care, anticipatory guidance, health teaching, and evaluating the results. Emerging problems are identified by comparing the woman's status against established standards.

I. **Biological foundations of the postpartal period**
  A. **Uterine involution**—integrated processes by which the uterus returns to nonpregnant size, shape, and consistency.
    ◆ 1. **Assessment:**
      a. Contractions ("afterpains")—shorten muscles, close venous sinuses, restore normal tone.
        (1) Frequency, intensity, and discomfort decrease after first 24 hr
        (2) More common in multiparas and after birth of a large baby; primiparous uterus remains contracted.
        (3) Increased by breastfeeding.
      b. Autolysis—breakdown and excretion of muscle protein (decreasing size of myometrial cells). Lochia—sloughing of decidua and blood.
      c. Formation of *new endometrium*—4–6 wk until placental site healed.
      d. *Cervix*
        (1) *Immediately following* birth—bruised, small tears; admits one hand.
        (2) *Eighteen hours* after birth—becomes shorter, firmer; regains normal shape.
        (3) *One week* postpartum—admits two fingers.
        (4) Never returns fully to prepregnant state.
          (1) Parous os is wider and not perfectly round.
          (2) Lacerations heal as scars radiating out from the os.
      e. *Fundal height and consistency*

    > (1) After birth—at umbilicus; size and consistency of firm grapefruit.
    > (2) Day 1 (first 12 hr)—one finger above umbilicus.
    > (3) Descends by one finger-breadth daily until day 10.
    > (4) Day 10—behind symphysis pubis, nonpalpable.

      f. *Lochia*
        (1) Character:

        > (a) Days 1-3: rubra (red).
        > (b) Days 3-7: serosa (pink to brown).
        > (c) Day 10: alba (creamy white).

        (2) Amount:
          (a) Moderate: 4–8 pads/day (average 6 pads/day).
          (b) Following cesarean birth: less lochia—due to manipulation during surgery.
        (3) Odor: normal lochia has characteristic "fleshy" odor; foul odor is characteristic of infection.
        (4) Clots: normal: a few small clots, most commonly on arising—due to pooling. *Note:* Clots and *heavy* bleeding are associated with uterine atony, retained placental fragments.
  B. **Birth canal**
    1. *Vagina*—never returns fully to prepregnant state.
      a. First few weeks postpartum—thin walled, due to lack of estrogen; few rugae.
      b. Week 3: rugae may reappear.
    2. *Pelvic floor*
      a. Immediately after birth—infiltrated with blood, stretched, torn.
      b. Month 6: considerable tone regained.
    3. *Perineum*
      a. Immediately following birth—edematous; may have episiotomy (or repaired lacerations); hemorrhoids.
      b. Healing, incisional line clean; no separation.
      c. Hematoma—blood in connective tissue beneath skin; complains of pain, unrelieved by mild analgesia or heat; perineal distention; painful, tense, fluctuant mass.
  C. **Abdominal wall**
    1. Overdistention during pregnancy may → rupture of elastic fibers, persistent striae, and diastasis of the rectus muscles.
    2. Usually takes 6–8 wk to retrogress, depending on previous muscle tone, obesity, and amount of distention during pregnancy.
    3. Strenuous exercises discouraged until 8 wk postpartum.
  D. **Cardiovascular system**—characteristic changes:
    1. Immediately after birth—*increased* cardiac load, due to:
      a. Return of uterine blood flow to general circulation.
      b. Diuresis of excess interstitial fluid.
    2. Volume—returns to prepregnant state (4 L) in about 3 wk. Major reduction—during first week, due to diuresis and diaphoresis.
    3. Blood values (see Table 4–5).

a. High WBC during labor (25,000–30,000/mm³), drops to normal level in first few days.
b. Week 1—Hgb, RBC, Hct, elevated fibrinogen return to normal.

4. Blood coagulation
   a. During labor: rapid consumption of clotting factors.
   b. During postpartum: increased consumption of clotting factors. Hypercoagulability maintained during first few days postpartum; predisposes to thrombophlebitis, pulmonary embolism.

◆ 5. **Assessment: potential complications**—vital signs:
   a. *Temperature*—elevated in:
      (1) Excessive blood loss, dehydration, exhaustion, infection.
      (2) Elevation: 100.4°F (38°C) after first day postpartum suggests puerperal infection.
   b. *Pulse*—physiological bradycardia (50–70) common through second day postpartum; may persist 7–10 days; etiology: unknown. *Tachycardia*—associated with: excessive blood loss, dehydration, exhaustion, infection.
   c. *Blood pressure*—generally unchanged. *Elevation*—associated with: preeclampsia, essential hypertension.

E. **Urinary tract**—characteristic changes:
   1. Output—increased due to: diuresis (12 hr to 5 days postpartum); daily output to 3000 mL.
   2. Urine constituents:
      a. Sugar—primarily lactose, usually not detected by conventional dipstick.
      b. Acetonuria—after prolonged labor; dehydration.
      c. Proteinuria—first 3 days in response to the catalytic process of involution ≤1⁺.
   3. Dilation of ureters—subsides in first few weeks.

◆ 4. **Assessment: potential complications**—measure first few voidings, palpate bladder to determine emptying.
   a. Edema, trauma, or anesthesia may → retention with overflow.
   b. Overdistended bladder—common cause of excessive bleeding in immediate postpartum.

F. **Integument (skin)**—characteristic changes:
   1. Striae—persist as silvery or brownish lines.
   2. Diastasis recti abdominis—some midline separation may persist.
   3. Diaphoresis—excessive perspiration for first few (approximately 5) days.
   4. Breast changes—see II.A.3. *Breasts.*
   5. Linea nigra and darkened areola fade.

G. **Legs**

1. Should have no redness, tenderness, local areas of increased skin temperature, or edema.
2. May have some soreness from birth position.
3. *Homans' sign* should be negative (no calf pain when knee is extended and gentle pressure applied to dorsiflex the foot).

H. **Weight**—characteristic changes:
   1. Initial weight loss—fetus, placenta, amniotic fluid, excess tissue fluid.
   2. Weighs more than in prepregnant state (weight maintained in breasts).
   3. Week 6—weight loss is individualized.

I. **Menstruation and ovarian function**—first menstrual cycle may be anovulatory.
   1. *Nonnursing*—ovulation at 4–6 wk; menstruation at 6–8 wk.
   2. *Nursing*—anovulatory period varies (39 days to 6 mo or more); some for duration of lactation; contraceptive value: *very unreliable.*

II. **Nursing management during the postpartal period**

◆ A. **Assessment**—minimum of twice daily.
   1. Vital signs.
   2. Emotional status, response to baby.
   3. *Breasts*
      a. Observe: size, symmetry, placement and condition of nipples, leakage of colostrum. Normal: although one breast is usually larger than the other, breasts are essentially symmetrical in shape; nipples: in breast midline, erectile, intact (no signs of fissure); bilateral leakage of colostrum is common.
      b. *Note:* reddened areas, elevations, supernumerary nipples, inverted nipples, cracks.
      c. Observe for signs of (normal) engorgement (i.e., tenderness, distention, prominent veins). Transient; normally occurs shortly before lactation is established—due to venous and lymphatic stasis.
      d. Palpate for: local heat, edema, tenderness, swelling (signs of localized infection).
   4. Fundus, lochia, perineum.
   5. Voiding and bowel function.
   6. Legs (see I.G., p. 154).
   7. Signs of complications.

◆ B. **Analysis/nursing diagnosis:** (See VI, Nursing actions during the fourth stage of labor, p. 133.)

◆ C. **Nursing care plan/implementation:**
   1. Goal: *comfort measures.*
   ▶ a. Perineal care—to promote healing, prevent infection.
      b. Sitz baths—to promote healing.
   ◐ c. Apply topical anesthetics, witch hazel to episiotomy area, hemorrhoids.
   ◐ d. Administer mild analgesia, as ordered.
      e. Instruct in tensing buttocks on position

change—to reduce stress on suture line, discomfort.

f. Breast care: *bottle-feeding mother*
   (1) Wash daily with clear water and mild soap.
   (2) Support with well-fitting brassiere.
   (3) For engorgement:
      (a) Prevent with tight binder.
      (b) Treat with ice pack and mild analgesic.
      (c) *Avoid* nipple stimulation.
   (4) Also see: Breastfeeding and lactation, p. 156.

2. Goal: *encourage normal bowel function.* (Normal to take 1–3 days for function to resume.)
   a. Administer stool softeners, as ordered.
   b. Encourage ambulation.
   c. Increase *dietary fiber* (salads, fresh fruit, vegetables, bran cereals).
   d. Provide adequate fluid intake.

3. Goal: *health teaching and discharge planning.*
   a. Reinforce appropriate perineal self-care.
   b. Reinforce hand washing (see VI. Nursing actions during the fourth stage of labor, p. 133.)
   ► c. *Infant care*
      (1) Bathing, cord care, circumcision care, diapering.
      (2) Feeding, burping, scheduling.
      (3) Assessment—temperature, skin color, newborn rash, jaundice.
      (4) Normal stool cycle and voiding pattern.
      (5) Common sleep/activity patterns.
      (6) Signs to report **immediately:**

   > (a) Fever, vomiting, diarrhea.
   > (b) Signs of inflammation or infection at cord stump.
   > (c) Bleeding from circumcision site.
   > (d) Lethargy, irritability.

   d. *Self-care*
      (1) Adequate rest, nutrition, hydration.
      (2) Breast self-examination; wear bra to support breasts and promote comfort.
      (3) Normal process of involution; lochial patterns.
   e. Resumption of intercourse approximately 4 wk postpartum (wait until lochia stops).
      (1) Explain that time interval varies as to first postpartal ovulation.
      (2) Family planning options may resume if desired:
         (a) If not breastfeeding, oral contraceptives (estrogen and progesterone); low-dose progesterone given to breastfeeding mothers (see Table 4–1).

(b) Long-acting progestins (subcutaneous implants or injectable). Safe to use during lactation.
(c) Use of IUD or diaphragm decided at postpartal check-up.
(d) Emphasize need to recheck size and fit of diaphragm.
(e) Other options: condom plus spermicides.

f. Exercises—to restore muscle tone, relieve tension.
   (1) Mild exercise during first few weeks.
      (a) Deep abdominal breathing.
      (b) Supine head-raising.
      (c) Stretching from head to toe.
      (d) Pelvic tilt.
      (e) Kegel—to regain perineal muscle tone.
   (2) Strenuous exercises (sit-ups, leg lifts)—deferred until later in postpartum.

g. Maternal signs to report **immediately:**

   > (1) Prolonged lochia rubra.
   > (2) Cramping.
   > (3) Signs of infection.
   > (4) Excessive fatigue, depression.
   > (5) Dysuria.

4. Goal: *anticipatory guidance*—discharge planning: mothers are discharged earlier in their postpartum recovery today—(6–48 hr after birth if asymptomatic).
   a. Discuss, assist in organizing time schedule. Nap, when possible, when infant asleep—to minimize fatigue.
   b. Common maternal emotional/behavior changes, feelings:
      (1) Jealous of infant; guilt feelings.
      (2) "Baby blues"—due to hormonal fluctuations, fatigue, change of lifestyle.
      (3) Feelings of inadequacy.
   c. Discuss support groups, aid in identifying supportive people.

◆ **D. Evaluation/outcome criteria:**
   1. Woman experiences normal, uncomplicated postpartal period. All assessment findings within normal limits.
   2. Woman returns demonstrations of appropriate self-care measures/techniques:
      a. Perineal care, pad change, hand-washing.
      b. Breast care, breast self-examination.
   3. Woman verbalizes understanding of:
      a. Need for adequate rest and diversion.
      b. Appropriate time for resumption of intercourse and exercise.
      c. Appropriate nutritional intake to meet needs (own and, if breastfeeding, infant's).
      d. Signs to be reported immediately.

e. Returns demonstration of appropriate infant care measures.

f. Evidences beginning comfort and increasing confidence in parenting role.

◆ **E. Postpartal assessment—6 or less wk after birth:**

1. Weight, vital signs, urine for protein, complete blood count (CBC).

2. Breast examination lactating or not.

3. Pelvic examination—involution and position of uterus; perineal healing; tone of pelvic floor.

4. Desire for selection of method of contraception.

III. Psychological/behavioral changes *Achievement of developmental tasks*—progress in assuming maternal role.

◆ **A. Assessment:**

1. *Taking-in* phase—1–3 days following birth.

   a. Talkative; verbally relives labor/birth experience.

   b. Passive, dependent, concerned with own needs (eating, sleeping, elimination).

2. *Taking-hold*—d 3 to 2 wk.

   a. Impatient to control own bodily functions, care for self.

   b. Expresses interest/concern in learning how to care for baby (desire to assume "mothering" role).

   c. Responds to positive reinforcement.

3. *Letting-go*—mother "lets go" of former self-concept, role, lifestyle; begins to integrate new role and self-concept as "mother."

   a. Feelings of insecurity, inadequacy.

   b. Hesitancy in approaching infant care tasks.

4. "Baby blues"—may appear on day 4 or 5. (*Note:* Often, father/partner experiences same feelings.)

   a. Thought to result from fatigue (sleep deprivation), realization of need for role change, recognition of new responsibilities, hormonal change.

   b. Mild depression, cries without provocation.

   c. Frightened—intimidated by own perceptions of responsibilities, hormonal changes.

5. Lag in experiencing "maternal feelings"—usually resolved within 6 wk.

   a. May contribute to "baby blues."

   b. Guilt regarding lack of "maternal feelings."

   c. Diminished by prompt bonding experience.

◆ **B. Analysis/nursing diagnosis:**

1. *Ineffective family coping: compromised,* related to achieving developmental tasks.

2. *Situational low self-esteem* related to perceived inadequacy in acceptance of maternal role.

3. *Ineffective individual coping* related to "baby blues," lag in experiencing maternal feelings.

◆ **C. Nursing care plan/implementation:**

1. *Taking-in.* Goal: *emotional support.*

   a. Encourage verbalization of labor/birth experiences; compliment parents on "how well" they did.

   b. Explore feelings of disappointment, if any.

   c. Meet dependency needs; comment on appearance, hair, personal gowns.

   d. Encourage rooming in.

2. *Taking-hold.* Goal: *health teaching.*

   a. Discuss self-care, postpartal physiological/psychological changes.

   b. Demonstrate infant care; mother returns demonstration.

◆ **D. Evaluation/outcome criteria:**

1. Woman demonstrates beginning comfort in maternal role.

2. Woman develops confidence and competence in infant care.

3. Woman expresses satisfaction with self, infant; eager to return home.

4. Woman succeeds in breastfeeding. (Tension inhibits let-down reflex; baby nurses poorly.)

IV. Breastfeeding and lactation

A. Biological foundations:

1. *Antepartal* alterations:

   a. High estrogen/progesterone levels—stimulate proliferation and development of breast ducts.

   b. High progesterone levels—also → development of mammary lobules and alveoli.

2. *Postpartum* alterations:

   a. Rapid drop in estrogen/progesterone levels.

   b. Increased secretion of prolactin—stimulates alveolar cells → milk.

   c. Suckling—stimulates release of oxytocin → contraction of ducts → milk ejection (let-down reflex).

   d. Engorgement—due to venous and lymphatic stasis.

      (1) Immediately precedes lactation.

      (2) Lasts about 24 hr

      (3) Frequent feeding reduces engorgement.

◆ **B. Assessment:**

1. Colostrum (yellowish fluid)—continues for first 2–3 days; has some antibiotic, immunologic, and nutritive value.

2. Milk (bluish-white, thin)—secreted on about third day.

◆ **C. Analysis/nursing diagnosis:**

1. *Knowledge deficit* related to breastfeeding techniques.

2. *Pain* related to engorgement.
3. *Personal identity disturbance* related to problems in breastfeeding.
4. *Sleep pattern disturbance* related to discomfort or infant care needs.
◆ **D. Nursing care plan/implementation:**
   1. Goal: *promote successful breastfeeding.*
      a. Encourage first feeding within 1 hr after giving birth.
      b. Encourage emptying both breasts at each feeding and before engorgement to stimulate milk production, prevent mastitis.
      c. Encourage rest, relaxation, fluids.
      d. *Nutritional* counseling (see **Unit 9**).
         (1) Additional 500 calories daily—may be supplied by one extra pint of milk, one extra egg, and one extra serving of meat, citrus fruit, and vegetable.
         (2) Increase fluid intake to 3000 mL daily.
   2. Goal: *prevent or relieve engorgement.*
      ▶ a. Pain: relieved by warm packs, emptying breasts.
      b. Wear good, supportive bra.
      c. Administer analgesics, as ordered/necessary.
   3. Goal: *health teaching.*
      ▶ a. Instruct, demonstrate *rooting reflex* and putting infant to breast. Infant must grasp nipple and areola over location of milk sinuses.
      b. Demonstrate burping techniques, what to do if infant chokes; removing infant from breast.
      ▶ c. Instruct in *basic nipple care.*
         (1) Teach good hand washing.
         (2) Nurse on each breast, making sure areola is in mouth, alternating position of infant.
         (3) Alternate "beginning" breast.
         (4) Break suction before removing infant from breast.
         (5) Air-dry nipples after each feeding and apply lanolin if abraded. *Note:* Creams, lotions, or ointments block secretion of a natural bacteriostatic oil by Montgomery glands—and infant may refuse breast until it is washed. Instead: expressed milk may be massaged gently around nipple.
         (6) Teach daily hygiene of breasts.
      d. Instruct in care of cracked or *fissured nipples.*
         (1) Encourage and support mothers.
         (2) Air-dry nipples after each feeding.
         (3) Use nipple shield if nipples extremely sore.
         (4) Discontinue nursing for 48 hr; maintain milk supply by expressing milk with pump.
      e. Discuss avoiding use of any drugs except under medical supervision—may affect infant or suppress lactation.
      f. Discuss possibility of sexual stimulation during breastfeeding.
         (1) Validate normalcy and acceptability.
         (2) *Note:* During orgasm, milk may squirt from nipples.
      g. Explain that contraceptive value of nursing is unpredictable; time ovulation is inhibited varies widely.
      h. Explain *contraindications to breastfeeding:*
         (1) Active tuberculosis.
         (2) Severe chronic maternal disease.
         (3) Mastitis (temporary interruption may be necessary).
         (4) Narcotic addiction, therapeutic drug dependence.
         (5) Severe cleft lip or palate in newborn (may pump and give in special bottles).
         (6) HIV-positive status; AIDS.
         (7) Drug abusers (must be drug-free 3 mo).
◆ **E. Evaluation/outcome criteria:**
   1. Woman verbalizes understanding of breastfeeding techniques, nutritional requirements for successful lactation.
   2. Woman successfully demonstrates breastfeeding; infant nurses well.
   3. Woman demonstrates appropriate burping techniques; clears excessive mucus from infant's mouth without incident.
   4. Woman verbalizes understanding of basic breast care techniques:
      a. Self-examination.
      b. Clear water bath.
      c. Drying nipples after bathing, feeding.
      d. Care of cracked or irritated nipples.
      e. Correct infant positioning for feeding.

Complications During the Postpartal Period

I. **Disorders affecting fluid-gas transport**
   A. **Postpartum hemorrhage**
      1. Definition—loss of 500 mL of blood or more during first 24 postpartal hr in vaginal birth; 1000 mL in cesarean birth.
      2. **Pathophysiology**—excessive loss of blood secondary to trauma, decreased uterine contractility; results in hypovolemia.
      3. **Etiology** (in order of frequency):
         a. Uterine atony
            (1) Uterine overdistention (multipregnancy, polyhydramnios, fetal macrosomia).
            (2) Multiparity.

(3) Prolonged or precipitous labor.

(4) Anesthesia—deep inhalation or regional (particularly saddle block).

(5) Myomata (fibroids).

(6) Oxytocin induction of labor.

(7) Overmassage of uterus in postpartum.

(8) Distended bladder.

b. Lacerations—cervix, vagina, perineum.

c. Retained placental fragments—usually delayed postpartum hemorrhage.

d. Hematoma—deep pelvic, vaginal, or episiotomy site.

◆ 4. **Assessment:**

a. Uterus—boggy, flaccid; excessive vaginal bleeding (dark; seepage, large clots) — due to uterine atony, retained placental fragments.

b. Late signs of shock—air hunger; anxiety/apprehension, tachycardia, tachypnea, hypotension.

c. Blood values (admission and postpartal)—hemoglobin (Hgb), hematocrit (Hct), clotting time.

d. Estimated blood loss: during labor/birth; in early postpartum.

e. Pain: vulvar, vaginal, perineal.

f. Perineum: distended—due to edema; discoloration—due to hematoma. May complain of rectal pressure.

g. Lacerations—bright red vaginal bleeding with firm fundus.

◆ 5. **Analysis/nursing diagnosis:**

a. *Fluid volume deficit* related to excessive blood loss secondary to uterine atony, retained placental fragments.

b. *Anxiety/fear* related to unexpected complication.

c. *Altered tissue perfusion* related to decreased oxygenation secondary to blood loss.

d. *Activity intolerance* related to fatigue.

◆ 6. **Nursing care plan/implementation:**

a. Medical management:

(1) IV oxytocin infusion; IV or oral ergot preparations (ergonovine [Ergotrate maleate]; methylergonovine [Methergine]; carboprost (Prostin/M15), an oxytocic; prostaglandin.

(2) Order blood work: clotting time, platelet count, fibrinogen level, Hgb, Hct, CBC.

(3) Type and crossmatch for blood replacement.

(4) Surgical:

(a) Repair of lacerations.

(b) Evacuation, ligation of hematoma.

(c) Curettage—retained placental fragments.

b. Nursing management:

(1) Goal: *minimize blood loss.*

(a) Notify physician promptly of abnormal assessment findings.

(b) Order lab work stat, as directed—to determine blood loss and etiology.

(c) Fundal massage.

(d) Administer medications to stimulate uterine tone. For ergot products and carboplast, monitor blood pressure (contraindicated in PIH).

(2) Goal: *stabilize status.*

(a) Establish IV line—to enable administration of medications and rapid absorption/action. Administer whole blood (with larger catheter).

(b) Administer medications, as ordered to control bleeding, combat shock.

(c) Prepare for surgery, as ordered.

(3) Goal: *prevent infection.* Strict aseptic technique.

(4) Goal: *continual monitoring.* Vital signs, bleeding (do pad count or weigh pads), fundal status.

(5) Goal: *prevent sequelae (Sheehan's syndrome).*

(6) Goal: *health teaching*—after episode: Reinforce appropriate perineal care and handwashing techniques.

◆ 7. **Evaluation/outcome criteria:**

a. Maternal vital signs stable.

b. Bleeding diminished or absent.

c. Assessment findings within normal limits.

B. Subinvolution—delayed return of uterus to normal size, shape, position.

1. **Pathophysiology**—inability of inflamed uterus (endometritis) to contract effectively → incomplete uterine involution; failure of contractions to effect closure of vessels in site of placental attachment → bleeding.

2. **Etiology:**

a. PROM with secondary amnionitis, endometritis.

b. Retained placental fragments.

c. Oxytocin stimulation or augmentation of labor of overdistended uterine muscle may interfere with involution.

◆ 3. **Assessment:**

a. Uterus: large, boggy; lack of uterine tone; failure to shrink progressively.

b. Discharge: persistent lochia; painless fresh bleeding, hemorrhagic episodes.

◆ 4. **Analysis/nursing diagnosis:**

a. *Pain* related to tender, inflamed uterus secondary to endometritis.

b. *Anxiety/fear* related to change in physical status.

c. *Knowledge deficit* related to diagnosis, treatment, prognosis.

d. *High risk for injury* related to infection.

e. *Fluid volume deficit* related to excessive bleeding.

◆ 5. **Nursing care plan/implementation:**

a. Medical management:

(1) Have woman void or catheterize; massage.

(2) Surgical (curettage)—to remove placental fragments.

⬤▷ (3) Antibiotic therapy—to treat intrauterine infection.

⬤▷ (4) Oxytocics—to stimulate/enhance uterine contractions.

b. Nursing management:

(1) Goal: *health teaching.*

(a) Explain condition and treatment.

(b) Describe, demonstrate perineal care, pad change, handwashing.

(2) Goal: *emotional support.* Encourage verbalization of anxiety regarding recovery, separation from newborn.

(3) Goal: *promote healing.*

(a) Encourage rest, compliance with medical/nursing regimen.

⬤▷ (b) Administer oxytocics, antibiotics, as ordered.

◆ 6. **Evaluation/outcome criteria:**

a. Verbalizes understanding of condition and treatment.

b. Complies with medical/nursing regimen.

c. Demonstrates normal involutional progress.

d. All assessment findings (vital signs, fundal height, consistency, lochial discharge) within normal limits.

e. Expresses satisfaction with care.

C. **Hypofibrinogenemia**

1. **Pathophysiology**—decreased clotting factors, fibrinogen; may be accompanied by DIC.

2. **Etiology:**

a. Missed abortion (retained dead fetus syndrome).

b. Fetal death, delayed emptying of uterine contents.

c. Abruptio placentae; Couvelaire uterus.

d. Amniotic fluid embolism.

e. Hypertension.

◆ 3. **Assessment:**

a. Observe for bleeding from injection sites, epistaxis, purpura.

b. See DIC assessment, p. 459, and **Unit 7.**

c. Maternal vital signs, color.

d. I&O.

e. Medical evaluation—procedures.

(1) Thrombin clot test—important: size and persistence of clot.

(2) Prothrombin time—prolonged.

(3) Bleeding time—prolonged.

(4) Platelet count—decreased.

(5) Activated partial thromboplastin time—prolonged.

(6) Fibrinogen (factor I concentration)—decreased.

(7) Fibrin degradation products—present.

◆ 4. **Analysis/nursing diagnosis:**

a. *Fluid volume deficit* related to uncontrolled bleeding secondary to coagulopathy.

b. *Anxiety/fear* related to unexpected critical emergency.

c. *Altered tissue perfusion* related to decreased oxygenation secondary to blood loss.

◆ 5. **Nursing care plan/implementation:**

a. Medical management:

(1) Replace platelets

(2) Replace blood loss

⬤▷ (3) IV heparin—to inhibit conversion of fibrinogen to fibrin.

b. Nursing management:

(1) Goal: *continuous monitoring.*

▶ (a) Vital signs.

(b) I&O hourly.

(c) Skin: color, emergence of petechiae.

(d) Note, measure (as possible), record, and report blood loss.

(2) Goal: *control blood loss.*

(a) Establish IV line, administer fluids or blood products as ordered.

◪ (b) *Position:* side-lying—to maintain blood supply to vital organs.

(3) Goal: *emotional support.*

(a) Encourage verbalization of anxiety, fear, concerns.

(b) Explain all procedures.

(c) Remain with woman continuously.

(d) Keep woman and family informed.

6. **Evaluation/outcome criteria:**

a. Bleeding controlled.

b. Laboratory studies—returning to normal values.

c. Status stable.

II. **Disorders affecting protective functions:** postpartal infection (Table 4–13).

A. **General aspects**

1. Definition—reproductive system infection occurring during the postpartal period.

2. **Pathophysiology**—bacterial invasion of birth canal; most common: localized infection of the lining of the uterus (endometritis).

3. **Etiology:**

a. Anaerobic nonhemolytic streptococci.

b. *E. coli.*

Table 4–13 **Postpartum Infections**

Condition/Etiology	◆ Assessment: Signs/Symptoms	◆ Nursing Interventions
Postpartum Infection Traumatic labor and birth and postpartum hemorrhage make woman more vulnerable to infection by such bacteria as non-hemolytic streptococci, *Escherichia coli*, and *Staphylococcus species*	Depends on location and severity of infection; usually include fever, pain, swelling, and tenderness Temperature of 100.4°F (38°C) or more after first 24 hr after birth on two or more occasions indicates puerperal infection ("childbed fever")	1. Monitor: Signs and symptoms, drainage (e.g., uterine) 2. Obtain culture and sensitivity 3. Administer *antimicrobial* agents and *analgesic* agents 4. Ensure comfort; encourage rest 5. Use standard precautions 6. Force *fluids* and provide *high*-calorie diet 7. Keep family informed of mother's and newborn's progress 8. Promote maternal-infant contact as soon as possible 9. Plan and implement discharge and follow-up care
Endometritis Microorganisms invade placental site and may spread to entire endometrium	Temperature, chills, anorexia, malaise, boggy uterus, foul-smelling lochia, and cramps	1. Administer *antimicrobial* agents and *analgesic* agents 2. Encourage *Fowler's position* to promote drainage 3. *Force fluids* 4. Take standard precautions
Pelvic Cellulitis or Parametritis Microorganisms spread through lymphatics and invade tissues surrounding uterus	Fever, chills, lower-abdominal pain, and tenderness	1. Administer *antimicrobial* agents and *analgesic* agents 2. Encourage bed rest 3. *Force fluids*
Perineal Infection Trauma to perineum makes woman more vulnerable to infection	Localized pain, fever, swelling, redness, and seropurulent drainage	1. Administer *antimicrobial* agents and *analgesic* agents 2. Provide sitz baths or heat/cold applications 3. Take standard precautions
Mastitis Lesions or fissure on nipples allow entry of microorganisms (e.g., *Staphylococcus aureus*) from infant's nose/mouth or mother's unwashed hands (Breast milk is a good medium for growth of organism)	Marked engorgement, pain, chills, fever, tachycardia If untreated, single or multiple breast abscesses may form	1. Order culture and sensitivity studies of mother's milk 2. Administer *antimicrobial* agents and *analgesic* agents 3. Apply heat or cold therapy 4. Assist with incising and draining abscesses 5. Use standard precautions and perform meticulous hand washing
Thrombophlebitis Infected pelvic or femoral thrombi Increased tendency to clot formation during pregnancy, trauma to tissues, and hemorrhage decrease new mother's resistance to infection	Pain, chills and fever *Femoral:* stiffness of affected area or part and positive *Homans'* sign *Pelvic:* severe chills and wide fluctuations in temperature	*Femoral:* 1. Rest and *elevate* leg 2. Administer *antimicrobial* agents, *analgesic* agents, and *anticoagulants* *Pelvic:* 1. Encourage bed rest 2. *Force fluids* 3. Administer *antimicrobial* agents and *anticoagulants*

c. *C. trachomatis* (bacteroides).

d. Staphylococci.

4. Predisposing conditions:

a. Anemia.

b. PROM.

c. Prolonged labor.

d. Repeated vaginal examinations during labor.

e. Intrauterine manipulation—e.g., manual extraction of placenta.

f. Retained placental fragments.

g. Postpartum hemorrhage.

◆ 5. **Assessment:**

a. Fever 38°C (100.4°F) or more on two or more occasions, after first 24 hr postpartum.

b. Other signs of infection: pain, malaise, dysuria, subinvolution, foul lochial odor.

◆ 6. **Analysis/nursing diagnosis:**

a. *Fluid volume deficit* related to excessive blood loss, anemia.

b. *Knowledge deficit* related to danger signs of postpartum period.

c. *High risk for injury* related to infection.

◆ 7. **Nursing care plan/implementation:** prevention

a. Goal: *prevent anemia.*

(1) Minimize blood loss—accurate postpartal assessment and management of bleeding.

(2) *Diet: high protein, high vitamin.*

(3) Vitamins, iron—suggest continuing prenatal pattern until postpartum checkup.

b. Goal: *prevent entrance/transport of microorganisms.*

▶ (1) *Strict aseptic technique* during labor, birth, and postpartum (standard precautions).

(2) Minimize vaginal examinations during labor.

(3) Perineal care.

c. Goal: *health teaching.*

(1) Hand washing—before and after each pad change, after voiding or defecating.

▶ (2) Perineal care—from front to back; use clear, warm water or mild antiseptic solution as a cascade; do *not* separate labia.

(3) Maintain sterility of pads; apply from front to back.

(4) *Avoid* use of tampons until normal menstrual cycle resumes.

◆ 8. **Evaluation/outcome criteria:**

a. Woman has assessment findings within normal limits:

(1) Vital signs.

(2) Rate of involution (fundal height, consistency).

(3) Lochia: character, amount, odor.

b. Woman avoids infection.

B. Endometritis—infection of lining of uterus.

1. **Pathophysiology**—see II. A. General aspects, p. 159.

2. **Etiology**—most common: invasion by normal body flora (e.g., anaerobic streptococci).

3. Characteristics:

a. Mild, localized—asymptomatic, or low-grade fever.

b. Severe—may lead to ascending infection, parametritis, pelvic abscess, pelvic thrombophlebitis.

c. If remains localized, self-limiting; usually resolves within 10 days.

◆ 4. **Assessment:**

a. Signs of infection: fever, chills, malaise, anorexia, headache, backache.

b. Uterus: large, boggy, extremely tender.

(1) Subinvolution.

(2) Lochia: dark brown; foul odor.

◆ 5. **Analysis/nursing diagnosis:**

a. *Anxiety/fear* related to effects on self and newborn.

b. *Self-esteem disturbance and altered role performance* related to inability to meet own expectations regarding parenting, secondary to unexpected hospitalization.

c. *Pain* related to inflammation/infection.

d. *Ineffective individual coping* related to physical discomfort and psychological stress associated with self-concept disturbance; worry, guilt, concern regarding newborn at home.

e. *Altered family processes*—interruption of adjustment to altered life pattern related to postpartal infection/hospitalization.

◆ 6. **Nursing care plan/implementation:**

▶ a. Goal: *prevent cross-contamination.* Contact-item isolation.

b. Goal: *facilitate drainage. Position:* semi-Fowler's.

c. Goal: *nutrition/hydration.*

(1) *Diet: high-calorie, high-protein, high-vitamin.*

(2) Push *fluids* to 4000 mL/day (oral or IV, or both, as ordered).

(3) I&O.

d. Goal: *increase uterine tone/facilitate involution.* Administer medications, as ordered (e.g., oxytocics, antibiotics).

e. Goal: *minimize energy expenditure*, as possible.

(1) Bed rest.

(2) Maximize rest, comfort.

f. Goal: *emotional support.*

(1) Encourage verbalization of anxiety, concerns.

(2) Keep informed of progress.

◆ 7. **Evaluation/outcome criteria:**

a. Vital signs stable, within normal limits.

b. All assessment findings within normal limits.

c. Unable to recover organism from discharge.

C. Urinary tract infections

1. **Pathophysiology**—normal physiological changes associated with pregnancy (e.g., ureteral dilation) and the postpartal period (e.g., diuresis, increased bladder capacity with diminished sensitivity of stretch receptors) → increased susceptibility to bacterial invasion and growth → ascending infections (cystitis, pyelonephritis).

2. **Etiology:** usually bacterial.

3. Predisposing factors:
   a. Birth trauma to bladder, urethra, or meatus.
   b. Bladder hypotonia with retention (due to intrapartal anesthesia or trauma).
   c. Repeated or prolonged catheterization, or poor technique.
   d. Weakening of immune response secondary to anemia, hemorrhage.

◆ 4. **Assessment:**
   a. Maternal vital signs (fever, tachycardia).
   b. Dysuria, frequency (flank pain—with pyelonephritis).
   c. Feeling of "not emptying" bladder.
   d. Cloudy urine; frank pus.

◆ 5. **Analysis/nursing diagnosis:**
   a. *Altered urinary elimination* related to diuresis, dysuria, inflammation/infection.
   b. *Pain* related to dysuria secondary to cystitis.
   c. *Knowledge deficit* related to self-care (perineal care).

◆ 6. **Nursing care plan/implementation:**
   a. Goal: *minimize perineal edema.* Perineal ice pack in fourth stage—to limit swelling secondary to trauma, facilitate voiding.
   b. Goal: *prevent overdistention of bladder.*
      (1) Monitor level of fundus, lochia, bladder distention. (*Note:* Distended bladder displaces uterus, limits its ability to contract → boggy fundus, increases its vaginal bleeding.)
      (2) Encourage *fluids* and voiding; I&O.
   ▶ (3) Aseptic technique for catheterization.
      (4) Slow emptying of bladder on catheterization—to maintain tone.
   c. Goal: *identification of causative organism—* to facilitate appropriate medication (antibiotics). Obtain clean-catch (or catheterized) specimen for culture and sensitivity.
   d. Goal: *health teaching.* See previous discussion of fluids, general hygiene, diet, and medications.

◆ 7. **Evaluation/outcome criteria:**
   a. Voiding: quantity sufficient (although small, frequent output may mean overflow with retention).

b. Urine character: clear, amber, or straw colored.

c. Vital signs: within normal limits.

d. No complaints of frequency, urgency, burning on urination, flank pain.

D. Mastitis—inflammation of breast tissue:

1. **Pathophysiology**—local inflammatory response to bacterial invasion; suppuration may occur; organism can be recovered from breast milk.

2. **Etiology**—most common: *Staphylococcus aureus;* source—most common: infant's nose, throat.

◆ 3. **Assessment:**
   a. Signs of infection (may occur several weeks: postpartum).
      (1) Fever.
      (2) Chills.
      (3) Tachycardia.
      (4) Malaise.
      (5) Abdominal pain.
   b. Breast
      (1) Reddened area(s).
      (2) Localized/generalized swelling.
      (3) Heat, tenderness, palpable mass.

◆ 4. **Analysis/nursing diagnosis:**
   a. *Impaired skin integrity* related to nipple fissures, cracks.
   b. *Pain* related to tender, inflamed tissue secondary to infection.
   c. *Disturbance in body image, self-esteem* related to association of breastfeeding with female identity and role.
   d. *Anxiety/fear* related to sexuality; impact on breastfeeding, if any.

◆ 5. **Nursing care plan/implementation:**
   a. Goal: *prevent infection.* Health teaching in early postpartum:
      (1) Hand washing.
      (2) Breast care—wash with warm water only (*no* soap)—to prevent removing protective body oils.
      (3) Let breast milk dry on nipples to prevent drying of tissue.
      (4) Clean bra (with no plastic pads or liners) to support breasts, reduce friction, minimize exposure to microorganisms.
      (5) Good breastfeeding techniques (see p. 157).
      (6) Alternate position of infant for nursing to change pressure areas.
   b. Goal: *comfort measures.*
      (1) Encourage bra or binder—to support breasts, reduce pain from motion.
   ▶ (2) Local heat or ice packs as ordered— to reduce engorgement, pain.
   ◗ (3) Administer analgesics, as necessary.
   c. Goal: *emotional support.*
      (1) Encourage verbalization of feelings, concerns.

(2) If breastfeeding is discontinued, reassure woman she will be able to resume breastfeeding.

d. Goal: *promote healing.*

(1) Maintain lactation (if desired) by manual expression or breast pump, q4h.

(2) Administer antibiotics as ordered.

◆ 6. **Evaluation/outcome criteria:**

a. Woman promptly responds to medical/nursing regimen.

(1) Symptoms subside.

(2) Assessment findings within normal limits.

b. Woman successfully returns to breastfeeding.

E. Thrombophlebitis

1. **Pathophysiology**—inflammation of a vein secondary to lodging of a clot.

2. **Etiology:**

a. Extension of endometritis with involvement of pelvic and femoral veins.

b. Clot formation in pelvic veins following cesarean birth.

c. Clot formation in femoral (or other) veins secondary to poor circulation, compression, and venous stasis.

◆ 3. **Assessment:**

a. Pelvic—pain: abdominal or pelvic tenderness.

b. Calf—pain: positive *Homans'* sign (pain elicited by flexion of foot with knee extended).

c. Femoral

(1) Pain.

(2) Malaise, fever, chills.

(3) Swelling—"milk leg."

◆ 4. **Analysis/nursing diagnosis:**

a. *Pain* in affected region related to local inflammatory response.

b. *Anxiety/fear* related to outcome.

c. *Ineffective individual coping* related to unexpected postpartum complications, hospitalization, separation from newborn.

d. *Impaired physical mobility* related to imposed bed rest to prevent emboli formation and dislodging clot (embolus).

◆ 5. **Nursing care plan/implementation:**

a. Goal: *prevent clot formation.*

(1) Encourage early ambulation.

(2) *Position: avoid* prolonged compression of popliteal space, use of knee gatch.

▶ (3) Apply thromboembolic disease (TED) hose, as ordered, preoperatively or postoperatively, or both, for cesarean birth.

b. Goal: *reduce threat of emboli.*

(1) Bed rest, with cradle to support bedding.

(2) Discourage massaging "leg cramps."

c. Goal: *prevent further clot formation.* Administer anticoagulants, as ordered.

d. Goal: *prevent infection.*

(1) Administer antibiotics, as ordered.

(2) Push *fluids.*

▶ e. Goal: *facilitate clot resolution.* Heat therapy, as ordered.

◆ 6. **Evaluation/outcome criteria:**

a. Symptoms subside; all assessment findings within normal limits.

b. No evidence of further clot formation.

III. Disorders affecting psychosocial-cultural functions—postpartum depression/psychosis

A. General aspects

1. Can occur in both new parents.

2. Usually occur within 2 wk of birth.

3. Increased incidence among single parents

4. Increased incidence among women with history of clinical depression.

5. Most common symptomatology: affective disorders.

6. Psychiatric intervention required if prolonged or severe; if underlying cause unresolved; increased risk in subsequent pregnancies.

B. Etiology—theory: birth of child may emphasize:

1. Unresolved role conflicts.

2. Unachieved normal development tasks.

◆ **C. Assessment:**

1. Withdrawal.

2. Paranoia.

3. Anorexia, sleep disturbance, mood swings.

4. Depression—may alternate with manic behavior.

5. Potential for self-injury or child abuse/neglect.

◆ **D. Analysis/nursing diagnosis:**

1. *Ineffective individual coping* related to perceived inability to meet role expectations ("mother") and ambivalence related to dependence/independence.

2. *Self-esteem disturbance and altered role performance* related to "femaleness" and reaction to responsibility for care of newborn.

3. *High risk for violence,* self-directed or directed at newborn, related to anger or depression.

4. *Ineffective family coping* related to lack of support system in early postpartum.

5. *Altered family processes* related to psychological stress, interruption of bonding.

6. *Altered parenting* related to hormonal changes and stress.

◆ **E. Nursing care plan/implementation:**

1. Goal: *emotional support.*

a. Encourage verbalization of feelings, fears, anxiety, concerns.

b. Support positive self-image, feelings of adequacy, self-worth.

(1) Reinforce appropriate comments and behaviors.

(2) Encourage active participation in self-care, comment on accomplishments.

(3) Reduce threat to self-image, fear of failure. Maintain support, gradually increase tasks.

2. Goal: *safeguard status of mother/newborn.*

   a. Unobtrusive, protective environment.

   b. Stay with woman when she is with infant.

3. Goal: *nutrition/hydration.*

   a. Encourage selection of favorite foods—to aid security in decision making; counteract anorexia (refusal to eat) by tempting appetite.

   b. Push *fluids* (juices, soft drinks, milkshakes) —to maintain hydration.

4. Goal: *minimize stress, facilitate effective coping.* Administer therapeutic medications, as ordered.

   a. Schizophrenia—phenothiazines.

   b. Depression—mood elevators.

   c. Manic behaviors—sedatives, tranquilizers.

◆ **F. Evaluation/outcome criteria:**

1. Woman increases interaction with infant.

2. Woman expresses interest in learning how to care for infant.

3. Woman evidences no agitation, depression.

4. Woman actively participates in caring for self and infant.

5. Woman demonstrates increasing comfort in mothering role.

6. Woman has positive family interactions.

CRITICAL PATHWAY for the Postpartal Period

Category	First 4 Hours	4–8 Hours Past Birth	8–24 Hours Past Birth
Referral	Report from labor nurse if not continuing in an LDR room	Lactation consultation as needed	Home nursing, WIC referral if indicated **Expected Outcomes:** Referrals made
Assessments ♦	Postpartum assessments q 30min × 2, q1h × 2, then q4h. Includes: ■ Fundus: firm, midline, at or below umbilicus ■ Lochia rubra <1 pad/hr; no free flow or passage of clots with massage ■ *Bladder:* voids large amounts of urine spontaneously; bladder not palpable following voiding ■ *Perineum:* sutures intact; no bulging or marked swelling; no c/o severe pain. Minimal bruising may be present. If hemorrhoids present, no tenseness or marked engorgement; <2 cm diameter ■ Breasts: soft, colostrum present Vital signs: ■ BP WNL; no hypotension; not >30 mm systolic or 15 mm diastolic over baseline ■ Temperature: <38°C (100.4°F) ■ Pulse: bradycardia normal, consistent with baseline ■ Respirations: 12–20/min; quiet, easy Comfort level: <3 on scale of 1–10	Continue postpartum assessment q4th × 2, then q8h *Breasts:* evaluate nipple status; should be no evidence of cracks or bruising Observe *feeding* technique with newborn *Vital signs:* assessment q8 hrs; all WNL; report temperature >38°C (100.4°F) Assess *Homan's sign* q8h Continue assessment of comfort level	Continue postpartum assessment q8h *Breasts:* nipples should remain free of cracks, fissures, bruising *Feeding* technique with newborn: should be good or improving *Vital signs:* assessment q8h; all WNL; report temperature >38°C (100.4°F) Continue assessment of comfort level **Expected Outcomes:** Vital signs medically acceptable, voids qs, postpartum assessment WNL; comfort level <3 on 1–10 scale, involution of uterus in process, demonstrates and verbalizes appropriate newborn feeding techniques
Teaching/ psychosocial	Explain postpartum assessments Teach self-massage of fundus and expected findings; rationale for fundal massage Instruct to call for assistance first time OOB and PRN Demonstrate peri-care, surgigator, sitz bath prn Explain comfort measures Begin newborn teaching; bulb suctioning, positioning, feeding, diaper change, cord care Orient to room if transferred from LDR room Provide information on early postpartal period Assess mother/infant attachment	Discuss psychological changes of postpartum period; facilitate transition through tasks of taking on maternal role Discuss peri-care/hygiene; encourage use of supportive brassiere for breast- or bottle-feeding Stress need for frequent rest periods Continue newborn teaching: soothing/comforting techniques, swaddling; return demonstrations indicate woman's understanding Provide opportunities for questions and review; reinforce previous teaching Breastfeeding: nipple care: air-drying, lanolin; proper latch-on technique; tea bags Bottle-feeding: supportive bra, ice bags, breast binder Assess mother/infant attachment	Reinforce previous teaching, complete teaching Discuss involution; anticipated physical changes in first 2 weeks postpartum; postpartal exercises; need to limit visitors Discuss postpartal nutrition; balanced diet **Breastfeeding:** ■ Increase calories by 500 kcal over non-pregnant state (200 kcal over pregnant intake) ■ Explain milk production, let-down reflex, use of supplements, breast pumping, and milk storage **Bottle-feeding:** ■ Return to nonpregnant caloric intake ■ Explain formula preparation and storage Discuss birth control options, sexuality Discuss sibling rivalry and plan for supporting siblings at home Discuss pets; suggestions for improving acceptance of infant by pets **Expected Outcomes:** Mother verbalizes teaching comprehension Positive bonding and emotional behaviors observed

Continued

Maternal-Infant

CRITICAL PATHWAY for the Postpartal Period—cont'd

Category	First 4 Hours	4–8 Hours Past Birth	8–24 Hours Past Birth
Nursing care management and reports ▶	Ice pack to perineum to decrease swelling and increase comfort Straight catheter prn × 1 if distended or voiding small amounts If continues unable to void or voiding small amounts, insert Foley catheter and notify CNM/physician	Sitz baths prn If woman Rh− and infant Rh+, RhoGAM work up; obtain consent; complete teaching Determine rubella status Obtain consent for rubella vaccine if indicated; explain purpose, procedure, implications of vaccine Obtain hematocrit	Continue sitz baths prn May shower if ambulating without difficulty DC saline lock if present Administer rubella vaccine as indicated **Expected Outcomes:** Using sitz bath; voids qs; lab work WNL; performs ADL without sequelae
Activity	Assistance when OOB first time, then prn Ambulate ad lib Rests comfortably between assessments	Encourage rest periods Ambulate ad lib; may leave birthing unit after notifying staff of plan to ambulate off unit	Up ad lib **Expected Outcomes:** Ambulates ad lib
Comfort ▶	Institute comfort measures: ■ *Perineal* discomfort: peri-care; sitz baths, topical analgesics ■ *Hemorrhoids:* sitz baths, topical analgesics, digital replacement of external hemorrhoids; side-lying or prone position ■ *Afterpains:* prone with small pillow under abdomen; warm shower or sitz baths; ambulation ■ Administer pain medication	Continue with pain management techniques *Offer alternative pain management options:* distraction with music, television, visitors; massage; warmed blankets or towels to affected area; using breathing techniques when infant latches on to breast and/or during cramping until medication's action is felt	Continue with pain management techniques **Expected Outcomes:** Comfort level <3 on 1–10 scale Verbalizes alternative pain management options
Nutrition	Regular diet Fluid ≥ 2000 ml/day	Continue diet and fluids	Continue diet and fluids **Expected Outcomes:** Regular diet/fluids tolerated
Elimination	Voiding large amounts straw-colored urine	Voiding large quantities May have bowel movement	Same **Expected Outcomes:** Voiding qs; passing flatus or bowel movement
Medications	Pain medications as ordered Methergine 0.2 mg q4th PO if ordered Stool softener Tucks pad prn, perineal analgesic spray	Continue meds Lanolin to nipples PRN; tea bags to nipples if tender; saline flush to Luer local adaptor (if present) q8h or as ordered May take own prenatal vitamins	Continue medications RhoGAM and rubella vaccine administered as indicated **Expected Outcomes:** Vaccines administered; pain controlled
Discharge planning/ home care	Evaluate knowledge of normal postpartum and newborn care Evaluate support systems	Discuss typical newborn schedule; plan for periods of rest Birth certificate paperwork completed Evaluate plans for transporting newborn; car seat available	Review discharge instruction sheet/checklist Describe postpartum warning signs and when to call CNM/physician Provide prescriptions. Gift packs given appropriate for bottle- or breast-feeding Arrangements for baby pictures as desired Postpartum and newborn visits scheduled **Expected Outcomes:** Discharged home; mother verbalizes postpartum warning s/s, follow-up appointment times/dates

Continued

CRITICAL PATHWAY for the Postpartal Period—cont'd			
Category	First 4 Hours	4–8 Hours Past Birth	8–24 Hours Past Birth
Family involvement	Identify available support persons Assess family perceptions of birth experience Parenting: demonstrates culturally expected early parenting behaviours	Involve support persons in care, teaching; answer questions Evidence of parental bonding behaviors present	Continue to involve support persons in teaching, involve siblings as appropriate Plans made for providing support to mother following discharge **Expected Outcomes:** Evidence of parental bonding behavior; support persons verbalize understanding of woman's need for rest, good nutrition, fluids and emotional support

Source: Maternal-Newborn Nursing (6th ed), by Olds, London, Ladewig © 2000. Pp. 933-934. Reprinted by permission of Prentice-Hall, Inc., Upper Saddle River, NJ.

Maternal-Infant

THE NEWBORN INFANT

General overview: Effective nursing care of the newborn infant is based on: (1) knowledge of the conditions present during fetal life; (2) requirements for independent extrauterine life; and (3) alterations needed for successful transition. *The first 24 hours are the most hazardous.*

I. **Biological foundations of neonatal adaptation—** *general aspects:*
   A. *Fetal anatomy and physiology*
      1. *Fetal circulation*—four intrauterine structures that differ from extrauterine structures (Figure 4–11):
         a. *Umbilical vein*—carries oxygen and nutrient-enriched blood from placenta to ductus venosus and liver.
         b. *Ductus venosus*—connects to inferior vena cava; allows most blood to bypass liver.
         c. *Foramen ovale*—allows fetal blood to bypass fetal lungs by shunting it from right atrium into left atrium.
         d. *Ductus arteriosus*—allows fetal blood to bypass fetal lungs by shunting it from pulmonary artery into aorta.
         e. *Umbilical arteries* (two) —allow return of deoxygenated blood to the placenta.

      2. *Umbilical cord*—extends from fetus to center of placenta: usually 50 cm (18–22 inches) long and 1–2 cm (½–1 inch) in diameter. Contains:
         a. *Wharton's jelly*—protects umbilical vessels from pressure, cord "kinking," and interference with fetal-placental circulation.
         b. Umbilical vein—carries oxygen and nutrients from placenta to fetus.
         c. Two umbilical arteries—carry deoxygenated blood and fetal wastes from fetus to placenta. *Note:* Absence of one artery indicates need to rule out intraabdominal anomalies.
      3. *Characteristics of fetal blood*
         a. Fetal hemoglobin (Hb_f)
            (1) Higher oxygen-carrying capacity than adult hemoglobin.
            (2) Releases oxygen easily to fetal tissues.
            (3) Ensures high fetal oxygenation.
            (4) Normal range at term: 12–22 g/dl; average: 15–20 g/dl.
         b. Total blood volume at term: 85 mL/kg body weight; Hct: 38–62%, average 53%; RBC 3–7 million, average 4.9 million/U.
   B. *Extrauterine adaptation: tasks*
      1. Establish and maintain ventilation, successful gas transfer—requires patent airway and adequate pulmonary surfactant.

FIGURE 4–11 Fetal circulation. (From Thomas, CL [ed]: Taber's Cyclopedic Medical Dictionary, ed. 18. FA Davis, Philadelphia, 1997.)

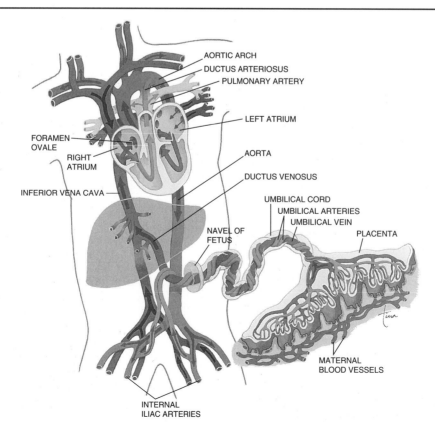

2. Modify circulatory patterns—requires closure of fetal structures.
3. Absorb and utilize fluids and nutrients.
4. Excrete body wastes.
5. Establish and maintain thermal stability.

◆ **C. Nursing care plan/implementation**
1. Facilitate successful transition to independent life.
2. Protect infant from physiological stress and environmental hazards.
3. Encourage development of a strong family unit.

II. Admission/assessment: 1–4 hours after birth
A. Admission assessment of normal, term neonate
1. Color and reactivity.
2. General appearance, symmetry.
3. Length and weight.
4. Head and chest circumferences.
5. Vital signs:
   a. Axillary temperature.
   b. Respirations (check rate, character, rhythm).
   c. Apical pulse.
6. General physical assessment (Table 4–14) and reflexes (Table 4–15).
7. Estimate of gestational age (Table 4–16).

◆ **B. Analysis/nursing diagnosis:**
1. *Altered health maintenance* related to separation from maternal support system.
2. *Impaired skin integrity* related to umbilical stump; incontinence of urine and meconium stool; skin penetration by scalp electrode, injections, heel stick, scalpel during cesarean birth; abrasion from obstetric forceps.
3. *Ineffective airway clearance* related to excessive mucus.
4. *Pain* related to environmental stimuli.
5. *Ineffective thermoregulation* related to immature temperature regulation mechanism.

◆ **C. Nursing care plan/implementation:**
1. Goal: *promote effective gas transport.*
   a. Maintain patent airway—to promote effective gas exchange and respiratory function.
   b. *Position:* right side-lying, head dependent (gravity drainage of fluid, mucus).
   c. Suction prn with bulb syringe for mucus.
2. Goal: *establish/maintain thermal stability.*
   a. *Avoid* chilling—to prevent metabolic acidosis.
   b. Dry, wrap, and apply hat.
   c. Place in heated crib.
   d. Monitor vital signs hourly until stable.
3. Goal: *reduce possibility of blood loss.*
   a. Check cord clamp for security.
   b. Administer vitamin K injection, as ordered, in anterior or lateral thigh muscle—to stimulate blood coagulability.

4. Goal: *prevent infection.*
   a. Administer antibiotic treatment to eyes (if not performed in birth room)—to prevent ophthalmia neonatorum.
   b. Treat cord stump (alcohol, Triple Dye antibiotic ointment), as ordered.
   c. Use standard precautions.
5. Goal: *promote comfort and cleanliness.* Admission bath when temperature stable.
6. Goal: *promote nutrition, hydration, elimination.*
   a. Encourage breastfeeding within 1 hr after birth.
   b. Check blood sugar (Dextrostix or Chemstrip) at 30 min, 1, 2, and 4 hr for infants at risk for hypoglycemia (e.g., SGA, LGA, IDM).
   c. First feeding at 1–4 hr of age with sterile water if permissible and if not breastfeeding.
   d. Note voiding or meconium stool; report failure to void or defecate within 24 hr.
7. Goal: *promote bonding.*
   a. Encourage parent-infant interaction (holding, touching, eye contact, talking to infant).
   b. Encourage breastfeeding within 1 hr of birth, if applicable.
   c. Encourage parent participation in infant care—to develop confidence and competence in caring for newborn.
      (1) Assist with initial efforts at feeding.
      (2) Discuss and demonstrate positioning and burping techniques.
      (3) Demonstrate/assist with basic care procedures, as necessary:
         (a) Bath.
         (b) Cord care.
         (c) Diapering.
         (d) Aid parents in distinguishing normal vs. abnormal newborn characteristics.
8. Goal: *health teaching*—to provide anticipatory guidance for discharge.
   a. Facilitate sibling bonding.
   b. Describe/discuss normal newborn behavior:

> (1) *Sleeping*—almost continual (wakes only to feed) or 12-16 hr daily.
> (2) *Feeding*—from every 2–3 hrs to longer intervals; establish own pattern; breast-fed babies feed more often.
> (3) *Weight loss*—5-10% in first few days; regained in 7-14 days.
> (4) *Stools*—Table 4–17.
> (5) *Cord care*—drops off in 7-10 days
>   (a) Keep clean and dry.
>   (b) Alcohol to stump.
>   (c) HIV precautions.
> (6) *Circumcision care*
>   (a) Keep clean and dry; heals rapidly.
>   *(Continued on page 172)*

TABLE 4–14 ◆ **Physical Assessment of the Term Neonate**

Criterion	Average Values and Normal Variations	Deviations from Normal
Vital Signs		
Heart rate	120–140/min, irregular, especially when crying, and functional murmur	Faint sound—pneumomediastinum; and heart rate <100 beats/min or >180 beats/min
Respiratory	30–60/min with short periods of apnea, irregular; vigorous and loud cry	Distress—flaring of nares, retractions, tachypnea, grunting, excessive mucus, <30 respirations/min or >60 respirations/min; cyanosis
Temperature	Stabilizes about 8–10 hr after birth; 36.5–37°C (97.7–98.6°F) axillary	Unreliable indicator of infection due to environmental influences
Blood pressure	60–80/40–50; varies with change in activity level	Hypotension: with RDS Hypertension: coarctation of aorta
Measurements		
Weight	3400 g (7½ lb); range: 5 lb 8 oz to 8 lb 13 oz	Birthweight <2500 g; preterm or SGA infant; >4000 g; LGA infant, evaluate mother for gestational diabetes
Length	50 cm (20 inches); range: 18–22 inches	
Chest circumference	2 cm (¾ inches) less than head circumference	If relationship varies, check for reason
Head circumference	33–35 cm (13–14 inches)	Check for microcephalus and macrocephalus
General Assessment		
Muscle tone	Good tone and generalized flexion; full range of motion; spontaneous movement	Flaccid, and persistent tremor or twitching; movement limited; asymmetrical
Skin color	Mottling, acrocyanosis, and physiologic jaundice; petechia (over presenting part), milia, mongolian spotting, lanugo, and vernix caseosa	Pallor, cyanosis, or jaundice within 24 hr of birth Petechiae or ecchymoses elsewhere; all rashes, except erythema toxicum; pigmented nevi; hemangioma; and yellow vernix
Head	Molding of fontanels and suture spaces; one-fourth of body length	Cephalhematoma, caput succedaneum, sunken or bulging fontanels, closed sutures; excessively wide sutures
Hair	Silky, single strands, lies flat; grows toward face and neck	Fine, wooly; unusual swirls, patterns, hair line; coarse
Eyes	Edematous eyelids, conjunctival hemorrhage; grayish-blue to grayish-brown; blink reflex, usually no tears; uncoordinated movements may focus for a few seconds; good placement on face; cornea is bright and shiny; pupillary reflex equal and reactive to light; eyebrows distinct	Epicanthal folds (in non-Asians); discharges; agenesis; opaque lenses; lesions; strabismus; "doll's eyes" beyond 10 days; absence of reflexes
Nose	Appears to have no bridge; should have no discharge; preferential nose breathers; sneezes to clear nose	Discharge and choanal atresia; malformed; flaring of nares beyond first few moments of life
Mouth	*Epstein's pearls* on gum ridges; tongue does not protrude and moves freely, symmetrically; uvula in midline; reflexes present; sucking, rooting, gag, extrusion	*Cleft lip or palate;* teeth, cyanosis, circumoral pallor; asymmetrical lip movement; excessive saliva; thrush; incomplete or absent reflexes
Ears	Well formed, firm; notch of ear should be on straight line with outer canthus	Low placement, clefts; tags; malformed; lack of cartilage
Face	Symmetrical movements and contours	*Facial palsy* (7th cranial nerve); looks "funny"
Neck	Short, freely movable; some head control	Wry neck, webbed neck; restricted movement; masses; distended veins; absence of head control
Chest	Enlarged breasts, *"witch's milk";* barrel shaped; both sides move synchronously; nipples symmetrical	Flattened, funnel-chested, asynchronous movement; lack of breast tissue; fracture of clavicle(s); supernumeray or widely spaced nipples; bowel sounds
Abdomen	Dome shaped, abdominal respirations, soft; may have small umbilical hernia; umbilical cord well formed, containing three vessels; dry around base; bowel sounds within 2 hr of birth; voiding; passage of meconium	Scaphoid shaped, omphalocele, diastasis recti, and distention; umbilical cord containing two vessels; redness or drainage around base of cord

TABLE 4–14   Physical Assessment of the Term Neonate—cont'd

Criterion	Average Values and Normal Variations	Deviations from Normal
General Assessment (continued)		
Genitalia		
Female	Large labia; may have pseudomenstruation, smegma; vaginal orifice open; increased pigmentation; ecchymosis and edema following breech birth; pink-stained urine (uric acid crystals)	Agenesis and imperforate hymen; ambiguous labia widely separated, fecal discharge per vagina; *epispadias or hypospadias*
Male	Pendulous scrotum covered with rugae, and testes usually descended; voids with adequate stream; increased pigmentation; edema and ecchymosis following breech birth	*Phimosis, epispadias,* or *hypospadias;* ambiguous; scrotum smooth and testes undescended *Hydrocele:* collection of fluid in the sac surrounding the testes
Extremities	Synchronized movements, freely movable through full range of motion; legs appear bowed, and feet appear flat; attitude of general flexion; arms longer than legs; grasp reflex; palmar and sole creases; normal contour	Fractures, brachial nerve palsy, *clubbed foot,* phocomelia or amelia, unusual number or webbing of digits, and abnormal palmar creases; poor muscle tone; asymmetry; hypertonicity; unusual hip contour and click sign *(hip dysplasia);* hypermobility of joints
Back	Spine straight, easily movable, and flexible; may have small pilonidal dimple at base of spine; may raise head when prone	Fusion of vertebrae: pilonidal dimple with tuft of hair; *spina bifida,* agenesis of part of vertebral bodies; limitation of movement; weak or absent reflexes
Anus	Patent, well placed; "wink" reflex	Imperforate, and absence of "wink" (absence of sphincter muscle); fistula
Stools	Meconium within first 24 hr; transitional—days 2–5; *breastfed:* loose, golden yellow; *bottlefed:* formed, light yellow (See Table 4–17)	Light-colored meconium (dry, hard), or absent with distended abdomen *(cyctic fibrosis* or *Hirschsprung's disease);* diarrhetic
Laboratory Values		
Hemoglobin (cord)	13.6–19.6 g/dl	Evaluate for anemia and persistent polycythemia
Serum bilirubin	2–6 mg/dl	Hyperbilirubinemia (*term:* 12 mg or more; *preterm:* 15 mg or more)
Blood glucose	40 mg/dl for *term;* >20 mg/dl for *preterm*	Identify hypoglycemia before overt or asymptomatic hypoglycemia—do Dextrostix on all suspects (LGA or SGA neonates, or neonates of diabetic mothers)
Neurologic Examination*	Specific to gestational age and state of wakefulness	
1. Behavioral patterns		
a. Feeding	Variations in interest, hunger; usually feeds well within 48 hr	Lethargic. Poor suck, poor coordination with swallow, choking, cyanosis
b. Social	Crying is lusty, strong, and soon indicative of hunger, pain, attention seeking. Responds to cuddling, voice by quietness and increased alertness	Absent; no focusing on person holding him/her; unconsolable
c. Sleep-wakefulness	Two periods of reactivity: at birth, and 6–8 hr later. Stabilization, with wakeful periods about every 3–4 hr	Lethargy, drowsiness Disorganized pattern
d. Elimination	Stooling: see Stools Urination First few days: 3–4 qd End of first week: 5–6 qd Later: 6–10 qd, with adequate hydration	See Stools Diminished number: dehydration
2. Reflex response	Bilateral, symmetrical response (see Table 4–15)	Absent, hyperactive, incomplete, asynchronous
3. Sensory capabilities		
a. Vision	Limited accommodation, with clearest vision within 7–8 inches. Focuses and follows by 15 min of age. Prefers patterns to plain.	Absence of these responses may be due to absence of or diminished acuity or to sensory deprivation
b. Hearing	By 2 min of age, can move in direction of sound: responds to high pitch by "freezing," followed by agitation; to low pitch (crooning) by relaxing	Absence of response: deafness

Continued

TABLE 4–14   Physical Assessment of the Term Neonate—cont'd

Criterion	Average Values and Normal Variations	Deviations from Normal
Neurologic Assessment (continued)		
c. Touch	Soothed by massaging, warmth, weightlessness (as in water bath)	Unable to be comforted: possible drug dependence Cocaine-addicted newborns avoid eye contact
d. Smell	By fifth day, can distinguish between mother's breasts and those of another woman	
e. Taste	Can distinguish between sweet and sour	
f. Motor	Coordinates body movement to parent's voice and body movement	Absence

*Based on Brazelton's method.

TABLE 4–15   ◆Assessment: Normal Newborn Reflexes*

Reflex	Description	Implications of Deviations from Normal Patterns
Moro (startle)	Symmetrical *abduction* and *extension* of arms with fingers extended in response to sudden movement or loud noise	Asymmetrical reflex may indicate brachial (Erb's) palsy or fractured clavicle
Tonic neck (fencing)	When head turned to one side, arm and leg on *that* side *extend,* and *opposite* arm and leg *flex*	Asymmetry may indicate cerebral lesion, if persistent
Rooting and sucking	With stimulus to cheek, turns *toward* stimulus, opens mouth, sucks	Absence of response may indicate prematurity, neurologic problem, or depressed infant (or not hungry)
Palmar grasp	If palm stimulated, fingers *curl;* holds adult finger briefly	Asymmetry may indicate neurological involvement
Plantar grasp	Pressure on sole will elicit *curling* of toes	Absence/asymmetry associated with defects of lower spinal column
Stepping/dancing	If held in upright position with feet in contact with hard surface, alternately raises feet	Asymmetry may indicate neurological problem
Babinski	Stroking the sole in a upward fashion elicits *hyper-extension* of toes	Same as for plantar grasp
Crawling	When placed in prone position, attempts to crawl	Absence may indicate prematurity or depressed infant

*Reflexes are good indicators of the neurological system in well infants but not in sick neonates. Infants with infections may not show normal reflexes yet have an intact neurological system.

(b) Watch for bleeding.
(c) Petroleum jelly, gauze prn, if ordered.
(d) Do *not* remove yellowish exudate.

(7) *Physiologic jaundice*—occurs 24-72 hr after birth.
   (a) Nonpathologic.
   (b) Need for hydration.

(8) Identify need for newborn screen after ingestion of milk (done routinely at 24 hr of age and later). Includes screen for congenital hypothyroidism and galactosemia. (See Table 11–2, **Unit 11,** for other newborn screening procedures.)

(9) Describe suggested sensory *stimulation* modalities (mobiles, color, music).

(10) Discuss *safety* precautions:
   (a) Position on back for sleep.
   (b) Infant seat for travel and home safety.
   (c) Maintaining contact/control over infant to prevent falls, drowning in bath.
   (d) Instruct parents in infant cardiopulmonary resuscitation (CPR).
   (e) *Hepatitis B vaccination*—first dose can be given 24–48 hr of life; second dose 1 mo; third dose 6 mo. If infant born to infected mother, hepatitis B vaccine and hepatitis B immune globulin should be administered within 12 hr of birth.

(11) Describe signs of *common health problems* to be reported promptly:
   (a) Diarrhea, constipation.
   (b) Colic, vomiting.

TABLE 4–16   Estimation of Gestational Age: Common Clinical Parameters

Characteristic	Preterm	Term
Head	Oval—narrow biparietal; large in proportion to body; face looks like "old man"	Square-shaped biparietal prominences; ¼ body length
Ears: form, cartilage	Soft, flat, shapeless	Pinna firm; erect from head
Hair: texture, distribution	Fine, fuzzy, or wooly; clumped; appears at 20 wk	Silk; single strands apparent
Sole creases	Starting at ball of foot: ⅓ covered with creases by 36 wk, ⅔ by 38 wk	Entire sole heavily creased
Breast nodules	0 mm at 36 wk; 4 mm at 37 wk	10 mm or more
Nipples	No areolae	Formed; raised above skin level
Genitalia		
Female	Clitoris large, labia gaping	Labia larger, meet in midline
Male	Small scrotum, rugae on inferior surface only, and testes undescended	Scrotum pendulous, covered with rugae; testes usually descended
Skin: texture, opacity	Visible abdominal veins; thin, shiny	Few indistinct larger veins; thick, dry, cracked, peeling
Vernix	Cover body by 31–33 wk	Small amount in creases or absent at term; postterm: dry, wrinkled
Lanugo	Apparent at 20 wk; by 33–36 wk, covers shoulders	Minimal or no lanugo (depends on parental ethnicity)
Muscle tone	Hypotonia; extension of arms and legs	Hypertonia; well flexed
Posture	Froglike	Attitude of general flexion
Head lag	Head lags; arms have little or no flexion	Head follows trunk; strong arm flexion
Scarf sign	Elbow can extend to opposite axilla	Elbow to midline only; infant resists
Square window	90 degrees	0 degrees
Ankle dorsiflexion	90 degrees	0 degrees
Popliteal angle	180 degrees	<90 degrees
Heel-to-ear maneuver	Touches ear easily	90 degrees
Ventral suspension	Hypotonia; "rag-doll"	Good caudal and cephalic tone
Reflexes		
Moro	Apparent at 28 wk; good, but no adduction	Complete reflex with adduction; disappears 4 mo postterm
Grasp	Fair at 28 wk; arm is involved at 32 wk	Strong enough to sustain weight for a few seconds when pulled up; hand, arm, shoulder involved
Cry	24 wk: weak; 28 wk: high-pitched; 32 wk: good	Lusty; can persist for some time
Length	Under 47 cm (18½ inches), usually	50 cm (20 in); range: 18–22 inches
Weight	Under 2500 g (5 lb 5 oz)	3400 g (7½ lb); range: 5 lb 8 oz to 8 lb 13 oz

TABLE 4–17   Infant Stool Characteristics

Age	Bottlefed	Breastfed	Implications of Abnormal Patterns
1 day	Meconium	Meconium	Absence may indicate obstruction, atresia
2–5 days (transitional)	Greenish yellow, loose	Greenish yellow, loose, frequent	*Note*—At any time:
>5 days	Yellow to brown, firm, 2–4 daily, foul odor	Bright golden yellow, loose, 6–10 daily	*Diarrhea*—greenish, mucus or blood tinged, or forceful expulsion, may indicate infection *Constipation*—dry, hard stools or infrequent or absent stools may indicate obstruction

    (c) Rash, jaundice.
    (d) Differentiation from normal patterns.

◆ **D. Evaluation/outcome criteria:**
    1. Infant demonstrates successful transition to independent life:

    a. Nurses well.
    b. Normal feeding, sleeping, elimination patterns.
    c. No evidence of infection or abnormality.
  2. Mother/family evidences bonding.
    a. Eye contact.

(continued on p. 176)

Maternal-Infant

CRITICAL PATHWAY for Newborn Care

Category	First 4 Hours	4–8 Hours Past Birth	8–24 Hours Past Birth
Referral	Review labor/birth record Review transitional nursing record Check ID bands PRN consults: orthopedics, genetics, infectious disease	Check ID bands Transfer to mother/baby care at 4–6 hours of age if stable As parents desire, obtain circumcision permit after their discussion with physician Lactation consult PRN	Check ID bands every shift **Expected Outcomes:** Mother/baby ID bands correlate at time of discharge; consults completed PRN
Assessments ◆	Continue assessments begun first hour after birth. Vital signs: TPR (q1h × 4), BP PRN (skin temp 97.8–98.6°F, resp may be irregular but within 30–60 per min)	Assess newborn's progress through periods of reactivity Vital signs: TPR q8h and PRN, BP PRN	VS q8h. Normal ranges: T, 97.5–99°F; P, 120–160; R, 30–60; BP, 60–80/40–45 mm Hg
	Newborn Assessments: ■ Respiratory status with resp distress scale × 1 then prn. If resp distress, assess q5–15min ■ Cord—bluish white color, clamp in place ■ Color: skin, mucous membranes, extremities; trunk pink with slight acrocyanosis of hands and feet ■ Wt (5 lb 8 oz–8 lb 13 oz), length (18–22 inches), HC (12.5–14.5 inches), CC (32.5 cm, 1–2 cm less than head) ■ Extremity movement—may be jerky or brief twitches ■ Gestational age classification—term AGA ■ Anomalies (cong. anomalies can interfere with normal extrauterine adaptation)	**Newborn Assessments:** ■ Skin color q4h prn (circulatory system stabilizing, acrocyanosis decreased) ■ Eyes for drainage, redness, hemorrhage ■ Ausculate lungs q4h (noisy, wet resp normal) ■ Increased mucus production (normal in second period of reactivity) ■ Check apical pulse q4h ■ Umbilical cord base for redness, drainage, foul odor, drying, clamp in place ■ Extremity movement q4h ■ Check for expected reflexes (suck, rooting, Moro, grasp, blink, yawn, sneeze, tonic neck, Babinski) ■ Note common normal variations ■ Assess suck and swallow during feeding ■ Note behavioral characteristics ■ Temp before and after admission bath	**Continue Newborn Assessments:** ■ Skin color q4h ■ Signs of drying or infection in cord area ■ Check cord clamp in place until removed before discharge ■ Check circ for bleeding after procedure, then q30min × 2, then q4h and PRN **Expected Outcomes:** Vital signs medically acceptable, color pink, assessments WNL, circ site without s/s infection, cord site without s/s infection and clamp removed; newborn behavior WNL
Teaching/ psychosocial	Admission activities performed at mother's bedside if possible, orient to nursery prn, hand washing, assess teaching needs Teach parents use of bulb syringe, signs of choking, positioning, and when to call for assistance Teach reasons for use of radiant warmer, infant hat, and warmed blankets when out of warmer Discuss/teach infant security, identification	Reinforce teaching about choking, bulb syringe use, positioning, temperature maintenance with clothing and blankets Teach infant positioning to facilitate breathing and digestion Teach new parents holding and feeding skills Teach parents soothing and calming techniques	**Final discharge teaching:** diapering, normal void and stool patterns, bathing, nail and cord care, circumcision/uncircumcised penis/genital care and normal characteristics, rashes, jaundice, sleep/wake cycles, soothing activities, taking temperatures, thermometer reading Explain s/s of illness and when to call health care provider Infant safety: car seats, immunizations, metabolic screening; on back for sleep **Expected Outcomes:** Mother/family verbalize comprehension of teaching; demonstrates care capabilities

CRITICAL PATHWAY **for Newborn Care—cont'd**

Category	First 4 Hours	4–8 Hours Past Birth	8–24 Hours Past Birth
Nursing care management and reports	Place under radiant warmer Place hat on newborn (decreases convection heat loss) Suction nares/mouth with ▶ bulb syringe prn Keep bulb syringe with infant Attach security sensor Obtain lab tests: blood glucose; as needed obtain blood type, Rh, Coombs on cord blood, HSV culture if parental hx Notify physician's office for exchange of infant's birth and status Maintain standard precautions	Wean from radiant warmer (T 98°F axillary) Chemstrips prn; BP prn Oxygen saturation prn Bathe infant if temp >97.8°F Position on side Suction nares prn (esp during ▶ second period of reactivity) Obtain peripheral Hct per protocol Cord care per protocol (alcohol or triple dye prn) Fold diaper below cord (for plastic diapers, turn plastic layer away from skin)	Check for hearing test results Weigh before discharge Cord care every shift DC cord clamp before discharge Perform newborn metabolic screening blood tests before discharge Circumcision if indicated. Circumcision care: ▶ change diaper prn noting ability to void, follow policy for Gomco or Plastibell care **Expected Outcomes:** Newborn maintains temp, lab test WNL, cord dry without s/s infection and clamp removed, screening tests accomplished, circ site without s/s infection or bleeding
Activity and comfort	Place under radiant warmer or wrap in prewarmed blankets until stable Soothe baby as needed with voice, touch, cuddling, nesting in warmer	Leave in warmer until stable, then swaddle Position on side after each feeding	Place in open crib Swaddle to allow movement of extremities in blanket, including hands to face **Expected Outcomes:** Infant maintains temp WNL in open crib; infant attempts self-calming
Nutrition	Assist newborn to breastfeed as soon as mother/baby condition allows Supplement breast only when medically indicated or per agency policy Initiate bottle-feeding within first hour Gavage feed if necessary to prevent hypoglycemia	Breastfeed on demand, at least q3–4h Teach positions, observe/assist with feeding, breast/nipple care, establishing milk supply, breaking suction, feeding cues, latching on techniques, nutritive suck, burping Bottlefeed on demand, at least q3–6h Determine readiness to feed and feeding tolerance	Continue breast/bottlefeeding pattern Assess feeding tolerance q4h Discuss normal feeding requirements, signs of hunger and satiation, handling feeding problems, and when to seek help **Expected Outcomes:** Mother verbalizes knowledge of feeding information; breastfeeds on demand without supplement; bottle—tolerates formula feeding, nipples without problems
Elimination	Note first void and stool if not noted at birth	Note all voids, amount and color of stools q4h	Evaluate all voids and stools color q8h **Expected Outcomes:** Voids qs; stools qs without difficulty; stool character WNL; diaper area without s/s skin breakdown or rashes
Medication	Prophylactic ophthalmic ointment OU after baby makes eye contact with parents within 1 hr after birth Administer Aquamephyton IM, dosage according to infant weight per MD/NP order	Hepatitis B injection as ordered by physician after consent signed by parents	Hepatitis B vaccine before discharge **Expected Outcomes:** Baby has received ophthalmic ointment and vitamin K injection; baby has received first hepatitis B vaccine if ordered and parental permission received
Discharge planning/home care	Hepatitis B consent signed Hearing screen consent signed	Review/reinforce teaching with mother and significant other Review home preparedness	Initial newborn screening tests (hearing, blood tests, PKU) before discharge Bath and feeding classes, videos, or written information given

Continued

CRITICAL PATHWAY	for Newborn Care—cont'd		
Category	First 4 Hours	4–8 Hours Past Birth	8–24 Hours Past Birth
Discharge planning/ home care— cont'd	Plan discharge call with parent or guardian in 24 hr to 2 days Assess parents' discharge plans, needs, and support systems	Obtain birth certificate information	Give written copy of discharge instructions Newborn photographs Set up appointment for follow-up PKU test Have car seat available before discharge All discharge referrals made, follow-up appt. scheduled **Expected Outcomes:** Infant discharged home with family; mother verbalizes follow up appt. time/date
Family involvement	Facilitate early investigation of baby's physical characteristics (maintain temp during unwrapping), hold infant en face Dim lights to help infant keep eyes open	Assess parents' knowledge of newborn behaviors, such as alertness, suck and rooting, attention to human voice, response to calming techniques	Assess mother-baby bonding/interaction Incorporate father and siblings in care Enhance parent-infant interaction by sharing characteristics and behavioral assessment Support positive parenting behaviors Identify community referral needs and refer to community agencies **Expected Outcomes:** Demonstrates caring and family incorporation of infant

Source: Maternal-Newborn Nursing (6th ed), by Olds, London, Ladewig © 2000. Pp. 754-755. Reprinted by permission of Prentice-Hall, Inc., Upper Saddle River, NJ.

b. Stroking, cuddling.
c. Crooning, calling baby by name, talking to infant.
3. Mother demonstrates comfort and skill in basic newborn care.
4. Mother verbalizes understanding of subjects discussed:
a. Safety precautions.
b. Health maintenance actions.
c. Signs of normal infant behavior and health.

Complications During the Neonatal Period: The High-Risk Newborn

I. General overview—successful newborn adaptation to the demands of independent extrauterine life may be complicated by environmental insults during the *prenatal* period or those arising in the period immediately surrounding birth. The nursing role focuses on minimizing the effect of present and emerging health problems and on facilitating and supporting a successful transition to extrauterine life.

II. General aspects—common neonatal risk factors:
A. Gestational age profile (see Tables 4-14 and 4-16):
1. Prematurity.
2. Dysmaturity.
3. Postmaturity.
B. Congenital disorders.

C. Birth trauma.
D. Infections.

III. Disorders affecting protective functions: neonatal infections
A. Assess for intrauterine infections.
B. Oral thrush (mycotic stomatitis).
1. **Pathophysiology**—local inflammation of oral mucosa due to fungal infection.
2. **Etiology:**
a. Organism—*Candida albicans.*
b. More common in vulnerable newborn, i.e., sick, debilitated; those receiving antibiotic therapy.
3. Mode of transmission—direct contact with:
a. Maternal birth canal, hands, and linens.
b. Contaminated feeding equipment, staff's hands.
◆ 4. **Assessment:**
a. White patches on oral mucosa, gums, and tongue that bleed when touched.
b. Occasional difficulty swallowing.
◆ 5. **Analysis/nursing diagnosis:**
a. *Pain* related to irritation of oral mucous membrane secondary to oral moniliasis.
b. *Altered nutrition, less than body requirements* related to irritability and poor feeding.
◆ 6. **Nursing care plan/implementation:**
Goal: *prevent cross-contamination.*
▶ a. Aseptic technique; good handwashing.
b. Give medications as ordered:
(1) Aqueous gentian violet, 1-2%: apply to infected area with swab.

(2) Nystatin (Mycostatin)—instill into mouth with medicine dropper, or apply to lesions with swab, *after* feedings. *Note:* Before medicating, feed sterile water to rinse out milk.

◆ 7. **Evaluation/outcome criteria:**
   a. Oral mucosa intact, lesions healed, no evidence of infection.
   b. Feeds well; maintains weight or regains weight lost, if any.

C. **Neonatal sepsis**
   1. **Pathophysiology**—generalized infection; may overwhelm infant's immature immune system.
   2. **Etiology:**
      a. Prolonged rupture of membranes.
      b. Long, difficult labor.
      c. Resuscitation procedures.
      d. Maternal infection (e.g., beta-hemolytic streptococcus vaginosis).
      e. Aspiration—amniotic fluid, formula, mucus.
      f. Iatrogenic (nosocomial)—caused by infected health personnel or equipment.

◆ 3. **Assessment:**
      a. Respirations—irregular, periods of apnea.
      b. Irritability or lethargy.

◆ 4. **Analysis/nursing diagnosis:**
      a. *Fatigue* related to increased oxygen needs.
      b. *High risk for infection* related to septic condition.

◆ 5. **Nursing care plan/implementation:**
      a. Cultures (spinal, urine, blood).
      b. Check vitals.
      c. Monitor respirations.
      d. Give medications, as ordered.

◆ 6. **Evaluation/outcome criteria:**
      a. Responds to medical/nursing regimen (all assessment findings within normal limits).
      b. Parent(s) verbalize understanding of diagnosis, treatment; demonstrate appropriate techniques in participating in care (as possible).
      c. Parent(s) demonstrate effective coping with situation; express satisfaction with care.

IV. **Disorders affecting nutrition: infant of the diabetic mother (IDM)**
   A. **Pathophysiology**—hyperplasia of pancreatic beta cells → increased insulin production → excessive deposition of glycogen in muscles, subcutaneous fat, and tissue growth. Results in fetal:
      1. *Macrosomia*—LGA infant.
      2. *Enlarged internal organs*—common.
         a. Cardiomegaly.
         b. Hepatomegaly.
         c. Splenomegaly.

   3. Neonatal—inadequate carbohydrate reserve to meet energy needs.
   4. Associated with *increased incidence of:*
      a. Congenital anomalies (five times average incidence with pregestational diabetes) includes cardiac, pelvic, and spinal anomalies.
      b. Preterm birth: respiratory distress syndrome (RDS); increased insulin needs prenatally lead to decreased surfactant production.
      c. Fetal dystocia—due to CPD.
      d. Neonatal metabolic problems:
         (1) Hypoglycemia.
         (2) Hypocalcemic tetany.
         (3) Metabolic acidosis.
         (4) Hyperbilirubinemia.

   B. **Etiology**—high circulating maternal glucose levels during fetal growth and development; loss of maternal glucose supply following birth; decreased hepatic gluconeogenesis.

◆ C. **Assessment:**
   1. Characteristics of IDM.
   2. Hypoglycemia—Dextrostix or Chem-strip to heel stick at:
      a. 30 min × 2.
      b. 1, 2, and 4 hr of age; before meals × 4 or until stable.
      c. Chemstrip: if <20 mg/dl, must draw glucose stat.
      d. Hypoglycemia laboratory values for term infant: under 40 mg/dl.
      e. Hypoglycemia laboratory values for preterm infant: under 40 mg/dl.
      f. Behavioral signs—tremors; twitching, hypotonia, seizures.
   3. Gestational age, since macrosomia may mask prematurity.
   4. Hypocalcemia—usually within first 24 hr
      a. Irritability.
      b. Coarse tremors, twitching, convulsions.
   5. Birth injuries.
      a. Fractures: clavicle, humerus, skull.
      b. Brachial palsy.
      c. Intracranial hemorrhage/signs of increased intracranial pressure.
      d. Cephalohematoma.
   6. Respiratory distress.
      a. Nasal flaring.
      b. Sternal retraction.
      c. Intercostal retractions.
      d. Cyanosis—central.
      e. Expiratory grunt.
   7. Jaundice.

◆ D. **Analysis/nursing diagnosis:**
   1. *High risk for injury* related to CPD, dystocia.
   2. *Altered cardiopulmonary tissue perfusion* related to placental insufficiency, RDS.
   3. *Impaired gas exchange* related to RDS.
   4. *Altered nutrition, less than body requirements,* related to hypoglycemia, hypocalcemia.

5. *Risk for altered endocrine/metabolic processes* related to hyperbilirubinemia and kernicterus.

◆ **E. Nursing care plan/implementation:**

💊 1. Hypoglycemia—administer formula or IV glucose, as ordered (may cause rebound effect).

2. Preterm/immature—institute preterm care prn.

💊 3. Hypocalcemia—administer oral or IV calcium gluconate, as ordered.

4. Inform pediatrician **immediately** of signs of:

> a. Jaundice.
> b. Hyperirritability.
> c. Birth injury.
> d. Increased intracranial pressure/hemorrhage

◆ **F. Evaluation/outcome criteria:**

1. Infant makes successful transition to extrauterine life.

2. Infant responds to medical/nursing regimen. Experiences minimal or no metabolic disturbances (hypoglycemia, hypocalcemia, hyperbilirubinemia).

3. Infant exhibits normal respiratory function and gas exchange.

V. Hypoglycemia

A. Pathophysiology—low serum-glucose level → altered cellular metabolism → cerebral irritability, cardiopulmonary problems.

B. Etiology:

1. Loss of maternal glucose supply.

2. Normal physiologic activities of respiration, thermoregulation, muscular activity exceed carbohydrate reserve.

3. Decreased hepatic ability to convert amino acids into glucose.

4. More common in:

a. Infants of diabetic mothers.

b. Preterm, postterm infants.

c. SGA infants.

d. Smaller twin.

e. Infant of mother with preeclampsia.

f. Birth asphyxia.

◆ **C. Assessment:**

1. Jitteriness, tremors, convulsions; lethargy and hypotonia.

2. Sweating; unstable temperature.

3. Tachypnea; apneic episodes; cyanosis.

4. High-pitched, shrill cry.

5. Difficulty feeding.

◆ **D. Analysis/nursing diagnosis:**

1. *Altered tissue perfusion (fetal)* related to placental insufficiency associated with maternal diabetes, PIH, renal or cardiac disorders; erythroblastosis.

2. *Risk for altered endocrine metabolic processes* related to high incidence of morbidity associated with birth asphyxia.

3. *Impaired gas exchange* related to coexisting RDS.

4. *Altered nutrition, less than body requirements,* related to hypoglycemia.

5. *High risk for injury* related to coexisting infection, metabolic acidosis.

◆ **E. Nursing care plan/implementation:** see IV. Infant of the diabetic mother, p. 177.

◆ **F. Evaluation/outcome criteria:** see IV. Infant of the diabetic mother, p. 177.

VI. Disorders affecting psychosocial-cultural functions: drug-dependent (heroin) neonate

A. General aspects

1. Maternal drug addiction has been associated with:

a. Prenatal malnutrition and vitamin deficiencies.

b. Increased risk of antepartal infections.

c. Higher incidence of antepartal and intrapartal complications.

2. Infant at risk for:

a. Intrauterine growth retardation (IUGR).

b. Prematurity.

c. Fetal distress.

d. Perinatal death.

e. Child abuse.

f. Sudden infant death syndrome (SIDS) (5-10 times higher than normal).

g. Learning and behavior disorders.

h. Poor social adjustment.

B. Pathophysiology—withdrawal of accustomed drug levels → physiological deprivation response.

C. Etiology—repeated intrauterine absorption of heroin/cocaine/methadone from maternal bloodstream → fetal drug dependency.

◆ **D. Assessment**—degree of withdrawal depends on type and duration of addiction and maternal drug levels at birth.

1. Irritability, hyperactivity, hypertonicity, exaggerated reflexes, tremors, high-pitched cry, difficult to comfort:

a. *"Step" reflex* (dancing)—infant places both feet on surface; assumes rigid stance—does not "step" or dance.

b. *"Head-righting" reflex*—holds head rigid; fails to demonstrate head-lag.

2. Nasal stuffiness and sneezing; respiratory distress, tachypnea, cyanosis or apnea.

3. Exaggerated acrocyanosis or mottling in the warm infant.

4. Sweating.

5. Hunger—sucks on fists; feeding problems—regurgitation, vomiting, poor feeding, diarrhea, and increased mucus production.

6. Convulsions with abnormal eye-rolling and chewing motions.

7. Developmental lags/mental retardation.

◆ **E. Analysis/nursing diagnosis:**

1. *High risk for injury* related to convulsions secondary to physiological response to withdrawal, CNS hyperirritability.

2. *Impaired gas exchange* related to respiratory distress secondary to inhibition of reflex clearing of fluid by the lungs.

3. *Altered nutrition, less than body requirements,* related to feeding problems secondary to respiratory distress and GI hypermotility.
4. *High risk for impaired skin integrity* related to scratching, secondary to withdrawal symptoms.

◆ **F. Nursing care plan/implementation:**
1. Goal: *prevent/minimize respiratory distress.*
   ◢ a. *Position:* side-lying, head dependent—to facilitate mucus drainage.
   ▶ b. Suction prn with bulb syringe for excess mucus—to maintain patent airway.
   c. Monitor respirations and apical pulse.
2. Goal: *minimize possibility of convulsions.*
   a. Decrease environmental stimuli—quiet, touch only when necessary, offer pacifier.
   b. Keep warm, swaddle for comfort.
3. Goal: *maintain nutrition/hydration.*
   a. Food/fluids—oral or IV, as ordered.
   b. I&O.
   c. Daily weight.
4. Goal: *assist in diagnosis of drug and drug level.* Collect all urine and meconium during first 24 hr for toxicologic studies.
5. Goal: *maintain/promote skin integrity.*
   a. Mitts over hands—to minimize scratching.
   b. Keep clean and dry.
   ◖▬ c. Medicated ointment/powder, as ordered, q2–4h, to excoriated areas.
   d. Expose excoriated areas to air.
◖▬ 6. Goal: *minimize withdrawal symptoms.* Administer medications, as ordered.
   a. Paregoric elixir—to wean from drug.
   b. Phenobarbital—to reduce CNS hyperirritability, hyperbilirubinemia.
   c. Chlorpromazine *(Thorazine),* diazepam *(Valium)* —to tranquilize, reduce hyperirritability. *Note: Valium* is **contraindicated** for jaundiced neonate because it predisposes to hyperbilirubinemia.
   d. Methadone.
7. Goal: *emotional support to mother.*
   a. Encourage verbalization of feelings of guilt, anxiety, fear, concerns.
   b. Refer to social service.

◆ **G. Evaluation/outcome criteria:**
1. Infant responds to medical/nursing regimen.
   a. Maintains adequate respirations.
   b. Feeds well, gains weight.
   c. No evidence of CNS hyperirritability. convulsions; demonstrates normal newborn reflexes.
2. Infant evidences bonding with parent(s). Responsive to mother's voice.

VII. Disorders affecting psychosocial-cultural function: fetal alcohol syndrome (FAS). *General aspects:*
A. Maternal alcohol abuse has been associated with:
1. Malnutrition, vitamin deficiencies.
2. Bone marrow suppression.
3. Liver disease.
4. Child abuse.
B. Infant at risk for:
1. Congenital anomalies.
2. Mental deficiency; learning disabilities.
3. IUGR.
C. **Pathophysiology**—permanent damage to developing embryonic/fetal structures; cardiovascular anomalies (ventricular septal defects).
D. **Etiology**—high circulating alcohol levels are lethal to the embryo; lower levels cause permanent cell damage.

◆ **E. Assessment:**
1. Characteristic craniofacial abnormalities:
   a. Short, palpebral fissure.
   b. Epicanthal folds.
   c. Maxillary hypoplasia.
   d. Micrognathia.
   e. Long, thin upper lip.
2. Short stature.
3. Irritable, hyperactive, poor feeding.
4. High-pitched cry, difficult to comfort.

◆ **F. Nursing care plan/implementation:**
1. Goal: *reduce irritability.*
   a. Reduce environmental stimuli.
   b. Wrap, cuddle.
   ◖▬ c. Administer sedatives, as ordered.
2. Goal: *maintain nutrition/hydration.*
3. Goal: *emotional support to mother.*

◆ **G. Evaluation/outcome criteria:** see VI. Drug-dependent (heroin) neonate, p. 178.
1. No respiratory distress.
2. Infant feeding properly.
3. Maternal bonding apparent.
4. Social service—home involvement.

VIII. Classification of infants by weight and gestational age
A. Terminology
1. *Preterm, or premature*—37 wk gestation or less (usually 2500 g [5 lb] or less).
2. *Term*—38-42 wk gestation.
3. *Postterm*—over 42 wk.
4. *Postmature*—gestation greater than 42 wk.
5. *Appropriate for gestational age (AGA)*—for each week of gestation, there is a normal range of expected weight (between 10th and 90th percentile).
   a. Term infants weighing 2500 g or more are usually mature in physiological functions.
   b. If respiratory distress occurs, it is usually related to meconium aspiration syndrome.
6. *SGA or dysmature*—weight falls below normal range for age (<10th percentile).
   a. Preeclampsia.
   b. Malnutrition.
   c. Smoking.
   d. Placental insufficiency.
   e. Alcohol syndrome.
   f. Rubella.

g. Syphilis.

h. Multifetal gestation (twins, etc.).

i. Genetic.

j. Cocaine abuse.

7. *LGA*—above expected weight for age (>90th percentile). *Note:* If **preterm**, at risk for **RDS.** If **postterm**, at risk for **aspiration** and **sudden intrauterine death.**

    a. *Etiology:*

      (1) Maternal diabetes or prediabetes.

      (2) Maternal weight gain over 35 lb.

      (3) Maternal obesity.

      (4) Genetic.

    b. *Associated problems:*

      (1) Hypoglycemia.

      (2) Hypocalcemia.

      (3) Hyperbilirubinemia.

      (4) Birth injury (e.g., fractures, Erb-Duchenne paralysis).

B. *Estimation of gestational age*—planning appropriate care for the newborn requires accurate assessment to differentiate between preterm and term infants.

Preterm Infant

Born at 37 weeks of gestation or less.

A. Pathophysiology—anatomical and physiological immaturity of body systems compromises ability to adapt to extrauterine environment and independent life.

1. *Interference with* **protective** *functions*

    a. *Temperature regulation*—unstable, due to:

      (1) Lack of subcutaneous fat.

      (2) Large body surface area in proportion to body weight.

      (3) Small muscle mass.

      (4) Absent sweat or shiver responses.

      (5) Poor capillary response to changes in environmental temperature.

    b. *Resistance to infection*—low, due to:

      (1) Lack of immune bodies from mother (these cross placenta *late* in pregnancy).

      (2) Inability to produce own immune bodies (immature liver).

      (3) Poor WBC response to infection.

    c. *Immature liver*

      (1) Inability to conjugate bilirubin liberated by normal breakdown of RBCs → increased susceptibility to hyperbilirubinemia and kernicterus.

      (2) Immature production of clotting factors and immune globulins.

      (3) Inadequate glucose stores → increased susceptibility to hypoglycemia.

2. *Interference with* **elimination:** immature *renal* function—unable to concentrate urine → precarious fluid/electrolyte balance.

3. *Interference with* **sensory-perceptual functions:** CNS—immature → weak or absent reflexes and fluctuating primitive control of vital functions.

B. Etiology: often unknown; preterm labor.

1. *Iatrogenic*—EDB miscalculated for repeat cesarean birth (rare).

2. *Placental factors*

    a. Placenta previa.

    b. Abruptio placentae.

    c. Placental insufficiency.

3. *Uterine factors*

    a. Incompetent cervix.

    b. Overdistention (multifetal gestation, polyhydramnios).

    c. Anomalies (e.g., myomas).

4. *Fetal factors*

    a. Malformations.

    b. Infections (rubella, toxoplasmosis, HIV-positive status, AIDS, cytomegalic inclusion disease).

    c. Multifetal gestations (twins, triplets).

5. *Maternal factors*

    a. Severe physical or emotional trauma.

    b. Coexisting disorders (PIH, hypertension, heart disease, diabetes, malnutrition).

    c. Infections (streptococcus, syphilis, bacterial vaginosis, pyelonephritis, pneumonia, influenza, leukemia, UTI).

6. *Miscellaneous factors*

    a. Close frequency of pregnancies.

    b. Advanced maternal age.

    c. Heavy smoking.

    d. High-altitude environment.

    e. Cocaine use.

C. Factors influencing survival:

1. Gestational age.

2. Lung maturity.

3. Anomalies.

4. Size.

D. Causes of mortality (in order of frequency):

1. Abnormal pulmonary ventilation.

2. Infection.

    a. Pneumonia.

    b. Septicemia.

    c. Diarrhea.

    d. Meningitis.

3. Intracranial hemorrhage.

4. Congenital defects.

E. Disorders affecting fluid-gas transport: RDS

1. **Pathophysiology**—insufficient pulmonary surfactant (lecithin) and insufficient number/maturity of alveoli predispose to atelectasis; alveolar ducts and terminal bronchi become lined with fibrous, glossy membrane.

2. **Etiology:**

    a. Primarily associated with prematurity.

    b. Other *predisposing* factors:

      (1) Fetal hypoxia—due to decreased placental perfusion secondary to maternal bleeding (e.g., abruptio) or hypotension.

(2) Birth asphyxia.

(3) Postnatal hypothermia, metabolic acidosis, or hypotension.

3. Factors *protecting* neonate from RDS:

   a. Chronic fetal stress—due to maternal hypertension, PIH, or heroin addiction.

   b. PROM.

   c. Maternal steroid ingestion (e.g., betamethasone).

   d. Low-grade chorioamnionitis.

◆ 4. **Assessment:**

   a. Usually appears during first or second day after birth.

   b. Signs of *respiratory distress:*
   > (1) Nasal flaring.
   > (2) Sternal retractions.
   > (3) Tachypnea (60 beats/min or more).
   > (4) Cyanosis—central.
   > (5) Expiratory grunt.
   > (6) Increasing number and length of apneic episodes.
   > (7) Increasing exhaustion.

   c. *Respiratory acidosis*—due to hypercapnea and rising CO_2 level.

   d. *Metabolic acidosis*—due to increased lactic acid levels and falling pH.

◆ 5. **Analysis/nursing diagnosis:**

   a. *Impaired gas exchange* related to lack of pulmonary surfactant secondary to preterm birth, intrapartal stress and hypoxia, infection, postnatal hypothermia, metabolic acidosis, or hypotension.

   b. *Altered nutrition, less than body requirements,* related to poor feeding secondary to respiratory distress, ↑ caloric demand.

◆ 6. **Nursing care plan/implementation:**

   a. Goal: *reduce metabolic acidosis, increase oxygenation, support respiratory efforts.*

   (1) Ensure warmth (isolette at 97.6°F).

   ▶ (2) Warmed, humidified O_2 at lowest concentration required to relieve cyanosis, through hood, nasal prongs, or endotracheal tube.

   ▶ (3) Monitor *continuous positive airway pressure (CPAP)*—oxygen–air mixture administered under pressure during inhalation *and* exhalation to maintain alveolar patency.

   ◤ (4) *Position:* side-lying or supine with neck slightly extended ("sniffing" position); arms at sides.

   ▶ (5) Suction prn with bulb syringe—for excessive mucus.

   ▶ b. Goal: *modify care for infant with endotracheal tube.*
   > (1) Disconnect tubing at adapter.
   > (2) Inject 0.5 mL sterile normal saline.
   > (3) Insert sterile suction tube, start suction, rotate tube, withdraw.

   > (4) Suction up to 5 sec.
   > (5) Ventilate with bag and mask during procedure.
   > (6) Reconnect tubing securely to adapter.
   > (7) Auscultate for breath sounds and pulse.

   c. Goal: *maintain nutrition/hydration.*

   (1) Administer fluids, electrolytes, calories, vitamins, minerals PO or IV, as ordered.

   (2) I&O.

   d. Goal: *prevent secondary infections.*

   ▶ (1) Strict aseptic technique.

   (2) Handwashing.

   e. Goal: *emotional support of infant.*

   (1) Gentle touching.

   (2) Soft voices.

   (3) Eye contact.

   (4) Rocking.

   f. Goal: *emotional support of parents.*

   (1) Keep informed of status and progess.

   (2) Encourage contact with infant—to promote bonding, understanding of treatment.

   g. Goal: *minimize possibility of iatrogenic disorders associated with oxygen therapy* (see **F.** and **G.**).

◆ 7. **Evaluation/outcome criteria:**

   a. Respiratory distress treated successfully; infant breathes without assistance.

   b. Infant completes successful transition to extrauterine life.

F. Iatrogenic (oxygen toxicity) disorders: retinopathy of prematurity

1. **Pathophysiology**—intraretinal hemorrhage → fibrosis → retinal detachment → loss of vision.

2. **Etiology**—prolonged exposure to high concentrations of oxygen.

3. **Assessment**—only perceptible retinal change is vasoconstriction.

> *Note:* Arterial blood (PaO_2) gas readings less than 50 or more than 80 mm Hg.

◆ 4. **Nursing care plan/implementation:** Goal: *prevent disorder.* Maintain PaO_2 of 50-70 mm Hg.

◆ 5. **Evaluation/outcome criteria:**

   a. Successful recovery from respiratory distress.

   b. No evidence of retinopathy.

G. Iatrogenic (oxygen toxicity) disorders: bronchopulmonary dysplasia (BPD)

1. **Pathophysiology**—damage to alveolar cells result in focal emphysema.

2. **Etiology**—positive pressure ventilation (CPAP and PEEP) and prolonged administration of high concentrations of oxygen.

◆ 3. **Assessment**—monitor for signs of:

   a. Tachypnea.

   b. Increased respiratory effort.

   c. Respiratory distress.

◆ 4. **Nursing care plan/implementation:**
Goal: *prevent disorder*
a. Use of *positive* pressure devices.
▶ b. Maintain oxygen concentration *below 80%*.
c. Supportive care.
d. Wean off ventilator, as possible.

◆ 5. **Evaluation/outcome criteria:**
a. Successful recovery from respiratory distress.
b. No evidence of disorder.

H. **Intraventricular hemorrhage**
1. **Pathophysiology**—rupture of thin, fragile capillary walls within ventricles of the brain (more common in preterm).
2. **Etiology:**
a. Hypoxia.
b. Respiratory distress.
c. Birth trauma.
d. Birth asphyxia.
e. Hypercapnia.

◆ 3. **Assessment:**
a. Hypotonia.
b. Lethargy.
c. Hypothermia.
d. Bradycardia.
e. Bulging fontanels.
f. Respiratory distress or apnea.
g. Seizures.
h. Cry: high-pitched whining.

◆ 4. **Nursing care plan/implementation:** Goal: *supportive care*—to promote healing.
a. Monitor vital signs.
b. Maintain thermal stability.
▶ c. Ensure adequate oxygenation (may be placed on CPAP).

◆ 5. **Evaluation/outcome criteria:**
a. Condition stable, all assessment findings within normal limits.
b. No evidence of residual damage.

I. **Disorders affecting nutrition**
1. **Pathophysiology**—underdeveloped feeding abilities, small stomach capacity, immature enzyme system, fat intolerance.
2. **Etiology**—immature body systems associated with preterm birth.

◆ 3. **Assessment:**
a. Weak suck, swallow, gag reflexes—tendency to aspiration.
b. Signs of malabsorption and fat intolerance (abdominal distention, diarrhea, weight loss, or failure to gain weight).
c. Signs of vitamin E deficiency (edema, anemia).

◆ 4. **Analysis/nursing diagnosis:**
a. *Altered nutrition, less than body requirements,* related to poor feeding reflexes, reduced stomach capacity, inability to absorb needed nutrients.

b. *Impaired gas exchange* related to aspiration.

◆ 5. **Nursing care plan/implementation:** Goal: *maintain/increase nutrition.*
a. Frequent, small feedings—to *avoid* exceeding stomach capacity, facilitate digestion.
b. Frequent "burping" during feeding—to *avoid* regurgitation/aspiration.
c. Supplement vitamin E (alpha-tocopherol) intake, as ordered, in formula-fed infants (*Note:* intake adequate in breastfed babies.) *Vitamin E actions:*
(1) Antioxidant.
(2) Maintains structure and function of smooth, skeletal, and cardiac muscle.
(3) Maintains structure and function of vascular tissue, liver, and RBC integrity.
(4) Coenzyme in tissue respiration.
(5) Treatment for malnutrition with macrocytic anemia.
d. Encourage parent/family participation.

◆ 6. **Evaluation/outcome criteria:**
a. Feeds well without regurgitation/aspiration.
b. Maintains/gains weight.
c. No evidence of malabsorption, vitamin deficiency.

J. **Disorders affecting nutrition/elimination: necrotizing enterocolitis (NEC)**
1. **Pathophysiology**—intestinal thrombosis, infarction, autodigestion of mucosal lining, and necrotic lesions; incidence increased in preterm.
2. **Etiology**—intestinal ischemia, due to blood shunt to brain and heart in response to:
a. Fetal distress.
b. Fetal/neonatal asphyxia.
c. Neonatal shock.
d. After birth, may result from:
(1) Low cardiac output.
(2) Infusion of hyperosmolar solutions.
e. Complicated by action of enteric bacteria on damaged intestine.

◆ 3. **Assessment**—early identification is **vital.**
a. Abdominal distention or erythema, or both.
b. Poor feeding, vomiting.
c. Blood in stool.
d. Systemic signs associated with sepsis that may need temporary colostomy or iliostomy:
(1) Lethargy or irritability.
(2) Hypothermia.
(3) Labored respirations or apnea.
(4) Cardiovascular collapse.
e. Medical diagnosis:
(1) Increased gastric residual.

(2) X-ray shows ileus, air in bowel wall.
◆ 4. **Analysis/nursing diagnosis:**
   a. *Altered nutrition, less than body requirements,* related to inability to tolerate oral feedings and gastrointestinal dysfunction secondary to ischemia, thrombosis, or necrosis.
   b. *Constipation* related to paralytic ileus with stasis; diarrhea related to water loss.
   c. *High risk for injury* related to infection, thrombosis, metabolic alterations (acidosis, osmotic diuresis, dehydration, hyperglycemia) due to parenteral nutrition.
   d. *Altered parenting* related to physiological compromise and prolonged hospitalization.
   e. *Impaired skin integrity* when colostomy is necessary.
◆ 5. **Nursing care plan/implementation:**
   a. Goal: *supportive care.*
      (1) Rest GI tract: *no oral intake*—to achieve gastric decompression.
      (2) IV fluids, as ordered—to maintain hydration.
   b. Goal: *prevent infection.* Administer antibiotics, as ordered.
   c. Goal: *prevent trauma to skin surrounding stoma.*
◆ 6. **Evaluation/outcome criteria:**
   a. Tolerates oral feedings.
   b. Demonstrates weight gain.
   c. Normal stool pattern.
   d. Parents are accepting and knowledgeable about care of infant.

Postterm Infant

Over 42 weeks of gestation.
A. General aspects
   1. Labor may be hazardous for mother and fetus because:
      a. Large size of infant contributes to cephalopelvic disproportion; obtain estimate of fetal weight (EFW) by ultrasound.
      b. Placental insufficiency → fetal hypoxia; diagnosis by:
         (1) Contraction stress test.
         (2) Nonstress test.
         (3) Amniotic fluid index (AFI).
      c. Meconium passage (common physiological response) increases chance of meconium aspiration.
◆ **B. Assessment:**
   1. If postmature skin: dry, wrinkled—due to metabolism of fat and glycogen reserves to meet in utero energy needs.
   2. Long limbs, fingernails, and toenails—due to continued growth in utero.
   3. Lanugo and vernix—absent.

4. Expression: wide-eyed, alert—probably due to chronic hypoxia (oxygen hunger).
5. Placenta—signs of aging.
◆ **C. Analysis/nursing diagnosis:** *High risk for injury* related to high incidence of morbidity and mortality due to dystocia or hypoxia.
◆ **D. Nursing care plan/implementation:**
   1. **During labor:**
      a. Goal: *emotional support of mother*—may require cesarean birth due to CPD or fetal distress.
      ▶ b. Goal: *continuous electronic monitoring of FHR.* Report *late* decelerations immediately (indicate fetal distress).
   2. **After birth:**
      a. Goal: *if born vaginally, prompt identification of birth injuries, respiratory distress.* Continual observation.
      b. goal: *early identification/treatment of emerging signs of complications.*
         (1) *Hypoglycemia*—Dextrostix readings and behavior.
         (2) Administer oral or intravenous glucose, as ordered.
   E. **Evaluation/outcome criterion:** successful transition to extrauterine life (all assessment findings within normal limits).

Congenital Disorders

   I. **General overview:** Genetic abnormalities and environmental insults often lead to congenital disorders of the newborn. Successful transition to independent extrauterine life may pose a major challenge to infants compromised by anatomical or physiological disorders. Knowledge regarding the implications of the neonate's structural or metabolic problems enables the nurse to identify early signs of health problems and to plan, provide, and evaluate appropriate outcome-directed care to safeguard the status of the infant with a congenital disorder.

  II. **Disorders affecting fluid-gas transport:** *congenital heart disease*
      A. **Pathophysiology**—altered hemodynamics, due to persistent fetal circulation or structural abnormalities.
         1. *Acyanotic defects*—no mixing of blood in the systemic circulation.
            a. *Patent ductus arteriosus.*
            b. *Atrial septal defect.*
            c. *Ventriclar septal defect.*
            d. *Coarctation of the aorta.*
         2. *Cyanotic defects*—unoxygenated blood enters systemic circulation.
            a. *Tetralogy of Fallot.*
            b. *Transposition of the great vessels.*

B. Etiology—unknown. Associated with maternal:
1. Prenatal viral disease (e.g., rubella, coxsackie).
2. Malnutrition; alcoholism.
3. Diabetes (poorly controlled).
4. Ingestion of lithium salts.

◆ **C. Assessment:**
1. *Patent ductus arteriosus* (see Figure 5–3, p. 222).
   a. Characteristic machine murmur, mid to upper left sternal border (cardiomegaly); persists throughout systole and most of diastole; associated with a "thrill."
   b. Widened pulse pressure.
   c. Bounding pulse, tachycardia, "gallop" rhythm.
2. *Atrial septal defect* (see Figure 5–1, p. 222).
   a. Characteristic crescendo/decrescendo systolic ejection murmur.
   b. Fixed S_2 splitting.
   c. Dyspnea, fatigue on normal activity.
   d. Medical diagnosis—cardiac catheterization, x-ray.
3. *Ventricular septal defect* (see Figure 5–2, p. 222).
   a. Loud, harsh, pansystolic murmur; heard best at left lower sternal border; radiates throughout precordium. (*Note:* may be absent—due to high pulmonary vascular resistance → equalization of interventricular pressure).
   b. Medical diagnosis—cardiac catheterization, ECG, chest x-ray.
4. *Coarctation of the aorta* (see p. 224).
   a. Absent femoral pulse.
   b. Late systolic murmur.
   c. Decreased blood pressure in *lower* extremities.
   d. Medical diagnosis: x-ray.
5. *Tetralogy of Fallot* ("blue" baby) (see Figure 5–4, p. 223).
   a. Acute hypoxic/cyanotic episodes.
   b. Limp, sleepy, exhausted; hypotonic extended position—postepisode.
   c. Medical diagnosis—cardiac catheterization.
6. *Transposition of the great arteries* (see Figure 5–5, p. 224).
   a. Cyanotic after crying or feeding.
   b. Progressive tachypnea—attempt to compensate for decreased PaO_2, metabolic acidosis.
   c. Heart sounds vary, consistent with defect.
   d. Signs of CHF.
   e. Medical diagnosis—cardiac catheterization, x-ray, ECG.

◆ **D. Analysis/nursing diagnosis:**
1. *Fluid volume excess* related to persistent fetal circulation, structural abnormalities.
2. *Impaired gas exchange* related to abnormal circulation, secondary to pathology.
3. *Altered nutrition, less than body requirements,* related to exhaustion, dyspnea.

◆ **E. Nursing care plan/implementation:**
1. Goal: *minimize cardiac workload.*
   a. Minimize crying—snuggle; pacifier—to meet psychological needs.
   b. Keep clean and dry.
2. Goal: *maintain thermal stability*—to reduce body need for oxygen.
3. Goal: *prevent infection.*
   a. Strict aseptic technique; standard precautions.
   b. Hand washing.
4. Goal: *parental emotional support.*
   a. Encourage verbalization of anxiety, fears, concerns.
   b. Keep informed of status.
5. Goal: *health teaching*—explain, discuss:
   a. Diagnostic procedures.
   b. Treatment procedures.
   c. Basic care modalities.
6. Goal: *promote bonding.* Encourage to participate in infant care, as possible.
7. Medical/surgical management: surgical intervention/repair of congenital cardiac abnormality.

◆ **F. Evaluation/outcome criteria:**
1. Experiences no respiratory distress in immediate postnatal period.
2. Completes transfer to high-risk center without incident, if applicable.
3. Surgical intervention successful, where applicable.

III. Disorders affecting fluid-gas transport: *hemolytic disease of the newborn*
   A. Rh incompatibility
   1. **Pathophysiology**—see p. 101.
   2. **Etiology**—see Rh isoimmunization, p. 102.
   ◆ 3. **Assessment:**
      a. *Prenatal*—maternal Rh titers, amniocentesis.
      b. *Intrapartal*—amniotic fluid color:
         (1) Straw-colored: mild disease.
         (2) Golden: severe fetal disease.
      c. Direct *Coombs' blood*; positive test demonstrates Rh antibodies in fetal blood.
   ◆ 4. **Nursing care plan/implementation—exchange transfusion:**
      a. Goal: *health teaching.*
         (1) Explain purpose and process to parents.
         (2) Removes anti-Rh antibodies and fetal cells that are coated with antibodies.
         (3) Reduces bilirubin levels—indicated when 20 mg/dl in term neonate and 15 mg/dl in preterm.

(4) Corrects anemia—supplies RBCs that will not be destroyed by maternal antibodies.

(5) Rh-negative type O blood elicits no reaction; maximum exchange is 500 mL; duration of exchange: 45–60 min.

▶ b. Goal: *minimize transfusion hazards.*

(1) Warm blood to room temperature, since cold blood may precipitate cardiac arrest.

(2) Use only fresh blood—to reduce possibility of hypocalcemia, tetany, convulsions.

(3) Give calcium gluconate, as ordered, after each 100 mL of transfusion.

c. Goal: *prepare for transfusion procedure.* Ready necessary equipment—monitor, resuscitation equipment, radiant heater, light.

d. Goal: *assist with exchange transfusion.*

(1) Continuous monitoring of vital signs; record baseline, and every 15 min during procedure.

(2) Record: time, amount of blood withdrawn; time and amount injected; medications given.

(3) Observe for dyspnea, listlessness, bleeding from transfusion site, cyanosis, cardiovascular irregularity or arrest; coolness of lower extremities.

e. Goal: *posttransfusion care.*

◆ (1) **Assessment:**

(a) Observe for dyspnea, cyanosis, cardiac arrest or irregularities, jaundice, hypoglycemia; frequent vital signs.

(b) *Signs of sepsis*—fever, tachycardia, dyspnea, chills, tremors.

◆ (2) **Nursing care plan/implementation:**

(a) Maintain thermal stability—to reduce physiological stress, possibility of metabolic acidosis.

▶ (b) Give oxygen—to relieve cyanosis.

(c) Keep cord moist—to facilitate repeat transfusion, if necessary.

(d) Maintain nutrition/hydration—feed per schedule.

◆ 5. **Evaluation/outcome criteria:**

a. Infant's hemolytic process ceases; bilirubin level drops.

b. Infant makes successful transition to extrauterine life.

c. Infant experiences no complications of therapeutic regimen.

d. Infant shows evidence of bonding.

B. **ABO incompatibility**

1. **Pathophysiology**—fetal blood carrying antigens A/B enters maternal type O bloodstream

→ antibody formation → antibodies cross placenta → hemolyze fetal RBCs. *Note:* less severe than Rh reaction.

2. **Etiology:**

a. Type O mother carries anti-A and anti-B antibodies.

b. Even first pregnancy is jeopardized if fetal blood enters maternal system.

c. Reaction possible if fetus is type A, type B, or type AB and mother is type O.

◆ 3. **Assessment:**

a. Jaundice within first 24 hr.

b. Rising bilirubin levels.

c. Enlarged liver and spleen.

◆ 4. **Nursing care plan/implementation:** Goal: *reduce hazard to newborn.*

▶ a. Prepare for exchange transfusion with O negative blood.

▶ b. Phototherapy may be ordered if bilirubin is 10 mg/dl, and anemia is mild or absent.

c. Close monitoring of status.

d. Supportive care.

◆ 5. **Evaluation/outcome criteria:**

a. Infant responds to medical/nursing regimen.

b. Infant's assessment findings within normal limits.

C. **Hyperbilirubinemia**

1. **Pathophysiology**—bilirubin, a breakdawn product of hemolyzed RBCs, appears at increased levels; exceeds 13–15 mg/dl. Bilirubin is safe when bound with albumin and conjugated by user for body excretion; danger is when unconjugated and deposits in CNS.

a. **WARNING:** There is no "safe" serum-bilirubin level; kernicterus is a function of the bilirubin level *and* neonatal age and condition; poor fluid-and-caloric balance subjects the infant (especially the preterm infant) to kernicterus at low serum-bilirubin levels.

b. *Kernicterus*—high bilirubin levels result in deposition of yellow pigment in basal ganglia of brain → irreversible retardation.

2. **Etiology:**

a. Rh or ABO incompatibility, during first 48 hr.

b. Resolution of an enclosed hemorrhage (e.g., cephalhematoma).

c. Infection.

d. Drug induced—vitamin K injection, maternal ingestion of sulfisoxazole (Gantrisin).

e. Bile duct blockage.

f. Albumin-binding capacity is exceeded.

g. "Breastfeeding jaundice" (e.g., pregnandiol in milk). Breastfeeding is *not* dangerous and not a cause of physiologic jaundice.

Maternal-Infant

h. Dehydration.

i. Immature liver (interferes with conjugation).

◆ 3. **Assessment:**

a. Jaundice noted after blanching skin to suppress hemoglobin color; noted in sclera or mucosa in dark-skinned neonates; make sure light is adequate; spreads from head down, with increasing severity.

b. Pallor.

c. Concentrated, dark urine.

d. Blood level determination—hemoglobin or indirect bilirubin (unconjugated, unbound bilirubin deposits in CNS).

e. *Kernicterus*—similar to intracranial hemorrhage.

(1) Poor feeding or sucking.

(2) Regurgitation, vomiting.

(3) High-pitched cry.

(4) Temperature instability.

(5) Hypertonicity/hypotonicity.

(6) Progressive lethargy; diminished Moro reflex.

(7) Respiratory distress.

(8) Cerebral palsy, mental retardation.

(9) Death.

◆ 4. **Analysis/nursing diagnosis:**

a. *Fluid volume (RBC) deficit* related to hemolysis secondary to blood incompatibility.

b. *High risk for injury* (brain damage) related to kernicterus.

c. *Altered thought processes* (mental retardation) related to brain damage secondary to kernicterus.

d. *Knowledge deficit (parental)* related to infant condition.

◆ 5. **Nursing care plan/implementation:**

a. Medical management:

(1) *Prenatal*—amniocentesis.

(2) *Postnatal*—exchange transfusion, phototherapy.

▶ b. Goal: *assist bilirubin conjugation through phototherapy.*

(1) Cover closed eyelids while under light; remove eyepads when not under light (feeding, cuddling, during parental visits)—to protect eyes.

(2) Expose as much skin as possible—to maximize exposure of circulating blood to light. Remove for only brief periods.

(3) *Change position* qlh—to maximize exposure of circulating blood to light.

(4) *Note:* any loose green stools as bile is cleared through gut; watch for skin breakdown on buttocks.

(5) Monitor temperature—to identify hyperthermia.

(6) *Push fluids* (to 25% more than average) between feedings—to counteract dehydration. Breast milk has natural laxative effects that help clear bile.

c. Goal: *health teaching.* Explain, discuss phototherapy, bilirubin levels, implications.

d. Goal: *emotional support.*

(1) Encourage verbalization of anxiety, fears, concerns.

(2) Encourage contact with infant.

(3) Reassure, as possible.

◆ 6. **Evaluation/outcome criteria:**

a. Infant's hemolytic process ceases; bilirubin level drops.

b. Infant makes successful transition to extrauterine life.

c. Infant experiences no complications of therapeutic regimen.

d. Infant shows evidence of effective bonding.

Emotional Support of the High-Risk Infant

I. **General aspects**

A. The high-risk infant has the same *developmental needs* as the healthy term infant:

1. Social and tactile stimulation.

2. Comfort and removal of discomfort (hunger, soiling).

3. Continuous contact with a consistent, parenting person.

B. Treatment for serious physiological compromise may result in:

1. Isolation.

2. Sensory deprivation or noxious stimuli.

3. Emotional stress.

◆ II. **Assessment—signs of neonatal emotional stress:**

A. Does not look at person performing care.

B. Does not cry or protest.

C. Poor weight gain; failure to thrive.

◆ III. **Analysis/nursing diagnosis:** *sensory/perceptual alterations* related to isolation in isolette, oxygen hood.

◆ IV. **Nursing care plan/implementation:**

A. Goal: *provide consistent parenting contact.* Assign same nurses whenever possible.

B. Goal: *emotional support.*

1. Comfort when crying.

2. Provide positive sensory stimulation. Arrange time to:

a. Stroke skin.

b. Hold hand.

c. Hum, sing, talk.

d. Hold in en-face position (nurse looking into infant's eyes).

e. Hold when feeding, if possible.

C. Goal: *encourage parents to participate in care*—to:

1. Reduce their psychological stress, anxiety, fear.

2. Promote bonding.

3. Reduce possibility of later child abuse (higher incidence of child abuse against children who have been high-risk infants).

◆ **V. Evaluation/outcome criteria:**

A. Infant demonstrates successful resolution of physiological problems.

B. Parents and infant evidence bonding.

C. Parents express satisfaction with care and result.

General Aspects: Nursing Care of the High-Risk Infant and Family

I. **General overview:** The birth of a physiologically compromised neonate is psychologically stressful for both infant and family and physiologically stressful for the neonate. Effective, goal-directed nursing care is directed toward:

A. Minimizing physiological and psychological stress.

B. Facilitating/supporting successful coping or adaptation.

C. Encouraging parental attachment/separation/grieving, as appropriate.

◆ II. **Assessment**—directed toward determining neonate's present and projected status:

A. Determine neonate's current physical status.

B. Identify specific status and diagnosis-related problems and needs.

C. Describe family psychological status, strengths, and coping mechanisms/skills.

D. Determine medical/surgical/nursing approach to problems—and prognosis.

◆ III. **Analysis/nursing diagnosis:**

A. Parental *anxiety/fear* related to physiological compromise of neonate.

B. *Self-esteem disturbance* related to feelings of guilt or anger.

C. *Ineffective individual coping* related to severe psychological stress.

D. *Knowledge deficit* related to diagnosis, treatment, prognosis of infant.

E. *High risk for altered parenting* related to concern about infant.

◆ IV. **Nursing care plan/implementation:**

A. Goal: *preoperative and postoperative care.*

1. Maintain/improve physiological stability.

a. Temperature stabilization—keep warm.

b. Oxygenation:

(1) Position.

▶ (2) Administer oxygen, as ordered or necessary.

c. Nutrition/hydration:

▶ (1) Administer/monitor IV fluids.

(2) Oral fluids, as ordered.

(3) Feed, as status permits.

2. Assist with diagnostic testing.

B. Goal: *emotional support of parents.*

1. Encourage exploring and ventilating feelings.

2. Involve parents in decision-making process.

C. Goal: *health teaching.*

1. Determine knowledge/understanding of problem.

2. Explain/simplify/clarify, as needed, physician's discussions with parents.

3. Describe/explain/discuss neonate's present status and any auxiliary equipment; teach CPR to family.

4. Refer, as needed, to hospital/community resources.

D. Goal: *promote bonding.* Encourage parental participation in care of the neonate.

◆ **V. Evaluation/outcome criteria:**

A. Parents verbalize understanding of relevant information; make informed decisions regarding infant care.

B. Parents demonstrate comfort and increasing participation in care of neonate.

C. Infant maintains/increases adequacy of adaptation to extrauterine life.

D. If relevant, parents demonstrate progress in grieving process.

Questions

Select the one answer that is best for each question.

1. Which contraceptive method is most appropriate for a woman whose history reveals two episodes of thrombophlebitis with her previous pregnancy, repeated *Candida* infections, and gestational diabetes and who wants to postpone pregnancy for at least 1 year?

1. Oral contraceptive pill.

2. Tubal ligation.

3. Diaphragm.

4. Intrauterine device.

2. Which of the following identifies the basal body temperature (BBT) change characteristic of ovulation?

1. Falls slightly, then increases by about 0.5°C.

2. Rises slightly, then falls by about 0.5°C.

3. Is affected by a surge of FSH.

4. Is due to an estrogen surge.

3. When calculating the 1-minute Apgar, the nurse adds the following assessment findings: heart rate—over 100; respiratory effort—slow and irregular; muscle tone—flaccid response to slap on soles of feet; weak cry; color—body pink, extremities blue. In view of these assessment findings, which Apgar score should the nurse record?
   1. 5.
   2. 6.
   3. 7.
   4. 8.

4. A woman 36 weeks pregnant is admitted directly from clinic, with a blood pressure of 146/98, puffy face and hands, and "awful headaches and problems seeing." Admission note states: Admit stat for preeclampsia. Which nursing order should be questioned?
   1. Assess reflexes and amount and distribution of edema every shift.
   2. Up as desired.
   3. Admission and daily weight.
   4. Test urine for protein every 4 hours.

5. Objectives for the initial prenatal visit include determining a woman's present health status, validating pregnancy, and identifying factors that may affect or be affected by a pregnancy. Which assessment finding indicates a need for further evaluation?
   1. Urinary frequency, nausea, fatigue.
   2. Vital signs—T 98.2, P 92, R 20, BP 110/70.
   3. Urine—negative for sugar, trace of protein.
   4. Marked vaginal discharge with itching for the past few days.

6. Health teaching about over-the-counter pregnancy test kits should include which of the following information?
   1. False-negative tests may be due to dilute urine secondary to diuresis and inaccurate technique.
   2. Urine tests are classed as presumptive signs of pregnancy.
   3. Levels of progesterone from the corpus luteum are sufficient to diagnose pregnancy as early as the fourth week.
   4. Urine tests are classed as positive signs of pregnancy.

7. A woman appears excited, euphoric, and eager to learn about her labor status. Her behavior supports the nursing assessment that she is progressing through which phase of labor?
   1. Latent.
   2. Active.
   3. Transitional.
   4. Prodromal.

8. Thirty minutes after the birth of twins, a new mother's fundus is "boggy" and her lochial flow increased. After massage to firm the fundus, and while supporting the uterus with a hand above the symphysis, the nurse expresses several large clots. Which action should the nurse take next?
   1. Notify the physician because the site of her bleeding must be located.
   2. Notify the physician because she needs surgery.
   3. Administer oxytocin according to prn order.
   4. Reapply perineal pad and tell her to keep her thighs together.

9. While performing a newborn assessment, the nurse notes yellowish vernix. The nurse promptly calls this to the physician's attention because this may be a sign of:
   1. Rh or ABO incompatibility or maternal ingestion of sulfisoxazole (Gantrisin).
   2. An intrauterine gonorrheal infection.
   3. Maternal diabetes mellitus.
   4. Fetal postmaturity.

10. Which plan should the nurse recommend to a pregnant woman for morning nausea?
    1. Eat a high-protein snack at bedtime.
    2. Eat two dry crackers or toast before arising.
    3. Eat a high-protein breakfast.
    4. Drink a glass of orange juice immediately on awakening.

11. Which of the following best explains indigestion, heartburn, and constipation during pregnancy?
    1. Progesterone, produced by the placenta, causes reduced motility of smooth muscle, e.g., intestinal tract.
    2. Stress due to developmental tasks of pregnancy results in increased gastric acidity and reflux.
    3. Pressure from the growing uterus displaces the stomach and intestines.
    4. Increased pancreatic activity results in digestive-tract fat intolerance.

12. When preparing the room for a woman with preeclampsia which equipment items are most important to have ready?
    1. Suction and oxygen apparatus.
    2. Urinary retention catheter and drainage bag.
    3. Electronic blood pressure monitor.
    4. Padded tongue blade and airway.

13. A mother who just gave birth saturates her perineal pad in 15 minutes. Her fundus is firm and smooth, and there is a constant trickle of blood from the vagina. No clots can be expressed when the fundus is massaged. On the basis of these findings, what should the nurse suggest?
    1. Atonic bleeding.
    2. Traumatic bleeding.
    3. Retained placental fragments.
    4. Inverted uterus.

14. Which nursing action *increases* a woman's discomfort during a pelvic examination?
    1. Explaining why the examination is being done and what she may expect.
    2. Offering the nurse's hand for her to squeeze.
    3. Suggesting breathing techniques to help her relax.
    4. Asking her to empty her bladder before the examination.

15. Which finding is inconsistent with an 8-week gestation?
    1. Chadwick's sign.
    2. Hegar's sign.
    3. Goodell's sign.
    4. Ballottement.

16. Four hours after birth, a newborn begins to show signs of respiratory distress. This newborn's history includes 42 weeks of gestation and two episodes of late FHR decelerations during labor. Which of the following should the nurse suspect?
    1. Aspiration syndrome.
    2. RDS.
    3. Oxygen toxicity.
    4. Bronchopulmonary dysplasia.

17. Plans to minimize symptoms of physiologic adaptations to pregnancy include suggesting which of the following?
    1. High-carbohydrate diet and decreased fluid intake, to stimulate peristalsis.
    2. Pelvic rock-and-tilt exercises, to increase tone of her abdominal muscles.
    3. Symptomatic relief by over-the-counter antacids and mild laxatives.
    4. Increased fluid intake and small, frequent, high-bulk meals.

18. Which theory provides the basis for the nurse's explanation and teaching regarding gestational diabetes?
    1. There is an anti-insulin effect of human placental lactogen (HPL).
    2. There is a proinsulin effect of HPL.
    3. Increased maternal tissue sensitivity to insulin.
    4. Diabetes is unrelated to pregnancy; size and production of the islets of Langerhans are unaffected.

19. A new mother wants to breastfeed. She has had no previous experience or instruction. Which of the following should the nurse include in teaching her about good nipple care?

1. Washing nipples and breasts every day with soap and water to prevent infection.
2. Keeping nipples clean with warm water and then air-drying to reduce irritation.
3. Applying dilute alcohol solution to nipples after each feeding, to toughen them.
4. Covering the nipples with a plastic-lined breast shield to protect clothing.

20. A woman in labor is becoming more serious, evidences a malar flush, and tends to hyperventilate with contractions. These signs occur most commonly during which phase?
    1. Latent.
    2. Active.
    3. Transitional.
    4. Pushing.

21. A newborn who weighed 7 lb at birth now weighs 6 lb 8 oz. Implementing health teaching, the nurse tells the mother the percentage of birthweight usually lost by normal, healthy babies. Which of the following represents the maximum amount of normal weight loss for this newborn?
    1. 6 oz (170 g).
    2. 8 oz (227 g).
    3. 11 oz (317 g).
    4. 16 oz (454 g).

22. For which reason must a preeclamptic woman be carefully assessed for fluid intake and urine output?
    1. Oliguria is a grave sign.
    2. Daily intake should never exceed 2000 mL.
    3. Sudden diuresis can precipitate convulsion.
    4. If urine output is less than 100 mL/4 hr, repeat dose of magnesium sulfate is needed.

23. A new mother saturates her perineal pad in 15 minutes. Her fundus is firm and smooth, and there is a constant trickle of blood from the vagina. No clots can be expressed when the fundus is massaged. Which action should the nurse take immediately?
    1. Notify the physician because she needs surgery.
    2. Notify the physician because the site of her bleeding must be located.
    3. Administer oxytocin according to prn order.
    4. Reapply perineal pad and evaluate bleeding in 15 minutes.

24. If a pregnant woman's vaginal discharge is thick, white, cheeselike, and pruritic, the nurse's therapeutic and educational actions should be based on which of the following?
    1. No action needed. This is normal leukorrhea of pregnancy.
    2. Metronidazole (Flagyl) is the drug of choice to treat this condition.
    3. Even if untreated, this condition presents no hazard to the neonate.
    4. This condition is more likely to occur in women who are pregnant or taking oral contraceptives or antibiotics or who are diabetic.

25. If a pregnant woman's last normal menstrual period started August 5, her EDB is:
    1. May 12.
    2. May 30.
    3. June 8.
    4. June 12.

26. A pregnant woman complains, "I waddle like a duck, and after even a short walk, my back and legs ache. Why? What can I do about that?" Which of the following provides the basis for appropriate health teaching?
    1. Relaxation of pelvic joint articulations and strain on supporting muscles due to the growing uterus cause these symptoms.
    2. An increased metabolic rate in pregnancy results in excess production of lactic acid in back muscles.

3. Progesterone causes striated muscle stretching and pain on motion.
4. Decreased venous return from the legs and the pressure of the heavy uterus cause waddling and discomfort.

27. Which action should the nurse recommend to reduce normal discomforts of pregnancy such as duck-waddle walk and back and leg ache?
    1. Avoid walking whenever possible; get bed rest in side-lying Sims' position several times daily.
    2. Perform pelvic tilt-and-rock exercises; get rest whenever possible, legs elevated.
    3. Wear a maternity girdle to provide support.
    4. Increase calcium intake, perform stretching exercises, and rest frequently during the day.

28. A new mother is distressed because her baby looks a little yellow. She says, "The other nurse said she has 'physical' jaundice. What's that? Is it bad?" The nurse's explanation is based on knowledge of the normal physiological changes of the newborn. Which of the following is responsible for a newborn's physiologic jaundice?
    1. Liver immaturity and fetal polycythemia.
    2. Oliguria and kidney immaturity.
    3. Infection.
    4. Dehydration.

29. When discussing common complaints arising from normal maternal adaptations to pregnancy, which normal physiologic change has greater implications for the woman with a history of diabetes mellitus and requires more teaching about warning signs and symptoms needing prompt medical evaluation?
    1. Increased venous pressure in lower extremities.
    2. Placental production of HPL (human placental lactogen).
    3. Increased cardiac output.
    4. Relaxation of the cardiac sphincter.

30. Close observation and continuous nursing assessment of a woman with severe preeclampsia are necessary to facilitate prompt identification and management of which of the following?
    1. Abruptio placentae.
    2. Placenta previa.
    3. Hydramnios.
    4. Hyperemesis gravidarum.

31. A pregnant woman is admitted for evaluation of her cardiac status at 24 weeks of gestation. During the evening, she complains of dyspnea and shortness of breath while ambulating. She has a moist cough. Her physician orders complete bed rest. Which nursing intervention is most appropriate to prevent further deterioration of her cardiac condition?
    1. Place her in Trendelenburg position to encourage venous return to the heart.
    2. Assist her with activities of daily living to reduce energy expenditures.
    3. Encourage frequent coughing and deep breathing to prevent pulmonary complications of immobility.
    4. Initiate a regimen of lower-limb exercises to prevent venous stasis and leg thrombosis.

32. A new mother tells the nurse she is breastfeeding because she can't stand the thought of the baby being vaccinated. Which response demonstrates effective health teaching?
    1. "That's great. Vaccinations aren't needed if you breast-feed him."
    2. "Oh, you still need to have him vaccinated against DPT, measles, and polio before he is 6 months old."
    3. "You can only give temporary protection to the infant against the diseases you have had yourself."
    4. "The most protection comes from colostrum just after birth. Unfortunately, you didn't start feeding him right away."

33. A woman says, "My doctor says I'm 5 months (20 weeks) pregnant. What does my baby look like now?" The nurse's response is based on knowledge of normal fetal development. Which of the following describes the average fetus at 20 weeks of gestation?
    1. Viable, able to survive outside of the uterus with minimal assistance.
    2. About 10 inches long, weight about 10 oz, and covered with fine, downy hair and vernix.
    3. Beginning sex differentiation, kidney function, and detectable movements.
    4. Shedding lanugo and vernix, growing rapidly, weighs about 1½ pounds.

34. In discussing "dos and don'ts," which health teaching aspect should be emphasized as important for health maintenance during pregnancy?
    1. Keeping appointments for prenatal visits, remembering to ask questions when necessary, and following the medical/nursing recommendations.
    2. Making preparation for childbirth classes.
    3. Moderate exercise, high-carbohydrate diet, and adequate rest.
    4. Taking multivitamins and iron, drinking six glasses of milk daily, and minimizing physical exertion.

35. Which response is appropriate to give to a pregnant woman who is worried about having urinary frequency?
    1. "Placental progesterone causes irritability of the bladder sphincter. Your symptoms will go away after the baby comes."
    2. "Frequency is due to bladder irritation from concentrated urine and is normal in pregnancy. Increase your daily fluid intake to 3000 mL."
    3. "Pregnant women urinate frequently to get rid of fetal wastes. Limit fluids to 1000 mL daily."
    4. "Try using Kegel (perineal) exercises and limiting fluids before bedtime. If you have frequency associated with fever, pain on voiding, or blood in the urine, call your doctor/nurse-midwife."

36. As a woman progresses through labor, she becomes increasingly irritable with her partner, complaining of lower-back pain and fatigue. Which nursing intervention is most appropriate now?
    1. Have the woman turn on her side and give her a back rub.
    2. Ask her if she would like the nurse to get an order for something for her discomfort.
    3. Reassure the partner that irritability is normal, and teach the partner to apply sacral pressure with contractions.
    4. Send the partner for a coffee break, and encourage the woman to try to get some rest.

37. At 37 weeks, a pregnant woman calls the office to say she awakened in a pool of blood and is dizzy and nauseated. She denies any abdominal pain or cramping. On the basis of this assessment, the nurse suggests she go to the hospital immediately. The nurse established a nursing diagnosis of *high risk for fluid volume deficit* associated with which of the following?
    1. Placenta previa.
    2. Abruptio placentae.
    3. Preeclampsia.
    4. Uterine rupture.

38. An expectant father says, "My wife is a heavy smoker—three packs a day. She won't listen to me. Will you talk to her?" Which nursing approach is appropriate to this problem?
    1. Tell the woman that, if she continues to smoke that much, the baby will be small and have a greater chance of childhood respiratory infections.
    2. Teach the woman to substitute snacking on cheese, dried apricots, or raisins to curb her desire to smoke.
    3. Discuss current thoughts about the effects of smoking during pregnancy with the woman, and ask her if she can think of ways to cut down.
    4. Ask the woman how she plans to cut down to 10 cigarettes daily.

39. Which signs and symptoms require immediate medical evaluation during pregnancy?
    1. Excessive saliva, "bumps" around the areolae, and increased vaginal mucus.
    2. Fatigue, nausea, and urinary frequency at any time during pregnancy.
    3. Ankle edema, enlarging varicosities, and heartburn.
    4. Severe abdominal pain or fluid discharge from the vagina.

40. Which signs and symptoms during pregnancy should the nurse teach as possible warning signs of potential problems?
    1. Edema of the lower extremities, vulvar varices, and copious, clear vaginal discharge.
    2. Heartburn, shortness of breath, change in appetite.
    3. Leg cramps, back pain, and increased pigmentation over the bridge of the nose and the cheeks.
    4. Headache, visual disturbances, or feeling of fullness in face and hands.

41. The pregnant woman who would likely be given a "trial of labor" for vaginal birth after cesarean (VBAC) is one who had a first:
    1. Cesarean through a classic uterine incision because of severe fetal distress.
    2. Low transverse cesarean for breech presentation; this pregnancy is in vertex presentation.
    3. Cesarean for fetopelvic disproportion.
    4. Low transverse cesarean for active vaginal/perineal herpes infection; culture at 39 weeks this pregnancy was positive for herpes.

42. A woman with a history of diabetes may require hospitalization during her pregnancy for treatment of any problems associated with her pregnancy or for diagnostic tests. When asked to verbalize her understanding of the discussion, which of this woman's responses indicates a need for further health teaching?
    1. "Pregnancy may change the amount of insulin I need for regulation of my diabetes."
    2. "I may need to be hospitalized to evaluate how well my placenta is functioning."
    3. "If this awful morning sickness keeps up, the doctor may put me in to control it."
    4. "The doctor may need to take a sample of my water (amniocentesis) to see if the baby has the gene for diabetes."

43. Assessment findings at 16 weeks of gestation include marked chloasma and secondary pigmented areolae; in addition, the woman's umbilicus is flush with her skin. During which trimester are these physical changes of pregnancy commonly found?
    1. First.
    2. Second.
    3. Third.
    4. Fourth.

44. A new mother tells the nurse, "I am afraid the baby will have something wrong with her because I was bad while I was carrying her. Is she really okay?" If observed, which of the following would the nurse note as unusual in a newborn girl?
    1. Enlarged breasts and some pink drainage from the baby's vagina.
    2. A dark line between the baby's umbilicus and symphysis.
    3. Little "blackheads" covering her nose and chin.
    4. A dark discoloration over her sacrum and lower back.

45. An infertility assessment begins with a thorough health history. Which factor is likely to be implicated in female infertility?
    1. Moderate alcohol intake.
    2. Menstrual cycle of 26 to 28 days.
    3. History of PID.
    4. Past use of diaphragm and spermicide for contraception.

46. Which nursing intervention is most likely to be included in the plan of care for a woman with heart disease during the first postpartum day?
    1. Push oral and IV fluid to stimulate diuresis and prevent fluid volume overload.
    2. Encourage early ambulation and exercise to reduce the risk of thrombophlebitis.
    3. Monitor vital signs, skin color, and pulmonary status to identify cardiac decompensation.
    4. Encourage her to defer breastfeeding on the first day to reduce the cardiac workload.

47. The nursing assessment of a newborn reveals a lump on one side of the head that does not cross suture lines. Which of the following should the nurse tell the mother is the cause of the lump?
    1. Bleeding between the periosteum and parietal bone occurred due to pressure against the bony pelvis during birth.
    2. Edema of the scalp occurred due to pressure of the vertex against the cervix during the first stage of labor.
    3. Intracranial hemorrhage occurred due to pressure from the forceps during birth.
    4. Simple swelling of a common hemangioma occurred due to prolonged pushing in the second stage of labor.

48. Assessing for the normal psychological changes in the third trimester, the nurse would expect a pregnant woman to exhibit which normal behavior?
    1. Ambivalence about the pregnancy.
    2. Eagerness to begin Lamaze classes.
    3. Fantasizing about her child.
    4. Withdrawal from other relationships.

49. In reviewing with a pregnant woman those symptoms that require prompt medical evaluation, which of the following would the nurse include?
    1. Increasing pedal edema.
    2. Feelings of dizziness on arising.
    3. Epigastric pain.
    4. Spotting within 24 hours of vaginal examination.

50. A pregnant woman's history reveals a pregnancy at age 15 that was terminated by elective abortion at 10 weeks, birth of twin girls at 37 weeks, and a spontaneous abortion at 12 weeks last year. Analyzing these data, the nurse selects which of the following to describe her present gravidity and parity?
    1. Gravida 5 para 2.
    2. Gravida 5 para 1.
    3. Gravida 4 para 2.
    4. Gravida 4 para 1.

51. The postovulation rise in BBT is due to the high blood level of which hormone?
    1. Follicle-stimulating hormone (FSH).
    2. Human placental lactogen (HPL).
    3. Estrogen.
    4. Progesterone.

52. Nursing assessment of a woman in labor notes marked introspection, irritability, and inability to focus. She is diaphoretic, and cries, "I can't take it!" These behaviors are characteristic of which stage or phase of labor?
    1. Active phase.
    2. Transitional phase.
    3. Second stage.
    4. Third stage.

53. During the last month of pregnancy, a pregnant woman comments, "I am sick and tired of this whole thing. I can hardly wait for it to be over." Comparing her statement to the normal psychological responses of other pregnant women during the last trimester, the nurse responds appropriately with which statement?
    1. "I think you should see the psychiatric social worker. You should be feeling more positive about the baby by now."
    2. "I know exactly how you feel. I've seen it a thousand times. It'll pass."
    3. "Well, sounds like you're ready for labor. Do you have any questions about your coming labor?"
    4. "Your pregnancy is getting a bit tiresome and the time is dragging?"

54. A 16-year-old, single woman wants to give her baby up for adoption. Which plan will be of most help to her?
    1. Provide a safe environment, encourage ventilation of her feelings, give no answers or direction so that she makes her own decisions.
    2. Provide the information she needs to understand the situation, place it in perspective in terms of her life goals, and begin to plan for the future.
    3. Support her choice whatever her decision.
    4. Help her see ways of not making the same error again so she can grow in self-esteem and self-respect.

55. The physician determines that a woman's inability to conceive is due to anovulatory cycles and discusses treatment options. An expected emotional response to this diagnosis and possible treatment indicating that the woman understands the underlying problem would be:
    1. Guilt for past sexual behaviors.
    2. Grief because she will never be able to conceive.
    3. Fears regarding the need for corrective surgery.
    4. Anxiety regarding the side effects of clomiphen citrate (Clomid).

56. A couple has been unable to conceive; the man is being evaluated for possible problems. A semen analysis is ordered. Which instruction regarding collection of a sperm specimen is appropriate?
    1. Collect specimen at night, refrigerate, and bring to clinic the next morning.
    2. Collect specimen in the morning after 24 hours of abstinence and bring to clinic immediately.
    3. Collect specimen after 48 to 72 hours of abstinence and bring to clinic within 2 hours.
    4. Collect a specimen at the clinic, place in iced container, and give to laboratory personnel immediately.

57. In health teaching for women who desire "natural childbirth," which statement should the nurse explain is a myth?
    1. Medication may be used to reduce tension and pain during labor.
    2. Labor and birth under Lamaze techniques are almost painless.
    3. Labor is easier for women who are self-assured, relaxed, and cooperative during the process.
    4. Preparation for childbirth may include body-building exercises, breathing techniques, and comfort aids.

58. A pregnant woman is told to increase her intake of foods high in iron. Which of the following foods should the nurse suggest as being the best source of iron?
    1. Lean red meat.
    2. Nuts.
    3. Shellfish.
    4. Dairy products.

59. Health teaching during the prenatal period should emphasize that expectant primigravida mothers should go to the hospital when which pattern is evident?
    1. Contractions are 2–3 minutes apart, lasting 90 seconds, and membranes have ruptured.

2. Contractions are 3–5 minutes apart, accompanied by rectal pressure and bloody show.

3. Contractions are 5 minutes apart, lasting 60 seconds, and increasing in intensity.

4. Contractions are 5–10 minutes apart, lasting 30 seconds, and are felt as strong menstrual cramps.

60. Assessment findings of Leopold's maneuvers reveal a soft, rounded mass in the fundus, irregular nodules on the right side, and a hard prominence on the right, just above the symphysis. Which of the following accurately describes the fetal presentation and position?
    1. Right sacrum posterior (RSP).
    2. Left sacrum anterior (LSA).
    3. Right occiput posterior (ROP).
    4. Left occiput anterior (LOA).

61. If the fetus is LOA, in which maternal location should the nurse anticipate finding the fetal heart tones (FHTs)?
    1. Below the umbilicus on the left side.
    2. Below the umbilicus on the right side.
    3. Above the umbilicus on the left side.
    4. Above the umbilicus on the right side.

62. Which normal assessment finding can the nurse expect in the 34th week of pregnancy?
    1. Braxton-Hicks contractions, joint hypermobility, and backache.
    2. Dysuria, constipation, hemorrhoids, and lightening.
    3. Feeling of tranquility and heightened introspection.
    4. Morning sickness, breast tenderness.

63. Which suggestion by the nurse may relieve a pregnant woman's heartburn symptoms?
    1. Eat dry bread products before rising.
    2. Bend at the knees when reaching down, not at the waist.
    3. Eat fewer, larger meals and avoid nibbling.
    4. Do pelvic-rock exercise.

64. A new mother complains of severe lower abdominal cramping after breastfeeding. Which would be the first action taken by the nurse to reduce her discomfort?
    1. Administer pain medication as per order.
    2. Have her lie on her abdomen with a rolled towel at the level of her fundus.
    3. Ask her to walk around for a few minutes.
    4. Ask her to empty her bladder.

65. In assessing a new mother's response to her son's birth on the first postpartum day, which behavior should the nurse expect to find present?
    1. Talkativeness, dependency, passivity.
    2. Autonomy and independence.
    3. Disinterest in her own body functions.
    4. Interest in learning to bathe the baby.

66. Which technique should the nurse use to assess the frequency, duration, and intensity of uterine contractions?
    1. Spread fingers of one hand lightly over the fundus.
    2. Move the fingers of one hand over the uterus, pressing into the muscle.
    3. Hold fingers and palm of one hand over the area just below the umbilicus.
    4. Indent the uterus in several places, during and between contractions.

67. Ongoing evaluation of a woman with severe preeclampsia reveals 4 plus deep-tendon patellar reflexes with two beats of clonus. The most appropriate nursing diagnosis related to her current status would be:
    1. *Pain* related to hyperreflexia and clonus.
    2. *Risk for injury* related to possible eclamptic seizures.
    3. *Impaired physical mobility* related to alterations in lower limbs.
    4. *Sensory/perceptual alterations* related to sensory overload.

68. Following a birth, after the physician or midwife has cut the cord, and before the baby is given to the mother, which should the nurse do first?
    1. Confirm identification of the infant and apply bracelets to mother and infant.
    2. Examine the infant for any observable abnormalities.
    3. Wrap the infant in a prewarmed blanket and cover the head.
    4. Instill prophylactic medication in the infant's eyes.

69. Which of the following should elicit the Moro reflex in healthy newborns?
    1. Sudden or loud noises.
    2. Stroking the soles of the feet.
    3. Turning a newborn's head to one side.
    4. Stroking a newborn's cheek.

70. Which assessment of a woman in labor can be determined by vaginal examination?
    1. Fetal weight.
    2. Cervical dilation.
    3. Strength of contractions.
    4. Fetal head circumference.

71. The decision is made to encourage a woman in early labor to walk around the unit for a while, and to then reassess her status. Which assessment distinguishes between true and false labor?
    1. Confirmation of spontaneous rupture of membranes.
    2. Signs and symptoms of increasing discomfort.
    3. Evidence of cervical dilation.
    4. Presence of copious bloody vaginal discharge.

72. Which of the following should be emphasized as the most important factor in safeguarding cardiac function during pregnancy, for a woman with rheumatic heart disease (RHD)?
    1. Adequate exercise.
    2. Adequate rest.
    3. Low-salt diet.
    4. Ferrous sulfate.

73. Late in pregnancy, which of the following is the most likely cause of groin pain that seems worse on the right side?
    1. Bladder infection.
    2. Constipation.
    3. Tension on the round ligament.
    4. Beginning of labor.

74. A pregnant woman's history reveals one pregnancy, terminated by elective abortion at 10 weeks; birth of twins at 37 weeks; and a spontaneous abortion at 12 weeks. According to the TPAL system, which of the following describes her present parity?
    1. 0-2-2-2.
    2. 2-0-2-2.
    3. 0-1-2-2.
    4. 1-0-2-2.

75. Which of the following influences the planning and implementation of postpartum care for a woman who has been diagnosed as severely preeclamptic?
    1. Even if she has had no convulsions during the antepartal and intrapartal periods, she remains at risk for convulsions for the first 48 hours postpartum.
    2. Preeclampsia is associated only with pregnancy. Once the baby has been born, she is cured.
    3. The woman should be advised she may be left with chronic renal damage.
    4. Since subsequent pregnancy is extremely hazardous, family planning should be implemented as soon as possible.

76. For which complication of pregnancy is an Rh-negative woman at risk?
    1. Spontaneous abortion.
    2. Preeclampsia.

3. Maternal anemia.

4. Erythroblastosis fetalis.

77. Which assessment findings indicate 20 weeks of gestation?
    1. Lightening, FHR audible by fetoscope, fundus palpable at the umbilicus.
    2. Braxton-Hicks contractions, ballottement, and fundus at umbilicus.
    3. Quickening noted, FHR audible by fetoscope, fundus at or just below the umbilicus.
    4. Goodell's, Hegar's, and Chadwick's signs present, fundus halfway between symphysis and umbilicus.

78. A new mother tells the nurse she is planning to breastfeed her son until he is 2 years old so she won't have to worry about getting pregnant. Which response demonstrates appropriate health teaching?
    1. "Lactation does suppress ovulation, so you'll be pretty safe."
    2. "You are safe only as long as you don't menstruate."
    3. "It's best to use some other form of birth control. You may not menstruate, hut you may ovulate and could get pregnant."
    4. "You'll find you won't be interested in intercourse until you wean your baby."

79. Nursing assessments during the fourth stage of labor following placenta previa will include close monitoring for signs of hemorrhage. This nursing decision is based on which rationale?
    1. Placenta was implanted in lower uterine segment, where there are fewer muscle fibers to contract the placental site.
    2. The area under an abrupted placenta never contracts as strongly as when there is no premature separation.
    3. Since the placenta was surgically removed, the uterine muscle does not contract as efficiently.
    4. The woman lost 250 mL of blood during the third stage of labor.

80. A woman in labor using the Lamaze technique is examined and found to be in transition. Which breathing pattern used at this time would indicate a need for nursing intervention?
    1. Rapid, shallow chest breathing.
    2. Slow, deep, abdominal breathing.
    3. Use of intercostal muscles with diaphragm relaxed.
    4. Beginning and ending each contraction with two cleansing breaths.

81. Which of these normal physiological changes has greater implications for the woman with a history of rheumatic fever at age 8, and requires more teaching about warning signs and symptoms needing prompt medical evaluation?
    1. Increased venous pressure in lower extremities.
    2. Placental production of HPL.
    3. Increased cardiac output.
    4. Relaxation of the cardiac sphincter.

82. Following an amniotomy, the nurse remains alert for any signs of complications. In addition to the FHR, which of the following may indicate fetal distress?
    1. Crowning and increased fetal activity.
    2. Crowning and hypotonic contractions.
    3. Increased fetal activity and meconium-stained amniotic fluid.
    4. Baseline variability on the monitor strip.

83. A woman in labor insists on remaining in a supine position in bed. Which response should the nurse make regarding this behavior?
    1. "It's best for the baby if you lie on your side."
    2. "These two pillows under your knees will be good for the baby and more comfortable for you."
    3. "You will get nauseated and light-headed if you stay in that position."

4. "This rolled-up towel under your hip will do the job just as well."

84. Which of the following would the nurse note as a deviation from the normal characteristics of the term neonate?
    1. Head circumference larger than chest circumference.
    2. Diaphragmatic breathing.
    3. Passage of meconium stool.
    4. Epicanthal folds and simian line.

85. The reason the nurse keeps the neonate in a neutral thermal environment is that when a newborn becomes too cool, he or she requires:
    1. Less oxygen, and the newborn's metabolic rate increases.
    2. More oxygen, and the newborn's metabolic rate decreases.
    3. More oxygen, and the newborn's metabolic rate increases.
    4. Less oxygen, and the newborn's metabolic rate decreases.

86. A mother is in the third stage of labor. The nurse is observing for signs of separation of the placenta, which include which of the following?
    1. The uterus becomes globular.
    2. The fundus appears at the introitus.
    3. The umbilical cord is shortened.
    4. Mucoid discharge is increased.

87. Immediately after a woman's membranes have ruptured, the first priority of nursing care is to:
    1. Take the woman's temperature.
    2. Time the woman's contractions.
    3. Check the fetal heart rate.
    4. Check the woman's blood pressure.

88. A woman in the postpartum stage has a low rubella titer and receives a rubella virus vaccine. Because she is being immunized, which instruction is most important for the nurse to include in health teaching?
    1. "Have your titers checked in two weeks."
    2. "Do not eat products that contain eggs for the next twenty-four hours."
    3. "Do not become pregnant for three months."
    4. "Expect to have a slight rash in a day or two."

89. A nurse's aide reports to the RN that a multigravida who is 6 hours postpartum has not voided and has not ambulated yet. The patient says she has no desire to void and says that with her last infant she needed to be catheterized. The RN should instruct the nurse's aide to:
    1. Ask the woman if she is bleeding heavily.
    2. Find out how much fluid the woman has consumed in the last 6 hours.
    3. Not be concerned because this is normal for this patient.
    4. Assist the woman to the bathroom.

90. A woman had previously used a diaphragm for contraception before her pregnancy. Now at 6 weeks postpartum, she asks the nurse if she needs to have her diaphragm refitted. The best response is:
    1. "Yes, it should be refitted after a pregnancy."
    2. "No, it is not necessary. Once involution is completed, it should fit as it did before."
    3. "It isn't advisable to use a diaphragm after giving birth to a baby."
    4. "Yes, but you should wait until you are 3 months postpartum."

91. The nurse should teach the parents' group that *Chlamydia trachomatis* is not only an intracellular bacterium that causes neonatal conjunctivitis, but it also can cause:
    1. Discoloration of baby and adult teeth.
    2. Snuffles and rhagades in the newborn.
    3. Pneumonia in the newborn.
    4. Central hearing defects in infancy.

92. A 13-year-old girl just delivered an infant who needs emergency surgery. The consent form should be signed by:
    1. The mother of the baby.
    2. The grandmother of the baby.
    3. The RN.
    4. The MD.

93. The nurse manager on a maternity unit is informed that a woman who is 36 weeks pregnant with severe preeclampsia is to be admitted to the unit. Which bed assignment is the best choice?
    1. Bed in a double room 50 feet from the nurse's station with a roommate who has rheumatic heart disease.
    2. Bed in a double room next to the nurse's station with a roommate who is a drug addict with withdrawal symptoms.
    3. Bed in a four-bed unit with all other women who are postpartum.
    4. Bed in a four-bed unit with other women who have pyelonephritis, diabetes, and premature rupture of membranes.

94. The nurse analyzes the following data: A woman in labor has remained at 6 cm dilation, −1 station (vertex presentation), with molding of the baby's head at +2 station for 3 hours. The baby's FHR has increased from a baseline of 140 to 170. The physician orders Pitocin augmentation of labor. The nurse's correct action would be to:
    1. Add Pitocin to the IV and label it correctly.
    2. Start the Pitocin drip using an IV pump.
    3. Accurately chart the Pitocin infusion.
    4. Refuse to carry out the order for Pitocin augmentation.

95. When forceps are used for the birth of an infant's head, the newborn should be assessed for:
    1. Torticollis.
    2. Facial paralysis.
    3. Fractured clavicle.
    4. Cephalhematoma.

96. Less than 24 hours after being discharged, a new postpartum mother calls the nurse on the mother/baby unit. She reports that she has very heavy, bright-red bleeding. What would be the best advice to give her?
    1. "Don't worry about it; it is normal."
    2. "Lie down for about an hour. Check your bleeding then, and if it is still as heavy, call me back."
    3. "Lie down, massage your uterus (lower abdomen). If it does not firm up and your bleeding does not decrease, come to the hospital immediately."
    4. "Call your doctor and ask what to do."

97. Of the following findings in a full-term newborn, which is not an expected outcome of maternal hormone influence, and therefore should be reported?
    1. "Witch's milk."
    2. Slight vaginal bleeding.
    3. Undescended testicles.
    4. Linea nigra.

98. The plan of care developed by nurses for parents of a drug-dependent baby includes:
    1. Recommendations for minimal contact between parents and the infant.
    2. Ways to encourage parent-infant bonding and any positive parental responses to the baby.
    3. Discouraging attachment between the parents and baby.
    4. Acknowledgment that drug-dependent parents are less likely to be interested in their babies.

99. The nurse is to assign a nurse's aide on the postpartum unit to care for patients. The aide has a cold that day, but no other problems. Which patient would the nurse not want to assign to this nurse's aide?
    1. Woman in renal failure.
    2. Woman who has hypertension.

3. Woman who had a prolonged labor.
4. Woman who has AIDS.

100. When teaching a woman about fertility awareness, the nurse should emphasize that the basal body temperature:
    1. Is the average temperature taken each morning.
    2. Should be recorded each morning before any activity.
    3. Has a lower degree of accuracy in predicting ovulation than the cervical mucus test.
    4. Can be done with a mercury thermometer but not a digital one.

101. A teaching plan to use in presenting information to parents about fetal development should include the fact that the embryonic membrane closest to the uterine lining, and the first to form, is called the:
    1. Amnion.
    2. Amniotic sac.
    3. Chorion.
    4. Mesoderm.

102. The amniotic fluid cushions the embryo/fetus against mechanical injury, controls the embryo/fetus' temperature, and:
    1. Creates adherence of the amnion.
    2. Provides for fetal respiration and metabolism.
    3. Provides a means of nutrient exchange for the embryo/fetus.
    4. Allows freedom of movement so the embryo/fetus can change position.

103. During a prenatal exam a patient asks the nurse, "How does my baby breathe inside?" The nurse's best response is:
    1. "The lungs of the fetus carry out respiratory gas exchange in utero."
    2. "The placenta assumes the function of the fetal lungs by supplying oxygen and allowing the excretion of carbon dioxide into your bloodstream."
    3. "The blood from the placenta is carried through the umbilical artery, which penetrates the abdominal wall of the fetus."
    4. "The fetus is able to obtain sufficient oxygen due to the fact that your hemoglobin concentration is 50% greater during pregnancy."

104. The hematocrit decreases an average of 7–10% during pregnancy. This is referred to as physiologic anemia of pregnancy. Which mechanism best explains this decrease?
    1. The total erythrocyte count increases about 30%; the plasma volume increases about 50%.
    2. The total erythrocyte count increases about 50%; the plasma volume decreases 30%.
    3. The total erythrocyte count decreases 30%; the plasma volume increases about 50%.
    4. The erythrocyte count remains the same; the plasma volume increases 50%.

105. Assessment data indicate an abnormality at 20 weeks of gestation when:
    1. The fundal height measurement is at 4 fingers below the umbilicus.
    2. Fetal movements are felt faintly on the right side of the abdomen.
    3. The woman complains of backache and fatigue.
    4. The fetal heart rate is 140 and sometimes is difficult to count.

106. During the postpartum period, the nurse should advise the breastfeeding adult woman to:
    1. Increase her calories by about 600 kcal/day over her pregnancy requirements.
    2. Return to prepregnancy requirements for protein.
    3. Increase her calories by about 500 kcal/day over her prepregnancy requirements.
    4. Decrease the amount of calcium that was consumed during pregnancy.

107. When responding to a question from a new mother about producing enough milk for the baby as the baby grows and needs more milk at each feeding, the nurse should explain that:
    1. The mother's milk supply will increase as the infant demands more at each feeding.
    2. The breast milk will gradually become richer to supply additional calories.
    3. Early addition of solid baby foods will ensure an infant's nutritional needs.
    4. As the infant requires more milk, feedings should be supplemented with cow's milk.
108. Which woman would be at highest risk for preterm labor?
    1. The pregnant woman who is working full-time at a sedentary job.
    2. The woman who is pregnant with twins.
    3. The woman who has gained 35 lb by 36 weeks of gestation.
    4. The woman who is pregnant with her first baby.
109. A woman gave birth to her second daughter. She tells the nurse, "I'm concerned my two-year-old daughter will not accept the new baby." The nurse should suggest that:
    1. The older daughter not have much interaction with the baby at the hospital, because she may harm her new sibling.
    2. The older daughter stay with her grandmother for a few days until the parents and new baby are settled at home.
    3. The older daughter be given more responsibility and assure her "that she is a big girl now, and doesn't need Mommy as much."
    4. The woman spend time alone with her older daughter when the baby is sleeping.

Answers/Rationale

1. **(3)** Of the family planning options presented, a diaphragm and jelly is the optimum choice for this woman. **Answer 1** is incorrect because oral contraceptives are contraindicated with a history of thrombophlebitis. **Answer 2** is incorrect because she is interested only in postponing pregnancy. **Answer 4** is incorrect because use of intrauterine devices is contraindicated for women with impaired responses to infection, such as diabetics.
    Test-taking tip—Select the option that is not a risk factor/contraindication with this woman's history.
    IMP, 5, HPM, Growth and Development
2. **(1)** Basal body temperature falls slightly immediately before ovulation, then rises approximately 0.5°C. This characteristic finding aids women in identifying the fertile period of their cycle. **Answer 2** is incorrect because the pattern described is reversed. **Answers 3** and **4** are wrong because ovulation is related to an LH surge.
    Test-taking tip—Remember the characteristic pattern: ↓T,↑T.
    AS, 5, HPM, Growth and Development

Key to codes following rationales   *Nursing process:* **AS,** assessment; **AN,** analysis; **PL,** plan; **IMP,** implementation; **EV,** evaluation. *Category of human function:* **1,** protective; **2,** sensory-perceptual; **3,** comfort, rest, activity, and mobility; **4,** nutrition; **5,** growth and development; **6,** fluid-gas transport; **7,** psychosocial-cultural; **8,** elimination. **Client need: SECE,** safe, effective care environment; **PhI,** physiological integrity; **PsI,** psychosocial integrity; **HPM,** health promotion/maintenance. See appendices for full explanation.

3. **(1)** Heart rate—2; respiratory effort—1; muscle tone—0; reflex response—1; color—1. Total Apgar score is 5. **Answers 2, 3,** and **4** are incorrect because of inaccurate allocation of points for behaviors described.
    💡 **Test-taking tip**—Use the acronym APGAR to help remember the five areas for assessment: A—Appearance, P—Pulse, G—Grimace, A—Activity, R—Respiratory effort.
    AS, 5, PhI, Physiological Adaptation
4. **(2)** If avoidable, women hospitalized for treatment of preeclampsia should be on bed rest in a quiet environment to minimize stimuli. **Answer 1** is incorrect because the nurse *should* assess the amount and distribution of edema. **Answer 3** is wrong because weight *is* an indicator of edema and diuresis and should be assessed in the preeclamptic woman. **Answer 4** is wrong because I & O relationships and the presence and amount of protein in the urine *are* important indicators of her status.
    Test-taking tip—This question asks for the *wrong* answer; three of the options *are* appropriate orders. Select the one that is not.
    IMP, 6, HPM, Prevention and Early Detection
5. **(4)** Marked vaginal discharge with itching for the past few days indicates a need for further assessment. Itching is most commonly associated with vaginal infections, and the cause should be identified and treated. Altered vaginal pH in pregnancy contributes to increased susceptibility to infection. **Answer 1** is incorrect because urinary frequency, nausea, and fatigue *are* common complaints in early pregnancy. **Answer 2** is wrong because vital signs *are* within normal limits. **Answer 3** is wrong because normally increased vaginal discharge in pregnancy may contaminate voided urine and result in a nonpathological trace of protein.
    Test-taking tip—Reword the question when the stem asks for "a need for further evaluation." The best answer will have an *incorrect* statement.
    AS, 1, HPM, Prevention and Early Detection
6. **(1)** The most common cause of false-negative findings in urine testing for signs of pregnancy (presence of HCG) is faulty technique; further, dilute urine secondary to diuresis may contain too little hormone to register in the routine over-the-counter (or office) pregnancy tests. *Note:* HCG levels peak approximately 50–60 days after conception. **Answer 2** is incorrect because urine tests are classed as "probable" signs of pregnancy. **Answer 3** is incorrect because pregnancy tests identify presence/levels of HCG (the biological marker for pregnancy). **Answer 4** is wrong because urine tests are classed as "probable" signs of pregnancy.
    Test-taking tip—Eliminate the two options that state that urine tests are presumptive and positive signs of pregnancy. Eliminate the incorrect marker of pregnancy (3).
    IMP, 5, HPM, Growth and Development
7. **(1)** These behaviors are typical of a woman during the latent phase of labor. **Answer 2** is incorrect because, as labor progresses, internal stimuli demand more focus. **Answer 3** is wrong because women in transitional phase are irritable and increasingly aware of their labor as contractions increase in strength, length, and discomfort. **Answer 4** is wrong because, in the prodromal period of labor, contractions are mild and irregular and her major question may be *"Am I really in labor?"*
    💡 **Test-taking tip**—A memory device to match expected behavior with correct phase of labor: latent = lively (i.e., excited, eager to learn).
    AN, 5, HPM, Growth and Development
8. **(3)** The most common cause of bleeding immediately postpartum is uterine *atony,* and bleeding may be controlled with fundal massage and oxytocin stimulation. **Answer 1** is incorrect because the patient has responded to the nursing measures. **Answer 2** is wrong because her bleeding does not

appear to be associated with lacerations that might require surgery. **Answer 4** is wrong because perineal pressure is effective only in treating *superficial tears*.

> **Test-taking tip**—Key word is "next" action. Eliminate the two options about notifying the MD when the problem is under control. Choose the only option that has a prn medication.

IMP, 6, PhI, Reduction of Risk Potential

9. **(1)** Yellow vernix results from the breakdown of hemoglobin or bile pigments in meconium. Both maternal anti-Rh-antigen antibodies and ingestion of sulfisoxazole (Gantrisin) are implicated in hemolysis of fetal RBCs. **Answer 2** is incorrect because gonorrheal infection is opaque, thick, and odorous *without* discoloring vernix. **Answer 3** is wrong because diabetes does *not* have any effect on the color of vernix. **Answer 4** is wrong because the postmature fetus does *not* have vernix.

> **Test-taking tip**—Eliminate the three options that have no effect on the vernix.

AN, 6, PhI, Physiological Adaptation

10. **(2)** Carbohydrates taken before arising seem to reduce symptoms of morning nausea; dry crackers may absorb stomach acid and raise blood sugar. **Answer 1** is incorrect because high-protein snacks at bedtime appear to have *no* effect on nausea in the morning. **Answer 3** is wrong because nausea is present before eating and may be severe enough to prevent eating. **Answer 4** is wrong because orange juice on an empty stomach may precipitate emesis in a woman with "morning sickness."

> **Test-taking tip**—Key point is *time*-frame: *before* getting out of bed. Choose dry over acidic fluid.

IMP, 4, PhI, Basic Care and Comfort

11. **(1)** The effects of progesterone on the GI tract include relaxation of the cardiac sphincter and delayed gastric emptying, which contribute to indigestion and heartburn, and slowed intestinal peristalsis, which increases water reabsorption and predisposes to constipation. **Answer 2** is incorrect because the major cause of symptoms is described in **Answer 1**. **Answer 3** is wrong because displacement due to pressure from the uterus is *secondary* to the effects of reduced smooth muscle tone. **Answer 4** is wrong because increased pancreatic activity does *not* cause fat intolerance.

> **Test-taking tip**—Select the option that explains hormonal influences.

AN, 4, HPM, Growth and Development

12. **(1)** is correct because the nurse's primary responsibility is to prepare for respiratory and cardiac support in case the woman experiences an eclamptic seizure. **Answer 2** is incorrect because not all preeclamptic women require bladder catheterization. **Answer 3** is incorrect because the nurse may monitor blood pressures using the standard sphygmomanometer and arm cuff. **Answer 4** is incorrect because tongue blades are never used to manage seizures today.

> **Test-taking tip**—Think airway first!

IMP, 2, PhI, Reduction of Risk Potential

13. **(2)** Traumatic bleeding (e.g., birth canal or cervical lacerations) is characterized by a firm, smooth uterus and a continuous trickle. **Answer 1** is incorrect because the uterus remains well contracted. **Answer 3** is wrong because bleeding from retained placental fragments occurs most commonly *later* in the postpartum period. **Answer 4** is wrong because an inverted uterus is characterized by profuse vaginal bleeding and maternal collapse.

> **Test-taking tip**—Narrow your choice by noting similarity in the use of the word "blood" in the stem and two of the options with "bleeding." Eliminate **(1)** because the fundus is *not* boggy, but firm.

AN, 6, PhI, Physiological Adaptation

14. **(2)** Offering your hand to squeeze encourages her to tense her muscles, including the pubococcygeus muscle of the pelvic floor increasing the discomfort of a pelvic examination. **Answer 1** is incorrect because explaining what she may expect and the reasons for examination procedures *is* an appropriate nursing action designed to *reduce* her anxiety and tension. **Answer 3** is wrong because suggesting and demonstrating breathing techniques *is* an appropriate nursing action designed to assist her to *relax* during the procedures. **Answer 4** is wrong because asking her to empty her bladder *is* appropriate anticipatory guidance designed to *reduce* the stress of the pelvic examination.

> **Test-taking tip**—Visualize what happens to the pelvic area when squeezing a hand; this may help you choose the best answer (i.e., what is helpful).

IMP, 3, PhI, Basic Care and Comfort

15. **(4)** The finding of ballottement is more consistent with a pregnancy of *19 or more weeks*. **Answer 1** is incorrect because Chadwick's sign (bluish discoloration of the vagina) *is* usually present at 8 weeks of gestation. **Answer 2** is wrong because Hegar's sign (softening of the lower uterine segment) *is* present by 8 weeks. **Answer 3** is wrong because Goodell's sign (softening of the cervix) *is* usually present at this point in gestation.

> **Test-taking tip**—Key words are "inconsistent" and "8 weeks of gestation." Three of the signs *are* present around 8 weeks; one is much later.

AS, 5, HPM, Growth and Development

16. **(1)** Aspiration syndrome occurs commonly among post-term newborns, especially if they are postmature. Hypoxia accompanies progressive placental insufficiency (evidenced by late FHR decelerations) with advancing gestational age. Physiological response to hypoxia is relaxation of the anal sphincter, with release of meconium into amniotic fluid, and the fetal gasp reflex. **Answer 2** is incorrect because RDS is associated most commonly with prematurity and insufficient pulmonary surfactant. **Answer 3** is wrong because oxygen toxicity occurs *after* a period of oxygen therapy. **Answer 4** is wrong because bronchopulmonary dysplasia (BPD) is associated with prolonged administration of oxygen at high concentrations; the time since birth is *too short* for the baby to develop BPD.

> **Test-taking tip**—The key element is a *time* factor: 42 weeks = *post*maturity.

AN, 6, PhI, Physiological Adaptation

17. **(4)** Increasing fluid and roughage intake will reduce symptoms of constipation. **Answer 1** is incorrect because a high-carbohydrate diet and reduced fluid intake may make constipation worse. **Answer 2** is wrong because exercise does not counteract the effects of progesterone. **Answer 3** is wrong because many over-the-counter antacids contain sodium and frequent use of laxatives may result in further loss of tone, leading to constipation.

> **Test-taking tip**—Because constipation is a common discomfort of pregnancy, focus on **(1)** and **(4)**, which relate to diet. Next, eliminate **(1)** because of decreased fluid.

IMP, 4, PhI, Basic Care and Comfort

18. **(1)** The anti-insulin effects of the placental hormone HPL (a growth hormone) and *reduced* maternal tissue sensitivity to insulin often may result in development of gestational diabetes in women who previously had no symptoms of diabetes. **Answer 2** is wrong because the effect of HPL is antagonistic to insulin, *not* proinsulin. **Answer 3** is wrong because there is *decreased* maternal tissue sensitivity to insulin. **Answer 4** is wrong because the size and production of the islets of Langerhans *increase* during pregnancy.

💡 **Test-taking tip**—Understand the mechanisms and risks for glucose intolerance/insulin resistance in pregnancy. To help remember the insulin requirements in pregnancy, use the following memory aid: trimester one:↓; trimester two: ↑; trimester three: ↑;postpartum:↓;

AN, 4, PhI, Physiological Adaptation

19. (2) Nipples cleansed with plain water and air-dried carefully are less likely to develop fissures. **Answer 1** is incorrect because soap is drying and removes natural oils. **Answer 3** is incorrect because alcohol would be too drying and promotes fissure development. **Answer 4** is wrong because a plastic shield would retain body heat and moisture, irritating nipples.

Test-taking tip—Three options have incorrect information. Eliminate the two options that may be too drying (soap, alcohol). Go for "water and air."

IMP, 5, PhI, Basic Care and Comfort

20. (2) These behaviors are characteristic of the active phase of the first stage of labor, at about 5 cm dilation. **Answer 1** is wrong because women are more excited and relaxed during the latent phase when labor is less uncomfortable. **Answer 3** is wrong because behaviors during transition reveal the woman's focus on completing the process rapidly; irritability is common. **Answer 4** is wrong because the woman uses sustained inhalations to increase the force of her pushing.

Test-taking tip—Recall stages and phases of labor and expected patient behaviors: *latent*—more relaxed, less uncomfortable; *active*—hyperventilation, flushed; *transitional*—irritable.

AN, 5, HPM, Growth and Development

21. (3) Term infants may lose 5-10% of their birth weight. Arithmetic: 7 × 16 oz = 112 oz; 10% of 112 = 11.2 oz (317.5 g). **Answers 1, 2,** and **4** are wrong because of inaccurate computation.

Test-taking tip—Accurate multiplication (16 oz = 1 pound) is the key. Remember that 5-10% loss is OK.

AN, 5, HPM, Growth and Development

22. (1) Oliguria is an ominous sign in preeclampsia. **Answer 2** is incorrect because daily intake is individualized for the preeclamptic woman. **Answer 3** is wrong because sudden diuresis is a *good* prognostic sign. **Answer 4** is wrong because urinary output *must equal or exceed* 120 mL/4 hr before magnesium sulfate, if needed, can be given again.

Test-taking tip—Scanty urine is a *critical* finding; lots of urine (diuresis) is a *good* sign (3).

AN, 8, PhI, Physiological Adaptation

23. (2) The laceration must be located and treated before bleeding will stop. **Answer 1** is incorrect because, if the laceration is accessible, bleeding may be controlled by insertion of vaginal packing. **Answer 3** is wrong because bleeding is not related to uterine atony. **Answer 4** is wrong because perineal pressure would be ineffective with a vaginal laceration.

Test-taking tip—Choose the answer that would be the *first* action; think assessment (by the MD) as the priority (i.e., "must be located").

IMP, 6, PhI, Reduction of Risk Potential

24. (4) Her discharge is characteristic of a monilial (yeast) infection. This infection is more common in women whose vaginal pH has changed because of pregnancy or diabetes or who are taking oral contraceptives. Antibiotic therapy is also associated with increased risk for developing an infection by *Candida albicans*. **Answer 1** is incorrect because normal leukorrhea associated with pregnancy is *thin, colorless,* and *nonpruritic*. **Answer 2** is wrong because *mycostatin (Nystatin)* is the drug of choice for treating vaginal yeast infections; metronidazole (Flagyl) is used in treating *trichomonal* infections. **Answer 3** is wrong because, if present during the baby's birth, this organism *causes neonatal thrush*.

Test-taking tip—Because these are the signs and symptoms of monilial infection, you can eliminate the first three options; this is *not* normal (1). The drug in **Answer 2** is incorrect, and there *is* a hazard to the neonate (3).

AN, 1, PhI, Reduction of Risk Potential

25. (1) Using Nägele's rule to calculate the EDB, the correct date is arrived at by taking the date of the first day of the last menstrual period (LMP) and subtracting 3 months and adding 7 days. **Answer 2** is wrong because 7 days have been *subtracted* from her LMP. **Answer 3** is wrong because calculations have erroneously included August as one of 3 months, and only 3 days have been added to the date of LMP. **Answer 4** is wrong because, although calculations added 7 days, August was again erroneously included as one of the 3 months subtracted.

💡 **Test-taking tip**—Use the memory aid for Nägele's formula: EDB = LMP – 3 months + 7 days.

AS, 5, HPM, Growth and Development

26. (1) Shifting the center of gravity to compensate for the weight of the growing uterus places strain on supporting musculature and contributes to low-back ache during pregnancy; relaxation of joint articulations is responsible for the waddling gait. **Answer 2** is wrong because *vigorous* exercise contributes to the production of lactic acid; the increased metabolic rate during pregnancy has no effect. **Answer 3** is wrong because progesterone affects *smooth* muscle. **Answer 4** is wrong because decreased venous return and pressure from the growing uterus contribute to development of varicosities.

Test-taking tip—Only (1) and (4) address *both* the "waddle" and back leg discomfort. Eliminate (4) because the explanation is for *varicosities*.

AN, 3, HPM, Growth and Development

27. (2) Exercises like the pelvic tilt slide and rock strengthen the abdominal and back muscles, which support the mother in an erect position—and the growing uterus; rest while elevating the legs reduces stress on these muscles and the legs and decreases symptoms. **Answer 1** is incorrect because walking *is* an excellent mild exercise recommended for the pregnant woman. **Answer 3** is wrong because a girdle may *contribute* to decreased venous return from the extremities. **Answer 4** is wrong because symptoms are due to strain on supporting muscles and are *unrelated* to the level of circulating calcium.

Test-taking tip—Choose the option that results in muscle strengthening.

IMP, 3, PhI, Basic Care and Comfort

28. (1) *Physiologic* jaundice is related to inability of the liver to conjugate bilirubin liberated by normal hemolysis of fetal RBCs and polycythemia. **Answer 2** is incorrect because jaundice associated with kidney immaturity is *pathological*. **Answer 3** is wrong because jaundice occurring secondary to infection is also *pathological*. **Answer 4** is wrong because, although dehydration may be associated with the jaundice, it also is *pathological*.

Test-taking tip—Identify physiologic vs. pathologic jaundice. *Pathological* is *not* normal. Note the words in the stem: "normal" physiological. Liver *immaturity* is *not* pathological, but oliguria, infection, and dehydration are.

AN, 6, PhI, Physiological Adaptation

29. (2) Human placental lactogen (HPL) is an insulin antagonist and may complicate management of diabetes during pregnancy. **Answer 1** is incorrect because fatigue and varicosities are common complaints associated with decreased venous return from the lower extremities. **Answer 3** is wrong because increased cardiac output places additional work on the heart. **Answer 4** is wrong because relaxation of the cardiac sphincter is associated with heartburn and gastric reflux.

Test-taking tip—By understanding the functions of HPL, you can see the connection with diabetes. **Answers 3 and 4** deal with cardiac problems, not diabetes.

AN, 4, HPM, Growth and Development

30. **(1)** Abruptio placentae may be a complication of severe preeclampsia and places both mother and fetus in jeopardy. **Answer 2** is incorrect because placenta previa is due to low implantation, not pathophysiological changes in preeclampsia. **Answer 3** is wrong because hydramnios is most commonly associated with maternal *diabetes*, and although it may coexist with preeclampsia, it is not a contributing factor. **Answer 4** is wrong because hyperemesis gravidarum occurs *earlier* in pregnancy and is *not* associated with development or progression of preeclampsia.

Test-taking tip—By recalling the definition of the four terms, identify the condition for which severe preeclampsia is a risk factor.

AS, 6, PhI, Reduction of Risk Potential

31. **(2)** Activities of daily living increase energy expenditures and may contribute to further cardiac decompensation. **Answer 1** is incorrect because dyspnea and shortness of breath will *be exacerbated* in Trendelenburg position. **Answer 3** is incorrect because any activity that causes her to perform a Valsalva maneuver (coughing) will cause a sudden increase in blood return to the heart, which is contraindicated in cardiac disease. **Answer 4** is incorrect because the major goal of care is to reduce all energy expenditures.

Test-taking tip—Look at the verbs: "place," "assist," "encourage," "initiate." Choose "assist" for preventing further cardiac decompensation.

IMP, 6, PhI, Reduction of Risk Potential

32. **(3)** Only disease-specific antibodies produced by the mother in response to that infection can be produced through breast milk to the baby. **Answer 1** is incorrect because vaccinations *would* be needed to develop active immunity. **Answer 2** is wrong because measles vaccination is not effective if given before *1 year* of age. **Answer 4** is wrong because maternal antibodies confer only short-lived passive immunity.

Test-taking tip—Understand the effects of antibodies on the infant who is breastfeeding. When a question asks for effective health teaching, three of the answers will not be accurate information. Choose the one that is.

IMP, 5, HPM, Prevention and Early Detection of Diseases

33. **(2)** These are the characteristics of the fetus at 20 weeks of gestation (22 menstrual weeks). **Answer 1** is incorrect because, although 20 weeks has been identified as viability, most such fetuses are too immature to survive independent extrauterine existence successfully. **Answer 3** is wrong because sex differentiation begins *at conception* and is discernible at 12 weeks, and kidneys begin secreting urine at 11 weeks. **Answer 4** is wrong because the fetus begins to exhibit these characteristics at 31 weeks.

Test-taking tip—Remember: 10 inches, 10 oz at 20 weeks. Review fetal development by trimester of pregnancy.

AS, 5, HPM, Growth and Development

34. **(1)** The most important factor in reducing morbidity and mortality associated with pregnancy is close health supervision and prompt management of emerging problems and complications. **Answer 2** is incorrect because the primary goal of prenatal classes is to prepare the couple for *labor and birth*. **Answer 3** is wrong because *high-protein* diets are recommended during pregnancy to reduce the possibility of preeclampsia. **Answer 4** is wrong because the pregnant woman should drink 1 quart of milk and increase her intake during lactation.

Test-taking tip—The best option relates to goals during pregnancy, not specifically for labor and delivery, as in **(2)**, for reduction of morbidity and mortality. When an answer has multiple points, be sure to read each of these carefully because *not all* points in the option are correct, such as **(3)** and **(4)**, making the option only partially accurate.

IMP, 5, HPM, Prevention and Early Detection

35. **(4)** Progesterone also reduces smooth muscle motility in the urinary tract and predisposes the pregnant woman to urinary tract infections. Women should contact their doctors if they exhibit signs of infection. Kegel exercises will help strengthen the perineal muscles; limiting fluids at bedtime reduces the possibility of being awakened by the necessity of voiding. **Answer 1** is incorrect because progesterone does *not* cause irritability of the bladder sphincter. **Answer 2** is wrong because frequency in early and late pregnancy is due to *pressure on the bladder from the growing uterus.* **Answer 3** is wrong because hydration is important in maintaining normal digestion and nutrient transport to body cells, removing wastes, and regulating body temperature. During pregnancy, eight 8 oz glasses of fluid daily are recommended.

Test-taking tip—When the question asks for an appropriate response, eliminate the theoretically incorrect responses first. Understand the effects of progesterone on smooth muscle (specifically the bladder).

IMP, 8, HPM, Prevention and Early Detection of Disease

36. **(3)** Reassurance that her behavior is normal for this point in labor helps reduce the partner's feelings of guilt and helplessness and fosters the sense of a mutual, shared experience; sacral pressure reduces her discomfort. **Answer 1** is wrong because it does not address the partner's feelings. **Answer 2** is wrong because it does not facilitate the shared experience and may result in feelings of failure in some women. **Answer 4** is wrong because she is progressing well and needs/wants her partner's support.

Test-taking tip—Note the pattern in the answers: three options do not involve the partner; one option does. In this case, choose the option that is different.

IMP, 5, PsI, Coping and Adaptation

37. **(1)** *Painless* vaginal bleeding is associated with placenta previa. **Answer 2** is wrong because abdominal *pain* and a tense abdomen are signs of possible *abruptio placentae.* **Answer 3** is wrong because painless vaginal bleeding is *not* indicative of preeclampsia. **Answer 4** is wrong because the uterine rupture is characterized by *sudden* sharp abdominal pain, signs of internal bleeding, and shock.

Test-taking tip—The key point is *painless*. Recall the differences between signs and symptoms of placenta previa and abruptio placentae. **Answers 2 and 4** involve pain and can be eliminated, and for one condition **(3)** pain is not relevant.

AN, 6, PhI, Physiological Adaptation

38. **(3)** Encouraging her to consider ways to reduce her smoking implies your respect for her ability to deal with the problem and encourages her active participation in her own pregnancy-related care. **Answer 1** is incorrect because such comments generate *guilt* and may threaten her self-image. **Answer 2** is wrong because telling her to substitute even "good foods" implies *lack of respect* for her judgment and assumes that she will comply with your choices for her behavior. **Answer 4** is wrong because it implies she has no choice in the matter; patient goals are best established mutually.

Test-taking tip—"Discuss" is better than "tell" or "teach" in this case.

IMP, 6, HPM, Prevention and Early Detection of Disease

39. **(4)** Severe abdominal pain may indicate complications of pregnancy such as abortion, ectopic pregnancy, or abruptio placentae; fluid discharge from the vagina may indicate pre-

mature rupture of the membranes. **Answer 1** is incorrect because ptyalism, elevated Montgomery tubercles, and leukorrhea *are normal* physiological responses during pregnancy. **Answer 2** is wrong because fatigue, nausea, and frequency *are normal* in early pregnancy. **Answer 3** is wrong because ankle edema, varicosities, and heartburn *are* normal during pregnancy.

> **Test-taking tip**—Select "severe pain" as the most critical finding. Know the signs of the most serious complications during pregnancy.

AS, 6, PhI, Reduction of Risk Potential

40. **(4)** Headache and feeling of fullness in face and hands may indicate preeclampsia. **Answer 1** is wrong because pedal edema, varicosities, and vaginal discharge are related to decreased venous return and increased vascularity in pregnancy. **Answer 2** is wrong because heartburn, shortness of breath, and change in appetite are *normal* responses in pregnancy. **Answer 3** is wrong because leg cramps, low-back ache, and chloasma are associated with *normal* physiological changes of pregnancy.

> **Test-taking tip**—Distinguish between common normal discomforts of pregnancy and more serious complications. Prioritize critical findings.

IMP, 2, PhI, Reduction of Risk Potential

41. **(2)** The reason for the first cesarean was a breech presentation, and that is not present in this pregnancy. Also, a low transverse uterine incision presents only a very slight risk for uterine rupture with subsequent VBAC deliveries. **Answer 1** is incorrect because the classic vertical incision through the uterus (and subsequent scar) is considered to weaken the uterus and compromise its ability to withstand stretching and contracting. **Answer 3** is incorrect because the original cause (fetopelvic disproportion) remains. **Answer 4** is incorrect because an infant may acquire herpes during passage through an infected birth canal.

> **Test-taking tip**—Visualize the common uterine incision used and why it would pose the greatest risk for uterine rupture. Eliminate **Answer 3** because the same condition exists *again* and eliminate **Answer 4** because there is maternal infection *now*. Review the risks of cesarean birth, and specifically the risks of a vaginal birth after a previous cesarean.

AN, 1, PhI, Reduction of Risk Potential

42. **(4)** Amniocentesis does not show whether the fetus is a potential diabetic, but it may be performed on diabetic women to test for *fetal lung maturity*. **Answer 1** is wrong because her statement indicates understanding of the interrelationship between her pregnancy and her diabetes. **Answer 2** is wrong because pregnant diabetics *may* be hospitalized for testing for placental function. **Answer 3** is wrong because nausea and vomiting in the pregnant diabetic *may* lead to acidosis.

> **Test-taking tip**—When a question asks for "need for further health teaching," the *best* answer will have an *incorrect* statement. Review the goals of care for a pregnant diabetic.

EV, 4, PhI, Reduction of Risk Potential

43. **(2)** Chloasma, secondary pigmented areolae, and umbilicus flush with the skin are characteristic changes in the second trimester. **Answer 1** is wrong because these signs are *not* present during the normal first trimester. **Answer 3** is wrong because, although present during the third trimester, these changes *begin* during the second. **Answer 4** is wrong because these signs *diminish* during the fourth trimester.

> **Test-taking tip**—Think *skin* (chloasma, pigmented areola) = *second*. Note the word "secondary" in the stem is similar to "second" in **(2)**.

AN, 5, HPM, Growth and Development

44. **(3)** is unusual because milia (unopened sebaceous glands) look like *white*heads. **Answer 1** *is typical* because enlarged breasts and pink spotting (pseudomenstruation) are effects of high circulating levels of maternal hormones. **Answer 2** is typical because the linea nigra is *evident* due to maternal hormones. **Answer 4** is *typical* because "mongolian spots" *are found* on the lower back and sacrum of darker-skinned people.

> **Test-taking tip**—Look for what is *not typical* after recalling normal assessment findings for a full-term neonate girl.

AS, 5, HPM, Growth and Development

45. **(3)** PID is associated with adhesions and blockage of the fallopian tubes, preventing transport and joining of the ovum and sperm. **Answer 1** is incorrect because moderate alcohol intake is *not* implicated in female infertility. **Answer 2** is incorrect because a normal menstrual cycle is *not* associated with infertility. **Answer 4** is incorrect because use of a diaphragm and spermicidal jelly is *not* implicated in infertility.

> **Test-taking tip**—Look for the risk factor that is a *common* cause of female infertility.

AN, 5, HPM, Prevention and Early Detection

46. **(3)** is correct because major cardiovascular changes that occur with the termination of pregnancy can result in sudden cardiac decompensation in the *first postpartum day*. **Answer 1** is incorrect because pushing fluids *can* result in fluid volume overload and cardiac decompensation. **Answer 2** is incorrect because the postpartum woman with heart disease is encouraged to *rest* on the first day to minimize cardiac stressors while major cardiovascular changes occur. **Answer 4** is incorrect because breastfeeding is *not* contraindicated.

> **Test-taking tip**—The emphasis is on a *time factor: first* postpartum day and the risks caused by heart disease during pregnancy and lactation.

IMP, 6, PhI, Reduction of Risk Potential

47. **(1)** Cephalohematoma is caused by subperiosteal bleeding, and the "lump" is limited by the suture lines. **Answer 2** is incorrect because edema of the scalp is *caput succedaneum*. **Answer 3** is wrong because a cephalohematoma is *outside the skull*. **Answer 4** is wrong because hemangiomas are *benign blood vessel tumors.*

> **Test-taking tip**—In this question, choose the answer that gives information but does not diagnose, for example, **Answers 3** and **4**. Recall *where* the problem is (i.e., outside of the skull and whether it crosses the suture line) to help focus on the difference between cephalohematoma and caput succedaneum.

IMP, 5, HPM, Growth and Development

48. **(2)** During the third trimester, the mother becomes ready to begin learning techniques for her use during labor. **Answer 1** is wrong because ambivalence about the pregnancy is usually seen in *early* pregnancy. **Answer 3** is wrong because fantasizing is most typical during the *second* trimester. **Answer 4** is wrong because the period of introspection and introversion occurs in the *second* trimester.

> **Test-taking tip**—*Time*-frame is the clue: *third* trimester. Three of the options occur earlier. Choose "eagerness" over "fantasizing." Note that the other two options, "ambivalence" **(1)** and "withdrawal" **(4)** are problematic. "Eagerness" comes through in the end (third trimester).

AS, 5, PsI, Coping and Adaptation

49. **(3)** Epigastric pain is associated with edema of the liver capsule in preeclampsia. **Answer 1** is incorrect because dependent edema is common in late pregnancy, due to reduced venous return from the lower extremities. **Answer 2** is wrong because orthostatic hypotension may be a common occurrence during the third trimester. **Answer 4** is wrong because brown spotting is a *normal* finding within 24 hours of vaginal examination, due to the increased friability of the cervix during pregnancy.

Test-taking tip—Think "most critical findings." "Prompt" = urgent. Pain is critical and urgent because of the signs/symptoms of preeclampsia.

AS, 2, PhI, Reduction of Risk Potential

50. **(4)** *Gravidity* is defined as the number of pregnancies; she has been pregnant three previous times and is now pregnant for the fourth time. *Parity* is defined as the number of *pregnancies* carried to viability (20 weeks since conception; 22 menstrual weeks). The woman has had two pregnancies terminated before viability (abortions) and has carried *one* pregnancy, which resulted in viable twin girls. **Answer 1** is incorrect because this counts the twins as two pregnancies carried to viability. **Answer 2** is wrong because, although it correctly identifies the twins as one parity, it counts them as two pregnancies. **Answer 3** is wrong because, although it correctly identifies the woman as gravida 4, it counts the twins twice.

Test-taking tip—Know definitions of *gravida* and *para* and how to determine a woman's obstetric history. Use the acronym GTPAL: G—Gravida; T—Term; P—Para; A—Abortions; L—Living children.

AN, 5, HPM, Growth and Development

51. **(4)** High circulating levels of progesterone released by the corpus luteum are thought to be responsible for the immediate postovulation rise in body temperature. **Answer 1** is wrong because FSH is responsible for *maturation* of the follicle before ovulation. **Answer 2** is wrong because HPL is produced by the placenta and is *not present* at this time. **Answer 3** is wrong because estrogen is *not* implicated in the rise in body temperature postovulation.

Test-taking tip—Think *P's*: postpovulation = progesterone. Recall female hormones and their functions related to the menstrual cycle.

AN, 5, HPM, Growth and Development

52. **(2)** These behaviors are characteristic of the transitional phase of labor, approaching 10 cm dilation. **Answer 1** is incorrect because the woman shows a more intense, *serious* demeanor and may *hyperventilate with contractions* in the active phase. **Answer 3** is incorrect because the *second* stage of labor is characterized by *expulsive* efforts. **Answer 4** is incorrect because in the third stage the placenta is expelled and the woman is *euphoric* and focuses on the infant.

Test-taking tip—The *three I's* (introspection, irritability, inability to...) are indicative of transition. Recall the phases and stages of labor and expected patient responses.

AN, 5, PsI, Coping and Adaptation

53. **(4)** She does need support for her feelings at this point in pregnancy and validation that they are *normal*. **Answer 1** is incorrect because she is evidencing only *normal* responses to late pregnancy. **Answer 2** is wrong because such statements tend to inhibit further exploration of her feelings and convey that such feelings are unimportant to the nurse. **Answer 3** is wrong because it neither validates the normalcy of her feelings nor encourages further ventilation.

Test-taking tip—Choose the most open-ended communication approach. The goal is to be supportive of *expected* psychological changes in the third trimester.

IMP, 7, PsI, Coping and Adaptation

54. **(2)** is correct because the nurse can best fulfill the role of advocate by providing all essential information the adolescent needs to make informed decisions; this allows opportunity for introspection and growth. **Answer 1** is incorrect because adolescents require and desire *some guidance* or assistance with major life decisions from supportive adults. **Answer 3** is incorrect because it may not be appropriate or ethical to support some decisions the adolescent makes. **Answer 4** is incorrect because such actions are judgmental, tend to destroy rapport, and nullify possible growth.

Test-taking tip—Select the answer that describes the advocacy role of the nurse in patient decision making (i.e., providing information for informed decision making by the patient).

PL, 7, PsI, Coping and Adaptation

55. **(4)** is correct because clomiphen citrate (Clomid) is used in infertility caused by anovulatory cycles. It increases the secretion of FSH and LH and stimulates ovulation. Side effects include vasomotor flushes, bloating, nausea, vomiting, headache, hair loss, and visual disturbances. **Answer 1** is incorrect because anovulatory cycles are *not* caused by past patterns of sexual behavior. **Answer 2** is incorrect because many women who experience anovulatory cycles *may* successfully conceive after treatment. **Answer 3** is incorrect because anovulatory cycles are *not* treated with surgical intervention.

Test-taking tip—The key word is *treatment* option. Narrow your focus to **(3)** or **(4)** because they are possible treatments for female infertility. Eliminate **(3)** because it is not a treatment for anovulatory cycles.

AS, 7, PsI, Coping and Adaptation

56. **(3)** is correct because semen analysis requires that a freshly masturbated specimen be obtained after a rest (abstinence) period of 48 to 72 hours. **Answer 1** is incorrect because an accurate sperm count and evaluation of motility require that the specimen be examined *within 2 hours*. Refrigeration will kill sperm. **Answer 2** is incorrect because 24 hours of abstinence is *insufficient* for adequate production of sperm. **Answer 4** is incorrect because ice will reduce motility and kill sperm.

Test-taking tip—Think: best is more rest (abstinence). Note the answer is *time* related: *when* in relation to abstinence, and *how*—that is, avoid ice, refrigeration as in **Answers 1** and **4**.

IMP, 1, HPM, Growth and Development

57. **(2)** Lamaze techniques, although helpful, do *not* guarantee freedom from discomfort throughout the labor process. **Answer 1** is incorrect because medication *may* be used to assist the woman in controlling her response to the childbearing process and to facilitate a successful experience. **Answer 3** is wrong because labor *is* easier for the woman who understands what is happening and is able to relax and cooperate. **Answer 4** is wrong because many preparation-for-childbirth courses *use* these aids.

Test-taking tip—When the question asks which one is a *myth*, choose the *incorrect* answer.

IMP, 5, PhI, Basic Care and Comfort

58. **(1)** Red meats, egg yolks, and organ meats are the best sources of iron. **Answers 2, 3,** and **4** are incorrect because they do not contain as much iron as red meat.

Test-taking tip—Knowing the best (highest) food sources of iron will help you choose the best answer.

IMP, 4, PhI, Basic Care and Comfort

59. **(3)** Although instructions vary among birth centers, primigravidas should seek care when regular contractions are felt about 5 minutes apart, becoming longer and stronger. **Answer 1** is incorrect because she should have sought care earlier. **Answer 2** is incorrect because she should have sought care earlier. Rectal pressure may be a sign of impending birth. **Answer 4** is incorrect because this pattern may reflect "false labor" or very early latent phase labor.

Test-taking tip—Think *time* factor: when, how long, "too late" vs. "too soon." Be aware of how to distinguish between **false** and **true** labor.

IMP, 5, HPM, Growth and Development

60. **(4)** Of the choices given, if the breech is in the fundus, the occiput must be the presenting part; if the irregular nodules (elbows, knees, feet) are on the right side, the fetal back is to the maternal left. **Answer 1** is incorrect because the "S"

refers to the fetal sacrum and describes a breech presentation. **Answer 2** is wrong because this also describes a breech presentation. **Answer 3** is wrong because the fetal back is on the maternal left side, as is the occiput.

> **Test-taking tip**—Visualize the fetal position described to help you choose the answer with the head (occiput) presenting.

AN, 5, HPM, Growth and Development

61. **(1)** FHR is heard best through the fetal back, which, in LOA presentations, is below the umbilicus on the maternal left side. **Answer 2** is incorrect because the fetal back is on the maternal left. **Answer 3** is wrong because, in a vertex presentation, the heart tones are more audible below the umbilicus. **Answer 4** is wrong because it describes the placement of FHTs in breech presentations.

> **Test-taking tip**—Visualize LOA fetal position and presentation. Think *left* side (1 and 3) for *left* occiput anterior (LOA).

AS, 5, HPM, Growth and Development

62. **(1)** Braxton-Hicks contractions, hypermobility of joints, and backache are all normal findings at this point in pregnancy. **Answer 2** is incorrect because complaints of dysuria should be explored due to the tendency to urinary tract infection in pregnancy. **Answer 3** is wrong because a feeling of tranquility and heightened introspection are common in the *second* trimester. **Answer 4** is wrong because these symptoms are most common in the *first* trimester.

> **Test-taking tip**—The clues in the stem are *normal* and *third* trimester. Match *time*-frame (later in pregnancy) with findings (contractions occur later in pregnancy).

AS, 3, HPM, Growth and Development

63. **(2)** Bending at the waist facilitates movement of food out of the stomach through a relaxed cardiac sphincter. **Answer 1** is incorrect because this is the treatment for *morning sickness.* **Answer 3** is wrong because this tends to *aggravate* heartburn. **Answer 4** is wrong because the pelvic rock relieves *backache, not* heartburn.

> **Test-taking tip**—Eliminate the two options about food and eating. Picture bending from the knees and the effect on cardiac sphincter/diagnosis.

IMP, 4, PhI, Basic Care and Comfort

64. **(4)** A full bladder may be the major source of her discomfort. **Answer 1** is incorrect because medication should be given for minor discomforts *only after* trying other comfort measures. **Answer 2** is wrong because this measure would be used *only after* she has voided. **Answer 3** is wrong because walking does *not* relieve afterpains.

> **Test-taking tip**—First eliminate the two options about position/activity because they are *secondary* measures. The question asks for the FIRST action. Because the discomfort is felt in the abdomen, choose the option with *bladder,* which is felt abdominally.

IMP, 3, PhI, Basic Care and Comfort

65. **(1)** Talkativeness, dependency, and passivity are all signs of the "taking-in" phase of the postpartum. **Answer 2** is incorrect because the mother needs to have her needs for nurturing and positive reinforcement met at this time. **Answer 3** is wrong because she is *most interested* in her own body functions, her return to normal, and her ability to void and defecate. **Answer 4** is wrong because she is *not* ready to "take hold."

> **Test-taking tip**—Taking-in phase **(1)** is before taking-hold phase **(4)**. **Answers 2 and 3** are theoretically incorrect (according to Reva Rubin's theories) because the opposite of these behaviors occur. Also note two options that are contradictory: *dependency* **(1)** vs. *independence* **(2)**. "Dependency" goes with taking-in.

AS, 7, PsI, Coping and Adaptation

66. **(1)** The frequency, duration, and intensity of uterine contractions are assessed by light palpation of the contractile part, i.e., the fundus. **Answer 2** is incorrect because moving the hand over the uterus may reduce the accuracy of perceiving contractions; pressure into the muscle may contribute to uterine dysfunction due to manipulation. **Answer 3** is wrong because the most contractile part of the uterus is the fundus, *not* the corpus. **Answer 4** is wrong because uterine manipulation between contractions may contribute to uterine dysfunction.

> **Test-taking tip**—Picture the actions (the position of the hands). Eliminate **Answers 2 and 4** because they may be harmful.

IMP, 5, HPM, Prevention and Early Detection

67. **(2)** is correct because deep-tendon reflexes indicate the degree of CNS irritability and the potential for seizure activity. **Answer 1** is incorrect because hyperreflexia and clonus are *not* associated with pain or discomfort. **Answer 3** is incorrect because hyperreflexia and clonus do *not* interfere with motor activity in the lower extremities. **Answer 4** is incorrect because women with preeclampsia are placed in environments with *reduced* stimuli to decrease the risk of seizure activity.

> **Test-taking tip**—Note the term *preeclampsia* in the stem and same term "eclamptic" in the correct option (2).

AN, 1, PhI, Physiological Adaptation

68. **(3)** The first priority (beside maintaining a newborn's patent airway) is body temperature. **Answer 1** is incorrect because, although important, identification of the newborn may be delayed until *after* the infant's status is stable. **Answer 2** is wrong because the *second* priority is to note any abnormalities. **Answer 4** is wrong because eye prophylaxis may be instilled 2 hours *later.*

> **Test-taking tip**—This question asks you to rank order of priority when all options are correct. Review protocols for newborn care immediately after birth.

IMP, 3, HPM, Prevention and Early Detection

69. **(1)** The Moro reflex occurs in response to sudden stimulation of the newborn's CNS by noise, falling, or jolting. **Answer 2** is incorrect because this action elicits the *Babinski reflex.* **Answer 3** is wrong because this action elicits the *tonic neck reflex.* **Answer 4** is wrong because this elicits *rooting.*

> **Test-taking tip**—Match common neurological reflexes of the newborn with the action described in each of the four options.

IMP, 5, HPM, Growth and Development

70. **(2)** Cervical dilation is determined by vaginal examination. **Answer 1** is incorrect because fetal weight can only be indirectly estimated by *fundal height* measurement and *sonography.* **Answer 3** is incorrect because strength of contractions is evaluated by *palpation* of the uterine fundus. **Answer 4** is incorrect because head circumference cannot be determined until *after* birth.

> **Test-taking tip**—Note the relationship between the word "vaginal" in the stem and the correct answer, "cervical."

AS, 5, HPM, Growth and Development

71. **(3)** The criterion used to distinguish true from false labor is evidence of cervical change. **Answer 1** is incorrect because spontaneous rupture of membranes can occur *before* initiation of labor. **Answer 2** is incorrect because women who are not in true labor may experience increasing pain due to obstetric *complications.* **Answer 4** is incorrect because copious bloody vaginal discharge can occur *without* labor (placental problems).

> **Test-taking tip**—True Labor = Cervical Changes (**TL = CC**).

AS, 5, HPM, Growth and Development

72. **(2)** The most important single factor in maintaining good health for the pregnant woman with heart disease is adequate rest. The woman should have approximately 8-10 hours rest each night and should lie down for 30 minutes

after each meal. **Answer 1** is incorrect because *reduced* activity reduces fatigue and supports preservation of cardiac reserve. **Answer 3** is wrong because *moderate* sodium intake (2000 mg) is allowable for the average class I cardiac; nutritional counseling focuses on increasing dietary intake of iron, protein, and essential nutrients to meet the increased demands of pregnancy. **Answer 4** is wrong because ferrous sulfate is prescribed to meet the increased demands for hemoglobin synthesis and to combat nutritional *anemia.*

> **Test-taking tip**—Note that two options are contradicting: exercise vs. rest. Think "rest the heart."

IMP, 6, PhI, Reduction of Risk Potential

73. **(3)** Tension on round ligaments occurs because of the erect human posture and pressure exerted by the growing uterus. **Answer 1** is incorrect because bladder infection is accompanied by *frequency and dysuria.* **Answer 2** is wrong because discomfort from constipation is accompanied by other symptoms, and the *location* of the discomfort differs. **Answer 4** is wrong because groin pain is *not* characteristic of beginning labor.

> **Test-taking tip**—The key is *time* and *place*. Note that the stem states *late* pregnancy and location is on the *right.*

AN, 3, HPM, Growth and Development

74. **(3)** 0-1-2-2 describes her present status. She has not carried a pregnancy to term **(T)**; one pregnancy terminated in the preterm **(P)** birth of twins, two pregnancies ended in abortion **(A),** and she has two living children **(L).** **Answer 1** is incorrect because only one was a preterm pregnancy. **Answer 2** is incorrect because it describes her as having delivered two term infants and no preterm infants. **Answer 4** is wrong because it describes her as having carried one pregnancy to term and having *no* preterm infants.

> **Test-taking tip**—Be able to determine an obstetric history using the **TPAL** system: T—Term; P—Preterm; A—Abortion; L—Living children.

AN, 5, HPM, Prevention and Early Detection

75. **(1)** The possibility of postpartum eclampsia, while high, is often overlooked. Nursing care is planned to maintain ongoing status assessments and minimize environmental stimuli. **Answer 2** is wrong because, although the risk decreases subsequent to birth, eclamptic convulsions have been known to occur in the *postpartum.* **Answer 3** is wrong because chronic renal disease is *not* a sequel to preeclampsia. **Answer 4** is wrong because preeclampsia does *not* necessarily occur in subsequent pregnancies.

> **Test-taking tip**—Narrow the choice to two contradictory options: "at risk" **(1)** vs. "cured" **(2).** Reduction of risk in the immediate postpartum period is the goal.

AN, 6, PhI, Reduction of Risk Potential

76. **(4)** Even Rh-negative women during their first pregnancy are at some risk for Rh incompatibility; erythroblastosis fetalis results from hemolysis of fetal cells by maternal antibodies. **Answers 1 and 2** are wrong because the Rh-negative woman is *not* more prone to spontaneous abortion or preeclampsia. **Answer 3** is wrong because *fetal, not* maternal, anemia results from Rh incompatibility.

> **Test-taking tip**—The focus should be on the potential risk for the fetus. Understand the pathophysiology of Rh isoimmunization.

AN, 6, PhI, Reduction of Risk Potential

77. **(3)** Quickening, audible FHR with fetoscope, and fundal height at just below the umbilicus are present in most women by the 20th week of pregnancy. **Answer 1** is wrong because lightening usually occurs at *36-38* weeks of gestation. **Answer 2** is wrong because Braxton-Hicks contractions are palpable around the *30th* week. **Answer 4** is wrong because Goodell's, Hegar's, and Chadwick's signs are first noted at *6-8* weeks of pregnancy, and this fundal height is consistent with the *16th* week of gestation.

> **Test-taking tip**—The best answer is derived from the correct *time-frame*—**(1)** and **(2)** occur *later* than 20 weeks; **(4)** occurs *earlier.*

AS, 5, HPM, Growth and Development

78. **(3)** Although lactation does suppress ovulation, time of ovulation varies widely, making this an unreliable birth control method (bottle-feeding mothers have ovulated as early as 36 days postpartum; breastfeeding mothers, as early as 39 days postpartum). **Answer 1** is incorrect because of *unpredictability* of the time of inhibition of ovulation. **Answer 2** is wrong because the mother may have anovulatory or ovulatory menses or may ovulate in the *absence* of menstruation. **Answer 4** is wrong because the woman may desire to resume intercourse when lochia stops.

> **Test-taking tip**—When a question asks which plan is *appropriate,* identify and eliminate the *inappropriate* statements first.

IMP, 5, HPM, Growth and Development

79. **(1)** The lower uterine segment does not contract as effectively as the fundus. Postpartum bleeding is more common in women with placenta previa. **Answer 2** is incorrect because the woman did *not* have abruptio placentae. **Answer 3** is wrong because surgical removal of the placenta does not inhibit uterine contraction. **Answer 4** is wrong because a loss of 250 mL during the third stage is within *normal* limits.

> **Test-taking tip**—The question is asking *why* hemorrhage may occur with placenta previa. **Answers 2** and **4** can be eliminated because they do not answer this question.

AN, 6, PhI, Reduction of Risk Potential

80. **(2)** is the best answer because *intervention is* needed. The breathing technique recommended for *transition* is rapid, shallow chest breathing. **Answer 1** is not the choice because rapid, shallow chest breathing is advised. **Answer 3** is not the choice because the use of intercostal muscles with a relaxed diaphragm *is recommended.* **Answer 4** is not the choice because each contraction *should* begin and end with two cleansing breaths in the Lamaze method.

> **Test-taking tip**—Look for the *inadvisable* breathing patterns. Narrow the choice to two contradictory breathing options: rapid and shallow chest vs. slow and deep abdominal. Note also that the question asks for *transition* phase breathing, not for latent and early active phase, where **Answer 2** *would* be appropriate.

EV, 3, PhI, Basic Care and Comfort

81. **(3)** Increased cardiac output has greater implications because her heart has been compromised by rheumatic fever. She should understand and be able to recognize signs of complications associated with her heart function. **Answer 1** is wrong because increased venous pressure in the lower extremities presents *little* more than an annoyance. **Answer 2** is wrong because placental production of HPL presents a greater problem for a woman with *diabetes.* **Answer 4** is wrong because relaxation of the cardiac results in *minor* complaints.

> **Test-taking tip**—Recall that the potential risk of rheumatic fever is *cardiac* problems.

EV, 6, HPM, Prevention and Early Detection

82. **(3)** Significantly increased fetal activity and meconium-stained amniotic fluid are signs of fetal distress. **Answer 1** is incorrect because crowning is followed rapidly by birth and because any fetal distress can be treated promptly. **Answer 2** is wrong because crowning is shortly followed by birth. **Answer 4** is wrong because baseline variability is a *normal* fetal pattern.

> **Test-taking tip**—Choose the *abnormal* fetal and amniotic fluid signs.

AS, 6, HPM, Prevention and Early Detection

83. **(4)** Tilting the hip moves the heavy uterus off the major blood vessels (the vena cava and aorta), preventing supine hypotension, reduced placental perfusion, and fetal bradycardia. **Answer 1** is incorrect because the statement denies the need for comfort at this time. **Answer 2** is wrong because the pillows may increase her comfort but will *not* prevent supine hypotension. **Answer 3** is wrong because the statement may be perceived as a threat and does not recognize the woman's need for comfort and emotional support.

    Test-taking tip—In positioning a patient, decide what you are trying to *prevent* or *promote*. Understand the effects of vena caval syndrome and preventive position changes.
    IMP, 6, Ph, I, Reduction of Risk Potential

84. **(4)** Epicanthal folds and simian lines are associated with a diagnosis of Down syndrome. **Answer 1** is incorrect because the head is the largest part of the newborn's body and *is* larger than the chest. **Answer 2** is wrong because diaphragmatic breathing *is* the normal newborn pattern of respiration. **Answer 3** is wrong because passage of meconium stool immediately following birth *is* within the normal pattern for newborns.

    Test-taking tip—"Deviation from normal" means look for what is *not* normal.
    AS, 5, HPM, Growth and Development

85. **(3)** When cold, the infant requires more oxygen and there is an increase in the newborn's metabolic rate. Nonshivering thermogenesis is a complex process that increases the metabolic rate and rate of oxygen consumption; therefore the newborn increases its heat production. **Answer 1** is incorrect because more oxygen is needed, *not* less. **Answer 2** is incorrect because the metabolic rate increases, *not* decreases. **Answer 4** is incorrect because *both* oxygen needs and metabolic rate *increase.*

    Test-taking tip—You can eliminate the two options with "less oxygen" first, because of the physiological responses of the newborn to thermoregulation. Recall complications associated with cold stress.
    AN, 6, PhI, Physiological Adaptation

86. **(1)** Signs of placental separation include a change in the shape of the uterus from ovoid to globular. **Answer 2** is incorrect because the placenta appears at the *introitus,* not the fundus of the uterus. **Answer 3** is incorrect because the umbilical cord *lengthens* with placental separation, not *shortens.* **Answer 4** is incorrect because there is often an increase in *bloody* discharge, not *mucoid.*

    Test-taking tip—Picture what happens to the *shape* of uterus as the placenta separates from it.
    AS, 5, HPM, Growth and Development

87. **(3)** Fetal heart rate is of primary concern, because the environment for the fetus has changed. There is an increased risk for prolapse of the umbilical cord immediately after rupture of membranes, especially if the presenting part is not engaged. **Answer 1** is incorrect because this is a *secondary* priority. The woman may develop an elevated temperature *later* because of increased risk of infection. **Answer 2** is incorrect because this is a *secondary* priority. **Answer 4** is incorrect because the woman's blood pressure will probably *not change* in response to the rupture of her membranes.

    Test-taking tip—Think heart rate first! *Study tip:* Review the assessment and nursing interventions for the emergency condition of prolapse of the umbilical cord.
    AS, 6, PhI, Reduction of Risk Potential

88. **(3)** Women who receive live rubella virus vaccine should be advised not to become pregnant for 3 months because of the potential risk to the fetus (congenital measles syndrome). **Answer 1** is incorrect because immunity is *not* established fully by 2 weeks. **Answer 2** is incorrect because dietary restrictions are *not* necessary following rubella vaccine.

Answer 4 is incorrect because mild symptoms may occur *11- 20 days* after vaccination, and are usually mild and transient. Breastfeeding is not contraindicated following vaccination.

    Test-taking tip—Focus on the two options about what *not* to do, and choose the one that deals with prevention of risk to the fetus.
    PL, 5, PhI, Pharmacological and Parenteral Therapies

89. **(4)** If a woman has not voided by 6 hours after delivery, she should be encouraged to ambulate to the bathroom. This may assist her in voiding. Catheterization may need to be done, but only after she is given the opportunity to void. **Answer 1** is incorrect because she should be encouraged to empty her bladder, and *then* her fundus should be assessed for firmness and position. Women who have distended bladders, however, may be at risk for uterine atony and increased bleeding. **Answer 2** is incorrect because her fluid intake is *not* likely to have an impact on her ability to void at this point in the postpartum period. Urinary retention is probably caused from birth trauma and effects of anesthesia. **Answer 3** is incorrect because a woman *should* void and empty her bladder within 6 hours postpartum. Women will begin to diurese in the postpartum period, and there is an increased risk of postpartum bleeding and rupture of the bladder.

    Test-taking tip—Choose the answer that delegates activities to LPN/LVN for stable patients with *predictable* outcomes, not assessment activities (**1, 2**).
    AS, 8, PhI, Basic Care and Comfort

90. **(1)** A diaphragm should be refitted after each pregnancy around 6 weeks postpartum. It should also be refitted if the woman loses or gains a significant amount of weight (15-20 lb) or has uterine or vaginal surgery. **Answer 2** is incorrect because a pregnancy *can* change the shape and size of the cervix and vagina. **Answer 3** is incorrect because women *may* use a diaphragm for postpartum contraception once involution is completed. **Answer 4** is incorrect because she does not need to wait until 3 months postpartum. Usually *6 weeks* is sufficient.

    Test-taking tip—It is a "yes" answer, but eliminate the option with the specific time frame (i.e., 3 months).
    AN, 5, HPM, Growth and Development

91. **(3)** Newborns can get pneumonia (tachypnea, mild hypoxia, cough, eosinophilia) and conjunctivitis from *Chlamydia.* **Answer 1** is incorrect because discolored teeth are caused by tetracycline. **Answer 2** is incorrect because snuffles is seen with *congenital syphilis.* Rhagades refers to circumoral radiating scars that result from cracked, rough mucocutaneous lesions of the lips. **Answer 4** is incorrect because congenital *rubella* causes central and peripheral hearing defects in infancy.

    Test-taking tip—Eliminate two of the options that are congenital (**2, 4**), and (**1**), which is caused by a medication.
    AN, 6, SECE, Safety and Infection Control

92. **(1)** Even though the mother is a minor, she is legally able to sign consent for her own child. **Answer 2** is incorrect because the baby's *mother* is able to give consent. The exception might be if the mother is unable and the baby's grandmother has power of attorney for her daughter. **Answer 3** is incorrect because the RN should *not* sign a consent form for treatment or surgery. **Answer 4** is incorrect because the physician *cannot sign* a consent form for treatment or surgery.

    Test-taking tip—Eliminate who should *not* sign the consent form (i.e., all but the patient should not).
    AN, 1, SECE, Management of Care

93. **(1)** A quiet room close to the nurse's station provides the best environment for treatment (observation and decreased stimulation). A private room is ideal, but of these choices,

Answer 1 is the best. **Answers 2, 3,** and **4** are incorrect because too much noise or stimulation can precipitate eclamptic seizures. All of these environments could be too noisy and too stimulating.

> **Test-taking tip**—Because of severe preeclampsia, choose the *least* stimulating environment (i.e., ↓ noise, ↓ number of people).

AN, 6, Reduction of Risk Potential

94. **(4)** The data indicate that the woman has an arrest of her labor (potentially cephalopelvic disproportion), and the fetus is developing a tachycardia (fetal distress). It would be contraindicated to augment labor under these circumstances. The nurse should emphasize the assessment findings to the physician. **Answers 1, 2,** and **3** are incorrect because augmentation of labor is *contraindicated* with the current situation.

> **Test-taking tip**—Because of the risk of hyperstimulation of the uterus, choose the *one* answer that does *not* give it. Think of patient safety, and think of the *legal* responsibility of the RN.

IMP, 1, PhI, Pharmacological Therapy

95. **(2)** Facial paralysis can occur when the forcep blades compress cranial nerve VII (facial) anterior to the ears. It is usually mild and temporary, lasting only a few days. **Answer 1** is incorrect. Torticollis, or wry neck, is caused by a shortened sternocleidomastoid *muscle* on one side of the fetal neck. **Answer 3** is incorrect. Fractured clavicle is usually caused when the *shoulders* are being born, when the infant is large, or when the mother's pelvis is small. **Answer 4** is incorrect. Cephalohematoma is *not caused* by properly placed forceps. This *bleeding* between the periosteum and one or more of the cranial bones (especially the parietal) is secondary to pressure from the maternal *pelvis.*

> **Test-taking tip**—Choose the one option that is related to *nerve* damage.

AS, 2, PhI, Reduction of Risk Potential

96. **(3)** This is subinvolution of the uterus and may cause postpartum hemorrhage. The uterus should firm up with massage. If it does not, or the bleeding continues to be heavy, she should go to the hospital immediately; she might need oxytocin and perhaps a D&C. She should also be checked for retained tissue, birth canal lacerations, or infection. **Answer 1** is incorrect because this is too much bleeding, and a return to bright-red, heavy bleeding postpartum, after the flow has decreased, is *not* normal. **Answer 2** is not correct because the woman could be hemorrhaging. She should *not wait* an hour for intervention. **Answer 4** is incorrect because the nurse's role after early discharge is to triage problems over the phone and prioritize which ones need immediate medical attention.

> **Test-taking tip**—Consider *time sequence* when advising patients (e.g., when is this taking place?).

AN, 6, PhI, Physiological Adaptation

97. **(3)** Undescended testicles are a condition unrelated to maternal hormonal influence. By 36-38 weeks of gestation, they should be descending through the inguinal canal and into the scrotal sac. **Answers 1, 2,** and **4** are incorrect. They are all a result of maternal hormonal influences and are considered *normal* findings in the full-term neonate.

> **Test-taking tip**—Eliminate the three options that are related to maternal hormone influence. Key concept is *time* related (i.e., at *term,* not at 36 weeks of gestation or earlier).

AS, 5, HPM, Growth and Development

98. **(2)** Positive parent-infant bonding and responses to the baby are encouraged; this may help motivate parents to enter drug rehabilitation. **Answer 1** is incorrect. Positive parental contact should be encouraged. **Answer 3** is incorrect. Positive parental contact should be encouraged. **Answer 4** is incorrect. The nurse cannot assume that drug-dependent parents are less likely to be interested in their babies.

> **Test-taking tip**—Choose the option that would reflect the nurse's *advocacy role* in fostering the well-being of the family. Because **Answers 1** and **3** are really saying the same thing, they cannot be correct. **Answer 2** is the opposite of the incorrect options (**1** and **3**). Choose the option that is different from the others.

PL, 7, PsI, Psychological Adaptation

99. **(4)** The woman with AIDS has compromised immunity. The nurse should not assign this patient to a health care provider who has a viral or infectious illness. **Answers 1, 2,** and **3** are incorrect. It would not be as great a risk for patients with renal failure, hypertension, or a prolonged labor to have contact with a health care provider who has a cold.

> **Test-taking tip**—Consider the nurse's role in *delegation of care,* and think about patient safety as the *priority* when there is a risk of exposure to infectious or viral agents for patients with compromised immunity.

PL, 6, SECE, Safety and Infection Control

100. **(2)** The basal body temperature (BBT) is the lowest body temperature of a healthy person that is taken immediately after waking and before getting out of bed. The BBT usually varies from 36.2°C to 36.3°C during menses and for about 5-7 days afterward. About the time of ovulation, a slight drop in temperature (approximately 0.05°C) may be seen; after ovulation, in concert with the increasing progesterone levels of the early luteal phase, the BBT rises 0.2°-0.4°C. This elevation remains until 2-3 days before menstruation, or if pregnancy has occurred. **Answer 1** is incorrect. The BBT is not an average temperature, but must be taken every day to assess for slight fluctuations. **Answer 3** is incorrect. Cervical mucus assessment is only one of the signs of approaching ovulation. Many things, such as semen, contraceptive gels, vaginal discharge from infection, and sexual arousal, can affect the amount and consistency of cervical mucus. Other factors, such as illness, can affect the BBT as well. **Answer 4** is incorrect. Either a mercury or digital thermometer may be used to accurately measure BBT; it is advisable that a woman uses the *same* thermometer the entire month, however, because the readings might vary slightly.

> **Test-taking tip**—The key is *when* (i.e., each morning before activity).

IMP, 5, HPM, Growth and Development

101. **(3)** At the time of implantation, two fetal membranes, which will surround the developing embryo, begin to form. The chorion develops from the trophoblast and contains chorionic villi on its surface. The villi burrowing into the decidua increase in size and complexity as the vascular processes develop into the placenta. The villi eventually atrophy and degenerate, leaving a smooth chorionic membrane. **Answer 1** is incorrect because the amnion is the other embryonic membrane, the inner cell membrane that develops from the interior cells of the blastocyst. The amnion eventually becomes the covering of the umbilical cord and covers the chorion on the fetal surface of the placenta. **Answer 2** is incorrect because the amniotic sac is the fluid-filled sac inside the membranes surrounding the embryo/fetus. **Answer 4** is incorrect because the mesoderm is a primary germ layer that develops into fetal bones, teeth, and muscles.

> **Test-taking tip**—The correct answer is based on knowing *when* the development of the embryo, including membranes, amniotic sac, and fluid, occurs.

AN, 5, HPM, Growth and Development

102. **(4)** Amniotic fluid allows freedom of movement for musculoskeletal development of the fetus, in addition to the other functions mentioned. **Answer 1** is incorrect because the amnion and chorion are formed and adhered *before* the development of the fluid. **Answer 2** is incorrect because the *placenta* provides for oxygen and carbon dioxide exchange.

Answer 3 is incorrect because one of the metabolic functions of the *placenta* is nutrient exchange.

> **Test-taking tip**—Visualize the fetus moving around in the fluid. Eliminate the two options that are functions of the *placenta*.

AN, 5, HPM, Growth and Development

103. (2) Oxygen diffuses from the maternal blood across the placental membranes into the fetal blood, and carbon dioxide diffuses in the opposite direction. In this way, the placenta functions as lungs for the fetus. **Answer 1** is incorrect because respiratory gas exchange does not occur in the fetal lung while in utero. **Answer 3** is incorrect because blood from the placenta is carried through the umbilical *vein*, not artery, to the fetus. **Answer 4** is incorrect because it is not the mother's hemoglobin that assists the baby to breathe; the *placenta* functions as the fetal lungs until birth.

> **Test-taking tip:** Remember—placenta = fetal "lungs."

AN, 5, HPM, Growth and Development

104. (1) Both red blood cells (RBCs) and plasma increase in pregnancy; but because the plasma increase exceeds the increase in RBC production, there is a decrease in both Hct and Hgb due to hemodilution. **Answers 2, 3,** and **4** are incorrect because the increases are not correct. Neither erythrocyte nor plasma volume decreases during pregnancy.

> **Test-taking tip:** The increases in both are a protective mechanism for both mother and fetus.

AN, 6, HPM, Growth and Development

105. (1) The height of the fundus (single pregnancy) should measure about 20 cm at 20 weeks (*at* the umbilicus). A measurement less than that might indicate inadequate fetal growth or an error in calculation of gestational age. **Answers 2, 3,** and **4** are all findings that would be considered *normal* during the second trimester of pregnancy.

> **Test-taking tip:** The key point is *when*—that is, when prenatal assessment findings are not normal during the second trimester.

AS, 5, HPM, Growth and Development

106. (3) The suggested RDA is an increase of 500 kcal more than the adult woman's nonpregnant intake. It is recommended that lactating women consume at least 1800 kcal/day because it becomes difficult to obtain adequate nutrients for the maintenance of lactation at levels below that. **Answer 1** is incorrect because this exceeds kcal requirements. It is recommended to increase 300 kcal/day for pregnancy and an additional 200 kcal/day (total 500 kcal) during lactation. **Answer 2** is incorrect because protein requirements increase in both pregnancy and lactation. RDA for magnesium, vitamin C, zinc, and protein is slightly to moderately higher than during pregnancy. **Answer 4** is incorrect because it is especially important that the calcium intake be adequate during pregnancy and lactation.

> **Test-taking tip:** First, decide if the RDA in the correct answer relates to *non*pregnancy time period or during pregnancy. Next, you can eliminate **Answers 1** and **4** because they relate to the time *during* pregnancy. Select **Answer 3** rather than (2) because of need to *increase* calories. Remember: ↑ calories, ↑ protein over *pre*pregnancy requirements.

AN, 4, PhI, Basic Care and Comfort

107. (1) As milk is removed from the breast, more is produced. **Answers 2, 3,** and **4** are incorrect because as the infant requires more milk with each feeding, the woman's breasts will meet the demands with adequate nutrition and volume if there is adequate maternal nutrition and hydration. Also, early introduction of solids (**Answer 3**) may make the infant more prone to food allergies. Regular feeding of solids may also lead to decreased intake of breast milk and has been associated with early cessation of breastfeeding.

> **Test-taking tip**—Remember the concept that milk production during lactation is a supply-demand system.

AN, 4, PhI, Basic Care and Comfort

108. (2) The considerable uterine distention involved with multiple gestation can place the woman at risk for premature contractions, cervical dilation, and delivery. If there are risk factors for preterm birth, abstinence from orgasm, nipple stimulation, and increased rest during the last trimester may be recommended to avoid preterm labor. **Answers 1, 3,** and **4** do not necessarily place a woman at increased risk for preterm labor. *Inadequate* weight gain is a risk factor, *not* extra weight gain. A history of preterm labor must always be considered a high-risk factor.

> **Test-taking tip**—Visualize what happens to the uterus with twins and what that can lead to.

AS, 1, PhI, Reduction of Risk Potential

109. (4) The introduction of a baby into a family with one or more children challenges parents to promote acceptance of the baby by siblings. The parents' attitudes toward the arrival of the baby can set the stage for the other children's reactions. Spending time with the older siblings alone will also reassure them of their place in the family, even though the older children will have to eventually assume new positions within the family hierarchy. **Answer 1** is incorrect because direct sibling contact does not place healthy newborns at risk for exposure to pathogenic organisms or for physical harm from siblings. It may facilitate the adjustment to the addition of a new family member. **Answer 2** is incorrect because parents need to assume the task of caring for a new child while *not* neglecting the others. A temporary separation might be necessary while the mother recovers, but involvement of the whole family is important. **Answer 3** is incorrect because the older child's goal is to maintain the lead position in a family. If the parents threaten that position even more by changing that child's status, it may delay adjustment to the new sibling. Allowing the older child to help with the new baby is positive.

> **Test-taking tip**—It is about the mother and 2-year-old first. Focus on the *age-appropriate* answer about reducing sibling rivalry.

PL, 7, HPM, Growth and Development

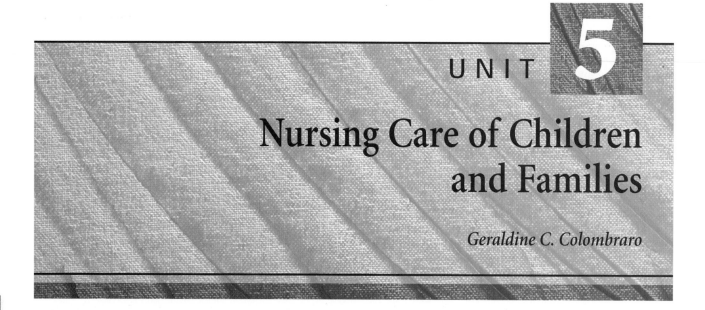

UNIT **5**

Nursing Care of Children and Families

Geraldine C. Colombraro

INTRODUCTION

The revised NCLEX-RN Test Plan includes content that has been covered in this unit, but often raises concern in candidates. This section assists NCLEX candidates to think about this content in terms of the current test plan, in a concrete and specific manner through the clinical examples given.

Management of Care of Infants, Children, and Adolescents

The role of the pediatric nurse in *management of care* includes the following:

1. Serving as an *advocate* for the child and family, such as informing child and family of all treatments and procedures.
2. Coordinating clinical *case management* to provide access to high-quality clinical resources appropriate to the level of care needed, such as referring child to acute rehabilitation facility following open heart surgery.
3. Coordinating *continuity of care* across the health care delivery continuum, such as discussing needs of child and family with home care nurse before child's discharge in a spica cast.
4. *Delegating* care to and *supervising* care among various members of the health care delivery team, such as assigning a float nurse to care for selected patients on the pediatrics unit.
5. Completing *incident/irregular occurrence/variance reports* as needed, including filing, monitoring, and analyzing reports of drug reactions to a new medication.

6. Working toward *continuous quality improvement*, such as studying incident reports of accidents on the pediatrics unit to determine what changes in practice are needed to increase patient safety.
7. Suggesting *organ donation* to selected families when appropriate—for example, asking the family whose 16-year-old has been declared brain dead about the possibility of organ donation.
8. Collaborating with other members of the health care team *in consultation and referrals*, such as requesting a psychiatric consultation for a child who is depressed.
9. Coordinating *resource management*, such as reminding the UAP to stamp all equipment charge forms used for each child.

Safety and Infection Control for Infants, Children, and Adolescents

The role of the pediatric nurse in *safety and infection control* includes the following:

1. Engaging in *disaster planning* activities—for example, the nurse reads and thoroughly reviews the disaster plan for the health care facility in which the nurse is practicing.
2. Engaging in activities designed to *prevent errors*, such as identifying pediatric patients only by their name bands or by a reliable adult who knows the child.
3. *Handling hazardous and infectious materials* appropriately—for example, always disposing of contaminated waste in a clearly marked biohazard container.
4. Using *medical and surgical asepsis*, such as using sterile gloves and technique when changing a surgical incision dressing.

Prevention and Early Detection of Disease in Infants, Children, and Adolescents

The role of the pediatric nurse in the *prevention and early detection of disease* includes the following:

1. Engaging in *disease prevention* activities (e.g., washing hands thoroughly before and after providing patient care).
2. Participating in *health promotion programs,* such as teaching a class on accident prevention to parents of infants and young children.
3. Conducting *health screening* as needed, such as performing Denver Developmental Screening Test (DDST) on age-appropriate patients (1 mo to 6 yr) in the pediatric clinic as part of routine screening.
4. Teaching families about and administering *immunizations* as ordered—signs/symptoms of reactions, providing parents with an immunization record card after administering immunization(s).

5. Discussing *lifestyle choices* with older children and adolescents, as appropriate (e.g., discussing risks associated with body piercing and tattooing).

Coping and Adaptation in Infants, Children, and Adolescents

The role of the pediatric nurse in *coping and adaptation* includes the following:

1. Understanding and respecting *religious and spiritual influences on children's health* (e.g., allowing families to engage in dying and death rituals according to their spiritual beliefs).
2. Helping patients engage in problem solving related to *situational role changes,* such as discussing transportation and child care issues with the parents of a child who is newly diagnosed with leukemia.

Pediatrics

GROWTH AND DEVELOPMENT

I. **Infant (28 days–1 year)**
   A. **Erikson's theory of personality development**
      1. *Central task:* basic trust vs. mistrust; central person: primary caretaker.
      2. *Behavioral indicators:*
         a. Crying is only means of communicating needs.
         b. Quieting usually means needs are met.
         c. Fear of strangers at 6–8 mo.
      3. **Parental guidance/teaching**
         a. Must meet infant's needs consistently—cannot "spoil" infant by holding, comforting.
      b. Neonatal *reflexes* fade between 4 and 6 mo, replaced with increase in purposeful behavior, e.g., babbling, reaching.
      c. *Fear of strangers* is normal—indicates attachment between infant and primary caretaker.
      d. Child may repeat over and over newly learned behaviors, e.g., sitting or standing.
      e. *Weaning* can begin around the time child begins walking.
      f. Review preventive care time line and Recommended Health Screenings (Tables 5–1 and 5–2) with parents of infants.
   4. For additional information about behavioral concerns for each age group, see Tables 5–3 and 5–4.
   B. **Physical growth** (by 1 year)
      1. *Height* (length): 50% increase by first birthday.

TABLE 5–1   Child Preventive Care Timeline

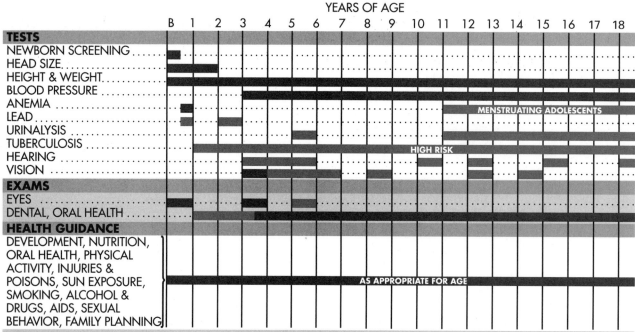

CHILD PREVENTIVE CARE TIMELINE

Check-up visits are important for your child's health. Some authorities recommend these visits at the following ages: 2-4 weeks; 2, 4, 6, 9, 12, 15, and 18 months; and 2, 3, 4, 5, 6, 8, 10, 12, 14, 16, and 18 years. Some authorities recommend yearly adolescent visits. Your child's doctor will discuss with you the individual needs of your child. At check-up visits, your child may receive a physical examination and the types of preventive care shown below.

■ Recommended by most major authorities
■ Recommended by some major authorities

Note: Children with special risk factors may need more frequent and additional types of preventive care. Some examples:

Risk Factor	Preventive Service(s) Needed
Exposure to TB	TB test
Sexually active	Pap test (women); syphilis, gonorrhea, chlamydia tests
High-risk sexual behavior	AIDS test, hepatitis immunization
Drug abuse	AIDS, TB tests, hepatitis immunization

Source: *Office of Disease Prevention and Health Promotion, in cooperation with the agencies of the Public Health Service, U.S. Department of Health and Human Services.*

TABLE 5–2 ▯ **Recommended Health Screenings for Infants, Children, and Adolescents: Specific Conditions**

Area of Concern	Screening Method	Recommendations
Neonatal metabolic and genetic screening: Hypothyroidism Sickle cell anemia PKU	Blood Tests: Serum T$_3$/T$_4$ levels ↓ Sickledex ↓ Phenylalanine levels ↓	All are done in immediate neonatal period, within first few days of life. Testing for PKU must be done after infant has ingested formula or breast milk for 48–72 hours.
Lead poisoning (see Table 5–1)	Blood-lead level (BLL)	Centers for Disease Control and Prevention (CDC) recommends universal or targeted screening for all children. At a minimum, all children should have BLL drawn between 1–2 yr, or earlier if needed. BLL should also be done on any child between 3–6 yr who has never been tested. Those children at high risk (e.g., live in older home with lead in paint and plumbing, have sibling or friend with lead poisoning) should be screened earlier and more frequently.
Hyperlipidemia	Serum cholesterol levels	Routinely at 2–4 yr, 6 yr, 10 yr, 11–14 yr, 15–17 yr, and 18–21 yr. May be done earlier or more frequently with risk factors such as diabetes, hypertension, parent with high cholesterol level.
Cystic fibrosis	Genetic studies, sweat test	Screen children who have sibling or other family members with CF. Screen family members of child with CF.
Tuberculosis (see Table 5–1)	Mantoux or PPD	First test done at age 12–15 mo; repeated prn based on risk and exposure.
Latex allergies	Health history	During each routine visit, but especially important preoperatively or before procedures or children with ongoing catheterizations.

TABLE 5–3 Pediatric Behavioral Concerns: Nursing Implications and Parental Guidance

Behavioral Concern	Nursing Implications/ Parental Guidance	Behavioral Concern	Nursing Implications/ Parental Guidance
Teething	Begins around age 4 mo—infant may seem unusually fussy and irritable but should *not* run a fever. Provide relief with teething rings, acetaminophen, topical preparations.	**Sibling rivalry**	Fairly common, normal. Allow older child to "help." Give each child "special" time, with individual attention.
Thumb sucking	Need to "suck" varies: may be due to hunger, frustration, loneliness. Do *not* stop *infant* from doing this—usually stops by preschool years. If behavior persists, evaluate need for attention, peer play.	**Masturbation**	Normal, common in *preschooler*. Set firm limits. *Avoid* overreacting.
		Lying	*In preschooler:* not deliberate; child is often unable to differentiate between "real" and "lie," and by speaking something often feels it makes a thing real. *In older child:* may indicate problems and need for professional attention if persists. Serve as role model—no "white lies."
Temper tantrums	Normal in the *toddler*—occurs in response to frustration. *Avoid* abrupt end to play or making excessive demands Offer only allowable choices. Once a decision is verbalized, *avoid* sudden changes of mind. Provide diversion to achieve cooperation. If it occurs, best means to handle is to *ignore* the outburst.	**Cursing**	*Avoid* overreacting. Defuse use of "the word" by simply stating "not here, not now." Distract, change subject, substitute activity. Serve as role model by own language.
Toilet training	Assess child for readiness: awareness of body functions, form of mutual communication, physical control over sphincters. Use child-size seat. *No* distractions (food, toys, books). Offer praise for success *or* efforts (never shame accidents).	**"Accidents" (enuresis)**	*Occasional*—common and normal through preschool. *If frequent*—need complete physical exam to rule out pathology. "Training": after dinner—*avoid* fluids; before bed—toilet (perhaps awaken once during night). *Never* put back into diapers or attempt to shame.
Discipline	*Not* for infant. Can begin with *toddler,* within limits. Be consistent and clear. *Avoid* excessively strict measures.	**Smoking/drinking**	May begin in *older school-age* child or adolescent. Serve as role model with own habits.

TABLE 5–4   Pediatric Sleep and Rest Norms: Nursing Implications and Parental Guidance

Pediatric Sleep and Rest Norms	Nursing Implications/Parental Guidance
INFANT: 16–20 hr/day	
3 mo: nocturnal pattern	No set schedule can be predetermined
6 mo: 1–2 naps, with 12 hr at night	If waking at night after age 3 mo, investigate hunger as a probable cause
12 mo: 1 nap, with 12 hr at night	Monitor behavior to determine sleep needs: alert and active? Growing, developing?
	Routine fairly well established
TODDLER: 12–14 hr/night	
"Dawdles" at bedtime	Set firm, realistic limits
Dependency on security object	Place favorite blanket or toy in crib/bed
May ask to sleep with bottle	**Avoid** "bottle mouth syndrome" (caries)
May rebel against going to sleep	Establish bedtime "ritual"
PRESCHOOL: 10–12 hr/night	
Gives up afternoon nap	Provide "quiet time" in place of nap;
	May regress in behavior when tired
Difficulty falling asleep/nighttime waking	**Avoid** overstimulation in evening
Fear of dark	Leave night-light on, door open
Enuresis	Occasional accidents are normal
May begin to have nightmares	Comfort child but leave in own bed
SCHOOL-AGE: 8–12 hr/night	
Nightmares common	Comfort child but leave in own bed
Awakens early in morning	Important that child play/relax after school
May not be aware he or she is tired	Remind about bedtime
Likes to stay up late	"Privilege" of later bedtime can be "awarded" as child gets older
Slumber parties	Permit, as good opportunity to socialize
ADOLESCENT: 10–14 hr/night	
Need for sleep increases greatly	Needs vary greatly among individuals
May complain of excessive fatigue	Rapid growth rate
	Related to rapid growth and overall increased activity

TABLE 5–5   Normal Vital Signs: Measurements and Variations with Age

Age (yr)	Heart (beats/min)	Respiratory Rate (breaths/min)	Blood Pressure (mm Hg)
Newborn	120–160	30–40	70/55
1	100–140	25–35	90/55
2	80–120	20–30	90/56
5	70–100	18–24	95/56
10	60–90	18–22	102/62
14	55–90	16–20	110/65
18	55–90	16–18	116/68

Source: Adapted from Wong, D: Whaley and Wong's Nursing Care of Infants and Children, ed 6. Mosby, St Louis, 1999.

2. *Weight:*
   a. Doubles by 4–7 mo, triples by 1 yr.
   b. Gains 5–7 oz/wk in first 6 mo of life.
   c. Gains 3–5 oz/wk in second 6 mo of life.
3. *Vital signs:* see Table 5–5.
4. *Cardiac system:*
   a. Heart begins to function effectively.
   b. Decreased heart rate, increased blood pressure from neonatal values.
5. *Pulmonary system:*
   a. Predisposed to upper respiratory infections due to anatomical differences (e.g., eustacian tube is shorter and straighter in infant).
   b. Decreased respiratory rate from neonatal values.
6. *Gastrointestinal system:*
   a. Swallowing improves.
   b. Stomach enlarges to hold greater volume.
   c. Digests more complex foods as enzymes increase (by 4–6 mo).
7. *Genitourinary system:*
   a. Immature; waste products poorly eliminated.
   b. Easily prone to fluid and electrolyte imbalances.
8. *Immune system:*
   a. Functional by 2 mo.
   b. Produces IgG and IgM antibiotics.
9. *Neurological system:*
   a. Fontanels:
      (1) Anterior—open or patent through first 12 mo.
      (2) Posterior—closed by 2 mo.
   b. Head circumference increases as brain grows rapidly.
   c. Neurological reflexes (e.g., Landau, parachute) appear; neonatal reflexes (e.g., Moro, rooting) disappear.
10. *Sensory:*
    a. Hearing improves from "quieting" to a sound, to locating a sound easily and turning toward it.

TABLE 5–6   Facts About the Denver Developmental Screening Test (DDST)

Parents' Questions	Nurse's Best Response
"Will this be used as a measure of my child's IQ?"	"No, it is a screening test for your child's development."
"What ages can be tested?"	"Infants through preschoolers, *or* from 1 month to 6 years."
"What will they test?"	"There are four areas: personal-social, fine motor-adaptive, language, gross motor."
"Can I stay with my child?"	"Yes, in fact it is preferred you be there."
"If my child fails, does it mean he is retarded?"	"No, this is not a diagnostic tool but rather a screening test."
"If he fails, what do we do?"	"Repeat the test in a week or two to rule out temporary factors."
"Why didn't my child accomplish everything?"	"He is not expected to."
"Why did my child score so poorly?"	"Perhaps it's a bad day for the child, he isn't feeling up to par, etc."

    b. Vision improves from 8–18 inches, to searching for hidden objects and following moving objects.

  11. *Teething:*
    a. Generally begins around 6 mo.
    b. First two teeth: lower central incisors.
    c. By 1 yr: six to eight teeth.

C. Denver Developmental Screening Test (DDST): Table 5–6
  1. *Birth—3 mo*
    a. Personal-social: smiles responsively, then spontaneously.
    b. Fine motor-adaptive:
      (1) Follows 180 degrees, past midline.
      (2) Grasps rattle.
      (3) Holds hands together.
    c. Language: laughs/squeals; vocalizes without crying.
    d. Gross motor: while on stomach, lifts head 45–90 degrees, able to hold head steady and erect; rolls over, from stomach to back.

  2. *4–6 mo*
    a. Personal-social: works for toy; feeds self (bottle).
    b. Fine motor-adaptive: palmar grasp, reaches for objects.
    c. Language: turns toward voice, imitates speech.
    d. Gross motor: some weight bearing on legs; no head lag when pulled to sitting; sits with support.

  3. *7–9 mo*
    a. Personal-social
      (1) Indicates wants
      (2) Plays pat-a-cake, waves bye-bye.
    b. Fine motor-adaptive: takes two cubes in hands and bangs them together; passes cube hand to hand; crude pincer grasp.
    c. Language: "dada," "mama," nonspecific, jabbers.
    d. Gross motor: creeps on hands and knees; gets self up to sitting; pulls self to standing; stands holding on.

  4. *10–12 mo*
    a. Personal-social
      (1) Plays ball.
      (2) Imitates activities.
      (3) Drinks from cup.
    b. Fine motor-adaptive: neat pincer grasp.
    c. Language: "dada," "mama," specific.
    d. Gross motor: stands alone well; walks holding on; stoops and recovers.

◆ **D. Nursing interventions/parental guidance, teaching:** *Infant*
  1. *Play*
    a. First year—generally solitary.
    b. Visual stimulation
      (1) Best color: red.
      (2) *Toys:* mirrors, brightly colored pictures.
    c. Auditory stimulation
      (1) Talk and sing to infant.
      (2) *Toys:* musical mobiles, rattles, bells.
    d. Tactile stimulation – *6 mon*
      (1) Hold, pat, touch, cuddle, swaddle/keep warm; rub body with lotion, powder.
      (2) *Toys:* various textures; nesting and stacking; plastic milk bottle with blocks to dump in, out.
    e. Kinetic stimulation
      (1) Cradle, stroller, carriage, infant seat, car rides, wind-up infant swing, jumper seat, walker, furniture strategically placed for walking.
      (2) *Toys:* cradle gym, push-pull.
  2. *Safety*
    a. Refer to Tables 5–7 and 5–8 for additional information on safety and infection control.
    b. *Note:* Most common accident during first 12 mo is the aspiration of foreign bodies.
      (1) Keep small objects out of reach.
      (2) Use one-piece pacifier only.
      (3) *No* nuts, raisins, hot dogs, popcorn.
      (4) *No* toys with small, removable parts.
      (5) *No* balloons or plastic bags.

[handwritten margin notes: Falls, Poisoning, Burns, MVA, Prevention]

[side tab:] **Pediatrics**

TABLE 5–7 Safety Considerations When Caring for Infants, Children, and Adolescents

Area of Concern	Safety Interventions
Security	■ Be alert to all visitors; restrict prn ■ Monitor/report suspicious visitors ■ Assess high-risk children (e.g., custody disputes) ■ Identify person to whom child is discharged ■ All staff to wear photo ID, especially when transporting child ■ Transport one child at a time; *never* leave child unattended during transport ■ Do *not* allow visitors to borrow scrubs or lab coat ■ Infants placed near nurses station, in direct line of vision ■ Access to pediatrics unit limited; doors alarmed to indicate when someone enters or leaves the unit
Electrical equipment (e.g., apnea monitor, ECG monitor, respirator)	■ Maintain all equipment in good working order ■ Remove leads when not attached to monitor ■ Unplug power cord when not connected to equipment ■ Keep equipment away from moisture (e.g., puddle of water, tub) ■ Do *not* turn off alarm for any reason ■ Always check the child when an alarm sounds; *never* ignore the alarm ■ Teach other children *not* to touch or play with the equipment **Home care:** ■ CPR guidelines posted near bed ■ Emergency numbers posted near phone ■ Notify electric company, get on priority service list in case of power outage ■ Use intercom or monitoring system
Environment	■ Keep unused electrical outlets covered with child-proof caps ■ Secure screens on all windows ■ Strap infant securely into infant seat, high chair, stroller ■ Discourage use of walkers ■ Crib rails up at all times when infant or young child is alone ■ When a crib rail is down, keep one hand on the infant or young child at all times ■ Keep plants or flowers out of the reach of infants or young children ■ *No* small or sharp objects within reach of infants or young children ■ *No* small or removable parts to toys of infants or young children ■ Keep all medications out of the reach of infants or young children ■ *Never* leave an infant or young child alone in a bath or near water

TABLE 5–8 Infection Control When Caring for Infants, Children, and Adolescents

Type	Definition	Equipment	Clinical Applications
↻ Standard precautions	Reduce the risk of transmission of infection from all recognized and unrecognized sources of infection (formerly termed *universal precautions*)	■ Gloves ■ Protective eyewear ■ Gown/apron ■ Mask	■ Blood ■ Body fluids ■ Secretions ■ Excretions ■ Any break in skin or mucous membranes
Airborne precautions	Reduce the risk of airborne transmission of infectious agents	■ Special air handling systems ■ Ventilation systems: HEPA filter masks, N95 Respirator	■ Measles ■ Varicella ■ Tuberculosis
Droplet precautions	Reduce the risk of airborne transmission of infectious agents transmitted by large particle droplets	■ Surgical mask	■ *Haemophilus influenzae* type B ■ Pertussis ■ Streptococcal pharyngitis ■ Scarlet fever
Contact precautions	Reduce the risk of transmission of infectious agents by direct patient contact or indirect contact with contaminated items in the patient's environment	■ Gloves ■ Gown	■ Enteric infections ■ Skin/wound infections ■ Respiratory syncytial virus (RSV) ■ Herpes simplex ■ Impetigo ■ Viral hemorrhagic conjunctivitis

c. *Falls*
(1) Raise crib rails.
(2) *Never* place child on high surface unsupervised.
(3) Use restraining straps in seats, swings, high-chairs, etc.

d. *Poisoning*
(1) Check that paint on toys/furniture is *lead-free.*
(2) Treat all medications as drugs, never as "candy."
(3) Store all poisonous substances in locked cabinet, closet.
(4) Have telephone number of poison control center on hand.
(5) Instruct in use of syrup of ipecac (see p. 254).

e. *Burns*
(1) Use microwave oven to heat refrigerated formula only; heat only 4 oz or more for about 30 sec. Test formula on top of your hand, not inside wrist.
(2) Check temperature of bath water; *never* leave infant alone in bath.
(3) Special care with cigarettes, hot liquids.
(4) Do *not* leave infant in sun.
(5) Cover all electrical sockets.
(6) Keep electrical wires out of sight/reach.
(7) *Avoid* tablecloths with overhang.
(8) Put guards around heating devices.

f. *Motor vehicles*
(1) Use only federally approved car seat for all car rides; safest position is rear-facing in middle of back seat (from *birth to 20 pounds,* and as close to *1 year* of age as possible)
(2) *Never* leave stroller behind parked car.
(3) Do *not* allow infant to crawl near parked cars or in driveway.

II. Toddler (1–3 yr)

A. Erikson's theory of personality development

1. *Central task:* autonomy vs. shame and doubt; central person(s): parent(s)
2. *Behavioral indicators*
   a. Does not separate easily from parents.
   b. Negativistic. "NO" (handwritten)
   c. Prefers rituals and routine activities.
   d. Active physical explorer of environment.
   e. Begins attempts at self-assertion.
   f. Easily frustrated by limits.
   g. Temper tantrums.
   h. May have favorite "security object."
   i. Uses "mine" for everything—does not understand concept of sharing.

3. **Parental guidance/teaching**
   a. *Avoid* periods of prolonged separation if possible.
   b. *Avoid* constantly saying "no" to toddler.
   c. *Avoid* "yes/no" questions.
   d. Stress that child may use "no" even when he or she means "yes."
   e. Establish and maintain rituals, e.g., toilet training, going to sleep.
   f. Offer opportunities for play, *with* supervision.
   g. Allow child to feed self.
   h. Offer only allowable choices.
   i. Best method to handle temper tantrums: ignore them.
   j. Keep security object with child, if so desired.
   k. Do not force toddler "to share."
   l. Review Recommended Health Screenings (see Tables 5–1 and 5–2) with parents of toddlers.

4. Additional information about behavioral concerns for each age group may be found in Tables 5–3 and 5–4.

B. Physical growth (by 3 years)

1. *Height*
   a. Slow, steady growth at 2–4 in/yr, mainly in *legs* rather than trunk.
   b. Adult height is roughly twice child's height at 2 years of age.
2. *Weight*
   a. Slow, steady growth at 4–6 lb/yr.
   b. Birth weight *quadruples* by 2.5 years of age.
3. *Vital signs:* refer to Table 5–5.
4. *Cardiac system*
   a. Heart begins to function more efficiently.
   b. Decreased heart rate, slight increase in blood pressure from infant values.
5. *Pulmonary system*
   a. Mainly abdominal breathing.
   b. Lumina of bronchial vessels ↑ in size → decrease in lower respiratory system infections.
   c. Decreased respiratory rate from infant values.
6. *Gastrointestinal system*
   a. Increased capacity → three meals a day feeding schedule.
   b. Gastric juices increase in acidity → decrease in GI infections.
   c. Possible voluntary control of anal sphincter.
7. *Genitourinary system*
   a. Bladder capacity increases; to determine bladder capacity in ounces, add 2 to the child's age (e.g., 2-year-old has a bladder capacity of 4 oz or 120 mL).
   b. Ability to "hold" urine increases.
   c. Possible voluntary control of urethral sphincter.
8. *Immune system*
   a. Possible immunity from intrauterine life/maternal transfer disappears.

b. Gradual increase in IgA, IgD, and IgE antibodies.

9. *Neurological system*
   a. Anterior fontanel closed by 18 mo.
   b. Brain increases to 90% of adult size.
   c. Progressive increase in intelligence.
   d. Myelinization of spinal cord is complete.

10. *Sensory system*
    a. Hearing evidences basic auditory skills.
    b. Vision shows evidence of convergence and accommodation; full binocular vision developed; visual acuity: 20/40.

11. *Teething*
    a. Introduce tooth brushing as a "ritual."
    b. By 30 mo: all 20 primary teeth present.
    c. First dental checkup should be between 12 and 18 mo.

12. *Musculoskeletal system*
    a. Lordosis: abdomen protrudes.
    b. Walks like a duck: wide-based gait, side-to-side.

C. **DDST** (see Table 5–6)
   1. *12–18 mo*
      a. Personal-social
         (1) Imitates housework.
         (2) Uses spoon, spilling little.
         (3) Removes own clothes.
         (4) Drinks from cup.
         (5) Feeds doll.
      b. Fine motor-adaptive
         (1) Scribbles spontaneously.
         (2) Builds tower with two to four cubes.
      c. Language
         (1) Three to six words other than "mama," "dada."
         (2) Points to at least one named body part.
      d. Gross motor
         (1) Kicks ball forward.
         (2) Walks up steps.
   2. *19–24 mo*
      a. Personal-social
         (1) Puts on clothing.
         (2) Washes and dries hands.
         (3) Brushes teeth with help.
      b. Fine motor-adaptive
         (1) Builds tower with four to six cubes.
         (2) Imitates vertical line.
      c. Language
         (1) Combines two or three words.
         (2) Speech partially understandable.
         (3) Names picture.
      d. Gross motor
         (1) Throws ball overhand.
         (2) Jumps in place.
   3. *2–3 yr*
      a. Personal-social
         (1) Puts on T-shirt.
         (2) Can name a friend.
      b. Fine motor-adaptive

(1) Thumb wiggles.
(2) Builds tower of eight cubes.
c. Language
   (1) Knows two verbs and two adjectives.
   (2) Names one color.
d. Gross motor
   (1) Balances on one foot briefly.
   (2) Pedals tricycle.

◆ **D. Nursing interventions/parental guidance:**
   1. *Play:* toddler years—generally parallel.
   2. *Toys*—stimulate multiple senses simultaneously:
      a. Push-pull.
      b. Riding toys, e.g., straddle horse or car.
      c. Small, low slide or gym.
      d. Balls, in various sizes.
      e. Blocks—multiple shapes, sizes, colors.
      f. Dolls, trucks, dress-up clothes.
      g. Drums, horns, cymbals, xylophones, toy piano.
      h. Pounding board and hammer, clay.
      i. Finger paints, chalk and board, thick crayons.
      j. Wooden puzzles with large pieces.
      k. Toy record player with kiddie records.
      l. Talking toys: dolls, See 'n Say, phones.
      m. Sand, water, soap bubbles.
      n. Picture books, photo albums.
      o. Nursery rhymes, songs, music.
   3. *Safety*
      a. Refer to Tables 5–7 and 5–8 for additional information on safety and infection control.
      b. Accidents are the leading cause of death among toddlers.
      c. *Motor vehicles:* most accidental deaths in children under age 3 are related to motor vehicles.
         (1) Use only federally approved car seat for all car rides, through age 6 or 60 lb.
         (2) Follow manufacturer directions carefully.
         (3) Make car seat part of routine for toddler.
      d. *Drowning*
         (1) Always supervise child near water: tub, pool, Jacuzzi, lake, ocean.
         (2) Keep bathroom locked to prevent drowning in toilet.
      e. *Burns*
         (1) Turn pot handles *in* when cooking.
         (2) Do *not* allow child to play with electrical appliances.
         (3) Decrease water temperature in house to avoid scald burns.
      f. *Poisonings:* most common in 2-year-olds.
         (1) Consider every nonfood substance a hazard and place out of child's sight/reach.

(2) Keep all medications, cleaning materials, etc. in clearly marked containers in locked cabinets.

(3) Instruct in use of syrup of ipecac (see p. 254).

g. *Falls*

(1) Provide barriers on open windows.

(2) *Avoid* gates on stairs—child can strangle on gate.

(3) Move from crib to bed.

h. *Choking: avoid* food on which child might choke:

(1) Fish with bones.

(2) Fruit with seeds or pits.

(3) Nuts, raisins.

(4) Hot dogs.

(5) Chewing gum.

(6) Hard candy.

III. Preschooler (3–5 yr)

A. Erikson's theory of personality development

1. *Central task:* initiative vs. guilt; central person(s): basic family unit.

2. *Behavioral indicators*

a. Attempts to perform activities of daily living (ADL) independently.

b. Attempts to make things for self/others.

c. Tries to "help."

d. Talks constantly: verbal exploration of the world ("Why?").

e. Extremely active, highly creative imagination: fantasy and magical thinking.

f. May demonstrate fears: "monsters," dark rooms, etc.

g. Able to tolerate short periods of separation.

3. **Parental guidance/teaching**

a. Encourage child to dress self by providing simple clothing.

b. Remind to go to bathroom (tends to "forget").

c. Assign small, simple tasks or errands.

d. Answer questions patiently, simply; do *not* offer child more information than he or she is asking for.

e. Normal to have "imaginary playmates."

f. Offer realistic support and reassurance with regard to fears.

g. Expose to a variety of experiences: zoo, train ride, shopping, sleigh riding, etc.

h. Enroll in preschool/nursery school program; kindergarten at 5 yr.

i. Review *Recommended Health Screenings* (see Tables 5–1 and 5–2) with parents of preschoolers.

4. Additional information about behavioral concerns for each age group may be found in Tables 5–3 and 5–4.

B. Physical growth (by 5 years)

1. *Height and weight*

a. Continued slow, steady growth.

b. Generally grows more in *height* than weight.

c. Posture: appears taller and thinner; "lordosis" of toddler gradually *disappears.*

2. *Vital signs:* see Table 5–5

3. *Cardiac system*

a. Increased heart size (4 times larger than at birth); heart function is comparable to a healthy adult (by 5 years).

b. Heart assumes vertical position in thoracic cavity.

c. May hear "splitting" of heart sounds, as well as innocent murmurs on auscultation.

d. Decreased heart rate, steady blood pressure from toddler values.

4. *Pulmonary system*

a. Increase in amount of lung tissue.

b. Adult-like lung sounds heard on auscultation.

c. Decreased respiratory rate from toddler values.

5. *Gastrointestinal system*

a. Continued increase in size.

b. Position is straighter and more upright than adult stomach → more rapid emptying (defecation, vomiting).

c. Lining still sensitive to roughage and spices.

d. Elimination controlled.

6. *Genitourinary systems*

a. Bladder remains palpable above symphysis pubis.

b. Needs to void frequently, or "accidents" may occur despite sphincter control.

c. Low-grade urinary tract infections common.

7. *Immune system*

a. Growth of lymphoid tissue (especially tonsils).

b. Illnesses (especially respiratory) tend to be more localized.

c. Continued increase in IgA and IgG.

8. *Neurological system*

a. "Handedness" (right or left) is established.

9. *Sensory*

a. Vision—far-sightedness is improving; visual acuity: 20/30.

b. Vision and hearing screening should be conducted before kindergarten, and annually thereafter.

10. *Teeth*

a. All 20 primary or deciduous teeth ("baby teeth") should be present.

b. Annual dental checkups; continue daily brushing.

C. DDST/developmental norms: Table 5–6

1. *3 yr*

a. Personal-social
   (1) Dresses without help.
   (2) Plays board/card games.
b. Fine motor-adaptive
   (1) Picks longer of two lines.
   (2) Copies circle, intersecting lines.
   (3) Draws person, three parts.
c. Language
   (1) Comprehends "cold," "tired," "hungry."
   (2) Comprehends prepositions: "over," "under."
   (3) Names four colors.
d. Gross motor
   (1) Pedals tricycle; hops, skips on alternating feet.
   (2) Broad jumps, jumps in place.
   (3) Balances on one foot.

2. *4 yr*
   a. Personal-social
      (1) Brushes own teeth, combs own hair.
      (2) Dresses without supervision.
      (3) Knows own age and birthday.
      (4) Ties own shoes.
   b. Fine motor-adaptive
      (1) Draws person with six body parts.
      (2) Copies square.
   c. Language
      (1) Knows opposite analogies (two of three).
      (2) Defines seven words.
   d. Gross motor
      (1) Balances on each foot for 5 sec.
      (2) Can walk heel-to-toe.

3. *5 yr*
   a. Personal-social
      (1) Interested in money.
      (2) Knows days of week, seasons.
   b. Fine motor-adaptive
      (1) Prints name.
   c. Language
      (1) Counts to 10.
      (2) Verbalizes number sequences (e.g., telephone number).
   d. Gross motor
      (1) Attempts to ride bike.
      (2) Rollerskates, jumps rope, bounces ball.
      (3) Backward heel-toe walk.

◆ **D. Nursing interventions/parental guidance:**
   1. *Play:* preschool years—associative and cooperative.
      a. Likes to play house, "work," school, firehouse.
      b. "Arts and crafts": color, draw, paint dot-to-dot, color by number, cut and paste, simple sewing kits.
      c. Ball, rollerskate, jump rope, jacks.
      d. Swimming.
      e. Puzzles, blocks (e.g., Lego blocks).
      f. Tricycle, then bicycle (with/without training wheels).
      g. Simple card games and board games.
      h. Costumes and dress-up: "make-believe."
   2. *Safety:* Emphasis shifts from protective supervision to teaching simple safety rules. Preschoolers are "the great imitators" of parents, who now serve as role models.
      a. Refer to Tables 5–7 and 5–8 for additional information on safety and infection control.
      b. Teach child car/*street* safety rules.
      c. Change to "child booster seat" in car at **6 yr or 60 lb.**
      d. Teach child not to go with strangers or accept gifts or candy from strangers.
      e. Teach child danger of *fire*, matches, flame: "drop and roll."
      f. Teach child rules of *water* safety; provide swimming lessons.
      g. Provide adult supervision, frequent checks on activity/location. Despite safety teaching, preschooler is still a child and may be unreliable.

IV. **School age (6–12 yr)**
   A. **Erikson's theory of personality development**
      1. *Central task:* industry vs. inferiority; central person(s): school, neighborhood friend(s).
      2. *Behavioral indicators*
         a. Moving toward complete independence in ADL.
         b. May be very competitive—wants to achieve in school, at play.
         c. Likes to be alone occasionally, may seem shy.
         d. Prefers friends and peers to siblings.
      3. **Parental guidance/teaching**
         a. Be accepting of the child as he or she *is*.
         b. Offer consistent support and guidance.
         c. *Avoid* authoritative or excessive demands on child.
         d. Respect need for privacy.
         e. Assign household tasks, errands, chores.
         f. Review *Recommended Health Screenings* (see Tables 5–1 and 5–2) with parents of school-age children.
      4. Additional information about behavioral concerns for each age group may be found in Tables 5–3 and 5–4.
   B. **Physical growth** (by 12 yr)
      1. *Height and weight*
         a. Almost *double* in weight from 6–12 yr.
         b. Period of slow, steady growth.
         c. 1–2 in/yr.
         d. 3–6 lb/yr.
         e. Girls and boys differ in size at end of school-age years.
      2. *Vital signs:* refer to Table 5–5.
      3. *Cardiac system*
         a. Increased size of left ventricle (to meet demands for increased blood to growing structures).

b. Decreased heart rate, increased blood pressure from preschool values.

4. *Pulmonary system*
   a. Front sinuses develop (by 7 yr).
   b. Lymphatic tissue completes growth (by 9 yr).
   c. Remains well oxygenated on exertion.
   d. Continued decrease in respiratory rate from preschool values; using intercostal muscles more effectively for breathing.

5. *Gastrointestinal system*
   a. Higher metabolic rate requires adequate food and fluids to ensure nutrition and hydration.
   b. Food retained in stomach for longer periods of time.

6. *Genitourinary system*
   a. Bladder capacity increase continues.
   b. Kidneys mature.
   c. Less likely to have fluid and electrolyte (F/E) imbalance as increased conservation of water occurs.

7. *Immune system*
   a. Growth of lymphoid tissue increases, then plateaus, then decreases.
   b. Continued improvement noted with body's increased ability to localize infections.

8. *Neurological system*
   a. Central nervous system matures.
   b. Myelinization continues → increase in both fine motor-adaptive and gross motor skills.

9. *Sensory*
   a. Vision: 20/20 vision well established between 9 and 11 yr.
   b. Should be screened for vision/hearing annually, usually in school.

10. *Teeth*
    a. Begins to lose primary teeth around sixth birthday.
    b. Eruption of permanent teeth, including molars; 28 permanent teeth (by 12 yr).
    c. Dental screening annually, daily brushing.

11. *Pubescence* (preliminary physical changes of adolescence)
    a. Average age of onset: girls at 10, boys at 12.
    b. Beginning of growth spurt.
    c. Some sexual changes may start to occur.

C. **Developmental norms**
   1. *6–8 yr*
      a. Dramatic, exuberant, boundless energy.
      b. Alternating periods: quiet, private behavior.
      c. Conscientious, punctual.
      d. Wants to care for own needs but needs reminders, supervision.
      e. Oriented to time and space.
      f. Learns to read, tell time, follow map.
      g. Interested in money—asks for "allowance."
      h. Eagerly anticipates upcoming events, trips.
      i. Can bicycle, swim, play ball.

   2. *9–11 years*
      a. Worries over tasks; takes things seriously, yet also developing sense of humor—likes to tell jokes.
      b. Keeps room, clothes, toys relatively tidy.
      c. Enjoys physical activity, has great stamina.
      d. Very enthusiastic at work and play; has lots of energy—may fidget, drum fingers, tap foot.
      e. Wants to work to earn money: mow lawn, babysit, deliver papers.
      f. Loves secrets (secret clubs).
      g. Very well behaved outside own home (or with company).
      h. Uses tools, equipment; follows directions, recipes.
      i. By twelfth birthday: paradoxical stormy behavior, onset of adolescent conflicts.

◆ D. **Nursing interventions/parental guidance:**
   1. *Play*
      a. Wants to win, likes competitive games.
      b. Prefers to play with same-sex children.
      c. Enjoys group, team play.
      d. Loves to do magic tricks and other "show-off" activities (e.g., puppet shows, plays, singing).
      e. Likes to collect things: cards, compact discs.
      f. Does simple scientific experiments, computer games.
      g. Has hobbies: needlework, woodwork, models.
      h. Enjoys pop music, musical instruments, radio, audiotapes, videos, posters.

   2. *Safety*—motor vehicles
      a. As passenger: teach to wear safety belt, not distract driver.
      b. As pedestrian: teach bike, street safety.
      c. Teach how to swim, rules of water safety.
      d. Sports: teach safety rules.
      e. Adult supervision still necessary; serve as role model for safe activities.
      f. Suggest Red Cross courses on first aid, water safety, babysitting, etc.
      g. Refer to Tables 5–7 and 5–8 for additional information on safety and infection control.

V. **Adolescent (12–18 yr)**
   A. **Erikson's theory of personality development**
      1. *Central task:* identity vs. role confusion; central person(s): peer group.
      2. *Behavioral indicators*
         a. Changes in body image related to sexual development.
         b. Awkward and uncoordinated in the beginning.
         c. Much interest in opposite sex: females become romantic.

d. Wants to be exactly like peers.

e. Becomes hostile toward parents, adults, family.

f. Concerned with vocation, life after high school.

3. **Parental guidance, teaching**
   a. Offer firm but realistic limits on behavior.
   b. Continue to offer guidance, support.
   c. Allow child to earn own money, control own finances.
   d. Assist adolescent to develop positive self-image.
   e. Review *Recommended Health Screenings* (see Tables 5–1 and 5–2) with parents of adolescents.

4. Additional information about behavioral concerns for each age group may be found in Tables 5–3 and 5–4.

B. **Physical growth** (by 18 yr)
   1. *Height and weight*
      a. Adolescent growth spurt lasts 24–36 mo.
      b. Growth in height commonly *ceases* at 16–17 yr in girls, 18-20 yr in boys.
      c. Boys gain more weight than girls, are generally taller and heavier.
   2. *Vital signs* approximately those of the adult. See Table 5–5. *close to adults*
   3. *Cardiac system*
      a. Increased heart size and strength to near-adult values.
      b. Decreased heart rate, increased blood pressure from school-age values.
   4. *Pulmonary system*
      a. Lungs increase in size to near-adult levels, but not as rapidly as other body systems (may explain lack of energy).
      b. System is "mature" by 12 yr.
      c. Continued decreased respiratory rate from school-age values.
   5. *Gastrointestinal system*
      a. Continued need for increased calories.
   6. *Genitourinary system*
      a. Fully developed; bladder can hold 700 mL.
   7. *Immune system*
      a. Fully developed; infections become increasingly rare in a healthy adolescent.
      b. Lymphoid tissue matures and regresses.
   8. *Neurological system*
      a. Fully developed.
   9. *Sensory*
      a. Fully developed.
   10. *Teeth:* 32 permanent teeth by 18–21 yr.
   11. *Sexual changes*
       a. *Girls*
          (1) Changes in nipple and areola; development of breast buds.
          (2) Growth of pubic hair.
          (3) Change in vaginal secretions.
          (4) Menstruation—12.8 yr (average); range 10.5–15 yr

          (5) Growth of axillary hair.
          (6) Ovulation.
       b. *Boys*
          (1) Enlargement of genitalia.
          (2) Growth of pubic, axillary, facial, and body hair.
          (3) Lowering of voice.
          (4) Production of sperm; nocturnal emission ("wet dreams").

C. **Developmental norms**
   1. *Motor development*
      a. *Early (12–15 yr)*—awkward, uncoordinated, poor posture, decrease in energy and stamina.
      b. *Later (15–18 yr)*—increased coordination and better posture; more energy and stamina.
   2. *Cognitive*
      a. Academic ability and interest vary greatly.
      b. "Think about thinking"—period of introspection.
   3. *Emotional*
      a. Same-sex best friend, leading to strong friendship bonds.
      b. Highly romantic period for boys and girls.
      c. May be moody, unpredictable, inconsistent.
   4. *Social*
      a. Periods of highs and lows, sociability and loneliness.
      b. Turmoil with parents—related to changing roles, desire for increased independence.
      c. Peer group is important socializing agent—conformity increases sense of belonging.
      d. Friendships: same-sex best friend advancing to heterosexual "relationships."

◆ D. **Nursing interventions/parental guidance:**
   1. *Play*
      a. School-related group activities and sports.
      b. Develops talents, skills, and abilities.
      c. Television—watches soap operas, romantic movies, sports.
      d. Develops interest in art, writing, poetry, musical instrument.
      e. Girls: increased interest in makeup and clothes.
      f. Boys: increased interest in mechanical and electronic devices.
   2. *Safety*—motor vehicles (cars and motorcycles)—as *passenger* or as *driver*
      a. Encourage driver education; serve as positive role model.
      b. Teach rules of safety for water sports.
      c. Wants to earn money but still needs guidance: advocate safe job, reasonable hours.
      d. Refer to Tables 5–7 and 5–8 for additional information on safety and infection control.

Developmental Disabilities

I. Down syndrome

    A. *Introduction:* Down syndrome (trisomy 21; mongolism) is a chromosomal abnormality involving an extra chromosome #21 and resulting in 47 chromosomes instead of the normal 46 chromosomes. As a consequence, the child usually has varying degrees of mental retardation, characteristic facial and physical features, and other congenital anomalies. Down syndrome is the most common chromosomal disorder, occurring in approximately 1 of 800 to 1000 live births. Perinatal risk factors include advanced maternal age, especially with the first pregnancy; paternal age is thought to be a related factor.

    ◆ **B. Assessment:**

      1. *Physical characteristics*

        a. Brachycephalic (small, round *head*) with oblique palpebral fissures (Oriental *eyes*) and Brushfield's spots (speckling of *iris*)—depressed *nasal* bridge ("saddle nose") and small, low-set *ears*.

        b. Mouth

          (1) Small oral cavity with protruding tongue causes difficulty sucking and swallowing.

          (2) Delayed eruption/misalignment of teeth.

        c. Hands

          (1) Clinodactyly—in-curved little finger.

          (2) Simian crease—transverse palmar crease.

        d. Muscles: hypotonic ("floppy baby") with hyperextensible joints.

        e. Skin: dry, cracked.

      2. Genetic studies reveal an extra chromosome #21 ("trisomy 21").

      3. *Intellectual characteristics*

        a. Mental retardation—varies from severely retarded to low-average intelligence.

        b. Most fall within "trainable" range, or IQ of 36–51 ("moderate mental retardation").

      4. *Congenital anomalies/diseases*

        a. 30–40% have congenital heart defects: mortality highest in patients with Down syndrome and cyanotic heart disease.

        b. GI: tracheoesophageal fistula (TEF), Hirschsprung's disease.

        c. Thyroid dysfunction, especially hypothyroidism.

        d. Visual defects: cataracts, strabismus.

        e. Hearing loss.

        f. Increased incidence of leukemia.

      5. *Growth and development*

        a. Slow growth, especially in height.

        b. Delay in developmental milestones.

      6. *Sexual development*

        a. Delayed or incomplete.

        b. Females—small number have had offspring (majority have had abnormality).

        c. Males—infertile.

      7. *Aging*

        a. Premature aging, with shortened life expectancy.

        b. Death—generally related to respiratory complications: repeated infections, pneumonia, lung disease.

    ◆ **C. Analysis/nursing diagnosis:**

      1. *Risk for aspiration* related to hypotonia.

      2. *Altered nutrition, less than body requirements,* related to hypotonia or congenital anomalies.

      3. *Altered growth and development* related to Down syndrome.

      4. *Self-care deficit* related to Down syndrome.

      5. *Altered family processes* related to birth of an infant with a congenital defect.

      6. *Knowledge deficit* related to Down syndrome.

    ◆ **D. Nursing care plan/implementation:**

      1. Goal: *prevent physical complications.*

        a. Respiratory

          (1) Use bulb syringe to clear nose, mouth.

          (2) Vaporizer.

          (3) Frequent position changes.

          (4) *Avoid* contact with people with upper-respiratory infections.

        b. Aspiration

          (1) Small, more frequent feedings.

          (2) Burp well during/after infant feedings.

          (3) Allow sufficient time to eat.

          (4) *Position after meals:* head of bed elevated, right side—or on stomach, with head to side.

        c. Observe for signs and symptoms of heart disease, constipation/GI obstruction, leukemia, thyroid dysfunction.

      2. Goal: *meet nutritional needs.*

        a. Suction (before meals) to clear airway.

        b. Adapt feeding techniques to meet special needs of infant/child; e.g., use long, straight-handled spoon.

        c. Monitor height and weight.

        d. As child grows, monitor caloric intake (tends toward obesity).

        e. Offer foods *high in bulk* to prevent constipation related to hypotonia.

      3. Goal: *promote optimal growth and development.*

        a. Encourage parents to enroll infant/toddler in early stimulation program and to follow through with suggested exercises at home.

        b. Preschool/school-age: special education classes.

        c. Screen frequently, using DDST to monitor development.

        d. Help parents focus on "normal" or positive aspects of infant/child.

e. Help parents work toward realistic goals with their child.
4. Goal: *health teaching.*
   a. Explain that tongue-thrust behavior is normal and that food should be refed.
   b. Before adolescence—counsel parents and child about delay in sexual development, decreased libido, marriage and family relations.
   c. In severe cases assist parents to deal with issue of placement/institutionalization.

◆ **E. Evaluation/outcome criteria:**
1. Physical complications are prevented.
2. Adequate nutrition is maintained.
3. Child attains optimal level of growth and development.

II. Attention deficit-hyperactivity disorder (ADHD); behavioral disorder (DSM-IV)

A. *Introduction:* As defined by the American Psychiatric Association (APA), this diagnostic term includes a persistent pattern of inattention or hyperactivity-impulsivity. The exact cause and pathophysiology remain unknown. The major symptoms include a greatly shortened attention span and difficulty in integrating and synthesizing information. This disorder is 10 times more common in boys than girls, with onset before age 7; the diagnosis is based on the child's history rather than on any specific diagnostic test.

◆ **B. Assessment:**
1. The behaviors exhibited by children with ADHD are not unusual behaviors seen in children. The behavior of children with ADHD *differs* from the behavior of non-ADHD children in both *quality* and *appropriateness:*
   a. Motor activity is excessive.
   b. Developmentally "younger" than chronological age.
2. Inattention
   a. Does not pay attention to detail.
   b. Does not listen when spoken to.
   c. Does not do what he or she is told to do.
3. Hyperactivity
   a. Fidgets and squirms excessively.
   b. Cannot sit quietly.
   c. Has difficulty playing quietly.
   d. Seems to be constantly in motion, moving or talking; always "on."
4. Impulsiveness
   a. Blurts out answers before question is completed.
   b. Has difficulty awaiting turn. Interrupts others.

◆ **C. Analysis/nursing diagnosis:**
1. *Altered thought processes* related to inattention and impulsiveness.

2. *Impaired physical mobility* related to hyperactivity.
3. *Risk for injury* related to impulsivity.
4. *Self-esteem disturbance* related to hyperactivity and impulsivity.
5. *Knowledge deficit* related to behavioral modification program, medications, and follow-up care.

◆ **D. Nursing care plan/implementation:**
1. Goal: *teach family and child about ADHD.*
   a. Provide complete explanation about disorder, probable course, treatment, and prognosis.
   b. Answer questions directly, simply.
   c. Encourage family to verbalize; offer support.
2. Goal: *provide therapeutic environment* using principles of behavior modification.
   a. Reduce extraneous or distracting stimuli.
   b. Reduce stress by decreasing environmental expectations (home, school).
   c. Provide firm, consistent limits.
   d. Special education programs.
   e. Special attention to safety needs.
3. Goal: *reduce symptoms by means of prescribed medication.*
   a. Medications: *Ritalin* and *Cylert*—both are CNS stimulants but have a paradoxical calming effect on the child's behavior. *Tofranil* and *Norpramin*—both are tricyclic antidepressants that stimulate the CNS, but also can have paradoxical calming effect on child's behavior; must monitor for arrhythmias.
   b. Health teaching (child *and* parents).
      (1) Need to take medication regularly, as ordered. *Avoid* taking medication late in the day because it may cause insomnia; monitor cardiac status.
      (2) Need for long-term administration, with decreased need as child nears adolescence.
4. Goal: *provide safe outlet for excess energy.*
   a. Alternate planned periods of outdoor play with schoolwork or quiet indoor play.
   b. Channel energies toward safe, large-muscle activities: running track, swimming, bicycling, hiking.

◆ **E. Evaluation/outcome criteria:**
1. Family and child verbalize understanding of "attention deficit disorders."
2. Therapeutic environment enhances socially acceptable behavior.
3. Medication taken regularly, with behavioral improvements noted.
4. Excess energy directed appropriately.
5. Dietary modification implemented.

PSYCHOSOCIAL-CULTURAL FUNCTIONS

Refer to Table 5–9 for information on the nursing care of hospitalized infants and children as it relates to key developmental differences.

TABLE 5–9   Nursing Care of Hospitalized Infants and Children: Key Developmental Differences

Age	◆ Assessment: Reaction to Hospitalization	◆ Nursing Care Plan/Implementation: Key Nursing Behaviors
INFANT	Difficult to assess needs, pain	Close observation, must look at behavioral cues
	Wants primary caretaker	Rooming-in
TODDLER	Separation anxiety	Rooming-in
	Frustration, loss of autonomy	Punching bag, pounding board, clay
	Regression	Behavior modification
	Fears intrusive procedures	Axillary temperatures
PRESCHOOLER	Fearful	Therapeutic play with puppets, dolls
	Fantasy about illness/hospitalization (may feel punished, abandoned)	Therapeutic play with puppets, dolls
	Peak of body mutilation fear	Care with dressings, casts, IMs
	Behavior problems: aggressive, manipulative	Clear, consistent limits
	Regression	Behavior modification
SCHOOL AGE	Cooperative	Use diagrams, models to teach
	Quiet, may withdraw	Indirect interview: tell story, draw picture
	May complain of being bored	Involve in competitive game with peer; encourage peers to call, send get well cards, and visit
ADOLESCENT	Fears loss of control	Provide privacy; allow to make some decisions
	Competitive—afraid of "failing"	Provide tutor prn; get books and homework
	Difficulty with body image	Provide own clothes; give realistic feedback
	Does not want to be separated from peers	Telephone in room; liberal visiting; teen lounge
	Rebellious behavior	Set clear rules; form teen "rap groups"

Pediatrics

DISORDERS AFFECTING FLUID-GAS TRANSPORT

Cardiovascular Disorders

Congenital Heart Disease (CHD)

I. *Introduction:* There are more than 35 documented types of congenital heart defects, which occur in 4 to 10 per 1000 live births. For the purpose of this review, only 5 *major* defects are given. These are presented in Figures 5–1 through 5–5. *Note:* The content has been synthesized for ease in review and recall; for additional study aids, the student may wish to refer to Tables 5–10 and 5–11. **Unit 7** also contains information on congestive heart failure, and **Unit 10** covers the most commonly used drugs, including digoxin and furosemide (*Lasix*).

◆ **II. Assessment:**
  A. Exact cause unknown, but related factors include:
   1. Familial history of CHD, especially in siblings, parents.
   2. Presence of other genetic defects in infant, e.g., Down syndrome, trisomy 13 or 18.
   3. History of maternal prenatal infection with rubella, cytomegalovirus, etc.
   4. High-risk maternal factors:
     a. Age: under 18 yr, over 40 yr.

   b. Weight: under 100 lb, over 200 lb.
   c. Maternal insulin-dependent diabetes.
  5. Maternal history of drinking during pregnancy, with resultant "fetal alcohol syndrome."
  6. Extracardiac defects including tracheoesophageal fistula, renal agenesis, and diaphragmatic hernia.

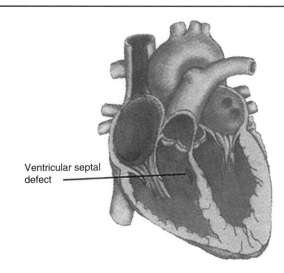

FIGURE 5–2 Ventricular septal defect. An opening between the two ventricles, allowing oxygenated and unoxygenated blood to mix. Shunting of blood occurs due to the higher pressure on the left side of the heart. Ventricular septal defects are classified as membranous or muscular according to location in the septum. (From Ashwill, JW, and Droske, SC: Nursing Care of Children: Principles and Practice. WB Saunders, Philadelphia, 1997.)

FIGURE 5–1 Atrial septal defect. An opening between the two atria, allowing oxygenated blood and unoxygenated blood to mix. Left-to-right shunting of blood occurs due to the higher pressure on the left side of the heart. (From Ashwill, JW, and Droske, SC: Nursing Care of Children: Principles and Practice. WB Saunders, Philadelphia, 1997.)

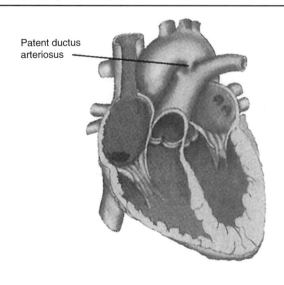

FIGURE 5–3 Patent ductus arteriosus. An artery that connects the aorta and the pulmonary artery during fetal life. It generally closes spontaneously within a few hours to several days after birth. Allows abnormal blood flow from the high-pressure aorta to the low-pressure pulmonary artery, resulting in a left-to-right shunt. (From Ashwill, JW, and Droske, SC: Nursing Care of Children: Principles and Practice. WB Saunders, Philadelphia, 1997.)

B. Most frequent parental complaint: *difficulty feeding.*
1. Infant must be awakened to feed.
2. Has weak suck.
3. May turn blue when eating, especially with cyanotic defects.
4. Infant takes overly long time to feed.
5. Falls asleep during feeding, without finishing.

◆ **C.** Nursing observations
1. *Most frequent symptom*—tachycardia, as body attempts to compensate for lack of oxygen (hypoxia), i.e., heart rate over 160 beats/min.
2. Tachypnea, corresponding to heart rate, i.e., respirations over 60 breaths/min.
3. Cyanosis due to hypoxia:
   a. *Not* with acyanotic defects (unless CHF is present).
   b. *Always* with cyanotic defects ("blue babies").
4. Failure to grow at a normal rate, i.e., slow weight gain, height and weight below the norm due to difficulty feeding and hypoxia.
5. Developmental delays related to weakened physical condition.
6. Frequent respiratory infections associated with increased pulmonary blood flow or aspiration.
7. Dyspnea on exertion due to hypoxia, shunting of blood.
8. Murmurs may or may not be present, e.g., patent ductus arteriosus (PDA) machinery murmur.
9. Changes in blood pressure, e.g., coarctation—increased blood pressure in arms; decreased blood pressure in legs.
10. Possible congestive heart failure—refer to **Unit 7.** *Note:* Infants may *not* demonstrate distended neck veins.
11. Cyanotic heart defects:
    a. **"Tet. spells"**—choking spells with paroxysmal dyspnea: severe hypoxia, deepening cyanosis; relieved by squatting, or placing infant in knee-chest position, which alters cardiopulmonary dynamics, thus increasing the flow of blood to the lungs.

TABLE 5–10   Comparison of Acyanotic and Cyanotic Heart Disease

Feature	Acyanotic	Cyanotic
Shunting of blood	L → R	R → L
Cyanosis	*Not usual* (unless congestive heart failure)	*Always;* "blue babies"
Surgery	Usually done in one stage—technically simple	Usually done in several stages—technically complex
Prognosis	Very good/excellent	Guarded
Major types	1. Atrial septal defect (ASD)	1. Tetralogy of Fallot
	2. Ventricular septal defect (VSD)	2. Transposition of the great vessels
	3. Patent ductus arteriosus (PDA)	
	4. Coarctation of the aorta	

FIGURE 5–4 Tetralogy of Fallot. Four cardiac anomalies make up tetralogy of Fallot: a ventricular septal defect, pulmonary stenosis, an overriding aorta, and right ventricular hypertrophy. There are other associated defects in certain cases. Pulmonary stenosis results in reduction of pulmonary blood flow; the ventricular septal defect allows mixing of oxygenated and unoxygenated blood. (From Ashwill, JW, and Droske, SC: Nursing Care of Children: Principles and Practice. WB Saunders, Philadelphia, 1997.)

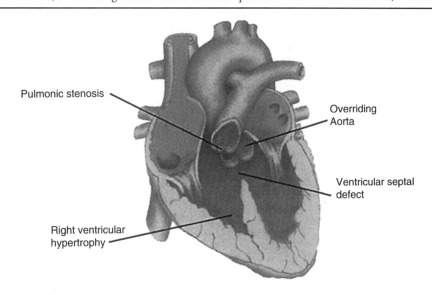

FIGURE 5–5 Transposition of the great arteries. The aorta and the pulmonary artery are reversed; i.e., the aorta rises from the right instead of the left ventricle, and the pulmonary artery arises from the left instead of the right ventricle. Systemic venous blood (unoxygenated blood) returns to the right side of the heart to pass through the aorta back to the body without being oxygenated because of bypassing the lungs. The pulmonary venous blood (oxygenated blood) enters the left side of the heart, returning to the lungs via the pulmonary artery. The systemic (unoxygenated) and pulmonary (oxygenated) circulations are totally separate. There must be some opening (i.e., patent ductus arteriosus or septal defect) to allow blood to mix. (From Ashwill, JW, and Droske, SC: Nursing Care of Children: Principles and Practice. WB Saunders, Philadelphia, 1997.)

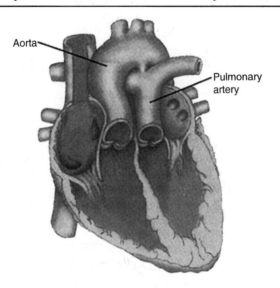

b. Clubbing of fingers and toes—due to chronic hypoxia.
c. Polycythemia (increased red blood cells [RBCs]) with possible thrombi/emboli formation.

◆ **III. Analysis/nursing diagnosis:**
    A. *Ineffective breathing pattern* related to tachypnea and respiratory infection.
    B. *Activity intolerance* related to tachycardia and hypoxia.
    C. *Altered nutrition, less than body requirements,* related to difficulty in feeding.
    D. *Risk for infection* related to poor nutritional status.
    E. *Knowledge deficit* related to diagnostic procedures, condition, surgical/medical treatments, prognosis.

◆ **IV. Nursing care plan/implementation:**
    A. Goal: *promote adequate oxygenation.*
      1. Administer oxygen per physician's order/prn.
      2. Use loose-fitting clothing; tape diapers loosely to *avoid* pressure on abdominal organs, which could impinge on diaphragm and impede respiration.
      3. *Position:* neck slightly hyperextended to keep airway patent; place in knee-chest (squatting) position to relieve "Tet. spell" (choking spell).
      4. Suction prn to clear the airway.
      5. Administer *digoxin,* per physician's order, to slow and strengthen heart's pumping action (refer to **Unit 10** and to Table 5–1 for pediatric pulse rate norms).
      6. Monitor pulse oximetry, as ordered.

TABLE 5–11   Overview of the Most Common Types of Congenital Heart Disease

Type of Defect	Medical Treatment	Surgical Treatment	Prognosis
ACYANOTIC			
Atrial septal defect (ASD)	Clinical trials using device closure during cardiac catheterization	Open chest/open heart surgery with closure through patch (recommended age: preschooler).	Excellent, with survival rate greater than 99%
Ventricular septal defect (VSD)	Clinical trials using device closure during cardiac catheterization	*Palliative treatment:* pulmonary banding; *definitive repair:* same as for **ASD**	Excellent, with 95% or greater survival rate
Patent ductus arteriosus (PDA)	In newborns—attempt pharmacological closure with indomethacin (prostaglandin inhibitor)	Open chest: surgical division or ligation of the patent ductus	Excellent, with survival rate greater than 99%
Coarctation of the aorta	Infants or children with CHF: digitalis and diuretics	Open chest: resection of coarcted portion of aorta with end-to-end anastomosis within first 2 years of life. Nonsurgical: balloon angioplasty	Fair—less than 5% mortality rate
CYANOTIC			
Tetralogy of Fallot	None—supportive prn	Often done in *stages* with definitive repair accomplished within first year of life	Fair—less than 5% mortality rate
Transposition of the great vessels	None—supportive prn	Arterial switch procedure during first weeks of life	Guarded—5–10% mortality rate

B. Goal: *reduce workload of heart to conserve energy.*

1. *Position:* infant seat, semi-Fowler's to promote maximum expansion of the lungs.
2. Provide pacifier to promote psychological rest.
3. Organize nursing care to provide periods of uninterrupted rest.
4. Adjust physical activity according to child's condition, capabilities to conserve energy.
5. Provide diversion, as tolerated, to meet developmental needs yet conserve energy.
6. *Avoid* extremes of temperature to avoid the stress of hypothermia/hyperthermia, which will increase the body's demand for oxygen.
7. Administer diuretics (*Lasix*), per physician's order, to eliminate excess fluids, which increase the heart's workload. *Note:* Refer to **Unit 10.**

C. Goal: *provide for adequate nutrition.*

1. Offer *low-sodium* formula (Lonalac) to minimize fluid retention.
2. Discourage foods with high or added sodium to minimize fluid retention.
3. I&O, daily/weekly weights, and monitor for rate of growth.
4. Limit PO feedings to 20 min to *avoid* overtiring infant. Supplement PO feeding with gavage feeding (prn with physician's order) to meet fluid and caloric needs.
5. Encourage foods *high in potassium* (prevent hypokalemia) and *high in iron* (prevent anemia). *Note:* Refer to **Unit 9.**

D. Goal: *prevent infection.*

1. Standard precautions to prevent infection.
2. Use good hand-washing technique.
3. Limit contact with staff/visitors (especially children) with infections.
4. Monitor for early symptoms and signs of infection; report stat.

E. Goal: *meet teaching needs of patient, family.*

1. Explain diagnostic procedures: blood tests, x-rays, urine, ECG, echocardiogram, cardiac catheterization.
2. Explain condition/treatment/prognosis. Refer to Table 5–11.
3. Review dietary restrictions, medications.
4. Discuss how to adjust realistically to life with congenital heart disease, activity restrictions, etc.

◆ **V. Evaluation/outcome criteria:**

A. Child's level of oxygenation is maintained, as evidenced by pink color in nailbeds and mucous membranes (for both light- and dark-skinned children) and ease in respiratory effort.

B. Energy is conserved, thus reducing the heart's workload as evidenced by vital signs within normal limits.

C. The child's fluid and caloric requirements are met, allowing for physical growth to occur at normal or near-normal rate.

D. The family (and child, when old enough) verbalize their understanding of the type of CHD, its treatment and prognosis.

E. The family and child demonstrate adequate coping mechanisms to deal with CHD.

Disorders of the Blood

I. Leukemia

A. *Introduction:* Known as "cancer of the blood," leukemia is the most common form of childhood cancer, with an incidence of 4/100,000. Acute leukemia is basically a malignant proliferation of white blood cell (WBC) precursors triggered by an unknown cause and affecting all blood-forming organs and systems throughout the body. The onset is typically insidious, and the disease is most common in preschoolers (age 2–6 yr), occurring more frequently in boys.

◆ **B. Assessment:**

1. Major problem—leukopenia: decreased WBC/increased blasts (overproduction of immature, poorly functioning white blood cells).
2. Bone marrow dysfunction results in:
   a. *Neutropenia:* multiple prolonged infections.
   b. *Anemia:* pallor, weakness, irritability, shortness of breath.
   c. *Thrombocytopenia:* bleeding tendencies (petechiae, epistaxis, bruising).
3. Infiltration of reticuloendothelial system (RES): hepatosplenomegaly, abdominal pain, lymphadenopathy.
4. Leukemic invasion of CNS: increased intracranial pressure/leukemic meningitis.
5. Leukemic invasion of bone: pain, pathological fractures, hemarthrosis.

◆ **C. Analysis/nursing diagnosis:**

1. *Risk for infection* related to neutropenia.
2. *Risk for injury* related to thrombocytopenia.
3. *Altered nutrition, less than body requirements,* related to loss of appetite, vomiting, mouth ulcers.
4. *Pain* related to disease process and treatments (e.g., hemarthrosis, bone pain, bone marrow aspiration).
5. *Activity intolerance* related to infection and anemia.
6. *Self-esteem disturbance* related to disease process and treatments (e.g., loss of hair with chemotherapy, moon face with prednisone).
7. *Anticipatory grieving* related to life-threatening illness.
8. *Knowledge deficit* related to diagnosis, treatment, prognosis.

◆ **D. Nursing care plan/implementation:**

1. Goal: *maintain infection-free state.*

Pediatrics

a. Standard precautions to prevent infection.

b. Use good hand-washing technique.

c. Ongoing evaluation of sites for potential infection, e.g., gums.

d. Provide meticulous oral hygiene.

e. Keep record of vital signs, especially temperature.

f. Provide good skin care.

g. Screen staff and visitors (especially children)—restrict anyone with infection.

▶ h. *Protective isolation/reverse isolation* to minimize exposure to potentially life-threatening infection.

i. Discharge planning: return to school, but isolate from chickenpox or known communicable diseases.

2. Goal: *prevent injury.*

a. *Avoid* IMs/IVs if possible, due to bruising and bleeding tendencies.

b. Do *not* give aspirin or medications containing aspirin, which will interfere with platelet formation, thus increasing the risk of bleeding.

c. Use soft toothbrush to *avoid* trauma to gums, which may cause bleeding and infection.

d. *Avoid* "per rectum" suppositories, due to probable rectal ulcers.

e. Supervise play/activity carefully to promote safety and prevent excessive bruising or bleeding.

3. Goal: *promote adequate nutrition.*

a. *Diet:* high *calorie*, high *protein*, high *iron.*

b. Encourage *extra fluids* to prevent constipation or dehydration.

c. I&O, daily weights, to monitor fluid and nutritional status.

d. Allow child to be involved with food selection/preparation; allow child almost any food he or she tolerates, to encourage better dietary intake.

e. Thoroughly wash/peel fresh fruits and vegetables, if child is neutropenic (or *avoid* eating these foods).

f. Serve frequent, small snacks to increase fluid and caloric consumption.

g. Offer dietary supplements to increase caloric intake.

h. Encourage local anesthetics such as dextromethorphan throat lozenges (*Chloraseptic*) before meals to allow child to eat without pain from oral mucous membrane ulcers.

4. Goal: *relieve pain.*

a. Offer supportive alternatives: extra company, back rub. Offer complementary therapies: meditation, visualization (if age appropriate).

b. Administer medications, regularly, before pain becomes excessive.

c. Use bean bag chair for positional changes.

d. *Avoid* excessive stimulation (noise, light), which may heighten perception of pain.

5. Goal: *promote self-esteem.*

a. Stress what child can still do to keep the child as independent as possible.

b. Encourage performance of ADL as much as possible to foster a sense of independence.

c. Provide diversion/activity as tolerated.

d. Give lots of positive reinforcement to enhance a sense of accomplishment.

e. Provide realistic feedback on child's appearance; offer suggestions, such as a wig or cap to cover alopecia secondary to chemotherapy.

f. Encourage early return to peers/school to avoid social isolation.

6. Goal: *prevent complications related to leukemia/prolonged immobility/treatments.*

a. Inspect skin for breakdown, especially over bony prominences, due to poor nutritional intake and limited mobility due to bone pain.

▶ b. Anticipate need for and administer (per physician's order) multiple transfusions of platelets, packed RBCs, etc.

c. Check for hemorrhagic cystitis; *push fluids* (especially with *cytoxan*).

d. Check for constipation or peripheral neuropathy (especially with vincristine). Refer to **Unit 10** for specific information on chemotherapy.

7. Goal: *assist child and parents to cope with life-threatening illness.*

a. Teach rationale for repeated hospitalizations, multiple invasive tests/treatments, long-term follow-up care.

b. Encourage compliance with all aspects of therapy, to increase chances of survival.

c. Support family and their coping mechanisms.

d. Offer factual information regarding ultimate prognosis ("70% cure" for acute lymphocytic leukemia [ALL]).

e. If death appears imminent, assist family to cope with dying and death.

◆ **E. Evaluation/outcome criteria:**

1. Child is maintained in infection-free state.

2. Injuries are prevented or kept to a minimum.

3. Adequate nutrition is maintained.

4. Child is free from pain or can live with minimum level of pain.

5. Child's self-esteem is maintained; child is treated as living (not dying).

6. Complications are prevented or kept to a minimum.

7. Child and family use positive coping mechanisms to deal with illness.

II. Sickle cell anemia

A. *Introduction:* Sickle cell anemia is a congenital hemolytic anemia resulting from a defective hemoglobin (Hgb) molecule (hemoglobin S). It is most common in African Americans (8% have sickle cell trait) and in people of Mediterranean, Hispanic, and Middle Eastern descent. The diagnosis is usually made during the toddler or preschool years, during the first crisis episode following an infection. There is also the need to differentiate between *sickle cell trait* (Sickledex test) and *sickle cell anemia* (hemoglobin electrophoresis). Sickle cell anemia has no known cure.

◆ **B. Assessment:**
1. Increased susceptibility to infection (cause: unknown; most common cause of death in children under 5).
2. Inherited as autosomal recessive disorder (Figure 5–6).
3. Precipitated by conditions of low oxygen tension, dehydration, vascular obstruction, increased blood viscosity.
4. Signs of anemia:
   a. Pallor (in dark-skinned children, do not rely on pallor alone—check hemoglobin [Hgb] and hematocrit [Hct]).
   b. Jaundice, due to excessive hemolysis.
   c. Irritability, lethargy, anorexia, malaise.
5. **Vaso-occlusive crisis:** severe pain (variable sites, e.g., chest, back, abdomen), fever, swelling of hands and feet, joint pain and swelling, all related to hypoxia, ischemia, and necrosis at the cellular level. Most common; usually non–life threatening.
6. **Splenic sequestration crisis:** blood is sequestered (pooled) in spleen; precipitous drop in hemoglobin levels and blood pressure, increased pulse rate, shock, and ultimately death from profound anemia and cardiovascular collapse.

◆ **C. Analysis/nursing diagnosis:**
1. *Altered tissue perfusion* related to anemia and occlusion of vessels.
2. *Pain* related to vaso-occlusion.
3. *Impaired physical mobility* related to pain, immobility.
4. *Knowledge deficit* related to disease process and treatment (e.g., prevention of sickling or infection; genetic counseling).

◆ **D. Nursing care plan/implementation:**
1. Goal: *prevent sickling.*
   a. *Avoid* conditions of low oxygen tension (hypoxia), which causes RBCs to assume a sickled shape.
   b. Provide continuous *extra fluids* to prevent dehydration, which causes sluggish circulation. Avoid temperature extremes.

[handwritten: Live to 40-50 yrs old. Chronic illness.]

FIGURE 5–6 Genetic transmission of sickle cell anemia.

(A) Normal parent and parent who carries trait	**(B)** Two parents who carry trait
A A A | AA | AA S | AS | AS 1:2 (or 2:4) chance offspring will carry trait.	A S A | AA | AS S | AS | SS 1:4 chance offspring will be normal. 1:4 chance offspring will have sickle cell anemia. 1:2 (or 2:4) chance offspring will carry trait.
(C) Normal parent and parent with sickle cell anemia	**(D)** Parent with sickle cell anemia and parent who carries trait
A A S | AS | AS S | AS | AS 4:4 (100%) chance offspring will carry trait.	A S S | AS | SS S | AS | SS 1:2 chance offspring will carry trait. 1:2 chance offspring will have sickle cell anemia.
(E) Two parents with sickle cell anemia	
S S S | SS | SS S | SS | SS 4:4 (100%) chance offspring will have sickle cell anemia.	*Key* AA = normal hemoglobin AS = sickle cell trait SS = sickle cell disease (anemia) *Note:* The odds cited here are for *each* pregnancy.

c. *Avoid* activities that may result in overheating, to prevent dehydration; suggest appropriate clothes; limit time in sun.

d. If dehydrated due to acute illness, supplement with IV fluids and additional oral fluids to reestablish fluid balance.

2. Goal: *maintain infection-free state.*

a. *Standard precautions* to prevent infection.

b. Use good hand-washing technique.

c. Evaluate carefully, check continually for potential infection sites, which may either lead to death due to sepsis or precipitate sickle cell crisis.

d. Teach importance of prevention of sickle cell crisis: adequate nutrition; frequent medical checkups; keep away from known sources of infection.

e. Stress need to report early signs of infection (Acute Chest Syndrome) promptly to physician.

f. Need to balance prevention of infection with child's need for a "normal" life.

g. Administer pneumococcal and influenza vaccines to prevent infection (ages 2, 6, and every 10 years).

3. Goal: *provide supportive therapy during crisis.*

a. Provide bed rest/hospitalization during crisis to decrease the body's demand for oxygen.

b. Relieve pain due to infarction of tissues by administering pain medications as ordered; handle gently and use proper positioning techniques.

c. Apply heat *(never cold)* to affected painful areas to increase blood flow (vasodilation) and oxygen supply.

d. Administer oxygen, as ordered, to relieve hypoxia and prevent further sickling.

e. Administer blood transfusions, as ordered, to correct severe anemia. *Complication:* If hypertransfusion programs are implemented, child may develop "iron overload." *Desferal* chelates the iron so that it can be excreted through the urine or bile to help reduce this complication.

f. Standard meds: hydroxyurea, folic acid.

g. Monitor fluid and electrolyte balance: I&O, weight, electrolytes.

h. Perform ADL for child if unable to care for own needs; encourage self-care as soon as possible to promote independence. *Avoid* stress and fatigue.

4. Goal: *teach child and family about sickle cell anemia.*

a. Provide factual information based on child's developmental level.

b. When asked, offer information regarding prognosis (no known cure).

c. Encourage child to live as normally as possible.

d. Genetic screening and counseling (Figure 5–6).

◆ **E. Evaluation/outcome criteria:**

1. Sickling is prevented or kept to a minimum.

2. Child is maintained in infection-free state.

3. Child/family verbalize that they can cope adequately with crisis.

4. Child/family verbalize their understanding about disease, its management, and its prognosis.

III. Hemophilia

A. *Introduction:* Hemophilia is a bleeding disorder inherited as a sex-linked (X-linked) recessive trait; i.e., it occurs only in males but is transmitted by symptom-free female carriers (Figure 5–7). Hemophilia results in a deficiency of one or more clotting factors, and it is necessary to determine which clotting factor is deficient and to what extent. Classic hemophilia (hemophilia A), a lack of clotting factor VIII, accounts for 75% of all cases of hemophilia.

◆ **B. Assessment:**

1. Major problem is bleeding.

a. In *newborn* male: abnormal bleeding from umbilical cord, prolonged bleeding from circumcision site.

b. In *toddler* male: excessive bruising, possible intracranial bleeding, prolonged bleeding from cuts or lacerations.

c. *General:* hemarthrosis, petechiae, epistaxis, frank hemorrhage anywhere in body, anemia.

2. Need to determine which clotting factor is deficient/missing and extent of deficiency:

a. *Mild:* child has 5–50% of normal amount of clotting factor.

b. *Moderate:* child has 1–5% of normal amount of clotting factor.

c. *Severe:* child has less than 1% of normal amount of clotting factor.

3. Definitive test: PTT

◆ **C. Analysis/nursing diagnosis:**

1. *Risk for injury* related to bleeding tendencies.

2. *Pain* related to hemarthrosis.

3. *Impaired physical mobility* related to bleeding and pain.

4. *Knowledge deficit* related to home care and follow-up.

◆ **D. Nursing care plan/implementation:**

1. Goal: *prevent injury and possible bleeding.*

a. Provide an environment that is as safe as possible, e.g., toys with no sharp edges, child's safety scissors.

b. Use soft toothbrush to prevent trauma to gums.

c. When old enough to shave, use only electric razor (no straight-edge razors).

d. *Avoid* IMs/IVs—but when absolutely necessary, treat as arterial puncture; that is, apply direct pressure to the site for at least 5 min after withdrawing needle.

e. Do **not** use aspirin or medication con-

FIGURE 5–7 Genetic transmission of hemophilia.

(A) "Normal" male and female with trait		
	X	Y
X*	X*X	X*Y
X	XX	XY

1:4 chance will be female with trait.
1:4 chance will be male with hemophilia.
1:2 (or 2:4) chance will be "normal" female/male.

(B) Male with hemophilia and "normal" female		
	X*	Y
X	XX*	XY
X	XX*	XY

1:2 (or 2:4) chance will be female with trait.
1:2 (or 2:4) chance will be "normal" male.

(C) Male with hemophilia and female with trait		
	X*	Y
X*	X*X*	X*Y
X	X*X	XY

1:2 (or 2:4) chance will be female with trait.
1:4 chance will be "normal" male.
1:4 chance will be male with hemophilia.

Key XY = normal male
X*Y = male with hemophilia
XX = normal female
X*X = female carrying hemophilia trait
X*X* = female with possible relative lack of clotting factor–*not* a true hemophiliac (von Willebrand's disease).

Note: The odds cited here are for *each* pregnancy.

taining aspirin (prolongs bleeding/clotting time).

2. Goal: *control bleeding episodes when they occur.*
   a. Local measures: apply direct pressure, elevate, apply ice (vasoconstriction), keep immobilized during acute bleeding episodes only. For epistaxis: child should sit up and lean slightly forward.
   b. Systemic measures: administer clotting *antihemophilic factor* (Factor VIII or DDVAP) via IV infusion. *Note:* These are blood products, so a transfusion reaction is possible.
   c. *Note:* cryoprecipitate (a blood product) is no longer used due to risk of transmission of hepatitis and HIV.
3. Goal: *prevent long-term disability related to joint degeneration.*
   a. Keep *immobilized* during period of acute bleeding and for 24–48 hr afterward to allow blood to clot and to prevent dislodging the clot.
   b. Administer prescribed pain medications *before* physical therapy sessions.
   c. Begin prescribed exercise program, starting with passive range of motion (ROM) and gradually advancing to active ROM, then full exercise program, as tolerated, to maintain maximum joint function.
   d. **Avoid:** prolonged immobility, braces, splints—which can lead to permanent deformities and loss of mobility.
4. Goal: *promote independence in management of own care.*
   a. Encourage child to assume responsibility for choosing safe activities.
   b. Encourage child to attend regular school as much as possible; provide support

through school nurse.
   c. Advise child to wear Medic Alert bracelet.
   d. Caution parents to *avoid* overprotecting child.
   e. Offer child chance to self-limit activities within appropriate limits (parents can offer guidance).
   f. Assist child to cope with life-threatening disorder with no known cure.
5. Goal: *health teaching.*
   a. Between 9 and 12 years of age: child can be taught to self-administer clotting factor IV (before this, family can perform).
   b. As child enters adolescence: begin to discuss issues such as realistic vocations, insurance coverage, genetic transmission (see Figure 5–7).

◆ **E. Evaluation/outcome criteria:**
1. Serious injuries are prevented; bleeding is kept to a minimum.
2. Episodes of bleeding controlled by prompt, effective intervention.
3. There are no long-term disabilities.
4. Child is able to manage own care independently, with minimum supervision.

Pulmonary Disorders

I. Cystic fibrosis
   A. *Introduction:* Cystic fibrosis is a generalized dysfunction of the exocrine glands that produces multisystem involvement. Although the disorder is inherited as an autosomal recessive defect, the basic biochemical defect is unknown. However, its probable cause is an alteration in a protein or an enzyme (e.g., pancre-

atic enzyme deficiency). The basic problem is one of *thick, sticky, tenacious mucous secretions that obstruct* the ducts of the exocrine glands, thus affecting their ability to function. Cystic fibrosis is found in all races and socioeconomic groups, although there is a significantly lower incidence in African Americans. It is a chronic disease with no known cure and guarded prognosis; median age at death in the United States is 27.6 years. Those born in the late 1990s can be expected to survive into their forties with new therapies.

◆ **B. Assessment:**
1. Newborn: *meconium ileus.*
2. Frequent, recurrent *pulmonary infections:* bronchitis, bronchopneumonia, pneumonia, and ultimately chronic obstructive pulmonary disease (COPD) due to mechanical obstruction of respiratory tract caused by thick, tenacious mucous gland secretions.
3. *Malabsorption syndrome:* failure to gain weight, distended abdomen, thin arms and legs, lack of subcutaneous fat due to disturbed absorption of nutrients that results from the inability of pancreatic enzymes to reach intestinal tract.
4. *Steatorrhea:* bulky, foul-smelling, frothy, fatty stools in increased amounts and frequency (predisposed to rectal prolapse).
5. Parents may note that child *"tastes salty"* when kissed, due to excessive loss of sodium and chloride in sweat.
6. *Sweat test* reveals high sodium and chloride levels in child's sweat, unique to children with cystic fibrosis.
7. Sexual development:
    a. *Male:* sterile (due to aspermia).
    b. *Female:* difficulty conceiving and bearing children (due to increased viscosity of cervical mucus, which acts as a plug in the cervical os and mechanically blocks the entry of sperm).

C. Analysis/nursing diagnosis:
1. *Ineffective breathing patterns* related to thick, viscid secretions.
2. *Altered nutrition, less than body requirements,* related to diarrhea and poor intestinal absorption of nutrients.
3. *Decreased cardiac output* related to COPD and decreased compliance of lungs.
4. *Activity intolerance* related to respiratory compromise.
5. *Self-esteem disturbance* related to body image changes.
6. *Knowledge deficit* related to disease process, treatments, medications, genetics.
7. *Noncompliance* (potential) related to complicated and prolonged treatment regimen.

◆ **D. Nursing care plan/implementation:**
1. Goal: *assist child to expectorate sputum.*
    ▶ a. Perform postural drainage as prescribed:

first thing in morning, between meals, before bedtime, *not* after meals to prevent aspiration.
    b. Administer nebulizer treatments, expectorants, mucolytics, bronchodilators. *Avoid* or limit use of medications that suppress cough mechanism.
    c. Provide for exercises that promote position changes and keep sputum moving up and out.
    d. Encourage *high fluid intake* to keep secretions liquefied.
    ▶ e. Suction, administer oxygen prn.
2. Goal: *prevent infection.*
    a. Standard precautions to prevent infection.
    b. Evaluate carefully, check continually for potential infection (especially respiratory); report to physician promptly.
    c. Limit contact with staff or visitors (especially children) with infection.
    d. Administer antibiotics as ordered, to *treat* respiratory infections and *prevent* overwhelming sepsis.
    e. May be placed on *prophylactic* antibiotic therapy *between* episodes of infection.
    f. Teach importance of prevention of infection at home: adequate nutrition, frequent medical checkups, stay away from known sources of infection.
3. Goal: *maintain adequate nutrition.*
    a. Diet: well balanced, *high calorie* and *protein* to prevent malnutrition.
    b. Administer *pancreatic enzyme* (viokase, pancreatin) immediately before *every* meal and *every* snack to enhance the absorption of vital nutrients, especially fats.
    c. If child is unable to swallow tablets, mix pancreatic enzyme powder with cold applesauce.
    d. Administer water-miscible preparations of *fat-soluble vitamins* (A, D, E, K), multivitamins, and iron.
    e. Encourage *extra salt* intake to compensate for excessive sodium losses in sweat (unless CHF is present).
    f. Encourage *extra fluid* intake (e.g., *Gatorade*) to prevent dehydration/electrolyte imbalance.
    g. Daily I&O and weights to monitor nutritional and hydration status.
    h. Encourage child to assume gradually increasing responsibility for choosing own foods within dietary restrictions.
4. Goal: *teach child and family about cystic fibrosis.*
    a. Discuss diagnostic procedures: sweat test, stool specimens.
    b. Review multiple medications: use, effects, side/toxic effects.
    c. Stress need to care for pulmonary systems (major cause of mortality/morbidity).

▶ d. Teach various treatments: postural drainage, nebulizers, oxygen therapy, breathing exercise.

e. Encourage child to assume as much responsibility for own care as possible: medications, treatments, diet.

f. Promote development of healthy attitude toward disease/prognosis (no known cure). Heart/lung transplant may be considered as an option.

g. Refer to appropriate community agencies for assistance with home care.

h. Assist with genetic counseling.

i. Discuss sexual concerns with adolescent.

5. Goal: *promote compliance with treatment regimen.*

a. Encourage child to verbalize anger or frustration at being "different"/body image alterations.

b. Suggest alternatives to postural drainage, e.g., yoga/standing on head.

c. Offer "rewards" for compliance: going swimming with friends or other types of peer activities.

◆ E. **Evaluation/outcome criteria:**

1. Child can clear own airway, expectorate sputum.

2. Child is maintained in infection-free state.

3. Adequate nutrition is maintained.

4. Child and family verbalize understanding of the disease.

5. Child complies with rigors of treatment.

II. Pediatric respiratory infections

◆ A. **Assessment:** general assessment of infant/child with respiratory distress. *Note:* Additional information about specific respiratory infections may be found in Table 5–12.

1. Restlessness—*earliest* sign of hypoxia.

2. Difficulty sucking/eating—parents may state the infant or child has "poor appetite."

3. Expiratory grunt, flaring of nasal alae, retractions.

4. Changes in vital signs: fever, tachycardia, tachypnea.

5. Cough: productive/nonproductive.

6. Wheeze; expiratory/inspiratory.

7. Hoarseness or aphonic crying.

8. Dyspnea or prostration.

9. Dehydration—related to increase in sensible fluid loss and poor PO intake.

10. Color change (pallor, cyanosis)—*later* sign of respiratory distress.

◆ B. **Analysis/nursing diagnosis:**

1. *Ineffective airway clearance* related to infection or obstruction.

2. *Fluid volume deficit* related to excessive losses through normal routes, discomfort and inability to swallow.

3. *Anxiety* related to hypoxia.

4. *Risk for injury* related to spread of infection.

5. *Knowledge deficit* related to disease process, infection control, home care, and follow-up.

◆ C. **Nursing care plan/implementation:**

1. Goal: *relieve respiratory distress by reducing swelling and edema and liquefying secretions.*

▶ a. Environment: cool, high-humidity mist (oxygen) tent (Table 5–13, p. 233).

b. Administer oxygen as ordered.

▰ c. *Position:* semi-Fowler's or in infant seat to promote maximum expansion of the lungs; small blanket or diaper roll under neck to keep airway patent; change position at least q2h to prevent pooling of secretions.

▶ d. Suction/postural drainage prn.

e. Tape diapers loosely and use only loose-fitting clothing to *avoid* pressure on abdominal organs, which could impinge on diaphragm and impede respirations.

◖ f. Administer medications: antibiotics, bronchodilators, steroids.

◖ ▶ g. Monitor temperature q4h/prn; reduce fever with acetaminophen, cool sponges, hypothermia blanket.

2. Goal: *observe for potential respiratory failure related to exhaustion or complete airway obstruction.*

a. Place in room near nurses' station for maximum observation.

b. Monitor vital signs: q1h during acute phase, then q4h.

▶ c. Place emergency equipment near bedside prn: endotracheal tube, tracheostomy set.

d. Monitor closely for signs of impending respiratory failure: increased rapid, shallow respirations, progressive hoarseness/aphonia, deepening cyanosis.

e. Report adverse changes in condition stat to physician.

3. Goal: *maintain normal fluid balance.*

a. May be NPO initially to prevent aspiration.

b. IVs until severe distress subsides and child is able to suck and swallow.

c. Monitor hydration status: I&O, urine specific gravity, weight.

◖ d. When resuming PO fluids—start with sips of clear liquids, advance slowly as tolerated: Pedialyte, clear broth, gelatin, popsicles, fruit juices, ginger ale, cola.

◖ e. **Avoid** milk/milk products, which may cause increased mucous production.

4. Goal: *provide calm, secure environment.*

a. During acute distress: remain with child/family (do not leave unattended).

b. Keep crying to a minimum to prevent severe hypoxia and to reduce the body's demand for oxygen.

c. *Avoid* painful/intrusive procedures if possible.

Pediatrics

TABLE 5–12 **Pediatric Respiratory Infections**

Name	Definition	Age Group	Etiology	◆ Assessment: Definitive Clinical Signs and Symptoms	◆ Plan: Specifics of Treatment	Prognosis
Bronchiolitis/ respiratory syncytial virus (RSV)	Acute viral infection of lower respiratory tract (small, low bronchioles), with resultant trapping of air	Infants 2–12 mo (peak at 2–5 mo)	Respiratory syncytial virus	Hyperinflation of alveoli Scattered areas of atelectasis Acute, severe respiratory distress for first 48–72 hr, followed by rapid recovery	Supportive care during acute phase: ■ Hospitalization ■ Croup tent ■ Clear liquids	Excellent (less than 1% mortality rate)
Croup (acute spasmodic laryngitis)	Paroxysmal attacks (spasms of larynx)	6 mo–3 yr	Viral (possible allergy or psychogenic)	Most common onset at night Inspiratory stridor "Croupy" barking cough Dyspnea Anxiety	Teach parents—turn on hot water in bathroom and close door (steam) Common to treat at home	Excellent (but likely to recur)
Laryngotracheo-bronchitis (LTB)	Acute infection of lower respiratory tract: larynx, trachea, and bronchi	Children less than 5 yr	Viral (possible secondary bacterial infection)	Inspiratory stridor High fever Signs and symptoms of severe respiratory distress Hoarseness, progressing to aphonia and respiratory arrest without treatment	Hospitalization: ■ Tracheostomy set at bedside ■ Racemic epinephrine/steroids ■ Antibiotics if cultures are positive	Good
Epiglottitis	Extremely acute, severe, and rapid, progressive swelling (due to infection) of epiglottis and surrounding tissue	2–5 yr	Bacterial (*H. influenzae* type b)	Abrupt onset—rapid progression; medical emergency Dyspnea, dysphagia Sit up/chin thrust/mouth open Thick muffled voice Cherry red, swollen epiglottis	Do *not* visualize epiglottis unless airway support is immediately available Will need endotracheal tube or tracheostomy for 24–48 hr to maintain patent airway ◖ IV ampicillin for 10–14 days to treat bacterial infection ◖ IV corticosteroids (e.g., Solu-Cortef) to reduce inflammation	Very good if detected and treated early Prevent via Hib immunization

TABLE 5–13   Nursing Care of the Child in a Mist (Oxygen) Tent

Nursing Actions	Rationale
1. Explain purpose of tent to parents and child; stress it is temporary, to make breathing easier.	1. Relieves anxiety
2. Inspect tent for cracks, tears. Repair or replace prn.	2. Leaks will allow oxygen to escape
3. Place unit at head of bed.	3. Child's upper torso and head must be inside tent
4. Cover bed with rubber/plastic sheet.	4. Keeps mattress dry
5. Apply extra linen to bed under tent.	5. Absorbs extra dampness, wetness
6. Secure metal frame to bedspring, and fasten tent to frame.	6. Prevents collapse of tent and keeps it open
7. Select "cool mode" by using the control switch.	7. Provides *cool air* to reduce swelling and edema
8. Close zippers and tuck in edges tightly.	8. Prevents loss of oxygen
9. "Flood" tent with oxygen for 5 min (flow rate = 15 L/min).	9. Raises oxygen concentration
10. Adjust flow rate per physician's order.	10. Usual flow rate is 8–10 L/min to maintain 35–40% oxygen concentration
11. Monitor pulse oximetry or use oxygen analyzer to check concentration at least q2h.	11. Achieves desired therapeutic O_2 levels
12. Place child in tent—stay with child.	12. Relieves anxiety
13. Place folded towel/blanket around child's head; stockinette cap for infant's head.	13. Keeps child dry and prevents heat loss
14. Cover child with blanket.	14. Avoids chilling
15. Selection of toys: (a) Nonflammable. (b) Items that can be wiped dry.	15. (a) Oxygen is highly combustible (b) Avoids bacterial growth
16. Change child's clothes and bed linens frequently (q4h or prn).	16. High humidity in tent will cause moisture to collect on these items

d. Organize nursing care to provide planned periods of uninterrupted rest.

e. Allow parents to room-in, and encourage their participation in care of their child to keep the child relatively calm and reduce anxiety.

f. Allow child to keep favorite toy or security object.

5. Goal: *provide parents with teaching, as necessary.*

   a. *Short term:* discuss equipment, treatments, procedures; offer frequent progress reports, answer parents' questions.

   b. *Long term:* how to handle recurrences, how to check temperature at home, medications for fever, when to call physician about respiratory problem.

◆ D. **Evaluation/outcome criteria:**

   1. No further evidence of respiratory distress.
   2. Resumption of normal respiratory pattern.
   3. Normal fluid balance maintained/restored.
   4. Parents verbalize their concerns and express confidence in their ability to care for their child after discharge.

III. **Apnea-related disorders**

   A. **Apnea of infancy**

   1. *Introduction:* Apnea of infancy is the unexplained cessation of breathing for 20 sec or longer in an apparently healthy, full-term infant who is more than 37 weeks of gestation.

It is usually diagnosed by the second month of life and is generally thought to resolve during the first 12–15 mo of life. The exact cause is unknown. The association between apnea of infancy and sudden infant death syndrome (SIDS) is still controversial. However, infants experiencing significant apnea without a known cause are thought to be at increased risk for SIDS and must be treated accordingly.

◆ 2. **Assessment:**

   a. Unexplained cessation of breathing (apnea) for 20 sec or longer.
   b. Bradycardia.
   c. Color change: cyanosis or pallor.
   d. Limp, hypotonic.
   e. Diagnostic tests including cardiopneumogram, pneumocardiogram, and polysomnography.

◆ 3. **Analysis/nursing diagnosis:**

   a. *Ineffective breathing patterns* related to apnea.
   b. *Anxiety, fear* related to apnea and threat of infant's death.
   c. *Knowledge deficit* regarding home care of infant on an apnea monitor and infant cardiopulmonary resuscitation (CPR).

◆ 4. **Nursing care plan/intervention:**

   a. Goal: *maintain effective breathing pattern.*
   ▶ (1) Apnea monitor on infant at all times, including at home.

(2) Place in room near nurses' station for maximum observation with a nurse or parent present at all times.

(3) Suction, oxygen, and resuscitation equipment readily available if needed.

(4) Observe for apnea or bradycardia; note duration and associated symptoms—color change, change in muscle tone.

▶ (5) If apnea occurs, use gentle stimulation to start infant breathing again. If ineffective, begin CPR (Figures 5–8 through 5–11).

▶ (6) If suctioning is needed, do it gently for the shortest time and least number of times possible to maintain patent airway. *Note:* Repeated, vigor-

FIGURE 5–8 One-rescuer CPR. *If victim is breathing or resumes effective breathing, place in recovery position: (1) move head, shoulders, and torso simultaneously; (2) turn onto side; (3) leg not in contact with ground may be bent and knee moved forward to stabilize victim; (4) victim should not be moved in any way if trauma is suspected and should not be placed in recovery position if rescue breathing or CPR is required. (Modified from Chandra, NC, and Hazinski, MF [eds]: Textbook of Basic Life Support for Healthcare Providers, American Heart Association, Dallas, 1997.)

	Objectives	**ACTIONS**		
		Adult (> 8 yr)	**Child (1–8 yr)**	**Infant (< 1 yr)**
A. AIRWAY	1. Assessment: determine unresponsiveness.	Tap or gently shake shoulder.		
		Say, "Are you okay?"		Speak loudly.
	2. Get help.	Activate EMS.	Shout for help. If second rescuer available, have person activate EMS.	
	3. Position the victim.	Turn on back as a unit, supporting head and neck if necessary (4–10 sec).		
	4. Open the airway.	Head tilt/chin lift.		
B. BREATHING	5. Assessment: determine breathlessness.	Maintain open airway. Place ear over mouth, observing chest. Look, listen, feel for breathing (3–5 sec).*		
	6. Give 2 rescue breaths.	Maintain open airway.		
		Seal mouth to mouth.		Mouth to nose/mouth.
		Give 2 slow breaths. Observe chest rise. Allow lung deflation between breaths.		
		1½–2 sec each	1–1½ sec each	
	7. Option for obstructed airway.	a. Reposition victim's head. Try again to give rescue breaths.		
			b. Activate EMS.	
		c. Give 5 subdiaphragmatic abdominal thrusts (the Heimlich maneuver).		c. Give 5 back blows.
				c. Give 5 chest thrusts.
		d. Tongue-jaw lift and finger sweep.	d. Tongue-jaw lift, but finger sweep only if you see a foreign object.	
		If unsuccessful, repeat a, c, and d until successful.		
C. CIRCULATION	8. Assessment: determine pulselessness	Feel for carotid pulse with one hand; maintain head tilt with the other (5–10 sec).		Feel for brachial pulse: keep head-tilt.
CPR	Pulse absent: begin chest compressions: 9. Landmark check.	Run middle finger along bottom edge of rib cage to notch at center (top of sternum).		Imagine a line drawn between the nipples.
	10. Hand position.	Place index finger next to finger on notch.		Place 2–3 fingers on sternum. 1 finger's width below line. Depress ½–1 in.
		Two hands next to index finger. Depress 1½–2 in.	Heel of one hand next to index finger. Depress 1–1½ in.	
	11. Compression rate.	80–100/min	100/min	At least 100/min
	12. Compressions to breaths.	2 breaths to every 15 compressions	1 breath to every 5 compressions	
	13. Number of cycles.	4	20 (approximately 1 min)	
	14. Reassessment.	Feel for carotid pulse.		Feel for brachial pulse.
		If no pulse, resume CPR, starting with compressions.	If alone, activate EMS. If no pulse, resume CPR, starting with compressions.	
	Pulse present; not breathing: begin rescue breathing.	1 breath every 5 sec (12/min)	1 breath every 3 sec (20/min)	

ous suctioning is associated with prolonged periods of apnea.

(7) Medications: respiratory stimulant drugs (such as caffeine) may be given until 2 to 3 months have passed without an episode of apnea.

(8) *Positions:* side-lying or supine, *never* prone, to prevent SIDS.

(9) Feedings: smaller and more frequent; *avoid* overfeeding, which can lead to reflux and apnea.

b. Goal: *teach parents how to care for their infant at home* (Table 5–14).

(1) Thoroughly explain discharge plans to parents; encourage questions and discussion.

FIGURE 5–9 Two-rescuer CPR. NOTE: Two-rescuer CPR for children ages 1 to 8 years can be performed similarly to that for adults with appropriate changes in chest compressions and ventilations. (Modified from Chandra, NC, and Hazinski, MF [eds]: Textbook of Basic Life Support for Healthcare Providers, American Heart Association, Dallas, 1997.)

Step	Objective	Actions
1. AIRWAY	**One rescuer (ventilator):** Assessment: determine unresponsiveness.	Tap or gently shake shoulder.
		Shout, "Are you okay?"
	Call for help.	Activate EMS.
	Position the victim.	Turn on back if necessary (4–10 sec).
	Open the airway.	Use a proper technique to open airway.
2. BREATHING	Assessment: determine breathlessness.	Look, listen, and feel (3–5 sec).
	Ventilate twice.	Observe chest rise: 1–1.5 sec/inspiration.
3. CIRCULATION	Assessment: determine pulselessness.	Feel for carotid pulse (5–10 sec).
	State assessment results.	Say, "No pulse."
	Other rescuer (compressor): Get into position for compressions.	Hand, shoulders in correct position.
	Locate landmark notch.	Landmark check.
4. COMPRESSION/ VENTILATION CYCLES	**Compressor:** begin chest compressions.	Correct ratio compressions/ventilations: 5:1
		Compression rate: 80–100/min (5 compressions/3–4 sec).
		Say any helpful mnemonic.
		Stop compressing for each ventilation.
	Ventilator: ventilate after every 5th compression and check compression effectiveness. (Minimum of 10 cycles.)	Ventilate 1 time (1.5–2 sec/inspiration).
		Check pulse occasionally to assess compressions.
5. CALL FOR SWITCH	**Compressor:** call for switch when fatigued.	Give clear signal to change.
		Compressor completes 5th compression.
		Ventilator completes ventilation after 5th compression.
6. SWITCH	Simultaneously switch:	
	Ventilator: move to chest.	Move to chest.
		Become compressor.
		Get into position for compressions.
		Locate landmark notch.
	Compressor: move to head.	Move to head.
		Become ventilator.
		Check carotid pulse (5 sec).
		Say, "No pulse."
		Ventilate once (1.5–2 sec/inspiration).
7. CONTINUE CPR	Resume compression/ventilation cycles.	Resume Step 4.

(2) Begin teaching use of apnea monitor and infant CPR techniques several days before discharge; allow parents to handle the monitor and become thoroughly familiar with its use.

(3) Provide parents with emergency response numbers and PHN referral.

(4) Stress need for at least *1 year of ongoing care* with constant use of monitor.

(5) Discuss need for support and refer to local self-help/support group.

(6) Encourage parents to take time for themselves if a reliable caregiver is available who is trained in use of monitor and infant CPR.

FIGURE 5–10 CPR and airway. Procedures for cardiopulmonary resuscitation (*A* through *H*) and clearing airway obstruction (*I* through *K*). (Modified from Chandra, NC, and Hazinski, MF [eds]: Textbook of Basic Life Support for Healthcare Providers, American Heart Association, Dallas, 1997.)

◆ 5. **Evaluation/outcome criteria:**
    a. Effective breathing pattern is established.
    b. Parents verbalize their concerns and express confidence in their ability to care for their infant at home.

B. Sudden infant death syndrome
    1. *Introduction:* SIDS is the *sudden, unexpected* death of an apparently healthy infant under 1 year of age, which remains *unexplained* after a complete postmortem examination. Various theories have been suggested, none proved; research is ongoing. It is the leading cause of death between 1 mo and 1 yr, affecting fewer than 3500 infants annually.

◆ 2. **Assessment:**
    a. Sudden, unexplained death in otherwise "normal" infant; occurs exclusively during sleep.

FIGURE 5–11 Foreign body airway obstruction management. (Modified from Chandra, NC, and Hazinski, MF [eds]: Textbook of Basic Life Support for Healthcare Providers, American Heart Association, Dallas, 1997.)

The truly choking child *cannot speak, becomes cyanotic, and collapses*

	Objectives	Actions		
		Adult (over 8 yr)	**Child (1 to 8 yr)**	**Infant (under 1 yr)**
CONSCIOUS VICTIM	1. Assessment: Determine airway obstruction.	Ask, "Are you choking?" Determine if victim can cough or speak.		Observe breathing difficulty, ineffective cough, no strong cry.
	2. Act to relieve obstruction.	Perform up to 5 subdiaphragmatic abdominal thrusts (Heimlich maneuver).		Give 5 back blows.
				Give 5 chest thrusts.
	Be persistent.	Repeat Step 2 until obstruction is relieved or victim becomes unconscious.		
VICTIM WHO BECOMES UNCONSCIOUS	3. Position the victim: call for help.	Turn on back as a unit, supporting head and neck, face up, arms by sides. Call out, "Help!" Activate EMS. If second rescuer available, have person activate EMS.		
	4. Check for foreign body.	Perform tongue-jaw lift and finger sweep.	Perform tongue-jaw lift. Remove foreign object only if you actually see it.	
	5. Give rescue breaths.	Open the airway with head-tilt/chin-lift. Try to give rescue breaths. If airway is obstructed, reposition head and try to ventilate again.		
	6. Act to relieve obstruction.	Perform up to 5 subdiaphragmatic abdominal thrusts (Heimlich maneuver).		Give 5 back blows.
				Give 5 chest thrusts.
	7. Be persistent.	Repeat steps 4-6 until obstruction is relieved.		
UNCONSCIOUS VICTIM	1. Assessment: Determine unresponsiveness.	Tap or gently shake shoulder. Shout, "Are you okay?"	Tap or gently shake shoulder.	
		If unresponsive, activate EMS.		
	2. Call for help: position the victim.	Turn on back as a unit, supporting head and neck, face up, arms by sides.		
			Call out for help.	
	3. Open the airway.	Head-tilt/chin-lift.		Head-tilt/chin-lift, but do not tilt too far.
	4. Assessment: Determine breathlessness.	Maintain an open airway. Ear over mouth; observe chest. Look, listen, feel for breathing (3-5 seconds).		
	5. Give rescue breaths.	Make mouth-to-mouth seal.		Make mouth-to-nose-and-mouth seal.
		Try to give rescue breaths.		
	6. If chest is not rising, try again to give rescue breaths.	Reposition head. Try rescue breaths again.		
	7. Activate the EMS system.		If airway obstruction not relieved after about 1 minute, activate EMS as rapidly as possible.	
	8. Act to relieve obstruction.	Perform up to 5 subdiaphragmatic abdominal thrusts (Heimlich maneuver).		Give 5 back blows.
				Give 5 chest thrusts.
	9. Check for foreign body.	Perform tongue-jaw lift and finger sweep.	Perform tongue-jaw lift. Remove foreign object only if you actually see it.	
	10. Rescue breaths.	Open the airway with head-tilt/chin-lift. Try again to give rescue breaths. If airway is obstructed, reposition head and try to ventilate again.		
	11. Be persistent.	Repeat steps 8-10 until obstruction is relieved.		

Pediatrics

b. Note overall appearance of infant (differentiate from child abuse).

c. Obtain history from parents—note affect or how parents are dealing with grief.

◆ 3. **Analysis/nursing diagnosis:**
   a. *Dysfunctional grieving* related to loss of infant.
   b. *Knowledge deficit* related to SIDS.

TABLE 5–14   Guidelines for Home Care of Infant on Apnea Monitor

1. Show the parents how to connect the monitor leads.
2. Remind parents to remove the leads unless they are connected to the infant.
3. Stress that the infant must be on the monitor whenever respirations are not being directly observed and that a trained person must be present in the home at all times in case the alarm sounds.
4. Teach parents **not** to adjust the monitor to eliminate false alarms.
5. Explain that the infant will need direct observation whenever loud noises could obscure the monitor alarm, e.g., dishwasher, vacuum.
6. Teach parents what to look for when the alarm sounds, i.e., loose monitor leads vs. apnea.
7. Teach parents how to assess the infant for an episode of apnea, i.e., lack of respirations, duration, color, muscle tone.
8. Teach the parents to first use gentle physical stimulation if the infant experiences an apnea spell, e.g., touching the face or stroking the soles of the feet.
9. Demonstrate infant CPR to be used if tactile stimulation is not effective in reestablishing respirations.
10. Encourage parents to keep emergency numbers posted near the telephone.
11. Explain that monitor will not interfere with normal growth and development. Encourage the parents to promote normal growth and development as much as possible.

Also refer to **Table 5–7: Safety Considerations.**

◆ 4. **Nursing care plan/implementation:**
   a. *Immediate goal:* support grieving parents.
      (1) Stress that nothing could have been done to prevent the death.
      (2) Allow parents to express grief emotions; provide privacy.
      (3) Offer parents opportunity to see, hold infant.
      (4) Explain purpose of autopsy (physician to obtain consent).
      (5) Contact spiritual advisor: priest, rabbi, minister.
      (6) Assist parents to plan what to tell siblings.
   b. *Ongoing goal:* provide factual information regarding SIDS.
      (1) Offer information that is known about SIDS in simple, direct terms (Table 5–15).
      (2) Answer questions honestly.
      (3) Give parents printed literature on SIDS.
      (4) Refer to local/national SIDS foundation group.
   c. *Long-term goal:* assist family to resolve grief.
      (1) Track progress of other siblings.
      (2) Refer to local perinatal bereavement group.
      (3) Consider subsequent pregnancy to be at risk for:
          (a) Attachment/bonding.
          (b) SIDS recurrence.

◆ 5. **Evaluation/outcome criteria:**
   a. Parents are able to express their grief and receive adequate support.
   b. Parents raise questions about SIDS and can understand answers.
   c. Family's grief is resolved; in time, normal family dynamics resume.

TABLE 5–15   SIDS: What To Tell Families

Concern	Facts
Cause	Unknown (possibly related to delayed maturation of cardiorespiratory system)
Incidence	Fewer than 3500 cases annually; leading cause of death between ages 1 mo and 1 yr
When	Occurs during *sleep* (nap, night)
Age	Peak at 2–4 mo; 95% of cases occur by age *6 mo*
Sex	More common in boys
Race	More common in African Americans and Native Americans
Season	More common in *winter,* peaks in January
Siblings	May have greater incidence
Perinatal	More common in preterm infants, in *multiple* births, and in infants with *low Apgar scores*
Socioeconomic	More common in lower socioeconomic classes
Feeding habits	More common in bottle-fed infants; less common in breast-fed infants.
Means of Prevention	Supine (on back) sleeping position prevention (mnemonic: "back to sleep")

DISORDERS AFFECTING PROTECTIVE FUNCTIONS

Immunity and Communicable Diseases

I. Recommended schedule for active immunization of healthy infants and children (Table 5–16).

◆ II. **Assessment:** common side effects of immunizations (occur 24–48 hr after immunization except as noted):
   A. Soreness, redness, tenderness, or lump at injection site.
   B. Fever: brief, mild to moderate.
   C. Crankiness and fussiness; anorexia; drowsiness.
   D. Measles—coryza and rash 7–10 days after immunization.
   E. Rubella—arthralgia and arthritis-like symptoms 2 weeks after immunization.

◆ III. **Nursing interventions/home care** for infant or child who has been immunized:
   A. Explain to parents the reason for each immunization and common side effects.
   B. Suggest acetaminophen for fever or discomfort.
   C. Extra affection and closeness—cuddling, soothing, rocking.
   D. Teach parents to notify MD of untoward, serious, or prolonged side effects.

IV. **Contraindications/precautions to immunizations:**
   A. Child who has a severe febrile illness (e.g., upper respiratory infection [URI], gastroenteritis, or any fever).
   B. Child with alteration in skin integrity: rash, eczema.

Pediatrics

TABLE 5–16

Recommended Childhood Immunization Schedule United States, 2002

		Range of recommended ages			Catch-up vaccination				Preadolescent assessment			
Vaccine ▼ Age ▶	Birth	1 mo	2 mos	4 mos	6 mos	12 mos	15 mos	18 mos	24 mos	4-6 yrs	11-12 yrs	13-18 yrs
Hepatitis B[1]	Hep B #1	only if mother HBsAg (-)									Hep B series	
			Hep B #2			Hep B #3						
Diphtheria, Tetanus, Pertussis[2]			DTaP	DTaP	DTaP		DTaP			DTaP	Td	
Haemophilus Influenzae Type b[3]			Hib	Hib	Hib	Hib						
Inactivated Polio[4]			IPV	IPV		IPV				IPV		
Measles, Mumps, Rubella[5]						MMR #1				MMR #2	MMR #2	
Varicella[6]						Varicella					Varicella	
Pneumococcal[7]			PCV	PCV	PCV	PCV				PCV	PPV	
Hepatitis A[8]											Hepatitis A series	
Influenza[9]						Influenza (yearly)						

— Vaccines below this line are for selected populations —

This schedule indicates the recommended ages for routine administration of currently licensed childhood vaccines, as of December 1, 2001, for children through age 18 years. Any dose not given at the recommended age should be given at any subsequent visit when indicated and feasible. ■ indicates age groups that warrant special effort to administer those vaccines not previously given. Additional vaccines may be licensed and recommended during the year. Licensed combination vaccines may be used whenever any components of the combination are indicated and the vaccine's other components are not contraindicated. Providers should consult the manufacturers' package inserts for detailed recommendations.

C. Child with alteration in immune system; steroids; chemotherapy, radiation therapy; human immunodeficiency virus (HIV)/acquired immunodeficiency syndrome (AIDS) (no live virus vaccine).

D. Child with a known allergic reaction to previous immunization or substance in the immunization.

E. Recent recipient of blood/blood products.

V. **Childhood communicable diseases** (Table 5–17). Basic principles of care:

  A. Standard precautions to prevent communicability/infection.

  B. Fever control with acetaminophen.

  C. Extra fluids for hydration.

  D. General home care procedures: comfort measures/supportive care.

Reye Syndrome

I. *Introduction:* Reye syndrome, first described as a disease entity in the mid-1960s, is a multisystem disorder primarily affecting children between 6 and 12 years of age. Although **not** truly a "communicable disease," studies have confirmed a relationship between aspirin administration during a viral illness (e.g., chickenpox, flu) and the onset of Reye syndrome. The exact cause remains unknown. Reye syndrome is characterized by acute metabolic encephalopathy and fatty degeneration of the visceral organs, particularly the liver. Earlier diagnosis, more sophisticated monitoring equipment, and more aggressive treatment have greatly improved the survival rate of children with Reye syndrome; recovery is generally rapid in those children who do survive.

(handwritten margin note: lapse into coma if not neurologically deficient.)

◆ II. **Assessment:**

A. Onset typically follows a viral illness, just as child appears to be recovering.

B. *Early signs and symptoms:*

  1. Rapidly progressing behavioral changes: irritability, agitation, combativeness, hostility, confusion, apathy, lethargy.

  2. Vomiting, which becomes progressively worse.

C. Rapidly progressive neurological deterioration:

  1. Cerebral edema and increased intracranial pressure.

  2. Alteration in level of consciousness from lethargy through coma, decerebrate posturing, and respiratory arrest.

D. Liver dysfunction, necrosis, and failure:

  1. Elevated serum alanine aminotransferase (ALT) (serum glutamic-oxaloacetic transaminase [SGOT]), aspartate aminotransferase (AST) (serum glutamate pyruvate transaminase [SGPT]), lactate dehydrogenase (LDH), serum-ammonia levels.

  2. Severe hypoglycemia.

  3. Increased prothrombin time, coagulation defects, and bleeding.

◆ III. **Analysis/nursing diagnosis:**

A. *Altered cerebral tissue perfusion* related to cerebral edema and increased intracranial pressure.

B. *Altered hepatic tissue perfusion* related to fatty degeneration of the liver.

C. *Risk for injury* related to coagulation defects and bleeding.

D. *Knowledge deficit* related to diagnosis, course of disease, treatment, and prognosis.

◆ IV. **Nursing care plan/implementation:**

A. Goal: *reduce intracranial pressure.*

  1. Child is admitted to pediatric intensive care unit (PICU) for intensive nursing care, continuous observation, and monitoring.

  2. Monitor neurological status and vital signs continuously.

  3. Assist with/prepare for numerous invasive procedures, including endotracheal (ET) tube/mechanical ventilation and intracranial pressure monitor.

  4. Monitor closely for the development of seizures; institute seizure precautions.

  5. *Position:* elevate head of bed (HOB) 30–45 degrees.

  6. Administer medications as ordered:

    a. Osmotic diuretics (e.g., mannitol) to decrease ICP.

    b. Diuretics (e.g., *Lasix*) to decrease CSF production.

    c. Anticonvulsants (e.g., *Dilantin*, phenobarbital).

B. Goal: *restore and maintain fluid and electrolyte balance, including perfusion of liver.*

  1. Administer IV fluids per physician's order—usually 10% glucose (or higher).

  2. Strict I&O.

  3. Prepare for/assist with Foley catheter placement, CVP, ICP monitor, NG tube, etc.

  4. Monitor serum electrolyte lab values.

C. Goal: *prevent injury and possible bleeding.*

  1. Observe child for petechiae, unusual bruising, oozing from body orifices or tubes, frank hemorrhage.

  2. Check all urine and stool for occult blood.

  3. Monitor lab values, including prothrombin time (PT), partial thromboplastin time (PTT), platelets.

  4. Administer blood products per physician's order.

D. Goal: *provide parents with thorough understanding of Reye syndrome.*

  1. Primary nurse assigned to provide care and follow through with teaching.

  2. Encourage parents' presence, even in PICU—explain all equipment and procedures in simple, direct terms.

  3. Provide factual, honest, and complete information regarding disease, diagnosis, and prognosis.

◆ **V. Evaluation/outcome criteria:**
  A. Intracranial pressure is reduced and normal neurological functioning is restored.
  B. Fluid and electrolyte balance is restored.
  C. No clinical evidence of bleeding is found.
  D. Parents express understanding of Reye syndrome.

Autoimmune Disorders

Streptococcus Infections/Sequelae

Introduction: Group A beta-hemolytic streptococcus is a common infectious organism that causes illness in children and is highly contagious. In themselves, the diseases caused by streptococcus do not seem very serious: e.g., strep throat, otitis media, impetigo, or scarlet fever. The most common treatment for strep is a full course of antibiotic therapy: 10 days of penicillin (or, if allergic, erythromycin). With adequate therapy, generally no sequelae are seen. If the strep is *not* treated, or is only partially treated, the sequelae include serious systemic diseases, with potentially long-term effects. If the effect is manifested primarily in the *heart (carditis),* it is acute rheumatic fever. If the effect is manifested primarily in the *kidneys,* it is *acute glomerulonephritis* (Figure 5–12).

I. Rheumatic fever
  A. *Introduction:* Rheumatic fever is an acute, systemic, inflammatory disease affecting multiple organs and systems: heart, joints, CNS, collagenous tissue, etc. Thought to be autoimmune in nature, it most commonly follows a streptococcus infection (see Figure 5–12) and occurs primarily in school-age children. In addition, it tends to recur, and the risk of permanent heart damage increases with each subsequent attack of rheumatic fever.
◆ **B. Assessment:**
  1. *Major manifestations* (modified Jones criteria)
     a. *Carditis:* tachycardia, cardiomegaly, murmur, congestive heart failure (CHF).
     b. *Migratory polyarthritis:* swollen, hot, red, and excruciatingly painful large joints; migratory and reversible.
     c. *Sydenham chorea* (St. Vitus Dance): sudden, aimless, irregular movements of the extremities; involuntary facial grimaces, speech disturbances, emotional lability, muscle weakness; completely reversible.
     d. *Erythema marginatum:* reddish pink rash most commonly found on the trunk; nonpruritic, macular, clear center, wavy but clearly marked border; transient.

Pediatrics

FIGURE 5–12 Sequelae of strep infections.

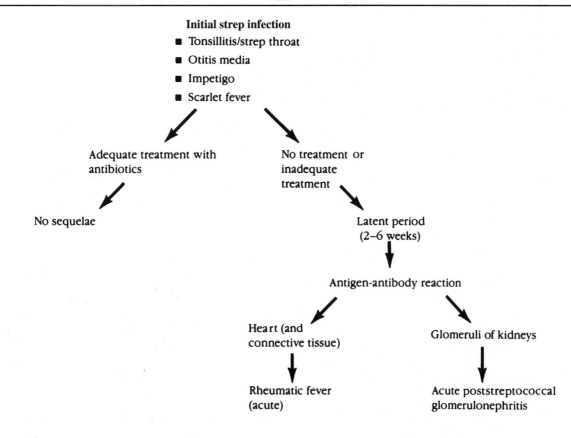

TABLE 5–17   Communicable Diseases of Childhood

Disease

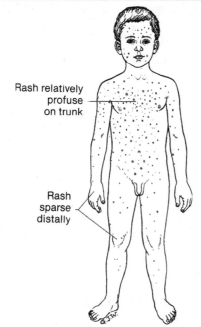

Rash relatively profuse on trunk

Rash sparse distally

Chickenpox (Varicella)

Agent: Varicella zoster virus (VZV)

Source: Primary secretions of respiratory tract of infected person and to a lesser degree skin lesions (scabs not infectious)

Transmission: Direct contact, droplet (airborne) spread, and contaminated objects

Incubation period: 2–3 wk, usually 13–17 days

Period of communicability: Probably 1 day before eruption of lesions (prodromal period) to 6 days after first crop of vesicles when crusts have formed

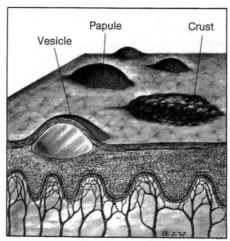

Simultaneous stages
of lesions in chickenpox

Chickenpox (varicella). (From Habif TP: Clinical Dermatology: a color guide to diagnosis and therapy, ed 3, St Louis, 1996, Mosby.)

Clinical Manifestations	Therapeutic Management/ Complications	Nursing Considerations
Prodromal stage: Slight fever, malaise, and anorexia for first 24 hours; rash highly pruritic; begins as macule, rapidly progresses to papule and then vesicle (surrounded by erythematous base, becomes umbilicated and cloudy, breaks easily and forms crusts); all three stages (papule, vesicle, crust) present in varying degrees at one time. *Distribution:* Centripetal, spreading to face and proximal extremities but sparse on distal limbs and less on areas not exposed to heat (i.e., from clothing or sun) *Constitutional signs and symptoms:* Elevated temperature from lymphadenopathy, irritability from pruritus	*Specific:* Antiviral agent acyclovir (Zovirax), varicella-zoster immune globulin (VZIG) after exposure in high-risk children *Supportive:* Diphenhydramine hydrochloride or antihistamines to relieve itching; skin care to prevent secondary bacterial infection *Complications:* Secondary bacterial infections (abscesses, cellulitis, pneumonia, sepsis) Encephalitis Varicella pneumonia Hemorrhagic varicella (tiny hemorrhages in vesicles and numerous petechiae in skin) Chronic or transient thrombocytopenia	▶ Maintain strict isolation in hospital Isolate child in home until vesicles have dried (usually 1 wk after onset of disease), and isolate high-risk children from infected children Administer skin care: give bath and change clothes and linens daily; administer topical calamine lotion; keep child's fingernails short and clean; apply mittens if child scratches Keep child cool (may decrease number of lesions) Lessen pruritus; keep child occupied Remove loose crusts that rub and irritate skin Teach child to apply pressure to pruritic area rather than scratch it If older child, reason with child regarding danger of scar formation from scratching *Avoid* use of aspirin; use of acetaminophen controversial

Continued

TABLE 5–17 Communicable Diseases of Childhood—cont'd

Disease

First day of rash | Third day of rash

Koplik spots on buccal mucosa (see inset)

Confluent maculopapules

Rash discrete

Discrete maculopapules

Measles (Rubeola)

Agent: Virus

Source: Respiratory tract secretions, blood, and urine of infected person

Transmission: Usually by direct contact with droplets of infected person

Incubation period: 10 to 20 days

Period of communicability: From 4 days before to 5 days after rash appears but mainly during prodromal (catarrhal) stage

Koplik spots

Mumps

Agent: Paramyxovirus

Source: Saliva of infected persons

Transmission: Direct contact with or droplet spread from an infected person

Incubation period: 14–21 days

Period of communicability: Most communicable immediately before and after swelling begins

Measles (rubeola). (From Seidel HM and others: Mosby's guide to physical examination, ed 3, St Louis, 1995, Mosby.)

Clinical Manifestations	Therapeutic Management/ Complications	Nursing Considerations
Prodromal (catarrhal) stage: Fever and malaise, followed in 24 hours by coryza, cough, conjunctivitis, *Koplik spots* (small, irregular red spots with a minute, bluish white center first seen on buccal mucosa opposite molars 2 days before rash); symptoms gradually increase in severity until second day after rash appears, when they begin to subside *Rash:* Appears 3–4 days after onset of pro-dromal stage; begins as erythematous maculopapular eruption on face and gradually spreads downward; more severe in earlier sites (appears confluent) and less intense in later sites (appears dis-crete); after 3–4 days assumes brownish appearance, and fine desquamation oc-curs over areas of extensive involvement *Constitutional signs and symptoms:* Anorexia, malaise, generalized lymphadenopathy	Vitamin A supplementation *Supportive:* Bed rest during febrile period Antipyretics Antibiotics to prevent secondary bacterial infection in high-risk children *Complications:* Otitis media Pneumonia Bronchiolitis Obstructive laryngitis and laryngotra-cheitis Encephalitis	Isolation until fifth day of rash; if hospital-ized, institute respiratory precautions Maintain bed rest during prodromal stage; provide quiet activity *Fever:* Instruct parents to administer an-tipyretics; *avoid* chilling; if child is prone to seizures, institute appropriate precautions (fever spikes to 104°F [40°C] between fourth and fifth days) *Eye care:* Dim lights if photophobia present; clean eyelids with warm saline solution to remove secretions or crusts; keep child from rubbing eyes; examine cornea for signs of ulceration *Coryza/cough:* Use cool mist vaporizer; pro-tect skin around nares with layer of petro-latum; encourage fluids and soft, bland foods *Skin care:* Keep skin clean; use tepid baths as necessary
Prodromal stage: Fever, headache, malaise, and anorexia for 24 hours, followed by "earache" that is aggravated by chewing *Parotitis:* By third day, parotid gland(s) (ei-ther unilateral or bilateral) enlarge(s) and reach(es) maximum size in 1–3 days; ac-companied by pain and tenderness *Other manifestations:* Submaxillary and sub-lingual infection, orchitis, and menin-goencephalitis	*Symptomatic and supportive:* Analgesics for pain and antipyretics for fever Intravenous fluid may be necessary for child who refuses to drink or vomits because of meningoencephalitis *Complications:* Sensorineural deafness Postinfectious encephalitis Myocarditis Arthritis Hepatitis Epididymo-orchitis Sterility (extremely rare in adult males)	Isolation during period of communicability; institute respiratory precautions during hospitalization Maintain bed rest during prodromal phase until swelling subsides Give analgesics for pain; if child is unwilling to chew medication, use elixir form Encourage fluids and soft, bland foods; *avoid* foods that require chewing Apply hot or cold compresses to neck, whichever is more comforting To relieve orchitis, provide warmth and local support with tight-fitting underpants (stretch bathing suit works well)

Pediatrics

Continued

TABLE 5–17 **Communicable Diseases of Childhood—cont'd**

Disease

Rubella (German Measles). **A,** Progression of rash. **B,** Appearance of rash. (Source: Habif TP: Clinical dermatology: a color guide to diagnosis and therapy, ed 3, St. Louis, 1996, Mosby.)

Rubella (German Measles)

Agent: Rubella virus

Source: Primarily nasopharyngeal secretions of persons with apparent or inapparent infection; virus also present in blood, stool, and urine

Transmission: Direct contact and spread via infected person; indirectly via articles freshly contaminated with nasopharyngeal secretions, feces, or urine

Incubation period: 14–21 days

Period of communicability: 7 days before to approximately 5 days after appearance of rash

Scarlet Fever

Agent: Group A β-hemolytic streptococci

Source: Usually from nasopharyngeal secretions of infected person and carriers

Transmission: Direct contact with infected person or droplet spread indirectly by contact with contaminated articles, ingestion of contaminated milk or other food

Incubation period: 2–4 days, with range of 1–7 days

Period of communicability: During incubation period and clinical illness approximately 10 days; during first 2 weeks of carrier phase although may persist for months

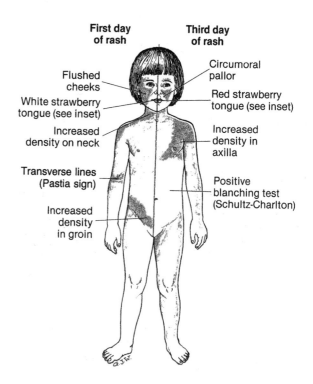

Scarlet fever.

Clinical Manifestations	Therapeutic Management/ Complications	Nursing Considerations
Prodromal stage: Absent in children, present in adults and adolescents; consists of low-grade fever, headache, malaise, anorexia, mild conjunctivitis, coryza, sore throat, cough, and lymphadenopathy; lasts for 1–5 days, subsides 1 day after appearance of rash *Rash:* First appears on face and rapidly spreads downward to neck, arms, trunk, and legs; by end of first day, body is covered with a discrete, pinkish red maculopapular exanthema; disappears in same order as it began and is usually gone by third day *Constitutional signs and symptoms:* Occasionally low-grade fever, headache, malaise, and lymphadenopathy	No treatment necessary other than antipyretics for low-grade fever and analgesics for discomfort *Complications:* Rare (arthritis, encephalitis, or purpura); most benign of all childhood communicable diseases; greatest danger is teratogenic effect on fetus	Reassure parents of benign nature of illness in affected child Use comfort measures as necessary Isolate child from pregnant women
Prodromal stage: Abrupt high fever, pulse increased out of proportion to fever, vomiting, headache, chills, malaise, abdominal pain *Enanthema:* Tonsils enlarged, edematous, reddened, and covered with patches of exudate; in severe cases appearance resembles membrane seen in diphtheria; pharynx is edematous and beefy red; during first 1–2 days tongue is coated and papillae become red and swollen (white strawberry tongue); by fourth or fifth day white coat sloughs off, leaving prominent papillae (red strawberry tongue); palate is covered with erythematous punctate lesions *Exanthema:* Rash appears within 12 hours after prodromal stage; red pinhead-sized punctate lesions rapidly become generalized but are absent on face, which becomes flushed with striking circumoral pallor; rash is more intense in folds of joints; by end of first week desquamation begins (fine, sandpaper-like on torso; sheetlike sloughing on palms and soles), which may be complete by 3 weeks or longer	Treatment of choice is a full course of penicillin (or erythromycin in penicillin-sensitive children); fever should subside 24 hr after beginning therapy Antibiotic therapy for newly diagnosed carriers (nose or throat cultures positive for streptococci) *Supportive measures:* Bed rest during febrile phase, analgesics for sore throat *Complications:* Otitis media Peritonsillar abscess Sinusitis Glomerulonephritis Carditis, polyarthritis (uncommon)	Institute respiratory precautions until 24 hr after initiation of treatment Ensure compliance with oral antibiotic therapy (intramuscular benzathine penicillin G [Bicillin] may be given if parents' reliability in giving oral drugs is questionable) Maintain bed rest during febrile phase; provide quiet activity during convalescent period Relieve discomfort of sore throat with analgesics, gargles, lozenges, antiseptic throat sprays (*Chloraseptic*), and inhalation of cool mist Encourage fluids during febrile phase; *avoid* irritating liquids (citrus juices) or rough foods; when child is able to eat, begin with soft diet Advise parents to consult practitioner if fever persists after beginning therapy Discuss procedures for preventing spread of infection

First day

White strawberry tongue

Third day

Red strawberry tongue

e. *Subcutaneous nodules:* small, round, freely movable, and painless swellings usually found over the extensor surfaces of the hands/feet or bony prominences; resolve without any permanent damage.

2. *Minor manifestations*
   a. Clinical
      (1) Previous history of rheumatic fever.
      (2) Arthralgia.
      (3) Fever—normal in morning, rises in mid-afternoon, normal at night.
   b. Laboratory
      (1) Increased erythrocyte sedimentation rate (ESR).
      (2) Positive C-reactive protein.
      (3) Leukocytosis.
      (4) Anemia.
      (5) Prolonged P-R/Q-T intervals on ECG.

3. Supportive evidence
   a. Recent history of streptococcus infection:
      (1) Strep throat/tonsilitis.
      (2) Otitis media.
      (3) Impetigo.
      (4) Scarlet fever.
   b. Positive throat culture for streptococcus.
   c. Increased ASO titer: indicates presence of streptococcus antibodies; begins to rise in 7 days, reaches maximum level in 4–6 wk.

C. Analysis/nursing diagnosis:
1. *Decreased cardiac output* related to carditis.
2. *Pain* related to migratory polyarthritis.
3. *Risk for injury* related to chorea.
4. *Diversional activity deficit* related to lengthy hospitalization and recuperation.
5. *Knowledge deficit* related to preventing cardiac damage, relieving discomfort, and preventing injury.
6. *Ineffective management of therapeutic regimen* with long-term antibiotic therapy and follow-up care.

D. Nursing care plan/implementation:
1. Goal: *prevent cardiac damage.*
   a. Hospitalization, with strict bed rest.
   b. Monitor apical pulse for changes in rate, rhythm, murmurs.
   c. Evaluate tolerance of increased activity by apical rate: if heart rate increases by more than 20 beats/min over resting rate, child should return to bed.
   d. Offer *low-sodium diet* to prevent fluid retention.
   e. Administer oxygen, digoxin/*Lasix* as ordered (if CHF develops). *Note:* Refer to **Unit 7** for additional information on CHF.
2. Goal: *relieve discomfort.*
   a. Use bed cradle to keep linens from resting on painful joints.
   b. Administer aspirin as ordered to relieve pain.

c. Move child carefully, minimally—support joints.
d. Do *not* massage; do *not* perform ROM exercises; do *not* apply splints; do *not* apply heat/cold. All these treatments will cause increased pain and are *not needed,* because *no* permanent deformities will result from this type of arthritis.

3. Goal: *promote safety and prevent injury related to chorea.*
   a. Use side rails: elevated, padded.
   b. Restrain in bed if necessary.
   c. *No* oral temperatures—child may bite thermometer.
   d. Spoon-feed—no forks or knives, to prevent injury to oral cavity.
   e. Assist with all aspects of ADL until child can care for own needs.

4. Goal: *provide diversion as tolerated.*
   a. Encourage quiet diversional activities: hobbies, reading, puzzles.
   b. Get homework, books; provide tutor as condition permits.
   c. Encourage contact with peers: telephone calls, letters, cards.

5. Goal: *encourage child and family to comply with long-term antibiotic therapy.*
   a. Begin antibiotics immediately, to eradicate any lingering streptococcus infection.
   b. Prepare child/family for minimum of 5 yr of IM injections of penicillin.
   c. Stress need for exact schedule: every 4 wk.
   d. Enlist child's cooperation with therapy, e.g., "hero" badge.

6. Goal: *health teaching.*
   a. To encourage compliance with prolonged bed rest—stress that ultimate prognosis depends on amount of cardiac damage.
   b. Teach necessity for long-term prophylactic therapy for 5 yr initially (with lifelong follow-up), e.g., during dental work, childbirth, surgery (to prevent subacute bacterial endocarditis [SBE]). Instruct adolescents to *avoid* body piercing and tattooing for same rationale.
   c. Teach rationale: permanent cardiac damage is more likely to occur with subsequent attacks of rheumatic fever.

E. Evaluation/outcome criteria:
1. No permanent cardiac damage occurs.
2. Child is free from discomfort or is able to tolerate discomfort.
3. Injuries are avoided.
4. Child's need for diversional activity is met.
5. Child/family comply with long-term antibiotic therapy/prophylactic therapy.

II. Acute poststreptococcal glomerulonephritis
   A. *Introduction:* Acute poststreptococcal glomerulonephritis (APSGN) is a bilateral inflammation

of the glomeruli of the kidneys and is the most common noninfectious renal disease of childhood. It occurs most frequently in early school-age children, with a peak age of onset of 6–7 yr; it is twice as common in boys as in girls. Like rheumatic fever, acute glomerulonephritis is thought to be the result of an antigen-antibody reaction to a streptococcus infection (see Figure 5–12); however, unlike rheumatic fever, it does *not* tend to recur, because specific immunity is conferred following the first episode of APSGN. (Further information about APSGN is found in Table 5–18.)

◆ **B. Assessment:**
1. Typical concerns from family about urine: change in color/appearance of urine (thick, reddish brown; decreased amounts).
2. *Acute edematous phase*—usually lasts 4–10 days.

a. Lab examination of urine:
(1) Severe **hematuria.**
(2) Mild proteinuria.
(3) Increased specific gravity.
b. **Hypertension**
(1) Headache.
(2) Potential hypertensive encephalopathy leading to seizures, increased intracranial pressure.
c. Mild-moderate edema: chiefly periorbital; increased weight due to fluid retention.
d. General:
(1) Abdominal pain.
(2) Malaise.
(3) Anorexia.
(4) Vomiting.
(5) Pallor.
(6) Irritability.

TABLE 5–18   Comparison of Nephrosis and Acute Poststreptococcal Glomerulonephritis

Factor	Nephrosis (Nephrotic Syndrome)	Acute Poststreptococcal Glomerulonephritis (APSGN)
Illness type	Chronic	Acute
Illness course	Characterized by periods of exacerbations and remissions during many years	Predictable, self-limiting, typically lasting 4–10 days (acute edematous phase)
Cause	Unknown	Group A β-hemolytic streptococci
Age at onset	2–4 yr	Early school-age children; peaks at 6–7 yr
Sex	More common among boys	More common among boys
Major signs and symptoms:		
General	Syndrome with variable pathology: massive proteinuria, hypoalbuminemia, severe edema, hyperlipidemia	Hematuria, hypertension
Blood pressure	Normal or decreased	Elevated
Edema	Generalized and severe	Periorbital and peripheral
Proteinuria	Massive	Moderate
Serum protein level	Decreased (6.1–7.9 g/dL)	Increased
Serum lipid level	Elevated	Normal
Potassium level	Normal (3.5–5 mEq/L)	Increased
Treatment	Symptomatic—no known cure; prednisone, cyclophosphamide, furosemide	Penicillin (EES), hydralazine, furosemide
Diet	Decrease sodium, increase protein	Decrease sodium, decrease potassium, increase protein
Fluid restrictions	Seldom necessary	Necessary if output is significantly reduced
Specific nursing care	Treat at home if possible; good skin care; prevent infection	Treat in hospital during acute phase; monitor vital signs, especially blood pressure; on discharge, stress need to restrict activity until microscopic hematuria is gone
Prognosis	Fair; subject to long-term steroid treatment and social isolation related to frequent hospitalizations/confinement during relapses; 20% suffer chronic renal failure	Good; stress that recurrence is *rare* because specific immunity is conferred

(7) Lethargy.
(8) Fever.
3. *Diuresis phase:*
   a. Copious diuresis.
   b. Decreased body weight.
   c. Marked clinical improvement.
   d. Decrease in gross hematuria, but microscopic hematuria may persist for weeks/months.

◆ **C. Analysis/nursing diagnosis:**
1. *Fluid volume excess* related to decreased urine output.
2. *Pain* related to fluid retention.
3. *Altered nutrition, less than body requirements,* related to anorexia and vomiting.
4. *Impaired skin integrity* related to immobility.
5. *Activity intolerance* related to fatigue.
6. *Knowledge deficit* related to disease process, treatment, and follow-up care.

◆ **D. Nursing care plan/implementation:**
1. Goal: *monitor fluid balance, observing carefully for complications.*
   a. Check and record blood pressure at least every 4 hr to monitor hypertension.
   b. Monitor daily weights.
   c. Urine: strict I&O; specific gravity and dipstick for blood every void.
   d. Note edema: extent, location, progression.
   e. Adhere to fluid restrictions if ordered.
   f. Bed rest, chiefly due to hypertension: monitor for possible development of hypertensive encephalopathy (seizures, increased intracranial pressure); report any changes stat to physician.
   g. Administer medications as ordered:
      (1) *Antibiotics*—eradicate any lingering streptococcus infection.
      (2) *Antihypertensives,* e.g., Apresoline.
      (3) Rarely use diuretics—limited value.
      (4) If CHF develops—may use digoxin.
      (5) Refer to **Unit 10** for additional information on medications.
2. Goal: *provide adequate nutrition.*
   a. *Diet: low sodium, low potassium*—to prevent fluid retention and hyperkalemia; *high protein* to replace protein being lost in the urine. Refer to **Unit 9** for additional information on diets.
   b. Stimulate appetite: offer small portions, attractively prepared; meals with family or other children; offer preferred foods, if possible; encourage parents to bring in special foods, e.g., culturally related preferences.
3. Goal: *provide reasonable measure of comfort.*
   a. Encourage parental visiting.
   b. Provide for positional changes, give good skin care.
   c. Provide appropriate diversion, as tolerated.

4. Goal: *prevent further infection.*
   a. Use good hand-washing technique.
   b. Screen staff, other patients, visitors (especially children) to limit contact with infectious persons.
   c. Administer antibiotics if ordered (usually only for children with positive cultures).
   d. Keep warm and dry, stress good hygiene.
   e. Note possible sites of infection: increased skin breakdown secondary to edema.
5. Goal: *teach child and family about APSGN/ discharge planning.*
   a. Teach how to check urine at home: dipstick for protein and blood. (*Note:* occult hematuria may persist for months.)
   b. Teach activity restriction: no strenuous activity until hematuria is completely resolved.
   c. Teach family how to prepare low-sodium, low-potassium diet.
   d. Arrange for follow-up care: physician, home health nurse.
   e. *Stress:* subsequent recurrences are *rare* because specific immunity is conferred.

◆ **E. Evaluation/outcome criteria:**
1. No permanent renal damage occurs.
2. Normal fluid balance is maintained/restored.
3. Adequate nutrition is maintained.
4. No secondary infections occur.
5. Child/family verbalize their understanding of the disease, its treatment, and its prognosis.

Kawasaki Disease (Mucocutaneous Lymph Node Syndrome)

I. *Introduction:* Kawasaki disease (mucocutaneous lymph node syndrome) is an acute, febrile, multisystem disorder believed to be autoimmune in nature. Affecting primarily the *skin* and *mucous membranes of the respiratory tract, lymph nodes,* and *heart,* Kawasaki disease has a low fatality rate (<2%), although vasculitis and cardiac involvement (coronary artery changes) may result in major complications in as many as 20–25% of children with this disease. The disease is not believed to be communicable, and the exact cause remains unknown; *geographic* (living near fresh water) and *seasonal* (late winter, early spring) outbreaks do occur. Kawasaki disease occurs in *both* boys and girls between 1 and 14 years of age; 80% of cases occur in children *under age 5 years.* It may be preceded by URI or exposure to a freshly cleaned carpet. A complete and apparently *spontaneous* recovery occurs within 3 to 4 wk in the majority of cases. Treatment, which is primarily symptomatic, does not appear to either enhance recovery or prevent complications, although recent research indicates that life-threatening complications and long-term disability may be avoided or minimized with early treatment (i.e., gamma globulin) to reduce cardiovascular damage.

◆ **II. Assessment:**

A. Abrupt onset with high fever (102°–106°F) lasting more than 5 days that does *not* remit with the administration of antibiotics and antipyretics.

B. Conjunctivitis—bilateral, nonpurulent.

C. Oropharyngeal manifestations:
 1. Dry, red, cracked lips.
 2. Oropharyngeal reddening and a "strawberry" tongue.

D. Peeling (desquamation) of the palms of the hands and the soles of the feet; begins at the fingertips and the tips of the toes; as peeling progresses, hands and feet become very red, sore, and swollen.

E. Cervical lymphadenopathy.

F. Generalized erythematous rash on trunk and extremities, without vesicles or crusts.

G. Irritability, anorexia.

H. Arthralgia and arthritis.

I. Panvasculitis of coronary arteries: formation of aneurysms and thrombi; CHF, myocarditis, pericardial effusion, arrhythmias, mitral insufficiency, myocardial infarction (MI).

J. Laboratory tests:
 1. Elevated: ESR.
 2. Elevated: WBC count.
 3. Elevated: platelet count.

◆ **III. Analysis/nursing diagnosis:**

A. *Hyperthermia* related to high, unremitting fever.

B. *Altered oral mucous membrane and impaired swallowing* related to oropharyngeal manifestations.

C. *Impaired skin integrity* related to desquamation.

D. *Fluid volume deficit* related to high fever and poor oral intake.

E. *Altered tissue perfusion* (cardiovascular, potential/actual) related to vasculitis or thrombi.

F. *Knowledge deficit* related to disease course, treatment, prognosis.

◆ **IV. Nursing care plan/implementation:**

A. Goal: *reduce fever.*
 1. Monitor rectal temperature every 2 hr or prn.
 2. Administer **aspirin** (*not* acetaminophen [Tylenol]) per physician's order. (*Note:* aspirin is the drug of choice to reduce fever; also has anti-inflammatory effect and antiplatelet effect. Dose is 100 mg/kg/day in divided doses q6h. Monitor for signs of salicylate toxicity.)
 3. Tepid sponge baths or hypothermia blanket per physician's order.
 4. Offer frequent cool fluids.
 5. Apply cool, loose-fitting clothes; use cotton bed linens only (no heavy blankets).
 6. Seizure precautions.

B. Goal: *provide comfort measures to oral cavity to ease the discomfort of swallowing.*
 1. Good oral hygiene with soft sponge and diluted hydrogen peroxide.
 2. Apply petroleum jelly to lips.
 3. *Bland* foods in small amounts at frequent intervals.
 4. *Avoid* hot, spicy foods.
 5. Offer favorite foods from home or preferred foods from hospital selection.

C. Goal: *prevent infections and promote healing of skin.*
 1. Monitor skin for desquamation, edema, rash.
 2. Keep skin clean, dry, well lubricated.
 3. *Avoid* soap to prevent drying.
 4. Gentle handling of skin to minimize discomfort.
 5. Provide sheepskin to lie on.
 6. Prevent scratching and itching—apply cotton mittens if necessary.
 7. Bed rest; *elevate* edematous extremities.

D. Goal: *prevent dehydration and restore normal fluid balance.*
 1. Strict I&O.
 2. Monitor urine specific gravity q8h for increase (dehydration) or decrease (hydration).
 3. Monitor vital signs for fevers, tachycardia, arrhythmia.
 4. Monitor skin turgor, mucous membranes, anterior fontanel for dehydration.
 5. "Force" fluids.
 6. IV fluids per physician's order.

E. Goal: *prevent cardiovascular complications.*
 1. ECG monitor—report arrhythmias or tachycardia.
 2. Administer aspirin (see goal A) and high-dose IV gamma globulin.
 3. Monitor for signs and symptoms of CHF: tachycardia, tachypnea, dyspnea, crackles, orthopnea, distended neck veins, dependent edema.
 4. Monitor circulatory status of extremities—check for possible development of thrombi.
 5. Stress need for long-term follow-up, including ECGs and echocardiograms.

◆ **V. Evaluation/outcome criteria:**

A. Fever returns to normal.

B. Oral cavity heals, and child is able to swallow.

C. Skin heals, and no infection occurs.

D. Normal fluid balance is restored.

E. Normal cardiovascular functioning is reestablished, and no complications occur.

F. Parents/child verbalize their understanding of Kawasaki disease.

Bacterial Infections

Introduction: Acute bacterial ear infection (*acute otitis media*) is common in young children, primarily because their eustachian tube is shorter and straighter than the adult's; this allows for ready drainage of infected mucus from URIs directly into the middle ear. In *some* cases, acute otitis media precedes the onset of *bacterial meningitis,* an extremely serious and potentially fatal disease. Bacterial meningitis is a *medical emergency,* requiring early detection and prompt, aggressive therapy to prevent permanent neurological damage or death. (Refer to section on hydrocephalus, p. 274). Serous otitis (chronic) may result in hearing impairment or loss but is not likely to result in meningitis. Refer to Myringotomy, Table 5–19.

I. Acute otitis media
◆ **A. Assessment:**
1. Fever.
2. Pain in affected ear. Infant may not complain of pain but may tug at ear, cry, shake head, refuse to lie down.
3. Malaise, irritability, anorexia (possibly vomiting).
4. May have symptoms and signs of URI: rhinorrhea, coryza, cough.
5. Diminished response to sound.

TABLE 5–19 Pediatric Surgery: Nursing Considerations

Surgical Procedure	Specific Nursing Care
TONSILLECTOMY (the most frequently performed pediatric surgical procedure)	*Preoperative:* check bleeding and clotting times *Postoperative:* ■ *Position*—place on abdomen or semiprone with head turned to side to prevent aspiration ■ *Observe for most frequent complication—hemorrhage* (frequent swallowing, emesis of bright red blood, shock) *Prevent bleeding:* ■ Do *not* suction—may cause bleeding ■ Do *not* encourage coughing, clearing throat, or blowing nose—may aggravate operative site and cause bleeding ■ Minimize crying *Decrease pain:* ■ Offer ice collar to decrease pain and for vasoconstriction, but do *not* force ■ Acetaminophen for pain (*no* aspirin) *Nutrition:* ■ NPO initially, then cool, clear fluids such as cool water, crushed ice, flavored icepops, dilute (noncitrus) fruit juice ■ No red or brown fluids (punch, Jell-O, icepops, colas), citrus juices, warm fluids (tea, broth), toast, milk/ice cream/pudding, carbonated sodas; progress to soft, bland foods; milk products can increase production of mucus *Teach parents/discharge planning:* ■ Signs and symptoms of infection; call physician promptly ■ 5–10 days postoperatively, expect slight bleeding ■ Continue soft, bland diet as tolerated
MYRINGOTOMY ("tubes")	*Postoperative:* ■ *Position*—place with operated ear down, to allow for drainage. Expect moderate amount of purulent drainage initially ■ Keep external ear canal clean and dry *Teach parents/discharge planning:* ■ Need to keep water out of ear—use special earplugs when bathing or swimming ■ "Tubes" will remain in place 3–7 mo and then fall out spontaneously (with healing of eardrum)
APPENDECTOMY	(Observe same principles of preoperative and postoperative care as for adult GI surgery) NPO until bowel sounds return (24–48 hr) If appendix ruptured preoperatively or intraoperatively, *position* in semi-Fowler's and implement wound precautions; administer antibiotics as ordered Monitor for signs and symptoms of peritonitis Typical course: speedy recovery, with discharge in about 2–3 days and excellent prognosis
HERNIORRHAPHY (umbilical/inguinal)	*Umbilical:* increased incidence in black infants *Inguinal:* increased incidence in boys *Preoperative:* monitor for possible complications of strangulation Routine postoperative GI surgery care Prognosis—excellent, with discharge 24–48 hr postoperatively

◆ **B. Analysis/nursing diagnosis:**

1. *Pain* related to pressure of pus/purulent material on eardrum.

2. *Risk for injury/infection* related to complication of meningitis.

◆ **C. Nursing care plan/implementation:**

1. Goal: *eradicate infection and prevent further complications (meningitis).* Administer antibiotics as ordered.

2. Goal: *relieve pain and promote comfort.*

   a. Administer decongestants as ordered.

   b. Offer analgesics/antipyretics to provide symptomatic relief and to decrease fever.

3. Goal: *health teaching.*

   a. Teach parents that the child needs to finish all medication, even though child will seem clinically better within 24–48 hr.

   b. Review appropriate measures to control fever: antipyretics, cool sponges.

◆ **D. Evaluation/outcome criteria:**

1. Infection is eradicated, no complications.

2. Child appears to be comfortable.

II. Bacterial meningitis

◆ **A. Assessment:**

1. Abrupt onset: initial sign may be a seizure, following an episode of URI/acute otitis media.

2. Chills and fever.

3. Vomiting; may complain of headache, neck pain.

4. Photophobia.

5. Alterations in level of consciousness: delirium, stupor, increased intracranial pressure.

6. Nuchal rigidity.

7. Opisthotonos position: head is drawn backward into overextension.

8. Hyperactive reflexes related to CNS irritability.

B. Analysis/nursing diagnosis:

1. *Risk for infection* related to communicability of meningitis.

2. *Risk for injury* related to CNS irritability and seizures.

3. *Pain* related to nuchal rigidity, opisthotonos position, increased muscle tension.

4. *Sensory/perceptual alterations* related to seizures and changes in level of consciousness.

5. *Altered nutrition, less than body requirements,* related to fever and poor oral intake.

6. *Knowledge deficit* regarding diagnostic procedures, condition, treatment, prognosis.

◆ **C. Nursing care plan/implementation:**

1. Goal: *prevent spread of infection.*

   a. Institute standard precautions.

   b. Enforce strict hand washing.

   c. Institute and maintain *respiratory isolation* for minimum of 24 hr after starting IV antibiotics, at which time child is no longer considered to be communicable and can be removed from isolation.

   d. Supervise all visitors in isolation techniques.

   e. Identify family members and others at high risk: do cultures (*Haemophilus influenzae, Escherichia coli,* etc.); possibly begin prophylactic antibiotics, e.g., rifampin.

   f. Treat with IV antibiotics (as ordered) as soon as possible after admission (after cultures are obtained); continue 10–14 days (until cerebrospinal fluid [CSF] culture is negative and child appears clinically improved).

   g. Anticipate large-dose IV medications only—administer *slowly* in *dilute* form to prevent phlebitis.

   ►h. Restrain as needed to maintain IV.

2. Goal: *promote safety and prevent injury/seizures.*

   a. Maintain seizure precautions. Give anticonvulsants, as ordered (e.g., phenytoin).

   b. Place child near nurses' station for maximum observation; provide private room for isolation.

   c. Minimize stimuli: quiet, calm environment.

   d. Restrict visitors to immediate family.

   e. *Position:* HOB slightly elevated to decrease intracranial pressure. (If opisthotonos: side-lying, for comfort and safety.)

3. Goal: *maintain adequate nutrition.*

   a. NPO or *clear liquids* initially; supplement with IVs, because child may be unable to coordinate sucking and swallowing.

   b. Offer diet for age, as tolerated—child may experience anorexia (due to disease) or vomiting (due to increased intracranial pressure).

   c. Monitor I&O, daily weights.

◆ **D. Evaluation/outcome criteria:**

1. No spread of infection noted; immunize all children against *H. influenzae* type B

2. Safety maintained.

3. Adequate nutrition and fluid intake maintained.

4. Child recovers without permanent neurological damage (e.g., seizure disorders, hydrocephalus).

III. Infestations

A. Lice (pediculosis)

1. *Introduction:* In children, the most common form of lice is pediculosis capitis, or head lice. This parasite feeds on the scalp, and its saliva causes severe itching. Head lice are frequently associated with the sharing of combs and brushes, hats, and clothing; thus, they are more common in girls, especially those with

long hair. Lice are also associated with over-crowded conditions and poor hair hygiene.

◆ 2. **Assessment:**
   a. Severe itching of scalp.
   b. Visible eggs/nits on shafts of hair.

◆ 3. **Analysis/nursing diagnosis:**
   a. *Impaired skin integrity* related to infestation of scalp with lice.
   b. *Risk for impaired skin integrity* related to severe pruritus of scalp.
   c. *Knowledge deficit* related to transmission and prevention of disease and treatment regimen.

◆ 4. **Nursing care plan/implementation:**
   a. Goal: *eradicate lice infestation.* Apply permethrin (*Nix*) as drug of choice for infants and children—rub shampoo in for 4–5 min, then comb with fine-tooth comb to remove dead lice and nits (eggs).
   b. Goal: *prevent spread of lice.*
     (1) Wear gloves and cap to protect self.
     (2) Inspect other family members; treat prn with pediculocide.
     (3) Wash all clothes and linens to kill any lice that may have fallen off the child's hair.
     (4) Encourage short hair, if acceptable.
     (5) Teach preventive measures: do *not* share comb, brushes, hats.

◆ 5. **Evaluation/outcome criteria:** lice are eradicated and do not spread.

B. Pinworms (enterobiasis)
   1. *Introduction:* In children, the most common helminthic infestation is pinworms. Infestation usually occurs when the child places fingers (and the pinworm eggs) into the mouth. Breaking the *anus-to-mouth* contamination cycle can best be accomplished by good hygiene, especially hand washing before eating and after toileting. If one family member has pinworms, it is highly likely that other family members are also infested; therefore, treat the entire family to eradicate the parasite. Pinworms are easily eradicated with antiparasitic medications.

◆ 2. **Assessment:**
   a. Intense perianal itching.
   b. Visible pinworms in the stool.
   c. Vague abdominal discomfort.
   d. Anorexia and weight loss.

◆ 3. **Analysis/nursing diagnosis:**
   a. *Risk for infection/injury* related to the anus-to-mouth contamination cycle of pinworm infestation, severe rectal itching.
   b. *Knowledge deficit* related to transmission and prevention of disease and treatment regimen.

◆ 4. **Nursing care plan/implementation:**
   a. Goal: *eradicate pinworm infestation.* Treat all family members simultaneously with an antiparasitic agent, e.g., *Vermox, Povan.*

   b. Goal: *prevent spread of pinworms.*
     (1) Launder all underwear, bed linens, and towels in hot soapy water to kill eggs.
     (2) Teach family members the importance of good hygiene, especially hand washing before eating (or preparing food) and after toileting. Stress to children to keep their fingers out of their mouths.

◆ 5. **Evaluation/outcome criteria:** Pinworms are eradicated and do not spread; reinfestation does not occur.

Accidents: Ingestions and Poisonings

I. **General principles** of treatment for ingestions and poisonings:
   A. *Prevention:* refer to section on toddler safety, p. 214.
   B. How to induce vomiting:
     1. Drug of choice—*syrup of ipecac* (available over the counter; does not require a physician's order). Families with young children should keep this medication on hand in case of accidental poisoning.
     2. Dose:
       a. 30 mL for adolescents over 12 yr; repeat dosage once if vomiting has not occurred within 20 min.
       b. 15 mL for children 1–12 yr; repeat dosage once if vomiting has not occurred within 20 min. *Note:* Do *not* administer to infants *less than 1 yr* of age without physician's order.
       c. 10 mL for infants 6–12 mo; do *not* repeat dosage.
     3. Follow dose of ipecac with 4–8 oz of tap water or as much water as child will drink. In young children, give water first because child may refuse to drink anything else after tasting the ipecac.
     4. The child *must* vomit the syrup of ipecac to avoid its being absorbed and causing potentially fatal cardiotoxicity (cardiac arrhythmias, atrial fibrillation, severe heart block). If child does not vomit within 20 min of second dose, manually stimulate gag reflex (use spoon to touch back of throat) or assist with gastric lavage.
   C. When **not** to induce vomiting:
     1. Child is stuporous or comatose.
     2. Poison ingested is a corrosive substance or petroleum distillate.
     3. Child is having seizures.
     4. Child is in severe shock.
     5. Child has lost the gag reflex.

II. **Salicylate poisoning**
  ◆ **A. Assessment:**
   1. Determine how much aspirin was ingested, when, which type.

2. Evaluate salicylate levels: normal, 0; therapeutic range = 15–30 mg/dL; *toxic,* >30 mg/dL.

3. *Early* identification of *mild toxicity:*
   a. Tinnitus (ringing in the ears).
   b. Changes in vision, dizziness.
   c. Sweating.
   d. Nausea, vomiting, abdominal pain.
4. *Immediate* recognition of salicylate *poisoning:*
   a. Hyperventilation (*earliest* sign).
   b. Fever—may be extremely high (105°–106°F).
   c. Respiratory alkalosis or metabolic acidosis.
   d. *Late* signs: bleeding tendencies, severe electrolyte disturbances, liver or kidney failure.

◆ B. **Analysis/nursing diagnosis:**
   1. *Ineffective breathing patterns* related to hyperventilation/respiratory alkalosis.
   2. *Fluid volume deficit* (dehydration) related to increased insensible loss of fluids through hyperventilation, increased loss of fluids through vomiting, and increased need for fluids due to hyperpyrexia (fever).
   3. *Risk for injury* related to bleeding.
   4. *Anxiety* related to parental/child feelings of guilt, uncertainty as to outcome, invasive nature of treatments.
   5. *Knowledge deficit* regarding accident prevention.

◆ C. **Nursing care plan/implementation:**
   1. Goal: *promote excretion of salicylates.*
   a. If possible, induce vomiting using syrup of ipecac (save, bring to emergency room).
   ▶ b. Assist with gastric lavage, if appropriate.
   c. Administer activated charcoal as early as possible.
   d. Assist with hemodialysis, as ordered, to promote excretion of salicylates and fluids.
   e. Administer IV fluids, as ordered.
   2. Goal: *restore fluid and electrolyte balance.*
   a. Monitor I&O, urinalysis, specific gravity.
   b. Prepare sodium bicarbonate, administer as ordered to correct metabolic acidosis.
   c. Monitor IV fluids and electrolytes.
   d. NPO initially (nasogastric [NG] tube).
   3. Goal: *reduce temperature.*
   a. **No** aspirin or acetaminophen, which might further complicate bleeding tendencies or lead to liver or kidney damage.
   ▶ b. Supportive measures: cool soaks, ice packs to armpits/groin, hypothermia blanket.
   4. Goal: *prevent bleeding and possible hemorrhage.*
   a. Monitor urine and stools for occult blood.
   ▶ b. Insert NG tube to detect gastric bleeding.
   c. Observe for petechiae, bruising; monitor laboratory values for Hct and Hgb.

   d. Administer vitamin K as ordered to correct bleeding tendencies.
   5. Goal: *health education to prevent another accidental poisoning:*
   a. Teach principles of poison prevention.
   b. Stress need to avoid accidental overdose with over-the-counter medications or dosage mix-ups.
   c. Allow child/parents to verbalize guilt, but *avoid* blaming or scapegoating.

◆ D. **Evaluation/outcome criteria:**
   1. Aspirin is successfully removed from child's body without permanent damage.
   2. Fluid and electrolyte balance is restored and maintained.
   3. Child is afebrile.
   4. Bleeding is controlled, no hemorrhage occurs.
   5. No further episodes of poisoning occur.

III. Acetaminophen poisoning
◆ A. **Assessment:**
   1. Determine how much acetaminophen was ingested, when, and which type.
   2. Evaluate acetaminophen levels: normal = 0; therapeutic range = 15–30 μg/mL; toxic = 150 μg/mL 4 hr after ingestion.
   3. *Initial period* (2–4 hr after ingestion): malaise, nausea, vomiting, anorexia, diaphoresis, pallor.
   4. *Latent period* (1–3 days after ingestion): clinical improvement with asymptomatic rise in liver enzymes.
   5. *Hepatic involvement* (may last 7 days or may be permanent): pain in right upper quadrant (RUQ), jaundice, confusion, hepatic encephalopathy, clotting abnormalities.
   6. Gradual recuperation.

◆ B. **Analysis/nursing diagnosis:**
   1. *Altered tissue perfusion* (liver) related to hepatic necrosis.
   2. *Fluid volume deficit* related to increased loss of fluids secondary to vomiting and diaphoresis.
   3. *Risk for injury* related to bleeding and clotting disorders.
   4. *Anxiety* related to parental/child feelings of guilt, uncertainty as to outcome, and invasive nature of treatments.
   5. *Knowledge deficit* regarding accident prevention.

◆ C. **Nursing care plan/implementation:**
   1. Goal: *promote excretion of acetaminophen.*
   a. If possible, induce vomiting; save, bring to emergency department.
   ▶ b. Assist with gastric lavage, if appropriate.
   c. Administer activated charcoal.
   d. Assist with obtaining acetaminophen level 4 hr after ingestion.
   2. Goal: *prevent permanent liver damage.*

a. Treatment must begin as soon as possible; therapy begun later than 10 hr after ingestion has no value.

b. Administer the antidote (acetylcysteine [*Mucomyst*]) per physician's order. Usually administered through NG tube because of offensive odor. Given as one loading dose and 17 maintenance doses.

c. Monitor hepatic functioning—assist with obtaining specimens and check results frequently; be aware that liver enzymes will rise and peak within 3 days and then should rapidly return to normal.

3. Goal: *restore fluid and electrolyte balance.*
   a. Monitor vital signs and perform neurological checks every 2–4 hr and prn.
   b. Monitor I&O; urine analysis, including specific gravity; and weight.
   c. Monitor IV fluids as ordered.

4. Goal: *prevent bleeding.*
   a. Assist in monitoring child's PT; notify physician of significant changes.
   b. Monitor urine and stool for occult blood.
   c. Observe for and report any petechiae or unusual bruising.

5. Goal: *health education to prevent another accidental poisoning.* (See goal 5, **Nursing care plan/implementation,** Salicylate poisoning.)

◆ **D. Evaluation/outcome criteria:**
   1. Acetaminophen is successfully removed from child's body.
   2. Normal liver functioning is reestablished.
   3. Fluid and electrolyte balance is restored and maintained.
   4. No further episodes of poisoning occur.

IV. Lead poisoning (plumbism)

A. *Introduction:* Lead poisoning is a heavy-metal poisoning that occurs from ingestion or inhalation of lead. In children, this is most common in the *toddler* age group (1–3 yr) and is usually a *chronic* type of poisoning that occurs as the result of repeated ingestions of lead. Children who engage in the practice of *pica,* the ingestion of nonnutritive substances, often ingest lead in flecks of lead-based paint from walls, furniture, or toys. In addition, research demonstrates that the parent-child relationship is a significant variable in lead poisoning; typically, there is a lack of adequate parental supervision that enables the child to engage in pica repeatedly over a fairly long time, until symptoms of lead poisoning become evident. (Figure 5–13 shows the pathophysiological effects of lead poisoning.)

◆ **B. Assessment:**
   1. Investigate history of pica (ingestion of nonnutritive substance).
   2. Evaluate parent-child relationship.
   3. *Chronic lead poisoning:* vague, crampy abdominal pain; constipation; anorexia and vomiting; listlessness.

4. Neurological, renal, hematological effects: see Figure 5–13.
5. "Blood-lead line"—bluish black line seen in gums.
6. X-rays: lead lines in long bones and flecks of lead in GI tract.
7. Elevated serum-blood-lead levels: ≥ 20 μg/dL requires clinical management; ≥ 45 μg/dL requires parenteral chelating therapy.

◆ **C. Analysis/nursing diagnosis:**
   1. *Altered thought processes* related to neurotoxicity.
   2. *Activity intolerance* (and *risk for infection*) related to anemia.
   3. *Altered urinary elimination* related to excretion of lead by kidneys.
   4. *Pain* related to lead poisoning and its treatment.
   5. *Knowledge deficit* related to etiology of lead poisoning.

◆ **D. Nursing care plan/implementation:**
   1. Goal: *promote excretion of lead.*
      a. Administer chelating agents (EDTA [IM or IV], BAL [IM only]) as ordered. Chelation therapy typically continues over several days, with multiple treatments daily.
      b. Monitor kidney function carefully: the treatment itself is potentially nephrotoxic. Maintain adequate oral intake of fluids.
      c. Institute seizure precautions.
   2. Goal: *prevent reingestion of lead.*
      a. Determine primary source of poisoning.
      b. Eliminate source from child's environment before discharge.
      c. Follow up with home care referral.
         (1) Screen other siblings prn.
         (2) Monitor "blood-lead level" of all children in the home.
   3. Goal: *assist child to cope with multiple painful injections when treated with IM chelation therapy.*
      a. Prepare child for treatment regimen.
      b. Stress that this is *not* a punishment.
      c. Rotate sites as much as possible.
      d. May use a local anesthetic, e.g., procaine, injected simultaneously with chelating agent to decrease pain of injections.
      e. Apply warm soaks to injection sites: may help lessen pain.
      f. Encourage child to self-limit gross muscle activity (which increases pain).
      g. Offer child safe outlets for anger, fear, frustration—punching bag, pounding board, clay.
      h. Offer opportunity for medical play with empty syringes, etc.
   4. Goal: *health teaching.*
      a. Stress (to child and parents) that removing the lead is the only way to prevent

FIGURE 5–13 Pathophysiological effects of lead poisoning.

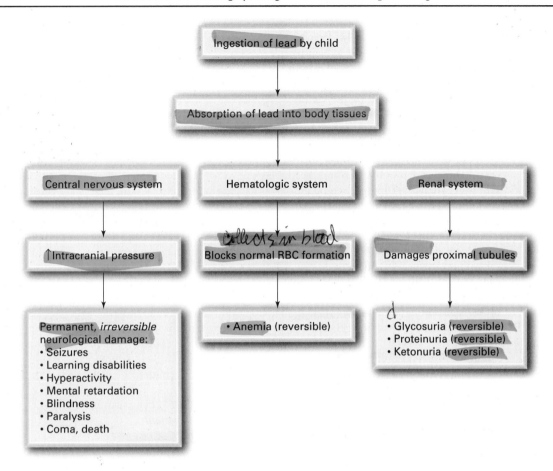

permanent, irreversible neurological damage (irreversible damage may have *already* occurred).

b. Teach that the chelating agent binds with the lead and promotes its excretion through the kidneys.

◆ **E. Evaluation/outcome criteria:**

1. Lead is successfully removed from child's body without permanent damage.
2. No further episodes of lead poisoning.
3. Child copes successfully with the disease and its treatment.

Allergic Response: Threats to Health Status

I. Infantile eczema (atopic dermatitis)

A. *Introduction:* Eczema is an allergic skin reaction, most commonly to foods (e.g., cow's milk, eggs). It is most common in *infants* and young children (under 2 yr). Infantile eczema generally undergoes permanent, spontaneous remission by age 3 years; however, approximately 50% of children who have had infantile eczema develop asthma during the preschool or school-age years.

◆ **B. Assessment:**

1. Erythematous lesions, beginning on cheeks and spreading to rest of face and scalp.
2. May spread to rest of body, especially in flexor surfaces, e.g., antecubital space.
3. Lesions may ooze or crust over.
4. Severe pruritus, which may lead to secondary infection.
5. Lymphadenopathy near site of rash.
6. Unaffected skin tends to be dry and rough.
7. Systemic manifestations are rare—but child may be irritable, cranky.

◆ **C. Analysis/nursing diagnosis:**

1. *Impaired tissue integrity* related to lesions.
2. *Pain* related to pruritus.
3. *Risk for (secondary) infection* related to breaks in the skin (first line of defense) and itching.
4. *Knowledge deficit* related to care of child with eczema, prognosis, how to prevent exacerbations.

◆ **D. Nursing care plan/implementation:**

1. Goal: *promote healing of lesions.*

Burow's solution

a. *Wet method:* frequent tepid baths (up to 4 times a day) followed by immediate application of a lubricant while the skin is still moist; **no soap** or very mild, nonperfumed soap is used (e.g., Dove, Neutrogena); most useful method if child lives in a *dry* climate.

b. *Dry method:* infrequent baths; cleanse skin with nonlipid, hydrophilic agent (e.g., cetaphil); most useful method if child lives in a *humid* climate.

c. Can add cornstarch to bath water to relieve itching and promote healing; keep skin well hydrated by applying emollients containing petrolatum or lanolin, which are occlusive and prevent evaporation of moisture.

d. Apply wet soaks with Burow's solution (aluminum acetate solution; topical astringent and antiseptic); wet soaks should not be used for more than 3 days at a time.

e. Protect child from possible sources of infection; standard precautions to prevent infection.

f. **Absolutely no** immunizations during acute exacerbations of eczema because of the possibility of an overwhelming dermatitis, allergic reaction, shock, or even death.

g. Apply topical creams/ointments as prescribed: A and D emollient ointment, hydrocortisone cream to promote healing.

2. Goal: *provide relief from itching/keep child from itching.*

a. Administer systemic oral antihistamines as ordered (e.g., *Benadryl* or *Atarax*) to break itch-scratch cycle. Most useful at bedtime when itching tends to increase.

b. Keep nails trimmed short—may need mittens (preferable not to use elbow restraints, because the antecubital space is a common site for eczema).

c. Use clothes and bedlinens that are nonirritating, i.e., pure cotton (**no** wool or blends).

d. Institute *elimination/hypoallergenic diet:*
   (1) *No* milk or milk products.
   (2) Change to lactose-free formula, e.g., Isomil. (soy base)
   (3) *Avoid* eggs, wheat, nuts, beans, chocolate.

e. *No* stuffed animals or hairy dolls.

3. Goal: *provide discharge planning/teaching for parents and child.*

a. Include all above information.

b. Include information on course of disease: characterized by exacerbations and remissions throughout early years.

c. Include information on prognosis: 50–60% will go into spontaneous (and permanent) remission during preschool years; 40–50% will develop asthma/hayfever during school-age years.

◆ **E. Evaluation/outcome criteria:**
1. Lesions heal well, without secondary infection.
2. Adequate relief from itching is achieved.
3. Parents verbalize understanding of eczema, prognosis, and how to prevent exacerbations.

II. Asthma

A. *Introduction:* Asthma is generally considered a chronic, lower airway disorder characterized by heightened airway reactivity with bronchospasm and obstruction. The exact cause of asthma is unknown; however, it is believed to include an allergic reaction to one or more allergens, or "triggers," that either precipitate or aggravate asthmatic exacerbation. The child usually exhibits other symptoms of allergy, such as infantile eczema or hayfever; in addition, 75% of children with asthma have a positive family history for asthma. The onset is usually before age 5 and remains with the child throughout life, although some children experience dramatic improvement in their asthma with the onset of puberty. Most children do *not* require continuous medication. Early relief of symptoms with a combination of drugs can reverse bronchospasm.

◆ **B. Assessment:**
1. Expiratory wheeze.
2. General signs and symptoms of respiratory distress, including anxiety, cough, shortness of breath, crackles, cyanosis due to obstruction within the respiratory tract, use of accessory muscles of respirations.
3. Cough: hacking, paroxysmal, nonproductive; especially at night.
4. *Position* of comfort for breathing: sitting straight up, leaning forward, which is the position for optimal lung expansion.
5. Peak Expiratory Flow Rate (PEFR) is in the yellow zone (50–80% of personal best) or in the red zone (<50% of personal best).

◆ **C. Analysis/nursing diagnosis:**
1. *Ineffective airway clearance* related to bronchospasm.
2. *Anxiety* related to breathlessness.
3. *Knowledge deficit,* actual or potential, related to disease process, treatment, and prevention of future asthmatic attacks.
4. *Activity intolerance* related to dyspnea and bronchospasm.

◆ **D. Nursing care plan/implementation:**
Treatment is aimed toward *improvement of ventilation, correction of dehydration and acidosis,* and *management of concurrent infection.*
1. Goal: *provide patent airway and effective breathing patterns.*
   ▶ a. Initiate oxygen therapy (by tent, face, mask or cannula), as ordered, to relieve

hypoxia, with high humidity (to liquefy secretions)

b. Administer corticosteroids as ordered (PO or IV) to reduce inflammation, relieve edema (prednisone, *Decadron*) and decrease bronchial hyperreactivity.

c. Administer bronchodilators, as ordered, to relieve the obstruction: epinephrine (1:1000), nebulized albuterol, *Brethine*. Inhalers may be used with metered dose inhalers (MDIs) to ensure proper delivery of the medication.

d. Administer antibiotics as ordered; infection is commonly either a trigger or complication of asthma.

e. *Note:* methylxanthines (theophylline, aminophylline) are third-line agents that are rarely used to treat asthma.

2. Goal: *relieve anxiety.*
   a. Provide relief from hypoxia (refer to goal 1), which is the chief source of anxiety.
   b. Remain with child, offer support.
   c. Administer sedation as ordered.
   d. Encourage parents to remain with child.

3. Goal: *teach principles of prophylaxis.*
   a. Review home medications, including cromolyn sodium. See **Unit 10.**
   b. Review breathing exercises.
   c. Discuss precipitating factors ("triggers") and offer suggestions on how to avoid them.
   ▶ d. Teach how to use peak expiratory flowmeter to monitor respiratory status and determine need for treatment.

e. Introduce need for child to assume control over own care.

◆ **E. Evaluation/outcome criteria:**
   1. Adequate oxygenation provided, as evidenced by pink color of nailbeds and mucous membranes and ease in respiratory effort.
   2. Anxiety is relieved.
   3. Child verbalizes confidence in, and demonstrates mastery of, skills needed to care for own asthma.

Pediatric Surgery: Nursing Considerations

I. In general, basic care principles for children are the same as for adults having surgery.

II. Exceptions:
   A. Children should be prepared according to their developmental level and learning ability.
   B. Children cannot sign own surgical consent form; to be done by parent or legal guardian.
   C. Parents should be actively involved in the child's care.

III. See Table 5–19, which reviews specific nursing care for the most common pediatric surgical procedures.

Pediatrics

DISORDERS AFFECTING NUTRITIONAL FUNCTIONING

Insulin-Dependent Diabetes Mellitus

Insulin-dependent diabetes mellitus (IDDM) was formerly called juvenile-onset diabetes. Diabetes mellitus is fully covered in **Unit 7.** Only the differences between the adult and the child are covered in Table 5–20.

Upper Gastrointestinal Anomalies

I. Cleft lip and cleft palate

  A. *Introduction:* Cleft lip and cleft palate are congenital facial malformations resulting from faulty embryonic development; there appear to be multiple factors involved in the exact etiology: mutant genes, chromosomal abnormalities, teratogenic agents, etc. The infant may be born with cleft lip alone, cleft palate alone, or with both cleft lip and cleft palate. Table 5–21 compares these conditions.

◆ **B. Assessment:**

  1. *Cleft lip*—obvious facial defect, readily detectable at time of birth.
  2. *Cleft palate*—must feel inside infant's mouth to check for presence of palatal defect and to note extent of defect: soft palate only or soft palate *and* hard palate.
  3. *Both*—major problems with feeding: difficult to feed, noisy sucking, swallows excessive amounts of air, prone to aspiration.
  4. *Parent-infant attachment (bonding)* may be adversely affected due to "loss of perfect infant," multiple hospitalizations; note amount and quality of parent-infant interaction.

◆ **C. Analysis/nursing diagnosis:**

  1. *Altered nutrition, less than body requirements,* related to physical defect.
  2. *Impaired physical mobility* (postoperative) related to postoperative care requirements.
  3. *Altered parenting* related to birth of child with obvious facial defect.
  4. *Knowledge deficit,* actual or potential, related to treatment and follow-up.

◆ **D. Nursing care plan/implementation:**

  1. Goal: *maintain adequate nutrition.*
    a. *Preoperative:* first encourage parents to watch nurse feed infant, then teach parents proper feeding techniques:

  ▶ (1) Use *Breck* feeder or Asepto syringe.
   (2) Deposit formula on back of tongue to facilitate swallowing and to prevent aspiration.
   (3) Rinse mouth with sterile water after feedings, to prevent infection.
   (4) Feed slowly, with child in sitting position, to prevent aspiration.
   (5) Burp frequently, because infant will swallow air along with formula due to the defect.

   (6) Monitor weight.
    b. *Postoperative*
   (1) Begin with *clear liquids* when child has fully recovered from anesthesia (see Table 5–21).
   (2) Monitor weight gain carefully, to ensure adequate rate of growth.
   (3) **No** sucking for either cleft lip or palate repair.

  2. Goal: *promote parent-infant attachment.*
    a. Show no discomfort handling infant; convey acceptance.
    b. Stay with parents the first time they see/hold infant.
    c. Offer positive comments about infant.
    d. Give positive reinforcement to parents' initial attempts at parenting.
    e. Encourage parents to assume increasing independence in care of their infant.
    f. Allow rooming-in on subsequent hospitalizations.

  3. Goal: *teach parents regarding feeding and need for long-term follow-up care.*
    a. Teach parents regarding long-term concerns (see Table 5–21).
    b. Make necessary *referrals* before discharge:
   (1) Specialists: speech, dentition, hearing.
   (2) Home health nurse.
   (3) Social service.
   (4) Disabled children's services for financial assistance.
   (5) Local facial-malformations support group.
    c. Refer parents to genetic counseling services because of mixed genetic/environmental etiology.
    d. Encourage parents to promote self-esteem in infant/child as child grows and develops.

◆ **E. Evaluation/outcome criteria:**

  1. Adequate nutrition is provided, and infant grows at "normal" rate for age.
  2. Parent-infant attachment is formed.
  3. Parents verbalize confidence in their ability to care for infant.

II. Tracheoesophageal fistula

  A. *Introduction:* Tracheoesophageal fistula (TEF) is a congenital anomaly resulting from faulty embryonic development; although there are nu-

TABLE 5–20   Differences Between Type 1 (Insulin-dependent) and Type 2 (Non–Insulin-dependent) Diabetes Mellitus

Variable	Type 1 (Insulin-dependent) Diabetes Mellitus	Type 2 (Non–Insulin-dependent) Diabetes Mellitus
Endogenous (naturally occurring) insulin	*Absolute* deficiency of insulin; pancreas produces no insulin	*Relative* insufficiency of insulin
Dependence on exogenous insulin	Total dependence on insulin injections for remainder of life	Varies; disease may be controlled by combination of: diet, exercise, oral hypoglycemics, and insulin injections
Typical onset	Abrupt	Insidious
Age at onset	Anytime during childhood years; usually before age 20	Most common between age 40 and 60 years
Weight at onset	Normal or sudden, unexplained loss of weight	Overweight or obese
Gender	Slightly more common in boys than girls	More common in women than men
Ethnicity	More common in Caucasians	More common in Hispanics and Native Americans
Ketoacidosis	Relatively common	Relatively rare
Ease of control/stability	Unstable, difficult to achieve steady blood sugar level	Stable, easier to achieve steady blood sugar level
Presenting symptoms	☼ Polyuria, polyphagia, polydipsia (**"three P's"**)	More commonly related to long-term complications (e.g., changes in vision or kidney function)
Complications	Occur more frequently and at relatively younger age because of younger age at onset of disease; rate 80% or greater	Occur less frequently, and often not seen until later adult years; rate is variable

TABLE 5–21   Comparison of Cleft Lip and Cleft Palate

Dimension	Cleft Lip Only	Cleft Palate Only	Both Cleft Lip and Cleft Palate
Incidence	1/1000 More common among boys	1/2500 More common among girls	Most common facial malformation More common among boys More common among Caucasians than African Americans
Surgical repair	"Cheiloplasty" (Logan bow)	Palatoplasty	Lip always repaired before palate to enhance parent-infant attachment, bonding
	Often done in a single stage Timing: age 6–12 wk	Often done in staged repairs Timing: age 12–18 mo	
◧ **Position postoperatively** ◖●◗ **Feeding postoperatively**	*Never* on abdomen *No* sucking Use Breck feeder or Asepto syringe	*Always* on abdomen *No* sucking Use wide-bowl spoon or plastic cup	
▶ **Nursing care postoperatively**	Elbow restraints Lessen crying Croup tent	Elbow restraints Lessen crying Croup tent	OK to show parents pictures of "before" and "after" repair
Long-term concerns	Bonding, attachment Social adjustment—potential threat to self-image	Defective speech—refer to speech therapist Abnormal dentition—refer to orthodontist Hearing loss—refer to pediatric eye, ear, nose, throat specialist/physician	

merous "types" of TEF, the major problem is an anatomical defect that results in an abnormal connection between the trachea (respiratory tract) and the esophagus (GI system) (Figure 5–14). No exact cause has been identified; however, infants born with TEF are often premature, with a maternal history of polyhydramnios. Diagnosis should be made immediately, within hours after birth, and preferably before feeding (to avoid aspiration pneumonia). Associated

FIGURE 5–14 Esophageal malformations. *(A)* The esophagus ends in a blind pouch with a fistula between the distal esophagus and trachea. *(B)* Esophageal atresia without fistula. *(C)* Tracheoesophageal fistula without esophageal atresia. (From Bowden, VR, Dickey, SB, and Greenberg, CS: Children and Their Families: The Continuum of Care. WB Saunders, Philadelphia, 1999, p 105.)

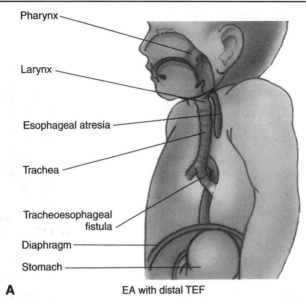

A   EA with distal TEF

B   EA without TEF   C   TEF without EA

anomalies include: CHD, anorectal malformations, and genitourinary anomalies.

◆ **B. Assessment:**
1. Perinatal history: maternal polyhydramnios, premature birth.
2. *Most important system* affected is *respiratory:*
   a. Shortly after birth, infant has excessive amounts of mucus.
   b. Mucus bubbles or froths out of nose and mouth as infant literally "exhales" mucus.
   c. **"Three C's": coughing, choking, cyanosis**—because mucus accumulates in respiratory tract.
   d. "Pinks up" with suctioning, only to experience repeated respiratory distress within a short time as mucus builds up again.
   e. Aspiration pneumonia occurs early.

f. Respiratory arrest may occur.
3. *Second* system affected is GI:
   a. Abdominal distention because excessive air enters stomach with each breath infant takes.
   b. Inability to aspirate stomach contents when attempting to pass NG tube.
   c. If all these signs are not correctly interpreted and feeding is attempted, infant takes two to three mouthfuls, coughs and gags, and forcefully "exhales" formula through nostrils.

◆ **C. Analysis/nursing diagnosis:**
1. *Ineffective breathing pattern/ineffective airway clearance* related to excess mucus.
2. *Altered nutrition, less than body requirements,* related to inability to take fluids by mouth.

3. *Anxiety* related to surgery, condition, preterm delivery, and uncertain prognosis.

4. *Knowledge deficit* regarding discharge care of infant related to gastrostomy tube, feeding.

◆ **D. Nursing care plan/implementation:**

1. Goal: *prepare neonate for surgery.*

   a. Stress to parents that surgery is *only* possible treatment.

   b. Allow parents to see neonate before surgery to promote bonding and attachment.

   c. Maintain NPO—provide IV fluids, monitor I&O, gastrostomy tube.

   d. *Position:* elevate HOB 20–30 degrees to prevent aspiration.

   ▶ e. Administer warmed, humidified oxygen, as ordered, to relieve hypoxia and to prevent cold stress.

2. Goal: *postoperative—maintain patent airway.*

   a. *Position:* elevate HOB 20–30 degrees.

   ▶ b. Care of chest tubes (open-chest procedure).

   ▶ c. Care of endotracheal tube/ventilator (neonate frequently requires ventilatory assistance for 24–48 hr postoperatively).

   d. Monitor for symptoms and signs of pneumonia (most common postoperative complication):

      (1) Aspiration.

      (2) Hypostatic, secondary to anesthesia.

   e. Monitor for symptoms and signs of respiratory distress syndrome (preterm infant).

   ▶ f. Use special precautions when suctioning: "suction with marked catheter" to avoid exerting undue pressure on newly sutured trachea.

   g. Administer prophylactic/therapeutic antibiotics, as ordered.

   ▶ h. Administer warmed, humidified oxygen, as ordered; monitor arterial blood gases (ABGs).

3. Goal: *maintain adequate nutrition.*

   a. Maintain NPO for 10–14 days, until esophagus is fully healed (offer pacifier).

   b. 48–72 hr postoperatively: IV fluids only.

   ▶ c. When condition is stable: begin gastrostomy tube (G-tube) feedings, as ordered.

      (1) Start with small amounts of clear liquids.

      (2) Gradually increase to full-strength formula.

      (3) *Postoperative:* leave G-tube open and elevated slightly above level of stomach to prevent aspiration if infant vomits.

      (4) Offer pacifier ad lib.

   d. Monitor weight, I&O.

   e. Between *10th and 14th postoperative day:* begin oral feedings.

      (1) Start with clear liquids again.

      (2) Note ability to suck and swallow.

      (3) Offer small amounts at frequent intervals.

      (4) May need to supplement postop feeding with G-tube feeding prn.

4. Goal: *prepare parents to successfully care for the infant after discharge.*

   a. Teach parents that infant will probably be discharged with G-tube in place; teach care of G-tube at home.

   b. Teach parents symptoms and signs of most common long-term problem, i.e., stricture formation.

      (1) Refusal to eat solids or swallow liquids.

      (2) Dysphagia.

      (3) Increased coughing or choking.

   c. Stress need for long-term follow-up care.

   d. Offer realistic encouragement, because prognosis is generally good.

◆ **E. Evaluation/outcome criteria:**

1. Neonate survives immediate surgical repair without untoward difficulties.

2. Patent airway is maintained; adequate oxygenation is provided.

3. Adequate nutrition is maintained; infant begins to gain weight and grow.

4. Parents verbalize confidence in ability to care for infant on discharge.

III. Hypertrophic pyloric stenosis

A. *Introduction:* Hypertrophic pyloric stenosis (HPS) causes obstruction of the upper GI tract, but the infant frequently does not have symptoms until 2 to 4 weeks of age. HPS results in thickening, or hypertrophy, of the pyloric sphincter located at the distal end of the stomach; this causes a mechanical intestinal obstruction that becomes increasingly evident as the infant begins to consume larger amounts of formula during the early weeks of life. Pyloric stenosis is five times more common in *boys* than girls and is most often found in full-term caucasian infants. The exact etiology remains unknown; however, there does seem to be a genetic predisposition.

◆ **B. Assessment:**

1. Classic symptom is *vomiting:*

   a. Begins as nonprojectile at age 2–4 wk.

   b. Advances to projectile at age 4–6 wk.

   c. Vomitus is non–bile stained (stomach contents only).

   d. Most often occurs shortly after a feeding.

   e. Major problem is the mechanical obstruction of the flow of stomach contents to the small intestine due to the anatomical defect of stenosis of the pyloric sphincter.

   f. *No* apparent nausea or pain, as evidenced by the fact that infant eagerly accepts a second feeding after episode of vomiting.

Pediatrics

g. Metabolic alkalosis develops due to loss of hydrochloric acid.

2. Inspection of abdomen reveals:
   a. Palpable olive-shaped *mass* in right upper quadrant.
   b. Visible peristaltic *waves,* moving from left to right across upper abdomen.
3. *Weight:* fails to gain or loses.
4. *Stools:* constipated, diminished in number and size—due to loss of fluids with vomiting.
5. Signs of *dehydration* may become evident (Table 5–22).
6. Upper GI series reveals:
   a. Delayed gastric emptying.
   b. Elongated and narrowed pyloric canal.

◆ **C. Analysis/nursing diagnosis:**
1. *Fluid volume deficit* related to vomiting.
2. *Altered nutrition, less than body requirements,* related to vomiting.
3. *Risk for injury/infection* related to altered nutritional state.
4. *Impaired skin integrity* related to dehydration and altered nutritional state.
5. *Knowledge deficit* related to cause of disease, treatment and surgery, prognosis, and follow-up care.

◆ **D. Nursing care plan/implementation:**
1. Goal (**preoperative**): *restore fluid and electrolyte balance.*
   a. Generally NPO, with IVs preoperatively to provide fluids and electrolytes.
   b. Observe and record I&O, including vomiting and stool.
   c. Weight: check every 8 hr or daily.
   d. Monitor laboratory data.

TABLE 5–22 ◆**Signs and Symptoms of Dehydration in Infants and Young Children**

■ *Weight loss* (most important variable to assess): *mild dehydration* (less than 5% weight loss); *moderate dehydration* (5–9% weight loss); *severe dehydration* (10–15% weight loss)

■ *Skin:* gray, cold to touch, poor skin turgor (check skin across abdomen)

■ *Mucous membranes:* dry oral buccal mucosa; salivation absent

■ *Eyes:* sunken eyeballs; absence of tears when crying

■ *Anterior fontanel* (in infant): sunken

■ *Shock:* increased pulse, increased respirations, decreased blood pressure

■ *Urine:* oliguria, increased specific gravity, ammonia odor

■ *Alterations in level of consciousness:* irritability, lethargy, stupor, coma, possible seizures

■ *Metabolic acidosis* (with diarrhea)

■ *Metabolic alkalosis* (with vomiting)

2. Goal: *provide adequate nutrition.*
   a. Maintain NPO with IVs for 4–6 hr postoperatively, as ordered (*can* offer pacifier).
   b. Follow specific feeding regimen ordered by doctor—generally start with clear fluids in small amounts hourly, increasing slowly as tolerated. Full feeding schedule reinstated within 48 hr. Offer pacifier between feedings.
   c. **Fed only by RN for 24–48 hr,** because vomiting tends to continue in immediate postoperative period.
   d. Burp well—before, during, and after feeding.
   e. *Position* after feeding: high Fowler, turned to right side; minimal handling after feeding to prevent vomiting.
3. Goal (**preoperative and postoperative**): *institute preventive measures to avoid infection or skin breakdown.*
   a. Use good hand-washing technique.
   ▶ b. Administer good skin care, especially in diaper area (urine is highly concentrated); give special care to any reddened areas.
   c. Give mouth care when NPO or after vomiting.
   d. Tuck diaper down below suture line to prevent contamination with urine (postoperatively).
   e. Note condition of suture line—report any redness or discharge immediately.
   f. Screen staff and visitors for any sign of infection.
4. Goal: *do discharge teaching to prepare parents to care for infant at home.*
   a. Teach parents that defect is anatomical and unrelated to their parenting behavior/skill.
   b. Demonstrate feeding techniques, and remind parents that vomiting may still occur.
   c. Stress that repair is complete; this condition will *never* recur.
   d. Instruct parents in care of the suture line: no baths for 10 days, tuck diaper down, report any signs of infection promptly.
   e. Offer follow-up referrals as indicated.

◆ **E. Evaluation/outcome criteria:**
1. Infant survives surgical repair without untoward difficulties (including infection/skin breakdown).
2. Adequate nutrition is maintained, and infant begins to grow and gain weight.
3. Parents verbalize confidence in their ability to care for their infant on discharge.

DISORDERS AFFECTING ELIMINATION

Gastrointestinal Disorders

I. Lower gastrointestinal anomalies/obstruction

A. **Hirschsprung's disease** (congenital aganglionic megacolon)

1. *Introduction:* Hirschsprung's disease is a congenital anomaly of the lower GI tract, but the diagnosis is often not established until the infant is 6–12 months old. The major problem is a functional obstruction of the colon caused by the congenital anatomical defect of lack of nerve cells in the walls of the colon, resulting in the *absence* of peristalsis. Hirschsprung's disease is four times more common in *boys* than girls and is frequently noted in children with *Down* syndrome.

◆ 2. **Assessment:**

a. In the newborn, failure to pass meconium (in addition to other signs and symptoms of intestinal obstruction).

b. *Obstinate constipation*—history of inability to pass stool without stool softeners, laxatives, or enemas; persists despite all attempts to treat medically.

c. *Stools* are infrequent and tend to be thin and ribbonlike.

d. *Vomiting:* bile stained, flecked with bits of stool (breath has fecal odor), due to GI obstruction and eventual backing up of stools.

e. Abdominal distention can be severe enough to impinge on respirations, due to GI obstruction and retention of stools.

f. Anorexia, nausea, irritability due to severe constipation.

g. Malabsorption results in *anemia, hypoproteinemia,* and loss of subcutaneous fat.

h. Visible peristalsis and palpable fecal masses may also be detected.

◆ 3. **Analysis/nursing diagnosis:**

a. *Constipation* related to impaired bowel functioning.

b. *Altered nutrition, less than body requirements,* related to poor absorption of nutrients.

c. *Risk for injury/infection* related to malnutrition.

d. *Pain* related to surgery and treatments.

e. *Knowledge deficit* regarding care of the child with a colostomy and follow-up care.

◆ 4. **Nursing care plan/implementation:**

a. Goal (**preoperative**): *promote optimum nutritional status, fluid and electrolyte balance.*

(1) Monitor for signs and symptoms of progressive intestinal obstruction: measure abdominal girth daily.

▶ (2) Administer IV fluids, as ordered—may include hyperalimentation or intralipids.

(3) Daily weights, I&O, urine specific gravity.

(4) Monitor for possible dehydration.

(5) *Diet: low* residue.

b. Goal (**preoperative**): *assist in preparing bowel for surgery.*

(1) Teach parents what will be done and why—enlist their cooperation as much as possible.

▶ (2) Insert NG tube, connect to low suction to achieve and maintain gastric decompression.

(3) *Position:* semi-Fowler's.

▶ (4) Bowel is cleansed with a series of isotonic saline (0.9%) enemas.

(5) Administer oral antibiotics and colonic irrigations to decrease bacteria.

(6) Take axillary temperatures *only.*

(7) If child can understand, prepare for probable colostomy using pictures, dolls (usual age at surgery is 10–16 mo).

c. Postoperative goals: same as for adult having major abdominal surgery or a colostomy (see **Unit 7**).

d. Goal (**postoperative**): *discharge teaching to prepare parents to care at home for infant with a colostomy.*

(1) Home care of colostomy of infant is essentially same as for adult (see **Unit 7**).

(2) Teach parents to keep written records of stools: number, frequency, consistency.

(3) Teach parents to tape diaper below colostomy to prevent irritation.

(4) Because colostomy is usually temporary, discuss:

(a) Second-stage repair (closure and pull-through) done when the child weighs approximately 20 lb.

(b) Possible difficulties in toilet training.

(5) Stress need for long-term follow-up care.

(6) Make referral to home care if indicated.

◆ 5. **Evaluation/outcome criteria:**
   a. Infant is prepared for surgery and tolerates procedure well.
   b. Postoperative recovery is uneventful.
   c. Parents verbalize confidence in ability to care at home for infant with a colostomy and verbalize their understanding that second surgery will be needed to close the colostomy.

B. Intussusception
   1. *Introduction:* Intussusception is the apparently spontaneous telescoping of one portion of the intestine into another, resulting in a mechanical obstruction of the lower GI tract. There is no known cause, and intussusception is three times more common in *boys* than girls; the child with intussusception is usually between 3 and 24 months of age.

◆ 2. **Assessment:**
   a. Typically presents with sudden onset in healthy, thriving child.
   b. *Pain:* paroxysmal, colicky, abdominal, with intervals when the child appears normal and comfortable.
   c. *Stools:* "currant-jelly," bloody, mixed with mucus.
   d. *Vomiting* due to intestinal obstruction.
   e. *Abdomen:* distended, tender, with palpable, sausage-shaped mass in RUQ.
   f. *Late signs:* fever, shock, signs of peritonitis as the compressed bowel wall becomes necrotic and perforates.

◆ 3. **Analysis/nursing diagnosis:**
   a. *Fluid volume deficit* related to diarrhea and vomiting.
   b. *Pain* related to bowel-wall ischemia, necrosis, and death.
   c. *Risk for injury/infection* related to bowel-wall perforation and peritonitis.
   d. *Knowledge deficit* regarding the disease, medical or surgical treatment, and prognosis.

◆ 4. **Nursing care plan/implementation:**
   a. Goal: *assist with attempts at medical treatment.*
      (1) Explain to parents that a barium enema will be given to the child in an attempt to reduce the telescoping through hydrostatic pressure (succeeds in 75% of cases).
      (2) Stress that, if this treatment is not successful, or if perforation of the bowel wall has already occurred, surgery will be necessary.
      (3) If medical treatment is apparently successful, monitor child for 24–36 hr for recurrence before discharge.
   b. *Preoperative and postoperative goals:* same as for adult with major abdominal surgery (see **Unit 7**).

   c. Goal: *discharge teaching to prepare parents for care of the child at home.*
      (1) Stress that recurrence is rare (10%) and most often occurs within the first 24–36 hr after reduction.
      (2) Other teaching: same as for adult going home after bowel surgery (see **Unit 7**).

◆ 5. **Evaluation/outcome criteria:**
   a. Infant tolerates medical-surgical treatment and completely recovers.
   b. Parents verbalize confidence in ability to care for infant after discharge.

II. Acute gastroenteritis (AGE)
   A. *Introduction:* In infants and young children, gastroenteritis is a common acute illness that can rapidly progress to dehydration, hypovolemic shock, and severe electrolyte disturbances.

◆ B. **Assessment:**
   1. Diarrhea: often watery, green, explosive, contains mucus and blood.
   2. Abdominal cramping and pain, often accompanied by bouts of diarrhea.
   3. Dehydration: see Table 5–22.
   4. Irritability, restlessness, alterations in level of consciousness.
   5. Electrolyte disturbances: see **Unit 7**.

◆ C. **Analysis/nursing diagnosis:**
   1. *Fluid volume deficit* related to vomiting and diarrhea.
   2. *Altered nutrition, less than body requirements,* related to AGE and its treatment, i.e., dietary restrictions.
   3. *Pain* related to abdominal cramping, diarrhea.
   4. *Impaired skin integrity* related to diarrhea.
   5. *Altered tissue perfusion* related to dehydration and hypovolemia.
   6. *Knowledge deficit* regarding diagnosis, dietary restrictions, treatment.

◆ D. **Nursing care plan/implementation:**
   1. Goal: *prevent spread of infection.*
      a. Standard precautions to prevent infection.
      b. Enforce strict hand washing.
      c. Institute and maintain *enteric precautions*—follow policies regarding linens, excretions, specimens ("double bag, special tag").
      d. Tape diapers snugly; keep hands out of mouth.
      e. Obtain stool culture to identify causative organism; then administer antibiotics as ordered.
      f. Identify family members and others at high risk, obtain cultures.
   2. Goal: *restore fluid and electrolyte balance.*
      a. Administer IV fluids and electrolytes as ordered.

b. Monitor for appropriate response to therapy: decreased specific gravity, good skin turgor, normal vital signs.

c. Monitor weight, I&O, specific gravity.

d. Oral feedings—oral rehydration therapy (ORT) with Pedialyte or comparable solution; resume normal diet as quickly as possible.

e. Ongoing assessment of stools: note **A**mount, **C**olor, **C**onsistency, **T**iming (**ACCT**).

3. Goal: *maintain or restore skin integrity.*
   a. Frequent diaper changes (use cloth diapers).
   b. Keep perineal area clean and dry.
   c. Apply protective ointments, e.g., petroleum jelly, A and D emollient ointment.
   d. If feasible, expose reddened buttocks to air (but *not* with explosive diarrhea).

4. Goal: *provide discharge teaching to parents.*
   a. Careful review of diet to be followed at home.
   b. Review principles of food preparation and storage to prevent infection.
   c. Instruct in disposal of stools at home.
   d. Emphasize importance of good hygiene.

◆ **E. Evaluation/outcome criteria:**
   1. No spread of infection noted.
   2. Fluid and electrolyte balance normal.
   3. No skin breakdown noted.
   4. Parents verbalize understanding of home care.

Genitourinary Disorders

I. Hypospadias

A. *Introduction:* Hypospadias is a congenital anatomical defect of the male genitourinary tract, readily detected at birth through simple visual examination. In hypospadias, the urethral opening is located on the ventral surface of the penile shaft; this makes voiding in the standing position virtually impossible, and serious psychological problems could therefore occur. Ideally, staged surgical repair should be completed *by 6–18 months of age,* before body image is developed or castration fears are evident.

◆ **B. Assessment:**
   1. Urethral opening is located on ventral surface of penis.
   2. May be accompanied by "chordee"—ventral curvature of the penis due to a fibrous band of tissue.
   3. Rare: ambiguous genitalia, resulting in need for chromosomal studies to determine sex of neonate.

◆ **C. Analysis/nursing diagnosis:**
   1. *Altered urinary elimination* related to congenital anatomical defect of penis.

2. *Pain* related to surgery and treatments.
3. *Self-esteem disturbance* related to anatomical defect in penis and resulting disturbance in ability to void standing up.
4. *Knowledge deficit* related to condition, surgeries, outcome.

◆ **D. Nursing care plan/implementation:**
   1. Goal: *promote normal urinary function.*
      a. Teach family that surgery is done in several stages, beginning in the early months of life and finishing by age 18 mo.
      b. Provide age-appropriate information to child regarding condition, surgery.
      c. *Preoperative* teaching with child: simulate anticipated postoperative urinary drainage apparatus and dressings on dolls; allow child to handle and play with them *now,* but stress need *not* to touch postoperatively.
      ▶ d. *Postoperatively:* Monitor urinary drainage apparatus; note hourly urine output, color, appearance (should be clear yellow, no blood).

   2. Goal: *promote self-esteem.*
      a. Do *not* scold child if he exposes penis, dressings, catheters, etc.
      b. Reassure parents that preoccupation with penis is normal and will pass.
      c. Encourage calm, matter-of-fact acceptance of, and *avoid* strict discipline for, this behavior, which could negatively affect the child.

◆ **E. Evaluation/outcome criteria:**
   1. Child is able to void in normal male pattern.
   2. Child does not experience disturbances in self-concept and has normal self-esteem.

II. Wilms' tumor (nephroblastoma)

A. *Introduction:* Wilms' tumor, a malignant tumor of the kidney, is the most common form of renal cancer in children. Peak incidence occurs at 3 years of age, with a slightly higher incidence in *boys* than girls. Ninety percent of the cases occur unilaterally; the treatment of choice is nephrectomy (and adrenalectomy) followed by chemotherapy and radiation.

◆ **B. Assessment:**
   1. Most common sign: abdominal mass (firm, nontender).
   2. Most often first found by parent changing diaper; felt as a mass over the kidney area.
   3. Intravenous pyelogram (IVP) confirms the diagnosis.
   4. Metastasis occurs most frequently to the lungs: pain in chest, cough, dyspnea.

◆ **C. Analysis/nursing diagnosis:** *altered urinary elimination* (other diagnoses depend on stage of tumor and presence of metastasis—similar to adult with cancer).

◆ **D. Nursing care plan/implementation:**

1. Goal: *promote normal urinary function.*

   a. Inform family that surgery is scheduled as soon as possible after confirmed diagnosis (within 24-48 hr).

   b. Explain to family that the preferred surgical approach is nephrectomy (and adrenalectomy).

   c. *Preoperative:* do *not palpate abdomen* because the tumor is highly friable, and palpation increases the risk of metastasis.

   d. *Postoperative nursing care:* similar to care of adult with nephrectomy (see **Unit 7**).

   e. *Postoperative care also includes long-term radiation* therapy and chemotherapy (actinomycin D, vincristine, adriamycin; see **Units 7** and **10**).

2. Goal: *discharge teaching to prepare parents to care for child at home.*

   a. Teach parents need for long-term follow-up care with specialists: oncologist, urologist.

   b. Answer questions regarding prognosis, offering realistic hope.

      (1) Children with localized tumor: 90% survival rate.

      (2) Children with metastasis: 50% survival rate.

◆ **E. Evaluation/outcome criteria:**

1. Child is able to maintain normal urinary elimination.

2. Parents verbalize their understanding of home care for the child.

III. Nephrosis. Nephrosis (idiopathic nephrotic syndrome) is a chronic renal disease having no known cause, variable pathology, and no known cure. It is thought that several different pathophysiological processes adversely affect the glomerular membranes of the kidneys, resulting in increased permeability to protein. This "leakage" of protein into the urine results in massive *proteinuria*, severe *hypoproteinemia*, and total body edema. A chronic disease, nephrosis often has its onset during the preschool years but is characterized by periods of exacerbation and remission throughout the childhood years.

The nursing care plan for the child with nephrosis is very similar to that for the adult with compromised renal functioning. Refer to **Units 9** and **10** for additional information about dietary restrictions and medications; refer to Table 5–18 for a chart comparing nephrosis and nephritis.

DISORDERS AFFECTING COMFORT, REST, ACTIVITY, AND MOBILITY

Musculoskeletal Disorders

Orthopedic conditions in infants and children are many and varied, but treatment is based on basic principles of nursing care. Table 5–23 and Figures 5–15 and 5–16 offer a quick review of the major pediatric orthopedic conditions.

Neuromuscular Disorders

I. **Cerebral palsy**
   A. *Introduction: Cerebral palsy (CP) is the most common permanent physical disability of childhood. It is a neuromuscular disorder of the* pyramidal motor system resulting in the major problem of impaired voluntary muscle control. The damage appears to be fixed and nonprogressive, and the cause is unknown. However, although a variety of factors have been implicated in the etiology of CP, it is now known that CP results more commonly from prenatal brain abnormalities.
   ◆ B. **Assessment:**
      1. Most common type of cerebral palsy—*spastic.*
         a. Delayed developmental milestones.
         b. Tongue thrust with difficulty swallowing and sucking. Poor weight gain. Aspiration may occur.
         c. Increased muscle tone: "scissoring" (legs crossed, toes pointed).
         d. Persistent neonatal reflexes.
         e. Associated problems:
            (1) Mental retardation in 30% of children with cerebral palsy (70% are normal).
            (2) Sensory impairment: vision, hearing.
            (3) Orthopedic conditions: congenital dysplasia of hip, clubfoot.
            (4) Dental problems: malocclusion.
            (5) Seizures.

Pediatrics

FIGURE 5–15 Signs of developmental *dysplasia of the hip.* *(A)* Asymmetry of gluteal and thigh folds. *(B)* Limited hip abduction as seen in flexion. *(C)* Apparent shortening of the femur, as indicated by the level of the knees in flexion. *(D)* Ortolani click (if infant is under 4 weeks of age). *(E)* Positive Trendelenburg sign or gait (if child is weight bearing). (From Wong, D: Whaley and Wong's Nursing Care of Infants and Children, ed 6. Mosby, St Louis, 1999, p 508.)

TABLE 5–23 **Common Pediatric Orthopedic Conditions**

Condition	Definition	Age at Onset/ Sex Difference	Treatment	Nursing Considerations
Clubfoot	Downward, inward rotation of one or both feet: talipes equinovarus (95%)	Newborn (congenital); twice as common in *boys*	Series of casts changed weekly followed by *Denis Browne splint* and then corrective shoes (severe cases—surgery)	Care of child in cast/brace Stress need for follow-up Encourage compliance
Developmental hip dysplasia (see Figure 5–15)	Abnormal development of hip joint (most frequently unilateral)	Newborn (congenital); more common in *girls*	*Newborn—Pavlik harness; older infant or toddler—*possible surgery, spica cast	Early identification Care of child in traction/cast: check circulation; turn q2h while cast is wet Encourage compliance Check for other anomalies (e.g., spina bifida)
Osteomyelitis	Most frequently occurring bone infection among children	5–14 yr; twice as common in *boys*	Blood cultures to diagnose causative organisms—select appropriate antibiotic; bed rest, immobilization with splint or cast	Care of child in splint/cast Provide diversion Pain medications/antibiotics per MD order
Legg-Calvé-Perthes	Aseptic necrosis of the head of the femur (cause unknown)	*Peak:* 4–8 yr; *range:* 3–12 yr; 5 times more common in *boys;* 10 times more common in whites than nonwhites	Conservative therapy lasts 2–4 yr, usually begins with bed rest and traction, followed by non–weight-bearing devices such as brace, cast	Early identification Care of child in traction/cast: check for frayed pulley ropes Provide diversion Assist child and family to cope with child's prolonged immobility
Juvenile rheumatoid arthritis	Chronic systemic inflammatory disease (cause unknown)	*Peak:* 2–5 yr and 9–12 yr; more common in *girls*	Prevent joint deformity by exercise, splints, medications (steroids, ASA); relieve symptoms (as per adult with arthritis)	Care of child in brace/splint Provide diversion Encourage compliance
Scoliosis (see Figure 5–16)	Lateral curvature of the spine (cause unknown)	Adolescence; more common in *girls*	*Milwaukee brace;* halo-pelvic traction; *Harrington rod*	Care of child in traction/cast/brace Teach that brace is worn 16–23 hr/day, 7 days/wk for 6 mo–2 yr Encourage compliance Promote positive self-image
Osteosarcoma	Most frequently occurring bone cancer among children	Adolescence (10–25 yr); more common in *boys* and men	Amputation→prosthesis; chemotherapy	Prepare child for loss of limb Help cope with prosthesis, life-threatening illness Assist with grieving process

◆ **C. Analysis/nursing diagnosis:**

1. *Ineffective airway clearance* related to hyperactive gag reflex and possible aspiration.
2. *Altered nutrition, less than body requirements,* related to difficulty sucking and swallowing.
3. *Fluid volume deficit* related to difficulty sucking and swallowing.
4. *Impaired verbal communication* related to difficulty with speech.
5. *Sensory/perceptual alterations* related to potential vision and hearing defects.
6. *Risk for injury* related to difficulty controlling voluntary muscles.
7. *Self-esteem disturbance* related to disability.
8. *Note:* Because the level of disabilities with CP can vary, the nurse must select those diagnoses that apply, and clearly specify the individual child's limitations in any diagnostic statements.

◆ **D. Nursing care plan/implementation:**

1. Goal: *maintain patent airway.*
   a. Have suction and oxygen readily available.

FIGURE 5–16 The four major curve patterns in idiopathic scoliosis. (From Bowden, VR, Dickey, SB, and Greenberg, CS: Children and Their Families: The Continuum of Care. WB Saunders, Philadelphia, 1999, p 1271.)

THORACIC

L   R

90% occur on the right side above T-11

LUMBAR

70% occur on the left side at L-1 or lower

THORACOLUMBAR

80% occur on the right side at T-11 – T-12

DOUBLE MAJOR

Usually involves right-sided and left-sided lumbar curves

Curve location is determined by the level of the apical vertebra

▶ b. Use feeding and positioning techniques to maintain patent airway.

c. Institute prompt, aggressive therapy for URIs, to prevent the possible development of pneumonia.

2. Goal: *promote adequate nutrition.*

⬤ a. *Diet: high* in *calories* (to meet extra energy demands).

b. Ensure balanced diet of basic foods that can be easily chewed. Refer to dentist for early dental care.

c. Provide feeding utensils that promote independence.

d. Relaxed mealtimes, decreased emphasis on manners, cleanliness.

e. Monitor I&O, weight gain.

3. Goal: *facilitate verbal communication.*

a. Refer to speech therapist.

b. Speak slowly, clearly to child.

c. Use pictures or actual objects to reinforce speech.

4. Goal: *prevent injury.* Refer to safety throughout growth and development sections, pp. 211–218.

a. Use individually designed chairs with restraints for positioning and safety.

b. Provide protective helmet to prevent head trauma.

c. Implement seizure precautions.

5. Goal: *provide early detection of and correction for vision and hearing defects.*
   a. Arrange for screening tests.
   b. Assist family with obtaining corrective devices: eyeglasses, hearing aids.

6. Goal: *promote locomotion.*
   a. Encourage "infant stimulation" program to assist infant in reaching developmental milestones.
   b. *Refer to physical therapy* for exercise program.
   c. Incorporate play into exercise routine.
   d. Use devices that promote locomotion: parallel bars, crutches, and braces.
   e. Surgical approach may be needed to relieve contractures.

7. Goal: *encourage independence in ADL.*
   a. Adapt clothing, feeding utensils, etc. to facilitate self-help.
   b. Encourage child to perform ADL as much as possible; offer positive reinforcement.
   c. Assist parents to have realistic expectations for their child; *avoid* excessively high expectations that might increase frustration.

8. Goal: *promote self-esteem.*
   a. Praise child for each accomplishment or for sincere effort.
   b. Help child dress and groom self daily in an attractive "normal" manner for developmental level and age.
   c. Encourage child to form friendships with children with similar problems.
   d. Enroll child in "special ed" classes to meet his or her needs.
   e. Encourage parents to expose child to wide variety of experiences.

▶ **E. Evaluation/outcome criteria:**

1. Patent airway and adequate oxygenation maintained.
2. Adequate nutrition maintained, and child begins to grow and gain weight.
3. Child has an acceptable means of verbal communication.
4. Safety is maintained.
5. Vision and hearing within normal limits using corrective devices prn.
6. Child is as mobile as possible, given disabilities.
7. Child is performing ADL, within capabilities.
8. Child has positive self-image/self-esteem.

II. Spina bifida (myelodysplasia)

A. *Introduction:* Three different types of spina bifida:

1. *Spina bifida occulta*—a "hidden" bony defect without herniation of the meninges or cord; not visible externally, no symptoms are present, no treatment is needed.
2. Spina bifida cystica—visible defect of the spine with external saclike protrusion.
   a. *Meningocele*—Table 5–24.
   b. *Myelomeningocele*—see Table 5–24. Most serious type of spina bifida cystica and also most common.

The remainder of this section deals with *myelomeningocele* exclusively.

▶ **B. Assessment:**

1. Congenital defect.
2. Readily detected by visual inspection in delivery room: round, bulging sac filled with fluid, usually in lumbosacral area.
3. Sensation and movement: complete lack below the level of the lesion.
4. Urinary: retention, with overflow incontinence.
5. Fecal: constipation, fecal impaction, oozing of liquid stool around impaction.

TABLE 5–24   Comparison of Two Major Types of Spina Bifida

Dimension	Meningocele	Myelomeningocele
Contents of sac	Meninges and cerebrospinal fluid	Meninges, cerebrospinal fluid, spinal cord
Transillumination	Present	Absent
Percentage of total cases	25%	75%
Motor function	Present	Absent
Sensory function	Present	Absent
Urinary/fecal incontinence	Absent	Present
Associated orthopedic anomalies	Rare	Developmental dysplasia of the hip, *clubfoot*
Other anomalies	Rare	*Hydrocephalus* (90–95%)
Treatment	Surgery	Surgery
Major *short-term* complication	Infection (meningitis)	Infection (meningitis)
Major *long-term* complication	None	Chronic urinary tract infection leading to renal disease/failure
Prognosis	Excellent	Guarded

6. 90–95% develop signs and symptoms of hydrocephalus (see p. 274).
7. May have associated orthopedic anomalies: clubfoot, developmental hip dysplasia.

◆ **C. Analysis/nursing diagnosis:**
 1. *Risk for injury/infection* related to rupture of the sac.
 2. *Altered urinary elimination* related to urinary retention and overflow incontinence.
 3. *Impaired skin integrity* related to immobility.
 4. *Constipation* related to fecal incontinence and impaired innervation.

◆ **D. Nursing care plan/implementation:**
 1. Goal: *prevent rupture of the sac and possible infection (preoperative).*
  a. *Position: no* pressure on sac; prone to prevent contamination with urine or stool.
  b. *No* clothing or diapers to *avoid* pressure on sac.
  ▶ c. Place in heated isolette to maintain body temperature. *Avoid* radiant heat, which can dry and crack the sac.
  d. Keep sac covered with sterile, moist, nonadherent dressing (sterile normal saline) to prevent drying, cracking, and leakage of CSF; change every 2–4 hr; document appearance of sac each dressing change to note signs and symptoms of infection, leaks, abrasions, or irritation.
  ▶ e. Enforce strict aseptic technique to prevent infection (leading cause of morbidity/mortality in neonatal period).
  f. *Avoid* repeated latex exposure (e.g., gloves, catheters) to decrease risk of latex allergy.
 2. Goal: *prevent infection in postoperative period.*
  a. *Position:* prone, side-lying, or partial side-lying.

 ▶ b. Use myelomeningocele apron (specific type of dressing) to prevent urine or stool from contaminating suture line.
 c. Administer antibiotics as ordered.
 d. Use strict aseptic techniques in dressing changes; standard precautions to prevent infection.
 3. Goal: *prevent urinary retention and UTI.*
  a. Monitor I&O, offer extra fluids to flush kidneys.
  b. Keep urethral meatus clean of stool to prevent ascending bacterial infection.
  c. Monitor urinary output for retention.
  d. Administer antibiotics/urinary tract antiseptics as ordered.
 4. Goal: *prevent complications of prolonged immobility or associated orthopedic anomalies.*
  a. *Position:* hips abducted.
  ▶ b. Use positional devices, rotating pressure mattress/flotation mattress.
  c. *Refer to physical therapy* for ROM exercises.
  d. Make necessary referrals for care of possible clubfoot/developmental hip dysplasia.
 5. Goal: *monitor for possible development of hydrocephalus.* Occurs in 90–95% of infants born with myelomeningocele.

● **E. Evaluation/outcome criteria:**
 1. Integrity of sac is maintained until surgery is done.
 2. No infection occurs.
 3. Adequate patterns of urinary and bowel elimination with necessary support.
 4. Complications of immobility, orthopedic anomalies are prevented or treated promptly.

Pediatrics

DISORDERS AFFECTING SENSORY-PERCEPTUAL FUNCTIONING

I. Hydrocephalus

A. *Introduction:* Hydrocephalus, known to the layperson as "water on the brain," is actually a syndrome resulting from disturbances in the dynamics of CSF. The accumulation of this fluid causes enlargement and dilation of the ventricles of the brain and increased intracranial pressure (ICP). If untreated, severe brain damage will result; treatment is a surgical shunting procedure that allows CSF to drain from the ventricles of the brain to another, less harmful area within the body: jugular vein, right atrium of the heart, or peritoneal cavity. Hydrocephalus can develop as the result of a *congenital malformation* (e.g., Arnold-Chiari malformation); can be *associated with other congenital defects* (e.g., spina bifida); or can be acquired secondary to infection (e.g., meningitis), trauma, or neoplasm.

◆ B. **Assessment:**

1. *Head:* increased circumference—earliest sign of hydrocephalus in the infant (more than 1 in/mo).
2. *Fontanels:* tense and bulging without head enlargement.
3. *Veins:* dilated scalp veins.
4. **"Setting-sun" sign:** sclera visible above pupil; pupils are sluggish with unequal response to light.
5. *Cry:* shrill, high pitched.
6. Developmental milestones: delayed.
7. *Reflexes:* persistence of neonatal reflexes; hyperactive reflexes.
8. Feeds poorly.
9. *Signs of increased ICP:*
   a. Vomiting.
   b. Irritability.
   c. Seizures.
   d. Decreased pulse.
   e. Decreased respirations.
   f. Increased blood pressure.
   g. Widened pulse pressure.
10. History may reveal other CNS defects (e.g., spina bifida), infection (e.g., meningitis), trauma, or neoplasm.

◆ C. **Analysis/nursing diagnosis:**

1. *Altered cerebral tissue perfusion* related to increased intracranial pressure.
2. *Impaired skin integrity* related to enlarged head size and lack of motor coordination.
3. *Altered nutrition, less than body requirements,* related to anorexia and vomiting.
4. *Anxiety* related to diagnosis and uncertain outcome.

5. *Knowledge deficit* regarding care of the child with a shunt and follow-up care.

◆ D. **Nursing care plan/implementation:**

1. Goal: *monitor neurological status.*
   a. Measure head circumference daily, and note any abnormal increase.
   ▶ b. Perform neurological checks at least every 4 hr to monitor for signs of increased ICP.
   c. Report signs of increased ICP **stat** to physician.
   d. Assist with diagnostic procedures/treatments: *ventricular tap, computed tomography* (CT) scan, etc.
2. Goal: *health teaching to reduce parental anxiety.*
   a. Do preoperative teaching regarding the shunt procedure: stress need to remove excessive CSF to relieve pressure on brain; done as soon as possible after diagnosis is established.
   b. Stress early diagnosis and prompt shunting procedure to minimize the risk of long-term neurological complications.
   c. Offer realistic information regarding prognosis:
      (1) Surgically treated, with continued follow-up care: 80% survival rate.
      (2) Of these survivors, 50% are completely normal and 50% have some degree of neurological disability (such as inattentiveness or hyperactivity).
3. Goal: *provide postoperative shunt care.*
   a. *Position:*
      (1) Flat in bed for 24 hr, to prevent subdural hematoma.
      (2) Gradually increase the angle of elevation of HOB, as ordered by surgeon.
      (3) On the *unoperative side,* to prevent mechanical pressure and obstruction to shunt.
   b. Monitor head circumference daily to note any abnormal increase that might indicate malfunctioning shunt.
   c. Monitor vital signs; monitor for signs of increased ICP.
   d. Monitor for possible complications:
      (1) Infection.
      (2) Malfunction of shunt: increased ICP.
4. Goal: *provide discharge teaching to parents regarding home care of the child with a shunt.*
   a. Stress need for long-term follow-up care.
   b. Discuss feeding techniques, care of skin (especially scalp), need for stimulation.
   c. Prepare parents for shunt revisions to be done periodically as child grows.
   d. Teach parents signs and symptoms of shunt malfunctioning (i.e., of increased ICP or infection) and to report these promptly to physician.
   e. Encourage parents to enroll infant in "early infant stimulation" program to maximize developmental potential.

f. Stress need to monitor development at frequent intervals, make referrals prn.

◆ **E. Evaluation/outcome criteria:**
1. Neurological functioning is maintained or improved.
2. Adequate nutrition is maintained.
3. No impairment of skin integrity occurs.
4. Parents' anxiety is relieved; they verbalize understanding of how to care for child after discharge.

II. Febrile seizures

A. *Introduction:* Febrile seizures are *transient* neurological disorders of childhood, affecting perhaps as many as 3% of all children. Although the exact cause of febrile seizures remains uncertain, they seem to be a relatively transient problem that occurs exclusively in the presence of high, spiked fevers. Children in the infant and toddler stages (6 mo–3 yr) appear to be most susceptible to febrile seizures, and they are twice as common in boys as in girls. There also appears to be an increased susceptibility within families, suggesting a possible genetic predisposition. *Note:* Epilepsy is discussed in **Unit 7.**

◆ **B. Assessment:**
1. History usually reveals presence of URI or gastroenteritis.
2. Occurs with a sudden rise in fever: often spiked and quite high (102°F or higher) vs. prolonged temperature elevation.

◆ **C. Analysis/nursing diagnosis:**
1. *Risk for injury* related to seizures.
2. *Knowledge deficit* related to prevention of future seizures, care of child having a seizure and possible long-term effects.

◆ **D. Nursing care plan/implementation:**
1. Goal: *reduce fever/prevent further increase in fever.*

a. Administer antipyretics, as ordered: acetaminophen only (*not* aspirin).
b. Use cool, loose, cotton clothes to decrease heat retention.
c. Sponge with tepid water 20–30 min; *avoid* shivering, which increases metabolic rate and temperature.
d. Encourage child to drink *cool fluids.*
e. Monitor temperature hourly.
f. Minimize stimulation, frustration for child.
2. Goal: *teach parents about care of child who experiences febrile seizure.*
a. Discuss how to prevent seizures from recurring: best method is to prevent temperature from rising over 102°F (see goal 1).
b. Discuss how to handle seizures if they do recur: prevent injury, maintain airway, etc.
c. Answer questions simply and honestly:
(1) 25% of children with one febrile seizure will experience a recurrence.
(2) 75% of recurrences occur within 1 year.
(3) Reassure parents of the benign nature of febrile seizures; 95–98% of children with febrile seizures do not develop epilepsy or neurological damage.

◆ **E. Evaluation/outcome criteria:**
1. Fever is kept below 102°F; additional seizures are prevented.
2. Parents verbalize their understanding of how to care for child at home.

Pediatrics

SELECTED PEDIATRIC EMERGENCIES

For a quick review; use this index to locate content on 19 pediatric emergencies that are covered in this book.

Questions

Select the one best answer for each question.

1. The best position for the delivery room nurse to place a newborn with myelomeningocele at the lumbosacral area in is:
   1. Prone.
   2. Supine.
   3. Side-lying.
   4. Trendelenburg.

2. A school-age child with rheumatic fever complains of severe joint pains in the knees and ankles. The best method to provide relief would be for the nurse to:
   1. Give a warm bath or shower.
   2. Apply splints to the affected joints.
   3. Refer the child to physical therapy.
   4. Place a bed cradle over the child's legs.

3. A hospitalized school-age child is very quiet and seldom talks to the staff. The nurse can best communicate with this child by saying:
   1. "I've noticed you seem very quiet. Is anything troubling you?"
   2. "Let's tell each other a secret; you start by telling me what you are thinking."
   3. "It must be awfully hard to be away from home. Let's call your mom!"
   4. "Draw me some pictures of the things you've seen and done while you've been in the hospital."

4. Three of the following signs or symptoms indicate an improvement in the condition of a toddler with laryngotracheobronchitis. Which one indicates a *worsening* and should be promptly reported to the physician?
   1. Apical pulse = 118.
   2. Increase in appetite.
   3. Progressive hoarseness.
   4. Pink nailbeds.

5. The nurse reviews a toddler's immunizations with the parents and finds that the child has had all immunizations recommended during the toddler years. The nurse should advise the parents that, at 4 to 6 years of age, the child should next receive:
   1. MMR (measles, mumps, rubella) and hepatitis B.
   2. Hepatitis B and varicella.
   3. *Haemophilus influenzae* type b and DTP.
   4. MMR (measles, mumps, rubella), polio, and DTP.

6. Which is the *most common* complaint by parents about infants with heart disease?
   1. Frequent, severe respiratory infections.
   2. "Slower" development.
   3. "Stunted" growth.
   4. Difficult to feed.

7. The nurse in the newborn nursery should plan any interventions with a newborn with myelomeningocele based on the knowledge that the major *short-term* complication the child is most likely to suffer is:
   1. Hydrocephalus.
   2. Meningitis.
   3. Mental retardation.
   4. Paraplegia.

8. The physician orders Tylenol elixir for a 14-month-old with a fever of 102°F. Considering this child's developmental level and diagnosis, which would be the best approach by the nurse?
   1. Use the medicine cup and tell the child the "pretty red syrup" will taste sweet like candy.
   2. Mix the medication with 4 oz of apple juice and allow the child to drink it through a "crazy straw."
   3. Put the medication into a brightly colored plastic cup and give the child a chance to drink it.
   4. Raise the child to a sitting position, bring the medicine cup to the lips, and tell the child kindly but firmly to drink it.

9. A toddler is to be placed in a croupette. The nurse should plan to perform which nursing action?
   1. Remove all toys from the crib.
   2. Withhold all liquids and solids temporarily.
   3. Monitor oxygen concentration daily and record in notes.
   4. Evaluate the toddler's reaction to oxygen therapy in terms of vital signs and color.

10. The nurse should review principles of care with a 12-year-old child with asthma. Which comment by the child would require additional teaching by the nurse?
    1. "I keep all my stuffed animals on my bookcase now."
    2. "I have vinyl miniblinds on the windows in my room."
    3. "I gave my cat to my best friend."
    4. "I joined the swim team at school."

11. A mother asks the nurse about the normal time for the onset of menstruation. The nurse would be most correct in advising her that menses usually begin at age:
    1. 11.2 years
    2. 12 years.
    3. 12.8 years.
    4. 13.5 years.

12. In doing an infant's admission examination, the nurse notes all the following abnormal findings. Which one is the *most common sign* of heart disease the nurse should assess?
    1. Circumoral cyanosis.
    2. Hypertension.
    3. Diastolic murmur.
    4. Tachycardia.

13. To "flood" the croupette with oxygen before placing a toddler in the tent, the nurse should initially adjust the oxygen flow rate to:
    1. 2–3 L/min.
    2. 4–5 L/min.
    3. 8–10 L/min.
    4. 15 L/min.

14. A toddler is admitted to the hospital with acute bilateral otitis media, with a temperature of 103°F and tremors in arms and legs. In addition to a spinal tap to rule out bacterial meningitis, the doctor orders all the following. Which order should the nurse perform *first?*
    1. Respiratory isolation.
    2. IV 5% dextrose in 0.45 normal saline solution at 35 mL/hr.
    3. Tylenol 120 mg PO q4h.
    4. Seizure precautions.

15. The doctor orders an IV to infuse at 35 mL/hr; a pediatric microdrip chamber is hanging. How many drops per minute should the nurse regulate the IV to infuse?
    1. 5–6.
    2. 7–8.
    3. 9–10.
    4. 35.

16. A 7-year-old who has had leukemia for 2 years was in primary remission for 18 months but recently experienced infections, epistaxis, and abdominal petechiae. The doctor suspects the child is no longer in remission and must be admitted to the hospital. In reviewing admitting blood work, the nurse notes all the following. Which finding should the nurse interpret as the probable cause of the infections?
    1. Anemia.
    2. Leukopenia.
    3. Neutropenia.
    4. Thrombocytopenia.

17. A school-age child with rheumatic fever develops heart failure and is placed on digoxin, Lasix, and potassium. The chief purpose for giving potassium is to:
    1. Enhance the cardiogenic effect of digoxin.
    2. Potentiate the diuretic action of Lasix.
    3. Prevent hypokalemia.
    4. Pharmacologically induce hyperkalemia.

18. Two hospitalized school-age children complain that they are "bored." The nurse should offer them:
    1. A game of Monopoly or Life.
    2. Workbooks, paper, and pencils.
    3. Some books from the hospital library.
    4. A chance to stay up late and watch TV.

19. A 12-year-old is admitted to the hospital in status asthmaticus, for the second time. In planning care for this child, the nurse must first assess:
    1. What she knows about asthma.
    2. How she usually cares for herself.
    3. What she knows about hospitalization.
    4. How she feels about becoming a teenager.

20. When the nurse begins teaching a teenager with diabetes about insulin, which one fact should be stressed to this teen and the family?
    1. Properly controlled dietary management, along with hypoglycemic agents, may eventually be used.
    2. Exogenous insulin will be necessary for the rest of the child's life.
    3. Activity level, nutritional intake, and state of health will necessitate daily modifications in the insulin dose.
    4. Due to the need for insulin, the child should no longer participate in active sports.

21. In doing a child's admission history, the nurse notes all the following signs of hemophilia. The hallmark, or classic sign, of hemophilia is:
    1. Excessive hematoma formation.
    2. Hemarthrosis.
    3. Prolonged bleeding from lacerations.
    4. Intracranial bleeding.

22. The nurse performs a Denver Developmental Screening Test (DDST) on a 3-year-old. Which behavior should the nurse expect this child to be capable of doing?
    1. Going up stairs on alternate feet.
    2. Pedaling a bicycle.
    3. Dressing without supervision.
    4. Tying shoelaces.

23. While admitting an infant, the nurse notes all the following abnormal findings. Which one is considered the classic sign of Hirschsprung's disease?
    1. Abdominal distention.
    2. Anorexia.
    3. Constipation.
    4. Vomitus flecked with feces.

24. The best way for a nurse to perform a DDST on a 9-month-old is to:
    1. Take the infant from the mother and ask her to wait in the child's room.
    2. Take the infant from the mother and ask her to come with them to the testing area.
    3. Briefly talk first with the mother, then take the infant to the testing area alone.
    4. Ask the infant's mother to carry the child to the testing area.

25. For an infant with severe chronic CHF, the formula the nurse should plan to offer would be:
    1. Isomil.
    2. Lofenalac.
    3. Lonalac.
    4. Similac 27 with iron.

26. The parents of a school-age child with leukemia tell the nurse that their daughter frequently has nightmares, and they wonder how to handle this. The nurse would be most correct in advising them to:
    1. Comfort her, but leave her in her own bed.
    2. Comfort her by bringing her into their bed.
    3. Consult a child psychologist to determine why she has recurring sleep disturbances.
    4. Encourage the child to keep a written record of her dreams and discuss them with her primary nurse during hospitalization.

27. Before giving a child digoxin, which pulse would the nurse be most correct in assessing?
    1. Apical.
    2. Brachial.
    3. Pedal.
    4. Radial.

28. A 20-month-old is admitted to the pediatrics unit for the third, and final, surgical procedure to correct his congenital hypospadias. When admitting this toddler to the hospital, the nurse should assess all of the following. Which information will be the most important to the nursing plan of care for this toddler?
    1. His developmental level.
    2. The parents' knowledge level regarding hypospadias.
    3. His previous experience with illness and hospitalization.
    4. The parents' plans for rooming-in.

29. A hospitalized preschooler wakes up crying at 2 A.M. and says, "I want my mommy now." The nurse should:
    1. Pick the child up and rock the child for a little while.
    2. Talk softly to the child while rubbing the back, but leave the child in the crib.
    3. Gently but firmly tell the child to go back to sleep.
    4. Call the mother and ask her to come to the hospital.

30. The nurse does discharge teaching with the mother of a preschooler with epiglottitis before discharge. Which statement by the mother indicates that she has *correctly* understood the nurse's teaching?
    1. "I'm so glad that my child is all better now."
    2. "I will keep my child home from preschool for the rest of this month."
    3. "I'm still worried that my child will get sick again when we get home."
    4. "I will get a portable tank of oxygen for my child before he comes home."

31. After flooding a croupette for 5 minutes, the nurse should readjust the flow rate of oxygen. To maintain an oxygen concentration of 35–40%, the nurse should now adjust the oxygen flow rate to:
    1. 2–3 L/min.
    2. 4–5 L/min.
    3. 8–10 L/min.
    4. 15 L/min.

32. A toddler tries to pull the IV out, and the nurse determines that the child must be restrained to maintain the IV site. Which restraint would the nurse be most correct in applying?
    1. Posey jacket.
    2. Elbow.
    3. Mummy.
    4. Clove-hitch.

33. A lumbar puncture is performed on a child by the doctor. After the procedure, the nurse should position the child:
    1. Flat in bed, with no pillow.
    2. Flat in bed, with a small pillow.
    3. In semi-Fowler's position.
    4. Semiprone, with head to the side.

34. When the parents of a newborn with myelomeningocele visit the nursery for the first time, they make no comments about the baby's spinal sac. Instead, they offer many positive observations about size, color, hair, and appearance. The nurse would be most correct in interpreting the parents' behavior as:
    1. Attachment.
    2. Denial.
    3. Immaturity.
    4. Love.

35. The pediatrician orders syrup of ipecac for a toddler who has ingested a harmful substance. Generally, the nurse *should* administer this medication only if the child is:
    1. Alert and reactive.
    2. Convulsing.
    3. Comatose.
    4. Known to have swallowed a corrosive substance.

36. The mother of a toddler who will have his third, and final, surgical procedure to correct congenital hypospadias questions the need for another surgical procedure while he is still so young. The nurse should stress that:
    1. It is the mother's right to refuse surgery at any time.
    2. It is in her son's best interest to follow the doctor's recommendations.
    3. He can have this third, and final, surgery any time before the onset of puberty.
    4. This type of surgery is usually timed to take place between 6 and 18 months of age.

37. After the nurse completes preoperative teaching with a preschooler, which would be the *best* method for evaluating the effectiveness of the teaching?
    1. Ask him to draw a picture of what he will look like after surgery.
    2. Using puppets, ask him to show the nurse what he has learned about his surgery.
    3. Tell him that this is a test and he must repeat what he has learned about his operation.
    4. Suggest his parents check on their child's level of understanding and report back to the nurse.

38. The nurse should withhold a 6-year-old's digoxin and notify the physician if the child's pulse was *below:*
    1. 80 beats/min.
    2. 90 beats/min.
    3. 100 beats/min.
    4. 110 beats/min.

39. An adolescent is admitted to the hospital in sickle cell crisis with severe pain in the legs and abdomen. The adolescent asks the nurse why the doctor ordered oxygen when there is no trouble breathing. The nurse would be *most* correct in stating that the main therapeutic effect of oxygen is to:
    1. Reverse sickling of RBCs.
    2. Prevent further sickling.
    3. Prevent respiratory complications.
    4. Increase the oxygen-carrying capacity of RBCs.

40. A child is admitted to the hospital with a second attack of rheumatic fever. In doing an admission assessment on this child, which group of symptoms would the nurse most likely find?
    1. Petechiae, malaise, and joint pain.
    2. Chorea, anemia, and hypertension.
    3. Tachycardia, erythema marginatum, and fever in late afternoon.
    4. Subcutaneous nodules, dependent edema, and conjunctivitis.

41. A school-age child has leukemia. Considering the diagnosis and health-teaching needs, the nurse would be most correct in advising this child to:
    1. Skip brushing the teeth at this time.
    2. Brush the teeth with a soft toothbrush only.
    3. Brush the teeth with a firm toothbrush only.
    4. Rinse the mouth with an antiseptic solution instead of brushing the teeth.

42. The mother of a hospitalized 3-year-old tells the nurse that he is a very poor eater at home. The best recommendation the nurse can make to increase his nutritional intake would be to:
    1. Provide him with a child-size table.
    2. Use plastic cups and plates with cartoon characters he likes.
    3. Offer him small portions of his favorite foods.
    4. Allow him to feed himself.

43. A 3-year-old with hemophilia is to be discharged, and the nurse has completed teaching with the child's parents. Which statement by the parents indicates they may have misunderstood the nurse's teaching regarding the care?
    1. "If our child gets a fever, we will only give acetaminophen, not aspirin."
    2. "We will be sure to supervise our child carefully so that our child doesn't experience another bleeding episode."
    3. "I'll order a Medic Alert bracelet for our child as soon as we get home."
    4. "It's a relief to know that our little daughter will not get this disease too."

44. An infant with CHF takes 1.25 oz of formula in 20 minutes. The doctor ordered 2 oz of formula q3h. The *best* action for the nurse to take at this time would be to:
    1. Ask the mother to feed the infant when she arrives.
    2. Burp the infant and try to stimulate sucking.
    3. Continue feeding slowly, allowing as much time as the infant needs to finish.
    4. Stop the feeding, and request an order for gavage feedings prn.

45. The mother of a child with epiglottitis tells the nurse that she does not even know what epiglottitis is. The nurse would be most correct in telling her that it is:
    1. An infection of the upper respiratory tract related to allergy and excessive mucous production.
    2. A potentially life-threatening infection that requires prolonged intensive care.
    3. A mild form of croup that is usually treated at home.
    4. A swelling in the throat that can lead to total airway obstruction if not treated promptly.

46. On admission, a preschooler is carrying a soiled and worn-looking stuffed animal. His mother states that this is his favorite toy. The most appropriate action for the nurse to take at this time is to:

1. Offer him a choice of another stuffed animal from the hospital playroom.
2. Place this stuffed animal somewhere in his room where he can see it but not touch it.
3. Suggest his mother bring him a new stuffed animal.
4. Tell him that he can keep this stuffed animal in the bed with him.

47. In reviewing a preschooler's admission history and laboratory results, the nurse should know that the two most common findings in children with nephrosis are:
1. Generalized edema and proteinuria.
2. Hyperlipidemia and periorbital edema.
3. Hypertension and hematuria.
4. Oliguria and anorexia.

48. The number one priority during the nurse's admission assessment of a school-age child with rheumatic fever is the child's:
1. Weight.
2. Apical pulse rate.
3. Developmental level.
4. ESR.

49. In planning care for a teenager in sickle cell crisis, the nurse should base any actions on the knowledge that pain in vaso-occlusive crisis is *primarily* due to:
1. Increased RBC destruction.
2. Hepatosplenomegaly.
3. Obstruction of small blood vessels.
4. Sequestration of blood.

50. A teenager is preparing the first dose of insulin. The physician orders 14 U of NPH insulin; the teen draws up 13 U and shows it to the nurse. The nurse should base any response on the knowledge that:
1. This is the first attempt and the teenager did come close to the exact dose.
2. At this age, the teenager cannot be expected to make such fine discriminations in dosage.
3. The teenager must draw up the exact amount before administration.
4. Teenagers often antagonize adults subconsciously.

51. Between feedings, the nurse should place an infant with CHF in which position?
1. In an infant seat with head elevated.
2. Prone with head turned to side.
3. Supine with head slightly hyperextended.
4. Side-lying with the head of the bed elevated 30 degrees.

52. The doctor attempts to shine a light through a myelomeningocele sac and notes "no transillumination." The nurse should interpret this finding to mean that the sac:
1. Can be easily repaired.
2. Cannot be evaluated by this technique.
3. Contains meninges and CSF.
4. Contains meninges, CSF, and the spinal cord.

53. After administering syrup of ipecac to a toddler, the nurse should also give:
1. Four ounces of warm milk.
2. Activated charcoal powder.
3. As much water as the child will drink.
4. A slice of dry toast.

54. After placing a toddler in a croup tent, the nurse should adjust the plastic canopy so that:
1. The edges are tucked tightly under the linen.
2. The edges are lying loosely on top of the linen.
3. The crib rails are raised and the canopy edges are over them.
4. The crib rails are lowered and the canopy edges are inside them.

55. In what position should the nurse place a child in status asthmaticus?
1. Knee-chest.
2. High Fowler's.
3. Lateral Sims'.
4. Supine, with neck hyperextended.

56. A teenager hospitalized with diabetes goes to the teen lounge and becomes very boisterous and aggressive, starting a fight with another teen. The *first* question the nurse should consider is:
1. "Should he be sent to his room?"
2. "Did he eat breakfast today?"
3. "What did the other teen do to him?"
4. "Does he miss his own friends?"

57. The nurse has completed discharge teaching with the parents of an infant with ventricular septal defect (VSD) and CHF. Which one statement by the mother would indicate the need for additional teaching by the nurse?
1. "I'll be sure to dress our baby in loose-fitting clothes."
2. "I'll try to keep my house as warm as I can for our baby."
3. "I'll be at the clinic in 3 days for the appointment."
4. "I'll put the baby in the playpen at least once a day."

58. A 7-month-old infant is admitted to the pediatrics unit with moderate dehydration secondary to acute gastroenteritis (AGE). The physician writes all the following orders for this infant. Which one should the nurse implement *first*?
1. Contact precautions.
2. IV of 5% dextrose in ⅓ normal saline solution at 25 mL/hr.
3. Urine specific gravity stat and q4h.
4. Stool culture every shift × 3.

59. The *best* advice the nurse can give to parents to handle a toddler's temper tantrums would be to:
1. Allow the toddler to make own choices.
2. Ignore this behavior.
3. Change the setting in which they occur.
4. Give in to the toddler's demands, to nurture autonomy.

60. A toddler is admitted to the hospital with classic hemophilia (factor VIII deficiency). Which admission procedure by the nurse will probably be the most frightening for this child?
1. Blood pressure.
2. Rectal temperature.
3. Urine specimen.
4. Weight.

61. In writing a nursing care plan for a child with leukemia, the nurse should include all of the following goals. Which goal is *most* important and should receive *top* priority?
1. Maintain infection-free state.
2. Prevent injury.
3. Promote adequate nutrition.
4. Meet developmental needs.

62. The physician orders sterile moist soaks to a myelomeningocele sac. The major reason for this treatment is to:
1. Promote comfort.
2. Prevent infection.
3. Relieve pressure.
4. Stimulate neural development.

63. The night before surgery, as he is getting ready for bed, a preschooler asks his father to "check under the bed for monsters." The nurse would be most correct in advising his father to:
1. Ask the child to talk more about these monsters.
2. Leave a light on and let the child check for himself.
3. Make a game of checking under his bed.
4. Tell him that monsters are only make-believe.

64. Following surgery to correct hypospadias, a toddler returns to the unit with a Foley catheter in place. The nurse should expect the drainage to have:
1. A clear yellow appearance.
2. Small clots of blood or mucus.
3. Gross hematuria in moderate amounts.
4. A brownish tinge.

65. A child with cystic fibrosis is to receive replacement pancreatic enzymes several times daily. The best time for the nurse to plan to administer this medication is:
    1. After every meal or snack.
    2. Between meals and after every snack.
    3. Immediately before meals or snacks.
    4. With meals and before snacks.

66. In addition to administering oxygen, the nurse can also relieve the pain experienced by a teenager in sickle cell crisis by:
    1. Applying warm compresses.
    2. Applying cold compresses.
    3. Performing passive ROM exercises.
    4. Performing ADL as needed.

67. The nurse observes a nursing student fastening an infant's diaper snugly around the abdomen; the infant has CHF. The nurse should:
    1. Ask the student to loosen the diaper.
    2. Do or say nothing, as this is expected behavior for a student.
    3. Loosen the diaper after the student leaves the room.
    4. Praise the student for outstanding attention to detail.

68. Which statement by the parents of a preschooler with nephrosis indicates that they have fully understood the nurse's teaching?
    1. "We will keep him away from other children so he doesn't get a relapse."
    2. "We're so glad this is all over and we don't have to worry any more."
    3. "When we get home, we're going to find it hard to keep him in bed."
    4. "We will watch him for any signs of this starting up again."

69. A child with leukemia is receiving vincristine. The nurse should observe this child closely for the side effect of:
    1. Diarrhea.
    2. Diplopia.
    3. Hemorrhagic cystitis.
    4. Peripheral neuropathy.

70. A 6-year-old with cystic fibrosis refuses to swallow the replacement pancreatic enzyme tablets. The best course of action for the nurse would be to:
    1. Check with the doctor about discontinuing this medication.
    2. Crush the tablets and mix with 1 teaspoon of cold applesauce.
    3. Dissolve the tablets in 4 oz of warm milk.
    4. Offer the child a "special treat" for swallowing the tablets "like a big kid."

71. A school-age child experiences the following signs or symptoms of rheumatic fever. The nurse should plan any interventions based on the knowledge that the only one that may result in *permanent* damage is:
    1. Sydenham's chorea.
    2. Migratory polyarthritis.
    3. Carditis.
    4. Erythema marginatum.

72. The best roommate for a 9-year-old girl with rheumatic fever would be:
    1. An 8-year-old girl with impetigo.
    2. A 9-year-old girl with a tonsillectomy.
    3. A 10-year-old girl with a concussion.
    4. An 11-year-old girl with a fractured elbow in skeletal traction.

73. The nurse should be aware that the most important nursing diagnosis in caring for a child with diabetes is:
    1. Risk for injury related to insulin deficiency.
    2. Altered family processes related to situational crisis (child with chronic disease).
    3. Knowledge deficit related to care of a child with diabetes.
    4. Altered body image related to treatment of diabetes.

74. An infant with myelomeningocele is scheduled to have surgery to close the sac. The mother asks the nurse if the baby will be able to move the legs following this operation. The best response for the nurse to make would be:
    1. "Not usually, although we can always hope for a miracle."
    2. "There is no way to predict. All we can do is watch the baby closely."
    3. "No, the surgery is done mainly to prevent infection."
    4. "Yes, the surgery will restore the ability to move the legs."

75. The best method to prevent the spread of infection from an infant with AGE to other staff members or visitors would be:
    1. Double-bagging all linens.
    2. Obtaining stool cultures.
    3. Strict hand washing.
    4. Wearing disposable gloves.

76. At 7 months of age, an infant exhibits the following skills. The nurse should know that the most recently acquired skill is probably the ability to:
    1. Roll over.
    2. Sit up.
    3. Bear some weight on legs.
    4. Pick up objects with palmar grasp.

77. The most appropriate person to administer a preoperative series of cleansing enemas to a 9-month-old with Hirschprung's disease would be the:
    1. Primary nurse.
    2. Mother.
    3. Nursing student.
    4. Nursing assistant.

78. On admission, the nurse would expect a toddler to demonstrate which two *early* signs of laryngotracheobronchitis (LTB)?
    1. Cyanosis and apnea.
    2. Hoarseness and croupy cough.
    3. Restlessness and tachypnea.
    4. Retractions and inspiratory stridor.

79. A diagnosis of bacterial meningitis is confirmed, and the child assumes an opisthotonos position. In which position should the nurse now place this child?
    1. Prone.
    2. Supine.
    3. Side-lying.
    4. Trendelenburg.

80. In planning a roommate for a hospitalized 12-year-old girl, the nurse should realize that a child of this developmental level will:
    1. Probably prefer another girl her own age.
    2. Most likely seek out opportunities to socialize with teenagers.
    3. Enjoy being with either a girl or boy, as long as they are the same age.
    4. Feel helpful if given the opportunity to look after a slightly younger child.

81. In teaching a teenager how to prevent further episodes of sickle cell crisis, the nurse should stress the need to *avoid:*
    1. Moderate emotional stress.
    2. Cool weather.
    3. Swimming in public pools.
    4. Extra fluid consumption.

82. If a child who was given syrup of ipecac has not vomited within 30 minutes, the nurse should:
    1. Stimulate the gag reflex using his or her fingers.
    2. Wait another 30 minutes before doing anything else.
    3. Assume the danger is past and no further treatment is needed at this time.
    4. Repeat the dose a second time.

83. The physician orders "increase activity as tolerated" for a school-age child with carditis associated with rheumatic

fever. After getting the child up into an armchair, the nurse should monitor how well this increase in activity is tolerated by checking the:
1. Apical pulse rate.
2. Breath sounds.
3. Degree of restlessness.
4. Lips and nailbeds.

84. About a week after discharge, a teenager newly diagnosed with diabetes and his mother return to the clinic for a checkup. His mother states, "I'm worried he will make a mistake, so I've been giving him his insulin." The nurse should:
1. Allow the teenager and his mother to work this out on their own.
2. Assist his mother to understand that he must assume this responsibility.
3. Encourage his mother to continue working closely with him.
4. Realize that this is an appropriate response by the mother.

85. The mother of a hospitalized infant with CHF asks the nurse why the baby is sucking on a pacifier. The nurse would be most correct in telling her:
1. "The baby seems to like it."
2. "Most infants prefer a pacifier to their thumb."
3. "This is to keep the baby from crying."
4. "We give all hospitalized infants a pacifier."

86. The first night in the hospital, a child with hemophilia suffers an episode of epistaxis. In which position should the nurse place this child?
1. Prone, with head turned to side.
2. Semi-Fowler's with two pillows.
3. Sitting up with head tilted backward.
4. Sitting up and leaning forward slightly.

87. Nursing care for a toddler in the croupette includes which of the following?
1. Giving a bald plastic doll.
2. Removing the blanket and pajamas.
3. Restraining the arms and legs.
4. Restricting visitors to the immediate family.

88. The mother of a child with cystic fibrosis tells the nurse that she is thinking of getting pregnant again but is worried that her next child might also have cystic fibrosis. Because her child does have this disease, the nurse should advise this mother that a second child:
1. Could be even more severely affected than her first child.
2. Might also have the disease.
3. Should be "normal," or disease free.
4. Would only carry the trait.

89. A child has had asthma since age 6. In reviewing this child's history, which one factor should the nurse realize may be related to the development of the asthma?
1. Strep throat/tonsillitis at age 2.
2. Eczema at age 3½.
3. Paternal death at age 5.
4. Pneumonia at age 7.

90. Which one behavior should the nurse expect a 5-month-old with CHF to be capable of demonstrating?
1. Rolling over from stomach to back.
2. Sitting with support.
3. Pincer grasp.
4. Bearing some weight on legs.

91. Following surgery to close the myelomeningocele sac, the nurse should place the infant on the:
1. Abdomen, with head 10 degrees lower than hips.
2. Abdomen, with head of bed elevated 30 degrees.
3. Abdomen, with hips 10 degrees lower than head.
4. Abdomen, flat in bed.

92. Parents of an infant with Hirschsprung's disease ask the nurse how their baby got the disease. The nurse would be most correct in advising them that:

1. Their baby was born with this condition.
2. It is the result of the meconium ileus the baby experienced as a newborn.
3. Their baby spontaneously developed this condition.
4. It often occurs following the introduction of solid foods due to a genetically inherited metabolic defect.

93. As a toddler recovers from meningitis, the nurse should watch carefully for which *long-term* complication?
1. Encephalitis.
2. Hydrocephalus.
3. Learning disabilities.
4. Mental retardation.

94. In reviewing what he would do if he experienced a hypoglycemic episode, a teenager correctly states that he would eat a piece of candy or drink a glass of orange juice. The nurse should then instruct him to follow this concentrated sweet with:
1. A blood glucose level.
2. A urine dipstick for glucose.
3. A glass of milk.
4. 5 U of regular insulin.

95. The mother of a child hospitalized with asthma asks the nurse what causes asthma. The nurse would be most correct in telling her the cause is:
1. Unknown.
2. Allergies.
3. Stress.
4. Multiple factors.

96. Long-term follow-up care is being planned for a school-age child with rheumatic fever before discharge from the hospital. This *must* include:
1. Indefinite antibiotic therapy.
2. Immunization against future attacks.
3. Cardiac rehabilitation program.
4. Home-bound tutoring.

97. A preschooler has been admitted with a tentative diagnosis of epiglottitis. A medical student wants to look down this child's throat to visualize the epiglottis. The nurse would be most correct in:
1. Asking the child's mother if she objects to the medical student checking her child.
2. Telling the medical student that this absolutely cannot be done.
3. Promising the child a special treat for "opening real wide for the doctor."
4. Helping restrain the child so the medical student can get a better look.

98. A preschooler with nephrosis is started on prednisone. If the prednisone is having the expected therapeutic effect, the nurse should expect that this child will:
1. Experience mood swings.
2. Have sugar in the urine.
3. Gain weight.
4. Feel better.

99. A toddler who is being placed in a croupette cries and tries to cling to the mother. The mother asks the nurse if she can climb into the crib and lie in the tent with the toddler. The nurse's best response would be:
1. "Do you always let your child behave this way?"
2. "I'll have to check with the doctor first."
3. "No, that would not be safe for you or the child."
4. "It may help the child calm down; let's give it a try."

100. In a 2-week-old infant, the earliest sign of hydrocephalus that the nurse would observe is:
1. Bulging anterior fontanel.
2. Increasing head circumference.
3. Shrill, high-pitched cry.
4. Sunset eyes.

101. A child with leukemia who is receiving chemotherapy develops oral ulcers. Three of the following are appropriate nursing interventions; which one is inappropriate?
    1. Encourage the child to use viscous lidocaine (Xylocaine) before meals.
    2. Offer the child a bland, moist, soft diet.
    3. Use a soft tooth brush.
    4. Provide frequent normal saline mouth rinses.

102. A child with nephrosis has a swollen scrotal sac. Which nursing action would be most effective in relieving discomfort?
    1. Apply zinc oxide to scrotum qid.
    2. Cleanse scrotum with warm water only.
    3. Sprinkle medicated powder on scrotum.
    4. Support scrotum on folded diapers.

103. The surgeon orders a preoperative series of cleansing enemas for an infant with Hirschsprung's disease. The nurse should expect the solution ordered for these enemas to be:
    1. Soapsuds enema (SSE).
    2. Normal saline.
    3. Pediatric Fleets.
    4. Tap water.

104. In doing the admission assessment, the nurse should expect to find which signs of dehydration in an infant?
    1. Fever and bradycardia.
    2. Irritability and sunken eyeballs.
    3. Hypotension and anuria.
    4. Dry mucous membranes and bulging anterior fontanel.

105. If a toddler were to develop hydrocephalus, which would be the *earliest* sign(s) the nurse would most likely note?
    1. Irritability and poor feeding.
    2. Increasing head circumference.
    3. Headache and diplopia.
    4. Ruptured retinal vessels.

106. The mother of a child with cystic fibrosis asks the nurse if the child will be allowed to participate in any team sports now that he is starting school. The nurse would be most correct in advising her that the child can participate in:
    1. Softball.
    2. Tennis.
    3. Soccer.
    4. Swimming.

107. Parents of a child with sickle cell anemia both have the sickle cell trait. In counseling these parents about having another child, the nurse would be most correct in telling them that future pregnancies will have a:
    1. 1:4 chance of producing a child with sickle cell anemia.
    2. 1:2 chance of producing a child with sickle cell anemia.
    3. 1:4 chance of producing a child with sickle cell trait.
    4. 4:4 chance of producing a child with sickle cell anemia.

108. A patient with hemophilia is to receive Factor VIII concentrate. During the infusion of this medication, the nurse should plan to observe this patient for which potential complications?
    1. Emboli formation.
    2. Fluid volume overload.
    3. Onset of AIDS.
    4. Transfusion reaction.

109. A preschooler with epiglottitis is admitted to the hospital and is to receive Solu-Cortef 100 mg IV q6h. The main purpose for this medication is to:
    1. Provide mild sedation.
    2. Reduce swelling.
    3. Relieve pain.
    4. Treat infection.

110. A child with leukemia is being discharged, and the doctor suggests an immediate return to school. The nurse should be sure to teach the parents to keep this child home if any classmates develop:
    1. Impetigo.
    2. Strep throat.
    3. Pneumonia.
    4. Chickenpox.

111. In discharge teaching with the parents of an infant with VSD and CHF, which one visitor should the nurse discourage from touching or holding this infant?
    1. An aunt, who has lupus.
    2. A grandmother, who has a slight cold.
    3. The father, who is a drug addict.
    4. A 3-year-old sister, who is in nursery school.

112. In monitoring a toddler for response to syrup of ipecac, the nurse should base any actions on the knowledge that ipecac is potentially:
    1. Cardiotoxic.
    2. Hepatotoxic.
    3. Nephrotoxic.
    4. Neurotoxic.

113. A mother who lost her first-born to SIDS tells the nurse that she plans to breastfeed her second baby to prevent this from happening again. The nurse should base any response on the knowledge that:
    1. The risk of SIDS is the same, however infants are fed.
    2. Breastfeeding *does* seem to prevent SIDS.
    3. SIDS occurs less frequently in infants who are bottlefed.
    4. Breastfeeding is contraindicated for *siblings* of infants who died from SIDS.

114. Normally, an infant's birth weight doubles by age 6 months and triples by age 1 year. By what age should the nurse expect the birth weight to *quadruple*?
    1. 18 months.
    2. 2 years.
    3. 2½ years.
    4. 3 years.

115. A mother asks the nurse how tall her child will be when grown up. What answer should the nurse offer?
    1. "This is virtually impossible to predict."
    2. "It will be double the child's height at 2 years of age."
    3. "It will be triple the child's height at 18 months of age."
    4. "Add 2 feet to the child's height at 4 years of age."

116. In teaching principles of poison control to a group of mothers, the nurse would be most correct in stressing that the age group most likely to suffer from accidental ingestions is:
    1. 6–18 mo.
    2. 12 mo–2½ yr.
    3. 2–4 yr.
    4. 3–5 yr.

117. In deciding which *one* type of accident prevention to discuss *first* with the parents of a toddler, the nurse should base the choice on the knowledge that most deaths in children under age 3 are caused by:
    1. Aspiration/suffocation.
    2. Falls.
    3. Motor vehicles.
    4. Poisonings.

118. The following four children are patients in the pediatrics unit. Which one should the nurse anticipate will be *most* affected by separation from parents?
    1. A 6-week-old with pyloric stenosis.
    2. A 19-month-old with salicylate poisoning.
    3. A 3½-year-old with hypospadias.
    4. A 5-year-old with hemophilia.

119. In assessing the development of a 5-year-old, the nurse would not expect the child to be able to:
    1. Name primary colors.
    2. Count to 100.
    3. Know the days of the week.
    4. Give telephone number and address.

120. An RN from the telemetry unit is floated to the pediatrics unit. The charge nurse must assign three patients to her. Which patient should *not* be assigned to the telemetry nurse?
    1. A 5-month-old with Kawasaki disease.
    2. A 9-year-old with rheumatic fever.
    3. A 4-year-old with VSD after cardiac catheterization.
    4. A 3-week-old after pyloromyotomy.

121. The nurse in the emergency department triage area must decide which of the following children should be examined first by the pediatrician. Which child requires immediate attention?
    1. A 3-year-old who fell off his bicycle and has several lower extremity lacerations requiring sutures.
    2. A 2-year-old with laryngotracheobronchitis who has wheezing on auscultation and a respiratory rate of 28 breaths per minute.
    3. A 6-month-old who fell from the sofa onto a carpeted floor, hitting her head.
    4. A 4-year-old with asthma who has diminished wheezing and is very irritable.

122. The RN is supervising a nurse's aide who is caring for a child with a multidrug-resistant respiratory infection. Which action by the aide would be unsafe and would require the nurse's immediate attention?
    1. The aide wears a gown and gloves when entering the child's room.
    2. The aide removes the gown and gloves before leaving the child's room.
    3. The aide leaves the sphygmomanometer, thermometer, and stethoscope in the child's room, out of the child's reach.
    4. The aide washes her hands after removing her gloves, and then leaves the child's room to care for another child in the next room.

123. The RN assigns an LPN/LVN to care for a child with Hirschsprung's disease; the child's abdomen is grossly distended. The RN directs the LPN/LVN to measure the child's abdominal girth. Which action by the LPN/LVN would require the RN's intervention and further direction? The LPN/LVN:
    1. Uses a cloth tape to measure the child's abdominal girth.
    2. Leaves the tape in place after measuring the child's abdominal girth.
    3. Measures the child's abdominal girth at the umbilicus.
    4. Pulls the tape snug, but not tight, around the abdomen when measuring girth.

124. A child with a diagnosis of "rule out meningitis" is admitted to the pediatrics unit. The RN assigns this child to an LPN/LVN. Admitting orders include the following: bed rest with vital signs q2h; CBC with chemistry and electrolytes; gentamicin 80 mg IVPB q8h; liquid diet as tolerated; nasopharyngeal culture; and droplet precautions. In what sequence should the RN instruct the LPN/LVN to implement these orders?
    1. Put the child to bed and check vitals, take culture, draw blood, start antibiotics, initiate droplet precautions, order diet.
    2. Offer fluids, draw blood, take culture, put the child to bed and check vitals, start antibiotics, initiate droplet precautions.
    3. Initiate droplet precautions, put child to bed and check vitals, take a culture, start antibiotics, draw blood, order diet.
    4. Draw blood, start antibiotics, initiate droplet precautions, take culture, offer fluids, put child to bed and check vitals.

125. The nursing student is teaching a newly diagnosed diabetic adolescent about the disease and its treatment. Which statement by the student would require the RN's intervention?
    1. "When you use the vial of insulin marked 'U80,' it means that there are 80 units of insulin in that vial."
    2. "Be sure to check in with your doctor right away if you develop a fever or have an infection. You could develop a complication called ketoacidosis."
    3. "When you are getting ready to give yourself insulin, first draw up the short-acting insulin and then draw up the intermediate-acting insulin."
    4. "You should check your blood sugar four times a day, just like the MD ordered. The supplies are easily transportable and can go with you wherever you go."

126. The RN instructs the aide to give a child with eczema her bath. Which action by the aide would require the RN to provide additional supervision? The aide:
    1. Adds bath oil to the water.
    2. Bathes the child for 15 to 20 minutes.
    3. Provides toys for water play.
    4. Applies Lubriderm to the skin immediately after the bath.

127. The nurse is caring for all of the following patients. Which patient should the nurse recognize is at the highest risk for fluid and electrolyte imbalance?
    1. Infant with acute gastroenteritis.
    2. Toddler with lead poisoning.
    3. Preschooler with leukemia.
    4. School-age child with multiple trauma.

128. The RN should instruct the LPN/LVN or UAP caring for a child with PKU to be sure *not* to give this child:
    1. Green grapes.
    2. Diet soda.
    3. Cheerios.
    4. Cranberry apple juice.

129. An RN can safely delegate three of the following tasks to an LPN/LVN caring for a child with Down syndrome. Which one task should the RN perform personally and not delegate to an LPN/LVN?
    1. Transporting the child to the cardiac catheterization lab.
    2. Taking the child's vital signs, including blood pressure.
    3. Listening to the child's breath sounds bilaterally.
    4. Assisting the child to eat meals and snacks.

130. During a routine physical examination, a healthy, well-nourished 16-year-old male tells the nurse that he feels like killing his girlfriend because she broke up with him. He then laughs, and asks the nurse to keep this a secret just between the two of them. The nurse reviews his chart and notes that there is no previous history of violence or psychiatric illness. All other findings are within normal limits. The best action for the nurse to take at this time would be to:
    1. Regard the comment seriously and notify the teen's primary health care provider and parents.
    2. Recall that teenage boys often say things they really do not mean, and ignore the comment.
    3. Suggest the teen meet with a counselor to discuss his feelings about the breakup with his girlfriend.
    4. Tell the teen that his feelings are normal, and recommend that he find another girlfriend to take his mind off the problem.

131. A nurse's aide is working with a group of children in the playroom. Which action by the aide would require the RN to intervene?
    1. The aide offers a pacifier to an infant who is NPO.
    2. The aide opens a can of Play-Doh and gives it to a toddler.
    3. The aide stops a preschooler with terminal cancer from pulling on the braids of another child who is ready to be discharged.
    4. The aide tells a school-age child that he is too big to be crying for his parents.

132. A nursing student has been assigned to plan the prehospitalization teaching for a group of preschoolers having elective surgery. The preceptor should correct the teaching plan if it included which of the following?
    1. Make a list of the things the children could bring from home.
    2. Show the children a video describing activities that will take place during their hospital stay.
    3. Provide a detailed explanation to the children of what they will experience during preadmission testing.
    4. Give the children a tour of the ambulatory surgery unit, followed by a light snack and a chance to talk with the staff.

133. Which of the following tasks could the RN safely delegate to a UAP?
    1. Give an oatmeal bath to a 1-year-old with eczema.
    2. Monitor the I&O of a comatose 3-year-old with salicylate poisoning.
    3. Perform a complete bed bath on a 2-year-old with multiple injuries from a serious multivehicle accident.
    4. Check the IV of a 4-year-old with Kawasaki disease.

134. A child with severe pain asks for pain medication. The team caring for this child includes an RN, an LPN/LVN, and a UAP. After assessing the child, the RN administers the pain medication. Who should subsequently evaluate the effectiveness of the pain medication?
    1. The RN only.
    2. The RN and the LPN/LVN.
    3. The LPN/LVN and the UAP.
    4. All of the members of the team caring for this child.

135. A 9-year-old child with a brain tumor refuses to take chemotherapy. Both parents are present and insist that the RN administer the chemotherapy. The RN should:
    1. Administer the medication as ordered.
    2. Hold the medication and discuss this as soon as possible with the charge nurse and the MD.
    3. Offer distraction and then proceed to put the medication into the child's IV line.
    4. Leave the parents and child alone for awhile, to discuss this important issue privately.

136. An RN from the obstetrics unit is floated to the pediatrics unit. Which patients could the charge nurse safely assign to this float nurse?
    1. A child who has had a nephrectomy for Wilms' tumor.
    2. A child receiving IV chelating therapy for lead poisoning.
    3. A child with Kawaski disease and cardiac complications.
    4. A child who suffered a closed head injury in a 10 ft fall from a tree.

137. A child with diabetes experiences a hypoglycemic episode while hospitalized. The RN instructs the UAP to give the child a glass of orange juice. The RN should then instruct the UAP to:
    1. Include this amount of liquid on the child's I&O sheet.
    2. Offer the child a choice of Jell-O or pudding.
    3. Bring the child several small cups of a variety of juices to keep at the bedside.
    4. Provide the child with a snack of peanut butter and crackers.

138. A 2-year-old patient has had an open reduction for a fractured femur; his current weight is 25 lb 7 oz. He is in skeletal traction, and the physician has ordered meperidine (Demerol) 50 mg IM q6h prn for severe pain and muscle spasms. The nurse should recognize that:
    1. This dose of Demerol is excessive for a child of this age and weight.
    2. This dose of Demerol is appropriate for a child of this age and weight.
    3. 2-year-old children usually do not require pain medication, and this order should be questioned.
    4. 2-year-old children usually do not require pain medication, but if the doctor ordered this drug for him, the nurse should give it as ordered.

139. An LPN/LVN is caring for a child who is postop and complaining of pain; the child asks for pain medication at 5 P.M. The LPN/LVN notes that the last dose was given at 11:30 A.M. The MD's order is for Demerol 25 mg IM q4–6h prn for pain. The RN supervising this LPN/LVN should expect the LPN/LVN to:
    1. Administer the Demerol as ordered and then ask the RN to monitor the child for pain relief.
    2. Report these findings to the RN.
    3. Notify the MD that the child may be developing a dependence on Demerol.
    4. Administer the Demerol as ordered, and then chart whether or not pain relief is noted.

140. When administering an IM injection to a young child, the nursing student aspirates before injecting and notices blood in the syringe. The RN should instruct the student to:
    1. Inject the drug and then complete an incident report.
    2. Withdraw, change needles, and inject the drug in another site.
    3. Inject the drug slowly, over a 2-minute interval, and watch for possible adverse reactions.
    4. Withdraw the needle one-quarter inch and aspirate again; if no further blood is obtained, inject the medication.

141. The LPN/LVN is assigned to administer both an aerosol bronchodilator and an aerosol steroid to a child with asthma. The RN should instruct the LPN/LVN to administer:
    1. Both inhalers simultaneously.
    2. The bronchodilator first and the steroid second.
    3. The steroid first and the bronchodilator second.
    4. Neither; the RN should question these orders with the MD.

142. The RN instructs the UAP to collect a routine urine specimen on an infant. Which action by the UAP would require the nurse's intervention and further direction?
    1. The UAP washes her hands and puts on gloves.
    2. The UAP cleanses and dries the infant's genital area.
    3. The UAP applies the bag directly to the infant's skin, with the urethral meatus in the center of the opening.
    4. The UAP leaves the bag in place until it is full of urine.

143. The RN assigns an LPN/LVN to care for a child who just had a spinal tap to rule out meningitis. Which observation(s), if reported by the LPN/LVN within the first hour after the tap, should the RN follow up on?
    1. The child refuses fluids after the tap.
    2. The child denies having a headache.
    3. The child is lying flat in bed and states that he does not have a headache.
    4. The child is resting quietly and vital signs are within normal limits.

144. The parents of a 12-year-old child call the clinic early one morning because they are concerned about their son. They report that he is refusing to go to school because he has a severe headache; he vomited once and the parents say that there has been a virus going around his class. The best advice for the clinic nurse to offer them over the phone should be:
    1. "Bring your son into the clinic as soon as you can."
    2. "Offer your son Tylenol or ibuprofen, and then drive him to school about an hour later."
    3. "Give your son Tylenol or ibuprofen every 4 hours and monitor for fever; keep him home today."
    4. "These symptoms are most likely due to the virus and should improve within 24 hours. Be sure he gets plenty of rest and fluids."

145. The RN caring for a child with acute lymphocytic leukemia is called to the phone to speak with a caller who claims to be the child's aunt and godmother and who lives in another country. The woman is clearly upset, and tearfully asks the nurse whether the child's leukemia has relapsed. From report, the nurse is aware that the child is out of remission and that chemotherapy was started within the past hour. The nurse should tell the caller:
    1. "Yes, unfortunately the child just began chemotherapy again."
    2. "I just came on duty and have not had a chance to review the child's chart yet."
    3. "I'm sorry, but I cannot give out that information over the phone."
    4. "You really need to speak with the doctor about the child's condition and treatment."

Answers/Rationale

1. **(1)** Place the infant with a myelomeningocele on her stomach in a prone position to avoid pressure on the sac, which could cause tears, leaks, and infection. The side-lying position (**Answer 3**) might be an acceptable second choice, depending on the exact size and location of the sac. Placing the infant on her back (**Answer 2**) is absolutely contraindicated, because this would lead to immediate rupture of the sac. Trendelenburg position (**Answer 4**) is unnecessary for this infant.
   Test-taking tip—Picture the anatomy where the problem is and avoid on the back positions (2, 4).
   IMP, 3, SECE, Safety and Infection Control

2. **(4)** For a child experiencing migratory polyarthritis secondary to rheumatic fever, even the weight of a single sheet can cause excruciating pain; therefore, a bed cradle will help keep the linens off the child's joints and provide symptomatic relief. This child is most likely on bed rest, thus making a bath or shower (**Answer 1**) out of the question. Splints or a referral to physical therapy (**Answers 2, 3**) is unnecessary, because this type of arthritis causes no permanent deformities.
   Test-taking tip—Comfort is the priority of care, because of pain associated with migratory polyarthritis.
   IMP, 1, PhI, Basic Care and Comfort

3. **(4)** Projective techniques seem to work best with school-age children in getting them to share their thoughts, feelings, and experiences. Direct questioning (**Answer 1**) often proves too threatening, causing the child to become even quieter. Challenging the child directly to "tell secrets" (**Answer 2**) is also too threatening and will likely cause the child to refuse to speak about anything. Calling the child's mother (**Answer 3**) will not necessarily assist the child to communicate with the nurse.
   Test-taking tip—Select the age-appropriate, nonthreatening approach. When in doubt, note the pattern in responses: three are verbal and one is nonverbal (draw). Choose the method that is different.

Key to codes following rationales: *Nursing process:* **AS,** Assessment; **AN,** Analysis; **PL,** Plan; **IMP,** Implementation; **EV,** Evaluation. *Category of human function:* **1,** Protective; **2,** Sensory-perceptual; **3,** Comfort, Rest, Activity, and Mobility; **4,** Nutrition; **5,** Growth and Development; **6,** Fluid-Gas Transport, **7,** Psychosocial-Cultural; **8,** Elimination. **Client need: SECE,** Safe, Effective Care Environment; **PhI,** Physiological Integrity; **PsI,** Psychosocial Integrity; **HPM,** Health Promotion/Maintenance. See appendices for full explanation.

IMP, 7, PsI, Coping and Adaptation

4. **(3)** Progressive hoarseness, followed by aphonia, is an ominous sign of impending airway obstruction and respiratory arrest secondary to edema and inflammation. This must be promptly reported to the physician, who will probably do an emergency tracheostomy. An apical pulse of 118 (**Answer 1**) is normal for a toddler; pink nailbeds (**Answer 4**) indicate a satisfactory level of oxygenation. As the toddler begins to improve, appetite should also pick up (**Answer 2**).
   Test-taking tip—The question calls for an option that is *not* normal (not OK) and possibly life threatening.
   EV, 6, PhI, Physiological Adaptation

5. **(4)** At preschool age (4–6 years), the child should receive immunizations for DTP, OPV, and MMR. MMR (**Answer 1**) is correct, but hepatitis B is not. Hepatitis (**Answer 2**) is completed by *18 months,* as is varicella. *Haemophilus influenzae* (**Answer 3**) is completed by *15 months,* although DTP is correct.
   Test-taking tip—The best answer is based on knowing the recommended schedule of immunizations.
   IMP, 1, HPM, Prevention and Early Detection of Disease

6. **(4)** Typically, the majority of parents of infants with CHD complain about the infant's being very difficult to feed: must be awakened to feed, has a weak suck, may turn blue with feeding, takes an overly long time to feed but falls asleep before finishing. Because of the weak suck and altered cardiopulmonary dynamics, the infant is also prone to aspiration, pneumonia, and various respiratory infections (**Answer 1**) as well, although parents often do not make the connection between these factors. In addition, because of the difficulty in feeding the infant, the infant typically has developmental delays (**Answer 2**) and a slow rate of growth (**Answer 3**), although again this is not what the majority of parents of infants with CHD complain about.
   Test-taking tip—Because all answers are correct and interrelated, the clue is in the stem. The parents are most likely to have a daily problem with feeding.
   AN, 6, PhI, Basic Care and Comfort

7. **(2)** The major short-term complication that infants with myelomeningocele face is infection following a tear or rupture of the sac. Hydrocephalus (**Answer 1**) does occur in 90% of these cases, usually following closure of the sac, but it is thought to be part of the CNS defect rather than a complication. Likewise, paraplegia (**Answer 4**) is part of the symptom complex these patients have, rather than a complication. Mental retardation (**Answer 3**) may or may not occur, but if it does occur it is a long-term complication.
   Test-taking tip—The question asks for a *short-term complication* rather than part of the symptoms (one that will be evident within 1–2 wk).
   AN, 3, SECE, Safety and Infection Control

8. **(4)** As a toddler, this child will probably assert autonomy by refusing to take this medication. The best approach is to be firm yet kind, and always calm. No child should be told that medicine is like candy (**Answer 1**). Medication should be mixed with no more than 1 teaspoon of any nonessential food or beverage (**Answer 2**). This toddler will probably not drink this medication (**Answer 3**), and the nurse should not offer this choice because, if the child refuses, a "power struggle" will follow.
   Test-taking tip—Look for the choice that addresses the major developmental task for toddler—autonomy.
   IMP, 5, HPM, Growth and Development

9. **(4)** If the toddler responds well to oxygen therapy, the child should show clinical improvement in terms of pink lips and nailbeds and normal vital signs, especially pulse. "All" toys do not have to be removed from the crib (**Answer 1**), nor will the child have to be NPO (**Answer 2**), although the child will probably be somewhat anorexic and prefer clear,

cool liquids initially. Oxygen concentrations should be monitored and recorded *at least every 2 hours* (**Answer 3**).

> **Test-taking tip**—Eliminate the two options with the absolute "all." Also, recall that in the nursing process, nursing interventions are followed by evaluation.

EV, 6, PhI, Physiological Adaptation

10. (1) Children with asthma should have *no stuffed* animals in their rooms, because they tend to collect dust; therefore more teaching would be needed. Additional measures to "allergy proof" the room and home should include using only washable miniblinds rather than curtains (**Answer 2**) and having no pets in the home (**Answer 3**). Moderate exercise such as swimming (**Answer 4**) is recommended.

> **Test-taking tip**—The question is asking for the *incorrect* response.

EV, 1, HPM, Prevention and Early Detection of Disease

11. (3) The *average* age for the onset of menstruation for American girls is 12.8 years of age; girls between 10.5 and 15 years *can* begin to menstruate within the normal range (**Answers 1, 2, 4**).

> **Test-taking tip**—"Normal," "usually," and "average" are used as synonyms here. Know age-typical prepubertal and pubertal developmental norms.

IMP, 5, HPM, Growth and Development

12. (4) The majority of infants with CHD have tachycardia, or a heart rate above 160 beats/min; this is often the *first* sign of CHD that the nurse can assess. Circumoral cyanosis (**Answer 1**), hypertension (**Answer 2**), and diastolic murmur (**Answer 3**) all *may or may not* be present, depending on the type and severity of the defect.

> **Test-taking tip**—Note the use of the words "most common sign" in this question. Eliminate the three others that *may not* be present.

AS, 6, PhI, Physiological Adaptation

13. (4) To "flood" the croupette with oxygen means to raise the oxygen concentration to that level ordered by the physician; in general, the flow rate should be adjusted to 15 L/min, the tent should be closed and tucked in, and the nurse should wait about 15 minutes before checking the concentration and readjusting the flow. Lower flow rates (**Answers 1, 2, 3**) would result in lower-than-required oxygen concentrations.

> **Test-taking tip**—Note the use of the words "initially adjust" in this question.

IMP, 6, PhI, Physiological Adaptation

14. (1) In caring for a patient with a potentially contagious condition such as meningitis, the first priority is protecting the nurse and other patients by observing appropriate infection control measures, in this case, respiratory isolation. All other nursing care measures would then follow in the appropriate order (**Answers 2, 3, 4**).

> **Test-taking tip**—Infection control is always a priority of care.

AN, 1, SECE, Safety and Infection Control

15. (4) With a pediatric microdrip chamber, the number of mL/hr = number of drops/min. Therefore, if the physician orders 35 mL/hr, the IV should infuse at 35 drops/min. Any other flow rate would be incorrect (**Answers 1, 2, 3**).

> **Test-taking tip**—The nurse must know how to calculate the rate of flow of IVs.

IMP, 1, PhI, Pharmacological and Parenteral Therapies

16. (3) Neutropenia is an abnormal decrease in the number of neutrophils, the specific type of WBC responsible for phagocytosis and bacterial destruction; as such, the infection in a patient with leukemia is most commonly related to neutropenia. These patients may also suffer from anemia (**Answer 1**), leukopenia (**Answer 2**), or thrombocytopenia (**Answer 4**), although these blood dyscrasias will result in other signs or symptoms of leukemia.

> **Test-taking tip**—Look for the cause that is *directly* related.

AN, 1, PhI, Reduction of Risk Potential

17. (3) Patients receiving digoxin in addition to Lasix are particularly prone to developing hypokalemia, which can result in digoxin toxicity and potentially fatal cardiac dysrhythmias. Potassium supplements are frequently administered to avoid this problem rather than for any of the other reasons cited here (**Answers 1, 2, 4**).

> **Test-taking tip**—It logically follows that if K$^+$ is given, the purpose is to *replace* K$^+$ and therefore to avoid *low* K$^+$.

AN, 1, PhI, Pharmacological and Parenteral Therapies

18. (1) School-age children are notoriously competitive, and they particularly enjoy the challenge of board games such as Monopoly or Life. Although schoolwork is important and should receive due consideration (**Answer 2**), it will not relieve their boredom. Likewise, books and TV (**Answers 3, 4**) are less effective diversions for the school-age child.

> **Test-taking tip**—Three options are passive, one is interactive. Remember that school-age children are highly competitive, enjoying interactive games with others.

IMP, 7, PsI, Coping and Adaptation

19. (3) In working with children in hospitals, the most important factor for the nurse to *assess first* is the child's experience with illness and hospitalization. This is of special importance with this child, who has been hospitalized previously. *After this* most important factor, the nurse would continue the admitting assessment by determining what she knows about asthma (**Answer 1**), how she usually cares for herself (**Answer 2**), and how she feels about becoming a teenager (**Answer 4**).

> **Test-taking tip**—A major principle of teaching-learning is to start where the client is.

AN, 7, PsI, Coping and Adaptation

20. (2) Because the beta cells of the islets of Langerhans of the pancreas will never again produce a sufficient quantity of insulin, this teenager will remain dependent on insulin injections (exogenous insulin) for the rest of his life. Patients with type 1 diabetes can never rely on hypoglycemic agents to control diabetes (**Answer 1**), because these drugs work by stimulating the pancreas, and in this case the stimulation would have absolutely no effect. *Daily* modifications would generally not be necessary (**Answer 3**), although *periodic* adjustments in insulin dosage would be needed as this teenager grows. The child can continue to participate in sports (**Answer 4**), but should be taught to take some extra foods on those days when actively participating in sports.

> **Test-taking tip**—To pick the most theoretically correct answer, pull apart the key points about a *time* element: eventually, *for life,* daily, never.

IMP, 4, PhI, Physiological Adaptation

21. (2) Hemarthrosis, or bleeding into a joint either spontaneously or following an injury, is considered the hallmark, or most typical sign, of hemophilia. If hemarthrosis is not treated properly or adequately, permanent joint deformities may result. Other signs of hemophilia include prolonged bleeding from a relatively minor injury (**Answer 3**), excessive or unusual hematoma formation (**Answer 1**), and intracranial bleeding following a closed head injury (**Answer 4**).

> **Test-taking tip**—When all are correct, choose the one most associated with pain (a classic symptom of hemophilia), such as pain due to bleeding into a joint.

AN, 6, PhI, Physiological Adaptation

22. (1) Three-year-olds should be able to coordinate the brain and gross motor activity necessary to go up stairs using alternate feet. They should also be able to pedal a Big Wheel or a tricycle but *not* a bicycle (**Answer 2**). Three-year-olds should also be able to get dressed *with* supervision but not without it (**Answer 3**). They should not be ready to master tying shoelaces (**Answer 4**) for another year or two.

Test-taking tip—Remember, *three years = three wheels;* a 3-year-old should be capable of pedaling a tricycle.
AN, 6, HPM, Growth and Development

23. **(3)** The classic sign of Hirschsprung's disease is obstinate constipation that persists despite all efforts at treatment. Other symptoms may also occur but are not generally considered *specific* to Hirschsprung's disease as much as they indicate intestinal obstruction: abdominal distention (**Answer 1**), anorexia (**Answer 2**), and vomiting (**Answer 4**).
Test-taking tip—Note the use of the words "classic sign" in this question, meaning *specific* to the condition.
AN, 8, PhI, Physiological Adaptation

24. **(4)** The instruction manual of the DDST clearly states that the parent should accompany the child who is to have the DDST and that the examiner should do everything possible to establish rapport with the parent and the child. With a 9-month-old, this should include allowing the parent to hold the child rather than separating them for the purpose of testing (**Answers 1, 2, 3**).
Test-taking tip—Fear of strangers peaks at 8–9 months of age (i.e., keep the mother and baby together). Therefore, eliminate **Answers 1, 3, and 4.**
IMP, 5, HPM, Growth and Development

25. **(3)** An infant with severe chronic CHF should be on a low-sodium formula, Lonalac. Isomil (**Answer 1**) is a lactose-free formula that contains a normal amount of sodium. Lofenalac (**Answer 2**) is the formula used to treat infants with PKU and also contains a normal amount of sodium. Similac 27 with iron (**Answer 4**) is most frequently used for preterm infants and also contains a normal amount of sodium.
Test-taking tip—Look at the name of the formula and try to think it through; *lo* = low, *na* = sodium, lac = sounds like simi*lac.* Thus, a low-sodium formula!
PL, 4, PhI, Basic Care and Comfort

26. **(1)** Most psychologists would recommend that a child be offered comfort in the form of a hug, kiss, or cuddle; however, the child should be left in his or her own bed to avoid overdependence on the parents or possible psychosexual conflicts caused by entering the parents' bed (**Answer 2**). For the school-age child, nightmares are a common occurrence and can be accepted as a *normal* part of growth and development; therefore, no professional intervention is necessary at this time (**Answer 3**). It could be very difficult for this child to keep written records of her dreams (**Answer 4**); in fact, such an expectation might lead to even more severe sleep disturbances for her.
Test-taking tip—Focus on two options with "comfort," which are better than "consult" or "written record." As a general rule, children should sleep in their own beds, not with parents.
IMP, 5, PsI, Coping and Adaptation

27. **(1)** Before administering digoxin to a child, the nurse should auscultate the apical pulse for a full minute to most accurately evaluate cardiac rate and rhythm. Other pulse sites (**Answers 2, 3, 4**) are less accurate in children.
Test-taking tip—In this case, the key words "most correct" mean *most accurate.* Infants' and childrens' pulses should always be checked apically.
AS, 6, PhI, Pharmacological Therapy

28. **(3)** In working with children in hospitals, the most important factor for the nurse to assess first is what that child's experience with illness and hospitalization has been thus far. This is of special importance with this child, who has previously had two hospitalizations and surgeries; the nurse needs to know if these were positive experiences for this child and how he was able to cope with them. After this, the nurse would continue the admitting assessment by determining the child's developmental level (**Answer 1**), what the parents already know about hypospadias (**Answer 2**), and

whether the child's parents plan to room-in with him (**Answer 4**).
Test-taking tip—An important principle of teaching-learning is to always start with what the client already knows.
PL, 8, PsI, Coping and Adaptation

29. **(2)** Hospitalized preschoolers often regress in their behavior and want "mommy," but this is obviously not practical all the time. The nurse should try to soothe the child back to sleep during the middle of the night. Calling the mother to come right in (**Answer 4**) would be inappropriate, because the family should not be called in the absence of a genuine emergency. The nurse should also not pick the child up (**Answer 1**), because hospitalized preschoolers frequently reject everyone except their "mommy." Simply insisting the child go back to sleep (**Answer 3**) is not enough, because the child needs some degree of comfort at this time.
Test-taking tip—Look at the verbs: "pick . . . rock," "talk softly . . . rubbing back," "firmly tell," "call . . . mother." Preschoolers will regress when stressed, and respond well to verbal and physical comfort ("talk softly . . . rubbing back.")
IMP, 7, PsI, Coping and Adaptation

30. **(1)** Although the abrupt onset and critical nature of this illness is very frightening for parents, the child is expected to make a total recovery before discharge. The parents should be aware of this very positive diagnosis. Although discharge instructions from the physician may include some rest at home, there is no need for the child to miss almost a month of school (**Answer 2**). The parents should not worry about the child's getting sick again (**Answer 3**) or having oxygen in the home again (**Answer 4**); the excellent prognosis should be stressed.
Test-taking tip—Eliminate the incorrect statement first. Note the use of the words "correctly understood" in this question.
EV, 6, HPM, Prevention and Early Detection of Disease

31. **(3)** To maintain an oxygen concentration of 35–40%, the flow rate should now be adjusted to 8–10 L/min; this is the usual concentration ordered for a croup tent. Other flow rates would result in higher or lower concentrations (**Answers 1, 2, 4**).
Test-taking tip—There is only one theoretically correct answer. Although respiratory therapy often sets up croupettes and other forms of oxygen therapy, the nurse should be thoroughly familiar with the usual rate of flow. In this case, pick the midrange response (not 2–5 or 15).
IMP, 6, PhI, Physiological Adaptation

32. **(4)** To restrain a toddler receiving IV therapy, clove-hitch restraint to two or more limbs is most effective in maintaining the IV site. A posey jacket (**Answer 1**) would allow the toddler use of hands with which to pull at the IV. Elbow restraints (**Answer 2**) would still allow the toddler to stand and twist at the IV tubing. A mummy restraint (**Answer 3**) would be unnecessarily restrictive for a toddler.
Test-taking tip—Choose the option that is effective while not restraining, by *visualizing* what these various restraints do and where they are placed.
IMP, 1, SECE, Safety and Infection Control

33. **(1)** The best position for patients who have had a spinal tap is perfectly flat in bed, with no pillow at all. Such patients are prone to headaches due to the loss of CSF during the spinal tap; until the fluid is naturally replaced by the body, a flat position will minimize cerebral irritation and minimize headache; thus, (**Answer 2**) is incorrect. Elevating the HOB (**Answer 3**) will increase headache and is not recommended. There is no need to place the child semiprone (**Answer 4**) at this time.
Test-taking tip—Focus on two options that are "flat." "Flat" is "flat," meaning *no* pillow. Following a spinal tap, all patients should be *flat* in bed.
IMP, 1, PhI, Reduction of Risk Potential

Answers/Rationale

34. (2) The usual response to the birth of a defective infant is denial, often manifest in the parents' "refusing" to acknowledge the problem; this is a normal response, at least initially. The parents' comments about their infant, in view of this serious defect, should not be interpreted as attachment (**Answer 1**), immaturity (**Answer 3**), or love (**Answer 4**).

   Test-taking tip—*Denying* (in this case, the obvious physical problem) is one of the most commonly seen defense mechanisms.

   EV, 7, PsI, Coping and Adaptation

35. (1) With a child who has suffered an ingestion, vomiting should be induced only if the child is fully alert and reactive. If the child has any alterations in level of consciousness, such as seizures (**Answer 2**) or coma (**Answer 3**), vomiting may cause an aspiration pneumonia. Further, if the child has swallowed a corrosive substance (**Answer 4**), the substance that burned once going down will burn a second time coming up if vomiting is induced.

   Test-taking tip—In this case, when one option (**1**) is different than two others (**2** and **3** = not alert), choose the one that is different; note the use of the words "*should* administer," implying that you can eliminate three contraindicated situations (**2, 3, 4**).

   AN, 1, PhI, Pharmacological Therapy

36. (4) The corrective surgery for hypospadias is usually timed to be completed before the child develops body image and castration anxiety, by 18 months of age. Developmental and psychological factors thus play a crucial role in the timing of this surgery, and other explanations (**Answers 1, 2, 3**) are either incorrect or inappropriate for this child.

   Test-taking tip—Note the two options with "time" (**3, 4**). Select the option that is age specific, not "anytime" (**3**).

   IMP, 8, SECE, Management of Care

37. (2) When doing preoperative teaching with preschoolers, the best method is to use puppets (doctor, nurse, hospital setup) to "act out" what the child can expect to happen. For evaluating the teaching, the nurse can then ask the child to use puppets to give a return demonstration of what was learned; this enables the nurse to clarify any misconceptions or answer any lingering questions the child might still have. Most preschoolers will not be able to *accurately* draw pictures regarding the factual information of preoperative teaching (**Answer 1**), although this might be a good way to get at feelings about the surgery or hospital. A preschooler probably has had limited experience with "tests" (**Answer 3**). The nurse should not rely on the parents to evaluate the preoperative teaching (**Answer 4**), because they are not professionals and are most likely too involved emotionally.

   Test-taking tip—Preschoolers respond best to *play*—therapeutic, or medical.

   EV, 1, PsI, Coping and Adaptation

38. (1) The lower limit of a normal pulse rate for a 6-year-old is 75–80 beats/min; the nurse would be most correct in withholding the child's digoxin and notifying the physician if the pulse were below 80. A pulse rate of from 90 to 110 (**Answers 2, 3, 4**) would be considered within normal limits for a 6-year-old, and the nurse would be correct in administering the medication as ordered.

   Test-taking tip—The nurse should know approximate pulse rate norms for children of varying age groups. Key word is *withhold* with age-relevant norm for bradycardia.

   EV, 6, PhI, Pharmacological Therapy

39. (2) Sickling of RBCs occurs under conditions of low oxygen tension; giving this adolescent oxygen will prevent further sickling of RBCs, but it will *not reverse* the sickling of cells that has already occurred (**Answer 1**). The oxygen is not given to prevent any respiratory complication (**Answer 3**), nor will the oxygen have an effect on the oxygen-carrying capacity of the RBCs (**Answer 4**).

   Test-taking tip—Focus on the two options with "prevent." Then note that the word "sickle" is in both the stem and **Answer 2** ("sickling").

   IMP, 6, PhI, Physiological Adaptation

40. (3) The most common symptom in children with rheumatic fever is tachycardia due to cardiac involvement; in addition, these children may develop a rash, "erythema marginatum," and a characteristic fever, which spikes in the late afternoon. They do not usually have petechiae (**Answer 1**), hypertension (**Answer 2**), or conjunctivitis (**Answer 4**).

   Test-taking tip—Remember that cardiac symptoms are associated with rheumatic fever; therefore, choose the option with tachycardia.

   AS, 6, PhI, Physiological Adaptation

41. (2) Children with leukemia often experience bleeding gums due to thrombocytopenia; in addition, chemotherapy may cause oral mucous membrane ulceration. Therefore, the nurse would be most correct in advising this child to use a soft toothbrush only. Using a firm toothbrush (**Answer 3**) might cause a break in the gums, leading to infection. Rinsing the mouth only (**Answer 4**) might also lead to infection, because this would not necessarily clean the gums and teeth adequately; likewise, infection might be caused by not brushing the teeth (**Answer 1**).

   Test-taking tip—Narrow your choices to two *contradictory* options about brushes (soft vs. hard) and choose soft, due to bleeding.

   IMP, 1, PhI, Reduction of Risk Potential

42. (4) For a child just leaving the toddler period of autonomy and just entering the preschool period of initiative, the best suggestion to improve his nutritional intake would be to allow the child to feed himself. Other suggestions would supplement and enhance this primary consideration (**Answers 1, 2, 3**).

   Test-taking tip—The major developmental task of the toddler is autonomy; the major developmental task of the preschooler is initiative. Look at the verbs: "provide," "use," "offer," and "allow." Choose "allow."

   IMP, 5, HPM, Growth and Development

43. (2) It would be impossible to supervise a child with hemophilia so carefully that any other bleeding episodes would be prevented; furthermore, to attempt to do so would cause the parents to restrict the child totally, resulting in extreme overprotection. An acceptable alternative response would be to prevent "major" episodes of bleeding or to promptly recognize signs of a bleeding episode that would require medical intervention. The other statements (**Answers 1, 3, 4**) *are all correct* responses by the parents, indicating they have probably *understood* the nurse's teaching regarding the child's care.

   Test-taking tip—Note the use of the word "misunderstood" in this question, meaning look for the *incorrect* statement.

   EV, 6, HPM, Prevention and Early Detection of Disease

44. (4) Infants with CHF should be given about 15–20 minutes per feeding; if the infant is unable to finish the feeding, or if the infant becomes cyanotic or experiences respiratory distress during the feeding, gavage feeding should be used to avoid exhausting the infant and possibly precipitating an episode of apnea. No attempts should be made to continue the feeding (**Answers 1, 2, 3**).

   Test-taking tip—Three options continue the feeding and one option stops the feeding. In this case, choose the option that is different.

   IMP, 4, PhI, Basic Care and Comfort

45. (4) Epiglottitis is a bacterial infection of the epiglottis resulting in rapid airway swelling and obstruction; without prompt, aggressive treatment, it can progress rapidly, resulting in respiratory arrest within 6 to 8 hours of onset. Although this condition does require hospitalization and is

potentially life-threatening, the ICU stay is usually short (**Answers 2, 3**). There is no allergic cause of epiglottitis (**Answer 1**).

> **Test-taking tip**—Of all the respiratory conditions of childhood, epiglottitis is the most *rapidly* progressive (i.e., *quickly* life threatening and *quick* to recover, hence *short* stay in ICU.)

IMP, 6, PhI, Physiological Adaptation

46. (4) When a preschooler has a favorite "security object," be it a blanket or a doll or a stuffed animal, that child should be allowed to keep the security object, even during hospitalization. This will promote the child's sense of trust and security, thus helping to make the hospitalization a more positive experience. Offering the child another toy (**Answer 1**), putting the toy where he can see it but not touch it (**Answer 2**), or giving him a new stuffed animal (**Answer 3**) will not take the place of the child's old but well-loved original stuffed animal.

> **Test-taking tip**—Preschoolers will regress when stressed. Note that two options allow the security object to remain—one at a distance and the other *close* by.

IMP, 7, PsI, Coping and Adaptation

47. (1) Nephrosis (nephrotic syndrome) is a *chronic* syndrome characterized by variable pathology and questionable prognosis. In general, most children with nephrosis have severe, total body edema and 4+ proteinuria, along with hypoproteinemia. Hypertension and hematuria (**Answer 3**), and hyperlipidemia and periorbital edema (**Answer 2**), are more common in *acute* glomerulonephritis. The child with nephrosis seldom has severe oliguria (**Answer 4**), although occasionally this may occur; anorexia (**Answer 4**) may or may not occur, depending on the severity of the exacerbation.

> **Test-taking tip**—Choose "generalized" edema over limited (periorbital) edema.

AN, 8, PhI, Reduction of Risk Potential

48. (2) Carditis is the only manifestation of rheumatic fever that can lead to permanent damage; the best way to evaluate a child for the presence of carditis is to monitor the apical pulse at least q4h. Growth and development (**Answers 1, 3**) and ESR (**Answer 4**) deserve *secondary* consideration after checking the apical pulse.

> **Test-taking tip**—When performing an assessment, *priority* always implies either heart or lungs.

AN, 1, PhI, Reduction of Risk Potential

49. (3) The pain in vaso-occlusive crisis is due primarily to the clumping together of RBCs, which blocks small blood vessels, thus causing tissue ischemia, necrosis, and death. Although there may be increased RBC destruction (**Answer 1**) and hepatosplenomegaly (**Answer 2**), this is *not* the *primary* cause of this child's pain. Sequestration of blood does not normally occur with sickle cell anemia (**Answer 4**).

> **Test-taking tip**—Vaso-*occlusive* crisis implies a blockage (obstruction) in blood flow. Note the similarity of the term in the stem and in option **3**.

PL, 6, PhI, Physiological Adaptation

50. (3) From the very first attempt by a child to administer his or her own insulin, the nurse should stress the need to administer exact amounts as ordered by the physician. The child should learn from the start that "close" is not "correct" (**Answer 1**). A teenager *can* and *should* be capable of drawing up the exact amount (**Answer 2**). Drawing up an incorrect dose does not mean this teen is trying to antagonize the nurse, consciously or subconsciously (**Answer 4**).

> **Test-taking tip**—Any medication administered must be in the *exact* amount ordered.

EV, 5, PhI, Pharmacological and Parenteral Therapies

51. (1) As with an adult with CHF, the infant should be positioned in a chair/infant seat, in semi-Fowler's position, to provide for maximum expansion of the lungs and to assist the heart. Placing the infant on the stomach (**Answer 2**) might be an acceptable second choice, providing the infant can tolerate this position. The infant should never be placed on the back (**Answer 3**), even with the head slightly hyperextended, because of the possibility of aspiration and other respiratory complications. A side-lying position (**Answer 4**) would not allow for maximum expansion of the lungs; an infant seat is more appropriate.

> **Test-taking tip**—Picture the various positions and eliminate options **2** and **3**. Cardiac rest is best promoted by a semi-Fowler's (i.e., head elevated) position, regardless of the patient's age or condition.

IMP, 6, PhI, Basic Care and Comfort

52. (4) Transillumination, or the procedure of shining a light through the sac, is the usual means for evaluating the contents of the sac. When there is "no transillumination" (the light cannot shine through the sac), this indicates the presence of solid material, or the spinal cord, within the sac. Thus **Answers 2** and **3** are incorrect. Transillumination has no bearing on determining whether the sac can be easily repaired (**Answer 1**).

> **Test-taking tip**—Break up the word *transillumination* into its respective parts, *trans* and *illumination,* to derive its meaning. Choose the option that is most inclusive (**3** is included in option **4**).

AN, 2, PhI, Reduction of Risk Potential

53. (3) Syrup of ipecac is an emetic used to induce vomiting following ingestion of a harmful substance; the usual dose in children is 10–15 mL PO followed by at least 200 mL of water. The water is thought to enhance the emetic effect of ipecac and stimulate emptying of the stomach, thus ridding the body of the harmful substance. Activated charcoal (**Answer 2**) will *neutralize* the emetic effect and should *not* be given with ipecac, although in some cases it may be given *after* vomiting has occurred. Milk or toast (**Answers 1, 4**) has *little or no effect* and will neither help nor harm; however, if the child does vomit, they may increase the risk of aspiration.

> **Test-taking tip**—Ipecac should always be administered with water.

IMP, 1, PhI, Pharmacological and Parenteral Therapies

54. (1) Because oxygen is heavier than room air, it will settle to the bottom of the croupette and leak out unless the edges are tucked in tightly. If the edges are lying loosely on top of the linens (**Answer 2**), the oxygen will escape, resulting in lower concentrations than ordered. The crib rails should be raised for safety, *not* lowered (**Answer 4**); and again the edges should be tucked in tightly, *not* draped over the rails (**Answer 3**).

> **Test-taking tip**—Focus on the two options about plastic canopy *edges* and select "tightly" over "loosely."

IMP, 6, PhI, Reduction of Risk Potential

55. (2) The preferred position for a child with asthma is high Fowler's, or sitting up straight, which allows for maximum expansion of the lungs. Other positions would *not* allow for the maximum expansion of the lungs (**Answers 1, 3, 4**) and would only contribute to this child's hypoxia.

> **Test-taking tip**—A full upright position allows for maximum expansion of the lungs.

IMP, 6, PhI, Basic Care and Comfort

56. (2) Juveniles with diabetes (type 1 diabetes) are extremely brittle, or difficult to control, and prone to episodes of hypoglycemia or ketoacidosis. If this teenager were to experience a hypoglycemic episode, the earliest symptoms would often be behavioral: irritability, personality changes, etc. If this teen becomes disruptive, the nurse should first ask if he has eaten his breakfast, how much he ate, and when; other areas (**Answers 1, 3, 4**) would be appropriate to explore *after* this primary consideration.

Answers/Rationale

Test-taking tip—An underlying physiological cause to a patient's behavior should be explored first, before looking at behavioral considerations.

AN, 4, PhI, Physiological Adaptation

57. **(2)** Extremes of temperatures, either too warm or too cold, should be avoided for infants with CHD, because this increases the body's demand for oxygen, thus increasing the workload of the heart. The mother would need no further teaching if she *correctly* stated that this infant should be dressed in loose-fitting clothing (**Answer 1**), should be brought back to the clinic for regularly scheduled appointments (**Answer 3**), and should be placed in a safe play area to stimulate development (**Answer 4**).

Test-taking tip—Note the use of the phrase "need for additional teaching" in this question (i.e., look for the incorrect statement).

EV, 6, HPM, Prevention and Early Detection of Disease

58. **(1)** With a patient with a potentially contagious infection such as AGE, the first priority is protection of the nurse and other patients by observing appropriate infection control measures, including contact precautions. Other interventions can *then* be safely implemented without risk of cross-contamination (**Answers 2, 3, 4**).

Test-taking tip—Infection control is always a priority of care.

AN, 1, SECE, Safety and Infection Control

59. **(2)** The general recommendation to make to parents on how to handle temper tantrums is to ignore this behavior. If a parent allows a child to make a choice (**Answer 1**) and then does not follow through with this choice either because of personal preference or because the choice is unsafe, tantrums will increase. Changing settings (**Answer 3**) is often a catalyst for a tantrum as the child is moved from one area to another (e.g., from the park to home). Giving in to a toddler's demands (**Answer 4**) is unrealistic; parents should offer only allowable choices to their toddler and then allow the toddler to follow through with these choices.

Test-taking tip—Paying attention to a temper tantrum will reinforce this behavior.

IMP, 5, HPM, Growth and Development

60. **(2)** Toddlers typically fear those procedures that are "intrusive," that is, where something goes into their bodies. Therefore, a rectal temperature would most likely evoke the most anxiety in a toddler. Generally, a toddler would be relatively cooperative with getting weighed (**Answer 4**) and giving a urine specimen (**Answer 3**), although having blood pressure taken might also be somewhat threatening (**Answer 1**).

Test-taking tip—Note the patterns in the answers: three options are nonintrusive procedures, one option *is* intrusive—and therefore most frightening.

AN, 7, HPM, Growth and Development

61. **(1)** The leading cause of morbidity and mortality in children with leukemia is infection; therefore, preventing infection is the most important nursing care plan goal. Preventing injury (**Answer 2**), promoting adequate nutrition (**Answer 3**), and meeting developmental needs (**Answer 4**) are less important goals for the child with leukemia.

Test-taking tip—Infection control is top *priority* of care when the immune system is compromised (e.g., in leukemia).

PL, 1, SECE, Safety and Infection Control

62. **(2)** The chief purpose of the moist soaks is to prevent tears or leaks in the sac, which could lead to infection, the number one cause of death during the neonatal period. Promoting comfort (**Answer 1**) and relieving pressure (**Answer 3**) are not reasons for ordering moist soaks for this infant. It is *not* possible to stimulate neural development (**Answer 4**), which is permanently and irreversibly arrested before birth.

Test-taking tip—Look at the verbs: "promote," "prevent," "relieve," and "stimulate." Choose "prevent."

AN, 1, SECE, Safety and Infection Control

63. **(3)** By making a game of "checking for monsters," a potentially frightening situation is relieved, and the child may even begin to realize that there "really" are no monsters. Asking the child to talk about his monsters (**Answer 1**) may make him believe they are real and that his father also believes in them. It would be too frightening to the child to have to look for these monsters by himself (**Answer 2**). Telling a preschooler that his fantasies are not real (**Answer 4**) would not be enough to convince him and might make him become even more convinced they are real.

Test-taking tip—Preschoolers are in the age of fantasy or magical thinking; therefore choose option 3, "make a game."

IMP, 5, HPM, Growth and Development

64. **(1)** The surgical repair for hypospadias is done on the urethra primarily and also on the urethral meatus. Postoperatively, a urinary drainage apparatus (Foley or suprapubic) will be in place, and the urine is expected to have a clear yellow appearance. There should normally be no blood or mucus (**Answers 2, 3, 4**), which would indicate hemorrhage or infection if present.

Test-taking tip—Choose the option that is different: three options indicate a problem, one says it is OK (yellow urine is normal).

EV, 8, PhI, Reduction of Risk Potential

65. **(3)** To be most effective, pancreatic enzymes should be administered immediately before every meal and every snack; this will facilitate the absorption of fats and proteins contained within the meal. The enzymes will have little or no therapeutic value if given at other times (**Answers 1, 2, 4**).

Test-taking tip—Key word is "replacement" of what is missing in CF; therefore, the best *time* to aid fat absorption is *before* eating.

PL, 6, PhI, Pharmacological and Parenteral Therapies

66. **(1)** Warmth causes vasodilation, thus relieving the occlusion of small vessels and preventing tissue damage. Cold (**Answer 2**) would never be used, because it causes vasoconstriction. Performing ROM exercises (**Answer 3**) or ADL (**Answer 4**) would not relieve pain.

Test-taking tip—Focus on two options that are contradictory: warmth → vasodilation; cold → vasoconstriction. Occluded blood vessels need vasodilation measures.

IMP, 6, PhI, Reduction of Risk Potential

67. **(1)** An infant with CHF should wear loose-fitting clothes, including diapers, to avoid pressure on the abdominal organs, which could impinge on the diaphragm and impede respiratory effort. The nursing student should loosen the diaper and should know the rationale for this action as well. The nurse should not take care of this after the student leaves (**Answer 3**), because the student will repeat the mistake without the nurse's intervention; in addition, pinning the diaper snugly is inappropriate for an infant with CHF (**Answers 2, 4**), and the nurse has the final responsibility for the care this infant receives.

Test-taking tip—Any patient with CHF, regardless of age, should wear *loose*-fitting clothes.

EV, 6, PhI, Reduction of Risk Potential

68. **(4)** Nephrosis is characterized by periods of exacerbations and remissions that occur throughout the childhood years. The child's parents should watch him closely for exacerbations, which should be reported promptly to the physician. The child should be encouraged to play with other children, not to stay away from them (**Answer 1**) to avoid feelings of social isolation. It is *not* "over" (**Answer 2**), and the child will need to be watched carefully for periods of exacerbation. Once the child is discharged, he will generally not need to remain in bed (**Answer 3**) but rather can convalesce at home with alternating periods of activity and rest.

Test-taking tip—Note the use of the words "fully under-stood" in this question; therefore, use a true-false approach to eliminate the three false statements.

EV, 8, HPM, Prevention and Early Detection of Disease

69. **(4)** Vincristine is an antineoplastic *Vinca* alkaloid, which causes numbness, tingling, footdrop, paresthesia, etc. In addition, vincristine may also cause constipation, *not* diarrhea (**Answer 1**). Hemorrhagic cystitis (**Answer 3**) may be caused by cyclophosphamide (Cytoxan), *not* vincristine. Vincristine does *not* cause visual changes (**Answer 2**).

Test-taking tip—Know the major side effects of vincristine (peripheral neuropathy).

IMP, 6, PhI, Pharmacological and Parenteral Therapies

70. **(2)** Pancreatic enzymes *are* enzymes; as such, they break down whatever food or liquid they are mixed with. However, for maximum therapeutic effect, the enzymatic action should be delayed until the medication reaches the stomach. The best food to mix with pancreatic enzyme tablets is the cold applesauce. The applesauce should be cold because cold delays the enzymatic action, which is most effective at 98.6°F. Applesauce is used because of its high fiber content, which also delays the enzymatic action of the medication. Any other foods or liquids the pancreatic enzymes might be mixed with (**Answer 3**) would be less than ideal. Pancreatic enzyme tablets cannot simply be discontinued (**Answer 1**) because a child has difficulty swallowing them; this medication must be taken for the rest of the child's life. It is not appropriate to bribe a child (**Answer 4**) with a reward for desired behavior; children should never be bribed or threatened into taking medication.

Test-taking tip—Focus on the two options with contradictory terms: cold vs. warm. Cold has the desired effect of delaying enzymatic action.

IMP, 4, PhI, Pharmacological and Parenteral Therapies

71. **(3)** Carditis can lead to permanent, irreversible cardiac damage, specifically, mitral valvular stenosis. The other manifestations of rheumatic fever (**Answers 1, 2, 4**) are *transient* and do not leave any permanent effects.

Test-taking tip—Key word is "permanent." Choose the option pertaining to the *heart*.

PL, 1, PhI, Physiological Adaptation

72. **(4)** A child with rheumatic fever will be in the hospital for a relatively longer time and will be confined to bed most of the time. The ideal roommate would be another child of the same sex and same developmental level who will also be in the hospital for some time and confined to bed. The best choice is the young girl with the fractured elbow, who will be in skeletal traction and also on bed rest. The child with a tonsillectomy (**Answer 2**) or the child with a concussion (**Answer 3**) will most likely be in the hospital for a very short time and will be out of bed. The child with impetigo, caused by streptococcus (**Answer 1**), would be a most unsatisfactory roommate for this child, because she might reinfect her with strep.

Test-taking tip—The ideal roommate for any child is another child of the same sex and developmental level.

IMP, 1, HPM, Growth and Development

73. **(1)** The most important nursing diagnosis relates to physiological integrity (i.e., maintaining a normal blood-sugar level). Other diagnoses (**Answers 2, 3, 4**) would be correct but not necessarily of primary concern.

Test-taking tip—Physiological integrity is always a priority of care.

EV, 4, PhI, Physiological Adaptation

74. **(3)** Parents often hope that the surgery done to close the sac will also help the infant move the legs. Surgery will *not* enable the infant to regain motor or sensory functioning; surgery is done primarily to prevent infection. Parents should not be told the infant will move the legs after surgery (**Answer 4**) or offered false hope (**Answers 1, 2**).

Test-taking tip—Myelomeningocele results in permanent, irreversible nerve damage.

IMP, 3, PsI, Coping and Adaptation

75. **(3)** The best means to prevent any type of infection in any type of setting is good hand washing. Other techniques are *secondary* (**Answers 1, 2, 4**).

Test-taking tip—Hand washing is the first line of defense in infection control.

AN, 8, SECE, Safety and Infection Control

76. **(2)** At 7 months of age, an infant may either sit with some support or sit alone; either behavior is commonly acquired at this age. Rolling over (**Answer 1**) is usually found in infants around 3 to 4 months of age, whereas weight bearing (**Answer 3**) and the palmar grasp (**Answer 4**) are commonly found in infants between ages 4 and 6 months.

Test-taking tip—Note the use of the phrase "most recently acquired skill" in this question.

AN, 5, HPM, Growth and Development

77. **(2)** As a 9-month-old with a chronic bowel problem, this infant has probably become accustomed to mother's administering suppositories or enemas. In addition, fear of strangers is common in this age group. Considering these factors, this infant's mother should at least be offered the opportunity to administer or assist with the enemas. If this is not feasible, another qualified person could take her place (**Answers 1, 3, 4**).

Test-taking tip—Look at the pattern of responses: three options are staff, one is the mother. Choose the one that is different, especially considering that fear of strangers peaks at 8–9 months.

AN, 6, HPM, Growth and Development

78. **(2)** LTB progresses through four distinct stages, with *early symptoms in the first* stage including fear, hoarseness, croupy cough, and inspiratory stridor only when disturbed. In the *second* stage, the stridor is constant and is accompanied by retractions (**Answer 4**). In the *third* stage, restlessness and tachypnea (**Answer 3**) are seen in addition to anxiety, pallor, and sweating. In the *fourth and final* stage, intermittent or constant cyanosis is followed by the cessation of breathing, or apnea (**Answer 1**).

Test-taking tip—Note the use of the words "early signs" in this question.

AN, 6, PhI, Physiological Adaptation

79. **(3)** The opisthotonos position occurs in children with severe meningitis due to the pressure on the spinal cord; the child's head is drawn back and the spine is arched backward in an attempt to minimize pressure on the cord. When the child assumes this position, the nurse should place the child in a side-lying position for safety and comfort. Any other position would not work as well (**Answers 1, 2, 4**).

Test-taking tip—Visualize the condition, and then visualize the options to identify the position for safety and comfort.

IMP, 1, PhI, Basic Care and Comfort

80. **(1)** Younger teenage girls in particular prefer the company of other young girls; they have a definite preference for same-sex, same-age companions. As such, this child would not necessarily seek out older or younger children (**Answers 2, 4**), nor would she have "no preference" regarding the sex of her companion (**Answer 3**).

Test-taking tip—Know age-relevant stages of psychosocial development. Young teenage girls generally prefer a same sex "best friend."

AN, 5, HPM, Growth and Development

81. **(3)** Crises are precipitated by conditions of low oxygen tension; this may include infection, which could easily be picked up by swimming in public pools. Other sources of low oxygen tension might include *severe* emotional stress (**Answer 1**), *extremely* cold or windy weather (**Answer 2**), or *dehydration* (**Answer 4**), as well as high altitudes.

Test-taking tip—Note the use of the word "avoid" in this question, and situations that may lead to infections.

IMP, 6, HPM, Prevention and Early Detection of Disease

82. **(4)** With children who have received a 10 mL dose of syrup of ipecac, if vomiting has not occurred within 30 minutes, the dose can and should be repeated once more. Although the first dose is generally effective in the majority of cases, a second dose is almost always 100% effective. If the child does not vomit *after* a second dose, manual stimulation of the gag reflex or gastric lavage must be promptly initiated to avoid toxic effects of ipecac. The nurse should *never use fingers* to stimulate the gag reflex (**Answer 1**), especially in a toddler, because of the danger of receiving a human bite. Ipecac works within 15–30 minutes, and waiting another 30 minutes will not be helpful (**Answer 2**). If the child does not vomit at all, thus not removing either the ipecac or the ingested substance(s), there is the danger of ipecac toxicity, as well as poisoning from the ingested substance (**Answer 3**).

Test-taking tip—Eliminate 2 (do *not* wait) and 3 (there *is* a danger) because ipecac is cardiotoxic and can cause complete heart block.

IMP, 1, PhI, Pharmacological and Parenteral Therapies

83. **(1)** Due to this child's carditis, the best means for the nurse to evaluate how well any increase in activity is tolerated would be by monitoring the apical pulse rate. Any increase in pulse rate over 15–20 beats/min would indicate that the increase in activity is not tolerated and would be an indication for returning the child to bed immediately. Any other method of evaluating tolerance of increasing activity would be less effective (**Answers 2, 3, 4**).

Test-taking tip—Activity tolerance in *heart* conditions (carditis in rheumatic fever) is best measured by *heart* rate.

IMP, 6, HPM, Prevention and Early Detection of Disease

84. **(2)** The teenager who is newly diagnosed with diabetes must assume responsibility for his own care as soon as possible; diabetes is a chronic disease with no known cure that this teen will have to live with for the rest of his life. The nurse should discourage his mother from being overly protective of him or from assuming this responsibility (**Answers 1, 3, 4**).

Test-taking tip—Self-care management is always a patient-centered goal.

IMP, 7, PsI, Coping and Adaptation

85. **(3)** The use of a pacifier for an infant with CHF will promote true psychological rest, thus reducing the body's demand for oxygen and reducing the workload of the heart. This is the *most* important reason that this infant should be offered the pacifier; although it may also be true that the infant seems to like the pacifier (**Answer 1**), this is not the main reason one should be given. **Answers 2** and **4** are too generalized and not necessarily true.

Test-taking tip—According to Freud, because infants are in the stage of oral gratification, a pacifier will reduce crying, which is medically significant in this case.

IMP, 6, PhI, Reduction of Risk Potential

86. **(4)** Contrary to popular belief, the best position for the nurse to place a child with a nosebleed in is sitting up and leaning forward slightly, with head remaining above the level of the heart; this position will allow the blood to drain freely from the nose and prevent aspiration. Sitting up with the head tilted backward (**Answer 3**) will predispose the child to swallowing or aspirating blood, as will a semi-Fowler's position (**Answer 2**). The prone position (**Answer 1**) might be an acceptable *second* choice if the child were too weak to sit up without assistance.

Test-taking tip—Preventing aspiration and maintaining a patent airway is always a priority of care.

IMP, 6, PhI, Reduction of Risk Potential

87. **(1)** While in the croupette, toddlers should be allowed only those toys that can be dried off easily; all stuffed animals, dolls with hair, etc. are not allowed, because they will harbor moisture and bacteria. While in the croupette, the child and the linens will also get damp or wet, and the nurse should implement measures to prevent chilling. Pajamas and blankets should be changed q4h or prn (**Answer 2**). There is no need to restrain a child in the croupette (**Answer 3**), because all working parts are safely outside the croupette. There is no need to restrict visitors (**Answer 4**).

Test-taking tip—Infection control is always a priority of care. Look at the verbs in the stem: "giving," "removing," "restraining," and "restricting." "Giving" is preferable; it sounds better than the 3 r's.

IMP, 6, SECE, Safety and Infection Control

88. **(2)** Cystic fibrosis is inherited as an autosomal recessive disorder. The fact that these parents have a child with CF means that they are carriers of the trait, and each subsequent pregnancy might result in a child who also has CF. It would not be correct to advise the mother that a second child would only carry the trait (**Answer 4**) or would be normal (**Answer 3**), although there is a possibility these might occur; the parents should be fully advised of the odds of this happening. In addition, it would needlessly worry the parents to tell them a second child might be more severely affected (**Answer 1**), although this is also a possibility.

Test-taking tip—Regardless of the genetics, having had one child with this disease, there is always a risk that subsequent children may also have this disease.

IMP, 1, HPM, Prevention and Early Detection of Disease

89. **(2)** About half the children who have eczema during the toddler or preschool years develop asthma during the school-age or teenage years. Asthma seems to have little or no relation to strep throat or tonsilitis (**Answer 1**). The father's death undoubtedly would have affected this child, but it occurred 1 year before the onset of the asthma (**Answer 3**). The pneumonia experienced at age 4 might have been related to the asthma, but was not the cause of it (**Answer 4**).

Test-taking tip—Although the etiology of asthma is multifactorial, there is thought to be an allergic predisposition.

AN, 1, HPM, Prevention and Early Detection of Disease

90. **(1)** Considering this infant's diagnosis, the nurse should anticipate that the infant will most likely have at least some developmental delays; most infants would begin to roll over by 3 months of age, but at 5 months the baby should be doing this now. Sitting (**Answer 2**) is normally found around 6 months of age; this infant will most likely *not* be capable of this behavior at 5 months. A pincer grasp (**Answer 3**) is normally found at 9–12 months of age, and this infant will most likely *not* be capable of this behavior. Weight bearing (**Answer 4**) is typically noted in healthy infants at 4–6 months of age; considering this infant's diagnosis, however, this baby may or may not be capable of this more strenuous behavior.

Test-taking tip—Infants learn to roll over at 3 months, sit at 6 months, and crawl at 9 months. Consider delayed development in congestive heart failure.

AS, 5, HPM, Growth and Development

91. **(1)** The infant is placed on the abdomen postoperatively to prevent trauma or pressure to the sutured area on the back. In addition, the infant's head should be positioned 10 degrees lower than the hips to prevent the pressure of circulating CSF from affecting the suture line on the lower back. An obvious contraindication to this position is the presence of increased intracranial pressure, in which case the infant would be positioned flat in bed (**Answer 4**). In general, the head is never higher than the hips (**Answers 2, 3**) during the immediate postoperative period for this type of surgery.

Test-taking tip—Visualize the positions; know postoperative objectives regarding preventing pressure to suture area.

IMP, 3, PhI, Reduction of Risk Potential

92. **(1)** Hirschsprung's disease is a congenital condition. It does not "develop spontaneously," although the diagnosis may not be made until symptoms have been present for several months and some attempts at conservative medical treatment (enemas, stool softeners, etc.) have been made (**Answer 3**). In the newborn with Hirschsprung's disease, there may be an episode of meconium ileus (**Answer 2**), but this occurs as a *result* of the Hirschsprung's disease *rather than as the cause of it*. There is no known metabolic defect (**Answer 4**).

> **Test-taking tip**—Narrow your option to the one that is different: congenital vs. acquired after birth.

IMP, 8, PsI, Coping and Adaptation

93. **(2)** As healing of the pathways of the CSF occurs following an episode of meningitis, scar tissue naturally forms; this may lead to noncommunicating hydrocephalus. The hydrocephalus might *then lead* to learning disabilities (**Answer 3**) or mental retardation (**Answer 4**). Encephalitis (**Answer 1**) may occur in *conjunction with* the meningitis, but it is *not* a complication.

> **Test-taking tip**—Note the use of the term *long-term complication* in this question, and select the option that incorporates (leads to two other conditions) or is in conjunction with the other options.

AS, 2, HPM, Prevention and Early Detection of Disease

94. **(3)** Because concentrated sweets will cause a rise in blood sugar, followed by a precipitous drop, the nurse should teach this patient that he should follow up this concentrated sweet with a complex carbohydrate such as a glass of milk. Any other action would be inappropriate at this time (**Answers 1, 2, 4**).

> **Test-taking tip**—The complex carbohydrate will help maintain a steady blood sugar level. Therefore, choose the only option that is not a diagnostic test or pharmacological agent.

IMP, 4, PhI, Reduction of Risk Potential

95. **(4)** There are multiple factors involved in the etiology of asthma, including an allergic predisposition (**Answer 2**), precipitation by severe emotional or physical stress (**Answer 3**), and other factors yet to be determined (**Answer 1**).

> **Test-taking tip**—When more than one option looks correct, choose the more comprehensive answer (multiple answers = "multiple factors").

IMP, 1, PsI, Coping and Adaptation

96. **(1)** Long-term follow-up care for children with rheumatic fever most frequently includes antibiotic therapy with penicillin or erythromycin on an exact schedule for an indefinite time. There is no way to immunize against future attacks (**Answer 2**). This child will be sent home on restricted activity, and cardiac rehabilitation programs are out of the question at this time (**Answer 3**). Home tutoring would be fine, but it is not a priority at this time (**Answer 4**).

> **Test-taking tip**—Medical prevention is the clue to the best choice.

IMP, 6, PhI, Reduction of Risk Potential

97. **(2)** In suspected cases of epiglottitis, the visualization of the epiglottis is strictly contraindicated, because it may precipitate laryngospasm and immediate respiratory arrest. It is a nursing responsibility to inform any less knowledgeable health care providers of this danger; any other action (**Answers 1, 3, 4**) would be inappropriate at this time.

> **Test-taking tip**—The nurse must always serve as a patient advocate. Also note that three responses allow the procedure, but one does not. Choose the one that is different from the others.

IMP, 6, PhI, Reduction of Risk Potential

98. **(4)** There is no known cure for nephrosis; rather, treatment is aimed at providing symptomatic relief. To that effect, prednisone—an anti-inflammatory corticosteroid—is given to relieve symptoms rather than effect a cure. If prednisone has the expected therapeutic effect, the patient should report "feeling better" as symptoms are relieved. *Side* effects of prednisone therapy may also include mood swings (**Answer 1**), glucosuria (**Answer 2**), and fluid retention with weight gain (**Answer 3**).

> **Test-taking tip**—Note the key words "expected therapeutic effects," *not* side effects.

EV, 8, PhI, Pharmacological and Parenteral Therapies

99. **(4)** Toddlers will suffer the most if separated from their mothers; a croupette is a particularly frightening experience, because explanations are difficult. If the toddler will calm down with the mother in the croupette, this will decrease the body's need for oxygen. There is no need to check with the physician (**Answer 2**), nor would it be "unsafe" (**Answer 3**). Considering that the child is hospitalized and most likely frightened by the strange equipment, there is no reason to question the parent's handling of the situation (**Answer 1**).

> **Test-taking tip**—First, decide if this is OK or not OK. Recall that toddlers are at a peak age for separation anxiety, and choose an "OK" answer.

IMP, 5, PsI, Coping and Adaptation

100. **(2)** In infants, the earliest sign of hydrocephalus is increasing head circumference, which occurs as the suture lines separate and the fontanels widen to accommodate the extra fluid within the skull. *Later* signs would indicate that no further accommodation can occur and brain tissue is being destroyed; these signs might include bulging anterior fontanel (**Answer 1**), shrill, high-pitched cry (**Answer 3**), and sunset eyes (**Answer 4**).

> **Test-taking tip**—Note the use of the term *earliest sign* in this question.

AN, 3, HPM, Prevention and Early Detection of Disease

101. **(1)** Viscous xylocaine is never recommended for children with mucosal ulcerations secondary to chemotherapy, because of the risk of a depressed gag reflex and aspiration. The other interventions (**Answers 2, 3, 4**) *are*, however, all *appropriate* nursing interventions.

> **Test-taking tip**—Note that this question is asking about an intervention that is *not* appropriate, meaning eliminate the correct statements.

IMP, 6, PhI, Pharmacological and Parenteral Therapies

102. **(4)** As generalized edema progresses, in males the scrotal sac can become extremely swollen, tender, and painful. The best nursing intervention is to place soft, folded diapers under the scrotum while the child is lying in bed. Zinc oxide (**Answer 1**) or medicated powder (**Answer 3**) will have little beneficial effect because the problem is *mechanical* rather than on the skin itself. Cleansing the scrotum (**Answer 2**) is important to prevent infection, because all edematous tissue needs special care to prevent skin breakdown; however, this will *not relieve* the child's discomfort.

> **Test-taking tip**—Providing comfort is the priority of care.

IMP, 8, PhI, Basic Care and Comfort

103. **(2)** The only solution that should be used in doing cleansing enemas for a child with Hirschsprung's disease is normal saline, because the child will retain some of this fluid, which will be absorbed through the bowel wall. As an isotonic solution, normal saline will not alter the fluid balance, as a non-isotonic solution almost certainly would (**Answers 1, 3, 4**).

> **Test-taking tip**—The choice is between isotonic and nonisotonic solutions. Select the isotonic solution.

AN, 8, PhI, Basic Care and Comfort

104. **(2)** Signs of dehydration in infants include irritability and sunken, dry eyeballs due to fluid loss. Fever may be present, and tachycardia, *not* bradycardia (**Answer 1**), is also common. Low blood pressure often results, followed by *oliguria*; anuria (**Answer 3**) is rare and would be an ominous sign of renal failure. The oral buccal mucosa may be quite dry, and the anterior fontanel may be *sunken, not* bulging (**Answer 4**).

Test-taking tip—If part of an answer is right but part of it is wrong, the answer must be wrong.
AS, 6, HPM, Prevention and Early Detection of Disease

105. (1) If a toddler were to develop hydrocephalus, the first sign would most likely be irritability and poor feeding due to increased intracranial pressure. The head circumference would *not increase* (**Answer 2**), because the fontanels have closed. Headaches or double vision might occur (**Answer 3**), but a toddler is not likely to complain of them. Ruptured retinal vessels (**Answer 4**) is a *later* sign of increased intracranial pressure.
Test-taking tip—Note the use of the word "toddler," not infant, in this question.
AN, 2, HPM, Prevention and Early Detection of Disease

106. (4) The best exercise for a child with cystic fibrosis is swimming, which provides needed exercise at an activity level that is not overly taxing for the child. Softball, tennis, and soccer (**Answers 1, 2, 3**) are all generally thought to be too strenuous for a child with CF.
Test-taking tip—"Swimming" is the option that is different from the others, which all call for ball playing.
IMP, 3, HPM, Prevention and Early Detection

107. (1) Because sickle cell anemia is inherited as an autosomal recessive disorder, if both parents have the trait, any future pregnancies would have a 1:4 (not 4:4 as in **Answer 4**) chance of producing a child *with* sickle cell anemia. **Answer 2** is incorrect because each pregnancy would have a 1:2 chance of producing a child *with the trait*. **Answer 3** is incorrect there is a 1:4 chance of producing a *normal* child. **Answer 4** is totally incorrect.
Test-taking tip—Autosomal recessive disorders have a 1:4 chance of occurring when both parents are carriers of the trait.
IMP, 6, HPM, Prevention and Early Detection of Disease

108. (4) Factor VIII concentrate is a blood product; a type and crossmatch may be ordered for the child before the IV administration of this medication. Given the relatively small volume of fluid to be administered, it would *not* usually cause fluid volume overload (**Answer 2**). Although there has been some discussion about administering multiple IV medications to a patient with hemophilia and the linkage to AIDS (**Answer 3**), this is *not* a concern *during* the actual administration of the medication but rather a long-term concern. Emboli formation (**Answer 1**) can occur with any IV administration and is *not specific* to cryoprecipitate, although the nurse would need to take the necessary precautions to prevent this possibility.
Test-taking tip—Any patient receiving blood or blood products should be closely monitored for a possible transfusion reaction.
PL, 6, PhI, Pharmacological and Parenteral Therapies

109. (2) Solu-Cortef is a corticosteroid/anti-inflammatory used in epiglottitis to relieve edema. Solu-Cortef does *not* provide sedation (**Answer 1**) or relieve pain (**Answer 3**), and the bacterial infection is treated with *antibiotics* (**Answer 4**).
Test-taking tip—Recall that this is a steroid; recall its function and recall that edema is a main concern in this condition. Therefore, reduction of swelling to keep airway patent is a priority.
AN, 6, PhI, Pharmacological and Parenteral Therapies

110. (4) Although any infection can be life-threatening to a child with leukemia, chickenpox presents a particular danger, because the child may develop encephalitis or sepsis. Infections such as impetigo (**Answer 1**), streptococcus (**Answer 2**), or pneumonia (**Answer 3**) are *less specific* dangers.
Test-taking tip—Choose the option that can result in encephalitis, a *specific* danger.
IMP, 1, SECE, Safety and Infection Control

111. (2) Because infants with VSD and CHF have a tendency toward respiratory infections, the infant should have limited contact with visitors with URIs, such as the grandmother with her slight cold. In fact, her slight cold might mean an episode of pneumonia for this infant. Lupus (**Answer 1**) in the aunt is not contagious, nor is the father's drug addiction (**Answer 3**). The sister (**Answer 4**) should be allowed to see and touch the infant, unless she herself is sick.
Test-taking tip—Respiratory infection control is the priority of care.
IMP, 6, SECE, Safety and Infection Control

112. (1) The chief danger of ipecac's being absorbed into the body is that it can cause cardiac arrhythmias, atrial fibrillation, or severe heart block. There is minimal effect on the liver (**Answer 2**), kidneys (**Answer 3**), or CNS (**Answer 4**).
Test-taking tip—Ipecac can cause cardiotoxicity.
AN, 1, PhI, Pharmacological and Parenteral Therapies

113. (2) The most recent research indicates that *infants who are breastfed do have a lower incidence of SIDS* than bottle-fed infants. It is not true that bottle-fed infants have a lower risk of SIDS (**Answer 3**), nor is it true that the risk of SIDS is the same (**Answer 1**) however infants are fed. Breastfeeding is not contraindicated for siblings of infants who died from SIDS (**Answer 4**); in fact, breastfeeding in this instance is recommended.
Test-taking tip—Breastfeeding is generally recommended for all infants whose mothers express an interest and willingness to do so.
IMP, 4, HPM, Prevention and Early Detection of Disease

114. (3) Generally, infants who weigh 7 lb at birth will weigh 28 lb, or quadruple their birthweight, by 2½ years of age. Consequently the other listed ages are incorrect (**Answers 1, 2, 4**).
Test-taking tip—Know growth and development milestones to choose the *only* correct answer.
EV, 5, HPM, Growth and Development

115. (2) The general rule of thumb to predict a child's height as an adult is to double the child's height at 2 years of age. The other answers (**Answers 1, 3, 4**) are incorrect.
Test-taking tip—Know developmental milestones to pick the only correct answer.
IMP, 5, HPM, Growth and Development

116. (2) Poisoning is most common in toddlers, who have the motor skills necessary to reach the poisons yet lack the intelligence to know not to ingest the poison. The other answers (**Answers 1, 3, 4**) are, therefore, incorrect.
Test-taking tip—Know age-relevant safety concerns.
AN, 1, SECE, Safety and Infection Control

117. (3) In children under 3 years, most accidental deaths are related to motor vehicles in which the child is a passenger; other types of accidents are not as common or not as likely to result in death (**Answers 1, 2, 4**).
Test-taking tip—Know age-typical cause of accidental death.
AN, 1, SECE, Safety and Infection Control

118. (2) Toddlers always suffer when separated from their parents, more so than any other age group (**Answers 1, 3, 4**). In fact, the years between ages 1 and 3 are when children are most likely to suffer separation anxiety.
Test-taking tip—It is the age, *not* the condition. Toddlers are at the peak age for separation anxiety.
AN, 5, PsI, Coping and Adaptation

119. (2) Five-year-olds may count up to 20 or 25, but seldom beyond this. They should be able to name colors such as red, green, and blue (**Answer 1**). In addition, they should be able to give their phone number and address (**Answer 4**) and have a better sense of temporal relationships, as evidenced by their ability to name days of the week, months of the year, and seasons (**Answer 3**).

Test-taking tip—The stem asks for what this child is *not* expected to do. The nurse should be familiar with developmental norms found in the DDST.

AS, 5, HPM, Growth and Development

120. **(4)** The RN floated from the telemetry unit would be least prepared to care for a young infant who has just had GI surgery and requires a specific feeding regimen. **Answer 1** is incorrect because the RN floated from the telemetry unit should be experienced in caring for patients with cardiac arrhythmias, a common complication of Kawasaki disease. **Answer 2** is incorrect because the RN floated from the telemetry unit should be experienced in caring for patients with carditis or congestive heart failure, common complications of patients with rheumatic fever. **Answer 3** is incorrect because the RN floated from the telemetry unit should be experienced in caring for patients who are post–cardiac catheterization.

Test-taking tip—"Least prepared" implies skills and knowledge that are not directly transferable. Look for the option that is different; in this question, the infant who is post-op pyloromyotomy is the only patient who does not have any *cardiac* involvement.

IMP, 1, SECE, Management of Care

121. **(4)** Diminished wheezing in a child with asthma indicates possible worsening of respiratory obstruction, especially when coupled with irritability, which is a sign of air hunger. **Answer 1** is incorrect because lacerations requiring sutures would not be a priority unless there was arterial hemorrhage. **Answer 2** is incorrect because these symptoms are consistent with a fairly mild case of laryngotracheobronchitis. **Answer 3** is incorrect because this type of fall onto a padded surface does not usually result in severe head trauma.

Test-taking tip—Note the use of the words "immediate attention" in this question, meaning potentially life threatening. Therefore, narrow the options to the two *respiratory* conditions.

AN, 6, PhI, Reduction of Risk Potential

122. **(2)** In addition to removing gown and gloves, the aide should wash her hands before leaving the child's room. **Answers 1, 3,** and **4** are incorrect because these actions *are* appropriate and would not require the nurse's immediate attention.

Test-taking tip—Key word: "unsafe." Use a true-or-false approach to rule out the three approaches that *are* OK.

EV, 1, SECE, Safety and Infection Control

123. **(1)** Cloth tape can stretch over time, eventually resulting in inaccurate measurements. The RN should intervene and direct the LPN/LVN to use paper tape instead of cloth tape. **Answers 2, 3,** and **4** are incorrect because these actions *are* appropriate and would *not* require intervention and further direction.

Test-taking tip—Key words: "intervention and further direction," implying that the best answer is the *incorrect* action.

EV, 8, SECE, Management of Care

124. **(3)** The nurse should always intiate infection control measures, such as droplet precautions, before administering any other care, in order to protect the nurse, other health care workers, and other patients and their families. **Answers 1, 2,** and **4** are not correct because the nurse is not initiating infection control measures first, but is checking vitals or offering fluids or drawing blood first.

Test-taking tip—Infection control is always a priority of care.

IMP, 1, SECE, Management of Care

125. **(1)** U80 means that there are 80 units of insulin per milliliter, not 80 units of insulin in the vial. **Answers 2, 3,** and **4** are incorrect because these statements *are true* and do not require the RN's intervention.

Test-taking tip—"U" (units) followed by a number always refers to the number of units of insulin per milliliter.

EV, 4, PhI, Pharmacological and Parenteral Therapies

126. **(1)** The child with eczema should be bathed in plain water, with no oils or soaps, to avoid further damage to the skin. **Answers 2, 3,** and **4** are incorrect because these actions *are* appropriate and require no additional supervision.

Test-taking tip—Note the use of the words "require . . . additional supervision" in this question, meaning *incorrect*, or *not* OK.

EV, 1, SECE, Management of Care

127. **(1)** Infants have the greatest percentage of fluid per pound of body weight than any other age group and are at highest risk for fluid and electrolyte imbalance. **Answers 2, 3,** and **4** are incorrect because none of the other conditions is at the *highest* risk for *fluid and electrolyte imbalance.*

Test-taking tip—It is not an age variable but the *condition* that is at risk.

AN, 6, PhI, Reduction of Risk Potential,

128. **(2)** Diet soda contains aspartame (NutraSweet), which metabolizes into phenylalanine. **Answers 1, 3,** and **4** are incorrect because these food items *are* allowed on a *low*-phenylalanine diet that this child is undoubtedly on.

Test-taking tip—Products containing aspartame (NutraSweet) should not be given to any patient with PKU. The stem calls for an elimination approach to what is OK to offer and what is not OK.

IMP, 4, PhI, Basic Care and Comfort

129. **(3)** This activity, auscultation of breath sounds, involves assessment skills. Patient transport (**Answer 1**), taking vital signs (**Answer 2**), and helping with activities of daily living (**Answer 4**) do *not* involve assessment and can therefore be safely delegated to an LPN/LVN.

Test-taking tip—Key concept in delegation: patient assessments can be done *only* by the RN.

IMP, 6, SECE, Management of Care

130. **(1)** Any threat to the safety of oneself or other should always be taken seriously and never disregarded by the nurse. **Answer 2** is incorrect because the nurse should never ignore threatening comments. **Answer 3** is incorrect because simply suggesting a meeting with a counselor at some vague point in time would not be sufficient. **Answer 4** is incorrect because this action is theoretically incorrect.

Test-taking tip—To narrow the choices, note two contradicting options: *not* OK (1) vs. OK (2). Choose the option in which safety is an issue. Safety is always a priority of care.

AN, 7, PsI, Psychosocial Adaptation

131. **(4)** No child or patient should be told not to express his or her feelings. Crying when upset is normal and healthy for any patient, regardless of age. **Answers 1, 2,** and **3** are incorrect because these actions *are* age and condition appropriate, and do not require the nurse to intervene.

Test-taking tip—Concept: therapeutic interventions/ communication calls for encouraging patients to express their feelings.

IMP, 7, SECE, Management of Care

132. **(3)** Preschoolers, who are at an age of fears and fantasies, should not be given detailed explanations of treatments. **Answers 1, 2,** and **4** are incorrect because these actions *are* age appropriate and do not require the preceptor to correct the teaching plan.

Test-taking tip—The concept here is an age-appropriate activity. Preschoolers should be given a simple and brief explanation, shortly before the intervention.

EV, 5, SECE, Management of Care

133. **(1)** Bathing a child with eczema can be safely delegated to an aide, who should be competent in performing this basic task. **Answer 2** is incorrect because only an RN can *monitor* an I&O, which is critical in a case of acute poisoning with an unpredictable outcome. **Answer 3** is incorrect because an RN should be caring for a child with *major* trauma. **Answer 4** is incorrect because only an RN can make an *assessment.*

Test-taking tip—Look for nonassessment, predictable outcome, stable condition, noncomplex care.

AN, 3, SECE, Management of Care

134. (1) Only the RN should evaluate the efficacy of pain medication or other treatments/medications. **Answers 2, 3,** and **4** are incorrect because the LPN/LVN and the UAP are not legally responsible for evaluating the efficacy of pain medication.

Test-taking tip—Recall that the concept of delegation sets responsibility for assessment/evaluation with the RN, not other assistive personnel.

PL, 1, SECE, Management of Care

135. (2) A 9-year-old child is within the age of reason, and his or her wishes regarding treatment must be considered by the health care team. The nurse, as part of the team, should consult with other team members before administering chemotherapy that the child refuses. **Answers 1** and **3** are incorrect because the nurse should not administer chemotherapy against the child's wishes. **Answer 4** is incorrect because the family should not make this important decision without the support and input of the health care team.

Test-taking tip—The best option involves the concept of patients' rights: patients have the right to refuse medication or treatment.

IMP, 1, SECE, Management of Care

136. (1) The RN floated from the obstetrics unit should be able to safely care for a patient with major abdominal surgery, because this nurse has cared for patients with cesarean births. **Answer 2** is incorrect because the RN floated from the obstetrics unit probably has not cared for patients receiving *chemotherapy.* **Answer 3** is incorrect because the RN floated from the obstetrics unit probably has limited experience with *cardiac* problems. **Answer 4** is incorrect because the RN floated from the obstetrics unit probably has limited experience with *neurological* injuries.

Test-taking tip—Look for the implied experience and skills that are applicable from one clinical area to another.

IMP, 1, SECE, Management of Care

137. (4) After administering a concentrated sugar to a patient with hypoglycemia, the nurse should be sure the child receives a complex carbohydrate, which will help maintain a steady blood sugar level. **Answer 1** is incorrect because simply adding this amount to the I&O is not sufficient. **Answers 2** and **3** are incorrect because offering more concentrated sweets will likely result in an unstable blood sugar level.

Test-taking tip—When two options are very similar (2, 3), neither option can be correct.

IMP, 4, PhI, Reduction of Risk Potential

138. (1) Although the nurse may not know the recommended dose, the nurse should recognize that 50 mg of Demerol is a normal *adult* dose. This would clearly be *unsafe* and inappropriate for a 2-year-old. **Answer 2** is incorrect because this is a normal adult dose and is *not* appropriate. **Answer 3** is incorrect because any patient may require pain medication, regardless of age. **Answer 4** is incorrect because the nurse should never administer medication simply because the doctor ordered it.

Test-taking tip—Narrow the choice to two contradicting options: in this situation, OK (2) vs. not OK (1), meaning it is excessive for a child.

AN, 3, PhI, Pharmacological and Parenteral Therapies

139. (2) The LPN/LVN should never give a prn medication unless the RN has completed an assessment of the patient to determine if it is safe and appropriate. **Answers 1** and **4** are incorrect because the LPN/LVN should never give a prn medication unless the RN has completed an assessment of the patient to determine if it is safe and appropriate. **Answer 3** is incorrect because the LPN/LVN should not contact the MD; this is the RN's responsibility.

Test-taking tip—Notice the pattern in the responses: two options *give* the drug, while two report/notify. Knowing role/responsibilities about assessment, eliminate the options that give the drug. Next, apply the lines of authority concept to arrive at the best answer.

AN, 3, PhI, Pharmacological and Parenteral Therapies

140. (2) Whenever the nurse aspirates blood when pulling back in giving an injection, the nurse must withdraw the needle and change it for another sterile needle. The nurse should then inject the medication in another site. **Answers 1, 3,** and **4** are incorrect because it is unsafe to inject when the nurse has aspirated blood; there is always the possibility of injecting the drug directly into the bloodstream.

Test-taking tip—Note the pattern in the responses: two options give the injection as is, and two do not. You must identify this as a *problem* and *not OK* to give this injection. Next, apply the concept of *sterile* technique to choose the best option.

EV, 1, PhI, Pharmacological and Parenteral Therapies

141. (2) By giving the bronchodilator first, this will help the air passages to open more fully. This enables the steroid to reach as deeply as possible into the bronchi, for maximum benefit to the patient. **Answers 1** and **3** are incorrect because the bronchodilator should be given first. **Answer 4** is incorrect because these medications *can* be given close to one another.

Test-taking tip—Remember: bronchodilator first, steroid second.

IMP, 6, PhI, Pharmacological and Parenteral Therapies

142. (4) Leaving the bag in place until it is full may cause tissue damage, as well as increase the likelihood of the bag pulling off and the specimen being lost. **Answers 1, 2,** and **3** are incorrect because these actions *are* appropriate and would not require the nurses's intervention and further direction.

Test-taking tip—The question is asking which action is *not* OK, *not* safe.

EV, 8, SECE, Safety and Infection Control

143. (1) After a spinal tap, patients should be encouraged to drink fluids to replace the circulating cerebrospinal fluid (CSF) and prevent a spinal headache. **Answers 2, 3,** and **4** are incorrect because these findings *are within normal* limits and require no follow-up.

Test-taking tip—Intervention is usually required for *abnormal* findings, *not* normal findings.

EV, 2, PhI, Reduction of Risk Potential

144. (1) These symptoms may indicate a potentially life-threatening infection such as bacterial meningitis, and the child should be evaluated promptly and thoroughly. **Answers 2** and **3** are incorrect because they would only cover up the symptoms. **Answer 4** is incorrect because this statement cannot be safely made on the basis of the information the parents have offered without first seeing the child.

Test-taking tip—When two answers (2, 3) are very similar, neither answer can be correct.

AN, 2, SECE, Management of Care

145. (3) Confidentiality precludes the nurse from giving this kind of information over the phone. **Answer 1** is incorrect because this is a breach of confidentiality. **Answer 2** is incorrect because it defers addressing the issue of confidentiality. **Answer 4** is incorrect because it disregards the caller's obvious distress. *After* directly answering the woman's question, the nurse might consider this as a possible follow-up statement.

Test-taking tip—The concept of confidentiality and *nurse*-appropriate role points to the best answer.

IMP, 1, SECE, Management of Care

Nursing Care of Behavioral and Emotional Problems Throughout the Life Span (Client Need: Psychosocial Integrity)

Sally L. Lagerquist

The chief *objective* of this unit is to highlight the most commonly observed behavioral and emotional problems and disorders in the mental health field. The emphasis is on (a) main points for *assessment,* (b) *analysis* of data based on underlying *basic concepts and general principles* drawn from a psychodynamic and interpersonal theoretical framework, and (c) *nursing interventions* based on the therapeutic use of self as the cornerstone of a helping process. Nursing actions are listed in *priority* whenever possible. Hence the **nursing process framework** is followed throughout. Note that nursing interventions are divided into *planning* and *implementation* (covering long-term and short-term *goals* and stressing *priority* of actions) and *health teaching. Evaluation* of results is listed separately, although this step of the nursing process is circular and relates back to "assessment" and "goals."

The categorization of psychiatric-emotional disorders can be complex and controversial. For purposes of clarity and simplicity, an attempt has been made here to capsulize many theoretical principles and component skills of the helping process that these disorders have *in common.* That

the term *client* is often used in place of *patient* reflects the interpersonal rather than medical model of psychiatric nursing. The diagnostic categorization of disorders (based on a synthesis of the North American Nursing Diagnosis Association [NANDA], Psychiatric Nursing Diagnosis [PND-I], and American Nurses Association [ANA] classification system for psychiatric nursing diagnoses) is included here to update the reader in current terminology in the mental health field.

The underlying organizational framework for this unit is based on applicable **categories of human functions** (Growth and Development; Protective Functions; Comfort, Rest, Activity, and Mobility; Sensory-Perceptual Functions; and Psychosocial-Cultural Functions; see **Appendices H** and **I**).

These categories have been incorporated into the diagnostic profile sent to the NCLEX-RN examinees as part of a report of their performance on the licensure exam. The categories reflect four **client needs** and are based on clusters of nursing activities designed to meet these needs (e.g., protecting clients, assisting clients with mobility needs).

GROWTH AND DEVELOPMENT

Major Theoretical Models

I. Psychodynamic model (Freud)
  A. Assumptions and key ideas
    1. No human behavior is accidental; each psychic event is determined by preceding ones.
    2. Unconscious mental processes occur with great frequency and significance.
    3. Psychoanalysis is used to uncover childhood trauma, which may involve conflict and repressed feelings.
    4. Psychoanalytic methods are used: therapeutic alliance, transference, regression, dream association, catharsis.
  B. *Freud*—shifted from classification of behavior to understanding and explaining in psychological terms and changing behavior under structured conditions.
    1. Structure of the mind: id, ego, superego; unconscious, preconscious, conscious.
    2. Stages of psychosexual development (Table 6–1).
    3. Coping mechanisms (see p. 373)

TABLE 6–1   Freud's Stages of Psychosexual Development

Stage	Age	Behaviors
Oral	Birth–1 yr	Dependency and oral gratification.
Anal	1–3 yr	Creativity, stinginess, cruelty, cleanliness, self-control, punctuality.
Phallic or oedipal	3–6 yr	Sexual, aggressive feelings; guilt.
Latency	6–12 yr	Reactivation of pregenital impulses; intellectual and social growth.
Genital	12–18 yr	Displacement of pregenital impulses; learns responsibility for self; establishes identity.

TABLE 6–2   Erikson's Stages of the Life Cycle

Age and Stage of Development	Conflict Areas Needing Resolution	Evaluation: Result of Resolution/Nonresolution
Infancy (birth–18 mo)	Trust vs.	Shows affection, gratification, recognition; trusts self and others; begins to tolerate frustrations; develops *hope*.
	Mistrust	Withdrawn, alienated.
Early childhood (18 mo–3 yr)	Autonomy vs.	Cooperative, self-controlled, self-expressive, can delay gratification; develops *will*.
	Shame and doubt	Exaggerated self-restraint; defiance; compulsive; overly compliant.
Late childhood (3–5 yr)	Initiative vs.	Realistic goals; can evaluate self; explorative; imitates adult, shows imagination; tests reality; anticipates roles; develops *purpose,* self-motivation.
	Guilt	Self-imposed restrictions relative to jealousy, guilt, and denial.
School age (5–12 yr)	Industry vs.	Sense of duty; acquires self-confidence from social and school *competencies;* persevering in real tasks.
	Inferiority	School and social dropout; social loner; incompetent.
Adolescence (12–18 yr)	Identity vs.	Has ideological commitments, self-actualizing; sense of self; experiments with roles; experiences sexual polarizations; develops *fidelity.*
	Role diffusion	Ambivalent, confused, indecisive; may act out (antisocial acts).
Young adulthood (18–25 yr)	Intimacy, solidarity vs.	Makes commitments to love, work relationships, a cause or creative effort; able to sustain mutual *love* relationships.
	Isolation	Superficial, impersonal, biased.
Adulthood (25–60 yr)	Generativity vs.	Productive, creative, procreative, concerned for others; develops *care.*
	Self-absorption, stagnation	Self-indulgent.
Late adulthood (60 yr–death)	Ego integrity vs.	Appreciates past, present, and future; self-acceptance of own contribution to others, of own *self-worth,* and of changes in lifestyle and life cycle; can face "not being"; develops *wisdom.*
	Despair	Preoccupied with loss of hope, of purpose; contemptuous, fears death.

Source: Lagerquist, S: Nursing Examination Review, ed 4. Addison-Wesley, Redwood City, Calif., 1992.

II. Psychosocial development model (Erikson, Maslow, Piaget, Duvall)

A. *Erik Erikson—Eight Stages of Man* (1963)

1. Psychosocial development—interplay of biology with social factors, encompassing total life span, from birth to death, in progressive developmental tasks.
2. *Stages of life cycle*—life consists of a series of developmental phases (Table 6–2 and Table 6–4).
   a. Universal sequence of biological, social, psychological events.
   b. Each person experiences a series of normative conflicts and crises and thus needs to accomplish specific psychosocial tasks.
   c. Two opposing energies (positive and negative forces) coexist and must be synthesized.
   d. How each age-specific task is accomplished influences the developmental progress of the next phase and the ability to deal with life.

B. *Abraham Maslow—Hierarchy of Needs* (1962)

1. Beliefs regarding emotional health based on a comprehensive, multidisciplinary approach to human problems, involving all aspects of functioning.
   a. *Premise:* mental illness cannot be understood without prior knowledge of mental health.
   b. *Focus:* positive aspects of human behavior (e.g., contentment, joy, happiness).
2. *Hierarchy of needs*—physiological, safety, love and belonging, self-esteem and self-recognition, self-actualization, aesthetic. As each stage is mastered, the next stage becomes dominant (Figure 6–1).
3. *Characteristics of optimal mental health*—keep in mind that *wellness is on a continuum with cultural variations.*
   a. *Self-esteem:* entails self-confidence and self-acceptance.
   b. *Self-knowledge:* involves accurate self-perception of strengths and limitations.
   c. *Satisfying interpersonal relationships:* able to meet reciprocal emotional needs through collaboration rather than exploitation or power struggles or jealousy; able to make full commitments in close relationships.
   d. *Environmental mastery:* can adapt, change, and solve problems effectively; can make decisions, choose from alternatives, and predict consequences. Actions are conscious, not impulsive.
   e. *Stress-management:* can delay seeking gratification and relief; does not blame or dwell on past; assumes self-responsibility; either modifies own expectations, seeks substitutes, or withdraws from stressful situation when cannot reduce stress.

C. *Jean Piaget—Cognitive and Intellectual Development* (1963)

1. **Assumptions**—child development is steered by interaction of environmental and genetic influences; therefore focus is on environmental and social forces. (See Table 6–4 for comparison with other theories.)
2. **Key concepts**
   a. *Assimilation:* process of acquiring new knowledge, skills, and insights by using what they already know and have.
   b. *Accommodation:* adjusts to change by solving previously unsolvable problems because of newly assimilated knowledge.
   c. *Adaptation:* coping process to handle environmental demands.
3. **Age-specific development levels**—sensorimotor, preconceptual, intuitive, concrete, formal operational thought (Table 6–3).

D. *E. M. Duvall—Family Development* (1971)—developmental tasks are family oriented, presented in eight stages throughout the life cycle (also see **Family Therapy,** p. 402).

1. *Married couple*
   a. Establishing relationship.
   b. Defining mutual goals.
   c. Developing intimacy: issues of dependence-independence-interdependence.
   d. Establishing mutually satisfying relationship.
   e. Negotiating boundaries of couple with families.
   f. Discussing issue of childbearing.
2. *Childbearing years*
   a. Working out authority, responsibility, and caretaker roles.

Mental Health

TABLE 6–3 Piaget's Age-Specific Developmental Levels

Age	Stage	Abilities
Infancy–2 yr	Sensorimotor	Preverbal; uses all senses; coordinates simple motor actions.
2–4 yr	Preconceptual	Can use language; egocentric; imitation in play, parallel play.
4–7 yr	Intuitive	Asks questions; can use symbols and associate subjects with concepts.
7–11 yr	Concrete	Sees relationships, aware of viewpoints; understands cause and effect, can make conclusions; solves concrete problems.
11 yr and older	Formal operational thought	Abstract and conceptual thinking; can check ideas, thoughts, and beliefs; lives in present and nonpresent; can use formal logic and scientific reasoning.

Source: Lagerquist, S: Nursing Examination Review, ed 4. Addison-Wesley, Redwood City, Calif., 1992.

FIGURE 6–1 Maslow's hierarchy of needs. (Modified from Townsend M: Essentials of Psychiatry/Mental Health Nursing. FA Davis, Philadelphia, 1999, p 5.)

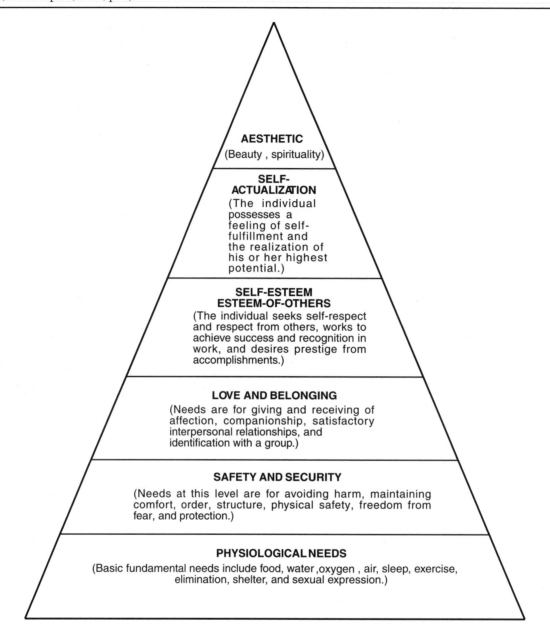

AESTHETIC
(Beauty , spirituality)

SELF-ACTUALIZATION
(The individual possesses a feeling of self-fulfillment and the realization of his or her highest potential.)

SELF-ESTEEM ESTEEM-OF-OTHERS
(The individual seeks self-respect and respect from others, works to achieve success and recognition in work, and desires prestige from accomplishments.)

LOVE AND BELONGING
(Needs are for giving and receiving of affection, companionship, satisfactory interpersonal relationships, and identification with a group.)

SAFETY AND SECURITY
(Needs at this level are for avoiding harm, maintaining comfort, order, structure, physical safety, freedom from fear, and protection.)

PHYSIOLOGICAL NEEDS
(Basic fundamental needs include food, water ,oxygen , air, sleep, exercise, elimination, shelter, and sexual expression.)

b. Having children and forming new unit.

c. Facilitating child's trust.

d. Need for personal time and space while sharing with each other and child.

3. *Preschool-age years*

   a. Experiencing changes in energy.

   b. Continuing development as couple, parents, family.

   c. Establishing own family traditions without guilt related to breaks with tradition.

4. *School-age years*

   a. Establishing new roles in work.

   b. Children's school activities interfering with family activities.

5. *Teenage years*

   a. Parents continue to develop roles in community other than with children.

b. Children experience freedom while accepting responsibility for actions.

c. Struggle with parents in emancipation process.

d. Family value system is challenged.

e. Couple relationships may be strong or weak depending on responses to needs.

6. *Families as launching centers*

   a. Young adults launched with rites of passage.

   b. Changes in couple's relationship due to empty nest and increased leisure time.

   c. Changes in relationship with children away from home.

7. *Middle-aged parents:* Dealing with issues of aging of own parents.

8. *Aging family members*

a. Sense of accomplishment and desire to continue to live fully.

b. Coping with bereavement and living alone.

III. Community mental health model (Gerald Kaplan)—levels of prevention

A. *Primary prevention*—lower the risk of mental illness and increase capacity to resist contributory influences by providing anticipatory guidance and maximizing strengths.

B. *Secondary prevention*—decrease disability by shortening its duration and reducing its severity through detection of early-warning signs and effective intervention following case-finding.

C. *Crisis intervention*—see p. 340.

D. *Tertiary prevention*—avoid permanent disorder through rehabilitation.

IV. Behavioral model (Pavlov, Watson, Wolpe, Skinner)

A. Assumptions

1. Roots in neurophysiology.
2. Stimulus-response learning can be *conditioned* through *reinforcement*.
3. Behavior is what one does.
4. Behavior is observable, describable, predictable, and controllable.
5. Classification of mental disease is clinically useless, only provides legal labels.

B. Aim: change *observable* behavior. There is *no underlying* cause, *no internal* motive.

V. Comparison of models—Table 6–4 compares four theories.

TABLE 6–4   Summary of Theories of Psychosocial Development Throughout the Life Cycle

Freud	Piaget	Sullivan	Erikson
Emphasis on			
Pathology (intrapsychic)	*Normal* children	Pathology (interpersonal)	Both health and illness
Anxiety	*No* emphasis on ego, anxiety, identity, libido	Anxiety	
Unconscious, uncontrollable drives	Cognitive development	Unconscious, uncontrollable drives	Problems are manageable and can be solved
Ego needing defense	Tasks can be accomplished through learning process	Self-system needing defense	Need to integrate individual and society
Pathological Development Influenced by			
Early feelings; repressed experiences in unconscious mind	Individual differences and social influences on the mind	Unconscious mind *and* interpersonal relationships (IPR)	Ego, anxiety, identity, libido concepts *combined* with social forces
Change Possible with			
Understanding content and meaning of unconscious	Socialization process to facilitate cognitive development	Improved IPR and understanding basic good-bad transformations	Integration of attitudes, libido, and social roles for strong ego identity
Age Group			
First 5 yr of life	Middle childhood years	Adolescence	Middle age, old age
Focus on			
Emotional development	Cognitive skills	Emotional and interpersonal development; relationships with opposite sex	Emotional, interpersonal, spiritual
Psychosexual aspects	Cognitive, interactive aspects	Psychosocial aspects; developing sense of identity	Psychosocial aspects
Cause of Conflicts and Problems			
Oral, anal, genital stage problems (especially unresolved oedipal/castration conflicts)	Faulty adaptation between individual and environment for intellectual development	Threats to self-system; disturbed communication process; 7 stages not complete	Unresolved conflicts, crises in 8 successive life cycle stages
Prognosis			
Few changes possible after age 5	Little change in adult cognitive structure after middle adolescence	Change usually possible with improved IPR	Change not only possible but *expected* throughout life
Sexual problems part of disturbed behavior	Sex as a variable in learning (age, IQ)	Sexual problems are only one type of faulty IPR affecting behavior	Sexual identity as one of many problems solved by interaction of desire and social process

Mental Health

Development of Body Image Throughout the Life Cycle

I. **Definition**—"Mental picture of body's appearance; an interrelated phenomenon which includes the surface, depth, internal and postural picture of the body, as well as the attitudes, emotions, and personality reactions of the individual in relation to his body as an object in space, apart from all others."*

II. **Operational definition†**
   A. Body image is created by social interaction.
      1. Approval given for "normal" and "proper" appearance, gestures, posture, etc.
      2. Behavioral and physical deviations from normality not given approval.
      3. Body image formed by the person's response to the approval and disapproval of others.
      4. Person's values, attitudes, and feelings about self continually evolving and unconsciously integrated.
   B. Self-image, identity, personality, sense of self, and body image are interdependent.
   C. Behavior is determined by body image.

III. **Concepts related to persons with problems of body image**
   A. Image of self changes with *changing posture* (walking, sitting, gestures).
   B. *Mental picture of self* may not correspond with the actual body; subject to continual but slow revision.
   C. The degree to which people like themselves (good self-concept) is directly related to how well defined they perceive their body image to be.
      1. *Vague, indefinite, or distorted body image* correlates with the following personality traits:
         a. Sad, empty, hollow feelings.
         b. Mistrustful of others; poor peer relations.
         c. Low motivation.
         d. Shame, doubt, sense of inferiority, poor self-concept.
         e. Inability to tolerate stress.
      2. *Integrated body image* tends to correlate positively with the following personality traits:
         a. Happy, good self-concept.
         b. Good peer relations.
         c. Sense of initiative, industry, autonomy, identity.

   d. Able to complete tasks.
   e. Assertive.
   f. Academically competent; high achievement.
   g. Able to cope with stress.
   D. Child's concept of body image can indicate degree of *ego strength* and personality integration; vague, distorted self-concept may indicate *schizophrenic* processes.
   E. *Successful* completion of various developmental phases determines body concept and degree of *body boundary definiteness.* (See Table 6–6.)
   F. *Physical changes* of height, weight, and body build lead to changes in perception of body appearance and of how body is used.
   G. Success in *using* one's body (motor ability) influences the value one places on self (self-evaluation).
   H. *Secondary sex characteristics* are significant aspects of body image (*too much, too little, too early, too late,* in the *wrong place,* may lead to disturbed body image). Sexual differences in body image are in part related to differences in anatomical structure and body function, as well as to contrasts in lifestyles and cultural roles.
   I. Different *cultures and families* value bodily traits and bodily deviations differently.
   J. Different *body parts* (for example, hair, nose, face, stature, shoulders) have varying personal significance; therefore there is variability in degree of threat, personality integrity, and coping behavior.
   K. *Attitudes* concerning the self will influence and be influenced by person's physical appearance and ability. Society has developed stereotyped ideas regarding outer body structure (body physique) and inner personalities (temperament). Current stereotypes are:
      1. *Endomorph*—talkative, sympathetic, good natured, trusting, dependent, lazy, fat.
      2. *Mesomorph*—adventuresome, self-reliant, strong, tall.
      3. *Ectomorph*—thin, tense and nervous, suspicious, stubborn, pessimistic, quiet.
   L. Person with a *firm ego boundary or body image* is more likely to be independent, striving, goal oriented, influential. Under stress, *may develop skin and muscle disease.*
   M. Person with *poorly integrated body image and weak ego boundary* is more likely to be passive, less goal oriented, less influential, more prone to external pressures. Under stress, *may develop heart and GI diseases.*
   N. Any situation, *illness,* or *injury* that causes a change in body image is a crisis, and the person will go through the *phases of crisis* in an attempt to reintegrate the body image (Table 6–5).

◆ IV. **Assessment—see Table 6–6.**

---

*Adapted from Kolb, L: Disturbances in body image. In Arieti, S (ed): American Handbook of Psychiatry. Basic Books, New York, 1959, pp 749–769.

†Adapted from Norris, C: Body image. In Carlson, C, and Blackwell, B (eds): Behavioral Concepts and Nursing Intervention, ed. 2. JB Lippincott, Philadelphia, 1978, p 6.

TABLE 6–5   Four Phases of Body Image Crisis

Phase	◆ Assessment	◆ Nursing Care Plan/Implementation
Acute shock	Anxiety, numbness, helplessness.	Provide sustained support, be available to listen, express interest and concern.
		Allow time for silence and privacy.
Denial	Retreats from reality; fantasy about the wholeness and capability of the body; euphoria; rationalization; refusal to participate in self-care.	Accept denial without reinforcing it. *Avoid* arguing and overloading with reality. Gradually raise questions, reply with doubt to convey unrealistic ideas.
		Follow client's suggestions for personal-care routine to help increase feelings of adequacy and to decrease helplessness.
Acknowledgment of reality	Grief over loss of valued body part, function, or role; depression, apathy; agitation, bitterness; physical symptoms (insomnia, anorexia, nausea, crying) serve as outlet for feeling; redefinition of body structure and function, with implications for change in lifestyle; acceptance of and cooperation with realistic goals for care and treatment; preoccupation with body functions.	Expect and accept displacement onto nurse of anger, resentment, projection of client's inadequacy.
		Examine own behavior to see if client's remarks are justified.
		Simply listen if this is the only way the client can handle feelings at this time.
		Offer sustained, nonjudgmental listening without being defensive or taking remarks personally.
		Help dispel anger by encouraging its ventilation.
		Encourage self-care activities.
		Support family members as they cope with changes in client's health or body image, role changes, treatment plans.
Resolution and adaptation	Perceives crisis in new light; increased mastery leads to increased self-worth; can look at, feel, and ask questions regarding altered body part; tests others' reactions to changed body; repetitive talk on painful topic of changed self; concentration on *normal* functions in order to increase sense of control.	Teaching and counseling by same nurse in warm, supportive relationship.
		Assess level of knowledge; begin at that level.
		Consider motivational state.
		Provide gradual, nontechnical medical information and specific facts.
		Repeat instructions frequently, patiently, consistently.
		Support sense of mastery in self-care; draw on inner resources.
		Do *not* discourage dependence while gradually encouraging independence.
		Focus on necessary adaptations of lifestyle due to realistic limitations.
		Provide follow-up care via referral to community resources after client is discharged.

Source: Lagerquist, S: Nursing Examination Review, ed 4. Addison-Wesley, Redwood City, Calif., 1992.

◆ **V. Analysis/nursing diagnosis—*body image development disturbance* may be related to:**
   A. *Obvious loss* of a major body part—amputation of an extremity, hair, teeth, eye, breast.
   B. Surgical procedures in which the relationship of body parts is *visibly* disturbed—colostomy, ileostomy, gastrostomy, ureteroenterostomy.
   C. Surgical procedures in which the loss of body parts is *not visible* to others—hysterectomy, lung, gallbladder, stomach.
   D. Repair procedures (plastic surgery) that do *not* reconstruct body image as assumed—rhinoplasty, plastic surgery to correct large ears, breasts.
   E. *Changes in body size and proportion*—obesity, emaciation, acromegaly, gigantism, pregnancy, pubertal changes (too early, too late, too big, too small, too tall).
   F. Other changes in *external body* surface—hirsutism in women, mammary glands in men.
   G. Skin *color* changes—chronic dermatitis, Addison's disease.
   H. Skin *texture* changes—scars, thyroid disease, excoriative dermatitis, acne.
   I. *Crippling* changes in bones, joints, muscles—arthritis, multiple sclerosis, Parkinson's.
   J. Failure of a body part to *function*—quadriplegia, paraplegia, cerebrovascular accident (CVA).
   K. Distorted ideas of structure, function, and significance stemming from *symbolism* of disease seen in terms of *life and death* when heart or lungs are afflicted—heart attacks, asthmatic attacks, pneumonia.
   L. *Side effects* of drug therapy—moon face, hirsutism, striated skin, changes in body contours.

Mental Health

TABLE 6–6   Body Image Development and Disturbance Throughout the Life Cycle: ◆Assessment

Age Group	Development of Body Image	Developmental Disturbances in Body Image
Infant and toddler	Becomes aware of body boundaries and separateness of own external body from others through sensory stimulation. Explores external body parts; handles and controls the environment and body through play, bathing, and eating. Experiences pain, shame, fear, and pleasure. Feels doubt or power in mastery of motor skills and strives for autonomy. Learns who one is in relation to the world.	*Infant* Inadequate somatosensory stimulation → impaired ego development, increased anxiety level, poor foundation for reality testing. Continues to see external objects as extension of self → unrealistic, *distorted* perceptions of significant persons, inability to form normal attachments to others (possessive, engulfing, autistic, withdrawn). *Toddler* If body fails to meet parental expectations → shameful, self-deprecating feelings. Failure to master environment and control own body → helplessness, inadequacy, and doubt.
Preschool and school age	Experiences praise, blame, derogation, or criticism for body, its part, or use (pleasure, pain, doubt, or guilt). Explores genitals—discovers anatomical differences between sexes with joy, pride, or shame. Begins awareness of *sexual identity.* Differentiates self as a body and self as a mind. Beginning of *self-concept;* of self as man or woman. Learns mastery of the body (to *do,* to protect *self,* to protect *others*) and environment (run, skip, skate, swim); feels pleasure, competence, worth, or inadequacy.	*Preschool* Distortion of body image of genital area due to conflict over pleasure versus punishment. If body build does not conform to sex-typed expectations and sex role identification → body image confusion. *School age* Physical impairments (speech, poor vision, poor hearing) → feelings of inadequacy and inferiority. Overly self-conscious about, and excessive focus on, body changes in puberty.
Adolescent	Physical self is of more concern than at any other time except old age. Forced body awareness due to physical changes (new senses, proportions, features); feelings of pleasure, power, confidence, or helplessness, pain, inadequacy, doubt, and guilt. Adult body proportions emerge. Anxiety over *ideal self versus emerging/emerged physical self;* body is compared competitively with same-sex peers. Use of body (adolescents' values and attitudes) to relate with opposite sex. Body image crucial for self-concept formation, status achievement, and adequate social relations. Physical changes need to be integrated into evolving body image (strong, competent, powerful, or weak and helpless).	Growth and changes may produce distorted view of self → overemphasis on defects with compensations; inflated ideas of body ability, beauty, perfection; preoccupation with body appearance or body processes, women more likely than men to see body fatter than it is; egocentrism.
Early adulthood	Learns to accept own body without undue preoccupation with its functions or control of these functions. Stability of body image.	
Middle age	New challenges due to differential rates of aging in various body parts. Body not functioning as well; unresolved fears, misconceptions, and experiences in relation to body image persist and become recognized.	Less dependable, less likable body → regression to adolescent behavior and dress due to denial of aging, defeat, depression, self-pity, egocentrism due to fear of loss of sexual identity, withdrawal to early old age. Women more likely to judge themselves uglier than do men or younger and older women.

TABLE 6–6   Body Image Development and Disturbance Throughout the Life Cycle: Assessment—cont'd

Age Group	Development of Body Image	Developmental Disturbances in Body Image
Old age	Accelerated physical decline with influence on self-concept and lifestyle. Can accept self and personality as a whole; continued emphasis on physical self, with increased emphasis on inner, emotional self.	Ill health → fear of invalidism, hypochondriasis. Denial related to feelings of threatened incapacity and fear of declining functions. Despair over loss of beauty, strength, and youthfulness, with self-disgust about body → projection of criticism onto others. Regression. Isolation (separation of affect and thought) leads to less intense response to death, disease, aging. Compartmentalization (focus on one thing at a time) causes narrowing of consciousness, resistance, rigidity, repetitiveness. Resurgence of egocentrism.

Source: Lagerquist, S: Nursing Examination Review, ed 4. Addison-Wesley, Redwood City, Calif., 1992.

M. *Violent attacks* against the body—incest, rape, shooting, knifing, battering.

N. *Mental, emotional disorders*—schizophrenia with depersonalization, somatic delusions, and hallucinations about the body; anorexia nervosa, hypochondriasis; hysteria, malingering.

O. *Diseases requiring isolation* may convey attitude that body is undesirable, unacceptable—tuberculosis, AIDS, malodorous conditions (e.g., gangrene, cancer).

P. *Women's movement and sexual revolution*—use of body for pleasure, not just procreation, sexual freedom, wide range of normality in sex practices, legalized abortion.

Q. *Medical technology*—organ transplants, lifesaving but scar-producing burn treatment, alive but hopeless, alive but debilitated with chronic illnesses.

◆ **VI. General nursing care plan/implementation:**

A. *Protect from psychological threat* related to impaired *self-attitudes*.
   1. Emphasize person's *normal* aspects.
   2. Encourage self-performance.

B. *Maintain warm, communicating relationship*.
   1. Encourage awareness of positive responses from others.
   2. Encourage expression of feelings.

C. *Increase reality perception*.
   1. Provide *reliable* information about health status.
   2. Provide *kinesthetic* feedback to paralyzed part; e.g., "I am raising your leg."
   3. Provide *perceptual* feedback; e.g., touch, describe, look at scar.
   4. Support a realistic assessment of the situation.
   5. Explore with the client his or her strengths and resources.

D. *Help achieve positive feelings about self, about adequacy*.
   1. Support strengths *despite* presence of handicaps.
   2. Assist client to look at self in *totality* rather than focus on limitations.

E. *Health teaching*:
   1. Teach client and family about expected changes in functioning.
   2. Explain importance of maintaining a positive self-attitude.
   3. Advise that negative responses from others be regarded with minimum significance.

VII. Evaluation:

A. Able to resume function in activities of daily living rather than prolonging illness.

B. Able to accept limits imposed by physical or mental conditions and not attempt unrealistic tasks.

C. Can shift focus from reminiscence about the healthy past to present and future.

D. Less verbalized discontent with present body; diminished display of self-displeasure, despair, weeping, and irritability.

Body Image Disturbance—Selected Examples

I. **Definition**—a body image disturbance arises when a person is unable to accept the body as is and to adapt to it; a conflict develops between the body as it actually is and the body that is pictured mentally, that is, the ideal self.

Mental Health

II. **Analysis/nursing diagnosis:** *body image disturbance* may be related to:

A. Sensation of *size change* due to obesity, pregnancy, weight loss.

B. Feelings of being *dirty*—may be imaginary due to hallucinogenic drugs, psychoses.

C. Dual change of body *structure and function* due to trauma, amputation, stroke, etc.

D. Progressive *deformities* due to chronic illness, burns, arthritis.

E. Loss of body boundaries and *depersonalization* due to sensory deprivation, such as blindness, immobility, fatigue, stress, anesthesia. May also be due to psychoses or hallucinogenic drugs.

◆ III. **Assessment—see Table 6–6.**

Body Image Disturbance Caused by Amputation

◆ A. **Assessment:**

1. Loss of self-esteem; feelings of helplessness, worthlessness, shame, and guilt.
2. Fear of abandonment may lead to appeals for sympathy by exhibiting helplessness and vulnerability.
3. Feelings of castration (loss of self) and symbolic death; loss of wholeness.
4. Existence of phantom pain (most clients).
5. Passivity, lack of responsibility for use of disabled body parts.

◆ B. **Nursing care plan/implementation:**

1. *Avoid* stereotyping person as being less competent now than previously by *not* referring to client as the "amputee."
2. Foster independence; encourage self-care by assessing what client *can* do for himself or herself.
3. Help person set *realistic* short-term and long-term goals by exploring with the client his or her strengths and resources.
4. *Health teaching:*
   a. Encourage family members to work through their feelings, to accept person as he or she presents self.
   b. Teach how to set realistic goals and limitations.
   c. Explain what phantom pain is; that it is a normal experience.
   d. Explain role and function of prosthetic devices, where and how to obtain them, and how to find assistance in their use.

◆ C. **Evaluation/outcome criteria:**

1. Can acknowledge the loss and move through three stages of mourning (shock and disbelief, developing awareness, and resolution).
2. Can discuss fears and concerns about loss of body part, its meaning, the problem of compensating for the loss, and reaction of persons (repulsion, rejection, and sympathy).

Body Image Disturbance in Cerebrovascular Accident (Stroke)

◆ A. **Assessment:**

1. Feelings of shame (personal, private, self-judgment of failure) due to loss of bowel and bladder control, speech function.
2. Body image boundaries disrupted; contact with environment is hindered by inability to ambulate or manipulate environment physically; may result in personality deterioration due to diminished number of sensory experiences. Loses orientation to body sphere; feels confused, trapped in own body.

◆ B. **Nursing care plan/implementation:**

1. Reduce frustration and infantilism due to communication problems by:
   a. Rewarding all speech efforts.
   b. Listening and observing for all nonverbal cues.
   c. Restating verbalizations to see if correct meaning is understood.
   d. Speaking slowly, using two- to three-word sentences.
2. Assist *reintegration* of body parts and function; help regain awareness of paralyzed side by:
   a. Tactile stimulation.
   b. Verbal reminders of existence of affected parts.
   c. Direct visual contact via mirrors and grooming.
   d. Use of safety features (e.g., Posey belt).
3. *Health teaching:* control of bowel and bladder function; how to prevent problems of immobility.

◆ C. **Evaluation/outcome criteria:** dignity is maintained while relearning to control elimination.

Body Image Disturbance in Myocardial Infarction

Emotional problems (e.g., anxiety, depression, sleep disturbance, fear of another myocardial infarction [MI]) during convalescence can seriously hamper rehabilitation. The adaptation and convalescence is influenced by the multiple symbolic meanings of the heart, for example:

1. Seat of emotions (love, pride, fear, sadness).
2. Center of the body (one-of-a-kind organ).
3. Life itself (can no longer rely on the heart; failure of the heart means failure of life).

◆ A. **Assessment:**

1. *Attitude*—overly cautious and restrictive; may result in boredom, weakness, insomnia, exaggerated dependency.
2. *Acceptance* of illness—Use of denial may result in noncompliance.
3. *Behavior*—self-destructive.
4. *Family conflicts*—related to activity, diet.
5. *Effects of MI on:*

a. *Changes in lifestyle*—eating, smoking, drinking; activities, employment, sex.

b. *Family members*—may be anxious, overprotective.

c. *Role in family*—role reversal may result in loss of incentive for work.

d. *Dependence-independence*—issues related to family conflicts (especially restrictive attitudes about desirable activity and dietary regimen).

e. *Job*—social pressure to "slow down" may result in loss of job, reassignment, forced early retirement, "has-been" social status.

◆ **B. Nursing care plan/implementation:**

1. Prevent "cardiac cripple" by shaping person's and family's attitude toward damaged organ.

   a. Instill optimism.

   b. Encourage *productive* living rather than inactivity.

2. Set up a physical and mental activity program with client and mate.

3. Provide anticipatory guidance regarding expected weakness, fear, uncertainty.

4. *Health teaching:* nature of coronary disease, interpretation of medical regimen, effect on sexual behavior.

◆ **C. Evaluation/outcome criteria:**

1. Adheres to medical regimen.

2. Modifies lifestyle without becoming overly dependent on others.

Body Image and Obesity

A. Definition: body weight exceeding 20% above the norm for person's age, sex, and height constitutes obesity. Body mass index (BMI) is also used. Although a faulty adaptation, obesity may serve as a protection against more severe illness; it represents an effort to function better, be powerful, stay well, or be less sick. The *problem* may *not* be difficulty in losing weight; reducing may *not* be the appropriate *cure*.

◆ **B. Assessment**—characteristics:

1. Age—one out of three persons under 30 years of age is more than 10% overweight.

2. Increase risks for CVA, MI, diabetes.

3. Feelings: self-hate, self-derogation, failure, helplessness; tendency to avoid clothes shopping and mirror reflections.

4. Viewed by others as ugly, repulsive, lacking in will power, weak, unwilling to change, neurotic.

5. Discrepancy between actual body size (real self) and person's concept of it (ideal self).

6. Pattern of successful weight loss followed quickly and repetitively by failure, that is, weight gain.

7. Eating in response to outer environment (e.g., food odor, time of day, food availability, degree of stress, anger); *not inner* environment (hunger, increased gastric motility).

8. Experiences less pleasure in physical activity; less active than others.

9. All obese people are *not* the same.

   a. In *obese newborns and infants,* there is an increased *number* of adipocytes via *hyperplastic* process.

   b. In *obese adults,* there may be increased body fat deposits, resulting in increased *size* of adipocytes via *hypertrophic* process.

   c. When an *obese infant becomes an obese adult,* the result may be an increased *number* of cells available for fat *storage.*

10. Loss of control of own body or eating behavior.

◆ **C. Analysis/nursing diagnosis:** *Defensive coping* related to eating disorder. Contributing factors:

1. Genetic.

2. Thermodynamic.

3. Endocrine.

4. Neuroregulatory.

5. Biochemical factors in metabolism.

6. Ethnic and family practices.

7. *Psychological:*

   a. Compensation for feelings of helplessness and inadequacy.

   b. Maternal overprotection; overfed and forcefed, especially formula-fed infants.

   c. Food offered and used to relieve anxiety, frustration, anger, and rage can lead to difficulty in differentiating between hunger and other needs.

   d. As a child, food offered instead of love.

8. *Social:*

   a. Food easily available.

   b. Use of motorized transportation and labor-saving devices.

   c. Refined carbohydrates.

   d. Social aspects of eating.

   e. Restaurant meals high in salt, sugar.

◆ **D. Nursing care plan/implementation:**

1. Encourage *prevention* of lifelong body image problems.

   a. Support *breastfeeding,* where infant determines quantity consumed, *not* mother; work through her feelings against breastfeeding (fear of intimacy, dependence, feelings of repulsion, concern about confinement, and inability to produce enough milk).

   b. Help mothers to *not overfeed* the baby if formula-fed: suggest water between feedings; do *not* start solids until 6 months old or 14 pounds; do *not* enrich the prescribed formula.

   c. Help mothers *differentiate* between hunger and other infant cries; help her to try out different responses to the expressed needs other than offering food.

2. Use *case findings* of obese infants, young children, and adolescents.

3. Assess current eating patterns.
4. Identify need to eat, and relate need to preceding events, hopes, fears, or feelings.
5. Employ behavior-modification techniques.
6. Encourage outside interests not related to food or eating.
7. Alleviate guilt, reduce stigma of being obese.
8. *Health teaching:*
   a. Promote awareness of certain *stressful* periods that can produce maladaptive responses such as obesity—e.g., puberty, postnuptial, postpartum, menopause.
   b. Assist in drawing up a meal plan for slow, steady weight loss.
   c. Advise eating five small meals a day.
◆ E. **Evaluation/outcome criteria:** goal for desired weight is reached; weight-control plan is continued.

Scope of Human Sexuality Throughout the Life Cycle

Human sexuality refers to all the characteristics of an individual (social, personal, and emotional) that are manifest in his or her relationships with others and that reflect gender-genital orientation.

I. **Components of sexual system**
   A. *Biological sexuality*—refers to chromosomes, hormones, primary and secondary sex characteristics, and anatomical structure.
   B. *Sexual identity*—based on own feelings and perceptions of how well traits correspond with own feelings and concepts of maleness and femaleness; also includes gender identity.
   C. *Gender identity*—a sense of masculinity and femininity shaped by biological, environmental, and intrapsychic forces, as well as cultural traditions and education.
   D. *Sex role behavior*—includes components of both sexual identity and gender identity. Aim: sexual fulfillment through masturbation, heterosexual, or homosexual experiences. Selection of behavior is influenced by personal value system and sexual, gender, and biological identity. Gender identity and roles are learned and constantly reinforced by input and feedback regarding social expectations and demands (Table 6–7).

II. **Concepts and principles of human sexual response**
   A. Human sexual response involves not only the genitals but the total body.
   B. Factors in early postnatal and childhood periods influence gender identity, gender role, sex typing, and sexual responses in later life.
   C. Cultural and personally subjective variables influence ways of sexual expression and perception of what is satisfying.

D. Healthy sexual expressions vary widely.
E. Requirements for human sexual response:
   1. Intact central and peripheral nervous system to provide *sensory* perception, *motor* reaction.
   2. Intact circulatory system to produce *vasocongestive* response.
   3. Desirable and interested partner, if sex outlet involves mutuality.
   4. *Freedom* from guilt, anxiety, misconceptions, and interfering conditioned responses.
   5. Acceptable physical *setting*, usually private.

Sexual-Health Counseling

General Issues

I. **Issues** in sexual practices with implications for counseling:
   A. *Sex education*—need to provide accurate and complete information on all aspects of sexuality to all people.
   B. *Sexual-health care*—should be part of total health care planning for all.
   C. *Sexual orientation*—need to avoid discrimination based on sexual orientation (such as homosexuality); the right to satisfying, nonexploitive relationships with others, regardless of gender.
   D. *Sex and the law*—sex between consenting adults not a legal concern.
   E. *Explicit sexual material* (pornography)—can be useful in fulfilling various needs in life, as in quadriplegia.
   F. *Masturbation*—a natural behavior at all ages; can fulfill a variety of needs (see **Masturbation**, p. 311).
   G. Availability of *contraception* for minors—the right of access to medical contraceptive care should be available to all ages.
   H. *Abortion*—confidentiality for minors.
   I. *Treatment for sexually transmitted disease (STD)*—naming of partners as part of STD control.
   J. *Sex and the elderly*—need opportunity for sexual expression; need privacy when in communal living setting.
   K. *Sex and the disabled*—need to have possible means available for rewarding sexual expressions.

II. **Sexual myths***
   A. *Myth:* Ignorance is bliss.
      Fact: What you don't know *can* hurt you (note the high frequency of STD and abortions); *myths* can perpetuate fears and such misinformation as:
      1. *Masturbation causes mental illness.*
      2. *Women don't or shouldn't have orgasms.*

---

*Adapted from Sedgwick, R: Myths in human sexuality: a social-psychological perspective. Nurs Clin North Am 10(3):539–550, 1975. WB Saunders, 1975.

TABLE 6–7 Sexual Behavior Throughout the Life Cycle

Age	Development of Sexual Behavior
First 18 mo	Major source of pleasure from touch and oral exploration.
18 mo–3 yr	Pleasurable and sexual feelings are associated with genitals (acts of urination and defecation). Masturbation without fantasy or eroticism.
3–6 yr	Beginning resolution of Oedipus and Electra complexes; foundation for heterosexual relationships; masturbation with curiosity about genitals of opposite sex.
6–12 yr	Peer relations with same sex; onset of sex play; morality and sexual attitudes taught and learned; phase of sexual tranquility.
12–18 yr (adolescence)	Onset of puberty with biological development of secondary sex characteristics; menstruation and ejaculation occur.
	Frequent masturbation. Intense anxiety and guilt may occur over heterosexual or homosexual behavior (petting, coitus, masturbation, STD, pregnancy, genital size).
18–23 yr (early adulthood)	Maximum interpersonal and intrapsychic self-consciousness about sexuality. Issues: premarital coitus, sexual freedom.
	Anxiety about: sexual competency, genital size, impotence, fear of pregnancy, rejection.
23–30 yr	Focus on sexual activity in coupling and parenthood; mutual masturbation.
30–45 yr (middle adulthood)	For women—peak sexuality without new sexual experiences. Conflict regarding extramarital sex may increase.

Purpose of Intercourse:

Need for body contact (and procreation until age 35+).

Physical expression of trust, love, and affection.

Reaffirmation of self-concept as sexually desirable and sexually competent due to worry about effects of aging.

Sexual Dysfunctions:

Men: erectile dysfunction, premature ejaculation, decreasing libido.

Women: intermittent lack of orgasmic response, vaginismus, dyspareunia.

For either or both: changes or divergences in degree of sexual interest.

Causes of Sexual Dysfunction (Men):

Overindulgence in food or drink.

Preoccupation with career and economic pursuits.

Mental or physical fatigue.

Boredom with monotony of relationship.

Drug dependency: alcohol, tobacco, certain medications.

Fear of failure.

Chronic illness: diabetes, alcoholism → peripheral neuropathy → impotence (smoking and drinking may result in decreased testosterone production); excessive smoking → vascular constriction → decreased libido; spinal cord injuries; prostatectomy, androgen deprivation therapy (for prostate cancer).

Self-devaluation due to accumulation of role function losses, sexual self-image, and body image.

Past history of lack of sexual enjoyment in younger years.

Causes of Sexual Dysfunction (Women):

Belief in myths regarding "shoulds and should nots" of frequency, variations, and enjoyment.

Widowhood: inhibition and loyalty to deceased.

45–65 yr (later adulthood)	Menopause occurs.
	Little or no fear of pregnancy; evidence of sexual activity differences in men and women: women may have increased pleasure, men take longer to reach orgasm; may prefer less strenuous mutual masturbation.
Over 65 yr (old age)	Activity depends on earlier sexual attitude.
	May suffer guilt and shame when engaging in sex.
	Can have active and enjoyable sex life with continuing sex needs.
	Age is not a barrier provided there is opportunity for sexual activity with a partner or for sublimated activities. Women in this age group outnumber men; single women outnumber single men by an even larger margin.

Source: Lagerquist, S: Nursing Examination Review, ed 4. Addison-Wesley, Redwood City, Calif., 1992.

Mental Health

3. *Tampons cause STD.*
4. *Plastic wrap works better than condoms.*
5. *Coca-Cola is an effective douche.*

Fact: Lack of knowledge during initial experiences may result in fear and set precedent for future sexual reactions.

B. *Myths:* The planned sex act is not OK and is immoral for "nice" girls. If a woman gets pregnant, it is her own fault. Contraceptives are solely a woman's responsibility.

Fact: Sex and contraception are the prerogative and responsibility of both partners.

C. *Myth:* A good relationship is harmonious, free of conflict and disagreement (which are signs of rejection and incompatibility).

Fact: Conflict can induce growth in self-understanding and in understanding of others.

D. *Myth:* Sexual deviance (such as homosexuality) is a sign of personality disturbance.

Fact: No single sexual behavior is the most desirable, effective, or satisfactory. Personal sexual choice is a fundamental right.

E. *Myth:* A woman's sexual needs and gratification should be secondary to her partner's; a woman's role is to satisfy others.

Fact: A woman has as much right to sexual freedom and experience as a man.

F. *Myth:* Menopause is an affliction signifying the end of sex.

Fact: Many women do not suffer through menopause, and many report renewed sexual interest.

G. *Myth:* Sexual activity past 60 years of age is not essential.

Fact: Sexual activity is therapeutic because it:
1. Affirms identity.
2. Provides communication.
3. Provides companionship.
4. Meets intimacy needs.

H. *Myth:* A woman's sex drive decreases in postmenopausal period.

Fact: The strength of the sex drive becomes greater as androgen overcomes the inhibitory action of estrogen.

I. *Myth:* Men over age 60 cannot achieve an erection.

Fact: According to Masters and Johnson, a major difference between the aging man and the younger man is the duration of each phase of the sexual cycle. The older man is slower in achieving an erection.

J. *Myth:* Regular sexual activity cannot help the aging person's loss of function.

Fact: Research is revealing that "disuse atrophy" may lead to loss of sexual capacity. Regular sexual activity helps preserve sexual function.

III. Basic principles of sexual-health counseling

A. There is *no* universal consensus about acceptable values in human sexuality. Each social group has very definite values regarding sex.

B. Counselors need to examine own feelings, attitudes, values, biases, knowledge base.

C. Help reduce fear, guilt, ignorance.

D. Offer guidance and education rather than indoctrination or pressure to conform.

E. Each person needs to be helped to make personal choices regarding sexual conduct.

IV. Counseling in sexual health

A. General considerations
1. Create atmosphere of *trust and acceptance* for objective, nonjudgmental dialogue.
2. Use *language* related to sexual behavior that is mutually comfortable and understood between client and nurse.
   a. Use alternative terms for definitions.
   b. Determine exact meaning of words and phrases because sexual words and expressions have different meanings to people with different backgrounds and experiences.
3. *Desensitize* own stress reaction to the emotional component of taboo topics.
   a. Increase awareness of own sexual values, biases, prejudices, stereotypes, and fears.
   b. *Avoid* overreacting, underreacting.
4. Become sensitively aware of *interrelationships* between sexual needs, fears, and behaviors and other aspects of living.
5. Begin with *commonly* discussed areas (such as menstruation) and progress to discussion of individual sexual experiences (such as masturbation). Move from areas where there is less voluntary control (nocturnal emissions) to more responsibility and voluntary behavior (premature ejaculation).
6. Offer *educational information* to dispel fears, myths; give tacit permission to explore sensitive areas.
7. Bring into awareness possibly *repressed* feelings of guilt, anger, denial, and suppressed sexual feelings.
8. Explore possible *alternatives* of sexual expression.
9. Determine *interrelationships* among mental, social, physical, and sexual well-being.

B. Assessment parameters:
1. Self-awareness of body image, values, and attitudes toward human sexuality; comfort with own sexuality.
2. Ability to identify sex problems on basis of own satisfaction or dissatisfaction.
3. Developmental history, sex education, family relationships, cultural and ethnic values, and available support resources.
4. Type and frequency of sexual behavior.
5. Nature and quality of sex relations with others.
6. Attitude toward and satisfaction with sexual activity.
7. Expectations and goals. See Table 6–8 for a guideline in conducting an *assessment* interview.

◆ **C. Nursing care plan/implementation:**
1. *Long-term goals*
   a. Increase knowledge of reproductive system and types of sex behavior.
   b. Promote positive view of body and sex needs.
   c. Integrate sex needs into self-identity.
   d. Develop adaptive and satisfying patterns of sexual expression.
   e. Understand effects of physical illness on sexual performance.
2. *Primary sexual health interventions*
   a. Goals: minimize stress factors, strengthen sexual integrity.
   b. Provide education to uninformed or misinformed.
   c. Identify stress factors (myths, stereotypes, negative parental attitudes).
3. *Secondary sexual health interventions:* identify sexual problems early and refer for treatment.

◆ **D. Evaluation/outcome criteria:**
1. Reduced impairment or dysfunction from acute sex problem or chronic, unresolved sex problem.
2. Evaluate how client's goals were achieved in terms of *positive* thoughts, feelings, and *satisfying* sexual behaviors.

Specific Situations

I. Masturbation
   A. Definition—act of achieving sexual arousal and orgasm through manual or mechanical stimulation of the sex organs.

B. Characteristics
1. Can be an interpersonal as well as a solitary activity.
2. "It is a healthy and appropriate sexual activity, playing an important role in ultimate consolidation of one's sexual identity."*
3. Accompanied by fantasies that are important for:
   a. Physically disabled.
   b. Fatigued.
   c. Compensation for unreachable goals and unfulfilled wishes.
   d. Rehearsal for future sexual relations.
   e. Absence or impersonal action of partner.
4. Can help release tension harmlessly.

C. Concepts and principles related to masturbation
1. Staff's feelings and reactions influence their responses to client and affect continuation of masturbation (that is, negative staff actions increase client's frustration, which increases masturbation).
2. Masturbation is normal and universal, *not* physically or psychologically harmful in itself.
3. Pleasurable genital sensations are important for increasing *self-pride,* finding *gratification* in *own* body, increasing sense of *personal value* of being lovable, helping to *prepare for adult* sexual role.

---

*Marcus, IM, and Francis, JJ: Masturbation from Infancy to Senescence. International Universities Press, New York, 1975.

TABLE 6–8   Suggested Format for Sexual Assessment Interview

Interview Step	Rationale
1. Open the discussion of sexual matters subtly with an open-ended question: "People with your illness or stresses often experience other difficulties, sometimes with sexual functioning."	This gentle opening lets the client know that other people have difficulties, too. It gives the client permission to talk with the nurse about sexual matters without labeling these matters as problems.
2. Follow up with another open-ended question about the client's current status: "Has your illness or stresses made any difference in what it's like for you to be a wife or husband (lover, boyfriend, girlfriend, sexual partner)?"	The phrasing of this question enables the client to acknowledge a problem without admitting a shortcoming.
3. If the client speaks of having a dysfunction, ask about its effect: "How does this affect you?" or "How do you feel about it?"	This indicates that the nurse is willing to explore sexual matters more completely.
4. Ask about the severity and duration of the dysfunction: "Is it always difficult to control your ejaculation?" "Tell me when you first noticed this."	These questions are directed at identifying the specific problem.
5. Ask about the effects on the client's sexual partner: "Has this affected your relationship with your partner?"	This question is directed toward exploring the interactional aspects of the identified problem.
6. Ask what the client has already done to alleviate the situation: "Have you made any adjustments in your sexual activity?"	This question yields data that will help the nurse to formulate an intervention plan.
7. Ask the client if and how he or she would like the situation changed: "How would you like to change the situation to make it more satisfying?"	This question conveys the negotiated nature of the therapeutic relationship, in which the client's own goals play an important part.

Source: Adapted from the classic article by Whitley, MP, and Willingham, W: Adding a sexual assessment to the health interview. Journal of Psychiatric Nursing and Mental Health Services, 16(4):17–27, 1978.

4. Excessive masturbation—some needs not being met through interpersonal relations; may use behavior to *avoid* interpersonal relations.
5. Activity may be related to:
   a. Curiosity, experimentation.
   b. Tension reduction, pleasure.
   c. Enhanced interest in sexual development.
   d. Fear and avoidance of social relationships.

◆ **D. Nursing care plan:**
1. *Long-term goals*
   a. Gain insight into *preference* for masturbation.
   b. Relieve accompanying guilt, worry, self-devaluation (Figure 6–2).
2. *Short-term goals*
   a. Clarify myths regarding masturbation.
   b. Help client see masturbation as an acceptable sexual activity for individuals of all ages.
   c. Set limits on masturbation in inappropriate settings.

◆ **E. Nursing implementation:**
1. Examine, control nurse's own negative feelings; show respect.
2. *Avoid:* reinforcement of guilt and self-devaluation; scorn; threats, punishment, anger, alarm reaction; use of masturbation for rebellion in power struggle between staff and client.
3. *Identify* client's unmet needs; consider purpose served by masturbation (may be useful behavior).
4. *Examine* pattern in which behavior occurs.
5. Intervene when degree of functioning in other daily life activities is *impaired.*
   a. Remain calm, accepting, but nonsanctioning.
   b. Promptly help clarify client's feelings, thoughts, at stressful time.
   c. Review precipitating events.
   d. Be a neutral "sounding board"; *avoid* evasiveness.
   e. If unable to handle situation, find someone who can.

6. For clients who masturbate at *inappropriate* times or in inappropriate places:
   a. Give special attention when they are not masturbating.
   b. Encourage new interests and activities, but *not* immediately after observing masturbation.
   c. Keep clients distracted, occupied with interesting activities.
7. *Health teaching:* explain myths and teach facts regarding cause and effects.

◆ **F. Evaluation/outcome criteria:**
1. Acknowledges function of own sexual organs.
2. States sexual experience is satisfying.
3. Views sexuality as pleasurable and wholesome.
4. Views sex organs as acceptable, enjoyable, and valued part of body image.
5. Self-image as fully functioning person is restored and maintained.

II. Homosexuality
   A. Definition—alternative sexual behavior; applied to sexual relations between persons of the same sex.
   B. Theories regarding causes
   1. Hereditary tendencies.
   2. Imbalance of sex hormones.
   3. Environmental influences and conditioning factors, related to learning and psychodynamic theories.
      a. Defense against unsatisfying relationship with father.
      b. Unsatisfactory and threatening early relationships with opposite sex.
      c. Oedipal attachment to parent.
      d. Seductive parent (incest).
      e. Castration fear.
      f. Labeling and guilt leading to sexual acting out.
      g. Faulty sex education.
   4. Preferred choice as a lifestyle.
   ◆ **C. Nursing care plan/implementation:**
   1. Nurse needs to be aware of and work through own attitudes that may interfere with providing care.

FIGURE 6–2 Operationalization of the behavioral concept of masturbation.

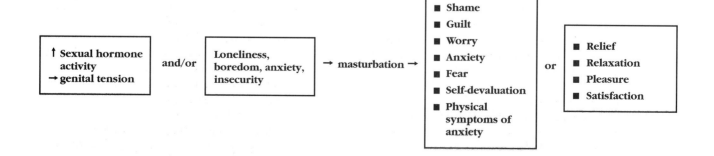

2. Accept and respect lifestyle of gay (male homosexual) or lesbian (female homosexual) client.
3. Assess and treat for possible sexually transmitted diseases and hepatitis.
4. *Health teaching:* assess and add to knowledge base about alternatives in sexual behavior.

◆ **D. Evaluation/outcome criteria:** expresses self-confidence and positive self-image; able to sustain satisfying sexual behavior with chosen partner and avoid at-risk behaviors for STDs.

III. Sex and the disabled person

◆ **A. Assessment parameters:**
1. Previous level of sex functioning and conflict.
2. Client's view of sex activity (self and mutual pleasure, tension release, procreation, control).
3. Cultural environment (influence on body image).
4. Degree of acceptance of illness.
5. Support system (partner, family, support group).
6. Body image and self-esteem.
7. Outlook on future.

◆ **B. Analysis/nursing diagnosis:** *Sexual dysfunction* associated with physical illness related to:
1. Disinterest in sexual activity.
2. Fear of precipitating or aggravating physical illness through sexual activity.
3. Use of illness as excuse to avoid feared or undesired sex.
4. Physical inability or discomfort during sexual activity.

◆ **C. Nursing care plan/implementation:**
1. Approach with nonjudgmental attitude.
2. Elicit concerns about current physical state and perceptions of changes in sexuality.
3. Observe nonverbal clues of concern.
4. Identify genital assets.
5. Support client and partner during adjustment to current state.
6. Explore culturally acceptable sublimation activities.
7. Promote adjustment to body image change.
8. *Health teaching:*
   a. Teach self-help skills.
   b. Teach partner to care for client's physical needs.
   c. Teach alternate sex behaviors and acceptable sublimation (touching, for example).

◆ **D. Evaluation/outcome criteria:** attains satisfaction with adaptive alternatives of sexual expressions; has a positive attitude toward self, body, and sexual activity.

IV. Inappropriate sexual behavior

◆ **A. Assessment:** public exhibitions of sexual behaviors that are offensive to others; making sexual advances to other clients or staff.

◆ **B. Analysis/nursing diagnosis:** *Conflict with social order* related to:
1. Acting out angry and hostile feelings.
2. Lack of awareness of hospital and agency rules regarding acceptable public behavior.
3. Variation in cultural interpretations of what is acceptable public behavior.
4. Reaction to unintended seductiveness by person's attire, posture, tone, or choice of terminology.

◆ **C. Nursing care plan/implementation:**
1. Maintain calm, nonjudgmental attitude.
2. Set firm limits on unacceptable behavior.
3. Encourage verbalization of feelings rather than unacceptable physical expression.
4. Reinforce appropriate behavior.
5. Provide constructive diversional activity for clients or patients.
6. *Health teaching:* explain rules regarding public behavior; teach acceptable ways to express anger.

◆ **D. Evaluation/outcome criteria:** verbalizes anger rather than acting out; accepts rules regarding behavior in public.

Concept of Death Throughout the Life Cycle

I. Ages 1–3

A. No concept per se, but experiences *separation anxiety and abandonment* any time significant other disappears from view over a period of time.

B. *Coping* means: fear, resentment, anger, aggression, regression, withdrawal.

◆ **C. Nursing care plan/implementation**—help the family:
1. Facilitate transfer of affectional ties to another nurturing adult.
2. Decrease separation anxiety of hospitalized child by encouraging family visits and by reassuring child that she or he will not be alone.
3. Provide stable environment through consistent staff assignment.

II. Ages 3–5

A. Least anxious about death.
B. Denial of death as inevitable and final process.
C. Death is separation, being alone.
D. Death is *sleep* and sleep is death.
E. "Death" is part of vocabulary; seen as real, gradual, *temporary*, not permanent.
F. Dead person is seen as alive, but in altered form, that is, lacks movement.
G. There are *degrees* of death.
H. Death means not being here anymore.
I. "Living" and "lifeless" are not yet distinguished.

Mental Health

J. Illness and death seen as *punishment* for "badness"; fear and guilt about sexual and aggressive impulses.

K. Death happens, but only to others.

◆ **L. Nursing care plan/implementation** (in addition to previous):

1. Encourage play for expression of feelings; use clay, dolls, etc.
2. Encourage verbal expression of feelings using children's books.
3. Model appropriate grieving behavior.
4. Protect child from the overstimulation of hysterical adult reactions by limiting contact.
5. Clearly state what death is—death is final, no breathing, eating, awakening—and that death is *not* sleep.
6. Check child at night and provide support through holding and staying with child.
7. Allow a choice of attending the funeral and, if child decides to attend, describe what will take place.
8. If parents are grieving, have other family or friends attend to child's needs.

III. Ages 5–10

A. Death is cessation of life; question of what happens after death.

B. Death seen as definitive, *universal,* inevitable, *irreversible.*

C. Death occurs to all living things, including self; may express, "It isn't fair."

D. Death is distant from self (an eventuality).

E. Believe death occurs by accident, happens only to the very *old* or very sick.

F. Death is personified (as a separate person) in fantasies and magical thinking.

G. Death anxiety handled by *nightmares, rituals,* and *superstitions* (related to fear of darkness and sleeping alone because death is an external person, such as a skeleton, who comes and takes people away at night).

H. Dissolution of bodily life seen as a perceptible result.

I. Fear of body mutilation.

◆ **J. Nursing care plan/implementation** (in addition to previous):

1. Allow child to experience the loss of pets, friends, and family members.
2. Help child talk it out and experience the appropriate emotional reactions.
3. Understand need for increase in play, especially competitive play.
4. Involve child in funeral preparation and rituals.
5. Understand and accept regressive or protest behaviors.
6. Rechannel protest behaviors into constructive outlets.

IV. Adolescence

A. Death seen as inevitable, *personal,* universal, and *permanent;* corporal life stops; body decomposes.

B. Does not fear death, but concerned with how to *live now,* what death feels like, *body changes.*

C. Experiences *anger, frustration, and despair* over lack of future, lack of fulfillment of adult roles.

D. Openly asks *difficult,* honest, *direct* questions.

E. Anger at healthy peers.

F. Conflict between *developing* body versus *deteriorating* body, *independent* identity versus *dependency.*

◆ **G. Nursing care plan/implementation** (in addition to previous):

1. Facilitate full expression of grief by answering direct questions.
2. Help let out feelings, especially through creative and aesthetic pursuits.
3. Encourage participation in funeral ritual.
4. Encourage full use of peer group support system, by providing opportunities for group talks.

V. Young adulthood

A. Death seen as *unwelcome* intrusion, *interruption* of what might have been.

B. Reaction: *rage, frustration, disappointment.*

◆ **C. Nursing care plan/implementation:** all of previous, especially peer group support.

VI. Middle age

A. Concerned with *consequences* of own death and that of significant others.

B. Death seen as disruption of involvement, responsibility, and *obligations.*

C. End of plans, projects, experiences.

D. Death is *pain.*

◆ **E. Nursing care plan/implementation** (in addition to previous): assess need for counseling when also in midlife crisis.

VII. Old age

A. *Philosophical* rationalizations: death as inevitable, final process of life, when "time runs out."

B. *Religious* view: death represents only the dissolution of life and is a doorway to a new life (a preparatory stage for another life).

C. Time of rest and peace, supreme refuge from turmoil of life.

◆ **D. Nursing care plan/implementation** (in addition to previous):

1. Help person prepare for own death by helping with funeral prearrangements, wills, and sharing of mementos.
2. Facilitate life review and reinforce positive aspects.
3. Provide care and comfort.
4. Be present at death.

Death and Dying

Too often the process of death has had such frightening aspects that people have suffered alone. Today there has been a vast change in attitudes; death and dying are no longer taboo topics. There is a growing realization that we need to accept death as a natural process. Elisabeth Kübler-Ross has written extensively on the process of dying, describing the stages of *denial* ("not me"), *anger* ("why me?"), *bargaining* ("yes me—but"), *depression* ("yes, me"), and *acceptance* ("my time is close now, it's all right"), with implications for the helping person.

I. Concepts and principles related to death and dying:
   A. Persons may know or *suspect* they are dying and may want to talk about it; often they look for someone to share their fears and the process of dying.
   B. Fear of death can be reduced by helping clients feel that they are *not alone.*
   C. The dying need the opportunity to live their final experiences to the fullest, in their *own* way.
   D. People who are dying remain more or less the *same* as they were during life; their approaches to death are consistent with their approaches to life.
   E. Dying persons' need to review their lives may be a purposeful attempt to reconcile themselves to what "was" and what "could have been."
   F. *Three ways* of facing death are (a) quiet acceptance with inner strength and peace of mind; (b) restlessness, impatience, anger, and hostility; and (c) depression, withdrawal, and fearfulness.
   G. *Four tasks* facing a dying person are (a) reviewing life, (b) coping with physical symptoms in the end stage of life, (c) making a transition from known to unknown state, and (d) reaction to separation from loved ones.
   H. Crying and tears are an important aspect of the grief process.
   I. There are many *blocks* to providing a helping relationship with the dying and bereaved:
      1. Nurses' unwillingness to share the process of dying—minimizing their contacts and blocking out their own feelings.
      2. Forgetting that a dying person may be feeling lonely, abandoned, and afraid of dying.
      3. Reacting with irritation and hostility to the person's frequent calls.
      4. Nurses' failure to seek help and support from team members when feeling afraid, uneasy, and frustrated in caring for a dying person.
      5. Not allowing client to talk about death and dying.
      6. Nurses' use of technical language or social chit-chat as a defense against their own anxieties.

◆ **II. Assessment** of death and dying:
   A. *Physical*
      1. Observable deterioration of physical and mental capacities—person is unable to fulfill physiological needs, such as eating and elimination.
      2. Circulatory collapse (blood pressure and pulse).
      3. Renal or hepatic failure.
      4. Respiratory decline.
   B. *Psychosocial*
      1. Fear of death is signaled by agitation, restlessness, and sleep disturbances at night.
      2. Anger, agitation, blaming.
      3. Morbid self-pity with feelings of defeat and failure.
      4. Depression and withdrawal.
      5. Introspectiveness and calm acceptance of the inevitable.

◆ **III. Analysis/nursing diagnosis:**
   A. *Terminal illness response.*
   B. *Altered feeling states* related to fear of being alone.
   C. *Altered comfort patterns* related to pain.
   D. *Altered meaningfulness* related to depression, hopelessness, helplessness, powerlessness.
   E. *Altered social interaction* related to withdrawal.

◆ **IV. Nursing care plan/implementation:**
   A. *Long-term goal:* foster environment where person and family can experience dying with dignity.
   B. *Short-term goals:*
      1. Express feelings (person and family).
      2. Support person and family.
      3. Minimize physical discomfort.
   C. Explore your own feelings about death and dying with team members; form support groups.
   D. Be aware of the *normal grief* process.
      1. *Allow* person and family to do the work of grieving and mourning.
      2. Allow crying and mood swings, anger, demands.
      3. Permit yourself to cry.
   E. Allow person to *express* feelings, fears, and concerns.
      1. *Avoid* pat answers to questions about "why."
      2. Pick up symbolic communication.
   F. Provide care and comfort with *relief from pain;* do not isolate person.
   G. Stay *physically close.*
      1. Use touch.
      2. Be available to form a consistent relationship.
   H. *Reduce isolation and abandonment* by assigning person to room in which isolation is less likely to occur and by allowing flexible visiting hours.
   I. Keep activities in room as *near normal* and *constant* as possible.

Mental Health

J. Speak in *audible* tones, not whispers.

K. Be alert to cues when person needs to be alone *(disengagement process).*

L. Leave room for *hope.*

M. Help person die with peace of mind by lending support and providing opportunities to express anger, pain, and fears to someone who will accept her or him and not censor verbalization.

N. *Health teaching:* teach grief process to family and friends; teach methods to relieve pain.

◆ **V. Evaluation/outcome criteria:**

A. Remains comfortable and free of pain as long as possible.

B. Dies with dignity.

Grief/Bereavement

Grief is a typical reaction to the loss of a source of psychological gratification. It is a syndrome with somatic and psychological symptoms that diminish when grief is resolved. Grief processes have been extensively described by Erich Lindemann and George Engle.*

I. Concepts and principles related to grief:

A. Cause of grief: reaction to loss (real or imaginary, actual or pending).

B. Healing process can be interrupted.

C. Grief is universal.

D. Uncomplicated grief is a self-limiting process.

E. Grief responses may vary in degree and kind (e.g., absence of grief, delayed grief, and unresolved grief).

F. People go through stages similar to stages of death described by Elisabeth Kübler-Ross.

G. Many factors influence successful outcome of grieving process:

1. The more *dependent* the person on the lost relationship, the greater the difficulty in resolving the loss.

2. A *child* has greater difficulty resolving loss.

3. A person with *few meaningful relationships* also has greater difficulty.

4. The *more losses* the person has had in the past, the more affected that person will be, because losses tend to be cumulative.

5. The more *sudden* the loss, the greater the difficulty in resolving it.

6. The more *ambivalence* (love-hate feelings, with guilt) there was toward the dead, the more difficult the resolution.

7. *Loss of a child* is harder to resolve than loss of an older person.

*Adapted from a classic article by George Engel: Grief and grieving. Am J Nurs 9(64):93–98, 1964. American Journal of Nursing.

◆ **II. Assessment—characteristic stages of grief responses:**

A. *Shock and disbelief* (initial and recurrent stage)

1. *Denial* of reality. ("No, it can't be.")

2. Stunned, *numb* feeling.

3. Feelings of loss, *helplessness,* impotence.

4. Intellectual acceptance.

B. *Developing awareness*

1. Anguish about loss.
   a. *Somatic* distress.
   b. Feelings of emptiness.

2. *Anger* and hostility toward person or circumstances held responsible.

3. Guilt feelings—may lead to self-destructive actions.

4. Tears (inwardly, alone; or inability to cry).

C. *Restitution*

1. Funeral *rituals* are an aid to grief resolution by emphasizing the reality of death.

2. Expression and sharing of feelings by gathered family and friends are a source of acknowledgment of grief and support for the bereaved.

D. *Resolving the loss*

1. Increased *dependency* on others as an attempt to deal with painful void.

2. More aware of own *bodily sensations*—may be identical with symptoms of the deceased.

3. Complete *preoccupation* with thoughts and memories of the dead person.

E. *Idealization*

1. All hostile and negative feelings about the dead are *repressed.*

2. Mourner may *assume* qualities and attributes of the dead.

3. Gradual lessening of preoccupation with the dead; *reinvesting* in others.

◆ **III. Analysis—see Table 6–9.**

◆ **IV. Nursing care plan/implementation in grief stages:**

A. *Apply crisis theory and interventions.*

B. *Demonstrate unconditional respect* for cultural, religious, and social mourning customs.

C. *Utilize knowledge of the stages of grief* to anticipate reactions and facilitate the grief process.

1. Anticipate and permit expression of different manifestations of shock, disbelief, and denial.
   a. News of impending death is best communicated to a family group (rather than an individual) in a private setting.
   b. *Let mourners see the dead or dying,* to help them accept reality.
   c. Encourage description of circumstances and nature of loss.

2. *Accept guilt, anger, and rage* as common responses to coping with guilt and helplessness.
   a. Be aware of potential suicide by the bereaved.

b. Permit crying; stay with the bereaved.
3. Mobilize social support system; promote hospital policy that allows gathering of friends and family in a private setting.
4. Allow dependency on staff for initial decision making while person is attempting to resolve loss.
5. Respond to somatic complaints.
6. Permit reminiscence.
7. Encourage mourner to relate accounts connected with the lost relationship that reflect positive and negative feelings and remembrances; *place loss in perspective.*
8. Begin to encourage and reinforce new interests and social relations with others by the end of the idealization stage, loosen bonds of attachment.
9. Identify high-risk persons for maladaptive responses. (See **I. G.** Many factors influence successful outcome of grieving process, earlier.)
10. *Health teaching:*
   a. Explain that emotional response is appropriate and common.
   b. Explain and offer hope that emotional pain will diminish with time.
   c. Describe normal grief stages.

◆ **V. Evaluation/outcome criteria:** outcome may take 1 yr or more—can remember comfortably and realistically both pleasurable and disappointing aspects of the lost relationship.
   A. Can express feelings of sorrow caused by loss.
   B. Can describe ambivalence (love, anger) toward lost person, relationship.
   C. Able to review relationship, including pleasures, regrets, etc.
   D. Bonds of attachment are loosened and new object relationships are established.

Mental and Emotional Disorders in Children and Adolescents

Children have certain developmental tasks to master in the various stages of development (e.g., learning to trust, control primary instincts, and resolve basic social roles; see **Unit 5**).

I. Concepts and principles related to mental and emotional disorders in children and adolescents
   A. Most emotional disorders of children are related to family dynamics and the place the child occupies in the family group.

TABLE 6–9 ◆**Analysis/Nursing Diagnosis:** *Altered Feeling States* **Related to Grief**

Problem Classification	Characteristics
1. Somatic distress	Occurs in waves lasting from 20 min to 1 hr
	Deep, sighing respirations most common when discussing grief
	Lack of strength
	Loss of appetite and sense of taste
	Tightness in throat
	Choking sensation accompanied by shortness of breath
2. Preoccupation with image of deceased	Similar to daydreaming
	May mistake others for deceased person
	May be oblivious to surroundings
	Slight sense of unreality
	Fear that he or she is becoming "insane"
3. Feelings of guilt	Accuses self of negligence
	Exaggerates existence and importance of negative thoughts, feelings, and actions toward deceased
	Views self as having failed deceased—"If I had only . . ."
4. Feelings of hostility	Irritability, anger, and loss of warmth toward others
	May attempt to handle feelings of hostility in formalized and stiff manner of social interaction
5. Loss of patterns of conduct	Inability to initiate or maintain organized patterns of activity
	Restlessness, with aimless movements
	Loss of zest—tasks and activities are carried on as though with great effort
	Activities formerly carried on in company of deceased have lost their significance
	May become strongly dependent on whomever stimulates him or her to activity

B. Children must be understood and treated within the context of their *families.*

C. Many disorders are related to the phases of development through which the children are passing. (Erik Erikson's developmental tasks for children are trust, autonomy, initiative, industry, identity, and intimacy.)

D. Table 6–10 summarizes key age-related disturbances, lists main *symptoms* and *analyses* of causes, and highlights *medical interventions* and *nursing plan/implementation.*

E. Children are not miniature adults; they have special needs.

F. Play and food are important media to make contact with children and help them release emotions in socially acceptable forms, prepare them for traumatic events, and develop skills.

G. Children who are physically or emotionally ill regress, giving up previously useful habits.

H. Adolescents have special problems relating to need for *control* versus need to *rebel, dependency* versus *interdependency,* and search for *identity* and *self-realization.*

I. Adolescents often *act out* their underlying feelings of insecurity, rejection, deprivation, and low self-esteem.

J. Strong feelings may be evoked in nurses working with children; these feelings should be expressed, and each nurse should be supported by team members.

◆ **II. Assessment** of *selected disorders:*

A. *Autistic disorders* (previously called childhood schizophrenia):
   1. Disturbance in how perceptual information is processed; normal abilities present.
      a. Behave *as though they cannot* hear, see, etc.
      b. Do *not react to external* stimulus.
      c. Mute or echolalic.
   2. Lack of self-awareness as a unified whole—may not relate bodily needs or parts as extension of themselves.
   3. Severe difficulty in communicating with others—may be mute and isolated.
   4. Bizarre postures and gestures (banging head, rocking back and forth).
   5. Disturbances in learning.
   6. *Etiology* is unknown.
   7. *Prognosis* depends on severity of symptoms and age of onset.

B. *Developmental disorders* (brain injury) characteristics:
   1. Hyperactivity.
   2. Explosive outbursts.
   3. Distractibility.
   4. Impulsiveness.
   5. Perceptual difficulties (visual distortions, such as figure-ground distortion and mirror reading; body-image problems; difficulty in telling left from right).

6. Receptive or expressive language problems.

C. *Elimination disorders* (functional enuresis)—related to feelings of insecurity due to unmet needs of attention and affection; important to preserve their self-esteem.

D. *Separation anxiety disorders of childhood* (school phobias)—anxiety about school is accompanied by physical distress. Usually observed with fear of leaving home, rejection by mother, fear of loss of mother, or history of separation from mother in early years.

E. *Conduct disorders*—include lying, stealing, running away, truancy, substance abuse, sexual delinquency, vandalism, and fire setting; chief motivating force is either overt or covert hostility; history of disturbed parent-child relations.

◆ **III. Analysis/nursing diagnosis:**

A. *Altered feeling states:* anxiety, fear, hostility related to personal vulnerability and poorly developed or inappropriate use of defense mechanisms.

B. *Risk for self-mutilation* related to disturbance in self-concept, abnormal response to sensory input, and history of abuse.

C. *Altered interpersonal processes:*
   1. *Impaired verbal communication* related to cerebral deficits, withdrawal into self, inability to trust other.
   2. *Altered conduct/impulse processes:* aggressive, violent behaviors toward self, others, environment related to feelings of distrust and altered judgment.
   3. *Dysfunctional behaviors:* age-inappropriate behaviors, bizarre behaviors; disorganized and unpredictable behaviors related to inability to discharge emotions verbally.
   4. *Impaired social interaction:* social isolation/withdrawal related to feelings of suspicion and mistrust, lack of bonding, inadequate sensory stimulation.

D. *Personal identity disturbance* related to lack of development of trust, organic brain dysfunction, maternal deprivation.

E. *Altered parenting* related to ambivalent or dissonant family relationships and failure of child to meet role expectations.

F. *Sensory/perceptual alterations:* altered attention related to disturbed mental activities.

G. *Altered cognition process:* altered decision making, judgment, knowledge, and learning processes; altered thought content and processes related to perceptual or cognitive impairment and emotional dysfunctioning.

◆ **IV. Nursing care plan/implementation** in mental and emotional disorders in children and adolescents:

A. *General goals:* corrective behavior—*behavior modification.*

TABLE 6–10   **Emotional Disturbances in Children**

Stage	Disturbance	Assessment: Symptoms ◆ or Characteristics	Analysis: Behavior ◆ Related To:	◆ Plan/Implementation
Oral (birth–1 yr)	Feeding disturbances	Refusal of food.	1. Rigid feeding schedule. 2. *Psychological* stress. 3. Incompatible formula. 4. *Physiological:* pyloric stenosis.	Pediatric evaluation, especially if infant is not gaining weight or is losing weight. Rule out physiological etiology or incompatible formula. Evaluate *feeding style* of caretaker. Is baby on demand feeding? Is caretaker sensitive to infant's needs or communications about holding, hunger, or satiation?
		Colic. Crying is usually confined to one part of day and starts after a feeding. Commonly lasts from first to third month.	Periodic tension in infant's immature nervous system, causing gas and sharp intestinal pains.	Reassure parents and teach about condition and how to relieve it with *hot water bottle, rocking, rubbing back, pacifier,* which may soothe infant.
	Sleeping disturbances	Infant resists being put down for sleep or going to sleep.	1. Need for parental attention. 2. A pattern formed during period of colic or other illness. 3. Emotional disturbance related to *anxiety.*	If it is attention-getting strategy, suggest parental lack of response for a few nights to break pattern. If emotional disturbance is suspected, evaluate *infant-caretaker interaction* and refer for psychotherapeutic intervention.
	Failure to thrive	Infant does not grow or develop over a period of time.	1. *Psychological:* inadequate caretaking. 2. *Physiological:* heart, kidneys, central nervous system (CNS) malfunction.	*Hospitalization* is essential. Assist in evaluation of physiological functioning, especially heart, kidneys, and CNS. *Nurturing plan* for infant, using specifically assigned personnel and the caretaker parent. If the infant grows and develops with nurturing, thus confirming problems of parenting as causative factor, psychotherapeutic and child protective interventions are necessary.
	Severe disturbances	**Autistic psychosis:** Very early onset; lack of response to others; bizarre, repetitive behavior; normal to above normal intelligence; failure to develop language or use communicative speech. Autism is one of the most severe and debilitating psychiatric disturbances.	1. Uncertain etiology; *regression* or *fixation* at earlier developmental stage, before child differentiates "me" from "not me." 2. A *"nature versus nurture"* controversy over the causative factors. These are variously thought to be: a. *Environment only:* Infant is tabula rasa and all disturbance is directly attributable to the environment (primarily the parenting). b. *Heredity only:* For genetic, biochemical, or other predetermined reasons, some infants will be psychotic regardless of the environment.	The severely disturbed child requires intensive psychotherapy and often milieu therapy available in residential or day care programs. Therapy is usually indicated for parents also. Nurses can work on a *primary level* of prevention by assessing parenting skills of prospective parents and *teaching* them these skills. On a *secondary level of prevention,* nurses can be knowledgeable about and *teach* others the early signs of childhood psychosis, making appropriate referrals. The earlier the intervention, the better the prognosis.

Continued

TABLE 6–10   Emotional Disturbances in Children—cont'd

Stage	Disturbance	◆ Assessment: Symptoms or Characteristics	◆ Analysis: Behavior Related To:	◆ Plan/Implementation
Oral—cont'd			c. *Combination of environment and heredity* plus *the interaction between them:* A *susceptible* infant, *less* than optimal parenting, and *negative* interaction between parent and infant will combine to produce disturbance.	On a *tertiary level of prevention,* nurses work with severely disturbed children and their families in child guidance clinics and residential and day care settings. *Health teaching* would include play activities that foster support, acceptance, and a nonthreatening mode of communication and interaction with a significant other.
		Symbiotic psychosis: Identified later than autistic type, usually between 2 and 5 years of age. These children seem to be unable to function independently of the caregiving parent. A situational stress, such as hospitalization of parent or child or entry into school, may precipitate a psychotic break in the child.	The same *"nature versus nurture"* controversy with respect to the origin of symbiotic psychosis. The child progresses beyond the self-absorbed autistic stage to form an object relationship with another (usually the mother). Having progressed to this stage, the child then *fails to differentiate his or her own identity* from that of the mother.	
Anal (1–3 yr)	Elimination disorders (disturbances related to toilet training)	*Constipation.*	1. *Diet.* 2. Child withholding due to history of one or two painful, *hard bowel movements.* 3. *Psychological* causation: child withholds from parents to *express anger, opposition,* or passage through a very *independent* development stage.	Evaluate *diet* and consistency of stools. Fecal softener may be prescribed if necessary. In all cases, *help parent avoid making* an issue of constipation with the child. Enemas are *contraindicated.* If child is withholding, *work with parents* around not forcing rigid toilet training on child. Most children are more cooperative about *toilet training* at 18–24 months.
		Encopresis (soiling).	Child's expression of anger or hostility. It is usually directed toward the parent with whom the child is experiencing conflict and is rarely physiological.	Medical evaluation, then assessment and intervention in the child-parent relationship. Therapy for child and parent may be indicated.
	Excessive rebelliousness	Frequent temper tantrums, fighting, destruction of toys and other objects, consistent oppositional behavior.	1. Fear caused by inconsistency in handling the child, the setting of rigid limits, or the parents' refusal or inability to set limits, which can all create insecurity and fear in the child. 2. Excessive rebelliousness, usually indicating a *frightened* child; should not be confused with expression of negativism normal at around age 2, which is a necessary (though trying) developmental stage.	The nurse should offer parent counseling if necessary. When working with the child, the nurse needs to be receptive and sympathetic while establishing and maintaining firm limits.

TABLE 6–10   Emotional Disturbances in Children—cont'd

Stage	Disturbance	◆ Assessment: Symptoms or Characteristics	◆ Analysis: Behavior Related To:	◆ Plan/Implementation
Anal—cont'd	Excessive conformity	Lack of spontaneity, anxious desire always to please all adult authority figures, timidity, refusal to assert own needs, passivity.	1. Very rigid control established in an attempt to handle fears. 2. Harsh *toilet training*, resulting in an overcompliant child. These children need help as much as overrebellious children, but they get it less frequently because their behavior is not a "problem"—that is, it is not difficult for parents to tolerate.	Excessive conformity can lead to *compulsive, ritualistic, or obsessive behavior* later. The nurse needs to be able to identify such a child, then work with the child and parents to encourage *self-expression* in the child. Referral for psychotherapy may be necessary to help the child deal with repressed anger.
		Enuresis. Ordinarily refers to wetting while asleep (nocturnal enuresis), though some enuretic children wet themselves during the day also. Enuresis is a *symptom*, not a diagnosis or disease entity.	1. *Faulty toilet training* (especially if child wets during the day also) or 2. *Psychological stress.* 3. *Physiological* etiology, such as genitourinary (GU) tract infections or CNS disease, is rare. The child *under 4 years* old is usually *not* considered enuretic but is included in this section because bladder training is part of toilet training. Etiology is uncertain.	Many approaches have been tried with varying degrees of success. These include *fluid restriction, behavioral intervention* (in which a buzzer wakes the child when the child starts to wet), and psychotherapy. *Educating parents in bladder training* techniques and attitudes can help solve the problem on a *primary* level. It is important when working with enuretic children or their parents to *suggest* ways to help the child *overcome feelings of shame and guilt.* These feelings are often exacerbated by well-meaning but misguided parents.
Oedipal (3–6 yr)	Excessive fears	Child will be frightened even in nonthreatening situations. *Nightmares and other sleep disturbances* occur. Usually, child will be very "clingy" with parents in an attempt to gain reassurance.	*Anxiety* as the causative factor. Anxiety can be induced by many things, such as: 1. Parental *failure to set appropriate limits.* 2. *Physical or psychological abuse.* 3. *Illness.* 4. Fear of *mutilation.* 5. *Imaginary* worries that are common at this age; e.g., a 4-year-old who is suddenly afraid of the dark, or dogs, or fire engines is not necessarily suffering from excessive fears.	If possible, identify and deal with the factors that are producing the anxiety. Offer child calm reassurance. *Night-light and open doors* can help allay night fears, but *counsel parents* that it is unwise to allow the child to sleep with the parents, which may make the child feel that the oedipal retaliation has succeeded. With the hospitalized child, the nurse needs to be aware of and work with the mutilation fears common at this age. Fears around certain procedures (e.g., injections) can often be resolved by helping the child *play out fears.*
	Excessive masturbation	Touching and fondling of genitals excessively, sometimes in a preoccupied or absentminded manner.	1. *Insecurity.* 2. Exploration and stimulation of the genital area, which is *normal* and common in this age group. However, if it is compulsive, the behavior is a signal that the child is *insecure.*	*Assess* the child's masturbating activity. When does it occur and why? Then help the child develop other *strategies* for coping with anxiety. *Answer questions about sexuality* in an open manner.

Continued

TABLE 6–10   Emotional Disturbances in Children—cont'd

Stage	Disturbance	◆ Assessment: Symptoms or Characteristics	◆ Analysis: Behavior Related To:	◆ Plan/Implementation
Oedipal— cont'd			3. Occasionally, a *specific fear.* For example, a boy viewing a baby sister's genitals may have castration fears. These can be dealt with directly.	*Counsel parents* that *threats and shaming are contraindicated,* and help parents deal with *their* feelings about masturbation.
	Regression	Resumption of activities (such as *thumb sucking, soiling and wetting, baby talk*) characteristic of earlier developmental levels.	1. Child's attempt to regain a more comfortable, previous level of development in response to a *threatening* situation (such as a new baby), or 2. A response to difficulty resolving oedipal *conflicts.*	*Counsel parents* not to make an issue of behavior. Offer child emotional support and acceptance, though not approval of regressive behavior.
	Stuttering	Articulation difficulty characterized by many stops and repetitions in speech pattern.	1. Anxiety. 2. Frustration. 3. Insecurity. 4. Excitement. Stuttering usually occurs when the affected child feels *anxious, frustrated, insecure,* or *excited.* Parental concerns and attention to stuttering focuses attention on it and increases anxiety. The origins of stuttering are not understood. It is *common around 2–3 years of age* and is *not* a cause for concern at that time.	Speech therapy is usually indicated. Psychotherapy may also be indicated, if stuttering is an expression of anxiety and conflict, persisting *beyond age 6.*
Latency (6–12 yr)	**Attention deficit disorder** (hyperactivity and hyperkinesis)	Both hyperactivity and hyperkinesis are occasionally observed in schoolchildren; characterized by a *short attention span,* restlessness, distractibility, and *impulsivity.*	1. An *organic disturbance* of the *CNS,* of uncertain origin, as the basis of *hyperkinesis.* Because the primary symptom—difficulty with attention span—is the same as that presented by the hyperactive child, the hyperactive child is frequently and incorrectly labeled hyperkinetic. 2. Attempts by *hyperactive child* to *control* anxiety through *reducement* (and *can* attend when interested or relaxed). Does not fit smoothly into environment, but problem may be with the environment *rather* than the child. In other words, the school situation requires a high degree of conformity. The child who does not fit the mold is *not* necessarily emotionally disturbed.	For the *hyperkinetic* child, psychopharmaceutical intervention—usually *Ritalin*—is most often employed. Psychotherapy and special education classes may also be indicated. Ritalin is also frequently prescribed for the *hyperactive* child—which raises the issue of whether an individual should be medicated to fit more smoothly into the environment. Therapy can help the hyperactive child *decrease anxiety* and *increase self-esteem,* thus reducing the symptoms.
	Withdrawal	Reduced body movement and verbalization, lack of close relationships, *detachment,* timidity, and seclusiveness.	Need to withdraw as a defensive behavior, through which the child controls anxiety by *reducing contact* with the outer world. Like	Offer *positive reinforcement* when child is more active. Help child *assert* self and *experience success* at certain tasks.

TABLE 6–10 Emotional Disturbances in Children—cont'd

Stage	Disturbance	Assessment: Symptoms ◆ or Characteristics	Analysis: Behavior ◆ Related To:	◆ Plan/Implementation
Latency— cont'd			the overcompliant child, the withdrawn child is frequently not identified as needing help because this behavior is not a "problem."	The nurse needs to work with parents who are overprotective. Therapy may be useful to work through anxiety and provide child with a chance to form a *trusting* relationship with another.
	Psychophysiological symptoms	The child experiences physical symptoms (such as *vomiting, headaches, eczema, asthma, colitis*) with no apparent physiologic cause.	*Conversion* of anxiety into physical symptoms.	After medical evaluation has established lack of physiological etiology, psychotherapy is usually indicated. Family therapy may be treatment of choice because *dysfunctional interpersonal family dynamics* are common in these cases. The nurse can also provide the child with a healthy interpersonal relationship. Nurses are frequently in a position to talk to parents and teachers about the importance of mental health counseling for children with physical symptoms.
	Separation anxiety disorders (school "phobia")	Sudden and seemingly inexplicable fear of going to school. These children often do not know what it is they fear at school. Frequently occurs *after an illness* and absence from school or birth of sibling.	An *acute anxiety reaction related to separation* from home (not actually a phobia).	If the child is allowed to stay home, the dread of returning to school usually increases. The child and parent should have psychiatric intervention quickly (before the problem becomes worse) to help the child separate from the parent.
	Learning disabilities	Failure or difficulty in learning at school	1. Emotional disorders, which cause school failure. 2. Feelings of *inferiority, discouragement,* and loss of confidence from school failure. Learning disabilities may be caused by many factors or combinations of factors, including *anxiety, poor sensory or sensorimotor integration, dyslexia, receptive aphasia.*	A comprehensive evaluation is essential. Ideally, this would include assessments by a pediatric neurologist, a mental health worker such as a psychiatric nurse or psychiatrist, a learning disabilities teacher specialist, and possibly an occupational therapist trained to work with sensory integration. Treatment is then based on the specific problem or problems.
	Conduct disorders	Behavior that is nonproductive; that is repeated in spite of threats, punishments, or rational argument; and that usually leads to punishment. Persistent *stealing and truancy* are examples.	*Conflicts* that are expressed and communicated through behavior rather than verbally. Child knows what he or she is doing but is unaware of the underlying motivations for the problem behavior.	Counseling or therapy for the child by a child psychiatric nurse or other mental health worker can allow the child to resolve the basic conflict, thus making the problem behavior unnecessary.

Source: Adapted from Wilson, HS, and Kneisl, CR: Psychiatric Nursing, ed 3. Addison-Wesley, Redwood City, Calif., 1988.

Mental Health

B. Help children gain self-awareness.

C. Provide *structured* environment to orient children to reality.

D. Impose *limits* on destructive behavior toward themselves or others without rejecting the children.
1. *Prevent* destructive behavior.
2. *Stop* destructive behavior.
3. *Redirect* nongrowth behavior into constructive channels.

E. Be *consistent*.

F. Meet *developmental and dependency* needs.

G. Recognize and encourage each child's strengths, growth behavior, and reverse regression.

H. Help these children reach the next step in social growth and development scale.

I. Use play and projective media to aid working out feelings and conflicts and in making contact.

J. Offer support to parents and strengthen the parent-child relationship.

K. *Health teaching:* teach parents methods of behavior modification.

◆ **V. Evaluation/outcome criteria:**

A. Destructive behavior is inhibited.

B. Demonstrates age-appropriate behavior on developmental scale.

Midlife Crisis: Phase of Life Problems

Midlife crisis is a time period that marks the passage between early maturity and middle age.

◆ **I. Assessment:**

A. Commonly occurs between ages 35 and 45.

B. Preoccupied with *visible* signs of aging, own mortality.

C. *Feelings: urgency* that time is running out ("last chance") for career achievement and unmet goals; *boredom* with present, *ambivalence, frustration, uncertainty* about the future.

D. Time of *reevaluation:*
1. Reassess: meaning of time and parental role (omnipotence as a parent is challenged).
2. Reexamine and contemplate change in career, marriage, family life.

E. *Personality changes* may occur. *Women:* traditional definitions of femininity may be challenged as become more assertive. *Males:* may be more introspective, sensitive to emotions, make external changes (younger mate, improve looks, new sports activity), mood swings.

F. Presence of *helpful elements* necessary to turn life's obstacles into opportunities.
1. Willingness to take risks.
2. Strong support system.
3. Sense of purpose.
4. Accumulated wisdom.

◆ **II. Analysis/nursing diagnosis:**

A. *Self-esteem disturbance (low self-esteem)* related to loss of youth, faltering physical powers, and facing discrepancy between youthful ambitions and actual achievement (no longer a promising person with potential).

B. *Altered role performance (role reversal):* related to parents who previously provided security and comfort but now need care.

C. *Altered feeling processes (depression):* related to disappointments and diminished optimism as life is reconsidered in light of the reality of aging and death.

◆ **III. Nursing care plan/implementation**—*long-term goal:* help individual to rebuild life structure.

A. Help client reappraise meaning of his or her life in terms of past, present, and future, and integrate aspects of time. Encourage introspection and reflection with questions.
1. What have I done with my life?
2. What do I really get from and give to my spouse, children, friends, work, community, and self?
3. What are my strengths and liabilities?
4. What have I done with my early dream, and do I want it now?

B. Assist client to complete *four major tasks:*
1. Terminate era of early adulthood by *reappraising* life goals identified and achieved during this era.
2. Initiate movement into middle adulthood by beginning to make *necessary changes* in *unsuccessful* aspects of the current life while trying out new choices.
3. Cope with *polarities* that divide life.
4. Directly confront *death of own parents.*

C. *Health teaching:* stress-management techniques; how to do self-assessment of aptitudes, interests; how to plan for retirement, aloneness, and use of increased leisure time; dietary modification and exercise program.

◆ **IV. Evaluation/outcome criteria:**

A. Gives up *idealized* self of early 20s for more *realistically* attainable self.
1. Talks *less* of early *hopes of eminence* and *more* on modest goal of *competence.*
2. Shifts values from sexuality to platonic relationships: replaces romantic dreams with *satisfying* friendships and companionships.
3. Modifies early illusions about own capacities.
4. Shifts values away from physical attractiveness and strength to *intellectual* abilities.

B. Comes to accept that life is finite and reconciles what *is* with what *might have been;* appreciates everyday human experience rather than glamor or power.

C. Through self-confrontation, self-discovery, and change, experiences time of restabilization; is reinvigorated, adventuresome.

D. Develops *alternative* abilities that release new energies.

E. Tries *less* to please everyone; others' opinions less important.

F. Makes more efficient and well-seasoned decisions from well-developed sense of judgment.

Mental Health Problems of the Aged

In general, problems affecting the elderly are *similar* to those affecting persons of *any* age. This section highlights the *differences* from the viewpoint of etiology, frequency, and prognosis.

I. **Concepts and principles related to mental health problems of the aged:**

A. The elderly *do* have capacity for growth and change.

B. Human beings, regardless of age, need sense of future and *hope* for things to come.

C. An inalienable right of all individuals should be to make or participate in all decisions concerning themselves and their possessions as long as they can.

D. Physical disability due to the aging process may enforce dependency, which may be unacceptable to elderly patients and may evoke feelings of anger and ambivalence.

E. In an attempt to *reduce feelings of loss,* elderly patients may *cling to concrete things* that most represent, in a *symbolic* sense, all that has been significant to them.

F. As memory diminishes, *familiar objects* in environment and *familiar routines* are important in helping *to keep clients oriented* and in contact with reality.

G. *Familiarity of environment brings security;* routines bring a sense of security about what is to happen.

H. If individuals feel unwanted, they may tell *stories* about their *earlier* achievements.

I. Many of the traits in the elderly result from *cumulative* effect of *past* experiences of frustrations and *present* awareness of limitations rather than from any primary consequences of physiological deficit.

◆ II. **Assessment:**

A. *Psychological characteristics of the aged:*

1. Increasingly *dependent* on others, not only for physical needs but also for emotional security.

2. Concerns focus more and more *inward,* with narrowed outside interests.

   a. Decreased emotional energy for concern with social problems unless these issues affect them.

   b. Tendency to *reminisce.*

   c. May appear selfish and unsympathetic.

3. Sources of pleasure and gratification are more childlike: *food, warmth, and affection,* for example.

   a. Tangible and frequent evidence of affection is important (e.g., letters, cards, and visits).

   b. May hoard articles.

4. *Attention span and memory are short;* may be forgetful and *accuse others of stealing.*

5. Deprivation of any kind is *not* tolerated:

   a. Easily frustrated.

   b. Change is poorly tolerated; need to have favorite chairs and established daily routine, for example.

6. Main *fears* in the aged include fear of *dependency,* chronic *illness, loneliness, boredom,* fear of being unloved, forgotten, *deserted* by those close to them, fear of *death;* fear of *loss of control* of one's own life; a failing *cognition;* loss of *purpose* and productivity.

7. *Nocturnal delirium* may be due to problems with night vision and inability to perceive *spatial* location.

B. *Psychiatric problems in aging*

1. *Loneliness*—related to *loss* of mate, diminishing circle of friends and family through death and geographic separation, *decline* in physical energy, loss of work (*retirement*), sharp loss of income, and loss of a lifelong lifestyle.

2. *Insomnia*—pattern of sleep changes in significant ways: disappearance of *deep* sleep, frequent *awakening, daytime* sleeping.

3. *Hypochondriasis*—anxiety may shift from concern with finances, job, or social prestige to concern about own bodily function.

4. *Depression*—common problem in the aging, with a *high suicide rate;* partly because of bodily changes that influence the *self-concept,* the older person may direct *hostility toward self* and therefore may be subject to feelings of depression and loneliness.

5. *Senility*—four early symptoms:

   a. Change in attention span.

   b. Memory loss for *recent* events and *names.*

   c. Altered intellectual capacity.

   d. Diminished ability to respond to others.

C. *Successful aging*

1. Being able to *perceive* signs of aging and limitations resulting from the aging process.

2. *Redefining* life in terms of effects on social and physical aspects of living.

3. Seeking *alternatives* for meeting needs and finding sources of pleasure.

4. Adopting a *different outlook* about self-worth.

5. *Reintegrating* values with goals of life.

D. *Causative factors* of mental disorder in the aged related to:

1. *Nutritional* problems and *physical ill health* related to *acute and chronic illness:*

   a. Cardiovascular diseases (heart failure, stroke, hypertension).

b. Respiratory infection.

c. Cancer.

d. Alcohol dependence and abuse.

e. Dentition problems.

2. Faulty adaptation related to *physical* changes of aging, e.g., depression, hypochondriases.

3. Problems related to *loss, grief, and bereavement.*

4. *Retirement* shock related to loss of status and financial security.

5. Social isolation and loneliness related to *inadequate sensory stimulation.*

6. *Environmental change* (relocation within a community or from home to institution): loss of family, privacy.

7. *Hopelessness, helplessness* related to condition and circumstances.

8. *Altered body image* (negative) related to aging process.

9. Depression related to *helplessness, inability to express anger.*

◆ **III. Analysis/nursing diagnosis:**

A. *Self-esteem disturbance* related to body-image disturbance and altered family role.

B. *Impaired social interaction* related to social isolation and environmental changes.

C. *Dysfunctional grieving* related to loss and bereavement.

D. *Altered feeling states and spiritual distress* related to hopelessness, anxiety, fear, powerlessness.

E. *Altered physical regulation processes* related to physical ill health.

F. *Sleep pattern disturbance* related to insomnia and altered sleep/arousal patterns.

◆ **IV. Nursing care plan/implementation:**

A. *Long-term goal:* to help reduce hopelessness and helplessness.

B. *Short-term goal:* to focus on ego assets.

C. Help elderly *preserve* what facet of life they can and *regain* that which has already been lost.

1. Help *minimize regression* as much as possible.

2. Help retain their *adult* status.

3. Help preserve their *self-image* as useful individuals.

4. Identify and *preserve their abilities* to perform, emphasizing what they *can* do.

D. Attempt to *prevent* loss of dignity and loss of worth—address them by titles, not "Gramps."

E. *Reduce* feelings of *alienation* and loneliness. Provide *sensory* experiences for those with visual problems:

1. Let them *touch* objects of various textures and consistencies.

2. Encourage heightened *use of remaining senses* to make up for those that are diminished or lost.

F. *Reduce* depression and feelings of isolation.

1. Allow time to *reminisce.*

2. *Avoid changes* in surrounding or routine.

G. *Protect* from rush and excitement.

1. Use simple, unhurried conversation.

2. Allow *extra* time to organize thoughts.

H. Be sensitive to *concrete* things they may want to *keep.*

I. *Health teaching:*

1. How to keep track of time (e.g., by marking off days on a calendar), to promote orientation.

2. How to keep track of medications.

3. Exercises to promote blood flow.

4. *Retirement counseling:*

a. Obtaining satisfaction from leisure time.

b. Nurturing relationships with younger generations.

c. Adjusting to changes: physical health, retirement, loss of loved ones.

d. Developing connections with own age group.

e. Taking on new social roles.

f. Maintaining a satisfactory and appropriate living situation.

g. Coping with dependence on others, especially one's children.

◆ **V. Evaluation/outcome criteria:**

A. Less confusion and fewer mood swings.

B. Increased interest in activities of daily living and interaction with others.

C. Lessened preoccupation with death, dying, physical symptoms, feelings of sadness.

D. Reduced insomnia and anorexia.

E. Expresses feelings of belonging and being needed.

PROTECTIVE FUNCTIONS

Common Behavioral Problems

I. Anger

A. **Definition:** feelings of resentment in response to anxiety when threat is perceived; need to discharge tension of anger.

◆ B. **Assessment:**

1. *Degree of anger and frequency:* scope of anger ranges on a continuum from *everyday mild annoyance* → *frustration* from interference with goal accomplishment → *assertiveness* (behavior used to deal with anger effectively) → *anger* related to helplessness and powerlessness that may interfere with functioning → *rage and fury,* when coping means are depleted or not developed.

2. *Mode of expression of anger*

   a. *Covert, passive* expression of anger: being overly nice; body language with little or no eye contact, arms close to body, soft voice, little gesturing; sarcasm through humor; *sublimation* through art and music; projection onto others; *denying* and pushing anger out of awareness; *psychosomatic* illness in response to internalized anger, e.g., headache.

   b. *Overt,* active expression of anger: physical activity to work off excess physical energy associated with biological response (e.g., hitting a punching bag, taking a walk); *aggression,* assertiveness.

3. *Physiological behaviors*—result of secretion of epinephrine and sympathetic nervous system stimulation preparing for fight-flight.

   a. *Cardiovascular* response: increased blood pressure and pulse, increased free fatty acid in blood.

   b. *Gastrointestinal* response: increased nausea, salivation, decreased peristalsis.

   c. *Genitourinary* response: urinary frequency.

   d. *Neuromuscular* response: increased alertness, increased muscle tension and deep-tendon reflexes, ECG changes.

4. *Positive functions of anger*

   a. Energizes behavior.

   b. Protects positive image.

   c. Provides ego defense during high anxiety.

   d. Gives greater control over situation.

   e. Alerts to need for coping.

   f. A sign of a healthy relationship.

◆ C. **Analysis/nursing diagnosis:** *defensive coping* related to source of stress (stressors):

1. *Biological stressors*—instinctual drives (Lorenz, on aggressive instincts, and Freud), *endocrine imbalances,* seizures, tumors, *hunger, fatigue.*

2. *Psychological stressors*—inability to resolve frustration that leads to aggression; real or imagined threatened loss of self-esteem; conflict, lack of control; anger as a learned expression and a reinforced response. Prolonged stress; an attempt to protect self; a desire for retaliation; a normal part of grief process.

3. *Sociocultural stressors*—lack of early training in self-discipline and social skills; crowding, personal space intrusion; *role modeling of abusive behavior* by significant others and by media personalities.

◆ D. **Nursing care plan/implementation**—*long-term goals:* constructive use of angry energy to accomplish tasks and motivate growth.

1. *Prevent* and *control* violence.

   a. Approach unhurriedly.

   b. Provide atmosphere of acceptance; listen attentively, refrain from arguing and criticizing.

   c. Encourage expression of feelings.

   d. Offer feedback of client's expressed feelings.

   e. Encourage mutual problem solving.

   f. Encourage realistic perception of others and situation and respect for the rights of others.

2. *Limit setting:*

   a. Clearly state *expectations* and *consequences* of acts.

   b. Enforce consequences.

   c. Encourage client to assume responsibility for behavior.

   d. Explore reasons and meaning of negative behavior.

3. Promote *self-awareness* and *problem-solving* abilities. Encourage and assist client to:

   a. Accept self as a person with a right to experience angry feelings.

   b. Explore reasons for anger.

   c. Describe situations where anger was experienced.

   d. Discuss appropriate alternatives for expressing anger (including assertiveness training).

   e. Decide on one feasible solution.

   f. Act on solution.

   g. Evaluate effectiveness.

4. *Health teaching:*

   a. Explore other ways to express feelings, and provide activities that allow appropriate expression of anger.

   b. Recommend that behavioral limits be set (by the family).

   c. Explain how to set behavioral limits.

d. Advise against causing defensive patterns in others.

◆ **E. Evaluation/outcome criteria:**
1. Demonstrates insight (awareness of factors that precipitate anger; identifies disturbing topics, events, and inappropriate use of coping mechanisms).
2. Uses appropriate coping mechanisms.
3. Reaches out for emotional support before stress level becomes excessive.
4. Evidence of increased reality perception and problem-solving ability.

II. Combative-aggressive behavior
A. Definition: *acting out* feelings of frustration, anger, anxiety, etc. through *physical or verbal* behavior.

◆ **B. Assessment:** recognize *precombative* behavior:
1. Demanding, fist clenching.
2. Boisterous, loud.
3. Vulgar, profane.
4. Limited attention span.
5. Sarcastic, taunting, verbal threats.
6. Restless, agitated, elated.
7. Frowning.

◆ **C. Analysis/nursing diagnosis:** *risk for self-injury* and *violence directed at others* related to:
1. Frustration as response to *breakdown of self-control* coping mechanisms.
2. Acting out as customary response to anger (*defensive coping*).
3. Confusion (*sensory/perceptual alterations*).
4. Physical restraints, such as when postoperative patient discovers wrist restraints.
5. Fear of intimacy, intrusion on emotional and physical space (*altered thought processes*).
6. Feelings of helplessness, inadequacy (*situational or chronic low self-esteem*).

◆ **D. Nursing care plan/implementation:**
1. *Long-term goal:* channel aggression—help person express feelings rather than act them out.
2. *Immediate goal: prevent injury to self and others.*
   a. Calmly call for assistance; do *not* try to handle *alone*.
   b. Approach cautiously. Keep client within *eye contact*, observing client's personal space.
   c. *Protect* against self-injury and injury to others; be aware of your position in relation to the weapon, door, escape route.
   d. *Minimize* stimuli, to control the environment—clear the area, close doors, turn off TV so person can hear you.
   e. *Divert* attention from the act; engage in talk and lead away from others.
   f. Assess *triggering* cause.
   g. Identify immediate problem.
   h. Focus on *remedy for immediate* problem.

i. Choose one calm, quieting individual to interact with person; nonauthoritarian, nonthreatening.
j. Maintain *verbal contact* to keep communication open; offer empathetic ear, but be firm and consistent in setting *limits* on dangerous behavior.
k. Negotiate, but do not make false promises or argue.
l. Restraints may be necessary as a *last* resort.
m. Place person in quiet room so he or she can calm down.
3. *Health teaching:*
   a. Explain how to obtain release from stress and how to rechannel emotional energy into acceptable activity.
   b. Advise against causing defensive responses in others.
   c. Explain what is justifiable aggression.
   d. Emphasize importance of how to recognize tension in self.
   e. Explain why self-control is important.
   f. Explain to family, staff, how to set behavioral limits.
   g. Explain causes of maladaptive coping related to anger.
   h. Teach how to use problem-solving method.

◆ **E. Evaluation/outcome criteria:**
1. Is aware of causes of anger; can recognize the feeling of anger and use alternative methods of expressing anger.
2. Expression of anger is appropriate, congruent with the situation.
3. Replaces aggression and acting out with assertiveness.

III. Confusion/disorientation
A. Definition: loss of reality orientation as to person, time, place, events, ideas.

◆ **B. Assessment:** note unusual behavior:
1. Picking, stroking movements in the air or on clothing and linens.
2. Frequent crying or laughing.
3. Alternating periods of confusion and lucidity (e.g., confused at night, when alone in the dark).
4. Fluctuating mood, actions, rationality (argumentative, combative, withdrawn).
5. Increasingly restless, fearful, leading to insomnia, nightmares.
6. Acts bewildered; has trouble identifying familiar people.
7. Preoccupied; irritable when interrupted.
8. Unresponsive to questions; problem with concentration and setting realistic priorities.
9. Sensitive to noise and light.
10. Has unrealistic perception of time, place, and situation.

11. Nurse no longer seen as supportive but as threatening.
◆ **C. Analysis/nursing diagnosis:** *Altered thought processes and sensory/perceptual alterations* related to:
1. *Physical and physiological disturbances*—metabolic (uremia, diabetes, hepatic dysfunction), fluid and electrolyte imbalances, cardiac arrhythmias, heart failure; anemia, massive blood loss with low hemoglobin; brain lesions; nutritional deficiency; pain; sleep disturbance; drugs (antidepressants, tranquilizers, sedatives, antihypertensives, diuretics, alcohol, PCP, street drugs).
2. *Unfamiliar environment*—unfamiliar routine and people; procedures that threaten body image; *noisy* equipment.
3. *Loss of sensory acuity* from partial or incomplete reception of orienting stimuli or information.
4. *Disability in screening out* irrelevant and excessive sensory input.
5. *Memory impairment.*
◆ **D. Nursing care plan/implementation:**
1. Check *physical signs,* e.g., vital signs, neurological status, fluid and electrolyte balance, and blood urea nitrogen.
2. Be calm; make contact to *reorient to reality:*
   a. *Avoid* startling if person is alone, in the dark, sedated.
   b. Make sure person can *see, hear, and talk* to you—turn off TV; turn on light, put on client's glasses, hearing aids, dentures.
   c. Call by name, clearly and distinctly.
   d. Approach cautiously, close to *eye* level.
   e. Keep your *hands visible;* for example, on bed.
3. *Take care of immediate problem,* e.g., disconnected IV tube or catheter.
   a. Give instructions slowly and distinctly; *avoid* threatening tone and comments.
   b. *Stay* with person until reoriented.
   c. Put *side rails* up.
4. Use conversation to *reduce* confusion:
   a. Use *simple, concrete phrases;* language the person can understand; *repeat* as needed.
   b. *Avoid:* shouting, arguing, false promises, use of medical abbreviations (e.g., NPO).
   c. Give *more time to concentrate* on what you said.
   d. Focus on *reality-oriented* topics or objects in the environment.
5. *Prevent confusion by establishing a reality-oriented relationship.*
   a. Introduce self by name.
   b. Jointly establish routines to prevent confusion from unpredictable changes and variations. Determine client's usual routine; attempt to incorporate this to lessen disruption in lifestyle.

   c. Explain what to expect in understandable words—where client is and why, what will happen, noises and activities client will hear and see, people client will meet, tests and procedures client will have.
   d. Find out what meaning hospitalization has to client; reduce anxiety related to feelings of apprehension and helplessness.
   e. Spend as much time as possible with client.
6. *Maintain orientation by providing nonthreatening environment.*
   a. Assign to room *near nurse's station.*
   b. Surround with *familiar* objects from home (e.g., photos).
   c. Provide *clock, calendar, and radio.*
   d. Have flexible visiting hours.
   e. Open curtain for *natural light.*
   f. Keep glasses, dentures, hearing aids nearby.
   g. Check client often, especially at night.
   h. *Avoid* using intercom to answer calls.
   i. *Avoid* low-pitched conversation.
7. *Take care of other needs.*
   a. Promote sleep according to usual habits and patterns to *prevent sleep deprivation.*
   b. *Avoid sedatives,* which may lead to or increase confusion.
   c. Promote independent functions, self-help activities, to *maintain dignity.*
   d. Encourage *nutritional* adequacy; incorporate familiar foods, ethnic preferences.
   e. Maintain *routine; avoid* being late with meals, medication, or procedures.
   f. Have *realistic expectations.*
   g. *Discover hidden fears.*
      (1) Do *not* assume confused behavior is unrelated to reality.
      (2) Look for clues to meaning from client's background, occupation.
   h. *Provide support to family.*
      (1) Encourage expression of feelings; avoid being judgmental.
      (2) Check what worked in previous situations.
8. *Health teaching:* explain possible causes of confusion. Reassure that it is common. Teach family, friends how to react to confused behavior.
◆ **E. Evaluation/outcome criteria:**
1. Less restlessness, fearfulness, mood lability.
2. More frequent periods of lucidity; oriented to time, place, and person; responds to questions.

IV. Demanding behavior
  A. Definition: a strong and persistent struggle to obtain satisfaction of self-oriented needs (such as control, self-esteem) or relief from anxiety.

◆ **B. Assessment:**

1. Attention-seeking behavior.
2. Multiple requests.
3. Frequency of questions.
4. Lack of reasonableness; irrationality of request.

◆ **C. Analysis/nursing diagnosis:** *defensive coping and impaired social interaction* related to:

1. Feelings of *helplessness* and *hopelessness*.
2. Feelings of *powerlessness* and *fear*.
3. A way of coping with anxiety.

◆ **D. Nursing care plan/implementation:**

1. *Control* own irritation; assess reasons for own annoyance.
2. *Anticipate* and meet client's needs; set time to discuss requests.
3. *Confront* with behavior; discuss reasons for behavior.
4. *Ignore* negative attention seeking and *reinforce appropriate* requests for attention.
5. Make plans with *entire staff* to set *limits*.
6. Set up *contractual* arrangement for brief, frequent, regular, uninterrupted attention.
7. *Health teaching:* teach appropriate methods for gaining attention.

◆ **E. Evaluation/outcome criteria:** fewer requests for attention; assumes more responsibility for self-care.

V. Denial of illness

A. Definition: an attempt or refusal to acknowledge some anxiety-provoking aspect of oneself or external reality. Denial may be an acceptable first phase of coping as an attempt to allow time for adaptation.

◆ **B. Assessment:**

1. Observe for *coping mechanisms* such as dissociation, repression, selective inattention, suppression, displacement of concern to another person.
2. Note behaviors that may indicate *denial of diagnosis*:
   a. Failure to follow treatment plan.
   b. Missed appointment.
   c. Refusal of medication.
   d. Inappropriate cheerfulness.
   e. Ignoring symptoms.
   f. Use of flippant humor.
   g. Use of second or third person in reference to illness.
   h. Flight into wellness, overactivity.
3. Use of earliest and most primitive defense by closing eyes, turning head away to separate from what is unpleasant and anxiety provoking.
4. Note *range* of denial: *explicit* verbal denial of obvious facts, disowning or *ignoring* aspects or *minimizing* by understatement.
5. Be aware of situations such as long-term physical disability that make people more prone to denial of anger. *Denial of illness protects the ego from overwhelming anxiety.*

◆ **C. Analysis/nursing diagnosis:** *ineffective denial* related to:

1. Untenable wishes, needs, ideas, deeds, or reality factors.
2. Inability to adapt to full realization of painful experience or to accept changes in body image or role perception.
3. Intense stress and anxiety.

◆ **D. Nursing care plan/implementation:**

1. *Long-term goal:* understand needs met by denial.
2. *Short-term goal: avoid* reinforcing denial patterns.
   a. Recognize behavioral cues of denial of some reality aspect; be aware of level of awareness and degree to which reality is excluded.
   b. Determine if denial interferes with treatment.
   c. Support moves toward greater reality orientation.
   d. Determine person's stress tolerance.
   e. Supportively help person discuss events leading to, and feelings about, hospitalization.
3. *Health teaching:*
   a. Explain that emotional response is appropriate and common.
   b. Explain to family and staff that emotional adjustment to painful reality is done at own pace.

◆ **E. Evaluation/outcome criteria:** indicates desire to discuss painful experience.

VI. Dependence

A. Definition: reliance on other people to meet basic needs, usually for love and affection, security and protection, and support and guidance; *acceptable in early phases* of coping.

◆ **B. Assessment:**

1. Excessive need for advice and answers to problems.
2. Lack of confidence in own decision-making ability and lack of confidence in self-sufficiency.
3. Clinging, too-trusting behavior.
4. Gestures, facial expressions, body posture, recurrent themes conveying "I'm helpless."

◆ **C. Analysis/nursing diagnosis:**

1. *Chronic low self-esteem* related to inability to meet basic needs or role expectations.
2. *Helplessness* and *hopelessness* related to inadvertent reinforcement by staff's expectations.
3. *Powerlessness* related to holding a belief that one's own actions cannot affect life situations.

◆ **D. Nursing care plan/implementation:**

1. *Long-term goal:* increase self-esteem, confidence in own abilities.

2. *Short-term goals:* provide activities that promote independence.
   a. *Limit setting*—clear, firm, consistent; acknowledge when demands are made; accept client but refuse to respond to demands.
   b. *Break cycle* of nurse avoids client when he or she is clinging and demanding → client's anxiety increases → demands for attention increase → frustration and avoidance on nurse's part increase.
   c. *Give attention before* demand exists.
   d. Use *behavior-modification* approaches:
      (1) *Reward* appropriate behavior (such as making decisions, helping others, caring for own needs) with attention and praise.
      (2) Give *no response* to attention-seeking, dependent, infantile behavior; goal is to increase incidence of mature behavior as client realizes little gratification from dependent behavior.
   e. *Avoid secondary gains* of being cared for, which impede progress toward aforementioned goals.
   f. Assist in developing *ability to control* panic by responding less to client's high anxiety level.
   g. Help client develop ways to seek gratification other than excessive turning to others.
   h. *Resist* urge to act like a parent when client becomes helpless, demanding, and attention seeking.
   i. *Promote decision making* by not giving advice.
   j. *Encourage accountability* for own feelings, thoughts, and behaviors.
      (1) Help identify feelings through nonverbal cues, thoughts, recurrent themes.
      (2) Convey expectations that client does have opinions and feelings to share.
      (3) Role model how to express feelings.
   k. *Reinforce self-esteem* and ability to work out problems independently. (Consistently ask: "How do you feel about . . ."; "What do you think?")
3. *Health teaching:*
   a. Teach family ways of interacting to enforce less dependency.
   b. Teach problem-solving skills, assertiveness.

◆ **E. Evaluation/outcome criteria:**
1. Performs self-care.
2. Asks less for approval and praise.
3. Seeks less attention, proximity, physical contact.

VII. Hostility

A. **Definition:** a feeling of *intense* anger or an attitude of antagonism or animosity, with the *destructive* component of intent to inflict harm and pain to another or to self; may involve *hate, anger, rage, aggression, regression.*

B. **Operational definition:**
1. Past experience of frustration, loss of self-esteem, unmet needs for status, prestige, or love.
2. Present expectations of self and others not met.
3. Feelings of humiliation, inadequacy, emotional pain, and conflict.
4. Anxiety experienced and converted into hostility, which can be:
   a. Repressed, with result of becoming withdrawn.
   b. Disowned to the point of overreaction and extreme compliance.
   c. Overtly exhibited: verbal, nonverbal.

C. **Concepts and principles:**
1. Aggression and violence are two *outward* expressions of hostility.
2. Hostility is often unconscious, automatic response.
3. Hostile wishes and impulses may be underlying motives for many actions.
4. Perceptions may be *distorted* by hostile outlook.
5. Continuum: from extreme politeness to *externalization* as murderous rage or homicide or *internalization* as depression or suicide.
6. Hostility seen as a defense *against* depression, as well as a *cause* of it.
7. Hostility may be repressed, dissociated, or expressed covertly or overtly.
8. *Normal* hostility may come from justifiable fear of *real* danger; *irrational* hostility stems from *anxiety.*
9. Developmental roots of hostility:
   a. *Infants* look away, push away, physically move away from threat; give defiant look. Role modeling by parents.
   b. *Three-year-olds* replace overt hostility with protective shyness, retreat, and withdrawal. Feel weak, inadequate in face of powerful person against whom cannot openly ventilate hostility.
   c. Frustrated or unmet needs for status, prestige, or power serve as a basis for *adult* hostility.

◆ **D. Assessment:**
1. Fault finding, scapegoating, sarcasm, derision.
2. Arguing, swearing, abusiveness, verbal threatening.
3. Deceptive sweetness, joking at other's expense, gossiping.
4. Physical abusiveness, violence, murder, vindictiveness.

◆ **E. Analysis/nursing diagnosis:**
1. *Causes*
    a. *Anxiety* related to a learned means of dealing with an interpersonal threat.
    b. *Risk for violence* related to a reaction to *loss of self-esteem* and *powerlessness.*
    c. *Defensive coping* related to intense frustration, insecurity, or apprehension.
    d. *Impaired social interaction* related to low anxiety tolerance.
2. *Situations with high potential for hostility:*
    a. *Enforced illness and hospitalization* cause anxiety, which may be expressed as hostility.
    b. Dependency feelings related to acceptance of illness may result in hostility as a coping mechanism.
    c. Certain illnesses or physical disabilities may be conducive to hostility:
        (1) *Preoperative cancer* client may displace hostility onto staff and family.
        (2) Postoperatively, if diagnosis is *terminal,* the family may displace hostility onto nurse.
        (3) Anger, hostility is a *stage of dying* the person may experience.
        (4) *Amputee* may focus frustration on others due to dependency and jealousy.
        (5) Patients on *hemodialysis* are prone to helplessness, which may be displaced as hostility.

◆ **F. Nursing care plan/implementation:**
1. *Long-term goal:* help alter response to fear, inadequacy, frustration, threat.
2. *Short-term goal:* express and explore feelings of hostility without injury to self or others.
    a. Remain calm, nonthreatening; endure verbal abuse in impartial manner, within limits; speak quietly.
    b. *Protect from self-harm,* acting out.
    c. Discourage hostile behavior while showing acceptance of client.
    d. Offer support to *express* feelings of frustration, anger, and fear *constructively, safely,* and *appropriately.*
    e. Explore hostile feelings *without* fear of retaliation, disapproval.
    f. *Avoid:* arguing, giving advice, reacting with hostility, punitiveness, finding fault.
    g. *Avoid* joking, teasing, which can be misinterpreted.
    h. *Avoid* words such as *anger, hostility;* use client's words *(upset, irritated).*
    i. Do *not* minimize problem or give client reassurance or hasty, general conclusions.
    j. *Do not stop verbal* expression of anger unless detrimental.
    k. Respond *matter-of-factly* to attention-seeking behavior, not defensively.
    l. *Avoid* physical contact; allow client to set pace in "closeness."
    m. Look for clues to antecedent events and focus *directly* on those areas; *do not evade* or ignore.
    n. Constantly focus on *here and now* and affective component of message rather than on content.
    o. Reconstruct what happened and why, discuss client's reactions; seek observations, *not* inferences.
    p. Learn how client would like to be treated.
    q. Look for ways to help client relate better without defensiveness, *when ready.*
    r. Plan to channel feelings into *motor* outlets (occupational and recreational therapy, physical activity, games, debates).
    s. Explain procedures beforehand; approach frequently.
    t. Withdraw attention, *set limits,* when acting out.
3. *Health teaching:* teach acceptable motor outlets for tension.

◆ **G. Evaluation/outcome criteria:** identifies sources of threat and experiences success in dealing with threat.

VIII. Manipulation
   A. Definition: process of playing on and using others by unfair, insidious means to serve own purpose without regard for others' needs; may take many forms; occurs consciously, unconsciously to some extent, in all interpersonal relations.
   B. Operational definition (Figure 6–3):
   1. Conflicting needs, goals exist between client and other person (e.g., nurse).
   2. Other person perceives need as unacceptable, unreasonable.
   3. Other person refuses to accept client's need.
   4. Client's tension increases, and he or she begins to relate to others as objects.
   5. Client increases attempts to influence others to fulfill his or her need.
       a. Appears unaware of others' needs.
       b. Exhibits excessive dependency, helplessness, demands.
       c. Sets others at odds (especially staff).
       d. *Rationalizes,* gives logical reasons.
       e. Uses deception, false promises, insincerity.
       f. Questions and *defies nurse's authority* and competence.
   6. Nurse feels powerless and angry at having been used.

◆ **C. Assessment:**
   1. Acts out sexually, physically.
   2. Dawdles, always last minute.
   3. Uses insincere flattery; expects special favors, privileges.
   4. Exploits generosity and fears of others.
   5. Feels no guilt.

FIGURE 6–3 Operationalization of the behavioral concept of manipulation.

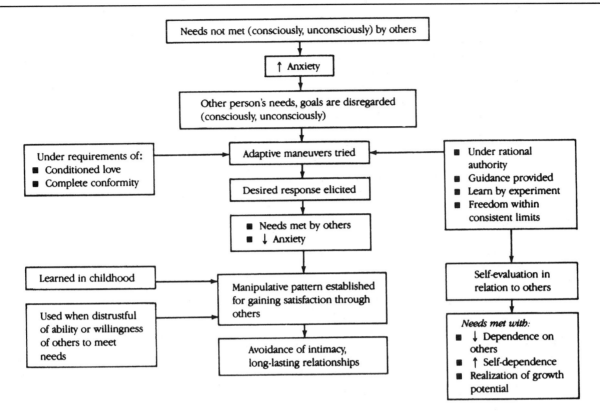

6. Plays one staff member against another.
7. *Tests limits.*
8. Finds weaknesses in others.
9. Makes excessive, unreasonable, unnecessary *demands* for staff time.
10. *Pretends* to be helpless, lonely, distraught, tearful.
11. Cannot distinguish between truth and falsehood.
12. *Plays on sympathy* or *guilt.*
13. Offers many excuses, lacks insight.
14. Pursues unpleasant issues without genuine regard for or feelings of individuals involved.
15. *Intimidates,* derogates, threatens, bargains, cajoles, violates rules to obtain reactions or privileges.
16. Betrays information.
17. Uses communication as a medium for manipulation, as verbal, nonverbal means to get others to cooperate, to behave in certain way, to get something from another for own use.
18. May be coercive, illogical, or skillfully deceptive.
19. *Unable to learn from experience,* i.e., repeats unacceptable behaviors despite negative consequences.

◆ **D. Analysis/nursing diagnosis:** *ineffective individual coping and impaired adjustment* related to:
   1. Mistrust and contemptuous view of others' motivations.

2. Life experience of rejection, deception.
3. Low anxiety tolerance.
4. Inability to cope with tension.
5. Unmet dependency needs.
6. Need to avoid anxiety when cannot obtain gratification.
7. Need to obtain something that is forbidden, or need for *instant gratification.*
8. Attempt to put something over on another when no real advantage exists.
9. *Intolerance of intimacy,* maneuvering effectively to keep others at a safe distance to dilute the relationship by withdrawing and frustrating others or distracting attention away from self.
10. Attempt to demand attention, approval, disapproval.

◆ **E. Nursing care plan/implementation:**
1. *Long-term goal:* define relationship as a mutual experience in *learning and trust* rather than a struggle for *power and control.*
2. *Short-term goals:* increase awareness of self and others; increase self-control; learn to accept limitations.
3. Promote use of **"three C's"**—*cooperation, compromise, collaboration*—rather than exploitation or deception.
4. *Decrease level and extent of manipulation.*
   a. Set *firm, realistic goals,* with clear, consistent expectations and limits.

b. *Confront* client regarding exploitation attempts; examine, discuss behavior.

c. Give *positive reinforcement* with concrete reinforcers for nonmanipulation, to lessen need for exploitive, deceptive, and self-destructive behaviors.

d. *Ignore* "wooden-leg" behavior (feigning illness to evoke sympathy).

e. *Allow verbal* anger; do *not* be intimidated; *avoid* giving desired response to obvious attempts to irritate.

f. Set *consistent, firm, enforceable limits* on *destructive,* aggressive behavior that impinges on others' health, rights, and interests, and on excessive dependency; *give reasons* when you cannot meet requests.

g. Keep staff informed of rules and reasons; obtain staff *consensus.*

h. Enforce *direct* communication; encourage openness about *real* needs, feelings.

i. Do *not* accept gifts, favors, flattery, or other guises of manipulation.

5. Increase responsibility for *self-control* of actions.

a. Decide who (client, nurse) is responsible for what.

b. Provide opportunities for *success* to increase self-esteem, experiencing acceptance by others.

c. Evaluate actions, *not* verbal behavior; point out the difference between talk and action.

d. Support efforts to be responsible.

e. Assist client to increase emotional repertoire; explore *alternative* ways of relating interpersonally.

f. *Avoid submission* to control based on fear of punishment, retaliation, loss of affection.

6. Facilitate awareness of, and *responsibility* for, manipulative behavior and its *effects on others.*

a. Reflect back client's behavior.

b. Discourage distortion and misuse of information.

c. *Increase tolerance* for differences and *delayed gratification* through behavior modification.

d. Insist on clear, consistent staff communication.

7. *Avoid:*

a. Labeling client as a "problem."

b. Hostile, negative attitude.

c. Making a public issue of client's behavior.

d. Being excessively rigid or permissive, inconsistent or ambiguous, argumentative or accusatory.

8. *Health teaching:* act as a role model; demonstrate how to deal with mistakes, human imperfections, by admitting mistakes in nonshameful, nonvirtuous ways.

◆ F. **Evaluation/outcome criteria:** accepts limits; able to compromise, cooperate rather than deceive and exploit; acts responsibly, self-dependent.

IX. **Noncompliance and uncooperative behavior**

A. **Definition:** consistently failing to meet the requirements of the prescribed treatment regimen, e.g., refusing to adhere to dietary restrictions or take required medications.

◆ B. **Assessment:**

1. Refuses to participate in routine or planned activities.

2. Refuses medication.

3. Violates rules, ignores limits, and abuses privileges; acts out anger and frustration.

◆ C. **Analysis/nursing diagnosis:** *noncompliance* related to:

1. *Psychological factors:* lack of knowledge; attitudes, beliefs, and values; denial of illness; rigid, defensive personality type; anxiety level (very high or very low); cannot accept limits or dependency (rebellious counterdependency).

2. *Environmental factors:* finances, transportation, lack of support system.

3. *Health care agent-client relationship:* client feels discounted and like an "object"; sees staff as uncaring, authoritative, controlling.

4. *Health care regimen:* too complicated; not enough benefit from following regimen; results in social stigma or social isolation; unpleasant side effects.

◆ D. **Nursing care plan/implementation:**

1. *General goal:* reduce need to act out by nonadherence.

a. Take *preventive* action—be alert to signs of noncompliance, such as intent to leave against medical advice.

b. *Explore* feelings and reasons for lack of cooperation.

c. Assess and *allay fears* in client in reassuring manner.

d. Provide *adequate* information about, and reasons for, rules and procedures.

e. *Avoid* threats or physical restraints; maintain calm composure.

f. Demonstrate *tact and firmness* when confronting violations.

g. Offer *alternatives.*

h. Firmly insist on cooperation in selected important activities but not all activities.

2. *Health teaching:* increase knowledge base regarding health-related problem, procedures, or treatments and consequences.

◆ E. **Evaluation/outcome criteria:** follows prescribed regimen.

Psychiatric Emergencies*

I. **Definition:** sudden onset (days or weeks, not years) of unusual (for that individual), disordered (without pattern or purpose), or socially inappropriate behavior caused by emotional or physiological situation. Examples include suicidal feelings or attempts, overdose, acute psychotic reaction, acute alcohol withdrawal, acute anxiety.

II. **General characteristics:**
◆ A. **Assessment:** the presence of great distress without reasonable explanation; *extreme* behavior in comparison with antecedent event.
  1. *Fear*—related to a particular person, activity, or place.
  2. *Anxiety*—fearful feeling without any obvious reason, not specifically related to a particular person, activity, or place (e.g., adolescent turmoil).
  3. *Depression*—continual pessimism, easily moved to tears, hopelessness, and isolation (e.g., student despondency around exam time, middle-aged crisis, elderly hopelessness).
  4. *Mania*—unrealistic optimism.
  5. *Anger*—many events seen as deliberate insults.
  6. *Confusion*—diminished awareness of who and where one is; memory loss.
  7. *Loss of reality contact*—hallucinations or delusion (as in acute psychosis).
  8. *Withdrawal*—neglect or giving away of belongings and neglect of appearance; loss of interest in activities; apathy.
◆ B. **Analysis/nursing diagnosis:** *ineffective individual coping* related to degree of seriousness:
  1. *Life-threatening emergencies*—violence toward self or others (e.g., suicide, homicide).
  2. *Serious emergencies*—confused and unable to care for or protect self from dangerous situations (as in substance abuse).
  3. *Potentially serious emergencies*—anxious and in pain; disorganized behavior; can become worse or better (as in grief reaction).
◆ C. **General nursing care plan/implementation:**
  1. *Remove* from stressful situation and persons.
  2. Engage in *dialogue* at a nonthreatening distance, to offer help.
  3. Use *calm, slow, deliberate* approach to relieve stress and disorganization.
  4. *Explain* what will be done about the problem and the likely outcome.
  5. *Avoid* using force, threat, or counterthreat.
  6. Use *confident, firm, reasonable* approach.
  7. Encourage client to relate.

*Adapted from Aguilera, D, and Messick, J: Crisis Intervention, ed. 5. Mosby, St. Louis, 1986.

  8. Elicit *details.*
  9. Encourage *ventilation* of feelings without interruption.
  10. Accept distortions of reality *without arguing.*
  11. Give form and *structure* to the conversation.
  12. Contact significant others to gain information and to be with client, including previous therapist.
  13. Treat emergency as *temporary* and *readily resolved.*
  14. Check every half hour if cannot remain with client.

III. **Categories of psychiatric emergencies:**
  A. *Acute nonpsychotic reactions,* such as acute anxiety attack or panic reaction (for symptoms, see **Anxiety and Anxiety Disorders,** pp. 371–373, 375–377).
  ◆ 1. **Assessment** includes differentiating hyperventilation that is anxiety—connected from asthma, angina, and heart disease.
  ◆ 2. **Nursing care plan/implementation** in hyperventilation syndrome—*goal:* prevent paresthesia, tetanic contractions, disturbance in awareness; reassure client that vital organs are not impaired.
    a. Increase CO_2 in lungs by rebreathing from paper bag.
    b. Minimize secondary gains; *avoid* reinforcing behavior.
    c. *Health teaching:* demonstrate how to slow down breathing rate.
  ◆ 3. **Evaluation/outcome criteria:** respirations slowed down; no evidence of effect of hyperventilation.
  B. *Delirium*—conditions produced by changes in the cerebral chemistry or tissue by metabolic toxins, direct trauma to the brain, drug effects, or withdrawal.
  1. *Acute alcohol intoxication* (see also **Alcohol Abuse and Dependence,** pp. 355–358).
    ◆ a. **Assessment:** signs of head or other injury (past and recent), emotional lability, memory defects, loss of judgment, disorientation.
    ◆ b. **Nursing care plan/implementation:**
      (1) Observe, monitor *vital signs.*
      (2) *Prevent aspiration* of vomitus by positioning.
      (3) *Decrease* environmental stimuli:
        (a) Place in quiet area of emergency department.
        (b) Speak and handle calmly.
      (4) Give medication (diazepam [Valium]) to control agitation.
    ◆ c. **Evaluation/outcome criteria:** oriented to time, place, person; appears calmer.
  2. *Hallucinogenic drug intoxication*—LSD, mescaline, amphetamines, cocaine, scopolamine, and belladonna.

◆ a. **Assessment:**
(1) Perceptual and cognitive distortions (e.g., feels heart stopped beating).
(2) Anxiety (apprehension → panic).
(3) Subjective feelings (omnipotence → worthlessness).
(4) Interrelationship of dose, potency, setting, expectations and experiences of user.
(5) Eyes: *red*—marijuana; *dilated*—LSD, mescaline, belladonna; *constricted*—heroin and derivatives.

◆ b. **Nursing care plan/implementation:**
(1) "Talk down."
(a) Establish *verbal* contact, attempt to have client verbally express what is being experienced.
(b) *Environment*—few people, normal lights, calm, supportive.
(c) Allay fears.
(d) Encourage to keep eyes *open*.
(e) Have client focus on *inanimate* objects in room as a bridge to reality contact.
(f) Use simple, *concrete, repetitive* statements.
(g) *Repetitively* orient to time, place, and temporary nature.
(h) Do *not* moralize, challenge beliefs, or probe into lifestyle.
(i) Emphasize confidentiality.
⬤ (2) *Medication (minor tranquilizer—diazepam [Valium], chlordiazepoxide HCl [Librium]):*
(a) Allay anxiety.
(b) Reduce aggressive behavior.
(c) Reduce suicidal potential; check client every 5–15 min.
(d) *Avoid* anticholinergic crisis (precipitated by use of phenothiazines, belladonna, and scopolamine ingestion) with 2–4 mg IM or PO of physostigmine salicylate.
(3) *Hospitalization:* if hallucinations, delusions last more than 12–18 hr; if client has been injecting amphetamines for extended time; if client is paranoid and depressed.

◆ c. **Evaluation/outcome criteria:** less frightened; oriented to time, place, person.

3. *Acute delirium*—seen in postoperative electrolyte imbalance, systemic infections, renal and hepatic failure, oversedation, metastatic cancer.

◆ a. **Assessment:**
(1) Disorientation regarding time, at night.
(2) Hallucinations, delusions, illusions.
(3) Alterations in mood.
(4) Increased emotional lability.

(5) Agitation.
(6) Lack of cooperation.
(7) Withdrawal.
(8) Sleep pattern reversal.
(9) Alterations in food intake.

◆ b. **Nursing care plan/implementation:**
(1) Identify and remove *toxic* substance.
(2) Reality orientation—well-lit room; constant attendance to inform *repetitively* of place and time and to *protect* from injury to self and others.
(3) Simplify environment.
⬤ (4) *Avoid* excessive medication and restraints; use low-dose phenothiazines; do *not* give barbiturates or sedatives (these increase agitation, confusion, disorientation).

◆ c. **Evaluation/outcome criteria:** oriented to time, place, person; cooperative; less agitated.

C. *Acute psychotic reactions*—disorders of mood or thinking characterized by hallucinations, delusions, excessive euphoria (mania), or depression.
1. *Acute schizophrenic reaction* (see also **Schizophrenic and Other Psychotic Disorders,** pp. 382–385, 386–387).

◆ a. **Assessment:**
(1) History of previous hospitalization, no illicit drug ingestion; use of major tranquilizers and recent withdrawal from them or alcohol.
(2) Auditory hallucinations and delusions.
(3) Violent, assaultive, suicidal behavior directed by auditory hallucinations.
(4) Assault, withdrawal, and panic related to paranoid delusions of persecution; fear of harm.
(5) Disturbance in mental status (associative thought disorder).

◆ b. **Nursing care plan/implementation** (see also **II. C. Hallucinations,** pp. 382–384):
(1) Hospitalization.
⬤ (2) Medication: phenothiazines.
(3) *Avoid* physical restraints or touch when fears and delusions of sexual attack exist.
(4) Allow client to *diffuse* anger and intensity of panic through talk.
(5) Use simple, *concrete* terms, *avoid* figures of speech or content subject to multiple interpretations.
(6) Do *not* agree with reality distortions; point out that client's thoughts are difficult to understand but you are willing to listen.

◆ c. **Evaluation/outcome criteria:** does not hear frightening voices; less fearful and combative behavior.

2. *Manic reaction* (see also **Bipolar Disorders,** pp. 391, 394–397).

◆ a. **Assessment:**
  (1) History of depression requiring antidepressants.
  (2) *Thought disorder* (flight of ideas, delusions of grandeur).
  (3) *Affect* (elated, irritable, irrational anger).
  (4) *Speech* (loud, pressured).
  (5) *Behavior* (rapid, erratic, chaotic).

◆ b. **Nursing care plan/implementation:**
  (1) Hospitalization to protect from injury to self and others.
  ▭ (2) Medication: *lithium carbonate.*
  (3) Same as for acute schizophrenic reaction, *except do not encourage talk,* because of need to decrease stimulation.
  ▯◖(4) Provide food and fluids that can be consumed while "on the go."

◆ c. **Evaluation/outcome criteria:** speech and activity slowed down; thoughts less disordered.

D. *Homicidal or assaultive reaction*—seen in acutely drug-intoxicated, delirious, paranoid, acutely excited manic, or acute anxiety-panic conditions.

◆ 1. **Assessment**—history of obvious antisocial behavior, paranoid psychosis, previous violence, sexual conflict, rivalry, substance abuse, recent moodiness, and withdrawal.

◆ 2. **Nursing care plan/implementation:**
  a. Physically restrain if client has a weapon; use group of trained people to help.
  b. Allow person to "save face" in giving up weapon.
  c. *Separate* from intended victims.
  d. Approach: calm, unhurried; *one person* to offer support and reassurance; use clear, unambiguous statements.
  e. Immediate and rapid admission procedures.
  f. Observe for *suicidal* behavior that may follow homicidal attempt.

◆ 3. **Evaluation/outcome criteria:** client regains impulse control.

E. *Suicidal ideation*—seen in anxiety attacks, substance intoxication, toxic delirium, schizophrenic auditory hallucinations, and depressive reactions.

  1. **Concepts and principles related to suicide:**
    a. *Based on social theory:* suicidal tendency is a result of collective social forces rather than isolated individual motives (Durkheim's *Le Suicide*).
      (1) Common factor: increased *alienation* between person and social group; psychological isolation, called "anomie," when links between groups are weakened.
      (2) "Egoistic" suicide: results from lack of integration of individual with others.

      (3) "Altruistic" suicide: results from insufficient individualization.
      (4) *Implication:* increase group cohesiveness and mutual interdependence, making group more coherent and consistent in fulfilling needs of each member.
    b. *Based on symbolic interaction theory:*
      (1) Person evaluates self according to *others' assessment.*
      (2) Thus, suicide stems from *social rejection* and disrupted social relations.
      (3) Perceived failure in relationships with others may be inaccurate but seen as real by the individual.
      (4) *Implication:* need to recognize difference in perception of alienation between own viewpoint and others'.
    c. *Based on psychoanalytic theory:*
      (1) Suicide stems mainly from the individual, with external events only as precipitants.
      (2) There is a strong life urge in people.
      (3) *Universal death instinct* is always present (Freud).
      (4) Person may be balancing life wishes and death wishes. When self-preservation instincts are diminished, death instincts may find direct outlet via suicide.
      (5) When *love instinct* is frustrated, *hate* impulse takes over (Menninger).
        (a) Desire to kill → desire to be killed → desire to kill oneself.
        (b) Suicide may be an act of extreme hostility, manipulation, and revenge to elicit guilt and remorse in significant others.
        (c) Suicide may also be act of self-punishment to handle own guilt or to control fate.
    d. *Based on synthesis of social and psychoanalytic theories:*
      (1) Suicide is seen as *running away* from an intolerable situation to interrupt it rather than *running to* something more desirable.
      (2) Process *defined in operational terms* involves:
        (a) Despair over inability to cope.
        (b) Inability to feel hope or adequacy.
        (c) Frustration with others when others cannot fill needs.
        (d) Rage and aggression experienced toward significant other is turned inward.
        (e) Psychic blow acts as precipitant.
        (f) Life seen as harder to cope with, with no chance of improvement in life situation.

Mental Health

(g) *Implication:* persons who experience suicidal impulses can gain a certain amount of control over these impulses through the support they gain from meaningful relationships with others.

e. *Based on crisis theory (Dublin):* concept of emotional disequilibrium:

(1) Everyone at some point in life is in a crisis, with temporary inability to solve problems or to master the crisis.

(2) Usual coping mechanisms do not function.

(3) Person unable to relate to others.

(4) Person searches consciously and unconsciously for useful coping techniques, with suicide as one of various solutions.

(5) With inadequate communication of needs and isolation, suicide is possible.

f. *Based on the view that suicide is an individual's personal reaction and decision, a final response to own situation:*

(1) *Process* of anger turned inward → self-inflicted, destructive action.

(2) *Definition* of concept in operational steps:

(a) Frustration of individual needs → anger.

(b) Anger turned inward → feelings of guilt, despair, depression, incompetence, hopelessness, and exhaustion.

(c) Stress felt and perceived as unbearable and overwhelming.

(d) Attempt to communicate hopelessness and defeat to others.

(e) Others do not provide hope.

(f) Sudden change in behavior, as noted when depression appears to lift, may indicate *danger,* as person has more energy to act on suicidal thoughts and feelings.

(g) Decision to end life → plan of action → self-induced, self-destructive behavior.

(3) May be *pseudosuicide* attempts, where there is no actual or realistic desire to achieve finality of death. Intentions or causes may be:

(a) "Cry for help," where nonlethal attempt notifies others of deeper intentions.

(b) Desire to *manipulate* others.

(c) Need for *attention and pity.*

(d) Self-punishment.

(e) Symbol of *utter frustration.*

(f) Wish to *punish* others.

(g) *Misuse* of alcohol and other drugs.

(4) Other reasons for self-destruction, where the individual *gives his or her life* rather than takes it, include:

(a) Strong parental love that can overcome fear and instinct of self-preservation to save child's life.

(b) "Sacrificial death" during war, such as kamikaze pilots in World War II.

(c) Submission to death for religious beliefs (martyrdom).

◆ 2. **Assessment of suicide:**

a. *Assessment of risk regarding statistical probability of suicide—composite picture:* male, older than 45 years, unemployed, divorced, living alone, depressed (weight loss, somatic delusions, sleep disturbance, preoccupied with suicide), history of substance abuse and suicide within family.

b. *Ten factors* to predict potential suicide and assess risk:

(1) *Age, sex, and race*—teenage, older age; more women make attempts; more men complete suicide act. *Highest risk:* older women rather than young boys; older men rather than young girls. Suicide occurs in all races and socioeconomic groups.

(2) *Recent stress*—family problems: death, divorce, separation, alienation; financial pressures; loss of job; loss of status; failing grades.

(3) *Clues to suicide:* suicidal thoughts are usually time limited and do not last forever. Early assessment of behavioral and verbal clues is important.*

(a) *Verbal clues—direct:* "I am going to shoot myself." *Indirect:* "It's more than I can bear." *Coded:* "This is the last time you'll ever see me." "I want you to have my coin collection."

(b) *Behavioral clues—direct:* trial run with pills or razor, for example. *Indirect:* sudden lifting of depression, buying a casket, giving away cherished belongings, putting affairs in order, writing a will.

(c) *Syndromes—dependent-dissatisfied:* emotionally dependent but dislikes dependent state, irritable, helpless. *Depressed:* detachment from life; feels life is a burden; hopelessness, futility. *Disoriented:* delusions or hallucinations, confusion, delirium tremens, organic

---

*Adapted from the classic article in the American Journal of Nursing, Vol. 65, No. 5. (c) May 1965, the American Journal of Nursing Company.

brain syndromes. *Willful-defiant:* active need to direct and control environment and life situation, with low frustration tolerance and rigid mind-set, rage, shame.

    (4) *Suicidal plan*—the more details about method, timing, and place, the higher the risk.

    (5) *Previous suicidal behavior*—history of prior attempt increases risk. Eight out of ten suicide attempts give verbal and behavioral warnings as listed previously.

    (6) *Medical status*—chronic ailments, terminal illness, and pain increase suicidal risk.

    (7) *Communication*—the more withdrawn and apathetic, the greater the potential for suicide, unless extreme psychomotor retardation is present.

    (8) *Style of life*—high risks include substance abusers, those with sexual-identity conflicts, unstable relationships (personal and job related). Suicidal tendencies are not inherited but learned from family and other interpersonal relationships.

    (9) *Alcohol*—can reinforce helpless and hopeless feelings; may be lethal if used with barbiturates; can decrease inhibitions, result in impulsive behavior.

    (10) *Resources*—the fewer the resources, the higher the suicide potential. Examples of resources: family, friends, colleagues, religion, pets, meaningful recreational outlets, satisfying employment.

  c. Assess *needs* commonly communicated by individuals who are suicidal:

    (1) To trust.

    (2) To be accepted.

    (3) To bolster self-esteem.

    (4) To "fit in" with groups.

    (5) To experience success and interrupt the failure syndrome.

    (6) To expand capacity for pleasure.

    (7) To increase autonomy and sense of self-mastery.

    (8) To work out an acceptable sexual identity.

◆ 3. **Analysis/nursing diagnosis:** *risk for self-directed violence* related to:

  a. Feelings of alienation.

  b. Feelings of rejection.

  c. Feelings of hopelessness, despair.

  d. Feelings of frustration and rage.

◆ 4. **Nursing care plan/implementation:**

  a. *Long-term goals*

    (1) Increase client's self-reliance.

    (2) Help client achieve more realistic and positive feelings of self-esteem, self-respect, acceptance by others, and sense of belonging.

    (3) Help client experience success, interrupt failure pattern, and expand views about pleasure.

  b. *Short-term goals*

▶ (1) Medical: assist as necessary with gastric lavage; provide respiratory and vascular support; assist in repair of inflicted wounds.

    (2) Provide protection from self-destruction until client is able to assume this responsibility.

    (3) *Allow outward* and *constructive* expression of hostile and aggressive feelings.

    (4) Provide for physical needs.

  c. *Suicide precautions* to institute under emergency conditions:

    (1) One-to-one supervision at *all* times for maximum precautions; check whereabouts every 15 min, if on basic suicide precautions.

    (2) Before instituting these measures, explain to client what you will be doing and why; MD must also explain; document this explanation.

    (3) Do *not* allow client to leave the unit for tests, procedures.

    (4) Look through client's belongings *with* the client and remove any potentially harmful objects, e.g., pills, matches, belts, razors, glass, tweezers.

    (5) Allow visitors and phone calls, but maintain one-to-one supervision during visits.

    (6) Check that visitors do not leave potentially harmful objects in the client's room.

    (7) Serve meals in an isolation meal tray that contains no glass or metal silverware.

    (8) Do *not* discontinue these measures without an order.

  d. *General approaches*

    (1) *Observe* closely at all times to assess suicide potential.

    (2) *Be available.*

      (a) Demonstrate concern for client as a person.

      (b) Be sensitive, warm, and consistent.

      (c) Listen with empathy.

      (d) *Avoid* imposing your own feelings of reality on client.

      (e) *Avoid* extremes in your own mood when with client (especially exaggerated cheerfulness).

(3) *Focus directly* on client's self-destructive ideas.

    (a) Reduce alienation and immobilization by discussing this "taboo" topic.

    (b) Acknowledge suicidal threats with calmness and without reproach—do *not* ignore or minimize threat.

    (c) *Find out details* about suicide plan and reduce environmental hazards.

    (d) Help client verbalize aggressive, hostile, and hopeless feelings.

    (e) *Explore death fantasies*—try to take "romance" out of death.

(4) Acknowledge that suicide is one of several options.

(5) *Make a contract* with the client, and structure a plan of alternatives for coping when next confronted with the need to commit suicide (e.g., the client could call someone, express feeling of anger outwardly, or ask for help).

(6) Point out client's *self-responsibility* for suicidal act.

    (a) *Avoid* manipulation by client who says, "You are responsible for stopping me from killing myself."

    (b) Emphasize protection against self-destruction *rather than* punishment.

(7) *Support* the part of the client that wants to live.

    (a) Focus on *ambivalence.*

    (b) Emphasize meaningful past relationships and events.

    (c) Look for reasons left for wanting to live. Elicit what is meaningful to the client at the moment.

    (d) Point out effect of client's death on others.

(8) *Remove sources of stress.*

    (a) Decrease uncomfortable feelings of *alienation* by initiating one-to-one interactions.

    (b) Make all *decisions* when client is in severe depression.

    (c) Progressively let client make simple decisions: what to eat, what to watch on TV, etc.

(9) *Provide hope.*

    (a) Let client know that problems can be solved with help.

    (b) Bring in new resources for help.

    (c) Talk about likely changes in client's life.

    (d) Review past effective coping behaviors.

(10) *Provide with opportunity to be useful.* Reduce self-centeredness and brooding by planning diversional activities within the client's capabilities.

(11) *Involve as many people as possible.*

    (a) Gradually bring in others, for instance, other therapists, friends, staff, clergy, family, co-workers.

    (b) Prevent staff "burnout," found when only one nurse is working with suicidal client.

(12) *Health teaching:* teach client and staff principles of crisis intervention and resolution. Teach new coping skills.

◆ 5. **Evaluation/outcome criteria:** physical condition is stabilized; client able to verbalize feelings rather than acting them out.

Crisis Intervention

Crisis intervention is a type of brief psychiatric treatment in which individuals or their families are helped in their efforts to forestall the process of mental decompensation in reaction to severe emotional stress by direct and immediate supportive approaches.

  I. Definition of crisis: sudden event in one's life that disturbs homeostasis, during which usual coping mechanisms cannot resolve the problem. Types of crisis:

    A. *Maturational* (internal): see Erik Erikson's eight stages of developmental crises anticipated in the development of the infant, child, adolescent, and adult (see **Unit 5**).

    B. *Situational* (external): occurs at any time, e.g., loss of job, loss of income, death of significant person, illness, hospitalization.

  II. Concepts and principles related to crisis intervention:

    A. Crises are turning points where changes in behavior patterns and lifestyles can occur; individuals in crisis are most amenable to altering old and unsuccessful coping mechanisms and are most likely to learn new and more functional behaviors.

    B. Social milieu and its structure are contributing factors in both the development of psychiatric symptoms and eventual recovery from them.

    C. If crisis is handled effectively, the person's mental stability will be maintained; individual may return to a precrisis state or better.

    D. If crisis is not handled effectively, individual may progress to a worse state with exacerbations of earlier conflicts; future crises may not be handled well.

    E. There are a number of universal developmental crisis periods (maturational crises) in every individual's life.

F. Each person tries to maintain equilibrium through use of adaptive behaviors.

G. When individuals face a problem they cannot solve, tension, anxiety, narrowed perception, and disorganized functioning occur.

H. *Immediate relief* of symptoms produced by crisis is more urgent than *exploring* their cause.

III. Characteristics of crisis intervention:

A. Acute, sudden onset related to a stressful precipitating event of which individual is aware but which immobilizes previous coping abilities.

B. Responsive to brief therapy with focus on immediate problem.

C. Focus shifted from the psyche in the individual to the *individual in the environment;* deemphasis on intrapsychic aspects.

D. Crisis period is *time limited* (usually up to 6 wk).

◆ **IV. Nursing care plan/implementation** in crises:

A. General goals:
1. *Avoid* hospitalization if possible.
2. Return to precrisis level and preserve ability to function.
3. Assist in problem solving, with *here-and-now* focus.

B. *Assess* the crisis:
1. Identify stressful *precipitating* events: duration, problems created, and degree of significance.
2. Assess *suicidal and homicidal risk.*
3. Assess amount of *disruption* in individual's life and effect on significant others.
4. Assess *current coping skills,* strengths, and general level of functioning.

C. *Plan* the intervention:
1. Consider *past coping* mechanisms.
2. Propose *alternatives* and untried coping methods.

D. *Implementation:*
1. Help client relate the crisis event to current feelings.
2. Encourage expression of all feelings related to disruption.
3. Explore past coping skills and *reinforce adaptive* ones.
4. Use all means available in *social network* to take care of client's *immediate needs* (e.g., significant others, law enforcement agencies, housing, welfare, employment, medical, and school).
5. Set limits.
6. *Health teaching:* teach additional problem-solving approaches.

◆ **V. Evaluation/outcome criteria:**

A. Client returns to precrisis level of functioning.

B. Client learns new, more effective coping skills.

C. Client can describe realistic plans for future in terms of own perception of progress, support system, and coping mechanisms.

Selected Specific Crisis Situations: Problems Related to Abuse

I. Domestic Violence: Battered Woman*

A. Characteristics
1. *Victims:* feel helpless, powerless to prevent assault; blame themselves; ambivalent about leaving the relationship.
2. *Abusers:* often blame the victims; have poor impulse control; use power (physical strength or weapon) to threaten and subject victims to their assault.
3. *Cycle* of stages, with increase in severity of the battering:
   a. *Buildup of tension* (through verbal abuse): abuser is often drinking or taking other drugs; victim blames self.
   b. *Battering:* abuser does not remember brutal beating; victim is in shock and detached.
   c. *Calm:* abuser "makes up," apologizes, and promises "never again"; victim believes and forgives the abuser, and feels loved.

B. Risk factors
1. *Learned responses:* abuser and victim have had past experience with violence in family; victim has "learned helplessness."
2. *Pregnant* women and those with one or more *preschool children,* who see no alternative to staying in the battering relationship.
3. Women who *fear* punishment from the abuser.

◆ **C. Assessment:**
1. Injury to parts of body, especially face, head, genitals (e.g., welts, bruises, fracture of nose).
2. Presents in the emergency department with report of "accidental injury."
3. Severe anxiety.
4. Depression.

◆ **D. Analysis/nursing diagnosis:**
1. *Risk for injury* related to physical harm.
2. *Posttraumatic response* related to assault.
3. *Fear* related to threat of death or change in health status.
4. *Pain* related to physical and psychological harm.
5. *Powerlessness* related to interpersonal interaction.
6. *Ineffective individual coping* related to situational crisis.
7. *Spiritual distress* related to intense suffering and challenged value system.

◆ **E. Nursing care plan/implementation:**
1. Provide safe environment; refer to community resources for shelter.
2. Treat physical injuries.

Source: Lagerquist, S: In Nursenotes Psychiatric-Mental Health, Lippincott, 1997.

Mental Health

3. Document injuries.
4. Supportive, nonjudgmental approach: identify woman's strengths; help her to accept that she cannot control the abuser; encourage description of home situation; help her to see choices.
5. Encourage individual and family therapy for victim and abuser.

◆ **F. Evaluation/outcome criteria:**
1. Physical symptoms have been treated.
2. Discusses plans for safety (for self and any children) to protect against further injury.

II. Rape-trauma Syndrome

A. Definition: forcible perpetration of an act of sexual intercourse on the body of an unwilling person.

◆ **B. Assessment:**
1. *Signs of physical trauma*—physical findings of entry.
2. *Symptoms of physical trauma*—verbatim statements regarding type of sexual attack.
3. *Signs of emotional trauma*—tears, hyperventilation, extreme anxiety, withdrawal, self-blame, anger, embarrassment, fears, sleeping and eating disturbances, desire for revenge.
4. *Symptoms of emotional trauma*—statements regarding method of force used and threats made.

◆ **C. Analysis/nursing diagnosis:** *rape-trauma syndrome* related to phases of response to rape:
1. *Acute response:* volatility, disorganization, disbelief, shock, incoherence, agitated motor activity, nightmares, guilt (should have been able to protect self), phobias (crowds, being alone, sex).
2. *Outward coping:* denial and suppression of anxiety and fear (silent rape syndrome), feelings appear controlled.
3. *Integration and resolution:* confronts anger with attacker; realistic perspective.

◆ **D. Nursing care plan/implementation** in counseling rape victims. Figure 6–4 is a summary of self-care decisions a victim faces the first night following a sexual assault.
1. Overall goals:
   a. Acknowledge feelings.
   b. Face feelings.
   c. Resolve feelings.
   d. Maintain and restore *self-respect, dignity, integrity,* and *self-determination.*
2. Work through issues:
   a. Handle *legal* matters and police contacts.
   b. Clarify facts.
   c. Get *medical* attention if needed.
   d. Notify *family and friends.*
   e. Understand emotional reaction.

FIGURE 6–4 Victim decisions following a sexual assault. (From the Rape Crisis Services of the YWCA, Greater Harrisburg, Pa.)

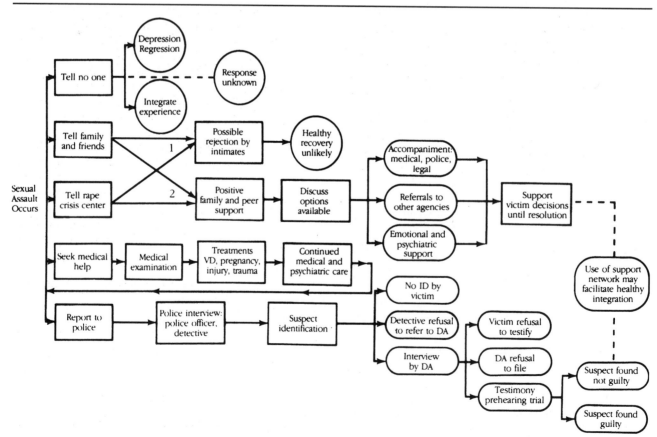

f. Attend to *practical* concerns.

g. Evaluate need for psychiatric consultations.

3. *Acute phase:*

   a. Decrease victim's stress, anxiety, fear.

   b. Seek medical care.

   c. Increase self-confidence and self-esteem.

   d. Identify and accept feelings and needs (to be in control, cared about, to achieve).

   e. Reorient perceptions, feelings, and statements about self.

   f. Help resume normal lifestyle.

4. *Outward coping phase:*

   a. Remain available and supportive.

   b. Reflect words, feelings, and thoughts.

   c. Explore real problems.

   d. Explore alternatives regarding contraception, legal issues.

   e. Evaluate response of family and friends to victim and rape.

5. *Integration and resolution phase:*

   a. Assist exploration of feelings (anger) regarding attacker.

   b. Explore feelings (guilt and shame) regarding self.

   c. Assist in making own decisions regarding health care.

6. Maintain confidentiality and neutrality—facilitate person's own decision.

7. Search for alternatives to giving advice.

8. *Health teaching:*

   a. Explain procedures and services to victim.

   b. Counsel to avoid isolated areas and being helpful to strangers.

   c. Counsel where and how to resist attack (scream, run unless assailant has weapon).

   d. Teach what to do if pregnancy or STD is outcome.

◆ **E. Evaluation/outcome criteria:** little or no evidence of possible long-term effects of rape (guilt, shame, phobias, denial).

III. Battered Child

◆ **A. Assessment**—clues to the identification of a battered child*

1. Clues in the *history*

   a. Significant *delay* in seeking medical care.

   b. Major *discrepancies* in the history:

     (1) Discrepancy between different people's versions of the story.

     (2) Discrepancy between the history and the observed injuries.

     (3) Discrepancy between the history and the child's developmental capabilities.

   c. History of multiple emergency department visits for various injuries.

   d. A story that is *vague* and *contradictory.*

2. Clues in the *physical examination*

   a. Child who seems withdrawn, apathetic, and *does not cry* despite his or her injuries.

   b. Child who *does not turn to parents for comfort;* or unusual desire to please parent; unusual fear of parent(s).

   c. *Child who is poorly nourished* and *poorly cared for.*

   d. The presence of *bruises: multiple bruises,* welts, and abrasions, especially around the trunk and buttocks; *old bruises in addition to fresh ones* (Table 6–11).

   e. The presence of *suspicious burns:*

     (1) Cigarette burns.

     (2) Scalds without splash marks or involving the buttocks, hands, or feet but sparing skinfolds.

     (3) Rope marks.

   f. Clues in parent behavior—exaggerate care and concern.

◆ **B. Analysis/nursing diagnosis:**

1. Same as for battered woman (see p. 341).

2. *Altered parenting* related to poor role model/identity, unrealistic expectations, presence of stressors and lack of support.

3. *Low self-esteem* related to deprivation and negative feedback.

◆ **C. Nursing care plan/implementation:**

1. Same as for battered woman (see p. 341).

2. Report suspected child abuse to appropriate source.

3. Conduct assessment interview in private, with child and parent separated.

4. Be supportive and nonjudgmental.

◆ **D. Evaluation/outcome criteria:**

1. Same as battered woman (see p. 341).

2. Child safety has been ensured.

3. Parent(s) or caregivers have agreed to seek help.

IV. Sexual Abuse of Children

◆ **A. Assessment**—characteristic behaviors:

1. *Relationship* of offender to victim: many filling paternal role (uncle, grandfather, cousin) with repeated, unquestioned access to the child.

2. Methods of *pressuring* victim into sexual activity: offering material goods, misrepresent-

---

*Adapted from Caroline, N: Emergency Care in the Streets, ed. 5. Little, Brown, Boston, 1995, p 761.

TABLE 6–11 Estimation of Time at Which Soft Tissue Injury Occurred

Injury Occurred	Color
0–2 hr	No discoloration (may have edema and pain)
1–5 days	Red/blue
5–7 days	Green
7–10 days	Yellow
10–14 days	Brown

ing moral standards ("it's OK"), exploiting need for human contact and warmth.

3. Method of pressuring victim to *secrecy* (to conceal the act) is inducing fear of punishment, not being believed, rejection, being blamed for the activity, abandonment.

4. Disclosure of sexual activity via:
   a. Direct visual or verbal confrontation and *observation* by others.
   b. *Verbalization* of act by victim.
   c. *Visible clues:* excess money and candy, new clothes, pictures, notes.
   d. *Signs and symptoms:* bed-wetting, excessive bathing, tears, avoiding school, somatic distress (*GI and urinary* tract pains).
   e. Overly solicitous parental attitude toward child.

◆ **B. Analysis/nursing diagnosis:**
   1. *Altered protection* related to inflicted pain.
   2. *Risk for injury* related to neglect, abuse.
   3. *Personal identity disturbance* related to abuse as child and feeling guilty and responsible for being a victim.
   4. *Ineffective individual coping* related to high stress level.
   5. *Sleep pattern disturbance* related to traumatic sexual experiences.
   6. *Ineffective family coping.*
   7. *Altered family processes* related to use of violence.
   8. *Altered parenting* related to violence.
   9. *Powerlessness* related to feelings of being dependent on abuser.
   10. *Social isolation/withdrawal* related to shame about family violence.
   11. *Risk for altered abuse response patterns.*

◆ **C. Nursing care plan/implementation:**
   1. Establish safe environment and the termination of trauma.
   2. Encourage child to verbalize feelings about incident to dispel tension built up by secrecy.
   3. Ask child to draw a picture or use dolls and toys to show what happened.
   4. Observe for symptoms over a period of time.
      a. *Phobic* reactions when seeing or hearing offender's name.
      b. *Sleep pattern* changes, recurrent dreams, nightmares.
   5. Look for *silent reaction* to being an accessory to sex (i.e., child keeping burden of the secret activity within self); help deal with unresolved issues.
   6. Establish therapeutic alliance with abusive parent.
   7. *Health teaching:*
      a. Teach child that his (her) body is private and to inform a responsible adult when someone violates privacy without consent.

   b. Teach adults in family to respond to victim with sensitivity, support, and concern.

◆ **D. Evaluation/outcome criteria:**
   1. Child's needs for affection, attention, personal recognition, or love met without sexual exploitation.
   2. Perpetrator accepts therapy.
   3. Conspiracy of silence is broken.

V. Elder Abuse/Neglect

   A. Definition: battering, psychological abuse, sexual assault, or any act or omission by personal caregiver, family, or legal guardian that results in harm or threatened harm.

   B. Concepts, principles, and characteristics:
   1. Elders who are currently being abused often abused their abusers—their offspring. Violence is a learned behavior.
   2. *Victim characteristics:* diminished self-esteem, feeling responsibility for the abuse, isolated.
   3. *Abuser characteristics:* usually has physical or psychosocial stressors related to marital or fiscal difficulties; substance abuse.
   4. *Legal:* most states have mandatory laws to report elder abuse, although many cases are not reported because of shame, fear of more abuse, cultural/religious beliefs, optimism, loyalty, financial dependency.
   5. Types of abuse:
      a. *Financial* abuse, e.g., fraudulent monetary schemes, theft (money, property, or both).
      b. *Neglect,* e.g., lack of food, clean clothing, medications; no provision for assistive devices (dentures, hearing aids, glasses, canes).
      c. *Psychological* abuse, e.g., verbal abuse.
      d. *Physical* abuse, e.g., beating, physical restraints, rape.

◆ **C. Assessment:**
   1. *Risk factors:*

Victim:	Abuser:
■ Poor health	■ Substance abuse
■ Isolated	■ Stressful life events
■ Impaired memory, thinking	■ Interpersonal problems
◄—— Hx: Mental illness ——►	
◄—— Hx: Family violence ——►	
◄—— Financial difficulties ——►	
◄——— Dependency ———►	
◄—— Share living space ——►	

   2. *Behavioral clues:* agitation, anger, denial, fear, confusion, depression, withdrawal, unbelievable stories about causes of injuries.
   3. *Physical indicators:* weight loss; unexplained cuts, bruises, puncture wounds; untreated injuries; unkempt; noncompliance with medical plan of care.
   4. *Financial matters:* e.g., recent changes in will;

unusual banking activity; missing checks, personal belongings; forged signatures; unwillingness to spend money on the elder.

◆ **D. Analysis/nursing diagnosis:**
1. *Risk for injury* related to neglect, abuse.
2. *Fear.*
3. *Powerlessness* related to dependency on abuser.
4. *Unilateral neglect.*
5. *Spiritual distress.*
6. *Altered family processes* related to use of violence.

◆ **E. Nursing care plan/implementation:**
1. *Primary prevention:*
   a. Early case finding; early treatment.
   b. Referral to community services for caregiver (e.g., respite care) before serious abuse occurs.

2. *Secondary prevention:*
   a. Report case to law enforcement agencies.
   b. Provide elder with phone number for confidential hotline.
   c. Plan for safety of elder (e.g., shelter).
3. *Tertiary prevention:*
   a. Counseling, support, and self-help groups for victim.
   b. Legal action against abuser.

◆ **F. Evaluation/outcome criteria:**
1. Elder develops trust in caregivers, without fear of further abuse.
2. Spiritual well-being is enhanced, with diminished feelings of guilt, hopelessness, and powerlessness.

Mental Health

COMFORT, REST, ACTIVITY, AND MOBILITY FUNCTIONS

Sleep Disturbance

I. Types of sleep:

A. *Rapid eye movement (REM) sleep:* colorful, dramatic, emotional, implausible dreams.

B. *Non-REM sleep—stages:*

1. Stage 1: lasts 30 sec–7 min—falls asleep, drowsy; easily awakened; fleeting thoughts.
2. Stage 2: more relaxed; no eye movements, clearly asleep but readily awakens; 45% of total sleep time spent in this stage.
3. Stage 3 (delta sleep): deep muscle relaxation; decreased temperature, pulse, respiration (TPR).
4. Stage 4 (delta sleep): very relaxed; rarely moves.

C. *Sleep cycle—common progression of sleep stages:*

1. Stages 1, 2, 3, 4, 3, 2, REM, 2, 3, 4, etc.
2. *Delta* sleep most common during first third of night, with *REM* sleep periods increasing in duration during night from 1–2 min at start to 20–30 min by early morning.
3. REM sleep varies.
   a. Adolescents spend 30% of total sleep time in REM sleep.
   b. Adults spend 15% of total sleep time in REM sleep.

II. Sleep deprivation (dyssomnias):

◆ **A. Assessment:**

1. *Non-REM sleep loss:* physical fatigue due to less time spent in normal deep sleep.
2. *REM sleep loss:* psychological effects—irritability, confusion, anxiety, short-term memory loss, paranoia, hallucinations.
3. *Desynchronized sleep:* occurs when sleep shifts more than 2 hr from normal sleep period. Irritability, anoxia, decreased stress tolerance.

◆ **B. Analysis/nursing diagnosis:** *sleep pattern disturbance* may be related to:

1. Interrupted sleep cycles before 90 min sleep cycle is completed.

2. Unfamiliar sleeping environment.
3. Alterations in normal sleep/activity cycles (e.g., jet lag).
4. Preexisting sleep deficits before hospital admission.
5. Medications, e.g., alcohol withdrawal or abruptly discontinuing the use of hypnotic or antidepressant medications.
6. Pain.

◆ **C. Nursing care plan/implementation:**

1. Obtain sleep history as part of nursing assessment. Determine normal sleep hours, bedtime rituals, factors that promote or interrupt sleep.
2. Duplicate normal bedtime rituals when possible.
3. Make *environment* conducive to sleep: lighting, noise, temperature.
   a. Close door, dim lights, turn off unneeded machinery.
   b. Encourage staff to muffle conversation at night.
4. Encourage *daytime* exercise periods.
5. Allow *uninterrupted periods of 90 min of sleep.* Group nighttime treatments and observations that require touching the client.
6. *Minimize* use of hypnotic medications.
   a. Substitute back rubs, warm milk, relaxation exercises.
   b. Encourage physician to consider prescribing hypnotics that minimize sleep disruption (e.g., chloral hydrate and flurazepam HCl [Dalmane]).
   c. *Taper* off hypnotics rather than abruptly discontinuing.
7. Observe client while asleep.
   a. Evaluate quality of sleep.
   b. It may be sleep apnea if client is extremely restless and snoring heavily.
8. *Health teaching: avoid* caffeine and hyperstimulation at bedtime; teach how to promote sleep-inducing environment, relaxation techniques.

◆ **D. Evaluation/outcome criteria:** verbalizes satisfaction with amount, quality of sleep.

EATING DISORDERS

Anorexia Nervosa/Bulimia Nervosa

Anorexia nervosa is an illness of starvation related to a severe disturbance of body image and a morbid fear of obesity; it is an eating disorder, usually seen in adolescence, when a person is underweight and emaciated and refuses to eat. It can result in death due to irreversible metabolic processes.

Bulimia nervosa is another type of eating disorder (binge-purge syndrome) also encountered primarily among older women and younger men. It is characterized by at least two binge-eating episodes of large quantities of high-calorie food over a couple of hours followed by disparaging self-criticism and depression. Self-induced vomiting, abuse of laxatives, and abuse of diuretics are commonly associated because they decrease physical pain of abdominal distention, may reduce postbinge anguish, and may provide a method of self-control. Bulimic episodes may occur as part of anorexia nervosa, but these clients rarely become emaciated, and not all have a body-image disturbance.

I. Concepts and principles related to anorexia nervosa:
- **A.** *Not* due to lack of appetite or problem with appetite center in hypothalamus.
- **B.** Normal stomach hunger is *repressed, denied, depersonalized;* no conscious awareness of hunger sensation.

◆ II. Assessment of anorexia nervosa:
- **A.** *Body-image disturbance*—delusional, obsessive (e.g., does not see self as thin and is bewildered by others' concern).
- **B.** Usually *preoccupied* with food, yet dreads gaining too much weight. *Ambivalence:* avoids food, hoards food.
- **C.** Feels ineffectual, with low sex drive. *Repudiation of sexuality.*
- **D.** *Pregnancy* fears, including misconceptions of oral impregnation through food.
- **E.** *Self-punitive* behavior leading to starvation; suppression of anger.
- **F.** *Physical signs and symptoms*
  1. Weight loss (20% of previous "normal" body weight).
  2. Amenorrhea and secondary sex organ atrophy.
  3. *Hyperactivity;* compulsiveness; excessive gum chewing.
  4. Constipation.
  5. *Hypotension, bradycardia,* hypothermia.
  6. Skin: hyperkeratosis, poor turgor, dry.

  7. Blood: leukopenia, anemia, hypoglycemia, hypoproteinemia, hypocholesterolemia, hypokalemia, hyponatremia, decreased magnesium, decreased chloride, increased BUN; ECG: T-wave inversion.

◆ III. Analysis/nursing diagnosis:
- **A.** *Altered nutrition, less than body requirements,* and *fluid volume deficit* related to attempts to vomit food after eating, overuse of laxatives/diuretics and refusal to eat, related to need to demonstrate control.
- **B.** *Risk for altered physical regulation processes/risk for or actual fluid volume deficit:* amenorrhea related to starvation; hypotension, bradycardia; metabolic alkalosis.
- **C.** *Risk for self-inflicted injury* related to starvation from refusal to eat or ambivalence about food.
- **D.** *Altered eating* related to altered thought processes: binge-purge syndrome.
- **E.** *Body-image disturbance/chronic low self-esteem* related to anxiety over assuming an adult role and concern with sexual identity; unmet dependency needs, personal vulnerability; perceived loss of control in some aspect of life; dysfunctional family system.
- **F.** *Compulsive behaviors* related to need to maintain control of self, represented by losing weight.

◆ IV. Nursing care plan/implementation:
- **A.** Help reestablish connections between body sensations (hunger) and responses (eating). Use *stimulus-response conditioning* methods to set up eating regimen.
  1. *Weigh* regularly, at same time and with same amount of clothing, with back to scale.
  2. Make sure water drinking is *avoided* before weighing.
  3. Give one-to-one supervision during and 30 min after mealtimes to *prevent* attempts to vomit food.
  4. Monitor exercise program and set limits in physical activity.
- **B.** *Monitor* physiological signs and symptoms (amenorrhea, constipation, hypoproteinemia, hypoglycemia, anemia, eroded tooth enamel, inflamed buccal cavity, brittle nails, dull hair, secondary sexual organ atrophy, hypothermia, hypotension, leg cramps and other signs of hypokalemia).
- **C.** *Health teaching:*
  1. Explain normal sexual growth and development to improve knowledge deficit and confront sexual fears.
  2. Use behavior modification to reestablish awareness of hunger sensation and to relate it to the clock and regular meal times.
  3. Teach parents skills in communication related to dependence/independence needs of

adolescent; allow patient to assume control in areas other than dieting, weight loss (e.g., management of daily activities, work, leisure choices).

◆ **V. Evaluation/outcome criteria:**
   A. Attains and maintains minimal normal weight for age and height.
   B. Eats regular meal (standard nutritional diet).
   C. No incidence of self-induced vomiting, bulimia, or compulsive physical activity.
   D. Acts on increased internal emotional awareness and recognition of body sensation of hunger (i.e., talks about being hungry and feeling hunger pangs).
   E. Relates increased sense of effectiveness with less need to control food intake.

VI. See sample **Critical Pathway: Eating Disorders**

CRITICAL PATHWAY | **Eating Disorders Program. Estimated Length of Stay: 28 Days Behavioral Unit**

Nursing Diagnosis and Categories of Care	Time Dimension	Goals/Actions	Time Dimension	Goals/Actions	Time Dimensions	Goals/Actions
Altered nutrition: less than body requirements R/T inadequate intake, self-induced vomiting, laxative use	Ongoing	Gain 3 lb/wk as indicated (or 0.5 lb/day)	Day 2–28	Consume at least 75% of food provided at each meal	Day 15–28	Demonstrate ability to select foods to meet at least 80% of nutritional needs
Risk for fluid volume deficit	Ongoing	Be free of signs/symptoms of dehydration Display balanced I&O	Day 2–28 / Day 3	Ingest at least 1000 mL fluid/day / Vital signs WNL	Day 22–28 / Day 28	Refrain from self-induced vomiting / Be free of signs/symptoms of malnutrition with all laboratory results WNL
Referral	Day 1 and prn	Dietitian				
Diagnostic studies	Day 1	Electrolytes, CBC, BUN/creatinine Thyroid function UA ECG as indicated	Day 14	Repeat selected studies		
Additional assessments	Day 1–2	Vital signs/I&O every shift	Day 3–7 qAM		Day 8–28	As indicated
	Day 1 / Day 1–28	Weight / Types and amount of food/fluid intake Behavior/purging following meals Level of activity	Day 7, 14	7:30 A.M., same clothes		
Medications Allergies:	Day 1–28	Periactin Tricyclic antidepressant Vitamin supplement				
Patient education	Day 1 and prn	Orient to unit and schedule Behavior modification program Minimum weight goal and initial nutritional needs	Day 7–14	Principles of nutrition; foods for maintenance of wellness	Day 21–28	Incorporate nutritional plan into lifestyle and home setting
Additional nursing actions	Day 1–3	Assist patient with formulation of behavioral contract and monitoring of cooperation	Day 7–28	Involve mother/significant other as appropriate in nutritional counseling and planning for future		
	Day 1–7	▶ Administer tube feeding/blenderized food as indicated				

Continued

Mental Health

CRITICAL PATHWAY	Eating Disorders Program. Estimated Length of Stay: 28 Days Behavioral Unit—cont'd						
Nursing Diagnosis and Categories of Care	Time Dimension	Goals/Actions	Time Dimension	Goals/Actions	Time Dimensions	Goals/Actions
Additional nursing actions—cont'd	Day 1–21	Bathroom locked for 1 hr after meals				
	Day 1–28	Provide social setting for meals				
Ineffective denial R/T presence of overwhelming anxiety-producing feelings, learned response pattern, personal/family value system	Ongoing	Participate in behavior modification program and adhere to unit policies	Day 8–28	Attend and contribute to group sessions	Day 18–28	Verbalize acceptance of reality that eating behaviors are maladaptive
			Day 14	Develop trusting relationship with at least one staff member on each shift		Demonstrate ability to cope more adaptively
	Day 2–28	Cooperate with therapy to restore nutritional well-being			Day 28	Identify ways to gain control in life situation
						Refrain from use of manipulation of others to achieve control
						Plan in place to meet postdischarge needs
Referrals	Day 5 (or when physical condition stable)	Psychologist Social worker Psychodramatist	Day 8–28	Group psychotherapy daily sessions	Day 25	Community resource contact person(s)
					Day 28	Verbalizes ways to gain control in life situation
Additional assessments	Day 1/ongoing	Degree and stage of denial Perception of situation	Day 5–7	Readiness to participate in group sessions		
	Day 1–17	Assess ability to trust; use of manipulation to achieve control	Day 7–28	Congruence between verbalizations and behaviors (insight)		
			Day 8–28	Degree/quality of nonmanipulative involvement in group sessions; trusting relationship with at least one staff member per shift		
Patient education	Day 1 and prn	Privileges and responsibilities of behavior modification Consequences of behaviors	Day 3/ongoing	Eating disorder and consequences of eating behavior	Day 21	Role of support groups/community resources
					Day 28	Patient and family verbalize intention to attend support group
Additional nursing actions	Day 1/ongoing	Encourage expression of feelings *Avoid* agreeing with inaccurate statements/perceptions Provide positive feedback for desired insight/behaviors	Day 5–28	Promote involvement in unit activities Support interactions with family members	Day 21–28	Involve family (as appropriate) in long-range planning for meeting individual needs
			Day 8–28	Encourage interactions in group sessions		

CRITICAL PATHWAY | Eating Disorders Program. Estimated Length of Stay: 28 Days Behavioral Unit—cont'd

Nursing Diagnosis and Categories of Care	Time Dimension	Goals/Actions	Time Dimension	Goals/Actions	Time Dimensions	Goals/Actions
Additional nursing actions—cont'd		Set limits on maladaptive behavior				
Body-image disturbance/chronic low self-esteem R/T perceived loss of control, unmet dependency needs, personal vulnerability, negative evaluation of self	Day 7	Acknowledge that attention will not be given to discussion of body image and food	Day 21	Acknowledge misperception of body image as fat Verbalize positive self-attributes	Day 28	Demonstrate realistic body image and self-awareness Verbalize acceptance of self, including "imperfections" Acknowledge self as sexual assault Not obsessed with food
Referrals	Day 1 (or when physical condition stable)	Therapists: occupational, recreational, music, art	Day 14	Image consultant	Day 28	Therapist to address issues of sexuality after discharge, as indicated
Additional assessments	Day 1–7	Suicidal ideation/behaviors	Day 8	Individual strengths/weaknesses		
	Day 3	Sexual history, including abuse	Day 8–28	Congruency of feelings/perceptions with actions		
	Day 3–28	Perceptions of body image Family patterns of interaction				
Patient education	Day 1–28	Responsibility for self in family setting	Day 8–10	General wellness needs	Day 21–28	Sex education reflecting individual sexuality and needs
	Day 7–28	Clarify misconceptions of body image	Day 8–28	Human behavior and interactions with family/others—transactional analysis (TA)		
			Day 14	Personal appearance and grooming		
			Day 14–28	Alternative coping strategies for dealing with feelings		
Additional nursing actions	Day 1	Develop therapeutic relationship	Day 7	Compare actual measurements of patient's body with patient's perceptions; clarify discrepancies	Day 14–28	Have patient keep diary of feelings, especially when thinking of food Role-play new behaviors for dealing with feelings and conflicts
	Day 1–28	Provide positive feedback for participation and independent decision making	Day 7–9	Assist with planning to meet individual goals		
	Day 3–5	Confront sabotage behavior by family members Encourage control in areas other than diet	Day 8–28	Involve in physical activity/exercise program	Day 28	Demonstrates adaptive coping strategies not related to eating and for dealing with feelings
	Day 4–6	Support development of goals and adaptive behaviors not related to eating				

Source: Adapted from Doenges, M: Nursing Care Plans, ed 4. FA Davis, Philadelphia, 1997, pp 400–403.

Mental Health

SENSORY-PERCEPTUAL FUNCTIONS

Sensory Disturbance

I. **Types** of sensory disturbance:
   A. *Sensory deprivation*—amount of stimuli *less* than required, such as isolation in bed or room, deafness, stroke victim.
   B. *Sensory overload*—receives *more* stimuli than can be tolerated, e.g., bright lights, noise, strange machinery, barrage of visitors.
   C. *Sensory deficit*—impairment in functioning of sensory or perceptual processes, e.g., blindness, changes in tactile perceptions.

◆ II. **Assessment**—based on awareness of behavioral changes:
   A. *Sensory deprivation*—boredom, daydreaming, increasing sleep, thought slowness, inactivity, thought disorganization, hallucinations.
   B. *Sensory overload*—same as sensory deprivation, plus restlessness and agitation, confusion.
   C. *Sensory deficit*—may not be able to distinguish sounds, odors, and tastes or differentiate tactile sensations.

◆ III. **Analysis/nursing diagnosis:** problems related to sensory disturbance:
   A. *Altered thought processes.*
   B. *Confusion.*
   C. *Anger, aggression.*
   D. *Body-image disturbance.*
   E. *Sleep pattern disturbance.*

◆ IV. **Nursing care plan/implementation:**
   A. *Management of existing* sensory disturbances in:
      1. *Acute sensory deprivation*
         a. Increase interaction with staff.
         b. Use TV.
         c. Provide touch.
         d. Help clients choose menus that have aromas, varied tastes, temperatures, colors, textures.
         e. Use light cologne or after-shave lotion, bath powder.
      2. *Sensory overload*
         a. Restrict number of visitors and length of stay.
         b. Reduce noise and lights.
         c. Reduce newness by establishing and following routine.
         d. Organize care to provide for extended rest periods with minimal input.
      3. *Sensory deficits*
         a. Report observations about hearing, vision.

   b. May imply need for new glasses, medical diagnosis, or therapy.
   B. *Health teaching: prevention* of sensory disturbance involves *education* of parents during child's growth and development regarding tactile, auditory, and visual stimulation.
      1. Hold, talk, and play with infant when awake.
      2. Provide bright toys with different designs for children to hold.
      3. Change environment.
      4. Provide music and auditory stimuli.
      5. Give foods with variety of textures, tastes, colors.

◆ V. **Evaluation/outcome criteria:**
   A. Client is oriented to time, place, person.
   B. Little or no evidence of mood or sleep disturbance.

Delirium, Dementia, and Amnestic and Other Cognitive Disorders

These disorders include etiology associated with (1) the *aging process* (dementias arising in the senium or presenium, including primary degenerative dementia of the Alzheimer type and multi-infarct dementia), (2) *substance-related disorders* (e.g., alcohol, barbiturates, opioids, cocaine, amphetamines, PCP, hallucinogens, *cannabis,* nicotine, and caffeine), and (3) general medical conditions.

I. **Concepts, principles, and subtypes:**
   A. Course may be progressive, with steady deterioration.
   B. Alternative pathways and compensatory mechanisms may develop to show a clinical picture of remissions and exacerbations.
   C. *Delirium* is characterized by a *disturbance of consciousness* with reduced ability to focus, sustain, or shift attention; and a *change in cognition* (e.g., memory deficit, disorientation [time and place], language disturbance); or *development of perceptual disturbance* (e.g., illusions, hallucinations) that develop over a *short* time (hours or days) and *fluctuate* during the course of the day. *Etiology:* a direct physiological consequence of a general medical condition, substance intoxication or withdrawal, use of a medication, or toxin exposure. *Diagnostic feature:* cannot repeat sequential string of information (e.g., digit span).
   D. *Dementia* is characterized by persistent *multiple cognitive deficits* (e.g., aphasia, apraxia, agnosia, disturbance in executive functioning) accompanied by memory impairment and mood and sleep disturbances. *Possible etiology:* vascular dementia, HIV infection, head trauma, Parkinson's disease, Pick's disease, Alzheimer's disease, Huntington's disease, substance induced, toxin

exposure, medication, infections, nutritional deficiencies (hypoglycemia), endocrine conditions (hypothyroidism) brain tumors, seizure disorders, hepatic and renal failure; cardiopulmonary insufficiencies; fluid and electrolyte imbalances. *Diagnostic features:* cannot learn (register) new information (e.g., a list of words), or retain, recall, or recognize information.

1. *Alzheimer's disease:* progressive; irreversible loss of cerebral function due to cortical atrophy; exists in 2–4% of people over age 65 yr; may have a genetic component; may begin at ages 40–65; may lead to death within 2 yr. Average duration from onset of symptoms to death: 8–10 yr.

   a. Progressive decline in intellectual capacity (recent and remote memory, judgment), affect and motor coordination (apraxia); loss of social sense; apathy or restlessness.

   b. *Problems with* speech (aphasia), recognition of familiar objects (agnosia), disorientation to self (even parts of *own* body).

2. *Pick's disease:* unknown cause; may have genetic component. Onset: middle age; women affected more than men. Pathology: atrophy in frontal and temporal lobes of brain. Clinical picture similar to Alzheimer's.

3. *Creutzfeldt-Jacobs disease:* uncommon, extremely rapid neurodegeneration caused by transmissible "slow" virus (prion); genetic component in 5–15%. Clinical picture: typical dementia, with muscle rigidity, ataxia, involuntary movements. Occurrence: ages 40–60 yr. Death within 1 yr.

E. *Amnestic disorder* is characterized by *severe* memory impairment *without* other significant impairments of cognitive functioning (i.e., without aphasia, apraxia, or agnosia). *Diagnostic features:* memory impairment is always manifested by impairment in the ability to learn *new* information and sometimes problems remembering previously learned information or past events. May result in *disorientation* to place and time, but *rarely* to self. Appears bewildered or befuddled.

1. *Etiology:* due to direct physiological effects of a general medical condition (e.g., physical trauma or vitamin deficiency) or due to persisting effects of a substance (e.g., drug of abuse, a medication, or toxin exposure).

2. Memory disturbance: sufficiently severe to cause marked impairment in social or occupational functioning and represents a significant decline from a previous level of functioning. May require supervised living situation to ensure appropriate feeding and care.

3. Lacks insight into own memory deficit and may explicitly deny the presence of severe memory impairment despite evidence to the contrary.

4. Altered personality function: apathy, lack of initiative, emotional blandness, shallow range of expression.

◆ **II. Assessment:**

A. *Most common areas of difficulty* can be grouped under the mnemonic term *JOCAM: J*—judgment, *O*—orientation, *C*—confabulation, *A*—affect, and *M*—memory.

   1. *Judgment:* impaired, resulting in socially inappropriate behavior (such as hypersexuality toward inappropriate objects) and inability to carry out activities of daily living.

   2. *Orientation:* confused, disoriented; perceptual disturbances (e.g., illusions, misidentification of other persons and objects; misperception to make unfamiliar more familiar; *visual, tactile, and auditory* hallucinations may appear as images and voices or disorganized light and sound patterns). *Paranoid delusions* of persecution.

   3. *Confabulation:* common use of this defense mechanism to fill in memory gaps with invented stories.

   4. *Affect:* mood changes and unstable emotions; quarrelsome, with outbursts of morbid anger (as in cerebral arteriosclerosis); tearful; withdrawn from social contact; *depression* is a frequent reaction to loss of physical and social function.

   5. *Memory:* impaired, especially for names and *recent* events; may compensate by confabulating and by using *circumstantiality and tangential* speaking patterns.

B. *Other areas of difficulty:*

   1. *Seizures* (e.g., in Alzheimer's disease and cerebral arteriosclerosis).

   2. *Intellectual capacities diminished.*

      a. Difficulty with *abstract* thought.

      b. Compensatory mechanism is to stay with familiar topics; repetition.

      c. Short concentration periods.

   3. *Personality changes.*

      a. Loss of ego flexibility; adoption of more rigid attitudes.

      b. *Ritualism* in daily activities.

      c. Hoarding.

      d. Somatic preoccupations (hypochondriases).

      e. *Restlessness,* wandering away.

      f. Impaired impulse control.

      g. *Aphasia* (in severe dementia).

      h. *Apraxia* (inability to carry out motor activities).

C. *Diagnostic tests:*

   1. *Neurological* exam: perform maneuvers or answer questions that are aimed at eliciting information about condition of specific parts of brain or peripheral nerves.

      a. Assessment of mental status and alertness.

b. Muscle strength and reflexes.

c. Sensory-perception.

d. Language skills.

e. Coordination.

2. *Laboratory* tests:

a. *Blood, urine* to test for: infections, hepatic and renal dysfunction, diabetes, electrolyte imbalances, metabolic/endocrine disorders, nutritional deficiencies, and presence of toxic substances (e.g., drugs).

b. Electroencephalography (EEG) to check brain's electrical activity.

c. Computed tomography (CT) scan—image of brain size and shape.

d. Positron emission tomography (PET)—reveals metabolic activity of brain (important for diagnosis of Alzheimer's).

e. Magnetic resonance imaging (MRI)—computerized image of soft tissue, with sharply detailed picture of brain tissues.

◆ **III. Analysis/nursing diagnosis:**

A. *Risk for trauma* related to cognitive deficits (inability to recognize/identify danger in the environment; confusion; impaired judgment) and altered motor behavior (restlessness, hyperactivity, muscular incoordination).

B. *Altered thought processes/confusion (altered abstract thinking and altered knowledge processes [agnosia])* related to destruction of cerebral tissue, inability to use information to make judgments and transmit messages, and memory deficits.

C. *Sensory/perceptual alterations:* visual, auditory, kinesthetic, gustatory, tactile, olfactory related to neurological deficit.

D. *Sleep pattern disturbance* resulting in disorientation at night, related to confusion; increased aimless wandering (day/night reversal).

E. *Self-care deficit* (feeding, bathing/hygiene, dressing, toileting) related to physical impairments (poor vision, uncoordination, forgetfulness), disorientation, and confusion.

F. *Altered nutrition, more or less than body requirements,* related to confusion.

G. *Total incontinence* related to sensory/perceptual alterations.

H. *Altered attention and memory* related to progressive neurological losses.

I. *Altered conduct/impulse processes* (irritability and aggressiveness) related to neurological impairment.

J. *Impaired communication* related to poverty of speech and withdrawal behavior, progressive neurological losses, and cerebral impairment.

K. *Caregiver role strain* related to long-term illness and complexity of home care needs.

L. *Relocation stress syndrome* related to separation from support systems, physical deterioration, and changes in daily routine.

◆ **IV. Nursing care plan/implementation:** Also see interventions in **III. Confusion/disorientation,** p. 328.

A. *Long-term goal:* minimize regression related to memory impairment.

B. *Short-term goal:* provide structure and consistency to increase security.

C. Make *brief, frequent* contacts, because attention span is short.

D. Allow clients *time* to talk and to complete projects.

E. Stimulate *associative* patterns to improve recall (by repeating, summarizing, and focusing).

F. Allow clients to *review* their lives and focus on the past.

G. Use *concrete* questions in interviewing.

H. *Reinforce* reality-oriented comments.

I. Keep environment structured the *same* as much as possible (e.g., same room and placement of furniture); *routine* is important to diminish stress.

J. Recognize the importance of *compensatory* mechanisms (e.g., confabulation) to increase self-esteem; build psychological reserve.

K. Give recognition for each accomplishment.

L. Use *recreational* and physical therapy.

M. *Health teaching:* give *specific* instructions for diet, medication (e.g., tacrine [Cognex], donepezil [Aricept] for improving cognition), and treatment; how to use many sensory approaches to learn new information; how to use existing knowledge, old learning, and habitual approaches to deal with new situations.

◆ **V. Evaluation/outcome criteria:**

A. Symptoms occur *less* frequently and are less severe in areas of: emotional lability and appropriateness; false perceptions; self-care ability; disorientation, memory, and judgment; and decision making.

B. Client is able to preserve optimum level of functioning and independence while allowing basic needs to be met.

C. Stays relatively calm and noncombative when upset or fearful.

D. Accepts own irritability and frustrations as part of illness.

E. Asks for assistance with self-care activities.

F. Knows and adheres to daily routine; knows own nurse, location of room, bathroom, clocks, calendars.

G. Uses supportive community services.

Substance-Related Disorders

I. **Definition:** ingesting in any manner a chemical that has an effect on the body.

◆ **II. General assessment:**

A. *Behavioral* changes exist while under the influence of substance.

B. Engages in regular *use* of substance.
1. *Substance abuse:*
   a. Pattern of *pathological* use (i.e., day-long intoxication; inability to stop use, even when contraindicated by serious physical disorder; overpowering need or desire to take the drug despite legal, social, or medical problems); daily need of substance for functioning; repeated medical complications from use.
   b. *Interference* with social, occupational functioning.
   c. Willingness to obtain substance by any means, including illegal.
   d. Pathological use for more than 1 mo.
2. *Substance dependence:*
   a. More severe than substance abuse; body *requires* substance to continue functioning.
   b. Physiological dependence (i.e., either develops a *tolerance*—must increase dose to obtain desired effect—or has *physical withdrawal symptoms* when substance intake is reduced or stopped).
   c. Person feels it is impossible to get along without drug.
C. Effects of substance on *central nervous system (CNS).*

◆ **III. General analysis:** only in recent years has substance abuse been viewed as an illness rather than moral delinquency or criminal behavior. The disorders are very complex and little understood. There are physiological, psychological, and social aspects to their causality, dynamics, symptoms, and treatment, where personality disorder has a major part.
A. *Physiological aspects*—current unproven theories include "allergic" reaction to alcohol, disturbance in metabolism, genetic susceptibility to dependency, and hypofunction of adrenal cortex. There are *organic effects* of chronic excessive use.
B. *Psychological aspects*—disrupted parent-child relationship and family dynamics; deleterious effect on ego function.
C. *Social and cultural aspects*—local customs and attitudes vary about what is excessive.
D. *Maladaptive behavior related to:*
1. Low self-esteem.
2. Anger.
3. Denial.
4. Rationalization.
5. Social isolation.
6. A rigid pattern of coping.
7. Poorly defined philosophy of life, values, mores.
◆ E. *Nursing diagnosis* in **acute phase of abuse, intoxication:**
1. *Risk for ineffective breathing patterns* related to pneumonia caused by aspiration, malnutri-

tion; depressed immune system.
2. *Risk for decreased cardiac output* related to effect of substances on cardiac muscle; electrolyte imbalance.
3. *Risk for injury* related to impaired coordination, disorientation, and altered judgment (worse at night).
4. *Risk for violence:* self-directed or directed at others, related to misinterpretation of stimuli and feelings of suspicion or distrust of others.
5. *Sensory/perceptual alterations:* visual, kinesthetic, tactile, related to intake of mind-altering substances.
6. *Altered nutrition,* less than body requirements.
7. *Altered thought processes* (delusions, incoherence) related to misinterpretation of stimuli due to severe panic and fear.
8. *Sleep pattern disturbance* related to mind-altering substance.
9. *Ineffective individual coping* related to inability to tolerate frustration and to meet basic needs or role expectations, resulting in unpredictable behaviors.
10. *Noncompliance* with abstinence and supportive therapy, related to inability to stop using substance because of dependence and refusal to alter lifestyle.
11. *Impaired communication* related to mental confusion or CNS depression related to substance use.
12. *Impaired health maintenance management* related to failure to recognize that a problem exists and inability to take responsibility for health needs.

Alcohol Use Disorders: Alcohol Abuse and Dependence

Alcohol dependence is a chronic disorder in which the individual is unable, for physical or psychological reasons or both, to refrain from frequent consumption of alcohol in quantities that produce intoxication and disrupt health and ability to perform daily functions.

◆ **I. Concepts and principles related to alcohol abuse and dependence:**
A. Alcohol affects cerebral cortical functions:
1. Memory.
2. Judgment.
3. Reasoning.
B. Alcohol as a *depressant:*
1. Relaxes the individual.
2. Lessens use of repression of unconscious conflict.
3. Releases inhibitions, hostility, and primitive drives.
C. Drinking represents a tension-reducing device and a relief from feelings of insecurity. Strength of drinking habit equals degree of anxiety and frustration intolerance.

D. Alcohol abuse and dependence is a *symptom* rather than a disease.

E. Underlying fear and anxiety, associated with inner conflict, motivate the alcoholic to drink.

F. Alcoholics can *never* be cured to drink normally; cure is to be a "sober alcoholic," with total abstinence.

G. The spouse of the alcoholic often unconsciously contributes to the drinking behavior because of own emotional needs (*co-alcoholic* or *co-dependent*).

H. Intoxication occurs with a blood-alcohol level of 0.08% or above. *Signs of intoxication* are:
1. Incoordination.
2. Slurred speech.
3. Dulled perception.

I. Tolerance occurs with alcohol dependence. Increasing amounts of alcohol must be consumed to obtain the desired effect.

◆ **II. Assessment:**

A. *Vicious cycle*—(a) low tolerance for coping with frustration; tension, *guilt* and shame, resentment; (b) uses alcohol for relief; (c) new problems created by drinking; (d) new anxieties; and (e) more drinking.

B. Coping mechanisms used: *denial, rationalization, projection*.

C. *Complications of abuse and dependence*.

1. *Alcohol withdrawal delirium (delirium tremens [DTs])* (Figure 6–5)—result of nutritional deficiencies and toxins; requires sedation and constant watchfulness against unintentional suicide and convulsions.
   a. *Impending* signs relate to *CNS*—marked nervousness and restlessness, increased irritability; gross tremors of hands, face, lips; weakness; also *cardiovascular*—increased blood pressure, tachycardia, diaphoresis, dysrhythmias; *depression; gastrointestinal*—nausea, vomiting, anorexia.
   b. *Actual*—*serious* symptoms of mental confusion, convulsions, hallucinations (visual, olfactory, auditory, tactile). Without treatment, *15–25%* may die due to cardiac dysrhythmias, respiratory arrest, severe dehydration, massive infection.

2. *Wernicke's syndrome*—a neurological disturbance manifested by confusion, ataxia, eye movement abnormalities, and memory impairment. Other problems include:
   a. Disturbed vision (diplopia).
   b. Wandering mind.
   c. Stupor and coma.

3. *Alcohol amnestic syndrome (Korsakoff's syndrome)*—degenerative neuritis due to *thiamine* deficiency.
   a. Impaired thoughts.

FIGURE 6–5 Symptoms associated with alcohol withdrawal. (Adapted from Wilson, HS, and Kneisl, CR: Psychiatric Nursing, ed 2. Addison-Wesley, Menlo Park, Calif., 1983, p 388.)

b. Confusion, loss of sense of time and place.

c. Use of confabulation to fill in severe recent memory loss.

d. Follows episode of *Wernicke's encephalopathy.*

4. *Polyneuropathy*—weak, irregular, rapid peripheral pulses; sensory and motor nerve endings are involved, causing pain, itching, and loss of limb control.

5. Related concerns—chronic heart failure (generalized tissue edema), *gastritis, esophageal varices, cirrhosis, pancreatitis, diabetes,* pneumonia, REM sleep deprivation, *malnutrition.*

D. Diagnostic tests

1. *Blood tests:*

a. *CBC: decreased* Hgb/Hct to detect iron-deficiency anemia or acute/chronic GI bleeding; *increased* WBC (infection); *decreased* WBC (if immunosuppressed).

b. *Glucose:* hyperglycemia/hypoglycemia may be present (pancreatitis, malnutrition, or depletion of liver glycogen stores).

c. *Electrolytes: decreased* potassium and magnesium.

d. *Liver function tests: increased* CPK, LDH, AST, ALT, and amylase (liver or pancreatic problem).

e. *Nutritional tests: decreased* albumin and total protein; *decreased* vitamins (malnutrition/malabsorption).

2. *Urinalysis:* infection; ketones due to breakdown of fatty acids in malnutrition (pseudo-diabetic condition).

3. *Chest x-ray:* rule out right lower lobe pneumonia (related to malnutrition, depressed immune system, aspiration).

4. *ECG:* dysrhythmias, cardiomyopathies, or ischemia due to direct effect of alcohol on the cardiac muscle or conduction system, as well as effects of electrolyte imbalance.

5. *Other screening studies* (e.g., hepatitis, HIV, TB): dependent on general condition, individual risk factors, and care setting.

◆ III. Analysis/nursing diagnosis:

A. *Risk for injury (self-directed violence):* tendency for *self-destructive* acts related to intake of mind-altering substances and chronic low self-esteem.

B. *Altered nutrition, less than body requirements,* related to a lack of interest in food, interference with absorption/metabolism of nutrients and amino acids.

C. *Ineffective individual coping: denial/defensive coping* related to tendency to be domineering and critical, with difficulties in *interpersonal* relationships.

D. *Conflict with social order* related to extreme dependence coupled with resentment of *authority.*

E. *Spiritual distress* or general dissatisfaction with life related to feelings of powerlessness, *low frustration* tolerance, and demand for immediate need satisfaction.

F. *Dysfunctional behaviors/sexual dysfunction* related to tendency for *excess* in work, sex, recreation, marked *narcissistic* behavior.

G. *Social isolation* related to use of coping mechanisms that are primarily *escapist.*

H. *Knowledge deficit* (learning need) regarding condition, prognosis, treatment, self-care, discharge needs.

◆ IV. Nursing care plan/implementation:

A. *Detoxification phase*—maintain physiological stability.

1. *Administer adequate sedation* to control anxiety, insomnia, agitation, tremors.

2. *Administer anticonvulsants* to prevent *withdrawal seizures* (Valium, Librium, phenobarbital, magnesium sulfate).

3. *Control nausea and vomiting* to avoid massive GI bleeding or rupture of esophageal varices (antiemetics, antacids).

4. *Assess for* hypertension, tachycardia, increased temperature, Kussmaul's respirations.

5. *Assess fluid and electrolyte balance* for dehydration (may need IV fluids) or overhydration (may need a diuretic).

6. *Reestablish proper nutrition: high protein* (as long as no severe liver damage), carbohydrate, thiamine, *vitamins B complex and C.*

7. *Promote patient safety—provide quiet, calm, safe environment:* bed rest *with rails,* and head of bed elevated; well-lit room to reduce illusions; constant supervision and reassurance about fears and hallucinations, assess depression for suicide potential.

B. *Recovery-rehabilitation phase:* encourage participation in *group* activities; *avoid sympathy* when client tends to rationalize behavior and seeks special privileges—use acceptance and a *nonjudgmental,* consistent, firm, but kind approach; *avoid* scorn, contempt, and moralizing or punitive and rejecting behaviors; do *not* reinforce feelings of worthlessness, self-contempt, hopelessness, or low self-esteem.

C. *Problem behaviors:*

1. *Manipulative*—be firm and consistent; *avoid* "bid for sympathy."

2. *Demanding*—set limits.

3. *Acting out*—set limits, enforce rules and regulations, strengthen impulse control and ability to delay gratification.

4. *Dependency*—place responsibility on client; *avoid* giving advice.

5. *Superficiality*—help client make realistic self-appraisals and expectations in lieu of grandiose promises and trite verbalizations; encourage formation of lasting interpersonal relationships.

D. *Common reactions among staff:*
1. Disappointment—instead, set realistic goals, take one step at a time.
2. Moral judgment—instead, support each other.
3. Hostility—instead, offer support to each other when feeling frustrated from lack of results.

E. Refer client from hospital to *community resources* for follow-up treatment with social, economic, and psychological problems, as well as to self-help groups, to reduce "revolving door" situation in which client comes in, is treated, goes out, and comes in again the next night.
1. *Alcoholics Anonymous (AA)*—a self-help group of addicted drinkers who confront, instruct, and support fellow drinkers in their efforts to stay sober 1 day at a time through fellowship and acceptance.
2. *Alanon*—support group for *families* of alcoholics. *Alateen*—support group for *teenagers* when parent is alcoholic.
3. *Aversion therapy*—client is subjected to revulsion-producing or pain-inducing stimuli at the same time he or she takes a drink, to establish alcohol rejection behavior. Most common is disulfiram *(Antabuse),* a drug that produces intense headache, severe flushing, extreme nausea, vomiting, palpitations, hypotension, dyspnea, and blurred vision when alcohol is consumed while person is taking this drug.
4. *Group psychotherapy*—the goals of group psychotherapy are for the client to give up alcohol as a tension reliever, identify cause of stress, build different means for coping with stress, and accept drinking as a serious symptom.

F. *Health teaching:* teach improved coping patterns to tolerate increased stress; teach substitute tension-reducing strategies; prepare in advance for difficult, painful events; teach how to reduce irritating or frustrating environmental stress.

◆ **V. Evaluation/outcome criteria:** complications prevented, resolved; everyday living patterns are restructured for a satisfactory life without alcohol; demonstrates feelings of increased self-worth, confidence, and reliance.

VI. See sample **Critical Pathway: Alcohol Withdrawal Program**

Other Substance-Related Disorders

I. Concepts and principles:
A. *Three* interacting key factors give rise to dependence—*psychopathology* of the individual; frustrating *environment;* and *availability* of powerful, addicting, and temporarily satisfying drug.

B. According to conditioning principles, substance abuse and dependence proceed in *several phases:*
1. *Use* of sedatives-hypnotics, CNS stimulants, hallucinogens and narcotics, for relief from daily tensions and discomforts or anticipated withdrawal symptoms.
2. Habit is *reinforced* with each relief by drug use.
3. Development of *dependency*—drug has less and less efficiency in reducing tensions.
4. Dependency is further reinforced as addict *fails* to maintain adequate drug intake—increase in frequency and duration of periods of tension and discomfort.

◆ **II. Assessment:**
A. Abuse
1. *Hallucinogens* (LSD, marijuana, STP, PCP, peyote): euphoria and rapid mood swings, flight of ideas; perceptual impairment, feelings of omnipotence, "bad trip" (panic, loss of control, paranoia), flashbacks, suicide.
2. *CNS stimulants (amphetamines* and *cocaine* abuse): euphoria, hyperactivity, hyperalertness, irritability, persecutory delusions; insomnia, anorexia → weight loss; tachycardia; tremulousness; hypertension; hyperthermia → convulsions.
3. *Narcotics (opium* and its derivatives, e.g., morphine, heroin, codeine, meperidine HCl [Demerol]): used by "snorting," "skin popping," and "mainlining." May lead to abscesses and hepatitis. Decreased pain response, respiratory depression; apathy, detachment from reality; impaired judgment; loss of sexual activity; pinpoint pupils.
4. *Sedatives-hypnotics (barbiturate abuse):* similar to alcohol-induced behavior, e.g., euphoria followed by depression, hostility; decreased inhibitions; impaired judgment; staggering gait; slurred speech; drowsiness; poor concentration; progressive respiratory depression.

B. *Withdrawal symptoms*
1. *Narcotics* (e.g., heroin): begins within 12 hr of last dose, peaks in 24–36 hr, subsides in 72 hr, and disappears in 5–6 days.
   a. Pupil *dilation.*
   b. Muscle: twitches, tremors, aches, pains.
   c. Goose flesh (piloerection).
   d. *Lacrimation, rhinorrhea, sneezing, yawning.*
   e. *Diaphoresis,* chills.
   f. Potential for fever.
   g. *Vomiting,* abdominal distress.
   h. Dehydration.
   i. Rapid weight loss.
   j. Sleep disturbance.
2. *Barbiturates:* may be gradual or abrupt ("cold turkey"); latter is dangerous or *life-threatening;* should be hospitalized.

CRITICAL PATHWAY	Alcohol Withdrawal Program. Estimated Length of Stay: 7 Days Behavioral Unit					

Nursing Diagnosis and Categories of Care	Time Dimension	Goals/Actions	Time Dimension	Goals/Actions	Time Dimensions	Goals/Actions
Risk for injury (varied autonomic and sensory responses)	Day 1	Verbalize understanding of unit policies, procedures, and safety concerns relative to individual needs Cooperate with therapeutic regimen	Day 3 Day 4	Vital signs stable I&O balanced Display marked decrease in objective symptoms	Day 7	Discharge: Be free of injury resulting from alcohol withdrawal Display no objective symptoms of withdrawal
Referrals	Day 1	RN-NP or MD If indicated: Internist Cardiologist Neurologist				
Diagnostic studies	Day 1	Blood alcohol level Drug screen (urine and blood) If indicated: Chest x-ray Pulse oximetry ECG	Day 2	SMA 20: serum Mg, amylase Urinalysis	Day 4	Repeat of selected studies as indicated
Additional assessments	Day 1 Day 1–4 Ongoing **Stage I** **Stage II** **Stage III**	VS, temperature, respiratory status/breath sounds q4h I&O q8h Motor activity, body language, verbalizations, need for/type of restraint **Withdrawal symptoms:** Tremors, N/V, hypertension, tachycardia, diaphoresis, sleeplessness Increased hyperactivity, hallucinations, seizure activity Extreme autonomic hyperactivity, profound confusion, anxiety, fever	Day 2–3	VS q8h if stable Marked decrease in objective symptoms	Day 4–7 Day 6	VS qd Discontinue I&O
Medications Allergies:	Day 1 Day 1–4 Day 2	Librium 200 mg PO Thiamine 100 mg IM Librium 160 mg PO	Day 3 Day 4	Librium 120 mg PO Librium 80 mg PO	Day 5	Librium 40 mg PO
Patient education	Day 1	Orient to room/unit, schedule, procedures	Day 5	Need for ongoing therapy Goals/availability of AA program	Day 7	Schedule of follow-up visits if indicated

Continued

CRITICAL PATHWAY — Alcohol Withdrawal Program. Estimated Length of Stay: 7 Days Behavioral Unit—cont'd

Nursing Diagnosis and Categories of Care	Time Dimension	Goals/Actions	Time Dimension	Goals/Actions	Time Dimensions	Goals/Actions
Additional nursing actions	Day 1	Bed rest 12 hr if in withdrawal ◢*Position* change, HOB elevated Cough, deep breathe Exercises if on bed rest	Day 3–7	Activity as tolerated		
	Day 1–2	Assist with ambulation, self-care as needed Encourage fluids if free of N/V				
	Ongoing	Provide environmental safety measures Seizure precautions as indicated Reorient as needed				
Ineffective individual coping R/T personal vulnerability, situational crisis, inadequate coping methods	Day 1–7	Participate in development/evaluation of treatment plan	Day 3	Verbalize understanding of relationship of alcohol abuse to current situation	Day 7	Plan in place to meet postdischarge needs
	Day 2–7	Interact in group sessions	Day 6	Identify/make contact with potential resources, support groups		
Referrals	Day 1	Psychiatrist	Day 5	Community classes: assertiveness training Stress management		
	Day 2–7	Group sessions				
Additional assessments	Day 1	Understanding of current situation Drinking pattern, previous withdrawal, other drug use, attitudes toward substance use	Day 2–3	Previous coping strategies/consequences Perception of drug use on life, employment, legal issues		
	Day 1–2	History of violence Relationships with others: personal, work/school Readiness for group activities	Day 3–7	Congruency of actions based on insight		
Medications			Day 5–7	Naltrexone 50 mg/day if indicated		
Patient education	Day 1	Physical effects of alcohol abuse	Day 3–7	Human behavior and interactions with others/ transactional analysis (TA)	Day 7	Medication dose, frequency, side effects Written instructions for therapeutic program
	Day 1–2	Types/use of relaxation techniques				
	Day 2	Consequences of alcohol abuse	Day 5–6	Community resources for self/ family		

CRITICAL PATHWAY	Alcohol Withdrawal Program. Estimated Length of Stay: 7 Days Behavioral Unit—cont'd					
Nursing Diagnosis and Categories of Care	**Time Dimension**	**Goals/Actions**	**Time Dimension**	**Goals/Actions**	**Time Dimensions**	**Goals/Actions**
Additional nursing actions	Day 1–7	Support patient's taking responsibility for own recovery Provide consistent approach/ expectations for behavior Set limits/confront inappropriate behaviors	Day 2–5 Day 2–7	Identify goals for change Discuss alternative solutions Provide positive feedback for efforts Support during confrontation by peer group Encourage verbalization of feelings, personal reflection		
Altered nutrition: less than body requirements R/T poor intake, effects of alcohol on digestive system, and hypermetabolic response to withdrawal	Day 2-7	Select foods appropriately to meet individual dietary needs	Day 4	Verbalize understandings of effects of alcohol abuse and reduced dietary intake on nutritional status	Day 7	Display stable weight or initial weight gain as appropriate, and laboratory results WNL
Referrals	Day 1 and prn	Dietitian				
Diagnostic studies	Day 1	CBC, liver function studies Serum albumin, transferrin	Day 2–7	Finger-stick glucose prn		
Additional assessments	Day 1 Day 1–2 Day 1–7	Weight, skin turgor, condition of mucous membranes, muscle tone Bowel sounds, characteristics of stools Appetite, dietary intake			Day 7	Weight
Medications	Day 1–7	Antacid ac and hs (e.g., Maalox) Imodium 2 mg prn	Day 2–7	Multivitamin tablet qd		
Patient education	Day 1–2	Individual nutritional needs	Day 4	Principles of nutrition, foods for maintenance of wellness		
Additional nursing actions	Day 1 Day 1–7	Liquid/bland diet as tolerated Encourage small, frequent, nutritious meals/ snacks Encourage good oral hygiene pc and hs	Day 2–7	Advance diet as tolerated		

Source: Adapted from Doenges, M: Nursing Care Plans, ed 4. FA Davis, Philadelphia, 1997, pp 859–861.

Mental Health

a. *Gradual* withdrawal reaction from barbiturates:
   (1) Postural hypotension.
   (2) Tachycardia.
   (3) Elevated temperature.
   (4) Insomnia.
   (5) Tremors.
   (6) Agitation, restlessness.

b. *Abrupt* withdrawal from barbiturates:
   (1) Apprehension.
   (2) Muscular weakness.
   (3) Tremors.
   (4) Postural hypotension.
   (5) Twitching.
   (6) Anorexia.
   (7) *Grand mal seizures.*
   (8) *Psychosis-delirium.*

3. *Amphetamines:* depression, lack of energy, somnolence.

C. *Difference* between alcohol and other abused substances (e.g., opioid).
   1. Other abused substances may need to be obtained by illegal means, making it a legal and criminal problem as well as a medical and social problem; *not* so with alcohol abuse and dependency.
   2. Opium and its derivatives *inhibit* aggression, whereas alcohol *releases* aggression.
   3. As long as she or he is on large enough doses to avoid withdrawal symptoms, abuser of narcotics, sedatives, or hypnotics is comfortable and functions well, whereas chronically intoxicated alcoholic *cannot* function normally.
   4. Direct physiological effects of long-term opioid abuse and dependence on other abused substances are much *less critical* than those with chronic alcohol dependence.

◆ **III. Analysis/nursing diagnosis:**
   A. *Risk for altered physical regulation processes* (cardiac, circulatory, gastrointestinal, sleep pattern disturbance) related to use of mind-altering drugs.
   B. *Risk for injury* due to *altered judgment* related to misinterpretation of sensory stimuli and low frustration tolerance.
   C. *Altered conduct/impulse processes* related to rebellious attitudes toward authority.
   D. *Altered social interaction* (manipulation, dependency) related to hostility and personal insecurity.
   E. *Altered feeling states* (denial) related to underlying self-doubt and personal insecurity.

◆ **IV. Nursing care plan/implementation:** generally the same as in treating antisocial personality and alcohol abuse and dependence.

A. Maintain *safety* and optimum level of *physical* comfort. Supportive physical care: vital signs, nutrition, hydration, seizure precautions.

B. *Assist with medical treatment* and offer support and *reality orientation* to reduce feelings of panic.
   1. *Detoxification (or dechemicalization)*—give medications according to detoxification schedule.
   2. *Withdrawal*—may be gradual (barbiturates, hypnotics, tranquilizers) or abrupt ("cold turkey" for heroin). Observe for symptoms and report immediately.
   3. *Methadone (Dolophine)*—person must have been dependent on narcotics at least 2 yr and have failed at other methods of withdrawal before admission to program of readdiction by methadone.
      a. *Characteristics:*
         (1) Synthetic.
         (2) Appeases desire for narcotics without producing euphoria of narcotics.
         (3) Given by mouth.
         (4) Distributed under federal control (**N**arcotic **A**ddict **R**ehabilitation **A**ct).
         (5) Given with urinary surveillance.
      b. *Advantages:*
         (1) Prevents narcotic withdrawal reaction.
         (2) Tolerance not built up.
         (3) Person remains out of prison.
         (4) Lessens perceived need for heroin or morphine.

C. *Participation in group therapy—goals:* peer pressure, support, and identification.

D. *Rehabilitation phase:*
   1. Refer to halfway house and group living (e.g., Day-top).
   2. Support *employment* as therapy (work training).
   3. Expand client's *range of interests* to relieve characteristic boredom and stimulus hunger.
      a. Provide *structured* environment and planned routine.
      b. Provide educational therapy (academic and vocational).
      c. Arrange activities to include current events discussion groups, lectures, drama, music, and art appreciation.

E. Achieve role of *stabilizer and supportive* authoritative figure; this can be achieved through frequent, regular contacts with the same client.

F. *Health teaching:* how to cope with pain, fatigue, and anxiety without drugs.

◆ **V. Evaluation/outcome criteria:** replaces addictive lifestyle with self-reliant behavior and a plan formulated to maintain a substance-free life.

PSYCHOSOCIAL-CULTURAL FUNCTIONS

Mental Status Assessment

I. Components of mental status exam
A. *Appearance*—appropriate dress, grooming, facial expression, stereotyped movements, mannerisms, rigidity.
B. *Behavior*—anxiety level, congruence with situation, co-operativeness, openness, hostility, reaction to interview, consistency.
C. *Speech characteristics*—relevance, coherence, meaning, repetitiveness, qualitative (*what* is said), quantitative (*how much* is said), abnormalities, inflections, affectations, congruence with level of education, impediments, tone quality.
D. *Mood*—appropriateness, intensity, hostility turned inwards or toward others, duration, swings.
E. *Thought content*—delusions, hallucinations, obsessive ideas, phobic ideas, themes, areas of concern, self-concept.
F. *Thought processes*—organization and association of ideas, coherence, ability to abstract and understand symbols.
G. *Sensorium:*
1. *Orientation* to person, time and place, situation.
2. *Memory*—immediate, rote, remote, and recent.
3. *Attention and concentration*—susceptibility to distraction.
4. *Information and intelligence*—account of general knowledge, history, and reasoning powers.
5. *Comprehension*—concrete and abstract.
6. *Stage of consciousness*—alert/awake, somnolent, lethargic, delirious, stuporous, comatose.
H. *Insight and judgment*
1. Extent to which client sees self as having problems, needing treatment.
2. Client awareness of intrapsychic nature of own difficulties.
3. Soundness of judgment.

◆ II. Individual assessment—consider the following (Table 6–12):
A. Physical and intellectual factors.
B. Socioeconomic factors.
C. Personal values and goals.
D. Adaptive functioning and response to present involvement.
E. Developmental factors.

◆ III. Cultural assessment (see Unit 3):
A. Knowledge of ethnic beliefs and cultural practices can assist the nurse in the planning and implementation of holistic care.
B. Consider the following:
1. *Demographic data:* is this an "ethnic neighborhood"?

Mental Health

TABLE 6–12 ◆Individual Assessment

Physical and Intellectual
1. Presence of physical illness or disability.
2. Appearance and energy level.
3. Current and potential levels of intellectual functioning.
4. How client sees personal world, translates events around self; client's perceptual abilities.
5. Cause-and-effect reasoning, ability to focus.

Socioeconomic Factors
1. Economic factors—level of income, adequacy of subsistence; how this affects lifestyle, sense of adequacy, self-worth.
2. Employment and attitudes about it.
3. Racial, cultural, and ethnic identification; sense of identity and belonging.
4. Religious identification and link to significant value systems, norms, and practices.

Personal Values and Goals
1. Presence or absence of congruence between values and their expression in action; meaning of values to individual.
2. Congruence between individual's values and goals and the immediate systems with which client interacts.
3. Congruence between individual's values and assessor's values; meaning of this for intervention process.

Adaptive Functioning and Response to Present Involvement
1. Manner in which individual presents self to others—grooming, appearance, posture.
2. Emotional tone and change or constancy of levels.
3. Style of communication—verbal and nonverbal; ability to express appropriate emotion, follow train of thought; factors of dissonance, confusion, uncertainty.
4. Symptoms or symptomatic behavior.
5. Quality of relationship individual seeks to establish—direction, purposes, and uses of such relationships for individual.
6. Perception of self.
7. Social roles that are assumed or ascribed; competence in fulfilling these roles.
8. Relational behavior:
   a. Capacity for intimacy.
   b. Dependence-independence balance.
   c. Power and control conflicts.
   d. Exploitiveness.
   e. Openness.

Developmental Factors
1. Role performance equated with life stage.
2. How developmental experiences have been interpreted and used.
3. How individual has dealt with past conflicts, tasks, and problems.
4. Uniqueness of present problem in life experience.

Adapted from Wilson, HS, and Kneisl, CR: Psychiatric Nursing, ed 2. Addison-Wesley, Menlo Park, Calif., 1983, pp 204–205.

2. *Socioeconomic status:* occupation, education (formal and informal), income level; who is employed?
3. *Ethnic/racial orientation:* ethnic identity, value orientation.
4. *Country of immigration:* date of immigration; where were the family members born? Where has the family lived?
5. *Languages spoken:* does family speak English? Language and dialect preferences.
6. *Family relationships:* what are the formal roles? Who makes the decisions within the family? What is the family lifestyle and living arrangements?
7. *Degree of acculturation* of family members: how are the family customs and beliefs similar to or different from the dominant culture?
8. *Communication patterns:* social customs, nonverbal behaviors.
9. *Religious preferences:* what role do beliefs, rituals, and taboos play in health and illness? Is there a significant religious person? Are there any dietary symbolisms or preferences or restrictions due to religious beliefs?
10. *Cultural practices related to health and illness:* does the family use folk medicine practices or a folk healer? Are there specific dietary practices related to health and illness?
11. *Support systems:* do extended family members provide support?
12. *Health beliefs:* response to pain and hospitalization; disease predisposition and resistance.
13. Other significant factors related to ethnic identity: what health care facilities does the family use?
14. Communication barriers:
    a. Differences in language.
    b. Technical languages.
    c. Inappropriate place for discussion.
    d. Personality or gender of the nurse.
    e. Distrust of the nurse.
    f. Time-orientation differences.
    g. Differences in pain perception and expression.
    h. Variable attitudes toward death and dying.

Interviewing

I. **Definition:** a goal-directed method of communicating facts, feelings, and meanings. For interviewing to be successful, interaction between two persons involved must be effective.

II. **Nine principles of verbal interaction**
   A. *Client's initiative* begins the discussion.
   B. *Indirect approach,* moving from the periphery to the core.
   C. *Open-ended* statements, using incomplete forms of statements such as "You were saying . . ." to prompt rather than close off an exchange.
   D. *Minimal verbal activity* in order not to obstruct thought process and client's responses.
   E. *Spontaneity,* rather than fixed interview topics, may bring out much more relevant data.
   F. *Facilitate expression of feelings* to help assess events and reactions by asking, for example, "What was that like for you?"
   G. *Focus on emotional areas* about which client may be in conflict, as noted by repetitive themes.
   H. *Pick up cues, clues, and signals from client,* such as facial expressions and gestures, behavior, emphatic tones, and flushed face.
   I. *Introduce material related to content* already brought up by client; do *not* bring in a tangential focus from "left field."

III. **Purpose and goals of interviewing**
   A. *Initiate and maintain a positive nurse-client relationship,* which can decrease symptoms, lessen demands, and move client toward optimum health when nurse demonstrates understanding and sharing of client's concerns.
   B. *Determine client's view of nurse's role* in order to utilize it or change it.
   C. *Collect information on emotional crisis* to plan goals and approaches in order to increase effectiveness of nursing interventions.
   D. *Identify and resolve crisis;* the act of eliciting cause or antecedent event may in itself be therapeutic.
   E. *Channel feelings directly* by exploring interrelated events, feelings, and behaviors in order to discourage displacement of feelings onto somatic and behavioral symptoms.
   F. *Channel communication* and transfer significant information to the physician and other team members.
   G. *Prepare for health teaching* in order to help the client function as effectively as possible.

General Principles of Health Teaching

One key nursing function is to promote and restore health. This involves teaching patients or clients new psychomotor skills, general knowledge, coping attitudes, and social skills related to health and illness (e.g., proper diet, exercises, colostomy care, wound care, insulin injections, urine testing). The teaching function of the nurse is vital in assisting normal development and helping patients and clients meet health-related needs.

I. **Purpose of health teaching**
   A. *General goal:* motivate health-oriented behavior.

B. *Nursing interventions*
1. Fill in *gaps* in information.
2. *Clarify* misinformation.
3. Teach necessary *skills.*
4. *Modify* attitudes.

II. Educational theories on which effective health teaching is based:
A. *Motivation theory*
1. Health-oriented behavior is determined by the degree to which person sees health problem as *threatening,* with *serious consequences, high probability of occurrence,* and *belief in availability of effective course of action.*
2. Non–health-related motives may *supersede* health-related motives.
3. Health-related motives may not always give rise to health-related behavior, and vice versa.
4. Motivation may be influenced by:
    a. *Phases of adaptation* to crisis (poor motivation in early phase).
    b. *Anxiety and awareness of need* to learn. (Mild anxiety is highly motivating.)
    c. *Mutual* versus externally imposed goal setting.
    d. Perceived *meaningfulness* of information and material. (If within client's frame of reference, both meaningfulness and motivation increase.)
B. *Theory of planned change*
1. *Unfreeze* present level of behavior—develop awareness of problem.
2. Establish *need* for change and relationship of trust and respect.
3. *Move* toward change—examine alternatives, develop intentions into real efforts.
4. *Freeze* on a new level—generalize behavior, stabilize change.
C. Elements of *learning theory*
1. *Drive* must be present based on experiencing uncertainty, frustration, concern, or curiosity; hierarchy of needs exists.
2. *Response* is a learned behavior that is elicited when associated stimulus is present.
3. *Reward and reinforcement* are necessary for response (behavior) to occur and remain.
4. *Extinction of response,* that is, elimination of undesirable behavior, can be attained through conditioning.
5. Memorization is the easiest level of learning, but least effective in changing behavior.
6. Understanding involves the incorporation of generalizations and specific facts.
7. After introduction of new material, there is a period of floundering when assimilation and insight occur.
8. Learning is a two-way process between learner and teacher; defensive behavior in either makes both activities difficult, if not impossible.

9. Learning flourishes when client feels respected, accepted by enthusiastic nurse; learning occurs best when differing value systems are accepted.
10. Feedback increases learning.
11. Successful learning leads to more successes in learning.
12. Teaching and learning should take place in the area where *targeted activity* normally occurs.
13. Priorities for learning are dependent on client's *physical and psychological status.*
14. Decreased visual and auditory perception leads to decreased readiness to learn.
15. Content, terminology, pacing, and spacing of learning must correspond to client's *capabilities, maturity level, feelings, attitudes, and experiences.*

III. Assessment of the client-learner:
A. *Characteristics:* age, sex, race, medical diagnosis, prognosis.
B. *Sociocultural-economic:* ethnic, religious group beliefs and practices; family situation (roles, support); job (type, history, options, stress); financial situation, living situation (facilities).
C. *Psychological:* own and family's response to illness; premorbid personality; current self-image.
D. *Educational:*
1. Client's *perception* of current situation: What is wrong? Cause? How will lifestyle be affected?
2. *Past experience:* previous hospitalization and treatment; past compliance.
3. *Level of knowledge:* What has client been told? From what source? How accurate? Known others with the same illness?
4. *Goals:* what client *wants* to know.
5. *Needs:* what nurse thinks client *should* know for self-care.
6. Readiness for learning.
7. *Educational* background; ability to read and learn.

IV. Analysis of factors influencing learning:
A. *Internal*
1. Physical condition.
2. Senses (sight, hearing, touch).
3. Age.
4. Anxiety.
5. Motivation.
6. Experience.
7. Values (cultural, religious, personal).
8. Comprehension.
9. Education and language deficiency.
B. *External*
1. Physical environment (heat, light, noise, comfort).
2. Timing, duration, interval.
3. Teaching methods and aids.
4. Content, vocabulary.

Mental Health

Mental Health

◆ **V. Teaching plan** must be:
A. Compatible with the *three* domains of learning:
1. *Cognitive* (knowledge, concepts): use written and audiovisual materials, discussion.
2. *Psychomotor* (skills): use demonstrations, illustrations, role models.
3. *Affective* (attitudes): use discussions, maintain atmosphere conducive to change; use role models.
B. Appropriate to educational material.
C. Related to client's abilities and perceptions.
D. Related to objectives of teaching.

◆ **VI. Implementation**—*teaching guidelines* to use with clients:
A. Select conducive *environment* and best *timing* for activity.
B. Assess the client's *needs*, interests, *perceptions*, motivations, and *readiness* for learning.
C. State purpose and *realistic goals* of planned teaching/learning activity.
D. Actually involve the client by giving him or her the opportunity to *do, react, experience*, and *ask questions*.
E. Make sure that the client views the activity as useful and worthwhile and that it is within the client's grasp.
F. Use comprehensible terminology.
G. Proceed from the *known to the unknown*, from *specific to general* information.
H. Provide opportunity for client to *see results* and progress.
I. Give *feedback* and *positive reinforcement*.
J. Provide opportunities to achieve *success*.
K. Offer repeated practice in *real-life* situations.
L. *Space and distribute* learning sessions over a period of time.

VII. Evaluation/outcome criteria
A. Client's deficit of knowledge is lessened.
B. Increased compliance to treatment.
C. Length of hospital stay is reduced.
D. Rate of readmission to hospital is reduced.

The Therapeutic Nursing Process*

A *therapeutic nursing process* involves an interaction between the nurse and client in which the nurse offers a series of planned, goal-directed activities that are useful to a particular client in relieving discomfort, promoting growth, and satisfying interpersonal relationships.

I. Characteristics of therapeutic nursing:
A. Movement from first contact through final outcome:

1. *Eight general phases* occur in a typical unfolding of a natural process of problem solving.
2. Stages are not always in the same sequence.
3. Not all stages are present in a relationship.
B. Phase†
1. *Beginning* the relationship. *Goal:* build trust.
2. *Formulating* and clarifying a problem and concern. *Goal:* clarify client's statements.
3. *Setting a contract* or working agreement. *Goal:* decide on terms of the relationship.
4. *Building* the relationship. *Goal:* increase depth of relationship and degree of commitment.
5. *Exploring goals* and solutions, gathering data, expressing feelings. *Goals:* (a) maintain and enhance relationship (trust and safety), (b) explore blocks to goal, (c) expand self-awareness, and (d) learn skills necessary to reach goal.
6. *Developing action plan. Goals:* (a) clarify feelings, (b) focus on and choose between alternative courses of action, and (c) practice new skills.
7. *Working through* conflicts or disturbing feelings. *Goals:* (a) channel earlier discussions into specific course of action and (b) work through unresolved feelings.
8. *Ending* the relationship. *Goals:* (a) evaluation of goal attainment; (b) pointing out assets and gains; and (c) leave-taking reactions (repression, regression, anger, withdrawal, acting out).

II. Therapeutic nurse-client interactions
◆ **A. Plans/goals:**
1. Demonstrate unconditional *acceptance*, interest, concern, and respect.
2. Develop trust—be *consistent and congruent*.
3. Make *frequent* contacts with the client.
4. Be *honest* and *direct, authentic* and spontaneous.
5. Offer support, security, and empathy, *not* sympathy.
6. Focus comments on concerns of client (*client centered*), not self (social responses). *Refocus* when client changes subject.
7. Encourage expression of *feelings;* focus on feelings and *here-and-now* behavior.
8. Give attention to a client who complains.
9. Give information at client's level of understanding, at appropriate time and place.
10. Use open-ended questions; ask *how, what, where, who,* and *when* questions; avoid *why* questions; avoid questions that can be answered by *yes* or *no.*
11. Use feedback or reflective listening.
12. Maintain hope, but *avoid* false reassurances, clichés, and pat responses.

---

*Source: Lagerquist, S: Addison-Wesley's Nursing Examination Review, ed 4. Addison-Wesley, Redwood City, Calif., 1992.

†Adapted from Brammer, LM: The Helping Relationship; Process and Skills. Prentice Hall, Englewood Cliffs, NJ, 1973, p 55.

13. *Avoid* verbalizing value judgments, giving personal opinions, or moralizing.
14. Do *not* change the subject *unless* the client is redundant or focusing on physical illness.
15. Point out *reality;* help the client leave "inner world."
16. Set *limits* on behavior when client is acting out unacceptable behavior that is self-destructive or harmful to others.
17. Assist clients in arriving at their own decisions by demonstrating problem solving or involving them in the process.
18. Do *not* talk if it is not indicated.
19. Approach, sit, or walk with agitated clients; stay with the person who is upset, if he or she can tolerate it.
20. Focus on nonverbal communication.
21. Remember the *psyche has a soma!* Do *not* neglect appropriate physical symptoms.

B. Examples of **therapeutic** responses as interventions:
1. Being *silent*—being able to sit in silence with a person can connote acceptance and acknowledgment that the person has the right to silence. (*Dangers:* The nurse may wrongly give the client the impression that there is a lack of interest, or the nurse may discourage verbalization if acceptance of this behavior is prolonged; it is not necessarily helpful with acutely psychotic behavior.)
2. Using *nonverbal communication*—for example, nodding head, moving closer to the client, and leaning forward; use as a way to encourage client to speak.
3. Give encouragement to continue with *open-ended leads*—nurse's responses: "Then what?" "Go on," "For instance," "Tell me more," "Talk about that."
4. *Accepting, acknowledging*—nurse's responses: "I hear your anger," or "I see that you are sitting in the corner."
5. *Commenting on nonverbal behavior* of client—nurse's responses: "I notice that you are swinging your leg," "I see that you are tapping your foot," or "I notice that you are wetting your lips." Client may respond with, "So what?" If she or he does, the nurse needs to reply why the comment was made—for example, "It is distracting," "I am giving the nonverbal behavior meaning," "Swinging your leg makes it difficult for me to concentrate on what you are saying," or "I think when people tap their feet it means they are impatient. Are you impatient?"
6. Encouraging clients to *notice with their senses* what is going on—nurse's response: "What did you see (or hear)?" or "What did you notice?"
7. Encouraging *recall and description* of details of a particular experience—nurse's response: "Give me an example," "Please describe the experience further," "Tell me more," or "What did you say then?"
8. *Giving feedback by reflecting, restating, and paraphrasing* feelings and content:

Client: I cried when he didn't come to see me.
Nurse: You cried. You were expecting him to come and he didn't?

9. *Picking up on latent content* (what is implied)—nurse's response: "You were disappointed. I think it may have hurt when he didn't come."
10. *Focusing, pinpointing,* asking "what" questions:

Client: They didn't come.
Nurse: Who are "they"?

Client: [Rambling.]
Nurse: Tell it to me in a sentence or two. What is your main point? What would you say is your main concern?

11. *Clarifying*—nurse's response: "What do you mean by 'they'?" "What caused this?" or "I didn't understand. Please say it again."
12. *Focusing on reality* by expressing doubt on "unreal" perceptions:

Client: Run! There are giant ants flying around after us.
Nurse: That is unusual. I don't see giant ants flying.

13. *Focusing on feelings,* encouraging client to be aware of and describe personal feelings:

Client: Worms are in my head.
Nurse: That must be a frightening feeling. What did you feel at that time? Tell me about that feeling.

14. Helping client to *sort and classify impressions, make speculations, abstract* and *generalize* by making connections, seeing common elements and similarities, making comparisons, and placing events in logical sequence—nurse's responses: "What are the common elements in what you just told me?" "How is this similar to . . . ?" "What happened just before?" or "What is the connection between this and . . . ?"
15. *Pointing out discrepancies* between thoughts, feelings, and actions—nurse's response: "You say you were feeling sad when she yelled at you; yet you laughed. Your feelings and actions do not seem to fit together."
16. *Checking perceptions* and *seeking agreement* on how the issue is seen, *checking* with the client to see if the message sent is the same one that was received—nurse's response: "Let me restate what I heard you say," "Are you saying that . . . ?" "Did I hear you correctly?" "Is this what you mean?" or "It seems that you were saying . . . ?"
17. *Encouraging client to consider alternatives*—nurse's response: "What else could you say?"

Mental Health

or "Instead of hitting him, what else might you do?"

18. *Planning a course of action*—nurse's response: "Now that we have talked about your on-the-job activities and you have thought of several choices, which are you going to try out?" or "What would you do next time?"

19. *Imparting information*—give additional data as new input to help client; e.g., state facts and reality-based data that client may lack.

20. *Summing up*—nurse's response: "Today we have talked about your feelings toward your boss, how you express your anger, and about your fear of being rejected by your family."

21. *Encouraging client to appraise and evaluate* the experience or outcome—nurse's response: "How did it turn out?" "What was it like?" "What was your part in it?" "What difference did it make?" or "How will this help you later?"

C. Examples of **nontherapeutic** responses:

1. *Changing the subject, tangential response,* moves away from problem or focuses on incidental, superficial content:

   Client: I hate you.
   Nurse: Would you like to take your shower now?

   Suggested responses: Use reflection: "You hate me; tell me about this," or "You hate me; what does hate mean to you?"

   Client: I want to kill myself today.
   Nurse: Isn't today the day your mother is supposed to come?

   Suggested responses: (a) give open-ended lead, (b) give feedback: "I hear you saying today that you want to kill yourself," or (c) clarifying: "Tell me more about this feeling of wanting to kill yourself."

2. *Moralizing:* saying with approval or disapproval that the person's behavior is good or bad, right or wrong; *arguing* with stated belief of person; directly opposing the person:

   Nurse: That's good. It's wrong to shoot yourself.
   Client: I have nothing to live for.

   Nurse: You certainly do have a lot!
   Suggested responses: similar to those in C. 1. above.

3. *Agreeing with client's autistic inventions:*

   Client: The eggs are flying saucers.
   Nurse: Yes, I see. Go on.

   Suggested response: use clarifying response first: "I don't understand," and then, depending on client's response, use either *accepting and acknowledging, focusing on reality,* or *focusing on feelings.*

4. *Agreeing with client's negative view of self:*

   Client: I have made a mess of my life.
   Nurse: Yes, you have.

Suggested response: use clarifying response about "mess of my life"—"Give me an example of one time where you feel you messed up in your life."

5. *Complimenting, flattering:*

   Client: I have made a mess of my life.
   Nurse: How could you? You are such an attractive, intelligent, generous person.

   Suggested response: same as in **C. 4.**

6. *Giving opinions and advice* concerning client's life situation—examples of poor responses include: "In my opinion . . ." "I think you should . . ." or "Why not?"

   Suggested responses: (a) encourage the client to consider alternatives ("What else do you think you could try?"); (b) encourage the client to appraise and evaluate for himself or herself ("What is it like for you?").

7. *Seeking agreement* from client with nurse's personal opinion—examples of poor responses include: "I think . . . Don't you?" and "Isn't that right?"
   Suggested responses: (a) it is best to keep personal opinion to oneself and only give information that would aid the client's orientation to reality; (b) if you give an opinion as a *model* of orienting to reality, ask client to *state his or her* opinion ("My opinion is . . . What is your opinion?").

8. *Probing* or *offering premature solutions and interpretations;* jumping to conclusions:

   Client: I can't find a job.
   Nurse: You could go to an employment agency.

   Client: I'd rather not talk about it.
   Nurse: What are you unconsciously doing when you say that? What you really mean is . . .

   Client: I don't want to live alone.
   Nurse: Are you afraid of starting to drink again?

   Suggested responses: use responses that seek clarification and elicit more data.

9. *Changing client's words* without prior validation:

   Client: I am *not feeling well* today.
   Nurse: What makes you feel so *depressed?*

   Suggested response: "In what way are you not feeling well?" Use the same language as the client.

10. *Following vague content* as if understood or *using vague global* pronouns, adverbs, and adjectives:

    Client: People are so *unfair.*
    Nurse: I know what you mean.

Suggested response: clarify vague referents such as "people" and "unfair."

Client: I feel sad.
Nurse: Everyone feels that way at one time or another.

Suggested response: "What are you sad about?"

11. *Questioning on different topics without waiting for a reply:*

Client: [Remains silent.]
Nurse: What makes you so silent? Are you angry? Would you like to be alone?

Suggested response: choose one of the above and wait for a response before asking the next question.

12. *Ignoring client's questions or comments:*

Client: Am I crazy, nurse?
Nurse: [Walking away as if he or she did not hear the client.]

Suggested responses: "I can't understand what makes you bring this up at this time," or "Tell me what makes you bring this up at this time." Ignoring questions or comments usually implies that the nurse is feeling uncomfortable. It is important not to "run away" from the client.

13. *Closing off exploration* with questions that can be answered by *yes* or *no:*

Client: I'll never get better.
Nurse: Is something making you feel that way?

Suggested response: "What makes you feel that way?" Use open-ended questions that start with *what, who, when, where,* etc.

14. *Using clichés* or stereotyped expressions:

Client: The doctor took away my weekend pass.
Nurse: The doctor is only doing what's best for you. Doctor knows best. [Comment: also an example of moralizing.]

Suggested response: "Tell me what happened when the doctor took away your weekend pass."

15. *Overloading:* giving too much information at one time:

Nurse: Hello, I'm Mr. Brown. I'm a nurse here. I'll be here today, but I'm off tomorrow. Ms. Anderson will assign you another nurse tomorrow. This unit has five RNs, three LVNs, and students from three nursing schools who will all be taking care of you at some time.

Suggested response: "Hello, I'm Mr. Brown, your nurse today." Keep your initial orienting information simple and brief.

16. *Underloading:* not giving enough information, so that meaning is not clear; withholding information:

Client: What are visiting hours like here?
Nurse: They are flexible and liberal.

Suggested response: "They are flexible and liberal, from 10 A.M. to 12 noon and from 6 to 8 P.M." Use specific terms and give specific information.

17. *Saying no without saying no:*

Client: Can we go for a walk soon?
Nurse: We'll see. Perhaps. Maybe. Later.

Suggested response: "I will check the schedule in the nursing office and let you know within an hour." Vague, ambiguous responses can be seen as "putting the client off." It is best to be clear, specific, and direct.

18. *Using double-bind communication:* sending conflicting messages that do not have "mutual fit," or are incongruent:

Nurse: [Continuing to stay and talk with the client.] It's time for you to rest.
Suggested response: "It's time for you to rest and for me to leave [proceeding to leave]."

19. *Protecting:* defending someone else while talking with client; implying client has no right to personal opinions and feelings:

Client: This hospital is no good. No one cares here.
Nurse: This is an excellent hospital. All the staff were chosen for their warmth and concern for people.

Suggested response: focus on feeling tone or on clarifying information.

20. *Asking "why" questions* implies that the person has immediate conscious awareness of the reasons for his or her feelings and behaviors. Examples of this include: "Why don't you?" "Why did you do that?" or "Why do you feel this way?"

Suggested response: ask clarifying questions using *how, what,* etc.

21. *Coercion:* using the interaction between people to force someone to do *your* will, with the implication that if he or she does not "do it for your sake," you will not love or stay with him or her:

Client: I refuse to talk with him.
Nurse: Do it for my sake, before it's too late.

Suggested response: "Something keeps you from wanting to talk with him?"

22. Focusing on *negative* feelings, thoughts, actions:

Client: I can't sleep; I can't eat; I can't think; I can't do anything.
Nurse: How long have you not been sleeping, eating, or thinking well?

Suggested response: "What *do* you do?"

23. *Rejecting* client's behavior or ideas:

   Client: Let's talk about incest.
   Nurse: Incest is a bad thing to talk about; I don't want to.

   Suggested response: "What do you want to say about incest?"

24. *Accusing, belittling:*

   Client: I've had to wait five minutes for you to change my dressing.
   Nurse: Don't be so demanding. Don't you see that I have several people who need me?

   Suggested response: "It must have been hard to wait for me to come when you wanted it to be right away."

25. *Evading a response* by asking a question in return:

   Client: I want to know your opinion, nurse. Am I crazy?
   Nurse: Do you think you are crazy?

   Suggested response: "I don't know. What do you mean by 'crazy'?"

26. *Circumstantiality:* communicating in such a way that the main point is reached only after many side comments, details, and additions:

   Client: Will you go out on a date with me?
   Nurse: I work every evening. On my day off I usually go out of town. I have a steady boyfriend. Besides that, I am a nurse and you are a client. Thank you for asking me, but no, I will not date you.

   Suggested response: abbreviate your response to: "Thank you for asking me, but no, I will not date you."

27. *Making assumptions* without checking them:

   Client: [Standing in the kitchen by the sink, peeling onions, with tears in her eyes.]
   Nurse: What's making you so sad?

   Client: I'm not sad. Peeling onions always makes my eyes water.
   Suggested response: use simple acknowledgment and acceptance initially, such as "I notice you have tears in your eyes."

28. *Giving false, premature reassurance:*

   Client: I'm scared.
   Nurse: Don't worry; everything will be all right. There's nothing to be afraid of.

   Suggested response: "I'd like to hear about what you're afraid of, so that together we can see what could be done to help you." Open the way for clarification and exploration, and offer yourself as a helping person—not someone with magic answers.

Alterations in Self-Concept

◆ **I. Assessment:**
   A. Self-derisive; self-diminution; and criticism.
   B. Denies own pleasure due to need to punish self; doomed to failure.
   C. Disturbed interpersonal relationships (cruel, demeaning, exploitive of others; passive-dependent).
   D. Exaggerated self-worth or rejects personal capabilities.
   E. Feels guilty, worries (nightmares, *phobias, obsessions*).
   F. Sets unrealistic goals.
   G. Withdraws from reality with intense self-rejection (*delusional, suspicious,* jealous).
   H. Views life as either-or, worst-or-best, wrong-or-right.
   I. Postpones decisions due to ambivalence (procrastination).
   J. Physical complaints (*psychosomatic*).
   K. Self-destructive (*substance abuse* or other destructiveness).

◆ **II. Analysis/nursing diagnosis:** *Altered self-concept may be related to:*
   A. *Low self-esteem* that is related to parental rejection, unrealistic parental expectations, repeated failures.
   B. *Altered personal identity (negative):* self-rejection and self-hate related to unrealistic self-ideals.
   C. *Identity confusion* related to role conflict, role overload, and role ambiguity.
   D. *Feelings of helplessness, hopelessness,* worthlessness, fear, vulnerability, inadequacy related to extreme *dependency* on others and *lack of personal responsibility.*
   E. *Disturbed body image.*
   F. *Depersonalization.*
   G. *Physiological factors* that produce self-concept distortions (e.g., fatigue, oxygen and sensory deprivation, toxic drugs, isolation, biochemical imbalance).

◆ **III. Nursing care plan/implementation:**
   A. *Long-term goal:* Facilitate client's self-actualization by helping him or her to grow, develop, and realize potential while compensating for impairments.
   B. *Short-term goals:*
   1. Expand client's *self-awareness:*
      a. Establish open, trusting relationship to *reduce fear* of interpersonal relationships.
         (1) Offer unconditional acceptance.
         (2) Nonjudgmental response.
         (3) Listen and encourage discussion of thoughts, feelings.
         (4) Convey that client is valued as a person, is responsible for self *and* able to help self.

b. Strengthen client's capacity for *reality-testing, self-control,* and *ego integration.*
  (1) Identify ego strengths.
  (2) Confirm identity.
  (3) Reduce panic level of anxiety.
  (4) Use undemanding approach.
  (5) Accept and clarify communication.
  (6) Prevent isolation.
  (7) Establish simple routine.
  (8) Set limits on inappropriate behavior.
  (9) Orient to reality.
  (10) Activities: gradual increase; provide positive experiences.
  (11) Encourage self-care; assist in grooming.
  c. Maximize *participation in decision making* related to self.
  (1) Gradually increase participation in own care.
  (2) Convey expectation of ultimate self-responsibility.
2. Encourage client's *self-exploration.*
  a. Accept client's feelings and assist *self-acceptance* of emotions, beliefs, behaviors, and thoughts.
  b. Help *clarify* self-concept and relationship to others.
  (1) Elicit client's perception of own strengths and weaknesses.
  (2) Ask client to describe: ideal self, how client believes he or she relates to other people and events.
  c. Nurse needs to be aware of *own* feelings as a model of behavior and to limit counter-transference.
  (1) Accept own positive and negative feelings.
  (2) Share own perception of client's feelings.
  d. Respond with *empathy,* not sympathy, with the belief that client is subject to own control.
  (1) Monitor sympathy and self-pity by client.
  (2) Reaffirm that client is *not* helpless or powerless but is responsible for own choice of maladaptive or adaptive coping responses.
  (3) Discuss: alternatives, areas of ego *strength,* available coping resources.
  (4) Use family and group-support system for self-exploration of client's conflicts and maladaptive coping responses.
3. Assist client in *self-evaluation.*
  a. Help to clearly *define* problem.
  (1) Identify relevant stressors.
  (2) Mutually identify: faulty beliefs, misperceptions, distortions, unrealistic goals, areas of strength.

b. Explore use of adaptive *and* maladaptive coping responses and their positive and negative *consequences:*
4. Assist client to formulate a *realistic action plan.*
  a. Identify alternative solutions to client's *inconsistent perceptions* by helping him or her to change:
  (1) Own beliefs, ideals, to bring closer to reality.
  (2) Environment, to make consistent with beliefs.
  b. Identify alternative solutions to client's *self-concept not consistent with his or her behavior* by helping him or her to change:
  (1) Own behavior to conform to self-concept.
  (2) Underlying beliefs.
  (3) Self-ideal.
  c. Help client set and clearly define *goals* with *expected concrete* changes. Use role rehearsal, role modeling, and role playing to see practical, reality-based, emotional consequences of each goal.
5. Assist client to become committed to decision to *take necessary action* to replace maladaptive coping responses and maintain adaptive responses.
  a. Provide opportunity for success and give assistance (vocational, financial, and social support).
  b. Provide positive reinforcement; strengths, skills, healthy aspects of client's personality.
  c. Allow enough time for change.
6. *Health teaching:* how to focus on strengths rather than limitations; how to apply reality-oriented approach.

◆ **IV. Evaluation/outcome criteria**
  A. Client able to discuss perception of self and accept aspects of own personality.
  B. Client assumes increased responsibility for own behavior.
  C. Client able to transfer new perceptions into possible solutions, alternative behavior.

Anxiety

Anxiety is a subjective warning of danger in which the specific nature of the danger is usually not known. It occurs when a person faces a new, unknown, or untried situation. Anxiety is also felt when a person perceives threat in terms of past experiences. It is a general concept underlying most disease states. In its milder form, anxiety can contribute to learning and is necessary for problem solving. In its severe form, anxiety can impede a client's treatment and recovery. The general feelings elicited on all levels of anxiety are nervousness, tension, and apprehension.

It is essential that nurses recognize their own sources of anxiety and behavior in response to anxiety, as well as help clients recognize the manifestations of anxiety in themselves.

◆ **I. Assessment:**

  A. *Physiological* manifestations:

    1. Increased heart rate and palpitations.

    2. Increased rate and depth of respiration.

    3. Increased urinary frequency and diarrhea.

    4. Dry mouth.

    5. Decreased appetite.

    6. Cold sweat and pale appearance.

    7. Increased menstrual flow.

    8. Increased or decreased body temperature.

    9. Increased or decreased blood pressure.

    10. Dilated pupils.

  B. *Behavioral* manifestations—stages of anxiety:

    1. *Mild anxiety:*

      a. Increased perception (visual and auditory).

      b. Increased awareness of meanings and relationships.

      c. Increased alertness (notice more).

      d. Ability to use problem-solving process.

    2. *Moderate anxiety:*

      a. Selective inattention (e.g., may not hear someone talking).

      b. Decreased perceptual field.

      c. Concentration on relevant data; "tunnel vision."

      d. Muscular tension, perspiration, GI discomfort.

    3. *Severe anxiety:*

      a. Focus on many fragmented details.

      b. Physical and emotional discomfort (headache, nausea, dizziness, dread, horror, trembling).

      c. Not aware of total environment.

      d. Automatic behavior aimed at getting immediate relief instead of problem solving.

      e. Poor recall.

      f. Inability to see connections between details.

      g. Drastically reduced awareness.

    4. *Panic state of anxiety:*

      a. Increased speed of scatter; does not notice what goes on.

      b. Increased distortion and exaggeration of details.

      c. Feeling of terror.

      d. Dissociation (hallucinations, loss of reality, and little memory).

      e. Inability to cope with any problems; no self-control.

  C. *Reactions in response to anxiety:*

    1. *Fight:*

      a. Aggression.

      b. Hostility, derogation, belittling.

      c. Anger.

    2. *Flight:*

      a. Withdrawal.

      b. Depression.

    3. *Somatization* (psychosomatic disorder).

    4. *Impaired cognition:* blocking, forgetfulness, poor concentration, errors in judgment.

    5. *Learning* about or searching for causes of anxiety, and identifying behavior.

◆ **II. Analysis/nursing diagnosis:** *Anxiety* related to:

  A. *Physical causes:* threats to biological well-being (e.g., sleep disturbances, interference with sexual functioning, food, drink, pain, fever).

  B. *Psychological causes: disturbance in self-esteem* related to:

    1. Unmet wishes or expectations.

    2. Unmet needs for prestige and status.

    3. *Impaired adjustment:* inability to cope with environment.

    4. *Altered role performance:* not using own full potential.

    5. *Altered meaningfulness:* alienation.

    6. *Conflict with social order:* value conflicts.

    7. Anticipated disapproval from a significant other.

    8. *Altered feeling states: guilt.*

◆ **III. Nursing care plan/implementation:**

  A. *Moderate to severe anxiety*

    1. Provide *motor outlet* for tension energy, such as working at a simple, concrete task, walking, crying, or talking.

    2. Help clients *recognize* their anxieties by talking about how they are behaving and by exploring their underlying feelings.

    3. Help clients *gain insight* into their anxieties by helping them to understand how their behavior has been an expression of anxiety and to recognize the threat that lies behind this anxiety.

    4. Help clients *cope* with the threat behind their anxieties by reevaluating the threats and learning new ways to deal with them.

    5. *Health teaching:*

      a. Explain and offer hope that emotional pain will decrease with time.

      b. Explain that some tension is normal.

      c. Explain how to channel emotional energy into activity.

      d. Explain need to recognize highly stressful situations and to recognize tension within oneself.

  B. *Panic state*

    1. Give simple, clear, *concise* directions.

    2. *Avoid* decision making by client. Do *not* try to reason with client, because he or she is irrational and cannot cooperate.

    3. *Stay* with client.

      a. Do *not* isolate.

      b. *Avoid* touching.

    4. Allow client to seek *motor* outlets (walking, pacing).

Mental Health

5. *Health teaching:* advise activity that requires no thought.

◆ **IV. Evaluation/outcome criteria:**
   A. Uses more positive thinking and problem-solving activities and is less preoccupied with worrying.
   B. Uses values clarification to resolve conflicts and establish realistic goals.
   C. Demonstrates regained perspective, self-esteem, and morale; expresses feeling more in control, more hopeful.
   D. Fewer or absent physical symptoms of anxiety.

Patterns of Adjustment (Coping Mechanisms)

Coping mechanisms (ego defense mechanisms or mental mechanisms) consist of all the *coping* means used by individuals to seek relief from emotional conflict and *to ward off excessive anxiety.*

I. Definitions

blocking a disturbance in the rate of speech when a person's thoughts and speech are proceeding at an average rate but are suddenly and completely interrupted, perhaps even in the middle of a sentence. The gap may last from several seconds up to a minute. Blocking is often a part of the thought disorder found in *schizophrenic* disorders.

compensation making up for real or imagined handicap, limitation, or lack of gratification in one area of personality by overemphasis in another area to counter the effects of failure, frustration, and limitation; e.g., the blind compensate by increased sensitivity in hearing; the unpopular student compensates by becoming an outstanding scholar; small men compensate for short stature by demanding a great deal of attention and respect; a nurse who does not have manual dexterity chooses to go into psychiatric nursing.

confabulating filling in gaps of memory by inventing what appear to be suitable memories as replacements. This symptom may occur in various *amnestic disorders* but is most often seen in *Korsakoff's syndrome* (deterioration due to alcohol) and in *dementia.*

conversion psychological difficulties are translated into physical symptoms **without conscious** will or knowledge; e.g., pain and immobility on moving your writing arm the day of the exam.

denial an intolerable thought, wish, need, or reality factor, is disowned automatically; e.g., a student, when told of a failing grade, acts as if he never heard of such a possibility.

displacement transferring the emotional component from one idea, object, or situation to another, more acceptable one. Displacement occurs because these are painful or dangerous feelings that cannot be expressed toward the original object; e.g., kicking the dog after a bad day at school or work; anger with clinical instructor gets transferred to classmate who was late to meet you for lunch.

dissociation splitting off or separation of differing elements of the mind from each other. There can be separation of ideas, concepts, emotions, or experiences from the rest of the mind. Dissociated material is deeply repressed and becomes encapsulated and inaccessible to the rest of the mind. This usually occurs as a result of some very painful experience, for example, split of affect from idea in *anxiety disorders* and *schizophrenia.*

fixation a state in which personality development is arrested in one or more aspects at a level short of maturity; e.g., "She is anally fixated" (controlling, stingy, holding onto things and memories).

idealization overestimation of some admired aspect or attribute of another person; e.g., "She was a perfect human being."

ideas of reference fixed, false ideas and interpretations of external events as though they had direct reference to self; e.g., client thinks that TV news announcer is reporting a story about client.

identification the wish to be like another person; situation in which qualities of another are unconsciously transferred to oneself; e.g., boy identifies with his father and learns to become a man; a woman may fear she will die in childbirth because her mother did; a student adopts attitudes and behavior of her favorite teacher.

introjection incorporation into the personality, without assimilation, of emotionally charged impulses or objects; a quality or an attribute of another person is taken into and made part of self; e.g., a girl in love introjects the personality of her lover into herself—his ideas become hers, his tastes and wishes are hers; this is also seen in *severe depression* following death of someone close—patient may assume many of deceased's characteristics; similarly, working in a psychiatric unit with a suicidal person brings out depression in the nurse.

isolation temporary or long-term splitting off of certain feelings or ideas from others; separating emotional and intellectual content; e.g., talking emotionlessly about a traumatic accident.

projection attributes and transfers own feelings, attitudes, impulses, wishes, or thoughts to another person or object in the environment, especially when ideas or impulses are too painful to be acknowledged as belonging to oneself; e.g., in *hallucinations* and *delusions* by alcoholics; or, "I flunked the course because the teacher doesn't know how to teach"; "I hate him" reversed into "He hates me"; or a student impatiently accusing an instructor of being intolerant.

rationalization justification of behavior by formulating a logical, socially approved reason for past, present, or proposed behavior. Commonly used, conscious or unconscious, with false or real reason; e.g., after losing a class election, a student states that she really did not want all the extra work and is glad she lost.

reaction formation   going to the opposite extreme from what one wishes to do or is afraid one might do; e.g., being overly concerned with cleanliness when one wishes to be messy, being an overly protective mother through fear of own hostility to child, or showing great concern for a person whom you dislike, going out of your way to do special favors.

regression   when individuals fail to solve a problem with the usual methods at their command they may resort to modes of behavior that they have outgrown but that proved successful at an earlier stage of development; retracing developmental steps; going back to earlier interests or modes of gratification; e.g., a senior nursing student about to graduate becomes dependent on a clinical instructor for directions.

repression   involuntary exclusion of painful and unacceptable thoughts and impulses from awareness. *Forgetting* these things solves the situation by not solving it; e.g., by not remembering what was on the difficult exam after it was over.

sublimation   channeling a destructive or instinctual impulse that cannot be realized into a *socially acceptable*, practical, and less dangerous outlet, with some relation to the original impulse for emotional satisfaction to be obtained; e.g., sublimation of sexual energy into other creative activities (art, music, literature) or hostility and aggression into sports or business competition; or an infertile person putting all energies into pediatric nursing.

substitution   when individuals cannot have what they wish and accept something else in its place for symbolic satisfaction; e.g., pin-up pictures in absence of sexual object, or a person who failed an RN exam signs up for an LVN/LPN exam.

suppression   a deliberate process of blocking from the conscious mind thoughts, feelings, acts, or impulses that are undesirable; e.g., "I don't want to talk about it," "Don't mention his name to me," or "I'll think about it some other time"; or willfully refusing to think about or discuss disappointment with exam results.

symbolism   sign language that stands for related ideas and feelings, conscious and unconscious. Used extensively by children, primitive peoples, and psychotic patients. There is meaning attached to this sign language that makes it very important to the individual; e.g., a student wears dark, somber clothing to the exam site.

undoing   a coping mechanism against anxiety, usually unconscious, designed to negate or neutralize a previous act; e.g., Lady Macbeth's attempt to wash her hands (of guilt) after the murder. A repetitious, symbolic acting out, in reverse of an unacceptable act already completed. Responsible for *compulsions* and magical thinking.

II. **Characteristics** of coping mechanisms:
   A. Coping mechanisms are used to some degree by everyone occasionally; they are normal processes by which the ego reestablishes equilibrium—unless they are used to an extreme degree, in which case they interfere with maintenance of self-integrity.
   B. Much overlapping:
      1. Same behavior can be explained by more than one mechanism.
      2. May be used in combination—e.g., isolation and repression, denial and projection.
   C. Common defense mechanisms compatible with mental well-being.
      1. Compensation.
      2. Compromise.
      3. Identification.
      4. Rationalization.
      5. Sublimation.
      6. Substitution.
   D. Typical coping mechanisms in:
      1. *Paranoid disorders*—denial, projection.
      2. *Dissociative disorders*—denial, repression, dissociation.
      3. *Obsessive-compulsive behaviors*—displacement, reaction-formation, isolation, denial, repression, undoing.
      4. *Phobic disorders*—displacement, rationalization, repression.
      5. *Conversion disorders*—symbolization, dissociation, repression, isolation, denial.
      6. *Major depression*—displacement.
      7. *Bipolar disorder, manic episode*—reaction-formation, denial, projection, introjection.
      8. *Schizophrenic disorders*—symbolization, repression, dissociation, denial, fantasy, regression, projection, insulation.
      9. *Dementia*—regression.

III. **Concepts and principles related to coping mechanisms:**
   A. Unconscious process—coping mechanisms are used as a substitute for more effective problem-solving behavior.
   B. *Main functions*—increase *self-esteem; decrease*, inhibit, minimize, alleviate, avoid, or eliminate *anxiety;* maintain feelings of personal worth and adequacy and soften failures; *protect the ego; increase security.*
   C. *Drawbacks*—involve high degree of self-deception and reality distortion; may be maladaptive because they superficially eliminate or disguise conflicts, leaving conflicts unresolved but still influencing behavior.

◆ IV. **Nursing care plan/implementation** with coping

mechanisms:

A. Accept coping mechanisms as normal, but not when overused.

B. Look beyond the behavior to the need that is expressed by the use of the coping mechanism.

C. Discuss alternative coping mechanisms that may be more compatible with mental health.

D. Assist the person to translate defensive thinking into nondefensive, direct thinking; a problem-solving approach to conflicts minimizes the need to use coping mechanisms.

Anxiety Disorders (Anxiety and Phobic Neuroses)

I. **Definition:** emotional illnesses characterized by *fear* and *autonomic nervous system symptoms* (palpitations, tachycardia, dizziness, tremor); related to *intrapsychic conflict* and psychogenic origin where instinctual impulse (related to sexuality, aggression, or dependence) may be in conflict with the ego, superego, or sociocultural environment; related to sudden object loss.

An *anxiety disorder* is a mild to moderately severe functional disorder of personality in which *repressed* inner conflicts between drives and fears are manifested in behavior patterns, including *generalized anxiety* and *phobic, obsessive-compulsive disorders.* (Other related disorders are *dissociative, conversion,* and *hypochondriasis.*)

II. **General concepts and principles related to anxiety disorders:**

A. Behavior may be an attempt to "bind" anxiety: to *fix* it in some particular area (hypochondriasis) or to *displace* it from the rest of personality (phobic, conversion, and dissociative disorders—amnesia, fugue, multiple personalities; obsessive-compulsive disorders).

B. *Purpose of symptoms:*
   1. To intensify *repression* as a defense.
   2. To exhibit some repressed content in *symbolic* form.

◆ III. **General assessment of anxiety disorders:**

A. Uses behavior to *avoid* tense situations.

B. Frightened, suggestible.

C. Prone to *minor* physical complaints (e.g., fatigue, headaches, and indigestion) and reluctance to admit recovery from physical illnesses.

D. Attitude of martyrdom.

E. Often feels helpless, insecure, inferior, inadequate.

F. Uses *repression, displacement,* and *symbolism* as key coping mechanisms.

Anxiety Disorders

I. *Generalized anxiety disorder:*

◆ A. **Assessment:**
   1. Persistent, diffuse, free-floating, painful anxiety for at least 1 mo.
   2. Motor tension, autonomic hyperactivity.
   3. Hyperattentiveness expressed through vigilance and scanning.

◆ B. **Analysis/nursing diagnosis:**
   1. *Anxiety/powerlessness: excessive worry* related to real or perceived threat to security, unmet needs.
   2. *Altered attention* related to overwhelming anxiety.
   3. *Fear* related to sudden object loss.
   4. *Guilt* related to inability to meet role expectations.
   5. *Risk for alteration in self-concept* related to feelings of inadequacy.
   6. *Altered role performance* related to inadequate support system.
   7. *Impaired social interaction* related to use of avoidance in tense situations.
   8. *Distractibility* related to pervasive anxiety.
   9. *Hopelessness* related to feelings of inadequacy.
   10. *Sleep pattern disturbance.*

◆ C. **Nursing care plan/implementation:**
   1. Fulfill needs as promptly as possible.
   2. Listen attentively.
   3. Stay with client.
   4. *Avoid* decision making and competitive situations.
   5. Promote rest; decrease environmental stimuli.
   6. *Health teaching:* teach steps of anxiety reduction.

◆ D. **Evaluation/outcome criteria:** symptoms are diminished.

II. *Panic disorder:*

◆ A. **Assessment:**
   1. Three acute, terrifying panic attacks within 3 wk period, *unrelated* to marked physical exertion, life-threatening situation, presence of organic illness, or exposure to specific phobic stimulus.
   2. Discrete periods of apprehension, fearfulness (lasting from few moments to an hour).
   3. *Mimics cardiac* disease: dyspnea, chest pain, smothering or choking sensations, palpitations, tachycardia, dizziness, fainting, sweating.
   4. Feelings of unreality, paresthesias.
   5. Hot, cold flashes and dilated pupils.
   6. Trembling, sense of impending death, fear of becoming insane.

◆ B. **Analysis/nursing diagnosis:**
   1. *Ineffective individual coping* related to undeveloped interpersonal processes.

2. *Altered comfort pattern:* distress, anxiety, fear related to threat to security.
3. *Decisional conflict* related to apprehension.
4. *Altered thought processes* related to impaired concentration.

◆ **C. Nursing care plan/implementation:**
   1. *Reduce immediate anxiety* to more moderate and manageable levels.
      a. Stay *physically close* to reduce feelings of alienation and terror.
      b. *Communication approach:* calm, serene manner; short, simple sentences; firm voice to convey that nurse will provide external controls.
      c. *Physical environment:* remove to smaller room to minimize stimuli.
   2. Provide *motor outlet* for diffuse energy generated at high anxiety levels, e.g., moving furniture, scrubbing floors.
   3. Administer *antianxiety medications* as ordered.
   4. *Health teaching:* recommend more effective methods of coping.

◆ **D. Evaluation/outcome criteria:** can endure anxiety while searching out its causes.

III. *Obsessive-compulsive disorder:*

◆ **A. Assessment**—chief characteristic: fear that client can harm someone or something.
   1. *Obsessions*—recurrent, persistent, involuntary, senseless *thoughts, images, ideas,* or *desires* that may be trivial or morbid, e.g., fear of germs, doubts as to performance of an act, thoughts of hurting family member, death, suicide.
   2. *Compulsions*—uncontrollable, persistent urge to perform repetitive, stereotyped *behaviors* that provide relief from unbearable anxiety, e.g., hand washing, counting, touching, checking and rechecking doors to see if locked, elaborate dressing and undressing rituals.

◆ **B. Analysis/nursing diagnosis:**
   1. *Ineffective individual coping* related to:
      a. *Intellectualization and avoidance* of awareness of feelings.
      b. Limited ability to express emotions (may be disguised or delayed).
      c. Exaggerated feelings of *dependence and helplessness.*
      d. High need to *control* self, others, and environment.
      e. Rigidity in thinking and behavior.
      f. Poor ability to tolerate anxiety and depression.
   2. *Social isolation* related to:
      a. Resentment.
      b. Self-doubt.
      c. Exclusion of pleasure.

◆ **C. Nursing care plan/implementation:**

1. *Accept* rituals permissively (e.g., excessive hand washing); stopping ritual will increase anxiety.
2. *Avoid* criticism or "punishment," making demands, or showing impatience with client.
3. *Allow* extra time for slowness and client's need for precision.
4. *Protect* from rejection by *others.*
5. *Protect* from *self-inflicted* harmful acts.
6. Engage in nursing therapy *after* the ritual is over, when client is most comfortable.
7. *Redirect* client's actions into substitute outlets.
8. *Health teaching:* teach how to prevent health problems related to rituals, e.g., use rubber gloves, hand lotion.

◆ **D. Evaluation/outcome criteria:** avoids situations that increase tension and thus reduces need for ritualistic behavior as outlet for tension.

IV. *Phobic disorders*—intense, *irrational, persistent* fear in response to *external* object, activity, or situation; e.g., *agoraphobia*—fear of being alone or in public places; *claustrophobia*—fear of closed places; *acrophobia*—fear of heights; *simple phobias* such as *mysophobia*—fear of germs. *Social phobias:* fear of situations that may be humiliating or embarrassing. *Dynamics: displacement* of anxiety from original source onto avoidable, *symbolic,* external, and specific object (or activity or situation); i.e., phobias help person control intensity of anxiety by providing specific object to attach it to, which he or she can then avoid.

◆ **A. Assessment:** same as for anxiety symptoms; fear that someone or something will harm them.

◆ **B. Analysis/nursing diagnosis:** *social isolation; avoidance; irrational *fear* out of proportion to actual danger; *defensive coping* with high need to control self, others, environment.

◆ **C. Nursing care plan/implementation:** promote psychological and physical calm:
   1. *Use systematic desensitization:* never force contact with feared object or situation.
   2. *Health teaching:* progressive relaxation, meditation, biofeedback training, or other behavioral conditioning techniques.

◆ **D. Evaluation/outcome criteria:** phobia is eliminated (i.e., able to come into contact with feared object with lessened degree of anxiety).

V. *Acute stress disorder and posttraumatic stress disorder:*

◆ **A. Assessment:**
   1. *Acute stress disorder:* symptoms occur *within 1 mo* of extreme stressor.
   2. *Posttraumatic stress disorder (PTSD):* symptoms occur *after* 1 mo.
   3. *Precipitant:* severe traumatic event (natural or man-made disaster) that is not an ordinary occurrence, e.g., rape, fire, flood, earthquake, tornado, bombing, torture, kidnapping.
   4. Self-report of reexperiencing incident; intrusive memories.

5. Numb, unresponsive, detached, estranged reaction to external world (unable to feel tenderness, intimacy).
6. Change in sleep pattern (insomnia, recurrent dreams, nightmares), memory loss, hyperalertness (startle response).
7. Guilt rumination about survival.
8. Avoids activities reminiscent of trauma; phobic responses.
9. Difficulty with task completion and concentration.
10. Depression.
11. Increased irritability may result in unpredictable, explosive outbursts.
12. Impulsive behavior, sudden lifestyle changes.

◆ **B. Analysis/nursing diagnosis:**
1. *Posttrauma response* related to overwhelming traumatic event.
2. *Anxiety* (severe to panic)/*fear* related to memory of environmental stressor, threat to self-concept, negative self-talk.
3. *Risk for violence directed at self/others* related to a startle reaction, use of drugs to produce a psychic numbing.
4. *Sleep pattern disturbance* related to fear and rumination.
5. *Decisional conflict (impaired decision making)* related to perceived threat to personal values and beliefs.
6. *Guilt* related to lack of social support system.
7. *Altered feeling-states:* emotional lability related to diminished sense of control over self and environment.

◆ **C. Nursing care plan/implementation:**
1. Crisis counseling (listen with concern and sympathy).
   a. Ease way for client to *talk out* the experience and express fear.
   b. Help client to become aware and accepting of what happened.
2. *Health teaching:* suggest how to resume concrete activity and reconstruct life with available social, physical, and emotional resources. Help make contact with friends, relatives, and other resources.

◆ **D. Evaluation/outcome criteria:** can cry and express anger, loss, frustration, and despair; begins process of social and physical reconstruction.

E. See **Critical Pathway for Posttrauma Client.**

Dissociative Disorders (Hysterical Neuroses, Dissociative Type)

◆ **I. Assessment:**
A. *Dissociative amnesia:* partial or total inability to recall the past; occurs during highly stressful events; client may have conscious desire to es-

cape but be unable to accept escape as a solution; uses *repression.*
B. *Dissociative fugue:* client not only forgets but also *flees* from stress.
C. *Dissociative identity disorder:* client exhibits two or more complete personality systems, each very different from the other; alternates from one personality to the other without awareness of change (*one* personality *may* be aware of others); each personality has well-developed emotions and thought processes that are in conflict; uses *repression.*
D. *Depersonalization disorder:* loss of sense of self; feeling of self-estrangement (as if in a dream); fear of going insane.

◆ **II. Analysis/nursing diagnosis:**
A. Sudden *alteration in:*
1. *Memory* (short- and *long-term memory loss:* cannot recall important personal events) related to repression.
2. *Personal and social identity* (amnesia: forgets own identity; becomes another identity) related to intense anxiety, childhood trauma/abuse, threat to physical integrity, underdeveloped ego.
B. *Sensory/perceptual alteration* of external environment related to repression and escapism.
C. *Confusion* related to use of repression.
D. *Spiritual despair* related to conversion of conflict into physical or mental flights.
E. *Altered meaningfulness* (hopelessness, helplessness, powerlessness) related to lack of control over situation.

◆ **III. Nursing care plan/implementation:**
A. *Remove* client from immediate environment to reduce pressure.
B. *Alleviate* symptoms using behavior-modification strategies.
C. *Divert* attention to topics other than symptoms (not remembering names, addresses, and events).
D. Encourage *socialization* rather than isolation.
E. *Avoid* sympathy, pity, and oversolicitous approach.
F. *Health teaching:* teach families to avoid reinforcing dissociative behavior; teach client problem solving, with goal of minimizing stressful aspects of environment.

◆ **IV. Evaluation/outcome criteria:** recall returns to conscious awareness; anxiety kept within manageable limits.

Somatoform Disorders

I. Main characteristic: involuntary, physical symptoms *without* demonstrable organic findings or

CRITICAL PATHWAY of Care for the Posttrauma Client

Estimated length of stay: 14 days—variations from designated pathway should be documented in progress notes

Nursing Diagnosis and Categories of Care	Time Dimension	Goals/Actions	Time Dimension	Goals/Actions	Time Dimensions	Discharge Outcome
Posttrauma response	Day 1	Reassurance of client safety	Ongoing	Environment is made safe for client.	Day 14	Client is able to carry out activities of daily living. Fewer flashbacks, nightmares.
Referrals	Day 1	Psychiatrist Psychologist Social worker Clinical nurse specialist Music therapist Occupational therapist Recreational therapist Chaplain			Day 14	Discharge with follow-up appointments as required.
Diagnostic studies	Day 1 Day 2–5	Drug screen ECG EEG MMPI Impact of event scale (IES)				
Medications	Day 1	Antidepressant medication as ordered (tricyclics or MAO inhibitors) Antianxiety medication, as ordered (benzodiazepines); may be given prn because of addictive quality Clonidine or propranolol (for intrusive thoughts and hyperarousal) Sedative-hypnotics for sleep disturbances; may be given prn	Day 1–14	Assess for effectiveness and side effects of medications. Administer addictive medications judiciously and taper dosage.	Day 14	Discharged with medications as ordered by MD (e.g., antidepressants, clonidine, propranolol).
Additional assessments	Day 1	VS every shift Assess: ■ Mental status ■ Mood swings ■ Anxiety level ■ Social interaction ■ Ability to carry out activities of daily living ■ Suicide ideation ■ Sleep disturbances	Day 2–14 Day 2–13	VS daily if stable. Ongoing assessments.	Day 14	Anxiety is maintained at manageable level. Mood is appropriate. Interacts with others. Carries out activities of daily living independently. Denies suicide ideation.

Mental Health

CRITICAL PATHWAY of Care for the Posttrauma Client—cont'd

Estimated length of stay: 14 days—variations from designated pathway should be documented in progress notes

Nursing Diagnosis and Categories of Care	Time Dimension	Goals/Actions	Time Dimension	Goals/Actions	Time Dimensions	Discharge Outcome
Additional assessments— cont'd		▪ Flashbacks ▪ Presence of guilt feelings				Sleeps without medication. Is able to interrupt flashbacks with adaptive, coping strategies. Has worked through feelings of guilt.
Diet	Day 1	▪ Client's choice or low-tyramine if taking MAO inhibitors	Day 2–14	Same.	Day 14	Client eats well-balanced diet.
Client education	Day 1	▪ Orient to unit	Day 5–12	Stages of grief. Side effects of medications. Coping strategies. Low-tyramine diet. Community resources. Support group. Importance of not mixing drugs and alcohol.	Day 14	Client is discharged. Verbalizes understanding of information presented before discharge.
			Day 12–13	Reinforce teaching.		

Source: Adapted from Townsend, M: Essentials of Psychiatric–Mental Health Nursing. FA Davis, Philadelphia, 1999, pp. 768–770.

identifiable physiological bases; involve psychological factors or nonspecific conflicts.

◆ **II. General assessment:**
   A. *Precipitant:* major emotional, interpersonal stress.
   B. Occurrence of secondary gain from illness.

◆ **III. General analysis/nursing diagnosis:**
   A. *Fear* related to loss of dependent relationships.
   B. *Powerlessness* related to chronic resentment over frustration of dependency needs.
   C. *Altered feeling states:* inhibition of anger, which is discharged physiologically and is related to control of anxiety.
   D. *Impaired judgment* related to denial of existence of any conflicts or relationship to physical symptoms.
   E. *Altered role performance:* regression related to not having dependency needs met.

Somatization Disorder

Repeated, multiple, vague or exaggerated physical complaints of several years' duration *without* identifiable physical cause; clients constantly seek medical attention, undergo numerous tests; at risk for unnecessary surgery or drug abuse.

◆ **A. Assessment:**
   1. Onset and occurrence—teen years, more common in women.
   2. Reports illness most of life.
      a. *Neuromuscular* symptoms—fainting, seizures, dysphagia, difficulty walking, back pain, urinary retention.
      b. *Gastrointestinal* symptoms—nausea, vomiting, flatus, food intolerance, constipation or diarrhea.
      c. *Female reproductive* symptoms—dysmenorrhea, hyperemesis gravidarum.
      d. *Psychosexual* symptoms—sexual indifference, dyspareunia.
      e. *Cardiopulmonary* symptoms—palpitations, shortness of breath, chest pain.
      f. *Rule out:* multiple sclerosis, systemic lupus erythematosus, porphyria, hyperparathyroidism.
   3. Appears anxious and depressed.

◆ **B. Analysis/nursing diagnosis:**
   1. *Anxiety* (severe) related to threat to security, unmet dependency needs, and inability to meet role expectations.
   2. *Self-care deficit* related to development of physical symptoms to escape stressful situations.

3. *Impaired social interaction* related to inability to accept that physical symptoms lack a physiological basis; preoccupation with self and physical symptoms, chronic pain; rejection by others.

4. *Body-image disturbance and altered role performance* related to passive acceptance of disabling symptoms.

Conversion Disorder (Hysterical Neuroses, Conversion Type)

Sudden symptoms of *symbolic* nature developed under *extreme* psychological stress (e.g., war, loss, natural disaster) that *disappear* through hypnosis.

◆ **A. Assessment:**

1. *Neurological* symptoms—paralysis, aphonia, tunnel vision, seizures, blindness, paresthesias, anesthesias.

2. *Endocrinological* symptoms—pseudocyesis.

3. Hysterical, dependent *personality profile:* exhibitionistic dress and language; self-indulgent; suggestible; impulsive and global impressions and hunches; little capacity to concentrate, integrate, and organize thoughts or plan action or outcomes; little concern for symptoms, despite severe impairment ("La Belle Indifference").

◆ **B. Analysis/nursing diagnosis:**

1. Prolonged *loss or alteration of physiological processes* related to severe psychological stress and conflict that results in disuse, atrophy, contractures. *Primary gain*—internal conflict or need is kept out of awareness; there is a close relationship in time between stressor and occurrence of symbolic symptoms.

2. *Impaired social interaction:* chronic sick role related to attention seeking.

3. *Noncompliance* with expected routines related to *secondary gain*—avoidance of upsetting situation, with support obtained from others.

4. *Impaired adjustment* related to *repression* of feelings through somatic symptoms, *regression, denial* and *isolation,* and *externalization.*

5. *Ineffective individual coping,* e.g., day-dreaming, fantasizing, superficial warmth and seductiveness related to inability to control symptoms voluntarily or to explain them by known physical disorder.

Hypochondriasis (Hypochondriacal Neurosis)

Exaggerated concern for one's physical health; *unrealistic* interpretation of signs or sensations as abnormal; *preoccupation with fear* of having serious disease, *despite* medical reassurance of no diagnosis of physical disorder.

◆ **A. Assessment:**

1. Preoccupation with symptoms; sweating, peristalsis, heartbeat, coughing, muscular soreness, skin eruptions.

2. Occurs in both men and women in adolescence, 30s, or 40s.

3. History of long, complicated shopping for doctors and refusal of mental health care.

4. *Organ neurosis* may occur (e.g., cardiac neurosis).

5. Personality trait: *compulsive.*

6. Prevalence of anxiety and depression.

7. *Controls* relationships through physical complaints.

◆ **B. Analysis/nursing diagnosis:**

1. *Personal identity disturbance* related to perception of self as ill in order to meet needs for dependency, attention, affection.

2. Displaced *anxiety* related to inability to verbalize feelings.

3. *Fear* related to not being believed.

4. *Powerlessness* related to feelings of insecurity.

5. *Altered role performance:* disruption in work and interpersonal relations related to regression and need gratification through preoccupation with fantasized illness; and related to control over others through physical complaints.

◆ **IV. General nursing care plans/implementation** for somatoform disorders:

A. *Long-term goals:*

1. Develop interests *outside* of self. Introduce to new activities and people.

2. Facilitate experiences of increased feelings of *independence.*

3. Increase *reality perception* and *problem-solving ability.*

4. Emphasize *positive* outlook and promote positive thinking. Reassure that symptoms are anxiety related, not a result of physical disease.

5. Develop mature ways for meeting *affection* needs.

B. *Short-term goals:*

1. *Prevent* anxiety from mounting and becoming uncontrollable by recognizing symptoms, for early intervention.

2. *Environment:* warm, caring, supportive interactions; instill hope that anxiety can be mastered.

3. Encourage client to *express* somatic concerns verbally. Encourage awareness of body processes.

4. Provide *diversional* activities.

5. Develop ability to relax rather than ruminate or worry. Help find palliative relief through anxiety reduction (slower breathing, exercise).

C. *Health teaching:*

1. Relaxation training as self-help measures.

2. Increase knowledge of appropriate and correct information on physiological responses that accompany anxiety.

◆ **V. General evaluation/outcome criteria:**

A. Does not isolate self.

B. Discusses fears, concerns, conflicts that are self-originated and not likely to be serious.

C. Decides which aspects of situation can be overcome and ways to meet conflicting obligations.

D. Looks for things of importance and value.

E. Deliberately engages in new activities other than ruminating or worrying.

F. Talks self out of fears.

G. Decrease in physical symptoms; is able to sleep, feels less restless.

H. Makes fewer statements of feeling helpless.

I. Can freely express angry feelings in *overt* way and not through symptoms.

Other Conditions in Which Psychological Factors Affect Medical Conditions (Psychophysiological Disorders)

This group of disorders occurs in various organs and systems, whereby emotions are expressed by affecting body organs.

I. **Concepts and principles related to psychological factors affecting physical conditions:**
   A. Majority of organs involved are usually under control of *autonomic* nervous system.
   B. Coping mechanisms
      1. *Repression or suppression* of unpleasant emotional experiences.
      2. *Introjection*—illness seen as punishment.
      3. *Projection*—others blamed for illness.
      4. *Conversion*—physical symptoms rather than underlying emotional stresses are emphasized.
   C. Clients often exhibit the following underlying *needs in excess:*
      1. Dependency.
      2. Attention.
      3. Love.
      4. Success.
      5. Recognition.
      6. Security.
   D. Need to distinguish between:
      1. Factitious disorders—deliberate, *conscious* exhibit of physical or psychological illness to avoid an uncomfortable situation.
      2. *Conversion disorder*—affecting *sensory* systems that are usually under *voluntary* control; generally *non–life-threatening;* symptoms are symbolic solution to anxiety; *no* demonstrable *organic* pathology.
      3. *Psychological factors affecting physical condition*—e.g., psychophysiological disorders; under *autonomic* nervous system control; structural *organic* changes; may be life threatening.
   E. A *decrease in emotional security* tends to produce an *increase in symptoms.*

F. When treatment is confined to physical symptoms, emotional problems are *not* usually relieved.

◆ II. **Assessment of physiological factors:**
   A. Persistent psychological factors may produce structural *organic* changes resulting in *chronic diseases*, which may be *life threatening* if untreated.
   B. *All* body systems are affected:
      1. Skin (e.g., pruritus, acne, dermatitis).
      2. Musculoskeletal (e.g., *backache*, muscle cramps, rheumatoid arthritis).
      3. Respiratory (e.g., *asthma*, hiccups, hay fever).
      4. Gastrointestinal (e.g., *ulcers*, ulcerative colitis, irritable bowel syndrome, heartburn, constipation, diarrhea).
      5. Cardiovascular (e.g., cardiospasm, angina, paroxysmal tachycardia, *migraines*, palpitations, hypertension).
      6. Genitourinary (e.g., impotence, enuresis, amenorrhea, dysuria, *dysmenorrhea*).
      7. Endocrine (e.g., hypoglycemia, hyperglycemia, hyperthyroidism).
      8. Nervous system (e.g., general fatigue, anorexia, exhaustion).

◆ III. **Analysis/nursing diagnosis:** *ineffective individual coping* related to inappropriate need-gratification through illness (actual illness used as means of meeting needs for attention and affection). Absence of life experiences that gratify needs for attention and affection.

◆ IV. **Nursing care plan/implementation** in disorders in which psychological factors affect physical conditions:
   A. *Long-term goal: release* of feelings through verbalization.
   B. *Short-term goals:*
      1. Take care of *physical* problems during acute phase.
      2. *Remove* client from anxiety-producing stimuli.
   C. Prompt attention in meeting clients' *basic needs*, to gratify appropriate needs for dependency, attention, and security.
   D. Maintain an attitude of *respect and concern;* clients' pains and worries are very real and upsetting to them; do *not* belittle the symptoms. Do *not* say, "There is nothing wrong with you" because emotions do in fact cause somatic disabilities.
   E. *Treat organic* problems as necessary, but without undue emphasis (i.e., do *not* reinforce preoccupation with bodily complaints).
   F. Help clients *express their feelings*, especially anger, hostility, guilt, resentment, or humiliation, which may be related to such issues as sexual difficulties, family problems, religious conflicts, and job difficulties. Help clients recognize that when stress and anxiety are not released

through some channel such as verbal expression, the body will release the tension through *"organ language."*

G. Provide *outlets* for release of tensions and diversions from preoccupation with physical complaints.

1. Provide social and recreational activities to decrease time for preoccupation with illness.
2. Encourage clients to use physical and intellectual capabilities in constructive ways.

H. *Protect* clients from any disturbing stimuli; help the healing process in the acute phase of illnesses (e.g., myocardial infarct).

I. Help clients feel *in control* of situations and be as independent as possible.

J. Be *supportive;* assist clients to bear painful feelings through a helping relationship.

K. *Health teaching:*

1. Teach how to express feelings.
2. Teach more effective ways of responding to stressful life situations.
3. Teach the family supportive relationships.

◆ **V. Evaluation/outcome criteria:** can verbalize feelings more fully.

Schizophrenia and Other Psychotic Disorders

Schizophrenia is a group of interrelated symptoms with a number of common features involving disorders of *mood, thought content, feelings, perception,* and *behavior.* The term means "splitting of the mind," alluding to the discrepancy between the content of *thought processes* and their emotional expression; this should *not* be confused with "multiple personality" (dissociative reaction).

Half of the clients in mental hospitals are diagnosed as schizophrenic; many more schizophrenics live in the community. The onset of symptoms for this disorder generally occurs between 15 and 27 years of age. Causes, psychodynamics, and psychopathology are still a matter of controversy.

I. Common subtypes of schizophrenia (without clear-cut differentiation):

disorganized type disordered, thinking ("word salad"), *inappropriate affect* (blunted, silly), regressive behavior, incoherent speech, preoccupied and withdrawn.

catatonic type disorder of muscle tension, with rigidity *waxy flexibility, posturing, mutism, violent rage* outbursts, negativism, and frenzied activity. Marked decrease in involvement with environment and in spontaneous movement.

paranoid type disturbed perceptions leading to disturbance in thought content of *persecutory, grandiose,* or hostile nature; *projection* is key mechanism, with religion a common preoccupation.

residual continued difficulty in thinking, mood, perception, and behavior after schizophrenic episode.

undifferentiated type unclassifiable schizophrenic-like disturbance with mixed symptoms of delusions, hallucinations, incoherence, gross disorganization.

II. Concepts and principles related to schizophrenic disorders:

A. *General:*

1. *Symbolic* language used expresses schizophrenic's life, pain, and progress toward health; all symbols used have meaning.
2. *Physical care* provides media for relationship; nurturance may be initial focus.
3. *Consistency, reliability,* and *empathic* understanding build trust.
4. *Denial, regression,* and *projection* are key defense mechanisms.
5. Felt anxiety gives rise to distorted thinking.
6. Attempts to engage in verbal communication may result in tension, apprehensiveness, and defensiveness.
7. Person *rejects real world* of painful experiences and *creates fantasy* world through illness.

B. *Withdrawal:*

1. Withdrawal from and resistance to forming relationships are attempts to reduce anxiety related to:
   a. Loss of ability to experience satisfying human relationships.
   b. Fear of rejection.
   c. Lack of self-confidence.
   d. Need for protection and restraint against potential destructiveness of *hostile* impulses (toward self and others).
2. *Ambivalence* results from need to *approach* a relationship and need to *avoid* it.
   a. Cannot tolerate swift emotional or physical closeness.
   b. Needs more time than usual to establish a relationship; time to test sincerity and interest of nurse.
3. Avoidance of client by others, especially staff, will reinforce withdrawal, thereby creating problem of mutual withdrawal and fear.

C. *Hallucinations:*

1. It is possible to replace hallucinations with satisfying interactions.
2. Person can relearn to focus attention on real things and people.
3. Hallucinations originate during *extreme* emotional stress when unable to cope.
4. Hallucinations are very real to client.
5. Client will react as the situation is perceived, *regardless* of reality or consensus.
6. Concrete experiences, *not* argument or confrontation, will correct sensory distortion.
7. Hallucinations are *substitutes* for human relations.

8. Purposes served by or expressed in falsification of reality:
   a. Reflection of problem in inner life.
   b. Statement of criticism, censure, self-punishment.
   c. Promotion of self-esteem.
   d. Satisfaction of instinctual strivings.
   e. Projection of unacceptable unconscious content in disguised form.
9. Perceptions *not* as *totally* disturbed as they seem.
10. Client attempts to restructure reality through hallucinations to *protect remaining ego integrity.*
11. Hallucinations may result from a variety of psychological and biological conditions (e.g., extreme fatigue, drugs, pyrexia, organic brain disease).
12. Person who hallucinates needs to feel free to describe his or her perceptions if he or she is to be understood by the nurse.

◆ **III. Assessment of schizophrenic disorders:**
A. Eugene Bleuler described four classic and *primary symptoms* as the **"four A's":**
   1. *Associative looseness*—impairment of logical thought progression, resulting in confused, bizarre, and abrupt thinking. *Neologisms*—making up new words or condensing words into one.
   2. *Affect*—exaggerated, apathetic, blunt, flat, inappropriate, inconsistent feeling tone that is communicated through face and body posture.
   3. *Ambivalence*—simultaneous, conflicting feelings or attitudes toward person, object, or situation; *need-fear* dilemma.
      a. Stormy outbursts.
      b. Poor, weak interpersonal relations.
      c. Difficulty even with simple decisions.
   4. *Autism*—*withdrawal* from external world; preoccupation with fantasies and idiosyncratic thoughts.
      a. *Delusions*—false, fixed beliefs, not corrected by logic; a defense against intolerable feeling. The two most common delusions are:
         (1) *Delusions of grandeur*—conviction in a belief related to being famous, important, or wealthy.
         (2) *Delusions of persecution*—belief that one's thoughts, moods, or actions are controlled or influenced by strange forces or by others.
      b. *Hallucinations*—false sensory impressions without observable external stimuli.
         (1) *Auditory*—affecting hearing (e.g., hears voices).
         (2) *Visual*—affecting vision (e.g., sees snakes).
         (3) *Tactile*—affecting touch (e.g., feels electric charges in body).
         (4) *Olfactory*—affecting smell (e.g., smells rotting flesh).
         (5) *Gustatory*—affecting taste (e.g., food tastes like poison).
      c. *Ideas of reference*—clients interpret cues in the environment as having reference to them. Ideas *symbolize guilt, insecurity,* and *alienation;* may become delusions, if severe.
      d. *Depersonalization*—feelings of strangeness and unreality about self or environment or both; difficulty in differentiating boundaries between self and environment.
B. *Regression*—extreme *withdrawal* and social isolation.
C. *Prodromal or residual symptoms:*
   1. Social isolation, *withdrawal.*
   2. Marked impairment in *role* functioning (e.g., as student, employee).
   3. Markedly *peculiar* behavior (e.g., collecting garbage).
   4. Marked impairment in personal *hygiene.*
   5. *Affect:* blunt, inappropriate.
   6. *Speech:* vague, overelaborate, circumstantial, metaphorical.
   7. *Thinking:* bizarre ideation or magical thinking, e.g., ideas of reference, "others can feel my feelings."
   8. Unusual *perceptual* experiences, e.g., sensing the presence of a force or person not physically there.
D. Rule out general medical conditions/substances that may cause psychotic symptoms.
   1. *Neurological* conditions: neoplasms, cardiovascular disease, epilepsy, Huntington's disease, deafness, migraine headaches, CNS infections.
   2. *Endocrine* conditions: hypothyroidism or hyperthyroidism, hypoparathyroidism or hyperparathyroidism, hypoadrenocorticism.
   3. *Metabolic* conditions: hypoxia, hypoglycemia, hypercarbia.
   4. *Autoimmune* disorders: SLE.
   5. *Other conditions:* hepatic or renal disease.
   6. *Substances: drugs of abuse* (alcohol, amphetamines, cannabis, cocaine, hallucinogens, inhalants); anesthetics; chemotherapeutic agents; corticosteroids; *toxins* (nerve gases, carbon monoxide, carbon dioxide, fuel or paint, insecticides).

◆ **IV. Analysis/nursing diagnosis:**
A. *Sensory/perceptual alterations* related to inability to define reality and distinguish the real from the unreal (hallucinations, illusions) and misinterpretation of stimuli, disintegration of ego boundaries.

Mental Health

B. *Altered thought processes* related to intense anxiety and blocking (delusions), ambivalence or conflict.

C. *Risk for violence to self or others* related to fear and distortion of reality.

D. *Altered communication process* with inability to *verbally* express needs and wishes related to difficulty with processing information and unique patterns of speech.

E. *Self-care deficit* with *inappropriate* dress and poor physical hygiene related to perceptual or cognitive impairment or immobility.

F. *Altered feeling states* related to anxiety about others (*inappropriate emotions*).

G. *Altered judgment* related to lack of trust, fear of rejection, and doubts regarding competence of others.

H. *Altered self-concept* related to *feelings of inadequacy* in coping with the real world.

I. *Body-image disturbance* related to inappropriate use of defense mechanisms.

J. *Disorganized behaviors:* impaired relatedness to others, related to withdrawal, distortions of reality, and lack of trust.

K. *Diversional activity deficit* related to personal ambivalence.

◆ **V. Nursing care plan/implementation in schizophrenic disorders:**

A. *General:*

1. Set *short-range* goals, realistic to client's levels of functioning.

2. Use *nonverbal* level of communication to demonstrate concern, caring, and warmth, because client often distrusts words.

3. Set climate for free expression of *feelings* in whatever mode, without fear of retaliation, ridicule, or rejection.

4. Seek client out in his or her own fantasy world.

5. Try to understand meaning of symbolic language; help him or her communicate less symbolically.

6. Provide *distance,* because client needs to feel safe and to observe nurses for sources of threat or promises of security.

7. Help client tolerate nurses' presence and learn to *trust* nurses enough to move out of isolation and share painful and often unacceptable (to client) feelings and thoughts.

8. Anticipate and accept negativism; do *not* personalize.

9. *Avoid* joking, abstract terms, and figures of speech when client's thinking is literal.

10. Give antipsychotic medications.

B. *Withdrawn behavior:*

1. *Long-term goal:* develop satisfying interpersonal relationships.

2. *Short-term goal:* help client feel safe in *one-to-one* relationship.

3. Seek client out at every chance, and establish some bond.

a. Stay with client, in silence.

b. Initiate talk when he or she is ready.

c. Draw out, but do *not* demand, response.

d. Do *not* avoid the client.

4. Use *simple language, specific words.*

5. Use an *object or activity* as medium for relationship; initiate activity.

6. Focus on *everyday* experiences.

7. *Delay* decision making.

8. *Accept one-sided* conversation, with silence from the client; *avoid* pressuring to respond.

9. Accept the client's outward attempts to respond and inappropriate social behavior, without remarks or disdain; teach social skills.

10. *Avoid* making demands on client or exposing client to failure.

11. *Protect* from aggressive persons and from impulsive attacks on self and others.

12. Attend to *nutrition, elimination, exercise,* hygiene, and signs of physical illness.

13. Add structure to the day; tell him or her, "This is your 9 A.M. medication."

14. *Health teaching:* assist family to understand client's needs, to see small sign of progress; teach client to perform simple tasks of self-care to meet own biological needs.

C. *Hallucinatory behavior:*

1. *Long-term goal:* establish satisfying relationships with *real* persons.

2. *Short-term goal:* interrupt *pattern* of hallucinations.

3. Provide a *structured* environment with routine activities. Use *real* objects to keep client's interest or to stimulate new interest (e.g., in painting or crafts).

4. *Protect* against injury to self and others resulting from "voices" client thinks he or she hears.

5. *Short, frequent* contacts initially, increasing social interaction gradually (one person → small groups).

6. Ask person to describe experiences as hallucinations occur.

7. *Respond to anything real* the client says, e.g., with acknowledgment or reflection. Focus more on *feelings,* not on delusional, hallucinatory content.

8. *Distract* client's attention to something real when he or she hallucinates.

9. *Avoid* direct confrontation that voices are coming from client himself or herself; do *not* argue, but listen.

10. *Clarify* who "they" are:

a. Use personal pronouns, *avoid* universal and global pronouns.

b. Nurse's own language must be clear and unambiguous.

11. Use one sentence, ask only one question, at a time.
12. Encourage *consensual validation*. Point out that experience is not shared by you; voice doubt.
13. *Health teaching:*
    a. Recommend more effective ways of coping (e.g., consensual validation).
    b. Advise that highly emotional situations be avoided.
    c. Explain the causes of misperceptions.
    d. Recommend methods for reducing sensory stimulation.

D. *Delusions* (see **IV. Nursing care plan/implementation in paranoid disorders,** p. 385, in following section).

◆ **VI. Evaluation/outcome criteria:**
   A. Small behavioral changes occur (e.g., eye contact, better grooming).
   B. Evidence of beginning trust in nurse (keeping appointments).
   C. Initiates conversation with others; participates in activities.
   D. Decreases amount of time spent alone.
   E. Demonstrates appropriate behavior in public places.
   F. Articulates relationship between feelings of discomfort and autistic behavior.
   G. Makes positive statements.

VII. See sample **Critical Pathway: Client with Schizophrenic Psychosis.**

Delusional (Paranoid) Disorders

Paranoid disorders have a concrete and pervasive delusional system, usually *persecutory*. *Projection* is a chief coping mechanism of this disorder.

I. Concepts and principles related to paranoid disorders:
   A. Delusions are attempts to cope with stresses and problems.
   B. May be a means of allegorical or symbolic communication and of testing others for their trustworthiness.
   C. Interactions with others and activities interrupt delusional thinking.
   D. To establish a rational therapeutic relationship, gross distortions, misorientation, misinterpretation, and misidentification need to be overcome.
   E. Delusional people have extreme need to maintain self-esteem.
   F. False beliefs cannot be changed without first changing experiences.
   G. A delusion is held because it *performs a function.*

H. When people who are experiencing delusions become at ease and comfortable with people, delusions will not be needed.
I. Delusions are misjudgments of reality based on a series of mental mechanisms: (a) *denial,* followed by (b) *projection* and (c) *rationalization.*
J. There is a *kernel of truth* in delusions.
K. Behind the anger and suspicion in a person who is paranoid, there is a *lonely, terrified* person who *feels vulnerable* and *inadequate.*

◆ **II. Assessment** of paranoid disorders:
   A. Chronically *suspicious,* distrustful (thinks "people are out to get me").
   B. Distant, but *not* withdrawn.
   C. Poor insight; blames others (*projects*).
   D. Misinterprets and *distorts reality.*
   E. Difficulty in admitting own errors; takes pride in intelligence and in being correct (superiority).
   F. Maintains false persecutory belief despite evidence or proof (may refuse food and medicine, insisting they are poisoned).
   G. Literal thinking (*rigid*).
   H. Dominating and provocative.
   I. Hypercritical and intolerant of others; *hostile,* quarrelsome, and aggressive.
   J. *Very sensitive* in perceiving minor injustices, errors, and contradictions.
   K. Evasive.

◆ **III. Analysis/nursing diagnosis:**
   A. *Altered thought processes* related to lack of insight, conflict, increased fear and anxiety.
   B. *Severe anxiety* related to projection of threatening, aggressive impulses and misinterpretation of stimuli.
   C. *Ineffective individual coping* (misuse of power and force) related to lack of trust, fear of close human contact.
   D. *Impaired cognitive functioning* related to rigidity of thought.
   E. *Chronic low self-esteem* related to feelings of inadequacy, powerlessness.
   F. *Impaired social interaction* related to lack of tender, kind feelings, feelings of grandiosity or persecution.

◆ **IV. Nursing care plan/implementation** in paranoid disorders:
   A. *Long-term goals:* gain clear, correct perceptions and interpretations through corrective experiences.
   B. *Short-term goals:*
      1. Help client recognize distortions, misinterpretations.
      2. Help client feel safe in exploring reality.
   C. Help client learn to *trust self;* help to develop self-confidence and ego assets through positive reinforcement.

Mental Health

CRITICAL PATHWAY of Care for Client with Schizophrenic Psychosis

Estimated length of stay: 14 days—variations from designated pathway should be documented in progress notes

Nursing Diagnosis and Categories of Care	Time Dimension	Goals/Actions	Time Dimension	Goals/Actions	Time Dimensions	Discharge Outcome
Alteration in thought processes/ sensory-perceptual alteration			Day 7	Client is able to differentiate between what is real and what is not.	Day 14	Client experiences no delusional thinking or hallucinations.
Referrals	Day 1	Psychiatrist Psychologist Social worker Clinical nurse specialist Music therapist Occupational therapist Recreational therapist			Day 14	Discharge with follow-up appointments as required.
Diagnostic studies	Day 1 Day 3–5	Drug screen CT, MRI, PET, EEG (may be ordered to examine structure and function of the brain)				
Additional assessments	Day 1	VS every shift Assess for: ■ Delusions ■ Hallucinations ■ Loose associations ■ Inappropriate affect ■ Excitement/stupor ■ Panic anxiety ■ Suspiciousness	Day 2–14 Day 2–5	Ongoing assessments. Establish trust with at least one person.	Day 2–14 Day 14	VS daily if stable. No evidence of delusions, hallucinations, loose associations, inappropriate affect, excitement/ stupor, panic anxiety, suspiciousness.
Medications	Day 1	Antipsychotic medication (scheduled and prn); may need order for concentrate and injectable form Antiparkinsonian medication prn	Day 1–14	Assess for effectiveness and side effects of medications.	Day 14	Client is discharged with medications.
Client education			Day 7 Day 10	Discuss correlation between increased anxiety and psychotic symptoms. Discuss ways to de-escalate anxiety. Discuss importance of taking medications regularly, even when feeling well.	Day 12–13 Day 14	Reinforce teaching. Client verbalizes understanding information presented before discharge.

CRITICAL PATHWAY of Care for Client with Schizophrenic Psychosis—cont'd

Estimated length of stay: 14 days—variations from designated pathway should be documented in progress notes

Nursing Diagnosis and Categories of Care	Time Dimension	Goals/Actions	Time Dimension	Goals/Actions	Time Dimensions	Discharge Outcome
Client education—cont'd				Discuss possible side effects of medications and when to see the doctor.		
Risk for violence: Self-directed or directed at others	Day 1	Environment safe for client and others	Ongoing	Client does not harm self or others.	Day 14	Client is discharged without harm to self or others.
Referrals	Day 1	Alert hostility management team for the admission of a potentially violent client For relaxation therapy: Music therapist Clinical nurse specialist Stress management specialist Psychiatrist: May give order for mechanical restraints to be used if needed			Day 14	Discharge with follow-up, appointments as required.
Additional assessments	Day 1	Assess for signs of impending violent behaviors: ■ Increase in psychomotor activity ■ Angry affect ■ Verbalized persecutory delusions or frightening hallucinations.	Day 2–14	Ongoing assessments.		
Medications	Day 1	Antipsychotic medications, prn, when signs of agitation begin	Day 1–14	Use of medications, isolation/seclusion, or mechanical restraints. If client refuses medications, administer after application of restraints.	Day 14	Client is discharged with medications.
Client education			Day 3–12	Teach relaxation techniques; discuss activities in which client could participate to relieve pent-up tension Discuss signs and symptoms of escalating anxiety.	Day 12–13 Day 14	Reinforce teaching. Client verbalizes understanding of information presented before discharge.

Source: Townsend, M: Essentials of Psychiatric–Mental Health Nursing. FA Davis, Philadelphia, 1999, pp 756–759.
CT, computed tomography; *EEG*, electroencephalogram; *MRI*, magnetic resonance imaging; *PET*, positron-emission tomography.

Mental Health

D. Help to *trust others.*
1. Be consistent and honest at all times.
2. *Do not whisper, act secretive, or laugh with others* in client's presence when he or she cannot hear what is said.
3. Do *not* mix medicines with food.
4. Keep promises.
5. Let client know ahead of time what he or she can expect from others.
6. Give *reasons* and careful, complete, and *repetitive* explanations.
7. Ask permission to contact others.
8. Consult client first about all decisions concerning him or her.

E. Help to *test reality.*
1. Present and repeat reality of the situation.
2. Do *not* confirm or approve distortions.
3. Help accept responsibility for own behavior rather than project.
4. *Divert* from delusions to reality-centered focus.
5. Let client know when behavior does not seem appropriate.
6. Assume nothing and leave no room for assumptions.
7. *Structure* time and activities to limit delusional thought, behavior.
8. Set limit for *not* discussing delusional content.
9. Look for underlying needs expressed in delusional content.

F. Provide *outlets* for anger and aggressive drives.
1. Listen matter-of-factly to angry outbursts.
2. *Accept* rebuffs and abusive talk as symptoms.
3. *Do not* argue, disagree, or debate.
4. *Allow* expression of negative feelings without fear of punishment.

G. Provide *successful group experience.*
1. *Avoid competitive* sports involving *close physical* contact.
2. Give recognition to skills and work well done.
3. Use *managerial* talents.
4. Respect client's intellect and engage him or her in activities with others requiring *intellect* (e.g., chess, puzzles, Scrabble).

H. *Limit* physical contact.

I. *Health teaching:* teach a more rational basis for deciding whom to trust by identifying behaviors characteristic of trusting and trustworthy people.

◆ **V. Evaluation/outcome criteria:** able to differentiate trustworthy from untrustworthy people; growing self-awareness, and able to share this awareness with others; accepting of others without need to criticize or change them; is open to new experiences; able to delay gratification.

Personality Disorders

Subtypes of personality disorders include *antisocial, histrionic, narcissistic, avoidant,* and *dependent personalities.* A *per-*sonality disorder* is a syndrome in which the person's inner difficulties are revealed through general behaviors and by a pattern of living that seeks *immediate gratification of impulses* and instinctual needs without regard to society's laws, mores, and customs and *without censorship* of personal conscience.

Borderline personality disorder is a subtype in which the client is unstable in many areas: she or he has unstable but intense interpersonal relationships, *impulsive* and unpredictable behavior, wide *mood swings,* chronic feelings of boredom or emptiness, intolerance of being alone, and uncertainty about identity, and is physically *self-damaging.*

I. Concepts and principles related to *antisocial personality disorders:*
A. One defense against severe anxiety is "acting out," or dealing with distressful feelings or issues through action.
B. Faulty or arrested emotional development in preoedipal period has interfered with development of adequate social control or superego.
C. Because there is a malfunctioning or *weakened superego,* there is little internal demand and therefore no tension between ego and superego to evoke guilt feelings.
D. The defect is *not* intellectual; person shows *lack of moral responsibility, inability to control emotions* and impulses, and *deficiency in normal feeling* responses.
E. "Pleasure principle" is dominant.
F. Initial stage of treatment is most crucial; treatment situation is very threatening because it mobilizes client's anxiety, and client ends treatment abruptly. Key underlying emotion: *fear of closeness,* with threat of *exploitation, control,* and *abandonment.*

◆ **II. Assessment** of antisocial personality disorders:
A. Onset *before* age 15.
B. History of behavior that *conflicts with society:* truancy, expulsion, or suspension from school for misconduct; delinquency, thefts, vandalism, running away from home; persistent lying; repeated substance abuse; initiating fights; chronic violation of rules at home or school; school grades below IQ level.
C. Inability to sustain consistent *work* behavior (e.g., frequent job changes or absenteeism).
D. Lack of ability to function as *responsible* parent (evidence of child's malnutrition or illness due to lack of minimal hygiene standards; failure to obtain medical care for seriously ill child; failure to arrange for caretaker when parent is away from home).
E. Failure to accept *social norms* with respect to *lawful* behavior (e.g., thefts, multiple arrests).
F. Inability to maintain enduring *intimate* relationship (e.g., multiple relations, desertion, multiple divorces); lack of respect or loyalty.
G. *Irritability* and *aggressiveness* (spouse, child abuse; repeated physical fights).

H. Failure to honor *financial* obligations.

I. Failure to *plan ahead.*

J. *Disregard for truth* (lying, "conning" others for personal gain).

K. *Recklessness* (driving while intoxicated, recurrent speeding).

L. *Violating* rights of others.

M. Does not appear to profit from experience; *repeats* same punishable or antisocial behavior; usually does not feel guilt or depression.

N. Exhibits *poor judgment;* may have intellectual, but not emotional, insight to guide judgments. Inadequate problem solving and reality testing.

O. Uses *manipulative* behavior patterns in treatment setting (see **VIII. Manipulation,** p. 332).

  1. Demands and controls.

  2. Pressures and coerces, threatens.

  3. Violates rules, routines, procedures.

  4. Requests special privileges.

  5. Betrays confidences and lies.

  6. Ingratiates.

  7. Monopolizes conversation.

◆ III. **Analysis/nursing diagnosis:**

A. *Ineffective individual coping* related to:

  1. Inability to tolerate frustration (altered conduct/impulse processes).

  2. Verbal, nonverbal manipulation *(lying).*

  3. Destructive behavior toward self (e.g., in borderline personality disorder) or others.

  4. Cognitive distortions (e.g., overuse of denial, projection, rationalization, intellectualization, persecutory thoughts).

  5. Inability to learn from experience.

B. *Personal identity disturbance* related to:

  1. *Self-esteem disturbance* as evidenced by grandiosity, depression, extreme mood changes.

  2. Lack of: responsibility, accountability, commitment, tolerance of rejection.

  3. Distancing relationships.

C. *Social intrusiveness* related to fear of real or potential loss.

D. *Noncompliance* related to excess need for independence.

◆ IV. **Nursing care plan/implementation** in personality disorders:

A. *Long-term goal:* help person accept responsibility and consequences of own actions.

B. *Short-term goal: minimize manipulation* and acting out.

C. Set *fair, firm, consistent limits and follow through on consequences* of behavior; let client know what she or he can expect from staff and what the unit's regulations are, as well as the consequences of violations. Be explicit.

D. *Avoid* letting staff be played against one another by a particular client; staff should present a unified approach.

E. Nurses should *control* their *own* feelings of anger and defensiveness aroused by any person's manipulative behavior.

F. Change focus when client persists in raising inappropriate subjects (such as personal life of a nurse).

G. Encourage expression of *feelings* as an alternative to acting out.

H. Aid client in realizing and accepting responsibility for own actions and *social responsibility* to others.

I. Use group therapy as a means of *peer control* and multiple feedback about behavior.

J. *Health teaching:* teach family how to use behavior-modification techniques to reward client's acceptable behavior (i.e., when he or she accepts responsibility for own behavior, is responsive to rights of others, adheres to social and legal norms).

◆ V. **Evaluation/outcome criteria:** less use of lying, blaming others for own behavior; more evidence of following rules; less impulsive, explosive behavior.

Mood Disorders

Mood disorders include (1) *depressive disorders* and (2) *bipolar disorders.* Bipolar disorders are further divided into (a) *manic,* (b) *depressed,* (c) *mixed,* or (d) *cyclothymia.* The mood disturbance may occur in a number of patterns of severity and duration, alone or in combination, where client feels extreme sadness and guilt, withdraws socially, expresses self-deprecatory thoughts *(major depression),* or experiences an elevated, expansive mood with hyperactivity, pressured speech, inflated self-esteem, and decreased need for sleep *(manic episode or disorder).*

Another specific mood disorder is *dysthymic* disorder (depressive neuroses), in which there is a chronic mood disturbance involving a depressed mood or loss of interest and pleasure in all usual activities, but not of sufficient severity or duration to be classified as a *major depressive episode.* Table 6–13 *summarizes* the main points of *difference between the two types of depression.*

These affective disorders should be *distinguished from grief.* Grief is *realistic* and proportionate to what has been *specifically* lost and involves *no loss of self-esteem.* There is a *constant* feeling of sadness over a period of 3–12 mo or longer, with good reality contact (no delusions).

Major Depressive Disorder

I. **Concepts and principles:**

A. Self-limiting factors—most depressions are self-limiting disturbances, making it important to look for a change in functioning and behavior.

B. *Theories of cause of depression:*

  1. Aggression turned inward—*self-anger.*

  2. Response to separation or object *loss.*

  3. *Genetic* or *neurochemical* basis—impaired neurotransmission of monoamine oxidase (MAO); high levels of catecholamines.

TABLE 6–13   Comparison of the Two Different Types of Depressive Disorders

Dimension	Major Depressive Disorder—Melancholic Type	Dysthymic Disorder
Cause	Primary disturbance in structure and function of brain and nervous system	Severe, prolonged stress, unresolved conflicts; chronic anxiety, fears, anger
Onset	Rapid and *without* apparent cause	Gradual
Form of depression	Restlessness and agitation, *or* psychomotor retardation; severe; tends to be *worse in morning* and better in evening	Mixed; mild to severe; unpredictable mood; usually optimistic in morning and *depressed in evening*
Sleep	Insomnia after being awakened; early-morning awakening	Easily awakened, but goes back to deep sleep in morning
Appetite	Anorexia leading to weight *loss*	Varied (anorexia leading to compulsive eating)
Activity	Chronically tired; needs structure at all times	Occasional energy bursts (feels embarrassed at lack of energy)
Self-esteem	Very low	Fluctuates from high to low
Fears	Intense fear of being alone	Multiple fears about present and future
Decision making	Totally indecisive	OK on minor decisions; indecisive on important decisions
Memory	Poor	Unreliable
Contact with reality	Poor; paranoid, self-deprecatory delusions, distorted judgment	Varies

4. *Cognitive*—negative mind-set of hopelessness toward self, world, future; overgeneralizes; focuses on single detail rather than whole picture; draws conclusions on inadequate evidence.
5. *Personality*—negative self-concept, low self-esteem affect belief system and appraisal of stressors; ambivalence, guilt, feeling of failure.
6. *Learned helplessness*—dependency; environment cannot be controlled; powerlessness.
7. *Behavioral*—loss of positive reinforcement; lack of support system.
8. *Integrated*—interaction of chemical, experiential, and behavioral variables acting on diencephalon.

◆ **II. General assessment:**
   A. *Physical:* early-morning awakening, *insomnia* at night, increased need for sleep during the day, fatigue, constipation, *anorexia* with weight loss, loss of sexual interest, *psychomotor retardation,* physical complaints, amenorrhea.
   B. *Psychological:* inability to remember, decreased *concentration,* slowing or blocking of thought, all-or-nothing thinking, *less interest in* and involvement with external world and own appearance, feeling worse at certain times of day or after any sleep, difficulty in enjoying activities, monotonous voice, *repetitive* discussions, *inability to make decisions* due to ambivalence, impaired coping with "practical problems."
   C. *Emotional:* loss of self-esteem, feelings of *hopelessness* and *worthlessness,* shame and self-derogation due to *guilt, irritability,* despair and *futility* (leading to *suicidal* thoughts), alienation,

helplessness, passivity, avoidance, *inertia,* powerlessness, denied anger; uncooperative, tense, crying, demanding, and *dependent* behavior.

◆ **III. Analysis/nursing diagnosis:**
   A. *Risk for violence* toward self (suicide) related to inability to verbalize emotions.
   B. *Sleep pattern disturbance* (insomnia or excessive sleep) related to unresolved fears and anxieties, biochemical alterations (decreased serotonin).
   C. *Impaired social interaction/social isolation/withdrawal* related to decreased energy/inertia, inadequate personal resources, absence of significant purpose in life.
   D. *Altered nutrition* (anorexia) related to lack of interest in food.
   E. *Self-care deficit* related to disinterest in activities of daily living.
   F. *Chronic low self-esteem* with self-reproaches and blame related to feelings of inadequacy.
   G. *Altered feeling states and meaning patterns* (sadness, loneliness, apathy) related to overwhelming feeling of unworthiness, hopelessness, and *dysfunctional grieving.*

◆ **IV. Nursing care plan/implementation:**
   A. Promote sleep and food intake: take nursing measures to ensure the *physical* well-being of the client.
   B. Provide steady company to assess *suicidal* tendencies and to diminish feelings of loneliness and alienation.
      1. Build trust in a one-to-one relationship.
      2. Interact with client on a nonverbal level if that is his or her immediate mode of commu-

nication; this will promote feelings of being recognized, accepted, and understood.

3. Focus on *today,* not the past or far into the future.

4. Reassure that present state is temporary and that he or she will be protected and helped.

C. Make the *environment* nonchallenging and non-threatening.

1. Use a kind, firm attitude, with warmth.

2. See that client has favorite foods; respond to other wishes and likes.

3. Protect from overstimulation and coercion.

D. Postpone client's *decision making* and resumption of duties.

1. Allow *more time* than usual to complete activity (dressing, eating) or thought process and speech.

2. Structure the environment for client to help reestablish a set schedule and predictable *routine* during ambivalence and problems with decisions.

E. *Provide nonintellectual activities* (e.g., sanding wood); *avoid* activities such as chess and crossword puzzles, because thinking capacity at this time tends to be circular.

F. Encourage expression of emotions, denial, hopelessness, helplessness, guilt, regret; provide *outlets for anger* that may be underlying the depression; as client becomes more verbal with anger and recognizes the origin and results of anger, help client resolve feelings—allow client to complain and be *demanding* in initial phases of depression.

G. Discourage *redundancy in speech and thought:* redirect focus from a monologue of painful recounts to an appraisal of more neutral or positive attributes and aspects of situations.

H. Encourage client to *assess own* goals, unrealistic expectations, and perfectionist tendencies.

1. May need to change goals or give up some goals that are incompatible with abilities and external situations.

2. Assist client to recapture what was lost through substitution of goals, sublimation, or relinquishment of unrealistic goals—reanchor client's self-respect to other aspects of his or her existence; help him or her free self from *dependency* on one person or single event or idea.

I. Indicate that success is possible and not hopeless.

1. Explore what steps client has taken to achieve goals and suggest new or alternative ones.

2. Set *small, immediate goals* to help attain mastery.

3. Recognize client's efforts to mobilize self.

4. Provide positive reinforcement for client through exposure to activities in which client can experience a sense of *success, achievement, and completion* to build *self-esteem* and self-confidence.

5. Help client experience *pleasure;* help client start good relationships in social setting.

J. *Long-term goal:* to encourage interest in external surroundings, outside of self, to increase and strengthen social relationships.

1. Encourage purposeful activities.

2. Let client advance to activities at own pace (graded task assignments).

3. Gradually encourage activities with others.

K. *Health teaching:* explain need to recognize highly stressful situation and fatigue as stress factor; advise that negative responses from others be regarded with minimum significance; explain need to maintain positive self-attitude; advise occasional respite from responsibilities; emphasize need for realistic expectation of others.

◆ **V. Evaluation/outcome criteria:** performs self-care; expresses increased self-confidence; engages in activities with others; accepts positive statements from others; identifies positive attributes and skills in self.

VI. See sample **Critical Pathway: Depressed Client.**

Bipolar Disorders

Bipolar disorders are major emotional illnesses characterized by mood swings, alternating from depression to elation, with periods of relative normality between episodes. Most persons experience a *single* episode of manic or depressed type; some have *recurrent* depression or recurrent mania or *mixed.* There is increasing evidence that a biochemical disturbance may exist and that most individuals with manic episodes eventually develop depressive episodes.

I. Concepts and principles related to bipolar disorders:

A. The psychodynamics of manic and depressive episodes are related to hostility and guilt.

B. The struggle between unconscious impulses and moral conscience produces feelings of *hostility, guilt,* and *anxiety.*

C. To relieve the internal discomfort of these reactions, the person *projects* long-retained hostile feelings onto others or onto objects in the environment during *manic* phase; during *depressive* phase, hostility and guilt are *introjected* toward self.

D. Demands, irritability, sarcasm, profanity, destructiveness, and threats are signs of the *projection of hostility;* guilt is handled through *persecutory delusions and accusations.*

E. Feelings of inferiority and fear of rejection are handled by being light and amusing.

F. Both phases, though appearing distinctly different, have the *same objective: to gain attention, approval, and emotional support.* These objectives and behaviors are unconsciously determined by the client; this behavior may be either biochemically determined or *both biochemically* and *unconsciously* determined.

CRITICAL PATHWAY of Care for the Depressed Client

Estimated length of stay: 14 days—variations from designated pathway should be documented in progress notes

Nursing Diagnosis and Categories of Care	Time Dimension	Goals/Actions	Time Dimension	Goals/Actions	Time Dimensions	Discharge Outcome
Risk for self-directed violence	Day 1	Environment safe for client	Ongoing	Client does not harm self.	Day 14	Client is discharged without harm to self.
Referrals	Day 1	Psychiatrist: May give order to isolate if risk is great or may do ECT For relaxation therapy: Music therapist Clinical nurse specialist Stress management specialist			Day 14	Discharge with follow-up appointments required.
Additional assessments	Day 1	Suicidal assessment: ■ Ideation ■ Gestures ■ Threats ■ Plan ■ Means ■ Anxiety level ■ Thought disorder	Day 2–14	Ongoing assessments.	Day 14	Client discharged. Denies suicidal ideations.
	Day 1	Secure no-suicide contract				
Medications	Day 1	Antidepressant medication, as ordered Antianxiety agents, prn	Day 1–14	Assess for effectiveness and side effects of medications. Be alert for sudden lifts in mood.	Day 14	Discharged with antidepressant medications.
Client education	Day 3–12	Teach relaxation techniques Discuss resources outside the hospital from whom client may seek assistance when feeling suicidal	Day 12–13	Reinforce teaching.	Day 14	Discharge with understanding of instruction given.
Dysfunctional grieving	Day 1	Assess stage of fixation in grief process			Day 14	Discharge with evidence of progression toward resolution of grief.
Referrals	Day 1	Psychiatrist Psychologist Social worker Clinical nurse specialist Music therapist Occupational therapist Recreational therapist Chaplain			Day 14	Discharge with follow-up appointments required.

Estimated length of stay: 14 days—variations from designated pathway should be documented in progress notes

Nursing Diagnosis and Categories of Care	Time Dimension	Goals/Actions	Time Dimension	Goals/Actions	Time Dimensions	Discharge Outcome
Diagnostic studies	Day 1 Day 2–3	Any of the following tests *may* be ordered: ■ Drug screen ■ Urine test for norepinephrine and serotonin ■ Dexamethasone suppression test ■ A measure of TSH response to administered TRH ■ Serum and urine studies for nutritional deficiencies				
Medications	Day 1	Antidepressant medication, as ordered Antianxiety agent, prn	Day 1–14	Assess for effectiveness and side effects of medications.	Day 14	Client is discharged with medications.
Diet	Day 1	If antidepressant medication is MAO inhibitor: *low tyramine*			Day 14	Client has experienced no symptoms of hypertensive crisis.
Additional assessments	Day 1	VS every shift Assess: ■ Mental status ■ Mood, affect ■ Thought disorder ■ Communication patterns ■ Level of interest in environment ■ Participation in activities ■ Weight	Day 2–14	VS daily if stable. Ongoing assessments.	Day 14	Mood and affect appropriate. No evidence of thought disorder. Participates willingly and appropriately in activities.
Client education	Day 1	Orient to unit	Day 8 Day 12–13	Discuss importance of taking medications regularly even when feeling well or if feeling medication is not helping. Discuss possible side effects of medication and when to see the physician. Teach which foods to eliminate from diet if taking MAO inhibitor. Reinforce teaching.	Day 14	Client is discharged. Verbalizes understanding of information presented before discharge.

Source: Townsend, M: Essentials of Psychiatric–Mental Health Nursing. FA Davis, Philadelphia, 1999, pp 760-763.

Mental Health

◆ **II. Assessment** of bipolar disorders:

A. Manic and depressed types are *opposite* sides of the *same* disorder.

1. Both are disturbances of mood and self-esteem.
2. Both have underlying aggression and hostility.
3. Both are intense.
4. Both are self-limited in duration.

B. Comparison of behaviors associated with mania and depression: see Table 6–14.

◆ **III. Analysis/nursing diagnosis:**

A. *Risk for violence directed at others/self* related to poor judgment, impulsiveness, irritability, manic excitement.

B. *Altered nutrition, less than body requirements,* related to inability to sit down long enough to eat, metabolic expenditures.

C. *Sleep pattern disturbance:* lack of sleep and rest related to restlessness, hyperactivity, emotional dysfunctioning, lack of recognition of fatigue.

D. *Self-care deficits* related to altered motor behavior due to anxiety.

E. *Sensory/perceptual alterations (overload)* related to endogenous chemical alteration, sleep deprivation.

F. *Altered feeling state* (anger), *judgment, thought content* (magical thinking), *thought processes* (altered concentration and problem solving) related to disturbance in self-concept.

G. *Altered feeling processes* (mood swings).

H. *Altered attention:* hyperalertness.

I. *Impaired social interaction* related to internal and external stimuli (overload, underload).

◆ **IV. Nursing care plan/implementation:**

A. *Manic:*

1. Prevent *physical* dangers stemming from suicide and exhaustion—promote rest, sleep, and intake of nourishment.

   a. Use *suicide* precautions.

   b. Reduce outside stimuli or remove to quieter area.

   c. *Diet:* provide *high-calorie beverages, finger foods within sight and reach.*

2. Attend to client's personal care.

3. Absorb with understanding and without reproach behaviors such as talkativeness, provocativeness, criticism, sarcasm, dominance, profanity, and dramatic actions.

   a. Allow, postpone, or partially fulfill demands and freedom of expression *within limits* of ordinary social rules, comfort, and safety of client and others.

   b. Do *not* cut off manic stream of talk, because this increases anxiety and need for release of hostility.

4. Constructively utilize excessive energies with *activities* that do *not* call for concentration or follow-through.

   a. Outdoor walks, gardening, putting, and ball tossing are therapeutic.

   b. Exciting, disturbing, and highly *competitive* activities should be *avoided.*

   c. Creative occupational therapy activities promote release of hostile impulses, as does creative writing.

5. Give tranquilizers as ordered until lithium affects symptoms *(3 wk);* then give lithium carbonate as ordered.

TABLE 6–14 Behaviors Associated with Mania and Depression

Mania (Periods of Predominantly and Persistently Elevated, Expansive, or Irritable Mood)	Depression (Loss of Interest or Pleasure in Usual Activities)
Affect	
Lack of shame or guilt; inflated self-esteem; euphoria; intolerance of criticism	Anger, anxiety, apathy, denial, delusions of guilt, helplessness, feelings of doom, hopelessness, loneliness, low self-esteem (self-degradation)
Physiology	
Insomnia; inadequate nutrition, weight loss	Insomnia; anorexia, constipation, indigestion, nausea, vomiting → weight loss
Cognition	
Denial of realistic danger *Thoughts:* flight of ideas, loose associations; illusions, delusions of grandeur; lack of judgment; distractibility	Ambivalence, confusion, inability to concentrate, self-blame; loss of interest and motivation; self-destructive (preoccupied with suicide)
Behavior	
Hyperactivity (social, sexual, work) → irrationality, aggressiveness, sarcasm, exhibitionism, and acting out in behavior and dress Hostile, arrogant, argumentative, demanding, and controlling *Speech:* rapid, rhyming, punning, witty, pressured	Altered activity level, social isolation, substance abuse, overdependency, underachievement, inability to care for self, *psychomotor retardation*

6. Help client to recognize and express *feelings* (denial, hopelessness, anger, guilt, blame, helplessness).
7. Encourage realistic self-concept.
8. *Health teaching:* how to monitor effects of lithium; instructions regarding salt intake.

B. *Depressed:*

1. Take routine *suicide* precautions.
2. Give attention to *physical* needs for food and sleep and to hygiene needs. Prepare warm baths and hot beverages to aid sleep.
3. Initiate *frequent* contacts:
   a. *Do not allow long periods of silence* to develop or client to remain withdrawn.
   b. Use a kind, understanding, but emotionally neutral approach.
4. *Allow dependency* in severe depressive phase. Because dependency is one of the underlying concerns with depressive persons, if nurse allows dependency to occur as an initial response, he or she must plan for resolution of the dependency toward himself or herself as an example for the client's other dependent relationships.

5. Slowly repeat simple, direct information.
6. *Assist in daily decision making* until client regains self-confidence.
7. Select *mild* exercise and diversionary *activities* instead of stimulating exercise and competitive games, because they may overtax physical and emotional endurance and lead to feelings of inadequacy and frustration.
8. Give antidepressive drugs.
9. *Health teaching:* how to make simple decisions related to health care.

◆ **V. Evaluation/outcome criteria:**

A. *Manic:* speech and activity are slowed down; affect is less hostile; able to sleep; able to eat with others at the table.

B. *Depressed:* takes prescribed medications regularly. Does not engage in self-destructive activities. Able to express feelings of anger, helplessness, hopelessness.

VI. See sample **Critical Pathway: Client Experiencing Manic Episode.**

Mental Health

Mental Health

CRITICAL PATHWAY of Care for the Client Experiencing a Manic Episode

Estimated length of stay: 14 days—variations from designated pathway should be documented in progress notes

Nursing Diagnosis and Categories of Care	Time Dimension	Goals/Actions	Time Dimension	Goals/Actions	Time Dimensions	Discharge Outcome
Risk for injury/ violence	Day 1	Environment is made safe for client and others.	Ongoing	Client does not harm self or others.	Day 14	Client has not harmed self or others.
Referrals	Day 1	Psychiatrist Clinical nurse specialist Internist (may need to determine if symptoms are caused by other illness or medication side effects) Neurologist (may want to check for brain lesion) Alert hostility management team			Day 14	Discharge with follow-up appointments as required.
Diagnostic studies	Day 1	Drug screen Electrolytes Lithium level	Day 5 Day 10	Lithium level. Lithium level.	Day 14	Lithium level and discharge with instructions to return monthly to have level drawn.
Additional assessments	Day 1 Ongoing Ongoing	VS q4h Restraints prn Assess for signs of impending violent behavior: ▪ Increase in psychomotor activity ▪ Angry affect ▪ Verbalized persecutory delusions or frightening hallucinations	Day 2–14	Ongoing assessments.		
Medications	Day 1	Antipsychotic medications, scheduled and prn Lithium carbonate, 600 mg tid or qid	Day 2–14	Administer medications as ordered and observe for effectiveness and side effects.	Day 14	Client is discharged on maintenance dose of lithium carbonate.
Client education			Day 9 Day 12	Teach about lithium: Continue to take medication even when feeling okay. Teach symptoms of toxicity. Emphasize importance of monthly blood levels. Reinforce teaching.	Day 14	Client is discharged with written instructions and verbalizes understanding of material presented.
Altered nutrition: less than body requirements					Day 14	Nutritional condition and weight have stabilized.

CRITICAL PATHWAY   of Care for the Client Experiencing a Manic Episode—cont'd

Estimated length of stay: 14 days—variations from designated pathway should be documented in progress notes

Nursing Diagnosis and Categories of Care	Time Dimension	Goals/Actions	Time Dimension	Goals/Actions	Time Dimensions	Discharge Outcome
Referrals	Day 1	Consult dietitian	Day 1–14	Fulfill nutritional needs.		
Diet	Day 1	High-*protein*, high-*calorie*, nutritious *finger* foods; juice and snacks as tolerated	As mania subsides	Regular diet with foods of client's choice.		
Diagnostic studies	Day 1	Chemistry profile Urinalysis	Day 2–13	Repeat of selected diagnostic studies as required.		
Additional assessments	Day 1–14	Weight I&O Skin turgor Color of mucous membranes				
Medications	Day 1–14	Multiple vitamin/ mineral tablet				
Client education			Day 9	Principles of nutrition, foods for maintenance of wellness, adequate sodium, 6–8 glasses of water per day. Contact dietitian if weight gain becomes a problem.	Day 12–14	Client demonstrates ability to select appropriate foods for healthy diet and verbalizes understanding of material presented.
			Day 12	Reinforce teaching.		

Source: Townsend, M: Essentials of Psychiatric–Mental Health Nursing. FA Davis, Philadelphia, 1999, pp 764–767.

Mental Health

TREATMENT MODES

Milieu Therapy

Milieu therapy consists of treatment by means of controlled modification of the client's environment to promote positive living experiences.

I. Concepts and principles related to milieu therapy:
  A. Everything that happens to clients from the time they are admitted to the hospital or treatment setting has a potential that is either therapeutic or antitherapeutic.
    1. Not only the therapists but all who come in contact with the clients in the treatment setting are important to the clients' recovery.
    2. Emphasis is on the social, economic, and cultural dimension, the interpersonal climate, and the physical environment.
  B. Clients have the right, privilege, and responsibility to make decisions about daily living activities in the treatment setting.

II. Characteristics of milieu therapy:
  A. Friendly, warm, trusting, secure, supportive, comforting atmosphere throughout the unit.
  B. An optimistic attitude about prognosis of illness.
  C. Attention to comfort, food, and daily living needs; help with resolving difficulties related to tasks of daily living.
  D. Opportunity for clients to take responsibility for themselves and for the welfare of the unit in gradual steps.
    1. Client government.
    2. Client-planned and client-directed social activities.
  E. Maximum individualization in dealing with clients, especially regarding treatment and privileges in accordance with clients' needs.
  F. Opportunity to live through and test out situations in a realistic way by providing a setting that is a microcosm of the larger world outside.
  G. Opportunity to discuss interpersonal relationships in the unit among clients and between clients and staff (decreased social distance between staff and clients).
  H. Program of carefully selected resocialization activities to prevent regression.

◆ **III. Nursing care plan/implementation** in milieu therapy:
  A. *New structured relationships*—allow clients to develop new abilities and use past skills; support them through new experiences as needed; help build liaisons with others; set limits; help clients modify destructive behavior; encourage group solutions to daily living problems.

  B. *Managerial*—inform clients about expectations; preserve orderliness of events.
  C. *Environmental manipulation*—regulate the outside environment to alter daily surroundings.
    1. Geographically move clients to units more conducive to their needs.
    2. Work with families, clergy, employers, etc.
    3. Control visitors for the benefit of the client.
  D. *Team approach* uses the milieu to meet each client's needs.

◆ **IV. Evaluation/outcomes criteria:**
  A. *Physical dimension:* order, organization.
  B. *Social dimension:* clarity of expectations, practical orientation.
  C. *Emotional dimension:* involvement, support, responsibility, openness, valuing, accepting.

Behavior Modification

Behavior modification is a therapeutic approach involving the application of learning principles so as to change maladaptive behavior.

I. Definitions:
  conditioned avoidance (also *aversion therapy*) a technique whereby there is a purposeful and systematic production of strongly unpleasant responses in situations to which the client has been previously attracted but now wishes to avoid.
  desensitization frequent exposure in small but gradually increasing doses of anxiety-evoking stimuli until undesirable behavior disappears or is lessened (as in phobias).
  token economy desired behavior is reinforced by rewards, such as candy, money, and verbal approval, used as tokens.
  operant conditioning a method designed to elicit and reinforce desirable behavior (especially useful in mental retardation).
  positive reinforcement giving rewards to elicit or strengthen selected behavior or behaviors.

II. Objectives and process of treatment in behavior modification:
  A. Emphasis is on changing unacceptable, overt, and observable behavior to that which is acceptable; emphasis is on changed way of *acting* first, not of thinking.
  B. Mental health team determines behavior to change and treatment plan to use.
  C. Therapy is based on the knowledge and application of *learning* principles, that is, *stimulus-response;* the unlearning, or *extinction,* of undesirable behavior; and the *reinforcement* of desirable behavior.
  D. Therapist identifies what events are important in the life history of the client and arranges situa-

tions in which the client is therapeutically confronted with them.

E. Two primary aspects of behavior modification:
1. *Eliminate* unwanted behavior by *negative reinforcement* (removal of an aversive stimulus, which acts to reinforce the behavior) and *ignoring* (withholding positive reinforcement).
2. *Create* acceptable new responses to an environmental stimulus by *positive* reinforcement.

F. Useful with: disturbed children, rape victims, dependent and manipulative behaviors, eating disorders, obsessive-compulsive disorders, sexual dysfunction.

III. Assumptions of behavioral therapy:
A. Behavior is what an organism does.
B. Behavior can be observed, described, and recorded.
C. It is possible to predict the conditions under which the same behavior may recur.
D. Undesirable social behavior is not a symptom of mental illness but is behavior that can be modified.
E. Undesirable behaviors are learned disorders that relate to acute anxiety in a given situation.
F. Maladaptive behavior is learned in the same way as adaptive behavior.
G. People tend to behave in ways that "pay off."
H. *Three ways* in which behavior can be reinforced:
1. *Positive* reinforcer (adding something pleasurable).
2. *Negative* reinforcer (removing something unpleasant).
3. *Adverse* stimuli (punishing).
I. If an undesired behavior is ignored, it will be extinguished.
J. Learning process is the same for all; therefore, all conditions (except organic) are accepted for treatment.

◆ **IV. Nursing care plan/implementation** in behavior modification:
A. Find out what is a "reward" for the person.
B. Break the goal down into small, successive *steps.*
C. Maintain *close* and continual observation of the selected behavior or behaviors.
D. Be *consistent* with on-the-spot, immediate intervention and correction of undesirable behavior.
E. Record focused observations of behavior frequently.
F. Participate in close teamwork with the *entire* staff.
G. Evaluate procedures and results continually.
H. *Health teaching:* teach preceding steps to colleagues and family.

◆ **V. Evaluation/outcome criteria:** acceptable behavior is increased and maintained; undesirable behavior is decreased or eliminated.

ACTIVITY THERAPY

Activity therapy consists of a variety of recreational and vocational activities (recreational therapy [RT]; occupational therapy [OT]; and music, art, and dance therapy) designed to test and examine social skills and serve as adjunctive therapies.

I. Concepts and principles related to activity therapy:
A. Socialization counters the regressive aspects of illness.
B. Activities must be selected for specific psychosocial reasons to achieve specific effects.
C. Nonverbal means of expression as an additional behavioral outlet add a new dimension to treatment.
D. Sublimation of sexual drives is possible through activities.
E. Indications for activity therapy: clients with *low self-esteem* who are socially *unresponsive.*

II. Characteristics of activity therapy:
A. Usually planned and coordinated by other team members, such as the recreational therapists or music therapists.
B. Goals:
1. Encourage socialization in community and social activities.
2. Provide pleasurable activities.
3. Help client release tensions and express feelings.
4. Teach new skills; help client find new hobbies.
5. Offer graded series of experiences, from passive spectator role and vicarious experiences to more direct and active experiences.
6. Free or strengthen physical and creative abilities.
7. Increase self-esteem.

◆ **III. Nursing care plan/implementation** in activity therapy:
A. Encourage, support, and cooperate in client's participation in activities planned by the adjunct therapists.
B. Share knowledge of client's illness, talents, interests, and abilities with others on the team.
C. *Health teaching:* teach client necessary skills for each activity (e.g., sports, games, crafts).

◆ **IV. Evaluation/outcome criteria:** client develops occupational and leisure-time skills that will help provide a smoother transition back to the community.

Group Therapy

Group therapy is a treatment modality in which two or more clients and one or more therapists interact in a helping process to relieve emotional difficulties, increase self-esteem and insight, and improve behavior in relations with others.

I. Concepts and principles related to group therapy:
  A. People's problems usually occur in a social setting; thus they can best be evaluated and corrected in a social setting (see Table 6–15 for summary of curative factors).
  B. *Not* all are amenable to group therapies. For example:
    1. Brain damaged.
    2. Acutely suicidal.
    3. Acutely psychotic.
    4. Persons with very passive-dependent behavior patterns.
    5. Acutely manic.
  C. It is best to match group members for *complementarity in behaviors* (verbal with nonverbal, withdrawn with outgoing) but for *similarity in problems* (obesity, predischarge group, cancer patients, prenatal group) to facilitate empathy in the sharing of experiences and to heighten group identification and cohesiveness.
  D. Feelings of *acceptance*, belonging, respect, and comfort develop in the group and facilitate change and health.
  E. In a group, members can *test reality* by giving and receiving *feedback*.
  F. Clients have a chance to experience in the group that they are not alone (concept of *universality*).
  G. Expression and *ventilation* of strong emotional feelings (anger, anxiety, fear, and guilt) in the safe setting of a group is an important aspect of the group process aimed at health and change.
  H. The group setting and the *interactions* of its members may provide *corrective emotional experiences* for its members. A key mechanism operating in groups is *transference* (strong emotional attachment of one member to another member, to the therapist, or to the entire group).
  I. To the degree that people modify their behavior through corrective experiences and identification with others rather than through personal-insight analysis, group therapy may be of special advantage over individual therapy, in that the possible number of interactions is greater in the group and the patterns of behavior are more readily observable.
  J. There is a higher client-to-staff ratio, and it is thus less expensive.

II. General group goals:
  A. Provide opportunity for self-expression of ideas and feelings.
  B. Provide a setting for a variety of relationships through group interaction.
  C. Explore current behavioral patterns with others and observe dynamics.
  D. Provide peer and therapist support and source of strength for the individuals to modify present behavior and try out new behaviors; made possible through development of identity and group identification.
  E. Provide on-the-spot, multiple feedback (i.e., incorporate others' reactions to behavior), as well as give feedback to others.
  F. Resolve dynamics and provide insight.

◆ **III. Nursing care plan/implementation** in group setting:
  A. Nurses need to fill different roles and functions in the group, depending on the type of group, its size, its aims, and the stage in the group's life cycle. The multifaceted roles may include:
    1. Catalyst.

TABLE 6–15 Curative Factors of Group Therapy

Factor	Definition
Instilling of hope	Imbuing the client with optimism for the success of the group therapy experience.
Universality	Disconfirming the client's sense of aloneness or uniqueness in misery or hurt.
Imparting of information	Giving didactic instruction, advice, or suggestions.
Altruism	Finding that the client can be of importance to others; having something of value to give.
Corrective recapitulation of the primary family group	Reviewing and correctively reliving early familial conflicts and growth-inhibiting relationships.
Development of socializing techniques	Acquiring sophisticated social skills, such as being attuned to process, resolving conflicts, and being facilitative toward others.
Imitative behavior	Trying out bits and pieces of the behavior of others and experimenting with those that fit well.
Interpersonal learning	Learning that the client is the author of his or her interpersonal world and moving to alter it.
Group cohesiveness	Being attracted to the group and the other members with a sense of "we"-ness rather than "I"-ness.
Catharsis	Being able to express feelings.
Existential factors	Being able to "be" with others; to be a part of a group.

Source: Adapted from Wilson, HS, and Kneisl, CR: Psychiatric Nursing, ed. 3. Addison-Wesley, Redwood City, Calif., 1988.

2. Transference object (of patient's positive or negative feelings)
3. Clarifier.
4. Interpreter of "here and now."
5. Role model and resource person.
6. Supporter.

B. During the *first sessions,* explain the purpose of the group, go over the "contract" (structure, format, and goals of sessions), and facilitate introductions of group members.

C. In *subsequent sessions,* promote greater group cohesiveness.
1. Focus on *group concerns* and group process rather than on intrapsychic dynamics of individuals.
2. Demonstrate nonjudgmental acceptance of behaviors within the limits of the group contract.
3. Help group members handle their anxiety, especially during the initial phase.
4. Encourage silent members to interact at their level of comfort.
5. Encourage members to interact verbally without dominating the group discussion.
6. Keep the focus of discussion on related themes; *set limits and interpret group rules.*
7. Facilitate sharing and *communication* among members.
8. Provide *support* to members as they attempt to work through anxiety-provoking ideas and feelings.
9. Set the expectation that the members are to take responsibility for carrying the group discussion and exploring issues on their own.

D. *Termination phase:*
1. Make early preparation for group termination (end point should be announced at the first meeting).
2. Anticipate common reactions from group members to separation anxiety and help each member to work through these reactions:
   a. Anger.
   b. Acting-out.
   c. Regressive behavior.
   d. Repression.
   e. Feelings of abandonment.
   f. Sadness.

◆ IV. **Evaluation/outcome criteria:**
A. *Physical:* shows improvement in daily life activities (eating, rest, work, exercise, recreation).
B. *Emotional:* asks for and accepts feedback; states feels good about self and others.
C. *Intellectual:* is reality-oriented; greater awareness of self, others, environment.
D. *Social:* willing to take a risk in trusting others; sharing self; reaching out to others.

Reality Orientation and Resocialization

See Table 6–16 for differences between these two modes therapy.

Mental Health

TABLE 6–16   Differences Between Reality Orientation and Resocialization

Reality Orientation	Resocialization
1. Maximum use of assets.	1. Reality living situation in a community.
2. Structured.	2. Unstructured.
3. Refreshments *may* be served.	3. Refreshments served.
4. Constant reminders of who the clients are, where they are, and why and what is expected of them.	4. Reliving happy experiences; encouragement to participate in home activities.
5. *Group size:* 3–5, depending on degree and level of confusion or disorientation.	5. *Group size:* 5–17, depending on mental and physical capabilities.
6. *Meetings:* 30 minutes daily, same time and place.	6. *Meetings:* 3 times per week for 30 minutes to 1 hour.
7. Planned topics: reality-centered objects.	7. *No* planned topic; group-centered feelings.
8. *Role of leader:* eliciting response of participants.	8. *Role of leader:* clarification and interpretation.
9. Periodic reality-orientation test of participants' level of confusion.	9. Periodic progress note of participants' enjoyment and improvements.
10. *Emphasis:* time, place, person orientation.	10. Any topic freely discussed.
11. Use of mind function still intact.	11. Rely on memories and experiences.
12. Participant is greeted *by name,* thanked for coming, extended a handshake or other physical contact.	12. Participant greeted on arrival, thanked, extended a handshake on leaving.
13. Conducted by trained aides and activity assistants.	13. Conducted by RN, LPN/LVN, aides, program assistants.

Source: Adapted, with permission, from the classic article by Barns, E, Sack, A, and Shore, H: *Gerontologist* 13:513, 1973.

Family Therapy

Family therapy is a process, method, and technique of psychotherapy in which the focus is not on an individual but the total family as an interactional system. See also Major Theoretical Models, p. 299.

I. Developmental tasks of North American family (Duvall, 1971):

   A. *Physical maintenance*—provide food, shelter, clothing, health care.

   B. *Resource allocation* (physical and emotional)—allocate material goods, space, and facilities; give affection, respect, and authority.

   C. *Division of labor*—decide who earns money, manages household, cares for family.

   D. *Socialization*—guidelines to control food intake, elimination, sleep, sexual drives, and aggression.

   E. *Reproduction, recruitment, release of family member*—give birth to, or adopt, children; rear children; incorporate in-laws, friends, etc.

   F. *Maintenance of order*—ensure conformity to norms.

   G. *Placement of members in larger society*—interaction in school, community, etc.

   H. *Maintenance of motivation and morale*—reward achievements, develop philosophy for living; create rituals and celebrations to develop family loyalty. Show acceptance, encouragement, affection; meet crises of individuals and family.

II. Basic theoretical concepts related to family therapy:

   A. The ill family member (called the *identified patient,* or *IP*), by symptoms, sends a message about the "illness" of the family as a *unit.*

   B. *Family homeostasis* is the means by which families attempt to maintain the status quo.

   C. *Scapegoating* is found in disturbed families and is usually focused on one family member at a time, with the intent to keep the family in line.

   D. Communication and behavior by some family members bring out communication and behavior in other family members.

   1. Mental illness in the IP is almost always accompanied by emotional illness and disturbance in other family members.

   2. Changes occurring in one member will produce changes in another; that is, if the IP improves, another IP may emerge, or family may try to place original person back into IP role.

   E. Human communication is a key to emotional stability and instability—to normal and abnormal health. *Conjoint* family therapy is a communication-centered approach that looks at interactions between family members.

   F. *Double bind* is a "damned if you do, damned if you don't" situation; it results in helplessness, insecurity; anxiety; fear, frustration, and rage.

   G. *Symbiotic tie* usually occurs between one parent and a child, hampering individual ego development and fostering strong dependence and identification with the parent (usually the mother).

   H. *Three basic premises* of communication:*

   1. One cannot *not* communicate; that is, silence is a form of communication.

   2. Communication is a *multilevel* phenomenon.

   3. The message sent is *not* necessarily the *same* message that is received.

   I. Indications for family therapy:

   1. Marital conflicts.

   2. Severe sibling conflicts.

   3. Cross-generational conflicts.

   4. Difficulties related to a transitional stage of family life cycle (e.g., retirement, new baby, death).

   5. *Dysfunctional family patterns:* overprotective mother and distant father, with timid child or destructive, acting-out teenager; overfunctioning "superwife" or "superhusband" and the underfunctioning, passive, dependent, and compliant spouse; child with poor peer relationships or academic difficulties.

◆ **III. Family assessment** should consider the following factors:

   A. *Family assessment: cultural profile* (see also **Unit 3**)

   1. *Communication style:*

      a. Language and dialect preference (understand concept, meaning of pain, fever, nausea).

      b. Nonverbal behaviors (meaning of bowing, touching, speaking softly, smiling).

      c. Social customs (acting agreeable or pleasant to avoid the unpleasant, embarrassing).

   2. *Orientation:*

      a. Ethnic identity and adherence to traditional habits and values.

      b. Acculturation: extent.

      c. Value orientations:

         (1) *Human nature:* evil, good, both.

         (2) *Relationship between humans and nature:* subjugated, harmony, mastery.

         (3) *Time:* past, present, future.

         (4) *Purpose of life:* being, becoming, doing.

         (5) *Relationship to one another:* lineal, collateral, individualistic.

   3. *Nutrition:*

      a. Symbolism of food.

      b. Preferences, taboos.

   4. *Family relationships:*

      a. Role and position of women, men, aged, boys, girls.

---

*Adapted from Watzlawick, P: An Anthology of Human Communication. Science and Behavior Books, Palo Alto, Calif., 1964.

b. Decision-making styles/areas: finances, child rearing, health care.

c. Family: nuclear, extended, or tribal.

d. Matriarchal or patriarchal.

e. Lifestyle, living arrangements (crowded; urban/rural; ethnic neighborhood or mixed).

5. *Health beliefs*

a. Alternative health care: self-care, folk medicine; cultural healer: herbalist, medicine man, curandero.

b. Health crisis and illness beliefs concerning causation: germ theory, maladaptation, stress, evil spirits, yin/yang imbalance, envy and hate.

c. Response to pain, hospitalization: stoic endurance, loud cries, quiet withdrawal.

d. Disease predisposition:

(1) *Blacks:* sickle cell anemia; cardiovascular disease, cerebrovascular accident, hypertension; high infant mortality rate; diabetes.

(2) *Asians:* lactose intolerance, myopia.

(3) *Hispanics:* cardiovascular, diabetes, cancer, obesity, substance abuse, TB, AIDS, suicide, homicide.

(4) *Native Americans:* high infant and maternal mortality rates, cirrhosis, fetal alcohol abnormalities, pancreatitis, malnutrition, TB, alcoholism.

(5) *Jews:* Tay-Sachs.

B. *Family as a social system:*

1. Family as responsive and contributing unit within network of other social units.

a. Family boundaries—permeability or rigidity.

b. Nature of input from other social units.

c. Extent to which family fits into cultural mold and expectations of larger system.

d. Degree to which family is considered deviant.

2. Roles of family members:

a. Formal roles and role performance (father, child, etc.).

b. Informal roles and role performance (scapegoat, controller, follower, decision maker).

c. Degree of family agreement on assignment of roles and their performance.

d. Interrelationship of various roles—degree of "fit" within total family:

3. Family rules:

a. Family rules that foster stability and maintenance.

b. Family rules that foster maladaptation.

c. Conformity of rules to family's lifestyle.

d. How rules are modified; respect for difference.

4. Communication network:

a. How family communicates and provides information to members.

b. Channels of communication—who speaks to whom.

c. Quality of messages—clarity or ambiguity.

C. *Developmental stage of family:*

1. Chronological stage of family.

2. Problems and adaptations of transition.

3. Shifts in role responsibility over time.

4. Ways and means of solving problems at earlier stages.

D. *Subsystems operating within family:*

1. Function of family alliances in family stability.

2. Conflict or support of other family subsystems and family as a whole.

E. *Physical and emotional needs:*

1. Level at which family meets essential physical needs.

2. Level at which family meets social and emotional needs.

3. Resources within family to meet physical and emotional needs.

4. Disparities between individual needs and family's willingness or ability to meet them.

F. *Goals, values, and aspirations:*

1. Extent to which family members' goals and values are articulated and understood by all members.

2. Extent to which family values reflect resignation or compromise.

3. Extent to which family will permit pursuit of individual goals and values.

G. *Socioeconomic factors* (see list in Table 6–12).

◆ **IV. Nursing care plan/implementation** in family therapy:

A. Establish a family *contract* (who attends, when, duration of sessions, length of therapy, fee, and other expectations).

B. Encourage family members to identify and clarify own *goals.*

C. *Set ground rules:*

1. Focus is on the family as a whole unit, *not* on the IP.

2. *No* scapegoating or punishment of members who "reveal all" should be allowed.

3. Therapists should *not* align themselves with issues or individual family members.

D. *Use self* to empathetically respond to family's problems; share own emotions openly and directly; function as a role model of interaction.

E. Point out and encourage the family to *clarify* unclear, inefficient, and ambiguous family communication patterns.

Source: Adapted from Topics in Clinical Nursing, Vol. 7, No. 3, p. 4, with permission of Aspen Publishers, Inc., (c) 1985.

Mental Health

F. Identify family *strengths*.

G. Listen for repetitive interpersonal *themes, patterns,* and *attitudes*.

H. *Attempt to reduce guilt and blame* (important to neutralize the scapegoat phenomenon).

I. Present possibility of *alternative* roles and rules in family interaction styles.

J. *Health teaching:* teach clear communication to all family members.

◆ **V. Evaluation/outcome criteria:** each person clearly speaks for self; asks for and receives feedback; communication patterns are clarified; family problems are delineated; members more aware of each other's needs.

Electroconvulsive Therapy

Electroconvulsive therapy (ECT) is a physical treatment that induces grand mal convulsions by applying electric current to the head. It is also called electric shock therapy (EST).

I. Characteristics of electroconvulsive therapy:

A. Usually used in treating: major depression with severe suicide risk, extreme hyperactivity, severe catatonic stupor, or those with bipolar affective disorders not responsive to psychotropic medication.

B. Consists of a series of treatments (6 to 25) over a period of time (e.g., three times per week).

C. Person is asleep through the procedure and for 20 to 30 minutes afterward.

D. Convulsion may be seen as a series of minor, jerking motions in extremities (e.g., toes). Spasms are reduced by use of muscle-paralyzing drugs.

E. Confusion is present for 30 minutes after treatment.

F. Induces loss of memory for *recent* events.

II. Views concerning success of electroconvulsive therapy:

A. Posttreatment sleep is the "curative" factor.

B. Shock treatment is seen as punishment, with an accompanying feeling of absolution from guilt.

C. Chemical alteration of thought patterns results in memory loss, with decrease in redundancy and awareness of painful memories.

◆ **III. Nursing care plan/implementation** in electroconvulsive therapy:

A. *Always* tell the client of the treatment.

B. Inform client about temporary memory loss for recent events after the treatment.

C. *Pretreatment care:*
   1. Take vital signs.
   2. See to client's toileting.
   3. Remove: client's dentures, eyeglasses or contact lenses, and jewelry.
   4. NPO for 8 hours beforehand.

5. Atropine sulfate subcutaneously 30 minutes before treatment to decrease bronchial and tracheal secretions.

6. Anesthetist gives anesthetic and muscle relaxant IV (succinylcholine chloride [*Anectine*]) and oxygen for 2 to 3 minutes and inserts airway. Often all three are given close together—anesthetic first, followed by another syringe with *Anectine* and atropine sulfate. Electrodes and treatment must be given within 2 minutes of injections, because *Anectine* is very short acting (2 minutes).

D. *During the convulsion* the nurse must make sure the person is in a safe position, to avoid dislocation and compression fractures (although *Anectine* is given to prevent this).

E. *Care during recovery stage:*
   1. Put up side rails while client is confused; side position.
   2. Take blood pressure, pulse (check for bradycardia) and respirations.
   3. Stay until person awakens, responds to questions, and can care for self.
   4. Orient client to time and place and inform that treatment is over when awakens.
   5. Offer support to help client feel more secure and relaxed as the confusion and anxiety decrease.
   6. Medication for nausea and headache, prn.

F. *Health teaching:* teach family members what to expect of client after ECT (confusion, headache, nausea); how to reorient the client.

◆ **IV. Evaluation/outcome criteria:** feelings of worthlessness, helplessness, and hopelessness seem diminished.

Glossary

affect *feeling* or *mood* communicated through the face and body posture. Can be blunted, blocked, flat, inappropriate, or displaced.

ambivalence coexisting *contradictory* (positive and negative) emotions, desires, or attitudes toward an object or person (e.g., love-hate relationship).

anhedonia inability to experience any pleasure.

amnesia loss of memory due to physical or emotion trauma.

anxiety state of uneasiness or response to a *vague*, unspecific danger cued by a threat to some value that the individual holds essential to existence (or by a threat of loss of control); the danger may be *real or imagined*. *Physiological* manifestations are increased pulse, respiration, and perspiration, with feeling of "butterflies."

associative looseness speaks with unconnected topics (e.g., "no one needs a bus; we all have heaven here").

autism self-preoccupation and absorption in fantasy, as found with schizophrenia, with a complete *exclusion of reality* and loss of interest in and appreciation of others.

catatonia type of schizophrenia characterized by muscular rigidity; alternates with periods of excitability.

circumstantiality speaks with too many unnecessary details.

compulsion an insistent, repetitive, intrusive, and unwanted urge to perform an *act* that is contrary to ordinary conscious wishes or standards.

concrete thinking difficulty with abstract concepts (e.g., "It's raining cats and dogs").

conflict emotional struggle resulting from *opposing* demands and drives of the id, ego, and superego.

coping mechanism device used to ward off anxiety or uncomfortable thoughts and feelings; an activity of the ego that operates outside of awareness to hold impulses in check that might cause conflict (e.g., repression, regression).

cyclothymia alterations in moods of elation and sadness, with mood swings out of proportion to apparent stimuli.

delusion a false fixed *belief*, idea, or group of ideas that are contrary to what is thought of as real and that cannot be changed by logic; arise out of the individual's needs and are maintained in spite of evidence or facts (e.g., grandeur and persecution).

depression morbid sadness or dejection accompanied by feelings of hopelessness, inadequacy, and unworthiness. *Distinguished from grief,* which is realistic and in proportion to loss.

disorientation loss of awareness of the position of self in relation to time, place, or person.

echolalia automatic repetition of heard *phrases or words.*

echopraxia automatic repetition of observed *movements.*

ego the "I," "self," and "person" as distinguished from "others"; that part of the personality, according to Freudian theory, that *mediates* between the primitive, pleasure-seeking, instinctual drives of the id and the self-critical, prohibitive, restraining forces of the superego; that aspect of the psyche that is *conscious* and most in touch with external reality and is directed by the *reality principle.* The part of the personality that has to make the *decision.* Most of the ego is conscious and represents the *thinking-feeling* part of a person. The *compromises* worked out on an unconscious level help to resolve intrapsychic conflict by keeping thoughts, interpretations, judgments, and behavior practical and efficient.

electroshock electroshock treatment (EST) or electroconvulsive treatment (ECT) is the treatment of certain psychiatric disorders (best suited for *depression*) by therapeutic administration of regulated electrical impulses to the brain to produce convulsions.

empathy an objective awareness of another's thoughts, feelings, or behaviors and their meaning and significance; intellectual identification versus emotional identification (sympathy).

euphoria exaggerated feeling of physical and emotional well-being *not* related to external events or stimuli.

flight of ideas a *thought disorder* in which one thought moves rapidly to another without reaching a main idea or point, as in manic behavior. The next sentence may be triggered by a word in the previous sentence or by something in the environment.

fugue dissociative state involving amnesia and actual *physical flight.*

hallucination *false sensory* perception in the absence of an actual external stimulus. May be due to chemicals or inner needs and may occur in any of the five senses. Seen in *psychosis* and *acute* and *chronic* brain disorder.

hypochondriasis state of morbid preoccupation about one's health (somatic concerns).

id psychoanalytic term for that division of the psyche that is unconscious, contains instinctual primitive drives that lead to immediate gratification, and is dominated by the *pleasure principle.* The id wants what it wants when it wants it.

illusion misinterpretation of a real, external sensory stimulus (e.g., a person may see a shadow on the floor and think it is a hole).

insanity *legal* term for mental defect or disease that is of sufficient gravity to bring person under special legal restrictions and immunities.

labile unstable and rapidly shifting (referring to emotions).

manipulation process of influencing another to meet one's own needs, *regardless* of the other's needs.

mental retardation term for mental deficiency or deficit in normal development of intelligence that makes intellectual abilities lower than normal for chronological age. May result from a condition present at birth, from injury during or after birth, or from disease after birth.

mutism inability or refusal to speak.

narcissism *exaggerated self-love* with all attention focused on own comfort, pleasure, abilities, appearance, etc.

neologism a newly coined word or condensed combination of several words not readily understood by others but with symbolic meaning for the person with *schizophrenia.*

neurosis *an older* term for mild to moderately severe illness in which there is a disorder of feeling or behavior but no gross mental disorganization, delusions, or hallucinations, as in serious psychoses. Typical reactions include disproportionate *anxiety, phobias,* and *obsessive-compulsive behavior.*

obsession persistent, unwanted, and uncontrollable *urge* or *idea* that *cannot* be banished by logic or will.

organic psychosis mental disease resulting from defect, damage, infection, tumor, or other *physical cause* that can be *observed* in the body tissues.

paranoid adjective indicating feelings of suspicion and persecution; one type of schizophrenia.

Mental Health

perseveration repeats same word or idea in response to different questions.

personality disorder broad category of illnesses in which inner difficulties are revealed not by specific symptoms but by *antisocial* behavior.

phobia *irrational, persistent,* abnormal, *morbid,* and unrealistic dread of external object or situation displaced from unconscious conflict.

premorbid personality state of an individual's personality *before* the onset of an illness.

psyche synonymous with mind or the *mental and emotional* "self."

psychoanalysis theory of human development and behavior, method of research, and form of treatment described by Freud that attributes abnormal behavior to repressions in the unconscious mind. Treatment involves dream interpretation and free association to bring into awareness the origin and effects of unconscious conflicts in order to eliminate or diminish them.

psychodrama a therapeutic approach that involves a structured, dramatized, and directed *acting-out* of emotional problems and troubled interactions by the client in order to gain insight into individual's own difficulties.

psychogenic symptoms or physical disorders caused by emotional or mental factors, as opposed to organic.

psychopath *older,* inexact term for one of a variety of *personality disorders* in which person has poor impulse control, releasing tension through immediate action, without social or moral conscience.

psychosis severe emotional illness characterized by a disorder of *thinking, feeling, and action* with the following symptoms: loss of contact, denial of reality, bizarre thinking and behavior, perceptual distortion, delusions, hallucinations, and regression.

regression retreat to earlier level of development.

schizoid form of personality disorder characterized by shyness, introspection, introversion, withdrawal, and aloofness.

schizophrenia severe functional mental illness characterized in general by a disorder in perception, thinking, feeling, behavior, and interpersonal relationships.

sociopathic pertaining to a disorder of behavior in which a person's feelings and behavior are asocial, with impaired judgment and inability to profit from experience; the intellect remains intact. This term is often used interchangeably with "antisocial personality."

soma term meaning the body or *physical* aspects.

superego in psychoanalysis, that part of the mind that incorporates the parental or societal values, ethics, and standards. It guides, restrains, criticizes, and punishes. It is unconscious and learned and is sometimes equated with the term *conscience.*

tangentiality speaks without getting to the point.

transference unconscious projections of feelings, attitudes, and wishes that were originally associated with early significant others onto persons or events in the present; may be positive or negative transference.

waxy flexibility psychomotor underactivity in which the individual maintains the posture in which he or she is placed.

word salad meaningless mixture of phrases and words often seen in *schizophrenic* behavior, e.g., "the rid jams frost wool mix."

Questions

Select the one best answer for each question.

1. A patient is in a withdrawn catatonic state and exhibits waxy flexibility. During the initial phase of hospitalization for this patient, the nurse's first priority is to:
   1. Watch for edema and cyanosis of the extremities.
   2. Encourage the patient to discuss concerns that led to the catatonic state.
   3. Provide a warm, nurturing relationship, with therapeutic use of touch.
   4. Identify the predisposing factors in the illness.
2. An elderly client who has dementia related to cerebral arteriosclerosis says to the nurse, "I'm going to the university today to be their guest lecturer on aerodynamics." Which response by the nurse would be most therapeutic?
   1. "Do you know that you are in the hospital now?"
   2. "Are you saying that you would like to be asked to give a lecture at the university?"
   3. "How about watching a movie on television instead?"
   4. "It's more important that you don't tire yourself out."
3. Which nursing approach would be best for a client with symptoms of severe depression?
   1. Allow the client time for quiet thought; remain silent.
   2. Ask the client to join the nurse and the other clients in the TV lounge.
   3. State that the nurse would like to go with the client for a short walk around the outside grounds, and assist the client with his or her coat.
   4. Give the client a choice of recreational activities.
4. When assessing clients who are exhibiting a depressed episode and those who are exhibiting a manic episode of bipolar mood disorders, which characteristic common to both episodes of the disorder is the nurse likely to note?
   1. Suicidal tendency.
   2. Underlying hostility.
   3. Delusions.
   4. Flight of ideas.
5. A patient who is overweight is referred by the physician to the nurse for diet counseling. What action would the nurse take?
   1. Develop a weight control plan, together with the patient, that will allow gradual weight loss.
   2. Ask the patient to describe his or her eating patterns.
   3. Support the patient's interests in other activities.
   4. Put the patient on a diet with very limited number of calories so he or she will have an immediate weight loss.
6. A patient begins having auditory hallucinations. When the nurse approaches, the patient whispers, "Did you hear that terrible man? He is scary!" Which would be the best response for the nurse to make initially?

1. "What is he saying?"
2. "I didn't hear anything. What scary things is he saying?"
3. "Who is he? Do you know him?"
4. "I didn't hear a man's voice, but you look scared."

7. After seeing a number of doctors for nonspecific complaints of chest pains, with no conclusive findings of organic disease, a client is referred to a local mental health center. The client has read extensively about coronary disease and talks continuously about the symptoms in great detail. Which approach by the nurse would be best when meeting this client for the first time?
   1. Allow the client to describe the physical problems to become familiar with them.
   2. Comment on a neutral topic instead of using the usual conversation opener of "How are you today?"
   3. Give the client a simple but direct explanation of the physiological basis for the symptoms.
   4. Let the client know that the nurse is familiar with the psychogenic problems and guide the discussion to other areas.

8. A 35-year-old married clerk had surgery for ulcerative colitis 3 days ago. The physical symptoms have abated, but he continues to complain angrily and to be demanding of the nursing staff. He makes numerous requests, such as to open or close the windows and to bring him fresh water. The nurse needs to understand that this behavior might be saying:
   1. "You aren't doing your job."
   2. "I am alone and helpless and need to depend on you to take care of me when I need you."
   3. "Everyone needs attention."
   4. "I'm going to get even with you for thinking I'm a crank by making you work."

9. The nurse is aware that the main function confabulation serves in clients, especially those with dementia, is to:
   1. Impress others.
   2. Protect their self-esteem.
   3. Control others by distance maneuvers.
   4. Maintain a sense of humor.

10. A 19-year-old patient is brought to the emergency department because she slashed her wrists. What is the nurse's first concern?
    1. Stabilization of physical condition.
    2. Determination of antecedent, causal factors relevant to the wrist slashing.
    3. Reduction of anxiety.
    4. Obtaining a detailed nursing history.

11. A patient who is agitated begins to shout insults and threats at others, and starts demolishing the recreation room. What is the best response or action by the nurse?
    1. Firmly set limits on the behavior.
    2. Allow the patient to continue, because the patient is seeking to express herself or himself.
    3. Tell the patient he or she is trying to intimidate other clients.
    4. Let the patient know that he or she does not need to express anger at the nurse by demolishing the recreation room.

12. A second-grade girl starts at a new school, and the child's grades suffer while focusing on adjusting to new peers. The father severely reprimands the child and forces the child to study after school rather than play with other children. These data indicate to the nurse that this child is deprived of forming which normal phase of development?
    1. A love relationship with the father.
    2. Close relationships with peers.
    3. Heterosexual relationships.
    4. A dependency relationship with the father.

13. The nurse is interviewing a teenage patient with acting-out behaviors. The teenager complains that no one will let

him "do his own thing," and sits glaring at the nurse. What is the nurse's best response?
   1. "I know you are angry, but how does being angry help?"
   2. "Stop being angry and tell me what is wrong."
   3. "I think you are angry because you feel you don't need any help?"
   4. "We have to meet because your parents are concerned about you."

14. A patient looks at a mirror and cries out, "I look like a bird. My face is no longer me." Which would be the best response by the nurse?
    1. "Which bird?"
    2. "That must be a distressing experience; your face doesn't look different to me."
    3. "Maybe it was the light at that particular time. Would you like to use another mirror?"
    4. "What makes you think that your face looks like a bird?"

15. A patient with ulcerative colitis and the patient's family are ready to make discharge plans jointly with the staff. Which assessment will have the greatest bearing on the patient's rehabilitation course?
    1. The amount of emotional support the family gives the patient.
    2. The spouse's interest in and ability to take care of the postoperative dietary needs.
    3. The family expectations of the patient to resume his or her role in the home.
    4. The spouse's understanding that the course of the illness may have exacerbations and remissions.

16. A 10-year-old child diagnosed with acute leukemia, terminal stage, asks the nurse one morning: "I am going to die, aren't I?" What would be the most appropriate response by the nurse?
    1. "No, you're not. You are getting the latest treatment available and you have a very good doctor. Your white count was better yesterday."
    2. "We are all going to die sometime."
    3. "What did the doctor tell you?"
    4. "I don't know. You have a serious illness. Do you have feelings that you want to talk about now?"

17. For a patient with a diagnosis of a somatoform disorder, which would be the appropriate initial nursing goal?
    1. Help the patient learn how to live with the functional organic disturbance without using the symptoms to control others.
    2. Assist the patient in developing new and varied interests outside of himself or herself at which he or she can be successful.
    3. Accept the patient as a person who is sick and needs help.
    4. Help the patient see how he or she uses the illness to avoid looking at or dealing with problems.

18. An acutely ill patient hospitalized with metastatic lung carcinoma begs for a pass to attend her son's high school graduation in a city 100 miles from the hospital. "If only I could do this one thing, then I'll be ready to die," the patient says. The nurse identifies this behavior as an example of:
    1. Being unrealistic and denying the degree of illness.
    2. Using bargaining as a reaction to death and dying.
    3. Being manipulative to get the patient's way.
    4. Being unaware of the diagnosis.

19. A patient who is overweight says to the nurse, "My therapist told me I eat because I didn't get enough love from my mother. What does the therapist mean?" What is the best response for the nurse to offer?
    1. "Tell me what you think the therapist means."
    2. "We are here to deal with your diet, not with your psychological problems."
    3. "You need to ask your therapist."
    4. "What do you think is the connection between your not getting enough love and your overeating?"

20. An elderly patient who is hard of hearing repeats, over and over again, the same story of the patient's family coming "out West" in a covered wagon. Which interpretation by the nurse would not demonstrate understanding of this behavior?
    1. The patient has better recall for past events than for recent ones.
    2. The patient enjoys reliving the pleasurable aspects of life, because the present and future are bleak.
    3. Repeating stories is one way of interacting, to compensate for a two-way conversation that is difficult for the patient to sustain.
    4. The patient wants to impress others.

21. A nursing care plan for a hospitalized hyperactive client in a manic episode must include:
    1. Involvement in a group activity and encouragement to talk.
    2. Attention to adequate food and fluid intake.
    3. Protection against suicide.
    4. Permissive acceptance of bizarre behavior.

22. The nurse finds an elderly patient with Alzheimer's in the hallway at 4:00 A.M., trying to open the door to the fire escape. Which response by the nurse would probably indicate the most accurate assessment of the situation?
    1. "You look confused. Would you like to sit down and talk with me?"
    2. "That door leads to the fire escape. Why do you want to go outside now?"
    3. "This is the fire escape door. Are you looking for the bathroom?"
    4. "Something seems to be bothering you. Let's go back to your room and talk about it."

23. Since the death of her baby, a woman has lost weight, will not eat, spends most of her time immobile, and speaks only in monosyllabic responses. She pays little attention to her appearance. One afternoon, this patient comes to lunch with her hair combed and traces of lipstick. What could the nurse say to reinforce this change of behavior?
    1. "What happened? You combed your hair!"
    2. "This is the first time I've seen you look so good."
    3. "You must be feeling better. You look much better."
    4. "I see that your hair is combed and you have lipstick on."

24. While the nurse is interviewing a teenage patient, the patient says, "I suppose you have to tell my parents everything." What would be the best response by the nurse?
    1. "What are you going to tell me that is so secret that I can't tell your parents?"
    2. "If you tell me you are going to do something to hurt yourself I will have to tell your parents, but I will tell you first before I tell them."
    3. "Everything you tell me is confidential. I will not tell your parents anything."
    4. "Everything you tell me I will need to tell your parents. They have a right to know."

25. In paranoid disorder, the part of the personality that is weak is called the:
    1. Id.
    2. Ego.
    3. Superego.
    4. "Not me."

26. A key consideration in planning the general care of clients with dementia is that:
    1. They be protected from suicide attempts.
    2. Their capacity for physical activity is diminished.
    3. Team effort be aimed at increasing their independence.
    4. The staff be sympathetic when clients mention their failing abilities.

27. A college student was doing exceptionally well and was complimented by her chemistry professor, who arranged for her to become his lab assistant and to do advanced research. Although very thorough in her work, when given constructive criticism this student becomes angry and stalks out of the lab for a few hours. The most plausible theoretical explanation is that the student:
    1. Knows she is right.
    2. Thinks the professor is jealous of her.
    3. Needs to feel and know that she is perfect.
    4. Feels anxiety as a result of a threat to her security and self-image.

28. One therapeutic nursing attitude is to be accepting and permissive. To convey this attitude most therapeutically, the nurse might:
    1. Wait for a client to initiate contact.
    2. Let the client make decisions.
    3. Ignore undesirable behavior.
    4. Meet the client at his or her level of functioning.

29. The basic goal of nursing in a mental health setting is to:
    1. Plan activity programs for clients.
    2. Maintain a therapeutic environment.
    3. Understand various types of family therapy and psychological tests and how to interpret them.
    4. Advance the science of psychiatry by initiating research and gathering data for current statistics on emotional illness.

30. Which nursing intervention is inappropriate with a person who is expressing anger?
    1. Stating observations of the expressed anger.
    2. Assisting the person to describe the feelings.
    3. Helping the person find out what preceded the anger.
    4. Helping the person refrain from expressing anger verbally.

31. The client tells the nurse about the client's parents' impending divorce. The client said, "I couldn't believe that he was going to leave us for someone else." Which would be best for the nurse to reply?
    1. "Was your mother expecting this to happen?"
    2. "Yes, go on."
    3. "Did you cry?"
    4. "I can understand how you must feel."

32. A crisis intervention nurse meets with a young patient who was admitted after attempting suicide by slashing the wrists. The nurse's initial goal at this time is to:
    1. Determine the precipitating event, determine how many people are involved in the incident, and determine how angry the patient is.
    2. Determine if the patient has an immediate support system, determine what the people in the support system think of the patient cutting the wrists, and determine how angry the patient is.
    3. Determine the precipitating event, determine if the patient has an immediate support system, and assess the likelihood of immediate recurrence of the suicidal act.
    4. Assess the likelihood of immediate recurrence of the suicidal act.

33. A client states, "The nofas are coming." In response to this neologism, it would be best for the nurse to:
    1. Divert the client's attention to an aspect of reality.
    2. State that what the client is saying has not been understood and then divert attention to something that is reality bound.
    3. Acknowledge that the word has some special meaning for the client.
    4. Try to interpret what the client means.

34. Which nursing approach is important in depression?
    1. Providing motor outlets for aggressive, hostile feelings.

2. Protecting against harm to others.

3. Reducing interpersonal contacts.

4. Deemphasizing preoccupation with elimination, nourishment, and sleep.

35. One evening the nurse sees a client in the dayroom without any clothes, shouting vulgarities and dancing wildly about the room while other clients are watching TV. The best initial response by the nurse at this time would be:

1. "Let's sit down with the others and watch TV; I'll put this blanket over you to keep you warm."

2. "We do not allow this behavior in the hospital. It is embarrassing the other clients."

3. "Please put your clothes on."

4. "Come put your clothes on. I will help you."

36. The nurse discovers a client crouched in a corner, looking pale and frightened, and holding a gushing wrist wound. A razor is nearby on the floor. What should the nurse do first?

1. Sit down on the floor, next to the client, and in a quiet, reassuring tone, say, "You seem frightened. Can I help?"

2. Ask the aide to watch the client and run to get the doctor.

3. Apply pressure on the wrist, saying to the client, "You are hurt. I will help you."

4. Go back down the hall to get the emergency cart.

37. Which characteristic should the nurse recognize as common in a person engaged in gradual self-destructive behavior (such as in obesity, drug addiction, and smoking)?

1. Acceptance of the death wish.

2. Denial of possibility of death.

3. Ability to control own behavior.

4. Ignorance of the consequences of own behavior.

38. A divorced woman learns that her ex-husband has died. Her reaction is stunned silence, followed by anger that he left no insurance money for their young children. The nurse should understand that:

1. The woman is experiencing a normal bereavement reaction.

2. To explain the woman's reaction, the nurse needs more information about the relationship and breakup.

3. The children and the injustice done to them by their father's death are the woman's main concern.

4. The woman is not reacting normally to the news.

39. What will the nurse most commonly note in the clinical picture of dementia?

1. Memory loss for events in the distant past.

2. Quarrelsome behavior directly related to the extent of lack of blood supply to the brain.

3. Increased resistance to change.

4. Insight into one's situation, its probable causes, and its logical consequences.

40. A man is hospitalized following a car accident in which his wife died, and he is unable to attend the funeral due to his severe chest injuries. What would the nurse consider in forecasting this surviving spouse's potential for difficulty with grief resolution?

1. Feelings of anger toward the hospital staff for keeping him hospitalized during the funeral.

2. Feelings of anger toward himself for having been injured but not killed in the accident.

3. His inability to participate in the cultural rituals of grief, wherein the reality of his wife's death is emphasized.

4. His preoccupation with his own physical distress at this time.

41. A patient who is depressed says, "I don't cry because my wife can't bear it." The nurse needs to be aware that this is an example of:

1. Suppression.

2. Undoing.

3. Repression.

4. Rationalization.

42. When interacting with clients who have autistic thinking and speaking patterns, what is likely to pose the *greatest difficulty* for the nurse?

1. Showing acceptance for their incomprehensible acts and verbalizations.

2. Ignoring their bizarre behavior.

3. Speaking in a way that clients can understand.

4. Determining which of the clients' needs are being met by their autistic expressions.

43. A patient refuses to eat meals in the hospital, stating that the food is poisoned. The nurse is aware that the patient is expressing an example of:

1. Hallucination.

2. Illusion.

3. Delusion.

4. Negativism.

44. An adolescent has a history of truancy from school, running away from home, and "borrowing" other people's things without their permission. The adolescent denies stealing, rationalizing instead that as long as no one was using the items, it was all right to borrow them. It is important for the nurse to understand that psychodynamically, this behavior may be largely attributed to a developmental defect related to the:

1. Id.

2. Ego.

3. Superego.

4. Oedipal complex.

45. What is the nurse likely to note in a patient being admitted for alcohol withdrawal?

1. Perceptual disorders.

2. Impending coma.

3. Recent alcohol intake.

4. Depression with mutism.

46. A patient says he must wash his hands from 9:00 to 9:45 A.M. each day and therefore cannot attend 9:00 A.M. group therapy sessions. Which concept does the nursing staff need to keep in mind in planning nursing interventions for this patient?

1. Fears and tensions are often expressed in disguised form through symbolic processes.

2. Unmet needs are discharged through ritualistic behavior.

3. Ritualistic behavior makes others uncomfortable.

4. Depression underlies ritualistic behavior.

47. To formulate an effective care plan for a client with a somatoform disorder, the nurse needs to have an understanding of which related psychodynamic principle?

1. The major fundamental mechanism is regression.

2. An extensive, prolonged study of the symptoms will be reassuring to the client, who seeks sympathy, attention, and love.

3. The symptoms of a somatoform disorder are an attempt to adjust to painful life situations or to cope with conflicting sexual, aggressive, or dependent feelings.

4. The client's symptoms are imaginary and the suffering is faked.

48. In evaluating a patient who has somatoform symptoms, the nurse is aware that the patient will probably show the most improvement when he or she:

1. Accepts the fact that the physical symptoms have an emotional component.

2. Finds more satisfying ways of expressing feelings through verbalization.

3. Becomes involved in group activities and focuses less on the symptoms.

4. Understands that the current way of reacting to stress is not healthy.

49. An important part of the nursing care for a client with dementia would be:
    1. Minimizing regression.
    2. Correcting memory loss.
    3. Rehabilitating toward independent functioning.
    4. Preventing further deterioration.

50. In explaining the goal of therapy in crisis intervention to a new colleague, the nurse states that the goal is to:
    1. Restructure the personality.
    2. Remove specific symptoms.
    3. Remove anxiety.
    4. Resolve immediate problems.

51. The steps in therapeutic nursing intervention with an angry client would be to describe the situation, then:
    1. Discuss alternative solutions, decide on several, try them out, and evaluate their effectiveness.
    2. Focus on one solution, try it out, and evaluate its effectiveness.
    3. Outline to the client exactly what to do about the anger.
    4. Discuss alternative solutions, decide on one, use it, evaluate its effectiveness, and continue repeating the process until the client is satisfied.

52. On a routine physical, a woman learns she has a lump in her breast. It is found to be malignant, and a modified mastectomy is performed. Immediately following the surgery, what behaviors could the nurse expect this patient to display?
    1. Signs of grief reaction.
    2. Signs of deep depression.
    3. Relief that the operation is over.
    4. Denial of the possibility of carcinoma.

53. A 19-year-old patient's overcompliance with his parents' expectations for his behavior could result in:
    1. Lack of development of a separate identity.
    2. Confusion of his sex role.
    3. Successful development of a separate identity.
    4. Identification of a weak superego.

54. A doctor asks the nurse to activate a patient who hears voices and is withdrawn and negativistic. What would be the nurse's best approach?
    1. Give the patient a long explanation of the benefits of activity.
    2. Tell the patient that the nurse needs a partner for an activity.
    3. Demand that the patient join a group activity.
    4. Mention that the "voices" would want the patient to participate.

55. When an experiment in the laboratory goes wrong, a researcher complains of a plot against her, and accuses the lab assistants of sending signals about her to each other. The nurse would determine that this behavior is related to:
    1. Delusions of grandeur.
    2. Illusion.
    3. Ideas of reference.
    4. Echolalia.

56. A teenager with acting-out behaviors says to the nurse, "I want you to go tell the teacher I am sick and I am to be allowed to do what I want." The nurse determines that this statement best represents:
    1. Insight.
    2. Manipulation.
    3. Dependency.
    4. Trust.

57. A 52-year-old patient who appears lucid learns that after surgery, he will wake up in the recovery room without his thick glasses and hearing aid. He immediately states that without these he will be confused and upset. The nurse determines that the patient is trying to say that he:
    1. Has periods of confusion and may have a psychiatric problem.

2. Is psychologically dependent on the hearing aid and glasses.
    3. Needs the hearing aid and glasses to correctly perceive what is going on around him, and misperception will cause confusion.
    4. Needs the hearing aid and glasses because he wants to be sure people are taking proper care of him.

58. A patient relates angrily to the nurse that his wife says he is selfish. Which would be the most helpful response by the nurse?
    1. "That's just her opinion."
    2. "I don't think you're that selfish."
    3. "Everybody is a little bit selfish."
    4. "You sound angry—tell me more about what went on."

59. When a client has dementia, it is most important that the nurse plan the daily activities to:
    1. Be highly structured.
    2. Be changed each day to meet the client's needs for variety.
    3. Be simplified as much as possible to avoid problems with decision making.
    4. Provide many opportunities for making choices to stimulate the client's involvement and interest.

60. A woman tells the nurse that she refuses to eat her husband's cooking because she thinks he is poisoning her. The nurse is aware that this behavior is related to:
    1. Delusion of persecution.
    2. Ideas of reference.
    3. Illusion.
    4. Hallucination.

61. The crisis nurse explains to a colleague that the focus of treatment in crisis intervention is on the:
    1. Present and on restoration to the usual level of functioning.
    2. Past and on freeing the unconscious.
    3. Past in relation to the present.
    4. Present and on the repression of unconscious drives.

62. A patient in the postoperative period following surgery for ulcerative colitis suddenly becomes angry with another patient who is monopolizing the group therapy meeting. Which interpretation of this noted change in behavior would indicate that the nurse understands the dynamics of this patient's somatoform disorder?
    1. The patient is intolerant of others.
    2. The patient has strong competitive drives.
    3. The patient has his or her own ideas of how the group members should act.
    4. The patient is repressing fewer feelings.

63. A client has a somatoform disorder, paralysis of the arm. It would not be helpful for the nurse to use logic and reason to divert this client's attention from this physical state because:
    1. The client is not in contact with reality and thus is unable to "hear" or understand the nurse.
    2. The client may need the symptoms to handle feelings of guilt or aggression.
    3. The nature of the client's particular illness makes the client suspicious of all medical personnel.
    4. Paralysis of the arm has become a habitual response to stress.

64. While communicating with a patient who is withdrawn, what would be important for the nurse to do at first?
    1. Remain silent and not encourage the patient to talk.
    2. Talk with the patient as one would to a normal person.
    3. Allow the patient to do all the talking.
    4. Use simple, concrete language in speaking to the patient.

65. The nurse bases a plan of care on the knowledge that persons engaged in gradual self-destructive behavior:
    1. Believe they can stop this behavior at any time.
    2. Have decreased anxiety when they stop the behavior.
    3. Believe the behavior controls them.
    4. Believe the behavior, in some manner, is "good" for them.

66. When a patient with symptoms of severe depression says to the nurse, "I can't talk; I have nothing to say," and continues being silent, what should the nurse do?
    1. Say, "All right. You don't have to talk. Let's play cards, instead."
    2. Explain that talking is an important sign of getting well and that the patient is expected to do so.
    3. Be silent until the patient speaks again.
    4. Say, "It may be difficult for you to speak at this time; perhaps you can do so at another time."

67. When talking with a client who is exhibiting a manic episode with flight of ideas, the nurse primarily needs to:
    1. Speak loudly and rapidly to keep the client's attention, because the client is easily distracted.
    2. Focus on the feelings conveyed rather than the thoughts expressed.
    3. Encourage the client to complete one thought at a time.
    4. Allow the client to talk freely.

68. A patient says to the nurse, "I was going to kill myself last night." What is the best initial response by the nurse?
    1. Say nothing. Wait for the patient's next comment.
    2. "What were you going to do this time?"
    3. "Have you felt this way before?"
    4. "You seem upset. I am going to be here with you; perhaps you will want to talk about it."

69. Which feeling is the nurse likely to identify as antecedent of self-destructive behavior?
    1. Omnipotence.
    2. Grandiosity.
    3. Low self-esteem.
    4. Self-satisfaction.

70. Resolution of grief related to death is likely to be complicated when:
    1. There are ambivalent feelings for the deceased.
    2. The death was due to a chronic illness.
    3. It is the first loss to be experienced.
    4. There was little emotional dependency on the deceased.

71. Which behavior might the nurse expect from a patient with congestive heart failure who is in the grief stage of developing awareness of the loss of a spouse?
    1. Crying, anger, or both.
    2. Appearing dazed and repeatedly saying, "No, it can't be."
    3. Preoccupation with thoughts of how ideal the marriage had been.
    4. Responding with a brief complaint about the patient's own physical pain.

72. What feeling tone is the nurse most likely to see the client demonstrate during major depression with psychotic features?
    1. Suspicion.
    2. Agitation.
    3. Loneliness.
    4. Worthlessness.

73. When a client's behavior is considered abnormal, the nurse first needs to:
    1. Ignore the client.
    2. Serve as a role model.
    3. Point out the client's disturbed behavior.
    4. Focus on the feelings communicated by the client's behavior.

74. A hospitalized patient cannot find his slippers and accuses other patients and staff of stealing them. The most therapeutic approach is to:
    1. Listen without reinforcing the patient's belief.
    2. Logically point out that the patient is jumping to conclusions.
    3. Inject humor to defuse the intensity.
    4. Divert the patient's attention.

75. In interacting with a patient with an antisocial personality disorder, what would be the most therapeutic approach?

1. Reinforce the patient's self-concept.
2. Gratify the patient's inner needs.
3. Give the patient opportunities to test reality.
4. Provide external controls.

76. To relate therapeutically with a patient who is dependent on alcohol, it is important that the nurse base his or her care on the understanding that alcohol dependence:
    1. Is hereditary.
    2. Is due to lack of willpower and true remorse.
    3. Results in always breaking promises.
    4. Cannot be cured.

77. A patient uses repetitive hand washing. To help the patient use less maladaptive means of handling stress, the nurse could:
    1. Provide varied activities on the unit, because change in routine can break this ritualistic pattern.
    2. Give the patient unit assignments that do not require perfection.
    3. Tell the patient of changes in routine at the last minute to avoid buildup of anxiety.
    4. Provide an activity in which positive accomplishment can occur so the patient can gain recognition.

78. The most common coping mechanisms used in somatoform disorders are:
    1. Repression and symbolism.
    2. Sublimation and regression.
    3. Substitution and displacement.
    4. Reaction formation and rationalization.

79. A patient who has been hospitalized with ulcerative colitis asks the doctor about the prognosis. The patient becomes alternately depressed and agitated when hearing of the impending discharge. Which nursing approach would be best at this time?
    1. "You *are* much better than when you first were hospitalized. You have to decide whether you need to be hospitalized longer or whether you are ready to go home."
    2. "You seem to have concerns about going home."
    3. "What is it about going home that bothers you?"
    4. "You seem sad about going home. Would you like to talk about it?"

80. It is important for the nurse to be aware that the mental health of an aged client is most directly influenced by:
    1. The attitude of relatives in providing for the client's needs.
    2. Societal factors such as role change, loss of loved ones, and loss of physical energy.
    3. The client's level of education and economic situation.
    4. The attitudes the client has toward life circumstances.

81. In crisis intervention therapy, the nurse plans her or his goals based on the principle that crises:
    1. May go on indefinitely.
    2. Seldom occur in normal people's lives.
    3. Usually are resolved in 4–6 weeks.
    4. Are related to deep, underlying problems.

82. The nurse can determine that the expression of hostility is appropriate and useful when the:
    1. Energy from anger is used to accomplish what needs to be done.
    2. Expression intimidates others.
    3. Degree of hostility is less than the provocation.
    4. Expression of anger dissipates the energy.

83. Two days after a mastectomy, a woman is crying and saying, "My husband won't love me anymore." The nurse is aware that this statement might stem from:
    1. The woman's deep insecurity about her marriage.
    2. Preexisting marital disharmony.
    3. The woman's concerns about her body and a resultant change in her beliefs about her own self-worth.
    4. A momentary fear about her husband's fidelity.

84. The nurse establishes a nurse-client relationship with a patient with a schizophrenic disorder. One of the goals is to help the patient develop a separate self-identity. One way to do this is to:
    1. Call the patient by a "pet" name frequently.
    2. Use "you" and "I" rather than "we."
    3. Correct the patient's opinions.
    4. Encourage "should" responses.

85. A patient is diagnosed as having a paranoid disorder. What implication might this have for the nurse?
    1. Let the patient talk about her or his suspicions without correcting misinformation.
    2. Avoid talking to other nurses when the patient can see them but cannot hear what is being said.
    3. Placate the patient by agreeing with what he or she says.
    4. Argue with the patient about his or her ideas.

86. A teenage patient says to the nurse, "I want you to go tell the teacher I am sick and I am to be allowed to do what I want." What is the nurse's best response?
    1. "Certainly. You are sick and need some relaxation of rules in the classroom."
    2. "I am glad you recognize you are sick."
    3. "No, you are expected to follow the rules of the class-room."
    4. "All teachers are too strict. I agree some rules need to be relaxed."

87. A 50-year-old patient says he needs his glasses and hearing aid with him in the recovery room after surgery, or he will be upset and confused. What is the nurse's best response?
    1. "You won't need your glasses or hearing aid. The nurses will take care of you."
    2. "I understand. You will be able to cooperate best if you know what is going on, so I will find out how I can arrange to have your glasses and hearing aid available to you in the recovery room."
    3. "I understand you might be more cooperative if you have your aid and glasses, but that is just not possible. Rules, you know."
    4. "Do you get upset and confused often?"

88. A mother talks about her daughter, who is mentally retarded: "She's really an inspiration to me, do you know what I mean?" Which would be the most appropriate initial comment by the nurse?
    1. "What makes her an inspiration?"
    2. "It seems to be important to you to find something positive about her."
    3. "No, explain more about what you mean."
    4. "Tell me more about her."

89. At the first therapy session with a patient who recently attempted suicide, what does the crisis nurse need to do?
    1. Discourage discussion of the suicide attempt.
    2. Encourage the patient to focus on feelings about how badly the patient was treated as a child.
    3. Encourage the patient to discuss the suicide attempt in detail.
    4. Help the patient see how the suicide attempt hurt others.

90. A mother says to the nurse, "When my baby had asthma 5 years ago, I thought he was going to die." What would be most appropriate for the nurse to say?
    1. "What made you think that he was going to die?"
    2. "What did you do?"
    3. "You thought he was dying?"
    4. "What were some of your feelings at that time?"

91. In preparing the nursing care plan for an elderly man, the *most* common basic need that must be met is:
    1. Sexual outlet and security.
    2. Unconditional acceptance by others of his impairments and deficits.
    3. Preservation of self-esteem.
    4. Socialization.

92. One effective way for a nurse to start an interaction with a client who is silent is to:
    1. Tell the client something about himself or herself and hope that the client does the same.
    2. Remain silent, waiting for the client to bring up a topic.
    3. Bring up a controversial topic to elicit the client's response.
    4. Introduce a neutral topic, giving the client a broad opening.

93. What would be the most realistic statement a nurse could make about a patient's prognosis after a course of necessary treatment for ulcerative colitis?
    1. The symptoms will recur.
    2. The ulcerative lesions will heal, but under stress the same symptoms will reappear.
    3. It is not possible to prognosticate the future course.
    4. Ongoing psychotherapy is essential for the patient to be free of symptoms.

94. What might be the most therapeutic response the nurse could make to a student who begins crying on hearing that he or she failed an exam?
    1. "You'll make it next time."
    2. "Failing an exam is an upsetting thing to happen."
    3. "How close were you to passing?"
    4. "It won't seem so important 5 years from now."

95. Which adaptive behavior by a client with somatoform disorders might indicate to the nurse the greatest improvement in the client's condition?
    1. The client recognizes that the behavior is unreasonable.
    2. The client agrees to go to occupational therapy and recreational therapy every day.
    3. The symptoms are replaced by expressions of hostility.
    4. The client is verbalizing feelings instead of demonstrating them by pathological body languages.

96. A client tells the nurse that he has something he wants to say but does not want the nurse to tell anyone else. The nurse should:
    1. Agree not to "tell."
    2. Refuse to agree to this.
    3. Say nothing, allowing him to go on.
    4. Let him know that the nurse cannot promise this.

97. Which is an example of *limit setting* as an effective nursing intervention in ritualistic hand-washing behavior?
    1. "I don't want you to wash your hands so often any-more."
    2. "If you continue to wash your hands so frequently, the skin on your hands will break down."
    3. "You may wash your hands before the group therapy meeting if you wish, but not during group therapy."
    4. "The doctor wrote an order that you are to stop washing your hands so often."

98. Which nursing intervention is effective when clients are severely anxious?
    1. Encourage group participation.
    2. Give detailed instructions before treatment procedures.
    3. Impart information succinctly and concretely.
    4. Increase opportunities for decision making.

99. A nursing care plan for a patient with a history of alcohol abuse and dependency must incorporate which physical consequence?
    1. Cardiac arrhythmia.
    2. Convulsive disorder.
    3. Psychomotor hyperactivity.
    4. Cirrhosis of the liver.

100. When a client tells the nurse that he or she cannot sleep at night because of fear of dying, what would be the best initial response?

1. "Don't worry, you won't die. You're just here for some tests."
2. "Why are you afraid of dying?"
3. "Try to sleep. You need the rest before tomorrow's test."
4. "It must be frightening for you to feel that way. Tell me more about it."

101. A new nurse is assigned to take clients for an outing. A patient with an antisocial disorder approaches the nurse and says, "I like you. I'm glad you'll be the one to take us out. My doctor told me that I can go too." Which initial response by the nurse is best?
    1. "Since I am new here and not familiar with unit routine, I will go check with the staff and be back."
    2. "It's a beautiful day, and I'm glad that you have ground privileges now."
    3. "When did the doctor tell you that?"
    4. "You seem pleased."

102. Which common physiological reaction occurring in response to anxiety is the nurse likely to note?
    1. Clammy hands and increased perspiration.
    2. Palpitations and pupillary constriction.
    3. Diarrhea and vomiting.
    4. Pupillary dilation and retention of feces and urine.

103. Clients with paranoid behavior use projection. The nurse is aware that this mechanism is chiefly a way to:
    1. Provoke anger in others.
    2. Control delusional thought.
    3. Handle their own unacceptable feelings.
    4. Manipulate others.

104. Which most characteristic behavior of a panic response is the nurse likely to note?
    1. Goal-directed behavior aimed at a "flight" from apparent threat.
    2. Automatic behavior with poor judgment.
    3. A severity of reaction that is not related to the severity of the threat to self-esteem.
    4. A delayed reaction in perceiving the danger.

105. At times, a client seems preoccupied with her own thoughts as she grins, giggles, grimaces, and frowns. Although she is 23 years old, her behavior seems childish and regressed. She is unkempt, voids on the floor, disrobes, and openly masturbates. The main nursing care at this time should be directed toward:
    1. Improving the client's social conduct to meet hospital standards.
    2. Controlling the narcissistic impulses.
    3. Finding out why the client is behaving this way.
    4. Showing acceptance of the client.

106. The nurse is aware that the two major types of precipitating factors in anxiety are:
    1. Fear of disapproval and shame.
    2. Conflicts involving avoidance and pain.
    3. Threats to one's biological integrity and threats to one's self-system.
    4. A person's poor health and poor financial condition.

107. After a patient with major depression visits with the spouse, the spouse reports that it was a stressful time. In an interview, the patient says, "We had a marvelous visit." The nurse is aware that this is an example of:
    1. Compensation.
    2. Denial.
    3. Symbolism.
    4. Identification.

108. Psychomotor manifestations of anxiety that a nurse may observe include:
    1. Decreased activity.
    2. Increased activity.
    3. Increased lability of emotions.
    4. Decreased lability of emotions.

109. A patient whose significant other recently died shows signs of grief resolution when he or she:
    1. Wants to enter into another relationship soon.
    2. Talks of both the positive and negative aspects of their relationship.
    3. Makes up for deficiencies in the relationship, saying, "Things would have been better if we had only had more time."
    4. Expresses anger toward the deceased.

110. The nurse needs to know that anxiety may increase intellectual functioning because anxiety may:
    1. Increase the perceptual field.
    2. Increase ability to concentrate.
    3. Decrease the perceptual field.
    4. Decrease random activity.

111. In planning patient care, a nurse needs to know that self-destructive behavior may be interpreted as the:
    1. Directing of hostile feelings toward self.
    2. Directing of hostile feelings toward others.
    3. Directing of hostile feelings toward an internalized love object.
    4. Internalization of the fear of death.

112. Based on knowledge of Erikson's stages of growth and development, the nurse determines that the task of old age is primarily concerned with:
    1. Ego integrity versus despair.
    2. Autonomy versus shame and doubt.
    3. Trust versus mistrust.
    4. Industry versus inferiority.

113. The nurse must assess for high risk of suicide when a patient's behavior suggests:
    1. Major depression with melancholia features.
    2. Schizophrenic disorders.
    3. Bipolar mood disorder, manic episode.
    4. Psychological factors affecting physical condition.

114. In working with clients who are depressed, the nurse must know that depression may stem from:
    1. A sense of loss—actual, imaginary, or impending.
    2. Revived memories of a painful childhood.
    3. A confused sexual identity.
    4. An unresolved oedipal conflict.

115. When working with a person who is anxious, what is the *overall* goal of nursing intervention?
    1. Remove anxiety.
    2. Develop the person's awareness of anxiety.
    3. Protect the person from anxiety.
    4. Develop the person's capacity to tolerate mild anxiety and to use it constructively.

116. In discussions between parents and adolescents about their relationship, a desired outcome is that adolescents benefit because they will be able to:
    1. See themselves as the victims.
    2. View their parents and themselves realistically.
    3. Enlist the therapist's aid as an ally against their parents.
    4. See their parents as victims.

117. The main nursing goal with clients with schizophrenic disorders is to:
    1. Set limits on their bizarre behavior.
    2. Establish a trusting, nonthreatening, reality-based relationship.
    3. Quickly establish a warm, close relationship to counteract their aloofness.
    4. Protect them from self-destructive impulses.

118. A patient is placed in isolation for seclusion due to agitated behavior. The nurse knows it is essential that:
    1. Restraints be applied.
    2. All the furniture be removed from the isolation room.
    3. A staff member have frequent contacts with the patient.
    4. The patient be allowed to come out after 4 hours.

119. Which activity would be best for the nurse to suggest to a client who is depressed?
    1. Folding laundry or stapling paper sheets for charts.
    2. Playing checkers.
    3. Doing a crossword puzzle.
    4. Ice skating.

120. A woman patient says to the nurse, "That patient over there is a lesbian." What is the best response by the nurse?
    1. "Are you afraid she will attack you?"
    2. "That woman is not a lesbian."
    3. "What did the woman do that makes you think she is a lesbian?"
    4. "Then stay away from her."

121. Which activity could a nurse suggest that would be best for a client with hyperactive behavior?
    1. Solitary activity, such as reading.
    2. Hammering on metal in a jewelry-making class.
    3. Playing chess.
    4. Competitive games.

122. A patient says to his mother, "You are controlling me." The mother asks the nurse what he may have meant. What is the best response by the nurse?
    1. "He is upset and thinks you are taking charge of him."
    2. "He resents always having to meet your expectations."
    3. "I can't tell you. You will have to ask him."
    4. "I think you can ask your son that. Do you want me to stay with you while you ask him?"

123. When a client exhibits signs of amnesia, the nurse knows that this behavior is probably related to:
    1. Selectively forgetting and storing unacceptable thoughts, wishes, and impulses in the unconscious mind.
    2. Conscious, deliberate forgetting.
    3. Transferring to another situation an emotion felt in a previous situation where its expression would not have been acceptable.
    4. Unconscious imitating of the manners, behavior, and feelings of another.

124. In caring for a patient at risk for suicide, the most important nursing action is to:
    1. Maintain constant awareness of the patient's where-abouts.
    2. Ignore the patient as long as he or she is talking about suicide, because a suicide attempt is unlikely.
    3. Relax vigilance when the patient seems to be recovering from depression.
    4. Administer medication.

125. A client who attempted suicide recently remarked to the nurse the next morning, "Let's not think about that now. Maybe I'll feel like thinking about it later." The nurse identifies this as:
    1. Blocking.
    2. Denial.
    3. Suppression.
    4. Repression.

126. After a mastectomy, a woman says, "My husband won't love me anymore." What would be the most therapeutic response by the nurse?
    1. "Of course your husband loves you."
    2. "Tell me what has happened that makes you think your husband won't love you anymore."
    3. "If you stop crying and fix yourself up, you will look good to your husband."
    4. "Do you think your husband won't love you because you have lost a breast?"

127. Repetitive hand washing is often seen when a client is experiencing guilt feelings. This ritualistic behavior can be described as a mechanism whereby the client attaches significance to the act of washing. The nurse would identify this behavior as:
    1. Symbolism.
    2. Fantasy.
    3. Isolation.
    4. Conversion.

128. In conducting an assessment interview, the nurse needs to be aware that self-destructive behavior is determined by:
    1. A variety of factors, with the same factors present in each individual.
    2. Genetic disturbances.
    3. Interpersonal disturbances.
    4. A variety of factors, different for each individual.

129. A client shouts at the nurse one morning, "Why do you waste your time on me? I'm not sick; I don't need you. Go talk to other patients. They are really sick!" The nurse identifies this as:
    1. Reaction formation.
    2. Denial.
    3. Intellectualization.
    4. Rationalization.

130. Which term would the nurse use to describe the experience of an individual who thought he heard a machine gun when his neighbor's lawnmower backfired as she was mowing the lawn?
    1. Delusion.
    2. Hallucination.
    3. Identification.
    4. Illusion.

131. It would be important for the nurse to implement definite suicide precautions for a patient who is depressed if the patient's mood changed suddenly to one of:
    1. Cheerfulness.
    2. Psychomotor retardation.
    3. Agitation.
    4. Hostility.

132. The nurse knows that the most characteristic task of puberty and adolescence, according to Erikson's stages of psychosexual development, is:
    1. Identity versus role confusion.
    2. Initiative versus guilt.
    3. Ego integrity versus despair.
    4. Intimacy versus isolation.

133. A patient recently attempted suicide by slashing the wrists. The crisis intervention nurse and physician agree that hospitalization is not necessary for this patient; therefore, the nurse needs to:
    1. Wish the patient luck and terminate the session.
    2. Make an appointment for tomorrow and give the patient a telephone number where the nurse can be reached tonight.
    3. Make an appointment for the patient in 2 weeks, when the wrists might be healed.
    4. Tell the patient to make an appointment when she or he wants to, at the local mental health clinic.

134. A 10-year-old boy was admitted to the hospital for a tonsillectomy. In the morning, the nurse notes that the bedding is wet. There are several boys his age in the room. Which initial approach would best demonstrate a nurse's understanding of enuresis and this patient's stage of growth and development?
    1. While proceeding to change the wet linens, ask him what sports he likes best, purposely ignoring the wet bed by staying on impersonal topics.
    2. Draw the curtains around his bed while changing the linen, saying, "I know that this must be embarrassing to you."
    3. Say nothing while changing the bed; return at another time, when the other boys are not in the room, and explain to him the medical-emotional reasons for enuresis.
    4. Sit down on the bed and convey acceptance of him as a person rather than focusing on the wet bed.

135. A patient with an antisocial personality disorder arouses anxiety and frustration in the staff and tends to intimidate by manipulative behaviors. One morning the patient shouts at the nurse, "Since you won't give me a pass, go away, you fat pig, or I'll hit you." What is the most effective response by the nurse to a client who threatens or derogates?
    1. "You are rude and I don't like it. It makes me not want to talk with you."
    2. "That kind of talk will keep you here longer."
    3. "What did I do wrong?"
    4. "I don't like to hear insults and threats. What is important about getting the pass today?"

136. In assessing the behavior of a child with autism, the nurse notes that a symptom that characteristically differentiates this child from one with Down syndrome is:
    1. Retardation of activity.
    2. Short attention span.
    3. Difficulty in responding to a nurturing relationship.
    4. Poor academic performance.

137. It is important for a nurse to understand that a patient's repetitive hand washing is probably an attempt to:
    1. Punish himself or herself for guilt feelings.
    2. Control unacceptable impulses or feelings.
    3. Do what the voices the patient hears tell him or her to do.
    4. Seek attention from the staff.

138. In establishing a therapeutic nursing approach with a client who abuses and is dependent on substances, the nurse primarily needs to:
    1. Promote a permissive, accepting environment.
    2. Use a straightforward and confronting approach.
    3. Meet the client's need for a chemical substitute for the drug.
    4. Prevent the client's use of the addictive drug.

139. At 2:30 A.M., a client walks out to the nurse's station complaining that he is choking, suffocating, weakening, and dying. He demands a cigarette. What is the best response by the nurse?
    1. Refuse and tell him it is against the rules.
    2. Call the doctor and inform the doctor of the client's request and behavior.
    3. Refuse and tell him the cigarettes are locked.
    4. Give him a cigarette and stay with him while he smokes.

140. What approach can the nurse use to best handle a client's disturbed behavior?
    1. Approve the behavior.
    2. Maintain consistency of approach.
    3. Encourage the client not to express negative opinions.
    4. Interpret for the client the reasons for the behavior.

141. The overall client goal in rape counseling is to help the victim:
    1. Forget the incident and repress her feelings in order to be able to carry on with her life.
    2. Identify the rapist in a court of law.
    3. Accept her part in the rape.
    4. Acknowledge, face, and resolve the reaction she is experiencing.

142. Which is the most appropriate response to a client who states emphatically, "I hate them"?
    1. "I will stay with you as long as you feel this way."
    2. "Tell me about your hate."
    3. "I understand how you can feel this way."
    4. "For whom do you have these feelings?"

143. The nurse observes for signs of heroin withdrawal, which may include:
    1. Rhinorrhea, sneezing, and high fever.
    2. Pupillary dilation, diaphoresis, and weight loss.
    3. Pupillary constriction, vomiting, and pruritus.
    4. Choreiform movements and frequent lip wetting.

144. The nurse will look for what likely outcome of methadone treatment for heroin abuse and dependence?
    1. Sedation.
    2. Euphoria.
    3. Neuritis.
    4. Blocking of the euphoric effect of heroin and elimination of craving.

145. An acutely agitated client becomes increasingly aggressive. The staff's verbal attempts to stop the aggressive behavior are not effective. The client begins to shout threats at the staff and other clients, throws furniture, breaks windows, and hits, kicks, and bites other clients and staff. The client has a prn order for medication when agitated. Which action should the nurse take initially?
    1. Orient the client to reality and place the client in a well-lit, quiet room.
    2. Give the ordered tranquilizer and put the client in bed with the side rails up.
    3. Lock the client in his or her room and call the doctor.
    4. Have at least two staff members physically restrain the client and take the client to a quiet room.

146. A teenage patient has a history of stealing cars and traffic violations. The home environment has been permissive, and the teenager has been overly familiar and obsequious with the nurses. A new nurse, about to leave the locked unit, is holding the key as the patient approaches and eagerly offers to unlock the door for the nurse, saying, "The other nurses let me." Which first response by the nurse would be most appropriate?
    1. Let the patient turn the key in the lock, but stay close while the patient does it.
    2. Ask the patient why he or she wants to unlock the door.
    3. Tell the patient in a nice way that this is not allowed.
    4. Go to the head nurse and ask if it is all right for the patient to unlock the door.

147. Several staff members voice their frustrations about a patient's constant questions, such as "Should I go to the dayroom or should I stay in my room?" and "Should I have a cup of tea or a cup of coffee?" Which interpretation about this behavior will help the nursing staff deal effectively?
    1. The patient's inability to make decisions reflects a basic anxiety about making a mistake and being a failure.
    2. The patient's indecisiveness is aimed at testing the staff's reaction and acceptance of him or her.
    3. The patient's dependence on others (staff) is a symptom that needs to be interrupted by firm limit setting.
    4. The patient's need to ask questions is a bid for attention.

148. In providing dietary instructions to an Orthodox Jewish client who is depressed, the nurse needs to know that which practice would be prohibited in dietary Kosher laws?
    1. Eating dairy products with meat.
    2. Eating meat from animals with cloven hoofs.
    3. Eating fish with scales and fins.
    4. Eating unleavened bread during the 8 days of Passover.

149. A patient with antisocial behavior flatters the nurse. What is the patient trying to do?
    1. The patient wants something in return.
    2. The patient wants the nurse to like him.
    3. The patient needs attention.
    4. The patient is trying to redirect the focus of the nurse-patient interaction.

150. A patient with schizophrenia is banging on the hallway door leading to the outside, saying he needs to go to an appointment. What nursing intervention is needed?
    1. Ask the patient to move away from the door.
    2. Ignore this behavior.
    3. Escort the patient back into the room.
    4. Tell the patient that he cannot bang on the door.

151. In preparing a patient for ECT, the nurse knows that succinylcholine (Anectine) will be administered for which therapeutic effect?
    1. Skeletal muscle paralysis.
    2. Short-acting anesthesia.
    3. Decreased oral and respiratory secretions.
    4. Analgesia.

152. The nurse can anticipate that the person most likely to be at risk for depression is:
    1. An elderly person with previous depressive episodes.
    2. A middle-aged man who is a moderate alcohol drinker.
    3. A housewife with three school-age children.
    4. A nursing student at exam time.

153. In admitting a patient with Alzheimer's to the unit, which placement variable would have the highest priority?
    1. Place the patient with a roommate.
    2. Place the patient without a roommate.
    3. Place the patient close to the nurses' station.
    4. Place the patient at a distance from the nurses' station.

154. During a home health assessment visit to an elderly patient living alone, which aspect of lifestyle noted by the nurse would be of greatest concern?
    1. The family visits only twice a month.
    2. The family maintains only phone contact daily.
    3. The patient uses a cordless telephone rather than a standard phone.
    4. The patient prefers not to attend a senior citizen center for meals and recreation.

155. A hospitalized patient with Alzheimer's disease is often found wandering in the streets. What measure(s) should be taken in the unit to prevent the patient from wandering off?
    1. Place the patient in daytime restraints.
    2. Place the patient in nighttime restraints.
    3. Provide a security guard at the door.
    4. Use electronic surveillance devices.

156. What parental behavior toward a child during admission procedure should cause the nurse to suspect child abuse?
    1. Acting overly solicitous toward the child.
    2. Ignoring the child.
    3. Expressions of guilt.
    4. Flat affect.

157. Which nursing action would be best for a hospitalized patient who is constantly upset with the staff, easily angers, and frequently shouts at the nurses?
    1. Request that the patient be moved to another unit.
    2. Schedule a conference with the MD, nurse manager, and patient about this behavior.
    3. Contact social services to meet with the patient and family about the problem.
    4. Involve the patient and family in the development of the care plan.

158. Which nursing action would be most appropriate for a nursing diagnosis of "self-esteem disturbance"?
    1. Compliment the patient as often as possible.
    2. Assist the patient to set reasonable, achievable goals.
    3. Assure the patient that all needs will be met.
    4. Encourage the patient's family to praise the patient verbally.

159. During a group education session on recovering from a myocardial infarction, one patient blurts out, "I don't agree with what you are saying." The best response would be:
    1. "Tell us where your information came from."
    2. "I'll talk to you after the class is over."
    3. "I've had patients say that before, but they were wrong."
    4. "Give us an example of what you feel is incorrect."

Answers/Rationale

1. **(1)** Circulation may be severely impaired in a patient with waxy flexibility who tends to remain motionless for hours unless moved. **Answer 2** is *not the first* priority. "Touch" is *not* used in this stage, as in **Answer 3**. **Answer 4** is incorrect because the patient is *mute* and also because intellectual discussion of predisposing factors *ignores* the *feelings* of the patient.
    Test-taking tip—Note the key words: "*first* priority."
    PL, 6, PhI, Physiological Adaptation

2. **(2)** The best of four poor choices here is an attempt to understand what the client means. The other choices are *not* helpful. **Answers 3** and **4** *switch* the focus and *ignore* the client's statement; **Answer 1** is too brusque an attempt to bring the client back to reality.
    Test-taking tip—Asking for clarification is a therapeutic communication technique.
    IMP, 2, PsI, Coping and Adaptation

3. **(3)** This will reduce the isolation and withdrawal while at the same time not putting the burden of decision making on the client. The client needs a structured routine that is simple. The client may not be able to handle close proximity to more than one person at this point, as in **Answer 2. Answer 1** incorrectly allows the client to *remain* isolated; **Answer 4** is incorrect because the client needs a *structured* routine until he or she can make decisions for himself or herself.
    Test-taking tip—Review theory on depression. Activity is a therapeutic intervention, on a 1:1 basis, and without requiring an answer or verbal interaction.
    IMP, 7, PsI, Psychosocial Adaptation

4. **(2)** In the depressed episode, anger is turned inward; in the manic, it is noted in sarcasm, demanding behavior, and angry outbursts. **Answers 3** and **4** occur in the manic episode. **Answer 1** is a particular problem in the depressed phase.
    Test-taking tip—Remember point of theory: depression may be anger turned *inward* as opposed to expressed *outwardly* (as in manic behavior).
    AS, 2, PsI, Coping and Adaptation

5. **(1)** The nurse should formulate a weight control plan, in *cooperation* with the patient, that allows for a *gradual* weight loss, *not immediate* loss as in **Answer 4**. **Answers 2** and **3** *are incorporated* into **Answer 1.**
    Test-taking tip—When three options are good, choose the one that covers them all. Also look at two contradictory options: "gradual" vs. "immediate" weight loss. Choose the more realistic option ("gradual").
    IMP, 4, PhI, Basic Care and Comfort

6. **(4)** This is a reality-based response, as well as one that acknowledges the patient's nonverbal reaction. The other choices are *not* the best because **Answers 1** and **3** focus on "voice," which reinforces the hallucination, and no doubt is placed; in **Answer 2** doubt is placed, but the focus is on "voice" and *not* on patient's *feelings*.
    Test-taking tip—Note the key word "initially," which includes reality orientation and patient's feelings.
    IMP, 2, PsI, Psychosocial Adaptation

Key to codes following rationales   *Nursing process:* **AS**, Assessment; **AN**, Analysis; **PL**, Plan; **IMP**, Implementation; **EV**, Evaluation. *Category of human function:* **1**, Protective; **2**, Sensory-perceptual; **3**, Comfort, Rest, Activity, and Mobility; **4**, Nutrition; **5**, Growth and Development; **6**, Fluid-Gas Transport; **7**, Psychosocial-Cultural; **8**, Elimination. **Client needs: SECE;** Safe, Effective Care Environment; **PhI**, Physiological Integrity; **PsI**, Psychosocial Integrity; **HPM**, Health Promotion/ Maintenance. See appendices for full explanation.

7. (1) It shows acceptance by listening to the client's initial account of the physical problems. Neither a superficial focus nor a technical explanation of physical problems (**Answers 2 and 3**) conveys acceptance of the client as a person; **Answer 4** is too abrupt for an initial response.

Test-taking tip—Look at the verbs: "allow," "comment," "give," "let (the patient know)." Choose the one that most conveys acceptance.

IMP, 7, PsI, Psychosocial Adaptation

8. (2) Characteristic underlying needs in somatoform disorders are dependency, attention, and the need for security through trust. **Answers 1 and 4** are incorrect because the patient's complaints are not aimed at blaming others or at seeking vengeance but at expressing dependency needs and seeking security. **Answer 3** is inappropriate because the patient is expressing his or her *own* need for attention; the patient is not speaking for everyone.

Test-taking tip—Apply the process of elimination. Eliminate the two hostile options (**1,4**); next eliminate the global "everyone."

AN,7,PsI, Coping and Adaptation

9. (2) Because confabulation is a coping mechanism, the best choice is the one that defines one of the main functions of coping mechanisms—to protect self-esteem. **Answers 1 and 3** are incorrect because they focus on *others*, not on self. **Answer 4** is completely *irrelevant*.

Test-taking tip—Choose the response that focuses on the *patients*, after eliminating two options that focus on *others* (**1, 3**). It's a "patient focus vs. others" type of test-taking tip.

AN,2,PsI, Coping and Adaptation

10. (1) Deal first with the *lifesaving* situation. **Answers 2 and 3** are incorrect because they are done *following* stabilization of physical condition. **Answer 4** is incorrect because it is *not* a necessary lifesaving concern.

Test-taking tip—Note key words "*first* concern," which is a priority on Maslow's hierarchy of human needs (e.g., physiological needs).

PL,7,PhI, Physiological Adaptation

11. (1) The nurse needs to set limits to ensure the safety of the patient and others. **Answer 2** is incorrect because the patient may hurt herself or himself or others. **Answers 3 and 4** are incorrect because they are interpretations that may or may not be correct, and they do *not control* the *unsafe* behavior.

Test-taking tip—Look at two options that are contradictory ("allow" and "limits"). Because the main concern is *safety* when a patient is agitated, select **Answer 1**. Avoid interpretive statements (**3, 4**).

IMP,1,SECE, Safety

12. (2) In second grade a person needs to form close relationships with *peers*. **Answer 1** needs to occur *earlier* than second grade or *later* in early teen years. **Answer 3** occurs *later*. **Answer 4** is incorrect because the father's actions *make* the child dependent on him rather than on peers.

Test-taking tip—Know normal age-appropriate growth and development.

AN,5,HPM, Growth and Development

13. (3) This tells the teenager the nurse heard his statement about "not doing his own thing" and *thinks* he is angry. **Answer 1** is incorrect because this states the nurse *knows* he is angry. **Answer 2** is incorrect because an angry person *cannot stop* being angry on command. **Answer 4** is incorrect because focusing on the parents puts the nurse on their side.

Test-taking tip—Choose a therapeutic communication response that focuses on the teenage *patient's feelings* (not "we," "your parents" as in **Answer 4**).

IMP,7,PsI, Coping and Adaptation

14. (2) This acknowledges the experience and points out reality as the nurse sees it. **Answers 1, 3, and 4** do not focus on the patient or attempt to explore feelings.

Test-taking tip—An effective response to hallucinatory behavior is to support the feeling aspect ("distressing") while also pointing out reality.

IMP,2,PsI, Psychosocial Adaptation

15. (1) Emotional support is a key need. **Answer 2** does *not* focus on emotional support. **Answer 3**, role expectation, in itself has *no* bearing; emotional support of role would. **Answer 4** would help the spouse and his or her own emotional reaction but would *not* help the patient.

Test-taking tip—Best answer focuses on *emotional* support for the *patient*. Eliminate the three other options because they focus on the spouse or family.

AS,7,PsI, Coping and Adaptation

16. (4) An honest, direct answer that focuses on feelings is the best approach. **Answers 1, 2, and 3** stop any further exploration of the client's feelings.

Test-taking tip—Choose the answer that helps *explore feelings*. Eliminate the other three options that close off communication and focus on facts, not feelings.

IMP,7,PsI, Coping and Adaptation

17. (3) Showing *acceptance* and gaining trust and confidence are usually the key initial nursing goals. You need to show acceptance before *helping* (**Answers 1 and 4**) or *assisting* (**Answer 2**).

Test-taking tip—Focus on the phrase "initial nursing goal," which is *acceptance*. Note the lead verb: *accept* before *help* or *assist*.

PL,7,PsI, Coping and Adaptation

18. (2) Refer to Elisabeth Kübler-Ross's emotional stages of death and dying. She is being neither unrealistic (**Answer 1**), manipulative (**Answer 3**), nor unaware of her diagnosis (**Answer 4**).

Test-taking tip—Select the response that typifies a common grief reaction ("bargaining"); eliminate the three responses that have a negative tone ("deny," "manipulative," "unaware").

EV,7,PsI, Coping and Adaptation

19. (1) This reply asks for information that the nurse can use. If the patient understands the statement, the nurse can support the therapist when focusing on connections between food, love, and mother. If the patient does not understand the statement, the nurse can help get clarification from the therapist. **Answer 2** alienates the client, and the nurse loses the chance for collaboration with the therapist. **Answer 3** shuts the patient off. **Answer 4** is incorrect because it is asked before the nurse is sure the patient understands the therapist's statement.

Test-taking tip—Choose a therapeutic communication response that helps the patient give the nurse *feedback* (on patient understanding of therapist statement).

IMP,7,PsI, Coping and Adaptation

20. (4) Redundancy is *not* meant to impress others but is aimed at *pleasure* gained through focus on the *past* and need to *control* the conversation when memory or hearing deficit is present. **Answers 1, 2, and 3** *would* demonstrate understanding of this behavior.

Test-taking tip—Focus on the key phrase "*not* demonstrate understanding"; use a true-or-false approach.

AN,5,HPM, Growth and Development

21. (2) During a manic episode, the client may be too busy to eat and sleep. **Answers 1 and 3** are more appropriate for a depressive episode; **Answer 4** is more appropriate for schizophrenia with bizarre behavior. Clients in manic episode exhibit hyperactive behavior.

Test-taking tip—Match characteristic behaviors with other main diagnostic categories: depression with **Answers 1 and 3** and schizophrenia with **Answer 4.**

PL, 2, PsI, Psychosocial Adaptation

22. (3) Nocturnal urination is a most common need, complicated by disorientation related to the patient's age, disorder, and unfamiliar environment at night. To sit down (**Answer**

1) or to go back to the patient's room and talk (**Answer 4**) does not take care of the possible problem, the need to urinate. Asking a person "why" questions (**Answer 2**) is not helpful and is too literal a response to the behavior.

> **Test-taking tip**—Confusion (Alzheimer's) and age-typical physiological need (nocturia) call for a response that is reality orientation and environmental redirection (to the location of the bathroom).

IMP, 7, HPM, Growth and Development

23. (**4**) A simple acknowledgment of what the nurse sees is the best response. **Answer 3** makes an assumption that the patient feels better if she looks better. **Answers 1 and 2** can be taken as a put-down.

> **Test-taking tip**—Eliminate put-downs and assumptions. Keep it simple (KIS) and simply acknowledge what the nurse observes.

IMP, 7, PsI, Coping and Adaptation

24. (**2**) Confidentiality cannot be guaranteed if there is a danger to the patient or to others. **Answer 1** is incorrect because it is a *sarcastic* response and *denies* that the patient has serious problems. **Answer 3** *contradicts* **Answer 2**. **Answer 4** is incorrect because parents do *not* have the right to know the content of therapy sessions except in the circumstances described in **Answer 2**.

> **Test-taking tip**—Eliminate two options with the global "everything" and one option that can be seen as a put-down.

IMP, 7, SECE, Management of Care

25. (**2**) A diagnosis of a paranoid disorder implies weak *ego* development. **Answers 1, 3, and 4** are incorrect because a client with a paranoid disorder might have *strong* id, super-ego, and "not me" components.

> **Test-taking tip**—Focus on the word "weak" in the stem.

AN, 5, PsI, Coping and Adaptation

26. (**2**) An important principle to remember here is that a program of care should not increase physiological losses by overtaxing the client's physical capacities. It is important to remember that suicide is the *main* concern of *depression* and *not* a key concern of dementia, as in **Answer 1**. Empathy *rather than* sympathy (**Answer 4**) is a helpful behavior. **Answer 3**, increasing independence, is *not realistic; maintaining* it *is*.

> **Test-taking tip**—Apply the process of elimination. Eliminate **Answer 4** because "sympathy" is not therapeutic; eliminate the unrealistic response in **Answer 3**; eliminate **Answer 1** because it applies to depression, not to general care in dementia.

PL, 2, PhI, Reduction of Risk Potential

27. (**4**) This is the all-inclusive answer. **Answers 1, 2, and 3** may be part of **Answer 4**.

> **Test-taking tip**—Choose the "umbrella" answer (i.e., most inclusive) when all four options are correct.

AN, 7, PsI, Coping and Adaptation

28. (**4**) If a particular client is nonverbal, for example, the nurse should not expect that client to function at a verbal level until ready. In **Answer 1**, if the nurse waits for a client who is withdrawn to make contact, it may not be helpful. In **Answer 2**, a client who is ambivalent may need assistance in making decisions. In **Answer 3**, the client's undesirable behavior may be adversely affecting others.

> **Test-taking tip**—Apply a reasoning "What if . . ." approach: "What if" a patient will *not* initiate, *can't* make decisions, and undesirable behavior *can't* be ignored?

IMP, 7, PsI, Coping and Adaptation

29. (**2**) This is the most neutral answer by process of elimination. **Answer 1** is *mainly* the function of a *recreational-occupational* therapist, although nurses participate. **Answer 3** is *usually* filled by *psychologists* and social workers, and **Answer 4** is carried out *primarily by psychologists* or *statisticians*, although nurses are involved. "Maintenance of a therapeutic environment" fits more readily into a nursing role by virtue

of the number of hours per day a nurse spends with the clients on a unit, in comparison with the number spent by other professionals.

> **Test-taking tip**—Keep it simple (KIS) response; a mental health setting should keep a therapeutic environment.

PL, 7, PsI, Psychosocial Adaptation

30. (**4**) A person needs to be allowed to express anger appropriately. **Answers 1, 2, and 3** are *incorrect* choices here because they *are* things the nurse assists a person to do when intervening in anger.

> **Test-taking tip**—Key word: "inappropriate."

IMP, 1, PsI, Psychosocial Adaptation

31. (**2**) Offering a broad opening by giving a general lead is most therapeutic to elicit further description of the client's reaction and to clarify feelings, which were vaguely stated. **Answer 1** is a *switch of focus* from the client to the mother. **Answer 3** is nontherapeutic because a question that can be *answered by yes or no* often closes off further exploration. **Answer 4** could be a helpful intervention but is *premature* acknowledgment before feelings have been elaborated.

> **Test-taking tip**—Choose the most therapeutic communication response: giving a broad opening, with a *general* lead to *clarify feelings*.

IMP, 7, PsI, Coping and Adaptation

32. (**3**) It incorporates all information a crisis intervention nurse needs immediately. **Answers 1 and 2** are incorrect because the nurse does not need to know about other people's involvement at this time. **Answer 4** is incorrect because it is *not as complete as* **Answer 3**.

> **Test-taking tip**—Key words: "initial goal."

PL, 7, PsI, Psychosocial Adaptation

33. (**3**) It is important to acknowledge a statement, even if it is not understood. **Answer 1** is not a *direct* response; **Answer 2** leaves out the importance of the meaning of the neologism to the client; and **Answer 4** is less valid and important than *acknowledgment* of the meaning to the client.

> **Test-taking tip**—Look at the verbs: "divert," "state," "acknowledge," "interpret." Select "acknowledge" as the first response.

PL, 2, PsI, Psychosocial Adaptation

34. (**1**) It is important to externalize the anger away from self. **Answer 2** is incorrect because usually the client is turning anger *inward*, toward the self. **Answer 3** increases the client's sense of isolation. The needs in **Answer 4** should be emphasized, *not deemphasized*, because the depressed client often has somatic delusions.

> **Test-taking tip**—Apply a commonly accepted point of theory about depression: anger turned inward that needs to be externalized.

PL, 7, PsI, Psychosocial Adaptation

35. (**4**) It is a matter-of-fact statement that is direct, while offering assistance and setting limits on inappropriate behavior. The other choices are not useful because **Answer 1** reinforces inappropriate social behavior; **Answer 2** sets limits but does not state a positive expectation for the client to follow; and **Answer 3** neither offers assistance nor sets limits, which the patient needs.

> **Test-taking tip**—Pay attention to the phrase "best initial response."

IMP, 2, PsI, Psychosocial Adaptation

36. (**3**) Take care of the bleeding (physical aspects of care) first. In **Answers 1 and 2** the client could suffer extensive blood loss if the nurse focuses on feelings at this point or leaves the client without first attempting to control the bleeding. In **Answer 4**, the client is left alone, bleeding, frightened, and with a razor still at the side.

> **Test-taking tip**—Be aware that the stem asks for *first* action.

AN, 7, PsI, Psychosocial Adaptation

37. (2) Persons engaged in self-destructive behavior other than active suicide behavior fantasize that *they can control* their behavior and deny the likelihood of death as a result. Thus **Answers 1, 3,** and **4** are incorrect.

    Test-taking tip—Know theory about gradual self-destructive behaviors and eliminate the three that are theoretically incorrect (**1, 3, 4**). Look at two options that are opposites (acceptance and denial) and choose a *most common* defense mechanism (denial).
    AN, 7, PsI, Coping and Adaptation

38. (1) Shock and anger are commonly the primary initial reactions. **Answer 2** is irrelevant. **Answer 3** is a literal, concrete interpretation of the patient's reaction, not aimed at the possible latent feelings. **Answer 4** is incorrect because it contradicts the correct answer, **Answer 1.**

    Test-taking tip—Look at two contradictory options (normal vs. not normal); review normal grief reactions and choose "normal."
    AN, 7, PsI, Coping and Adaptation

39. (3) One of the main needs experienced by most clients with dementia is the need for most things to be the same. The other choices are wrong for the following reasons: there has been no demonstrable evidence of relationship between any behavior symptom and the extent or severity of pathophysiological condition (**Answer 2**); intellectual *blunting* usually occurs, which interferes with ability to deal with insight and abstract thoughts (**Answer 4**); and memory loss is for *recent* events and names, *not* those in the distant past, as in **Answer 1.**

    Test-taking tip—Key words: "most commonly."
    AS, 2, PsI, Coping and Adaptation

40. (3) One way to enhance the development of unresolved grief is *not* to participate in activities that demonstrate death. **Answers 1, 2,** and **4** may occur, but they are *not* the best predictors of grief resolution difficulties.

    Test-taking tip—Apply theory about unresolved grief (which may be related to lack of culturally sanctioned rituals for "letting go").
    AN, 7, PsI, Coping and Adaptation

41. (4) *Rationalization* is the process of constructing plausible reasons for one's responses. **Answer 1,** *suppression,* is the intentional exclusion of material from consciousness. **Answer 2,** *undoing,* is an act that partially negates a previous one. **Answer 3,** *repression,* is the involuntary exclusion of painful or conflicting thoughts or feelings from awareness.

    Test-taking tip—Review definitions with clinical application of defense mechanisms.
    AN, 7, PsI, Coping and Adaptation

42. (4) Decoding symbolic, autistic expressions calls for skill and sensitivity in understanding latent messages. **Answer 1** is not a good choice, because showing "acceptance" is a basic, initial nursing goal that does not require a complexity of skills. **Answer 2** points out a nontherapeutic nursing action, which is best not to use at all. **Answer 3** implies that the nurse use short sentences with clear, concise, unambiguous meaning; this *can* be accomplished with practice. **Answers 1** and **3** must be accomplished before **Answer 4** is possible.

    Test-taking tip—"Greatest difficulty" is the key phrase to keep in mind.
    IMP, 7, PsI, Psychosocial Adaptation

43. (3) This is a false belief developed in response to an emotional need. In **Answer 1,** the situation is *not* a perceptual disorder. In **Answer 2,** the situation is *not* a misperception. In **Answer 4,** although the patient refuses meals, the reason for this is a false belief (delusion).

    Test-taking tip—Know the difference between a false belief, a misinterpretation, and misperception.
    AN, 7, PsI, Coping and Adaptation

44. (3) This shows a weak sense of moral consciousness. According to Freudian theory, personality disorders stem from a *weak* superego. **Answer 1** is incorrect, because the id is *strong.* These disorders are *not* characterized by a weak ego, as in **Answer 2,** whereas schizophrenia is. **Answer 4** is of relevance in sexual-identity difficulties rather than in personality disorders.

    Test-taking tip—Sociopathic behavior and weak superego can be matched. Key word: "defect."
    AN, 5, PsI, Coping and Adaptation

45. (1) Frightening visual hallucinations are especially common. **Answer 2** is incorrect because coma is usually *not* an immediate consequence of alcohol withdrawal. **Answer 3** is incorrect because the diagnosis is *withdrawal* from alcohol, not alcohol intoxication (intake). **Answer 4** is incorrect because the patient will be *agitated* and *rambling* in conversation, not mute and depressed.

    Test-taking tip—Key words: "likely," "on admission," and "withdrawal."
    AS, 7, PsI, Psychosocial Adaptation

46. (1) Anxiety is generated by group therapy at 9 A.M. The ritualistic behavioral defense of hand washing decreases anxiety by avoiding group therapy. **Answer 2** is incorrect because *tension,* not unmet needs, is discharged through ritualistic behavior. **Answer 3** may be true, but it is not essential to planning care. **Answer 4** is incorrect, because depression is *not* characteristic of ritualism.

    Test-taking tip—Apply theory about ritualistic behavior (also called obsessive-compulsive disorder, which is an *anxiety* disorder). "Fears" and "tensions" are similar to "anxiety."
    AN, 7, PsI, Coping and Adaptation

47. (3) Somatoform disorders provide a way of coping with conflicts. **Answer 1** is incorrect because conversion, *not regression,* is the major coping mechanism. **Answer 2** is incorrect because if a possible cause is identified and treatment relieves the discomfort, the client often develops another symptom. Frequently, clients do not want to be cured of their symptoms because they *need* the symptoms to control the behavior of others or because they do not know how else to get attention. In **Answer 4,** the converse is true: the symptoms *are* real, not imagined or faked.

    Test-taking tip—When in doubt as to the most theoretically correct answer, choose the option that has "feelings" in it.
    AN, 7, PsI, Coping and Adaptation

48. (2) All the other choices (**1, 3, 4**) are correct but can be dovetailed into **Answer 2.**

    Test-taking tip—Choose the "umbrella" answer that encompasses the other three choices.
    EV, 7, PsI, Coping and Adaptation

49. (1) Use of regression as a coping response *can* be minimized. Memory loss is usually permanent, not correctable; thus **Answer 2** is wrong. However, disorientation attributed to loss of memory can be minimized. Clients usually become *more* dependent in the course of illness *and* deteriorate progressively. Thus **Answers 3** and **4** are incorrect.

    Test-taking tip—Know what can and cannot be ameliorated. Whereas the nurse cannot stop the pathological course of Alzheimer's disease (i.e., memory loss is *permanent;* deterioration is *progressive* and rehabilitation is *not* possible), use of a coping mechanism (regression) *can* be minimized.
    PL, 2, PsI, Psychosocial Adaptation

50. (4) The major goal of crisis intervention is to resolve immediate problems. **Answer 1** is incorrect because restructuring personality is the goal of *psychoanalytic* therapy. **Answers 2** and **3** are incorrect because they are goals of *brief* psychotherapy, and although they may occur in the resolution of immediate problems, they are *not the* goal.

    Test-taking tip—Note the similarity between the word "crisis" in the stem and "immediate" in the correct option.
    IMP, 7, PsI, Coping and Adaptation

Answers/Rationale

51. **(4)** It provides the complete steps. **Answer 1** is incorrect because of the phrase "decide on *several*"; it should be *one* solution at a time. **Answer 2** is incorrect because it does *not* include "discuss alternative solutions." **Answer 3** is incorrect because it does not describe a requested *series* of steps and because *giving* a person one answer is untherapeutic.

     Test-taking tip—The best answer meets the condition of the stem: a series of *steps* in the *therapeutic* process. **Answer 2** would be also a good choice, but it is incomplete (misses one step). Eliminate **Answer 1** because it is an overload (i.e., *several* solutions); and eliminate **Answer 3** because it is dictatorial, not a discussion. Therefore, first focus on the two options that have "discuss" and choose "one solution" at a time.
     IMP, 7, PsI, Psychosocial Adaptation

52. **(1)** It is most likely that grief would be expressed because of object loss. **Answer 2** is incorrect because deep depression, if it occurs, would be the result of *lack* of resolution of grief over object loss. **Answer 3** is incorrect because relief is *not part* of the grief process. **Answer 4** is incorrect because the question asks for the client's *immediate* response. Denial of carcinoma, if it occurs, would probably occur *later*.

     Test-taking tip—Note the word "immediately" following the surgery.
     AS, 7, PsI, Coping and Adaptation

53. **(1)** Overcompliance leads to lack of development of self-identity, one of the major problems in schizophrenic disorders. **Answer 2** is incorrect because there are *no substantiating data*. **Answer 3** is incorrect because it *contradicts* the correct statement in **Answer 1. Answer 4** is incorrect because the patient probably has a *strong* superego due to an implied "should" system (overcompliance with parents' expectations of behavior).

     Test-taking tip—Look at two contradictory options: "lack of separate identity" vs. "a separate identity."
     AN, 7, HPM, Growth and Development

54. **(2)** The nurse helps to activate by doing something with the patient. **Answer 1** is incorrect because the patient will not hear a long explanation. **Answer 3** is incorrect because demanding will not work; the patient cannot join in unless you are with the patient (as in **Answer 2**). **Answer 4** is incorrect because you should not produce psychosis to motivate a person.

     Test-taking tip—Look at key words in the options and eliminate the three worst: "long explanation"; "demand"; "voices want the patient."
     IMP, 7, PsI, Psychosocial Adaptation

55. **(3)** The meaning of "ideas of reference" is that all that goes on is somehow connected to a person. **Answer 1** is incorrect because delusions of grandeur mean a person has an *exalted* opinion of self. **Answer 2** is incorrect because illusion is a false perceptual experience occurring in response to a stimulus. **Answer 4** is incorrect because echolalia is a person's automatic *repetition* of what is said.

     Test-taking tip—You can apply the correct term if you understand what the terms mean.
     AN, 7, PsI, Coping and Adaptation

56. **(2)** Manipulation is the attempt to control the behavior of others to achieve one's own goals. **Answer 1,** *insight,* is understanding and using understanding to correct one's behavior. **Answers 3** and **4** are incorrect because although the client may be trying to con the nurse into believing he or she *needs* the nurse to do something for him or her and the client *trusts* the nurse, the *real* purpose of the request is manipulation.

     Test-taking tip—Review the concept of manipulation. Eliminate three options that have *no* relationship to "acting out" (insight, dependency, trust).
     AN, 7, PsI, Coping and Adaptation

57. **(3)** A person with limited hearing and sight becomes confused and disturbed. **Answers 1** and **4** are *unwarranted*

assumptions. **Answer 2** is incorrect because the patient's situation is *not psychological* dependency but actual *sensory* need.

     Test-taking tip—Choose the most reasonable explanation and avoid making assumptions (1, 4).
     AN, 2, PhI, Basic Care and Comfort

58. **(4)** It is important to pick up on a feeling tone and encourage exploration of the feelings and the situation. **Answer 1** *stops* exploration of the patient's feeling. **Answers 2** and **3** *shift* the focus away from feelings to content of selfishness.

     Test-taking tip—Focus on *feelings* and encourage elaboration, with an open-ended statement ("tell me more about . . .").
     IMP, 7, PsI, Coping and Adaptation

59. **(1)** Clients with dementia feel more secure when they can count on their environment being the same, predictable, and consistent in detail from day to day (hence, structured) to compensate for feelings of loss of the familiar in terms of body functions, social environment, and so on. **Answers 2** and **4** imply change, not routine. **Answer 3**, although correct, is not the *most* important.

     Test-taking tip—Two options are correct (1, 3). When the activities are *structured* (the best response), they are usually also *simplified* and avoid decision-making problems. This is a "telescope" answer, in which a broader option subsumes a narrower one.
     PL, 6, SECE, Safety

60. **(1)** The patient has ideas that someone (her husband) is out to kill her. **Answer 2** is incorrect because the problem is *beyond* just an "idea of reference" (she fears bodily harm). **Answer 3** is incorrect because illusion is a false perceptual experience occurring in response to a stimulus. **Answer 4** is incorrect because a hallucination is a sensory experience triggered by a person's inner needs, functioning independently of stimulation from the environment.

     Test-taking tip—Know your terminology to spot the only correct answer.
     AN, 7, PsI, Coping and Adaptation

61. **(1)** To resolve immediate problems, focus on a person's ability to cope and usual level of functioning. **Answer 2** is incorrect because it is a *psychoanalytic* focus. **Answers 3** and **4** are incorrect because they are the focus of *brief* psychotherapy.

     Test-taking tip—Crisis focuses on the *present* and restoration of *here-and-now* coping.
     IMP, 7, PsI, Psychosocial Adaptation

62. **(4)** One coping mechanism often seen in somatoform disorders is repression. As the patient is better able to handle the anxiety connected with underlying feelings, the *need for repression lessens*. **Answers 1, 2,** and **3** may be the content of the patient's feelings, but they do not explain the dynamics, the *reason* the patient is expressing more feelings.

     Test-taking tip—Note the key word: "dynamics." Separate content from dynamics to choose the best answer.
     AN, 7, PsI, Coping and Adaptation

63. **(2)** This disorder is an attempt to cope with stress and is a better choice than **Answer 4,** which may be true but is a tangential and irrelevant reason. **Answer 1** is not correct because the client *is* aware of reality but may not understand the *cause* for the somatoform disorder. **Answer 3** is more relevant in a *paranoid* reaction.

     Test-taking tip—Look for the statements that correctly explain somatoform disorders (2, 4); eliminate **Answer 4** because it is incorporated in **Answer 2**.
     AN, 7, PsI, Coping and Adaptation

64. **(4)** Patients with withdrawn behavior in schizophrenic disorders tend to think in concrete terms. Therefore, use of simple language enables them to grasp meaning. **Answer 1** is incorrect because if the nurse remains silent the patient will remain silent. **Answer 2** is incorrect because if the nurse is

not concrete the patient might have trouble understanding some terms in normal conversation. **Answer 3** is incorrect because the patient has difficulty talking.

Test-taking tip—KIS means keep it simple—i.e., "simple . . . language."

PL, 7, PsI, Psychosocial Adaptation

65. (1) These persons have not faced up to the idea that they are controlled by their behavior, and this relieves their anxiety. Contrary to **Answer 2**, persons have *increased* anxiety if they stop the behavior. **Answer 3** is also incorrect because they fantasize that *they* control their behavior. **Answer 4** is incorrect because these persons *know* the behavior is not "good" for them.

Test-taking tip—Eliminate the three options that are *opposite* of correct points of theory.

AN, 7, PsI, Psychosocial Adaptation

66. (4) Meet the patient at her or his level of functioning, and provide support and encouragement for a higher level in the near future. **Answer 1** implies that the nurse agrees that the patient has nothing to say. **Answer 2** conveys no empathy or understanding. **Answer 3** is incorrect because silence reinforces silence and a sense of isolation.

Test-taking tip—The best answer acknowledges feelings and is supportive, without reinforcing the silence.

IMP, 7, PsI, Psychosocial Adaptation

67. (2) Often the verbalized ideas are jumbled, but the underlying feelings are discernible and must be acknowledged. Flight of ideas should be *curtailed;* thus **Answer 4** is incorrect. The client may not be able to control the internal stimuli to focus on one idea at a time as in **Answer 3**. A louder and more rapid tone by the nurse may only increase the external stimuli for the client, making **Answer 1** incorrect.

Test-taking tip—Choose the answer that focuses on *feelings.*

PL, 2, PsI, Psychosocial Adaptation

68. (4) The patient needs to have his or her feelings acknowledged, with encouragement to discuss feelings, and be reassured about the nurse's presence. The patient may interpret the nurse's silence as discomfort in talking about suicidal feelings and thoughts (**Answer 1**). **Answer 2** focuses on facts too swiftly without providing an opportunity for the patient to express feelings. Also, **Answer 2** would be most appropriate in *crisis* intervention when the patient is *first* admitted, *not* the next morning. **Answer 3** moves away from focus on here-and-now to focus on the past.

Test-taking tip—Choose the answer that focuses on acknowledging *feelings.*

IMP, 7, PsI, Psychosocial Adaptation

69. (3) When feelings of low self-esteem are prevalent, self-destructive behavior reaches its peak. Hence, **Answers 1, 2,** and **4** are incorrect.

Test-taking tip—*Low* self-esteem is the option that is different from the three other options (omnipotence, grandiosity, self-satisfaction).

AN, 7, PsI, Coping and Adaptation

70. (1) Love-hate feelings take longer to resolve. Reactions to loss tend to be cumulative in effect, in that the more loss experienced in the past, the greater the reaction the next time; thus **Answer 3** is wrong. Reactivation of feelings connected with previous losses by the current loss accounts for the increased intensity of the reaction. Sudden, unexpected death, *rather* than death due to a chronic illness, as in **Answer 2**, is harder to resolve, and strong, *not little,* emotional dependency (as in **Answer 4**) also complicates grief resolution.

Test-taking tip—Apply your knowledge about grief theory to choose the only correct answer.

AN, 7, PsI, Coping and Adaptation

71. (1) These behaviors are correct according to Lindemann's and Engle's grief stages. Hence, incorrect are **Answer 2** ("shock" stage), **Answer 3** ("idealization" stage), and **Answer 4** ("resolving the loss" stage).

Test-taking tip—Review stages of grief to choose the correct stage.

AS, 7, PsI, Coping and Adaptation

72. (4) Feelings of worthlessness or low self-esteem are the underlying problem in depression. **Answers 1, 2,** and **3** may occur but are *not most* apt.

Test-taking tip—Note key phrase: "*most* likely to see."

AN, 7, PsI, Coping and Adaptation

73. (4) Focusing on feelings is usually the best choice. Ignoring the client is rarely an acceptable intervention (**Answer 1**). Pointing out disturbed behavior and role modeling by the nurse are valid, but *not* as first interventions (**Answers 2** and **3**).

Test-taking tip—Key words: "*first* need."

PL, 7, PsI, Psychosocial Adaptation

74. (1) Listening is probably the most effective response of the four choices. A key consideration in interacting with patients who are suspicious is to *avoid* the use of logic and argument; thus **Answer 2** is incorrect. Humor usually intensifies the anger and suspicion; thus **Answer 3** is incorrect. Changing the topic, as in **Answer 4**, may serve to reinforce the patient's belief in the guilt of others.

Test-taking tip—Choose the term that involves the least action and does not *reinforce* suspicious behavior.

PL, 7, PsI, Psychosocial Adaptation

75. (4) Personality disorders stem from a weak superego, implying a lack of adequate controls. **Answer 1** is not relevant, as the patient's *self-identity* is *not* a focus here. **Answer 2** is incorrect because the patient typically gratifies his or her own inner needs; this is part of the difficulty with a strong id, and requires external controls as in **Answer 4**. **Answer 3** is incorrect because the patient is *not* psychotic, but has a personality disorder for which reality testing is *not* impaired. The patient *is* aware of reality.

Test-taking tip—Apply knowledge about antisocial behavior to select the *only* correct answer, and to eliminate the three that are theoretically incorrect.

PL, 7, PsI, Psychosocial Adaptation

76. (4) Arrest of the disease is possible through abstinence, not through change in psychophysiological response to alcohol. **Answers 1, 2,** and **3** are stereotyped statements, not generally or universally accepted.

Test-taking tip—Choose the *least* controversial belief: that alcohol dependence cannot be cured. Eliminate the option that has "always"; eliminate the option that is a cliché (**Answer 2**); it has not been universally accepted that alcohol dependency is hereditary.

AN, 7, PsI, Psychosocial Adaptation

77. (4) The *opposite* of what is stated in the first three choices is true. The patient seems to do best when *routine* activities are set up and anxiety-provoking changes are avoided (**Answer 1**); *perfection-type* activities bring satisfaction (e.g., cleaning and straightening a linen closet) (**Answer 2**); and the patient knows *ahead of time* about changes in routine (**Answer 3**).

Test-taking tip—By knowing, understanding, and applying theory about dynamics of ritualistic behavior, you can eliminate three options that are theoretically inaccurate. You can also make an educated guess and choose as the best option the answer that includes the phrase "*positive* accomplishment can occur."

IMP, 7, PsI, Psychosocial Adaptation

78. (1) The original source of conflict, pain, or guilt is repressed (pushed out of awareness), only to surface in a symbolic way. **Answers 2, 3,** and **4** are only partially correct: in somatoform disorders, regression is common, *not sublimation;* displacement is common, *not substitution;* reaction formation is common, *not rationalization.*

Test-taking tip—To serve as the best answer, *all* parts must be correct, not just partially correct. Review coping mechanisms as they relate to somatoform disorders.

AN, 7, PsI, Coping and Adaptation

79. **(2)** It reflects the patient's underlying concerns in the *most* open-ended manner. **Answer 1** is incorrect because the nurse cannot say how the patient is feeling; this assumes here that the patient *is* better, which is inappropriate. **Answer 4** focuses on only *one* aspect: sadness. What about the *agitation* the patient *also* expresses? **Answer 3** is not incorrect, but it is also not the *best* choice because it asks a direct question when a simple acknowledgment (as in **Answer 2**) would be better *initially*.

    Test-taking tip—KIS (Keep It Simple); a simple acknowledgment is the most open-ended communication approach. Eliminate **Answers 3** and **4** because they *require* the patient to answer. Eliminate **Answer 1** because it is an overload.
    IMP, 7, PsI, Psychosocial Adaptation

80. **(4)** Although all the other choices (**1, 2, 3**) *are* valid and important, **Answer 4** encompasses them all and is therefore the most *comprehensive* answer.

    Test-taking tip—When all four options are correct, choose the "umbrella" answer that includes them all.
    AN, 7, HPM, Growth and Development

81. **(3)** Part of the definition of a crisis is a time span of 4–6 weeks. **Answer 1** is incorrect because by definition, crises do *not* continue indefinitely. **Answer 2** is incorrect because *all* people have crises, and having crises does not determine abnormality. **Answer 4** is incorrect because although crises may be related to deep, underlying problems, one of the principles of crisis intervention therapy is to deal with the immediate situation, not the underlying problem.

    Test-taking tip—By definition, crisis are short term. Look at two contradictory options: "indefinitely" vs. short term ("4–6 weeks").
    PL, 7, PsI, Psychosocial Adaptation

82. **(1)** This is the proper use of anger. **Answer 2** is incorrect because although anger can be used to intimidate others, that use creates interpersonal problems. **Answer 3** is incorrect because in order for hostility to be a helpful communication mechanism, the degree of hostility must be *appropriate* to the provocation. **Answer 4** is incorrect because this expression of anger does not produce positive accomplishment.

    Test-taking tip—The best answer is usually the most *understandable*, with a positive tone, and free of jargon. **Answer 2** has a negative tone ("intimidate others"); **Answers 3** and **4** are confusing as to meaning.
    EV, 7, PsI, Coping and Adaptation

83. **(3)** A change in body image has made the patient feel unloved and unworthy of love. **Answers 1, 2,** and **4** are incorrect because there are *no supporting data*.

    Test-taking tip—Eliminate the three options in which there is lack of information in the stem to support data about problems in the marriage. The best option centers on the *patient* and *her* self-concept.
    AN, 7, PsI, Coping and Adaptation

84. **(2)** Use of "you" and "I" forces the patient to acknowledge separate identities. **Answer 1** is incorrect because "pet" names are usually not a person's choice. The patient needs to be called by his or her real name. **Answer 3** is incorrect because the patient has no identity if he or she cannot have his or her own opinions. **Answer 4** is incorrect because "should" responses imply others' ideas, not the patient's.

    Test-taking tip—The best answer ("you" and "I") reflects the stem: *separate* self-identity. Keep it simple (KIS) by selecting the *obvious* answer.
    IMP, 7, PsI, Psychosocial Adaptation

85. **(2)** A patient with paranoid disorder is suspicious, so a nurse must make every effort not to engage in behavior the patient can misinterpret. **Answers 1** and **3** are incorrect because a nurse *should* give correct information about what the patient says and *not* placate him or her (the patient will sense the

falseness). **Answer 4** is incorrect because arguing just solidifies the patient's ideas. In a neutral voice, the nurse should give correct information.

    Test-taking tip—Review interventions with paranoid behavior to choose a response that minimizes distortions and avoids reinforcing the pathology.
    IMP, 7, PsI, Psychosocial Adaptation

86. **(3)** This response *stops* the manipulation and suggests the patient is responsible for his or her own behaviors. **Answers 1, 2,** and **4** are incorrect because they indicate that the nurse has been conned and manipulated.

    Test-taking tip—First, recognize manipulative behavior; next, rule out the three options that may play into this.
    IMP, 5, PsI, Psychosocial Adaptation

87. **(2)** The patient will be easier to care for if he has his hearing aid and glasses. In **Answer 1,** the nurse is *denying* the patient his right to the full information of his senses. **Answer 3** is incorrect because the nurse has the responsibility to change rules for clearly therapeutic reasons. **Answer 4** does *not* respond to the patient's needs.

    Test-taking tip—Choose the option that starts with "I understand" and in which the nurse takes on a patient advocacy role.
    IMP, 2, PsI, Coping and Adaptation

88. **(3)** An appropriate direct response to a "you know what I mean" comment is to say you do *not* automatically know what is meant. **Answers 1, 2,** and **4** are not the best response because they *shift the focus* from the client's experience to the characteristics of the *other* person.

    Test-taking tip—First, choose the answer that directly relates to the mother's question; *then,* seek clarification.
    IMP, 7, PsI, Coping and Adaptation

89. **(3)** The patient needs to be aware of his or her actions and the possible ramifications of those actions. **Answer 1** is incorrect because the patient *needs to discuss* the actions. **Answer 2** is incorrect because the purpose of crisis intervention is to deal with the *present* problem and situation, *not* the past. **Answer 4** is incorrect because the focus must be on the patient, *not* on others.

    Test-taking tip—First note the two options that are similar ("encourage") and one that is the opposite ("discourage"). Next, compare the difference between the two "encourage" options: one focuses on the past ("as a child") and the other on the here-and-now (recent suicide attempt). Choose the latter option.
    PL, 7, PsI, Psychosocial Adaptation

90. **(4)** Attempts to focus on encouraging the client to describe feelings are important. **Answers 1** and **2** ask for facts rather than focusing on feelings, and **Answer 3** is an example of reflecting—a therapeutic response, but in this case it only reflects a *thought*, not a feeling.

    Test-taking tip—Choose the *feelings*-oriented option.
    IMP, 7, PsI, Coping and Adaptation

91. **(3)** Self-esteem is *the most basic* psychological need at *any* age, especially so for the elderly. **Answers 1, 2,** and **4,** although also important, are not the most basic needs.

    Test-taking tip—When you see an option that has "self-esteem," go for it!
    PL, 7, HPM, Growth and Development

92. **(4)** This is the least threatening. **Answer 2** is incorrect because the nurse *needs* to intervene into a pattern of silence. It is not therapeutic for the focus to be on the *nurse*, as in **Answers 1** and **3**, and bringing up a *controversial* topic (such as religion or politics) usually results in an exchange of opinions and arguments.

    Test-taking tip—The words "neutral" and "broad opening" in **Answer 4** lead you to the best answer.
    PL, 7, PsI, Coping and Adaptation

93. **(3)** This answer is the best choice because the other choices (**1, 2, 4**) seem *too certain* for a disorder that, although it has a

pattern, can be altered *if* and *when* the patient adopts different outlets for expressing emotions.

Test-taking tip—Choose the most *plausible, tentative* response here rather than the three definitive ones ("will," "essential").

EV, 7, PhI, Basic Care and Comfort

94. (2) This response picks up a "here-and-now" underlying feeling tone. **Answers 1** and **4** focus on "there-and-then" rather than "here-and-now" feelings and events, and **Answer 3** is *irrelevant* because the focus is on a *fact* rather than a feeling.

Test-taking tip—Focus on feelings. Eliminate two options with clichés (**1, 4**) and the option that avoids feelings by asking a factual question.

IMP, 7, PsI, Coping and Adaptation

95. (4) Expressing feelings *in general* through verbalization is a desired outcome. This answer also incorporates a *specific* feeling in **Answer 3.** Agreement to attend activities (**Answer 2**) does not indicate the *greatest* improvement. The client *already* recognizes that the behavior is irrational but cannot understand the cause or banish the behavior by will, as in **Answer 1.**

Test-taking tip—When two answers could be correct, choose the one that incorporates both.

EV, 7, PsI, Coping and Adaptation

96. (4) Information that is given to the nurse that may interfere with the client's recovery must be related to other team members. The other choices are not the best response because **Answer 1** is withholding information from other staff members who are also responsible for care and may interfere with recovery needs; **Answer 2** is a refusal that may stop the interaction—a negotiation is needed; and **Answer 3** does not provide a client with the clear feedback needed to work through conflict.

Test-taking tip—The best answer calls for knowledge about the concept of confidentiality.

IMP, 7, SECE, Management of Care

97. (3) This is the best example of setting limits on the behavior. **Answers 1** and **4** may be closely linked to nontherapeutic use of power. **Answer 2** is more of an example of a punishment approach.

Test-taking tip—You can readily eliminate the three negative options (nurse power in **Answer 1**; threatening sounding in **Answer 2**; MD power in **Answer 4**).

IMP, 7, PsI, Psychosocial Adaptation

98. (3) Brief and specific information *can* be processed during severe anxiety. In severe anxiety, the person cannot respond to the social environment (as in **Answer 1**); giving detailed information results in overload, because the client cannot retain and recall data (as in **Answer 2**). Only directive information that is brief and specific is effective when the client cannot focus on what is happening. Decision making needs to be postponed until the person is less anxious; hence, **Answer 4** is wrong.

Test-taking tip—The severely anxious person needs to have "KISS" communication—Keep It Simple and Succinct.

PL, 7, PsI, Coping and Adaptation

99. (4) The liver is affected by both the direct effect of alcohol and nutritional deficiencies associated with alcohol abuse and dependence. **Answers 1, 2,** and **3** are areas not usually affected by alcohol abuse and dependence.

Test-taking tip—Review physiological consequences of alcohol abuse.

AN, 7, PhI, Reduction of Risk Potential

100. (4) Acknowledging a feeling tone is the most therapeutic response and provides a broad opening for the client to elaborate feelings. The other choices are not the best response because **Answer 1** is false *reassurance* that does not allay feelings; **Answer 2** is asking a *"why"* question, which is confrontative and may increase anxiety; and **Answer 3** gives *advice,* which stops exploration of underlying feelings.

Test-taking tip—The best answer focuses on feelings. Review and eliminate examples of nontherapeutic communication.

IMP, 3, PsI, Coping and Adaptation

101. (1) This response aims to prevent use of manipulative patterns. In **Answers 2, 3,** and **4,** the nurse needs to seek validation, and these responses indicate acceptance without validation.

Test-taking tip—The team approach for consistent reinforcement of rules is needed when interacting with patients who display manipulative behavior.

IMP, 7, SECE, Management of Care

102. (1) **Answer 1** is the best choice because these are typical symptoms/responses to anxiety. Other common reactions are pupillary dilation, *not* constriction (**Answer 2**); diarrhea, *not* constipation (**Answer 4**). Vomiting is not typical of an anxiety response (**Answer 3**).

Test-taking tip—Review physiological manifestations of anxiety.

AS, 7, PhI, Physiological Adaptation

103. (3) This response refers to the definition of *projection* as a coping mechanism (attributing one's own unacceptable thoughts, feelings, and behaviors to another). **Answers 1, 2,** and **4** are incorrect because they have nothing to do with the coping mechanism of projection. Coping mechanisms in general function in the service of "self"—that is, they protect the ego and preserve self-esteem in an effort to cope with anxiety; the focus is *not* on *others,* as in **Answers 1** and **4.** Symptoms of projection do in fact *express* delusional thought rather than *control* it, contrary to **Answer 2.**

Test-taking tip—Select the option that has "feelings."

AN, 7, PsI, Coping and Adaptation

104. (2) In panic, a person is highly suggestible and follows "herd instinct" rather than exercising independent judgment and goal-directed problem solving (**Answer 1**). **Answer 3** is incorrect because the severity of the reaction *is* related to the severity of the threat. The more severe the perceived threat (actual or imaginary), the more intense the reaction to the danger, and *not* delayed as in **Answer 4.**

Test-taking tip—Apply knowledge about panic reaction.

AN, 7, PsI, Coping and Adaptation

105. (4) The primary initial focus of the nurse-client relationship is in showing the client, through acceptance, that it is the *client* one is concerned about, *not* the *symptoms.* **Answers 1** and **2** are incorrect because the focus of *initial* nursing care is on the client, not on meeting hospital standards or controlling impulses. **Answer 3** is incorrect because it is an attempt to analyze the *whys* of behavior, which is not an appropriate *basic* nursing intervention and *not* an initial aspect of care.

Test-taking tip—The key word is "acceptance," a basic tenet of the nurse-patient relationship.

PL, 7, PsI, Psychosocial Adaptation

106. (3) This is the most inclusive answer. **Answers 1, 2,** and **4** are all *incorporated* into **Answer 3.**

Test-taking tip—When all answers are correct, choose the "umbrella" answer that covers them all.

AN, 7, PsI, Coping and Adaptation

107. (2) *Denial* is the act of avoiding disagreeable realities by ignoring them. **Answer 1** is incorrect because *compensation* is the process by which a person makes up for a deficiency in self-image by emphasizing an asset. **Answer 3,** *symbolism,* is the use of one mental image to represent another. **Answer 4,** *identification,* is the process of taking on another person's attribute.

Test-taking tip—Knowledge of coping mechanisms is necessary to select the only correct answer. Review definitions and examples of the most common coping mechanisms.

AN, 7, PsI, Coping and Adaptation

108. (2) Research shows that *increased* activity is a psychomotor manifestation of anxiety; therefore, **Answer 1** is wrong. **Answers 3** and **4** are incorrect because emotion is *not* a psychomotor manifestation.

    Test-taking tip—Note the *similarity* between the word "psychomotor" in the stem and the word "activity" in **Answers 1** and **2**. Next decide on "increased activity" by applying theory about anxiety.
    AS, 3, PhI, Physiological Adaptation

109. (2) When the mourner can pass through the idealization stage and be more realistic about the positive and negative aspects of the loss, resolution of grief is beginning. **Answers 3** and **4** occur in *earlier* stages of grief. **Answer 1** could be a sign of denial of grieving, an initial grief reaction.

    Test-taking tip—Because all of the answers could be acceptable, you need to review the *stages* of grief to identify the best answer in relation to a *time sequence*. The other three options relate to *earlier* stages.
    EV, 7, PsI, Coping and Adaptation

110. (3) Research shows that anxiety *decreases* the perceptual field; therefore, **Answer 1** is incorrect. Research also shows that anxiety *decreases* the ability to concentrate and *increases* random activity; therefore, **Answers 1, 2,** and **4** are incorrect.

    Test-taking tip—Note the two *contradictory* options: "increase perceptual field" vs. "decrease perceptual field." Next, apply knowledge about anxiety to select the *theoretically* correct answer. **Answers 2** and **4** are theoretically incorrect.
    AN, 7, PsI, Coping and Adaptation

111. (3) This is correct by Freudian theory. **Answers 1, 2,** and **4** are incorrect because they are incomplete.

    Test-taking tip—The correct answer directly stems from a particular theoretical viewpoint—Freudian, which you will need to review.
    AN, 7, PsI, Coping and Adaptation

112. (1) This is correct according to Erickson. **Answer 2** relates to toddler; **Answer 3,** to infancy; **Answer 4,** to latency period in childhood.

    Test-taking tip—Review and apply your knowledge of the *age-related* stages, which will lead to the only correct answer.
    AN, 5, HPM, Growth and Development

113. (1) Another name for major depression is depression with psychotic features. Suicide risk is a part of all depressions. **Answers 2, 3,** and **4** are incorrect because these diagnoses alone do not indicate suicide risk as does the diagnosis of depression.

    Test-taking tip—Depression is the *most common* direct risk factor for suicide.
    AN, 7, PsI, Coping and Adaptation

114. (1) "Loss" is *most basic* to the development of depression. **Answers 2, 3,** and **4** are *not essential* to development of depression.

    Test-taking tip—When in doubt, choose the *least controversial,* more *general* answer ("a sense of loss") rather than pinpointing specific causal factors (e.g., "painful childhood," "confused sexual identity," "unresolved oedipal conflict").
    AN, 7, PsI, Coping and Adaptation

115. (4) Some anxiety is necessary to learn. **Answer 2** is incorrect because it is *incomplete.* **Answers 1** and **3** are incorrect because anxiety *is necessary* for learning and growth.

    Test-taking tip—When two answers seem right, choose the answer that incorporates the other (i.e., capacity to tolerate anxiety would *also mean* developing awareness of anxiety).
    PL, 7, PsI, Psychosocial Adaptation

116. (2) Part of maturing is learning to view one's parents *and* oneself realistically. **Answers 1, 3,** and **4** are incorrect because they represent the *misinformation* that creates problems between individuals.

    Test-taking tip—The key word in the correct option is "realistically."
    EV, 7, HPM, Growth and Development

117. (2) A permissive atmosphere is the key, as well as a *slowly* evolving relationship (not quickly evolving, as in **Answer 3**) with room for *distance*. Self-destruction is *not a persistent* problem requiring *major* focus for concern, as in **Answer 4. Answer 1** is not the best response because "acceptance" of *bizarre* behavior is more important than setting limits.

    Test-taking tip—Note the key words in the correct answer: "trusting, nonthreatening, reality-based relationship."
    PL, 7, PsI, Psychosocial Adaptation

118. (3) Frequent contacts at times of stress are important, especially when a patient is isolated. The other choices are not useful because **Answer 1,** *isolation,* does not automatically imply the use of restraints; *all* furniture need not be removed (**Answer 2**), depending on the institution and the type of behavior exhibited by the patient; and there is *no specific* time limit (**Answer 4**), because time depends on individual behavior and the patient's individual needs.

    Test-taking tip—Eliminate the option with the global word "all." Next, eliminate the too-specific time frame ("4 hours") that is not based on the patient's behavior or safety. Then eliminate the option on restraints, which is a last-resort action. Now you can readily choose the simple, most obvious option about "frequent contacts."
    PL, 1, SECE, Safety

119. (1) An undemanding task that the client could finish would allow a feeling of successful accomplishment. **Answers 2** and **3** require intellectual activity, which is usually slowed down during a depressive phase. **Answer 4** requires a skill that the client may not have and that might frustrate the client to learn; also, the client may not have the psychomotor energy for ice skating.

    Test-taking tip—Apply the process of elimination. Eliminate the two activities that call for intact cognitive functioning (which is slowed down in depression). The best answer does not involve a great deal of physical exertion, either (**Answer 4**).
    IMP, 3, PsI, Psychosocial Adaptation

120. (3) The nurse should encourage the patient to *explain* her statement in order to understand the experience she is having. **Answer 1** is incorrect because it offers an *interpretation* that may or may not be true. **Answer 2** is incorrect because it denies the patient's perception without clarification. **Answer 4** is incorrect because the nurse agrees with an unsupported statement.

    Test-taking tip—When none of the options is appropriate, *sound out* the responses, and choose the option closest to an attempt to seek clarification.
    IMP, 7, PsI, Coping and Adaptation

121. (2) It will provide energy release without the external stimuli and pressure of *competitive games* (**Answers 3** and **4**). Reading (**Answer 1**) usually requires sitting, which a client who is hyperactive cannot readily do.

    Test-taking tip—Apply theory about manic behavior (hyperactivity) and select the only option that helps the patient to externalize the energy (**Answer 2**), without additional stimuli (competitive games).
    IMP, 3, PsI, Psychosocial Adaptation

122. (4) The mother needs to ask the patient, not the nurse, but the nurse should also support the mother and encourage her to interact with her son. **Answers 1** and **2** are incorrect because they are *interpretations* that state opinions about the patient without his participation. **Answer 3** is incorrect because *no support is given* to the mother.

Test-taking tip—First, eliminate the two options that are interpretive (**Answers 1** and **2**); then choose the option that *redirects* the mother to the patient while providing *support* to the mother (**Answer 4**).
IMP, 7, PsI, Coping and Adaptation

123. (1) By definition, this is repression. **Answer 2** is suppression; **Answer 3** is displacement; and **Answer 4** is identification.
Test-taking tip—Review definitions of defense mechanisms in order to select the only correct answer.
AN, 2, PsI, Coping and Adaptation

124. (1) The patient must be constantly observed. **Answer 2** is incorrect because all suicidal talk and gestures are to be taken seriously. If the patient *talks* about suicide, there *may* be an attempt. **Answer 3** is incorrect because suicide risk is greater when depression is lifting, requiring greater vigilance. **Answer 4** is incorrect because medication for depression may take up to 2 weeks to decrease symptoms, and the patient needs vigilant surveillance *now*.
Test-taking tip—Key words: "*most* important nursing action." Eliminate the option that is a myth (**Answer 2**). Focus on the contradictory options: "constant awareness" vs. "ignore the patient" and "relax vigilance." Choose "constant awareness." Giving medications is *not* the most important nursing action.
PL, 7, PsI, Psychosocial Adaptation

125. (3) By definition, this is the conscious, deliberate effort to avoid talking or thinking about painful, anxiety-producing experiences. **Answers 1, 2,** and **4** are incorrect terms for the example given in the stem.
Test-taking tip—Review definitions of coping mechanisms in order to select the correct answer.
AN, 7, PsI, Coping and Adaptation

126. (2) This question attempts to get a specific description of what has happened and will allow the client to describe grief and feelings of low self-worth because of loss of a breast. **Answer 1** is incorrect because it offers *false* reassurance. **Answer 3** is incorrect because it is a *stereotyped* response to a woman and denies the client's actual loss. **Answer 4** is incorrect because it is an *interpretation* that, although possibly true, the client may reject. Resolution of grief is better achieved if the client can state a connection.
Test-taking tip—First, eliminate the options that give false reassurance (**Answer 1**), offer a stereotyped response (**Answer 3**), and are interpretive (**Answer 4**). Then, select the option that is an example of therapeutic communication, which helps the patient to elaborate and look for connections between feelings/belief and events.
IMP, 7, PsI, Coping and Adaptation

127. (1) Symbolism is the most clearly descriptive mechanism. **Answer 2**, *fantasy*, is a mental activity; **Answer 3**, *isolation*, is the exclusion from awareness of a feeling; **Answer 4**, *conversion*, is a disruption of motor or sensory functioning.
Test-taking tip—Review definitions of defense mechanisms to select the only correct answer.
AN, 7, PsI, Coping and Adaptation

128. (4) A variety of factors can cause self-destructive behavior, and these differ for each individual. Hence, **Answers 2** and **3** are not the best choices because, although correct, they are *examples* of a *variety* of factors; **Answer 1** is the opposite of the correct answer.
Test-taking tip—Choose the most inclusive answer when two options are *examples* of a *main* point. Eliminate **Answer 1**, which is partially the same as **Answer 4** but also the opposite ("same" vs. "different" factors).
AS, 7, PsI, Coping and Adaptation

129. (2) Denial is the mind's way of protecting the self-system from a disturbing reality. **Answer 1**, *reaction formation*, is an expression of an attitude opposite to unconscious feelings;

Answer 3, *intellectualization*, is giving rational reasons without expression of underlying feelings; **Answer 4**, *rationalization*, is the attempt to make one's behavior look like the result of logical thinking.
Test-taking tip—Review defense mechanisms to select the only correct answer.
AN, 7, PsI, Coping and Adaptation

130. (4) This is correct by definition. **Answer 1** is incorrect because delusion is a fixed *idea* arising out of a person's inner needs and contrary to observed facts. **Answer 2** is incorrect because a hallucination is a misperception that is *unrelated to an external stimulus*. **Answer 3** is incorrect because identification is the process of taking on another person's attribute.
Test-taking tip—Apply knowledge about adaptive and maladaptive coping mechanisms. Notice the option that is different (i.e., not a coping mechanism—**Answer 4**). For an educated guess, ask yourself: "Which of the following is not like the others?" Then, select it (this helps to focus on patterns.)
AN, 7, PsI, Coping and Adaptation

131. (1) A person who has settled on a plan for suicide may become more cheerful. **Answer 2** is incorrect because a person who is severely retarded in the psychomotor area cannot carry out a suicide act. **Answers 3** and **4** are incorrect because the patient is more likely to be hostile and agitated if he or she does not have a suicide plan. Agitated behavior can also represent the need to "repent" for sins thought to be committed.
Test-taking tip—Look at the two sets of contradictory options: "cheerfulness" (**1**) vs. "hostility" (**4**); "psychomotor retardation" (i.e., slowing down) (**2**) vs. "agitation" (**3**). Hostility and agitation can be paired and, therefore, ruled out; that leaves "cheerfulness" as the option that is different, and the one to select ("which of the following is not like the others?").
EV, 7, PsI, Psychosocial Adaptation

132. (1) This is the correct match between age period and developmental task. **Answer 2** refers to preschool age, **Answer 3** is characteristic of "maturity" in later years of life, and **Answer 4** refers to young adulthood.
Test-taking tip—Review *age*-related psychosocial growth and development stages according to Erikson.
AN, 7, HPM, Growth and Development

133. (2) On principle, the crisis intervention nurse needs to be *immediately* available to the patient. **Answer 1** is incorrect because it abandons the patient. **Answer 3** is incorrect because the patient needs to deal with the situation *immediately*. **Answer 4** is incorrect because the patient might decide that the crisis intervention nurse is not interested in helping, and the patient needs *immediate* assistance.
Test-taking tip—Continuity of care is the concept to apply in selecting the next step in time sequence.
IMP, 7, SECE, Management of Care

134. (4) The goal is to preserve ego strength through acceptance and respect of the patient as a person. **Answer 1** focuses on the tangential and irrelevant; **Answer 2** makes the problem more obvious to others in the room and makes an assumption without validation about how the patient must feel; **Answer 3** is incorrect because it is usually not helpful to give a rational explanation for an emotional difficulty related to enuresis.
Test-taking tip—Focus on the option with the key word "acceptance."
IMP, 7, PhI, Basic Care and Comfort

135. (4) The nurse must state feelings, without anger; show no intimidation; and then help the patient examine what he or she is doing and why. **Answer 1** is incorrect because it points the finger in an angry, accusatory way and labels the patient

in turn ("*You* are rude"). **Answer 2** sounds like "Big Nurse"—authoritarian and punitive. **Answer 3** may place the nurse in a position to be intimidated and "kicked" by the patient.

> **Test-taking tip**—Sounding out the response may help eliminate the threatening-sounding answers (**1, 2**) and the apologetic-sounding response (**3**). The better response to choose is one in which the nurse gives feedback and uses open-ended communication to seek clarification (**4**).

IMP, 7, PsI, Psychosocial Adaptation

136. **(3)** Most children with Down syndrome are affectionate and enjoy being held and cuddled, whereas the *opposite* is usually the case with a child who is autistic. All other responses (**1, 2,** and **4**) may apply to *both* Down syndrome and autism.

> **Test-taking tip**—Apply knowledge about characteristics of Down syndrome and autism to select an important difference related to *interpersonal* behavior.

AS, 5, PsI, Coping and Adaptation

137. **(2)** A ritual, such as compulsive hand washing, is an attempt to allay anxiety caused by unconscious impulses that are frightening. **Answer 1** is incorrect because it is the opposite of what the hand-washing ritual is intended to do—the ritual is aimed at *absolving* guilt, not *punishing*. **Answer 3** is related to *psychotic* symptoms and not at all relevant to symptoms of ritualism. **Answer 4** is incorrect because hand washing is aimed at relief of guilt and self-help to reduce anxiety, *not* at seeking attention from staff.

> **Test-taking tip**—Apply theory about psychodynamics underlying ritualistic behavior: getting a handle on and seeking *relief* from anxiety (rather than punishment). Eliminate the two other options because they do not relate to ritualism.

AN, 7, PsI, Coping and Adaptation

138. **(2)** It is important to provide external support in helping develop the superego. **Answer 1** may promote manipulative behavior in the client. **Answer 3** may foster additional dependence. Preventing the client's use of drugs (**Answer 4**) is *not* the primary step in building a nurse-client relationship based on therapeutic communication.

> **Test-taking tip**—Note the key word, "primarily"; then, focus on two contradictory options: permissive vs. confronting. Next, apply theory regarding addictive personalities and select "confronting" (**Answer 2**).

PL, 7, PsI, Psychosocial Adaptation

139. **(4)** The client is anxious and needs someone with him. **Answer 1** is incorrect because it *ignores* the client's anxiety and needs. **Answer 2** is incorrect because it also *ignores* the client's anxiety, and uses the doctor as an excuse to ignore his needs. **Answer 3** is incorrect because it also *ignores* the client's anxiety and needs, and gives a poor reason for refusal.

> **Test-taking tip**—First, recognize symptoms of anxiety; then, choose the only answer that appears to focus on the patient's anxiety (although you may not like this answer).

IMP, 7, PsI, Coping and Adaptation

140. **(2)** Consistency lets clients know consequences of behavior and develops trust. **Answer 1** is incorrect because the nurse *cannot approve all* behavior (e.g., destructive behavior). **Answer 3** is incorrect because it can be therapeutic *to express* negative opinions. **Answer 4** is incorrect because interpretation of behavior is *not* always advisable. Clients may use interpretations of behavior to avoid consequences of behavior or may see them as an excuse not to change behavior.

> **Test-taking tip**—Look at the option with the key word, "consistency," as the better answer. Eliminate **Answers 3** and **4** because they are examples of *nontherapeutic* approaches.

PL, 7, PsI, Coping and Adaptation

141. **(4)** The victim needs to engage in *expression* of the experience, which will assist her to work through her feelings so that the experience may not interfere in future interpersonal

relations. To repress the incident, as in **Answer 1**, would make it continually interfere in her relationships. **Answer 2** is done only *after* **Answer 4** has been accomplished. **Answer 3** is incorrect because the rape victim has *no* "part" in the rape.

> **Test-taking tip**—Focus on the key words in the stem: "*overall* client goal."

PL, 1, PsI, Psychosocial Adaptation

142. **(2)** The nurse is asking the client to clarify and further discuss feelings. **Answer 1** is incorrect because while staying with the client *might* convey acceptance, it does *not help* the client clarify or deal with feelings. **Answer 3** is incorrect because it cuts off any further response from the client and because it is *doubtful* that the nurse can understand this person's feelings without clarification. **Answer 4** is incorrect because it is *more* important to *clarify* the client's *feelings* than it is to understand the *object* of hate.

> **Test-taking tip**—Best answer is an attempt to clarify *feelings*, rather than to focus on facts ("For whom . . .").

IMP, 7, PsI, Coping and Adaptation

143. **(2)** Note the eyes: when a person is *on* heroin, the pupils are constricted; during *withdrawal*, they are dilated. Withdrawal does *not* usually include high fever, pupillary constriction, or choreiform movements, as in **Answers 1, 3,** and **4**.

> **Test-taking tip**—Note two *contradictory* options about the eyes ("dilation" vs. "constriction"), and know which applies to *withdrawal* vs. being *on* heroin.

AS, 7, PsI, Psychosocial Adaptation

144. **(4)** Methadone is a synthetic narcotic and has no euphoric effect. Methadone does not produce sedation (**Answer 1**), euphoria (**Answer 2**), or neuritis (**Answer 3**).

> **Test-taking tip**—Eliminate the three options that are not related to methadone. Review effects of methadone.

EV, 7, PhI, Pharmacological Therapy

145. **(4)** With concern for danger to the other clients, staff, and the environment, it is essential for the client to be restrained at this time. The other choices are incorrect because orientation and a quiet environment *alone* do *not* provide for safety when the client's agitation is out of control (**Answer 1**); the initial *delay* in onset of effectiveness of the tranquilizer does not *immediately* provide for the safety needs of other clients, staff, and the environment (**Answer 2**); and locking the client in his or her room eliminates only the danger to others—additional measures would be needed to provide for the safety of this *client* (**Answer 3**).

> **Test-taking tip**—Note the key word, "initially." Know *when* it is acceptable to use restraints.

IMP, 1, SECE, Safety

146. **(4)** Based on the patient's history of antisocial behavior, he or she is probably attempting to use the nurse for his or her own purpose and is not truthful. Therefore, it is best that the new nurse on the unit go directly to the head nurse to check on what is permissible and not accept the patient's word that it is permissible. **Answer 1** is not helpful because allowing the patient to unlock the door may feed into the manipulative attempt by the patient to get off the unit. **Answer 2** is incorrect because asking a "why" question is not a therapeutic communication. **Answer 3** is incorrect because this option places the new nurse in an argumentative position with the patient, who is likely to become defensive and say, "Oh, yes. I *am* allowed to open doors."

> **Test-taking tip**—Note the key word: "new" nurse. Review the theory about acting-out and manipulative behavior. Select the answer that calls for consistency among staff (**4**).

IMP, 7, PsI, Psychosocial Adaptation

147. **(3)** Limit setting is an important intervention with a patient who exhibits excessive, constant dependence on others for simple, seemingly inconsequential decisions in everyday life. The other choices are wrong because the situation presented provides insufficient data on which to base interpretations

related to fear of failure (**Answer 1**), a need to test for staff acceptance (**Answer 2**), or a bid for attention (**Answer 4**).

> **Test-taking tip**—Eliminate the three options for which there are no data in the stem to validate the interpretations (**Answers 1, 2,** and **4**).

AN, 7, PsI, Psychosocial Adaptation

148. (1) This is the only correct answer regarding dietary prohibitions. **Answers 2, 3,** and **4** *are allowed.*

> **Test-taking tip**—Knowledge regarding Orthodox Jewish dietary laws is needed to select the correct option. Note the key word: "prohibited" (i.e., not *not* allowed).

AN, 4, PsI, Coping and Adaptation

149. (1) Manipulation is a characteristic antisocial behavior. Flattery is a form of manipulation—with hidden agenda, to get what the patient wants, whatever that may be. **Answer 2** may or may not be the agenda behind the flattery. **Answers 3** and **4** are also possible examples of what the patient wants.

> **Test-taking tip**—When more than one answer is plausible, choose the one that covers them all—the "umbrella" answer (**1**).

AN, 7, PsI, Coping and Adaptation

150. (3) Gentle but firm guidance and nonverbal direction is needed to intervene when a patient with schizophrenic symptoms is being disruptive. **Answer 1** requires the patient to listen and respond accordingly. This behavior *is* disruptive and should not be ignored (**Answer 2**). **Answer 4** says only what cannot be done, without providing an alternative activity.

> **Test-taking tip**—Knowing the theory about characteristics of schizophrenia (e.g., autistic behavior, thought disorders) would help eliminate **Answers 1** and **4**. Ignoring disruptive behavior is not appropriate. The process of elimination leads to **Answer 3** as the best answer.

IMP, 7, PsI, Psychosocial Adaptation

151. (1) is correct because it is a depolarizing muscle relaxant causing paralysis. It is used to reduce the intensity of muscle contractions during the convulsive stage, thereby reducing the risk of bone fractures or dislocation. **Answer 2** is incorrect because it describes the action of methohexital (Brevital), which is administered in the treatment room before ECT. **Answer 3** is incorrect because it describes the action of atropine sulfate, given IM 30 minutes before treatment, to decrease secretions and counteract vagal stimulation effects induced by ECT. **Answer 4** is incorrect because analgesia is not required in ECT (before, during, or after), and it is *not* related to Anectine.

> **Test-taking tip**—Knowledge of the three standard drugs used in ECT and their effects will lead to the best answer.

IMP, 3, PhI, Pharmacological Therapy

152. (1) is correct because depressive episodes are often *recurrent.* **Answers 2, 3,** and **4** may or may not experience depression. **Answers 2** and **4** are more likely to experience anxiety. There does not appear to be any reason to expect that a housewife with three children in school would be at risk for any particular emotional distress (**Answer 3**).

> **Test-taking tip**—Match the key word in the *answers,* "depressive," with the key word in the *stem,* "depression."

AN, 7, PsI, Coping and Adaptation

153. (3) Nursing observation is easier if the patient with Alzheimer's is *nearby.* Therefore, **Answer 4** is incorrect. A roommate may (**Answer 1**) or may not (**Answer 2**) be all right, but facilitating nursing observations is the highest priority for a patient with memory problems and confusion who is a safety risk for wandering off the unit.

> **Test-taking tip**—Focus in on the best option by first narrowing choices to two that are contradictory (with/without a roommate; near/at distance from the nurses' station). Then ask, Is it roommate or proximity to nurses' station that is the

priority? Next, consider what goal is met by being near the *nurses' station* rather than a roommate. Answer: *safety* from wandering.

AN, 1, SECE, Management of Care

154. (1) This is the correct answer because it lets the nurse know that contacts with the elderly person are infrequent and that ongoing assessment of needs and health concerns is not likely to occur. **Answer 2** is incorrect because it is *not the greatest concern,* as long as there is the opportunity for assessment by phone. A cordless phone is a *good* idea rather than a great concern (**Answer 3**). Although isolation is further increased by not wanting to go to a senior citizen center, it is not of greatest concern (**Answer 4**).

> **Test-taking tip**—Put logic and reasoning to work here. Look at patterns in the stem: two options focus on family (**1, 2**), one option focuses on a phone instrument (**3**), and another option focuses on a community agency (**4**).

AN, 1, SECE, Management of Care

155. (4) This answer is concerned with accident prevention and is a means of observation of the patient. **Answers 1** and **2** are incorrect because the use of restraints is inappropriate and not justified. Having a security guard is not realistic (**Answer 3**).

> **Test-taking tip**—Use the process of elimination. Eliminate the two options dealing with restraints; eliminate the most unlikely option (**Answer 3**); **Answer 4**, therefore, is the best answer.

IMP, 1, SECE, Safety and Infection Control

156. (1) This is an example of reaction formation, a coping mechanism. **Answer 2** is incorrect because "ignoring" is the *opposite* of **Answer 1**, the correct choice. **Answer 3** is incorrect because guilt may be *manifested* by being overly solicitous (**Answer 1**). **Answer 4** is incorrect because "flat" is the *opposite* of an emotional reaction/action (overly solicitous).

> **Test-taking tip**—Remember Shakespeare: "Methinks the (lady) doth protest too much"—showing care and concern (love) but inflicting harm (hate).

AN, 1, PsI, Psychosocial Adaptation

157. (4) The patient is probably experiencing a loss of control over the hospitalization situation. Initially the patient and family should be included in planning care, which returns decision making to the patient and decreases frustration. **Answers 1** and **3** shift the problem rather than attempt to resolve the issue. **Answer 2** involves the patient but brings in an authority figure (the MD), which may be seen as punishment or "parental" by the patient.

> **Test-taking tip**—Look for the choice that gives the patient the most control; do not "pass the buck" to someone else (MD, social services, etc.)

PL, 7, SECE, Management of Care

158. (2) The patient needs to experience personal success. Setting reasonable and achievable goals will affirm the patient's value and ability to succeed. **Answers 1, 3,** and **4** will most likely be meaningless to a patient who does not feel important or successful. The choices are all verbal with no active participation by the patient.

> **Test-taking tip**—Maximize the patient's actions. Choose an option that "assists" the patient to do something.

PL, 7, PsI, Coping and Adaptation

159. (4) It is important to recognize differences of opinion and clarify patient perceptions of information presented without appearing defensive or putting the patient on the defensive. The patient may be anxious following an MI, and the outburst may be an indication of fear and anxiety. **Answers 1, 2,** and **3** are defensive or avoiding responses by the nurse.

> **Test-taking tip**—Only one option acknowledges the patient's statement as important to address.

IMP, 7, PsI, Coping and Adaptation

Nursing Care of the Acutely Ill and the Chronically Ill Adult

Robyn Nelson and Janice Stecchi

ASSESSMENT, ANALYSIS, AND NURSING DIAGNOSIS OF THE ADULT

Assessment is the process of gathering a comprehensive database about the patient's present, past, and potential health problems, as well as a description of the patient as a whole in his or her environment. It includes a comprehensive nursing history, a physical examination, and laboratory/x-ray data, and it concludes with the formulation of nursing diagnoses.

Subjective Data

Nursing History

The nursing history obtains data for planning and implementing nursing actions.

 I. **General health information:** reason for admission; duration of present illness; previous hospitalization; history of illnesses; diagnostic procedures before admission; allergies—type and severity of reactions; medications taken at home—over-the-counter and prescription medications.

 II. **Information relative to growth and development:** age; menarche—age at onset; heavy menses; dysmenorrhea; vaginal discharge; date of last Pap smear; pregnancies; abortions; miscarriages.

 III. **Information relative to psychosocial functions:** feelings (anger, denial, fear, anxiety, guilt, lifestyle changes); language barriers; family support; spiritual needs; history of trauma/rape.

 IV. **Information relative to nutrition:** appetite—normal, changes; dietary habits; food preferences or intolerances; difficulty swallowing or chewing; dentures; use of caffeine/alcohol; weight changes; excessive thirst, hunger, sweating.

 V. **Information relative to fluid and gas transport:** difficulty breathing; shortness of breath; history of cough/smoking; colds; sputum; swelling of extremities; chest pain; palpitations; varicosities; excessive bruising; blood transfusions; excessive bleeding.

 VI. **Information relative to protective functions:** skin problems—rash, itch; current treatment; unusual hair loss.

 VII. **Information relative to comfort, rest, activity, mobility:** usual activity (activities of daily living [ADL]); present ability and restrictions; rest and sleep pattern; weakness; joint or muscle stiffness, pain, or swelling; occupation; interests.

VIII. **Information relative to elimination:** bowel habits; changes—constipation, diarrhea; ostomy; emesis; nausea; voiding—retention, frequency, dysuria, incontinence.

 IX. **Information relative to sensory/perceptual functions:** pain—verbal report; quality, location; precipitating factors; duration; limitations in vision (glasses), hearing, touch, smell; orientation to person, place, time; confusion; headaches; fainting; dizziness; convulsions.

Adult

Objective Data

◆ **I. General**—provides information on the patient as a whole.

 A. *Race, sex, apparent age* in relation to stated age.

 B. *Nutritional status*—well hydrated and developed or obesity, cachexia—include weight.

 C. *Apparent health status*—general good health or mild, moderate, severe debilitation.

 D. *Posture and motor activity*—erect, symmetrical, and balanced gait and muscle development or ataxic, circumducted, scissor, or spastic gait; slumped or bent-over posture; mild, moderate, or hyperactive motor responses.

 E. *Behavior*—alert; oriented to person, time, place; hears and comprehends instructions, or tense, anxious, angry; uses abusive language; slightly or largely unresponsive; delusions, hallucinations.

 F. *Odors*—noncontributory, or acetone, alcohol, fetid breath, incontinent of urine or feces.

◆ **II. Physical assessment**—requires knowledge of normal findings, organization, and keen senses, i.e., visual, auditory, touch, smell. For abnormal findings, refer to the *Assessment* section of each health problem discussed under the categories of human functioning.

 A. *Components*

  1. Inspection—uses observations to detect deviations from normal.

  2. *Auscultation*—used to perceive and interpret sounds arising from various organs, particularly heart, lungs, and bowel.

  3. *Palpation*—used to assess for discomfort, temperature, pulsations, size, consistency, and texture.

  4. *Percussion*—technique used to elicit vibrations produced by underlying organ structures; used less frequently in nursing practice.

   a. Flat—normal percussion note over muscle or bone.

   b. Dull—normal percussion note over organs such as liver.

   c. Resonance—normal percussion note over lungs.

   d. Tympany—normal percussion note over stomach or bowel.

 B. *Approach*—head to toe

  1. *General appearance*—well or poorly developed or nourished. Color (black, white, jaundiced, pale). In distress (acutely or chronically)?

  2. *Vital signs*—blood pressure (which arm or both, orthostatic change). Pulse (regular or irregular, orthostatic change). Respirations (labored or unlabored, wheeze). Temperature (axillary, rectal, tympanic membrane, or oral). Weight. Height.

  3. *Skin, hair, and nails*—pigmentation, scars, lesions, bruises, turgor. Describe or draw rashes.

   a. Skin color:

    (1) Red—fever, allergic reaction, carbon monoxide (CO) poisoning.

    (2) White (pallor)—excessive blood loss, fright.

    (3) Blue (cyanosis)—hypoxemia, peripheral vasoconstriction.

    (4) Mottled—cardiovascular embarrassment.

   b. Skin temperature:

    (1) Hot, dry—excessive body heat (heatstroke).

    (2) Hot, wet—reaction to increased internal or external temperature.

    (3) Cool, dry—exposure to cold.

    (4) Cool, clammy—shock.

  4. *Head*—scalp, skull (configuration), scars, tenderness, bruits.

  5. *Neck*—suppleness. Trachea, larynx, thyroid, blood vessels (jugular veins, carotid arteries).

  6. *Nodes*—any cervical, supraclavicular, axillary, epitrochlear, inguinal lymphadenopathy? If so, size of nodes (in centimeters), consistency (firm, rubbery, tender), mobile or fixed.

  7. *Eyes:*

   a. **External eye.** Conjunctivae, sclerae, lids, cornea, pupils (including reflexes), visual fields, extraocular motions.

   b. **Fundus.** Disk, blood vessels, pigmentation.

  8. *Ears*—shape of pinnae, external canal, tympanic membrane, acuity, air conduction versus bone conduction *(Rinne test)*, lateralization *(Weber's test)*.

  9. *Nose*—septum, mucosa, polyps.

  10. *Mouth and throat*—lips, teeth, tongue (size, papillation), buccal mucosa, palate, tonsils, oropharynx.

  11. *Chest*

   a. **Inspection.** Contour, symmetry, expansion.

   b. **Palpation.** Expansion, rib tenderness, tactile fremitus.

   c. **Percussion.** Diaphragmatic excursion, dullness.

   d. **Auscultation.** Crackles, rubs, wheezes, egophony, pectoriloquy.

    (1) Use diaphragm or bell. Normal sounds over alveoli—*vesicular.* Large airway or abnormal sounds—*bronchial or bronchovesicular.* Adventitious sounds—*crackles or wheezes.*

    (2) *Crackles*—discontinuous noises heard on auscultation; caused by popping open of air spaces; usually associated with increased fluid in the lungs; *formerly called rales and rhonchi.*

    (3) *Wheezes*—high-pitched, whistling sounds made by air flowing through narrowed airways.

  12. *Breasts*—symmetry, retraction, lesions, nipples (inverted, everted), masses, tenderness, discharge.

Adult

13. *Heart:*
    a. **Inspection.** Point maximal impulse, chest contour.
    b. **Palpation.** Point maximal impulse, thrills, lifts, thrusts.
    c. **Auscultation.** Heart sounds, gallops, murmurs, rubs. Use diaphragm for high-pitched sounds of normal heart sounds (S_1 and S_2) and bell for abnormal sounds (S_3 and S_4).
14. *Abdomen:*
    a. **Inspection.** Scars (draw these), contour, masses, vein pattern.
    b. **Auscultation.** Bowel sounds, rubs, bruits. Use diaphragm. Auscultate *after* inspection and *before* palpation and percussion. Listen to each quadrant for at least 1 min. If bowel sounds are present, they will be heard in lower right quadrant (area of ileocecal valve).
    c. **Percussion**—organomegaly, hepatic dullness.

d. **Palpation**—tenderness, masses, rigidity, liver, spleen, kidneys.
    e. **Hernia**—femoral, inguinal, ventral.
15. *Genitalia:*
    a. **Male.** Penile lesions, scrotum, testes. Circumcised?
    b. **Female.** Labia, Bartholin's and Skene's glands, vagina, cervix. Bimanual examination of internal genitalia.
16. *Rectum*—perianal lesions, sphincter tone, tenderness, masses, prostate, stool color, occult blood.
17. *Extremities*—pulses (symmetry, bruits, perfusion). Joints (mobility, deformity). Cyanosis, edema. Varicosities. Muscle mass.
18. *Back*—contour spine, tenderness. Sacral edema.
19. *Neurological:*
    a. **Mental status.** Alertness, memory, judgment, mood.
    b. **Cranial nerves** (I–XII). See Figure 7–1.
    c. **Cerebellum.** Gait, finger-nose, heel-shin, tremors.

FIGURE 7–1 Cranial nerves and their distributions. (From Thomas, CL [ed]: Taber's Cyclopedic Medical Dictionary, ed 18. FA Davis, Philadelphia, 1997, p 457.)

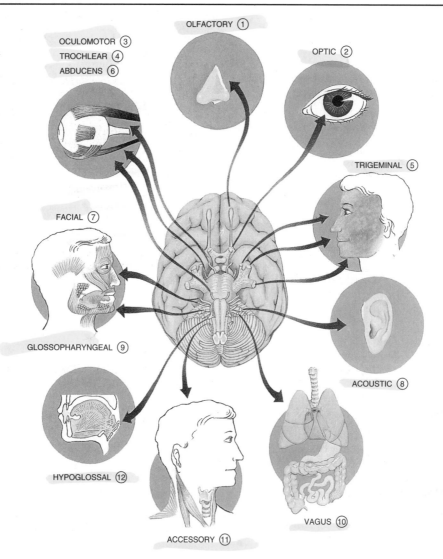

d. **Motor.** Muscle mass, strength; deep-tendon reflexes. Pathological or primitive reflexes.

e. **Sensory.** Touch, pain, vibration. Heat and cold as indicated.

III. Routine laboratory studies—see **Appendix A** for normal ranges.

A. *Hematology:*
1. Complete blood count—detects presence of anemia, infection, allergy, and leukemia.
2. Prothrombin time—increase may indicate need for vitamin K therapy.
3. Serology (VDRL)—determines presence of syphilis; false-positive result may indicate collagen dysfunction.

B. *Urinalysis:*
1. Specific gravity—measures ability of kidney to concentrate urine. Fixed specific gravity indicates renal tubular dysfunction.

2. Albumin and pus—indicate renal infection.
3. Sugar and acetone—presence indicates metabolic disorder.

C. *Chest x-ray*—detects tuberculosis or other pulmonary dysfunctions, as well as changes in size or configuration of heart.

D. *Electrocardiogram (ECG)*—detects rhythm and conduction disturbances, presence of myocardial ischemia or necrosis, and ventricular hypertrophy.

E. *Blood chemistries*—detect deviation in electrolyte balance, presence of tissue damage, and adequacy of glomerular filtration.

IV. Preventive Care

A. Checkup visits recommended every 1 to 3 years until age 65 and then yearly thereafter. See Table 7–1 for suggested timelines.

B. Individuals with *special risk factors* may need more frequent and additional types of preventive care.

TABLE 7–1 Preventive Care Timelines

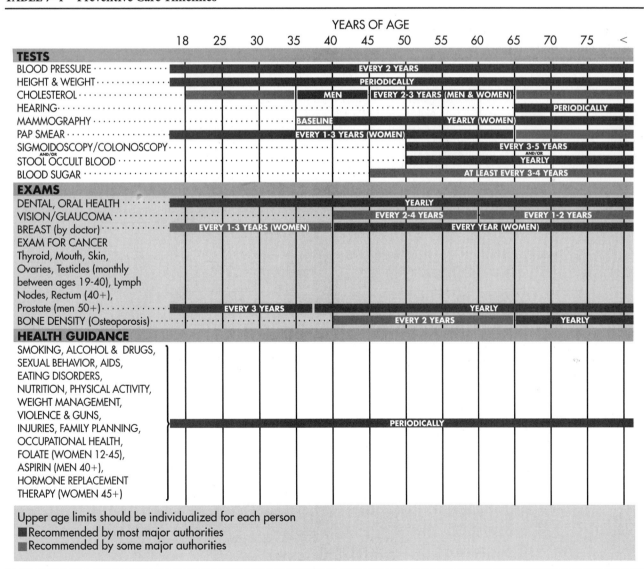

Source: Office of Disease Prevention and Health Promotion, in cooperation with the agencies of the Public Health Service, U.S. Department of Health and Human Services.

1. *Diabetes*—eye, foot exams; urine, blood sugar tests.
2. *Drug abuse*—AIDS, TB tests; hepatitis immunization.
3. *Alcoholism*—influenza, pneumococcal immunizations; TB test.
4. *Overweight*—blood sugar test.
5. *Homeless, recent refugees or immigrant*—TB test.
6. *High-risk sexual behavior*—AIDS, syphilis, gonorrhea, chlamydia (every year for sexually active women), hepatitis tests.
7. *Pregnancy*—Rubella blood test (prior to first pregnancy).

C. *Adult immunizations*—prevention of disease and reduction in the severity of disease (Table 7–2).

Assessment is followed by analysis of data and formulation of a nursing diagnosis. Possible nursing diagnoses for each category of human functioning are given in the following sections.

TABLE 7–2   Summary of Recommendations for Adult Immunization ●

Vaccine Name and Route	For Whom It Is Recommended	Schedule	Contraindications and Precautions (Mild Illness Is Not a Contraindication)
Influenza ("flu shot")— give IM	■ Adults who are 60 years of age or older. ■ People 6 mo–65 yr of age with medical problems such as heart disease, lung disease, diabetes, renal dysfunction, hemoglobinopathies, immunosuppression, or those living in chronic care facilities. ■ People (≥6 mo of age) working or living with at-risk people. ■ All health care workers and those who provide key community services. ■ Healthy pregnant women who will be in their 2nd or 3rd trimesters during the influenza season. ■ Pregnant women who have underlying medical conditions should be vaccinated before the flu season, regardless of the stage of pregnancy. ■ Anyone who wishes to reduce the likelihood of becoming ill with influenza. ■ Travelers to areas where influenza activity exists or when traveling among people from areas of the world where there is current influenza activity.	■ Given *every year.* ■ October through November is the optimal time to receive an annual flu shot to maximize protection, but the vaccine may be given at any time during the influenza season (typically December through March) or at other times when the risk of influenza exists. ■ May be given anytime during the influenza season. ■ May be given with all other vaccines but at a separate site.	■ Previous anaphylactic reaction to this vaccine, to any of its components, or to eggs. ■ Moderate or severe acute illness.
Pneumococcal—give IM or SC	■ Adults who are 65 years of age or older. ■ People 2 yr–65 yr of age who have chronic illness or other risk factors including chronic cardiac or pulmonary diseases, chronic liver disease, alcoholism, diabetes mellitus, CSF leaks, as well as persons living in special environments or social settings (including Alaska natives and certain American Indian populations). Those at highest risk of fatal pneumococcal infection are persons with anatomical or functional asplenia (including sickle cell disease); immunocompromised persons, including those with HIV infection, leukemia, lymphoma, Hodgkin's disease, multiple myeloma, generalized malignancy, chronic renal failure, or nephrotic syndrome; those receiving immunosuppressive chemotherapy (including corticosteroids); and those who received an organ or bone marrow transplant.	■ Routinely given as a *one-time* dose; administer if previous vaccination history is unknown. ■ One-time revaccination is recommended 5 years later for people at highest risk of fatal pneumococcal infection or rapid antibody loss (e.g., renal disease) and for people ≥65 years if the 1st dose was given before age 65 and ≥5 years have elapsed since previous dose. ■ May be given with all other vaccines but at a separate site.	■ Previous anaphylactic reaction to this vaccine or to any of its components. ■ Moderate or severe acute illness.

Hepatitis B (hep-B)— give IM; brands may be used interchangeably	■ High-risk adults including household contacts and sex partners of HBsAg-positive persons; users of illicit injectable drugs; heterosexuals with more than one sex partner in 6 months; men who have sex with men; people with recently diagnosed STDs; patients in hemodialysis units and patients with renal disease that may result in dialysis; recipients of certain blood products; health care workers and public safety workers who are exposed to blood; clients and staff of institutions for the developmentally disabled; inmates of long-term correctional facilities; and certain international travelers. *Note:* Prior serological testing may be recommended depending on the specific level of risk or likelihood of previous exposure.
	■ *All adolescents.*
	Note: In 1997, the NIH Consensus Development Conference, a panel of national experts, recommended that hepatitis B vaccination be given to all persons infected with hepatitis C virus. *Do serologic screening for people who have emigrated from endemic areas. When HBsAg-positive persons are identified, offer them appropriate disease management. In addition, screen their household members and intimate contacts and, if found susceptible, vaccinate.*
		■ *Three* doses are needed on a *0, 1, 6 mo* schedule.
		■ Alternative timing options for vaccination include:
		      0, 2, 4 months
		      0, 1, 4 months
		■ There must be 4 wk between doses #1 and #2, and 8 wk between doses #2 and #3. Overall there must be at least 4 mo between doses #1 and #3.
		■ **Schedule for those who have fallen behind:** If the series is delayed between doses, do *not* start the series over. Continue from where you left off.
		■ May be given with all other vaccines but at a separate site.
			■ Previous anaphylactic reaction to this vaccine or to any of its components.
			■ Moderate or severe acute illness.

Continued

Adult

Adult

TABLE 7–2   Summary of Recommendations for Adult Immunization—cont'd

Vaccine Name and Route	For Whom It Is Recommended	Schedule	Contraindications and Precautions (Mild Illness Is Not a Contraindication)
Hepatitis A (hep-A)— give IM; brands may be used interchangeably	▪ People who travel outside of the United States (except for Northern and Western Europe, New Zealand, Australia, Canada, and Japan). ▪ People with chronic liver disease, including people with hepatitis C virus infection; people with hepatitis B who have chronic liver disease; illicit drug users; men who have sex with men; people with clotting-factor disorders; people who work with hepatitis A virus in experimental lab settings (this does not refer to routine medical laboratories); and food handlers where health authorities or private employers determine vaccination to be cost-effective. *Note:* Prevaccination testing is likely to be cost-effective for persons >40 yr of age, as well as for younger persons in certain groups with a high prevalence of hepatitis A virus infection.	▪ *Two doses are needed.* ▪ The minimum interval between dose #1 and #2 is 6 mo. ▪ If dose #2 is delayed, do *not* repeat dose #1. Just give dose #2. ▪ May be given with all other vaccines but at a separate site.	▪ Previous anaphylactic reaction to this vaccine or to any of its components. ▪ Moderate or severe acute illness. ▪ Safety during pregnancy has not been determined, so benefits must be weighed against potential risk.

Td (tetanus, diphtheria)—give IM	▪ *All adolescents and adults.*
	▪ After the primary series has been completed, a booster dose is recommended every 10 years. Make sure your patients have received a primary series of 3 doses.
	▪ A booster dose as early as 5 years later may be needed for the purpose of wound management, so consult ACIP recommendations.
		▪ Booster dose *every 10 years* after completion of the primary series of three doses.
		▪ **For those who have fallen behind:** The primary series is three doses:
		  ▪ Give dose #2 four weeks after #1.
		  ▪ #3 is given 6–12 months after #2.
		▪ May be given with all other vaccines but at a separate site.
			▪ Previous anaphylactic or neurological reaction to this vaccine or to any of its components.
			▪ Moderate or severe acute illness.

MMR (measles, mumps, rubella)—give SC	▪ Adults born in 1957 or later who are ≥18 yr of age (including those born outside the United States) should receive at least one dose of MMR if there is no serological proof immunity or documentation of a dose given on or after 1st birthday. ▪ Adults in high-risk groups, such as health care workers, students entering colleges and other post-high school educational institutions, and international travelers should receive a total of two doses. ▪ All women of childbearing age (i.e., adolescent girls and premenopausal adult women) who do not have acceptable evidence of rubella immunity or vaccination. *Note:* Adults born before 1957 are usually considered immune, but proof of immunity may be desirable for health care workers.	▪ *One or two doses are needed.* ▪ If dose #2 is recommended, give it no sooner than 4 wk after dose #1. ▪ May be given with all other vaccines but at a separate site. ▪ If varicella vaccine and MMR are both needed and are not administered on the same day, space them at least 4 wk apart.	▪ Previous anaphylactic reaction to this vaccine or to any of its components. (Anaphylactic reaction to eggs is *no longer* a contraindication to MMR.) ▪ Pregnancy or possibility of pregnancy within 3 months. ▪ HIV positivity is *not* a contraindication to MMR except for those who are severely immunocompromised. ▪ Immunocompromised persons due to cancer, leukemia, lymphoma, immunosuppressive drug therapy, including high-dose steroids or radiation therapy. ▪ If blood products or immune globulin has been administered during the past 11 months, consult the ACIP recommendations regarding time to wait before vaccinating. ▪ Moderate or severe acute illness. *Note:* MMR is *not* contraindicated if a PPD test was done recently. PPD should be delayed for 4–6 weeks after an MMR has been given.

Vaccine	Recommendation	Contraindications/Precautions
Varicella (var), "chicken-pox shot"—give SC	*All* susceptible adults and adolescents should be vaccinated. Make special efforts to vaccinate susceptible persons who have *close contact with persons at high risk for serious complications* (e.g., health care workers and family contacts of immunocompromised persons) and susceptible persons who are at *high risk of exposure* (e.g., teachers of young children, day care employees, residents and staff in institutional settings such as colleges and correctional institutions, military personnel, adolescents and adults living with children, nonpregnant women of childbearing age, and international travelers who do not have evidence of immunity). *Note:* People with reliable histories of chickenpox (such as self or parental report of disease) can be assumed to be immune. For adults who have no reliable history, serological testing may be cost-effective because most adults with a negative or uncertain history of varicella are immune.	■ Previous anaphylactic reaction to this vaccine or to any of its components. ■ Pregnancy, or possibility of pregnancy within 1 month. ■ Immunocompromised persons due to malignancies and primary or acquired cellular immunodeficiency, including HIV/AIDS. Note: For those on high-dose immunosuppressive therapy, consult ACIP recommendations regarding delay time. ■ If blood products or immune globulin have been administered during the past 5 months, consult the ACIP recommendations regarding time to wait before vaccinating. ■ Moderate or severe acute illness. *Note:* Manufacturer recommends that *salicylates be avoided for 6 weeks after* receiving varicella vaccine because of a theoretical risk of Reye syndrome.
	■ *Two* doses are needed. ■ Dose #2 is given *4–8 wk after* dose #1. ■ May be given with all other vaccines but at a separate site. ■ If varicella vaccine and MMR are both needed and are not administered on the same day, space them at least 4 wk apart. ■ If the second dose is delayed, do *not* repeat dose #1. Just give dose #2.	
Polio (IPV)—give IM or SC	■ *Not routinely recommended* for persons 18 years of age and older. *Note:* Adults living in the United States who never received or completed a primary series of polio vaccine need *not* be vaccinated unless they intend to travel to areas where exposure to wild-type virus is likely. Previously vaccinated adults should receive *one booster dose if traveling to polio en-demic areas.*	■ *Four* doses of inactivated polio vaccine (IPV) at 2, 4, and 6–18 mo, and 4–6 yr. ■ May be given with all other vaccines but at a separate site.
Lyme disease—give IM	■ Consider for persons 15–70 years of age who reside, work, or recreate in areas of high or moderate risk and who engage in activities that result in frequent or prolonged exposure to tick-infested habitat. ■ Persons with a history of previous uncomplicated Lyme disease who are at continued high risk for Lyme disease. (See description in the first bullet.) ■ See ACIP statement for a definition of high and moderate risk.	■ Previous anaphylactic reaction to this vaccine or to any of its components. ■ Pregnancy. ■ Moderate or severe acute illness. ■ Persons with treatment-resistant Lyme arthritis. ■ There are not enough data to recommend Lyme disease vaccine to persons with these conditions: immunodeficiency, diseases associated with joint swelling (including rheumatoid arthritis) or diffuse muscular pain, chronic health conditions due to Lyme disease.
	■ *Three* doses are needed. Give at intervals of 0, 1, and 12 mo. Schedule dose #1 (given in year 1) and dose #3 (given in year 2) to be given several weeks before tick season. See ACIP statement for details. ■ Safety of administering Lyme disease vaccine with other vaccines has not been established. ■ ACIP says if it must be administered concurrently with other vaccines, give it at a separate site.	

Source: Adapted from the Advisory Committee on Immunization Practices (ACIP), Centers for Disease Control, by the Immunization Action Coalition, 1999.

Adult

GROWTH AND DEVELOPMENT

Young Adulthood (20–30 Years of Age)

I. Stage of development—psychosocial stage: intimacy versus isolation.

II. Physical development
   A. *At the height* of bodily vigor.
   B. *Maximum* level of strength, muscular development, height, and cardiac and respiratory capacity; also, period of peak sexual capacity for men.

III. Cognitive development
   A. Close to *peak* of intelligence, memory, and abstract thought.
   B. Maximum ability to solve problems and learn new skills.

IV. Socialization
   A. Has a vision of the future and imagines various possibilities for self.
   B. Defines and tests out what can be accomplished.
   C. Seeks out a mentor to emulate as a guiding, though transitional, figure; the mentor is usually a mixture of parent, teacher, and friend who serves as a role model to support and facilitate the developing vision of self.
   D. Grows from a beginning to a fuller understanding of own authority and autonomy.
   E. Transfers an interest into an occupation or profession; crucial work choice may be made after one has knowledge, judgment, and self-understanding, usually at the end of young adulthood; when the choice is deferred beyond these years, valuable time is lost.
   F. Experiments with and chooses a lifestyle.
   G. Forms mature peer relationships with the opposite sex.
   H. Overcomes guilt and anxiety about the opposite sex and learns to understand the masculine and feminine aspects of self, as well as the adult concept of roles.
   I. Learns to take the opposite sex seriously and may choose someone for a long-term relationship.
   J. Accepts the responsibilities and pleasures of parenthood.

Adulthood (31–45 Years of Age)

I. Stage of development—psychosocial stage: generativity versus self-absorption.

II. Physical development
   A. Gradual decline in biological functioning, although in the late 30s the individual is still near peak.
   B. Period of peak sexual capacity for women occurs during the mid-30s.
   C. Distinct sense of bodily decline occurs around 40 years of age.
   D. *Circulatory* system begins to slow somewhat after 40 years of age.

III. Cognitive development
   A. Takes longer to memorize.
   B. Still at peak in abstract thinking and problem solving.
   C. Generates new levels of awareness.
   D. Gives more meaning to complex tasks.

IV. Socialization
   A. Achieves a realistic self-identity.
   B. Perceptions are based on reality.
   C. Acts on decisions and assumes responsibility for actions.
   D. Accepts limitations while developing assets.
   E. Delays immediate gratification in favor of future satisfaction.
   F. Evaluates mistakes, determines reasons and causes, and learns new behavior.
   G. Struggles to establish a place in society.
      1. Begins to settle down.
      2. Pursues long-range plans and goals.
      3. Has a stronger need to be responsible.
      4. Invests self as fully as possible in social structure, including work, family, and community.
   H. Seeks advancement by improving and using skills, becoming more creative, and pursuing ambitions.

Middle Life (46–64 Years of Age)

I. Stage of development—psychosocial stage: continuation of generativity versus self-absorption.

II. Physical development
   A. Failing *eyesight*, especially for close vision, may be one of the first symptoms of aging.
   B. Hearing loss is very gradual, especially for low sounds; hearing for *high-pitched* sounds is impaired more readily.
   C. There is a gradual loss of *taste* buds in the 50s and gradual loss of sense of *smell* in the 60s, causing the individual to have a diminished sense of taste.
   D. *Muscle strength* declines because of decreased levels of estrogen and testosterone; it takes more time to accomplish the same physical task.
   E. *Lung* capacity is impaired, which adds to decreased endurance.
   F. The *skin* begins to wrinkle, and hair begins graying.
   G. *Postural changes* take place because of loss of calcium and reduced activity.

III. Cognitive development

A. *Memory* begins to decline slowly around age 50 years.

B. It takes longer to *learn* new tasks, and old tasks take longer to perform.

C. *Practical judgment* is increased due to experiential background.

D. May tend to withdraw from mental activity or overcompensate by trying the impossible.

IV. Socialization

A. The middle years can be very rewarding if previous stages have been fulfilled.

B. The years of responsibility for raising children are over.

C. Husbands and wives usually find a closer bond.

D. There is less financial strain for those with steady employment.

E. Individuals are usually at the height of their careers; the majority of leaders in their field are in this age group.

F. Self-realization is achieved.
   1. There is more inner direction.
   2. There is no longer a need to please everyone.
   3. Individual is less likely to compare self with others.
   4. Individual approves of self without being dependent on standards of others.
   5. There is less fear of failure in life because past failures have been met and dealt with.

Early Late Years (65–79 Years of Age)

I. Stage of development—psychosocial stage: ego integrity and acceptance versus despair and disgust.

II. Physical development

A. Continues to decrease in vigor and capacity.

B. Has more frequent aches and pains.

C. Likely to have at least one major illness.

III. Cognitive development

A. Mental acuity continues to slow down.

B. Judgment and problem solving remain intact, but the processes may take longer.

C. May have problems in remembering *names and dates.*

IV. Socialization

A. Individual is faced with the reality of the experience of physical decline.

B. Physical and mental changes intensify the feelings of aging and mortality.

C. Increasing frequency of death and serious illness among friends, relatives, and associates further reinforces the concept of mortality.

D. Constant reception of medical warnings to follow certain precautions or run serious risks adds to general feeling of decline.

E. Individual is less interested in obtaining the rewards of society and is more interested in using own inner resources.

F. Individuals feel that they have earned the right to do what is important for self-satisfaction.

G. Retirement allows time for expression of own creative energies.

H. Overcomes the splitting of youth and age; gets along well with adolescents.

I. Learns to deal with the reality that only old age remains.

J. Provides moral support to grandchildren; more tolerant of grandchildren than was of own children.

K. Tends to release major authority of family to children while holding self in the role of consultant.

Later Years (80 Years of Age and Older)

I. Stage of development—psychosocial stage: continuation of ego integrity and acceptance versus despair and disgust.

II. Physical development

A. Additional sensory problems occur, including diminished sensation to *touch and pain.*

B. Increase in loss of muscle tone occurs, including *sphincter* (urinary and anal) control.

C. Individual is insecure and unsure about orientation to *space* and sense of *balance*, which may result in falls and injury.

III. Cognitive development

A. Has better memory for the *past* than the present.

B. *Repetition* of memories occurs.

C. Individual may use *confabulation* to fill in memory gaps.

D. Forgetfulness may lead to serious *safety* problems, and individual may require constant supervision.

E. Increased arteriosclerosis may lead to mental illness (dementia and other cognitive disorders).

IV. Socialization

A. Few significant relationships are maintained; deaths of friends, family, and associates cause isolation.

B. Individual may be preoccupied with immediate bodily needs and personal comforts; the *gastrointestinal tract* frequently becomes the major focus.

C. Individuals see that they can provide others with an example of wisdom and courage.

D. Individuals come to terms with themselves.

E. Individuals are concerned with own immortality.

F. Individuals come to terms with the process of dying and prepare for own death.

Adult

FLUID-GAS TRANSPORT

Conditions Affecting Fluid Transport

I. **Hypertension:** sustained, elevated, systemic, arterial blood pressure; diastolic elevation more serious, reflecting pressure on arterial wall during resting phase of cardiac cycle (Table 7–3).
  A. **Pathophysiology:** increased peripheral resistance leading to thickened arterial walls and left ventricular hypertrophy.
  B. **Risk factors:**
    1. Black race (2:1).
    2. Use of birth control pills.
    3. Overweight.
    4. Smoking.
    5. Stress.
    6. Excessive sodium intake or saturated fat.
    7. Lack of activity.
  C. **Classifications:**
    1. *Essential* (primary or idiopathic): occurs in 90–95% of patients; etiology unknown; diastolic pressure is ≥90 mm Hg, and other

causes of hypertension are absent. *Benign* hypertension (diastolic pressure ≤120 mm Hg) considered controllable; asymptomatic until complications develop.
    2. *Secondary:* occurs in remaining 5–10%; usually renal, endocrine, neurogenic, or cardiac in origin.
    3. *Malignant hypertension* (systolic >140–150 mm Hg); uncontrollable. May arise from both types.
    4. *Labile* (prehypertensive): a fluctuating blood pressure; increases during stress, otherwise normal or near normal.
  ◆ D. **Assessment:**
    1. *Subjective data:*
      a. Early-morning headache, usually occipital.
      b. Light-headedness, tinnitus.
      c. Palpitations.
      d. Fatigue, insomnia.
      e. Forgetfulness, irritability.
      f. Altered vision: white spots, blurring, or loss.
    2. *Objective data:*
      a. Epistaxis (nosebleeds).
      b. Elevated blood pressure: systolic >140 mm Hg, diastolic >90 mm Hg; narrowed pulse pressure. Rise in diastolic from sit-

TABLE 7–3   Imbalances in Blood Pressure: Comparative Assessment of Hypotension and Hypertension

	Hypotension	Hypertension
Common Causes		
	Angina pectoris	Essential hypertension
	Myocardial infarction	Iron deficiency anemia
	Acute and chronic pericarditis	Pernicious anemia
	Valvular defects	Arteriosclerosis obliterans
	Heart failure	Polycythemia vera
◆ **Assessment**		
Behavior	Anxiety, apprehension, decreasing mentation, confusion	Nervousness, mood swings, irritability, difficulty with memory, depression, confusion
Neurological	Essentially noncontributory	Decreased vibratory sensations, increased/decreased reflexes, Babinski reflex, changes in coordination
Head/neck	Distended neck veins, worried expression	Bruits over carotids, distended neck veins, epistaxis, diplopia, ringing in ears, dull occipial headaches on arising
Skin	Pale, cool, moist	Dry, pale, glossy, flaky, cold; decreased or absent hair
GI	Anorexia, nausea, vomiting, constipation	Anorexia, flatulence, diarrhea, constipation
Respiratory	Dyspnea, orthopnea, paroxysmal nocturnal dyspnea, tachypnea, moist crackles, cough	Dyspnea, orthopnea, crackles
Cardiovascular	Tires easily	Decreased exercise tolerance, weakness, palpitations
	Blood pressure—decreased systolic, decreased systolic/diastolic	Blood pressure—increased systolic, increased systolic and diastolic
	Pulse—increased/decreased, weak, thready, irregular, arrhythmias	Decreased or absent pedal pulses
Renal	Oliguria	Oliguria, nocturia, proteinuria
Extremities	Dependent edema	Tingling, numbness, or cold hands and feet, dependent edema, ulcers of legs or feet

ting to standing with *essential;* fall in BP from sitting to standing with *secondary.*

  c. Retinal changes; papilledema.

  d. Shortness of breath on slight exertion.

  e. Cardiac, cerebral, and renal changes.

  f. *Lab data:* UA, ECG, chest x-ray to rule out complications of hypertension.

◆ **E. Analysis/nursing diagnosis:**

  1. *Knowledge deficit* (learning need) regarding condition, treatment plan, and self-care and discharge needs.

  2. *Risk for decreased cardiac output* related to ventricular hypertrophy, vasoconstriction, or myocardial ischemia.

  3. *Risk for injury* related to complications of hypertension.

  4. *Impaired adjustment* related to required lifestyle changes.

  5. *Activity intolerance* related to weakness, fatigue.

◆ **F. Nursing care plan/implementation:**

  1. Goal: *provide for physical and emotional rest.*

    a. Rest periods before/after eating, visiting hours; *avoid* upsetting situations.

    b. Give tranquilizers, sedatives, as ordered.

  2. Goal: *provide for special safety needs.*

    a. Monitor blood pressure: both arms; standing, sitting, lying positions.

    b. Limit/prevent activities that increase pressure (anxiety, anger, frustration, upsetting visitors, fatigue).

    c. Assist with ambulation; change position gradually to prevent dizziness and lightheadedness (postural hypotension).

    d. Monitor for electrolyte imbalance when on low-sodium diet, diuretic therapy; I&O to prevent fluid depletion and arrhythmias from potassium loss.

    e. Observe for signs of hemorrhage, shock, stroke, which may occur following surgery.

  3. Goal: *health teaching* (patient and family).

    a. Procedures to decrease anxiety; relaxation techniques, stress management.

    b. Side effects of hypotensive drugs: initial therapy includes *diuretics* and *beta blockers;* if response inadequate may use *ACE inhibitors, adrenergic blockers, vasodilators, calcium channel blockers* (faintness, nausea, vomiting, hypotension, sexual dysfunction). See **Unit 10** for specific pharmacological actions.

    c. Weight control to reduce arterial pressure.

    d. Restrictions: stimulants (tea, coffee, tobacco), sodium, calories, fat.

    e. *Lifestyle adjustments:* daily exercise needed; reduce occupational and environmental stress; importance of rest.

    f. Blood pressure measurement: daily, same conditions, position preference of physician; use of self-monitoring cuff; check at least twice per week.

  g. Signs, symptoms, complications of disease (headache, confusion, visual changes, nausea/vomiting, convulsions).

  h. Causes of intermittent hypotension: alcohol, hot weather, exercise, febrile illness, hot bath.

◆ **G. Evaluation/outcome criteria:**

  1. Blood pressure within normal range for age (diastolic <90 mm Hg)—stable.

  2. Minimal or no pathophysiological or therapeutic complications (e.g., visual changes, stroke, drug side effects).

  3. Reduces weight to reasonable level for height, bone structure.

  4. Takes prescribed medications regularly, even after symptoms have resolved.

  5. Complies with restrictions: no smoking, restricted sodium, fat.

  6. Exercises regularly—program compatible with personal and health care goals.

II. Cardiac arrhythmias (dysrhythmias): any variations in normal rate, rhythm, or configuration of waves on ECG (Figure 7–2).

  A. Pathophysiology

    1. Dysfunction of SA node, atria, AV node, or ventricular conduction.

    2. Primary heart problem or secondary systemic problem.

  B. Risk factors

    1. Myocardial infarction.

    2. Drug toxicity.

    3. Stress.

    4. Cardiac surgery.

    5. Hypoxia.

    6. Congenital.

    7. See Table 7–4.

◆ **C. Assessment:** see Table 7–4 for specific dysrhythmias.

◆ **D. Analysis/nursing diagnosis:**

  1. *Decreased cardiac output* related to abnormal ventricular function.

  2. *Altered tissue perfusion* related to inadequate cardiac functioning.

  3. *Knowledge deficit* (learning need) regarding cause/treatment of condition, self-care, and discharge needs.

  4. *Anxiety* related to dependence, fear of death.

◆ **E. Nursing care plan/implementation:**

  1. Goal: *provide for emotional and safety needs.*

    a. Document ECG tracing for presence of life-threatening arrhythmia.

    b. Encourage discussion of fears, feelings (patient and significant other).

    c. *Bed rest:* restricted activities; quiet environment; limit visitors.

    d. Oxygen, if ordered.

    e. Check vital signs frequently for shock, HF, drug toxicity.

    f. Prepare for cardiac emergency: CPR.

g. Give cardiac medications; check lab tests for digitalis and potassium levels, to prevent drug toxicity.

2. Goal: *prevent thromboemboli.*
   ▶ a. Apply antiembolic stockings (TED hose).
   b. Give anticoagulants as ordered. (Check for bleeding—gums, urine; monitor *lab tests*—Lee White clotting time and activated partial thromboplastin time with heparin; prothrombin time with coumarin.)
   c. Encourage flexion-extension of feet.

3. Goal: *prepare for cardioversion with atrial fibrillation if indicated* (usually if pulse greater than 140 beats/min, symptomatic, or no conversion after 3 days of drug therapy).
   a. Give quinidine as ordered at least 24 hr before.
   b. NPO 8 hr before.
   c. Hold digoxin morning of cardioversion per order.

4. Goal: *provide for physical and emotional needs with pacemaker insertion.*
   a. *General concerns:*
      (1) Report excessive bleeding/infection at insertion site—hematoma may contribute to wound infection.
      (2) Encourage verbalization of feelings.
      (3) Report prolonged hiccoughs, which may indicate pacemaker failure.
      (4) Know pacing mode: fixed-rate or demand (most common); type of insertion (temporary or permanent).
   b. *Temporary pacemaker:*
      (1) Limit excessive activity of extremity if antecubital insertion, to prevent displacement; subclavian insertion increases catheter stability.
      (2) Secure wires to chest to prevent tension on catheter.
      (3) Do *not* defibrillate over insertion site, to avoid electrical hazards.
      (4) Electrical safety (grounding; disconnect electric beds/call lights; use battery-operated equipment).
   c. *Permanent pacemaker:*
      (1) Limit activity of shoulder for 48–72 hr with transvenous catheter to prevent dislodgement; *avoid* extending arms over head for 8 wk.
      (2) Postinsertion ROM (passive) at least once per shift after 48 hr to prevent frozen shoulder.
      (3) If defibrillation is required, place paddles at least 4 inches from pulse generator.

FIGURE 7–2 Interpretation of normal cardiac cycle. (From Thomas, CL [ed]: Taber's Cyclopedic Medical Dictionary, ed 18. FA Davis, Philadelphia, 1997, p 612.)

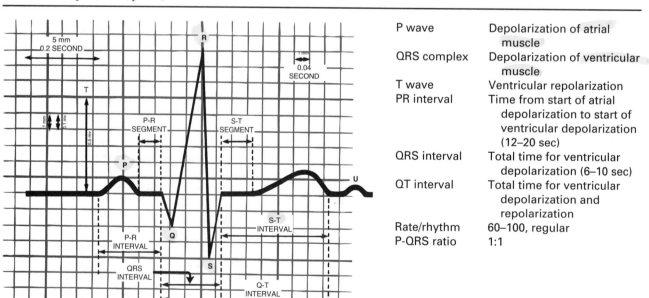

P wave	Depolarization of atrial muscle
QRS complex	Depolarization of ventricular muscle
T wave	Ventricular repolarization
PR interval	Time from start of atrial depolarization to start of ventricular depolarization (12–20 sec)
QRS interval	Total time for ventricular depolarization (6–10 sec)
QT interval	Total time for ventricular depolarization and repolarization
Rate/rhythm	60–100, regular
P-QRS ratio	1:1

TABLE 7–4   Comparison of Selected Cardiac Dysrhythmias

Dysrhythmia	Description	Etiology	Symptoms/ Consequences	Treatment
Dysrhythmias of Sinus Node				
Sinus dysrhythmia	Phasic shortening then lengthening of P-P and R-R interval	Respiratory variation in impulse initiation by SA node	Usually none	Usually none ⬤▭ Atropine if rate below 40 beats/min
Sinus tachycardia	P waves present followed by QRS Rhythm regular Heart rate 100–150 beats/min	Increased metabolic demands Decreased oxygen delivery, heart failure, shock, hemorrhage, anemia	May produce palpitations Prolonged episodes may lead to decreased cardiac output	Treat underlying cause Occasionally sedatives
Sinus bradycardia	P waves present followed by QRS Rhythm regular Heart rate <60 beats/min	Physical fitness Parasympathetic stimulation (sleep) Brain lesions Sinus dysfunction Digitalis excess	Very low rates may cause decreased cardiac output: light-headedness, faintness, chest pain	⬤▭ Atropine if cardiac output is decreased Pacemaker Treat underlying cause if necessary
Atrial Dysrhythmias				
Premature atrial beats	Early P wave QRS may or may not be normal Rhythm irregular	Stress, ischemia, atrial enlargement, caffeine, nicotine	May produce palpitations Frequent episodes may decrease cardiac output Is sign of chamber irritability	Sedation ⬤▭ Quinidine May require no other treatment
Atrial tachycardia	P wave present (may merge into previous T wave), QRS usually normal; rapid heart rate usually >150 beats/min	Sympathetic stimulation, chemical stimuli (caffeine, nicotine), drug toxicity	Palpitations Possible anxiety	Usually none Prolonged episodes may require carotid artery pressure, vagal stimulation, ver- ⬤▭ apamil, digitalis, or beta blockers
Atrial fibrillation	Rapid, irregular P waves (>350/min) Ventricular rhythm irregularly irregular Ventricular rate varies, may increase to 120–150/min if untreated	Rheumatic heart disease Mitral stenosis Atrial infarction Coronary atherosclerotic heart disease Hypertensive heart disease Thyrotoxicosis	Palpitations Pulse deficit Decreased cardiac output if rate is rapid Promotes thrombus formation in atria	⬤▭ Digitalis ⬤▭ Quinidine Cardioversion
Ventricular Dysrhythmias				
Premature ventricular beats (PVBs)	Early wide bizarre QRS, not associated with a P wave Rhythm irregular	Stress, acidosis, ventricular enlargement Electrolyte imbalance Myocardial infarction Digitalis toxicity Hypoxemia, hypercapnia	Same as for premature atrial beats	⬤▭ MEDS: Procainamide Quinidine Disopyramide (Norpace) Lidocaine Mexiletine Sodium bicarbonate Potassium Oxygen Treat heart failure
Ventricular tachycardia	No P wave before QRS; QRS wide and bizarre; ventricular rate >100, usually 140–240	PVB striking during vulnerable period; hypoxemia; drug toxicity; electrolyte imbalance; bradycardia	Decreased cardiac output, hypotension, loss of consciousness, respiratory arrest	⬤▭ MEDS: Lidocaine Procainamide Bretylium Mexiletine Cardioversion

Adult

Continued

TABLE 7–4   Comparison of Selected Cardiac Dysrhythmias—cont'd

Dysrhythmia	Description	Etiology	Symptoms/Consequences	Treatment
Ventricular Dysrhythmias—cont'd				
Ventricular fibrillation	Chaotic electrical activity No recognizable QRS complex	Myocardial infarction Electrocution Freshwater drowning Drug toxicity	No cardiac output Absent pulse or respiration Cardiac arrest	Defibrillation ⬤▷ MEDS: Epinephrine Lidocaine Sodium bicarbonate Bretylium ▶ CPR
Pulseless electrical activity (PEA)	Organized ECG rhythm	Electromechanical dissociation Escape rhythms	Pulseless Minimal or no perfusion	▶ CPR ⬤▷ Epinephrine
Ventricular standstill	Can be distinguished from ventricular fibrillation only by ECG P waves *may* be present No QRS "Straight line"	Myocardial infarction Chronic diseases of conducting system	Same as for ventricular fibrillation	▶ CPR Pacemaker ⬤▷ Intracardiac epinephrine ⬤▷ Atropine
Impulse Conduction Deficits				
First-degree atrioventricular (AV) block	PR interval prolonged, >0.20 sec	Rheumatic fever Digitalis toxicity Degenerative changes of coronary atherosclerotic heart disease Infections (e.g., Lyme carditis) Decreased oxygen in AV node	Warns of impaired conduction	Usually none as long as it occurs as an isolated deficit ⬤▷ Atropine if PR interval > 0.26 sec or bradycardia
Bundle branch block	Same as normal sinus rhythm (NSR) except QRS duration > 0.10 sec	Hypoxia, acute myocardial infarction, heart failure, coronary atherosclerotic heart disease, pulmonary embolus, hypertension	Same as first-degree AV block	Usually none unless severe blockage of left posterior division (see text)
Second-degree AV blocks	P waves usually occur regularly at rates consistent with SA node initiation (not all P waves followed by QRS; PR interval may lengthen before nonconducted P wave or may be consistent; QRS may be widened)	Acute myocardial infarction Same as first-degree AV block	Serious dysrhythmia that may lead to decreased heart rate and cardiac output	May require temporary pacemaker If symptomatic (e.g., dizziness), atropine ⬤▷ 1 mg
Complete third-degree AV block	Atria and ventricles beat independently P waves have no relation to QRS Ventricular rate may be as low as 20–40 beats/min	Digitalis toxicity Infectious disease Coronary artery disease Myocardial infarction	Very low rates may cause decreased cardiac output: light-headedness, fainting, chest pain	Pacemaker ⬤▷ Isoproterenol to increase heart rate ⬤▷ Epinephrine if isoproterenol ineffective

Source: Phipps, W, Long, B, Woods, N, and Cassmeyer, V (eds): Medical-Surgical Nursing, ed 5. Mosby, St. Louis.

d. *Health teaching* following permanent pacemaker:
  (1) Explain procedure: duration, equipment, purpose, type of pacemaker.
  (2) Medic Alert bracelet; pacemaker information card.
  (3) Daily pulse taking on arising (report variation of ±5 beats).
  (4) Signs, symptoms of *malfunction* (vertigo, syncope, dyspnea, slowed speech, confusion, fluid retention); *infection* (fever, heat, pain, skin breakdown at insertion site).
  (5) **Restrictions:** contact sports; electromagnetic interferences (few)—TV/radio transmitters, improperly functioning microwave oven (maintain distance of 3 ft), certain cautery machines; may trigger airport metal-detector alarm.

◆ **F. Evaluation/outcome criteria:**
  1. Regular cardiac rhythm, monitors own radial pulse.
  2. No complications (e.g., pacemaker malfunction).
  3. Returns for regular follow-up of pacemaker function.
  4. Tolerates physical or sexual activity.
  5. Wears identification bracelet; carries pacemaker identification card.
  6. Reports anxiety is reduced to manageable level.

III. Cardiac arrest: sudden unexpected cessation of heartbeat and effective circulation leading to inadequate perfusion and sudden death.
  A. Risk factors:
  1. Myocardial infarction.
  2. Multiple traumas.
  3. Respiratory arrest.
  4. Drowning.
  5. Electrical shock.
  6. Drug reactions.

◆ **B. Assessment**—*objective data:*
  1. Unresponsive to stimuli (i.e., verbal, painful).
  2. Absence of breathing, carotid pulse.
  3. Pale or bluish: lips, fingernails, skin.
  4. Pupils: dilated.

◆ **C. Analysis/nursing diagnosis:**
  1. *Decreased cardiac output* related to heart failure.
  2. *Impaired gas exchange* related to breathlessness.
  3. *Altered tissue perfusion* related to pulselessness.

◆ **D. Nursing care plan/implementation:**
  1. Goal: *prevent irreversible cerebral anoxic damage:* initiate CPR within 4–6 min; continue until relieved; document assessment factors,

effectiveness of actions; presence or absence of pulse at 1 min and every 4–5 min.
  2. Goal: *establish effective circulation, respiration:* see **Emergency Nursing Procedures,** Table 7–46, p. 628, for complete protocols.

◆ **E. Evaluation/outcome criteria:**
  1. Carotid pulse present; check after 1 min and every few minutes thereafter.
  2. Responds to verbal stimuli.
  3. Pupils constrict in response to light.
  4. Return of spontaneous respiration; adequate ventilation.

IV. Arteriosclerosis: loss of elasticity, thickening, hardening of arterial walls; symptoms depend on organ system involved; common type—atherosclerosis. Atherosclerosis (coronary heart disease) precedes angina pectoris and myocardial infarction.
  A. Pathophysiology:
  1. Atherosclerotic plaque, discrete lumpy thickening of arterial wall; cholesterol-lipid-calcium deposits in lining.
  2. Narrows lumen, can occlude vessel.
  B. Risk factors:
  1. Increased serum cholesterol (low-density lipids ≥160 mg/dL).
  2. Hypertension.
  3. Cigarette smoking.
  4. Diabetes mellitus.
  5. Family history of premature CHD.

(See **V. Angina pectoris,** and **VI. Myocardial infarction,** following sections, for nursing implications.)

V. Angina pectoris: transient paroxysmal episodes of substernal or precordial pain. Types: *stable* (follows an event, same severity); *unstable* (at rest or minimal exertion, recent onset, increasing severity); *Prinzmetal's variant* (at rest, caused by coronary spasms).
  A. Pathophysiology:
  1. Insufficient blood flow through coronary arteries. Oxygen demand exceeds supply.
  2. Temporary myocardial ischemia.
  B. Risk factors:
  1. Cardiovascular:
    a. Atherosclerosis.
    b. Thromboangiitis obliterans.
    c. Aortic regurgitation.
    d. Hypertension.
  2. Hormonal:
    a. Hypothyroidism.
    b. Diabetes mellitus.
  3. Blood disorders:
    a. Anemia.
    b. Polycythemia vera.
  4. *Lifestyle choices:*
    a. Smoking.
    b. Obesity.
    c. Cocaine use.
    d. Inactivity.

◆ **C. Assessment:**
   1. *Subjective data*
      a. Pain (Table 7–5).
         (1) *Type:* squeezing, pressing, burning.
         (2) *Location:* retrosternal, substernal, left of sternum, radiates to left arm (Figure 7–3).
         (3) *Duration:* short, usually 3–5 min, <30 min.
         (4) *Cause:* emotional stress, overeating, physical exertion, exposure to cold; may occur at rest.
         (5) *Relief:* rest, nitroglycerin.
      b. Dyspnea.
      c. Palpitations.
      d. Dizziness; faintness.
      e. Epigastric distress; indigestion; belching.
   2. *Objective data*
      a. Tachycardia.
      b. Pallor.
      c. Diaphoresis.
      d. ECG changes during attack.
◆ **D. Analysis/nursing diagnosis:**
   1. *Altered cardiopulmonary tissue perfusion* related to insufficient blood flow.
   2. *Pain* related to myocardial ischemia.
   3. *Activity intolerance* related to onset of pain.
◆ **E. Nursing care plan/implementation:**
   1. Goal: *provide relief from pain.*
      a. Rest until pain subsides.
      b. Nitroglycerin or amyl nitrite, beta-adrenergic blockers, as ordered.
      c. Identify precipitating factors: large meals, heavy exercise, stimulants (coffee, smoking), sex when fatigued, cold air.
      d. Vital signs: hypotension.
      e. Assist with ambulation; dizziness, flushing occurs with nitroglycerin.
   2. Goal: *provide emotional support.*
      a. Encourage verbalization of feelings, fears.
      b. Reassurance; positive self-concept.
      c. Acceptance of limitations.
   3. Goal: *health teaching.*
      a. Pain: alleviation, differentiation of angina from myocardial infarction, precipitating factors (see Table 7–5).
      b. Medication: frequency, expected effects (headache, flushing); carry fresh nitroglycerin; loses potency after 6 mo ("stings" under tongue when potent); may use nitroglycerin paste—instruct how to apply.
      c. *Diet:* restricted calories if weight loss indicated; restricted fat, cholesterol, gas-producing foods; small, frequent meals.
      d. *Diagnostic tests* if ordered (e.g., thallium stress test, cardiac catheterization; see pp. 450–451 and **Unit 11**).
      e. Exercise: regular, graded, to promote coronary circulation.

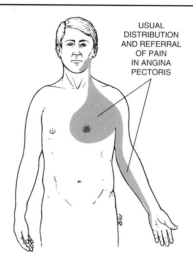

FIGURE 7–3 Angina pectoris. (From Thomas, CL [ed]: Taber's Cyclopedic Medical Dictionary, ed 18. FA Davis, Philadelphia, 1997, p 104.)

USUAL DISTRIBUTION AND REFERRAL OF PAIN IN ANGINA PECTORIS

ANGINA PECTORIS

      f. Prepare for coronary bypass surgery, if necessary.
      g. Behavior modification to assist with lifestyle changes, e.g., stress reduction, stop smoking.
◆ **F. Evaluation/outcome criteria:**
   1. Relief from pain.
   2. Fewer attacks.
   3. No myocardial infarction.
   4. Alters lifestyle; complies with limitations.
   5. No smoking.

VI. Myocardial infarction (MI, heart attack): localized area of necrotic tissue in myocardium from cessation of blood flow; leading cause of death in North America.
   A. Pathophysiology:
      1. Coronary occlusion due to thrombosis, embolism, or hemorrhage adjacent to atherosclerotic plaque.
      2. Insufficient blood flow from cardiac hypertrophy, hemorrhage, shock, or severe dehydration.
   B. Risk factors:
      1. Age (35–70 yr).
      2. Men more than women until menopause.
      3. Lifestyle: obesity, smoking, sedentary, amphetamine or cocaine use.
      4. Stress or type A personality.
      5. High-cholesterol, low-density lipoproteins, and serum triglyceride levels.
      6. Chronic illness (diabetes, hypertension).
   ◆ **C. Assessment:**
      1. *Subjective data*
         a. Pain (see Table 7–5).
            (1) *Type:* sudden, severe, crushing, heavy tightness. May be absent in elderly or diabetics.

TABLE 7–5   Comparison of Physical Causes of Chest Pain

Characteristic	Myocardial Infarction	Pericarditis	Gastric Disorders	Angina Pectoris	Dissecting Aneurysm	Pulmonary Embolism
Onset	Gradual or sudden	Sudden	Gradual or sudden	Gradual or sudden	Abrupt, without prodromal symptoms	Gradual or sudden
Precipitating factors	Can occur at rest or after exercise or emotional stress	Breathing deeply, rotating trunk, recumbency, swallowing or yawning	Inflammation of stomach or esophagus; hypersecretion of gastric juices; some medications	Usually after physical exertion, emotional stress, eating, exposure to cold, or defecation; unstable angina occurs at rest	Hypertension	Immobility or prolonged bedrest following surgery; trauma, hip fracture, HF, malignancy, oral contraceptives
Location	Substernal, anterior chest, or midline; rarely back; radiates to jaw or neck	Precordial; radiates to neck or left shoulder and arm	Xiphoid to umbilicus	Substernal, anterior chest; poorly localized	Correlates with site of intimal rupture; anterior chest or back; between shoulder blades	Pleural area, retrosternal area
Quality	Crushing, burning, stabbing, squeezing or vicelike	Pleuritic, sharp	Aching, burning, cramp-like, gnawing	Squeezing, feeling of heavy pressure; burning	Sharp, tearing or ripping sensation	Sharp, stabbing
Intensity	Asymptomatic to severe; increases with time	Mild to severe	Mild to severe	Mild to moderate	Severe and unbearable; maximal from onset	Aggravated by breathing
Duration	30 min to 1–2 hr; may wax and wane	Continuous	Periodic	Usually 2–10 min; average 3–5 min	Continuous; does not abate once started	Variable
Relief	Narcotics	Sitting up, leaning forward	Physical and emotional rest, food, antacids, H₂-receptor antagonists	Nitroglycerin, rest	Large, repeated doses of narcotics	O₂; sitting up, morphine
Associated symptoms	Nausea, fatigue, heartburn; peripheral pulses equal	Fever, dyspnea, nausea, anorexia, anxiety	Nausea, vomiting, dysphagia, anorexia, weight loss	Belching, indigestion, dizziness	Syncope, loss of sensations or pulses, oliguria; discrepancy between BP in arms; decrease in femoral or carotid pulse	Dyspnea, tachypnea, diaphoresis, hemoptysis, cough, apprehension

(2) *Location:* substernal; radiates to one or both arms, jaw, neck. May be confused with indigestion.

(3) *Duration:* >30 min.

(4) *Cause:* unrelated to exercise; frequently occurs when sleeping (REM stage).

(5) *Relief:* oxygen, narcotics; *not* relieved by rest or nitroglycerin.

b. Nausea.

c. Shortness of breath.

d. Apprehension, fear of impending death.

e. History of cardiac disease (family); occupational stress.

2. *Objective data*

a. Vital signs: shock; rapid (>100), thready pulse; fall in blood pressure; S$_3$ gallop; tachypnea, shallow respirations; elevated temperature within 24 hr (100°–103°F).

b. Skin: ashen or clammy; diaphoretic.

c. Emotional: restless.

d. Lab data: *increased*—WBC (12,000–15,000/μL), serum enzymes (CK-MB, LDH$_1$ > LDH$_2$—"flipped LDH"); *changes*—ECG (elevated ST segment, inverted T wave, arrhythmia).

D. **Analysis/nursing diagnosis:**

1. *Decreased cardiac output* related to myocardial damage.

2. *Impaired gas exchange* related to poor perfusion, shock.

3. *Pain* related to myocardial ischemia.

4. *Activity intolerance* related to pain or inadequate oxygenation.

5. *Fear* related to possibility of death.

E. **Nursing care plan/implementation** (see **Clinical Pathway for Acute MI,** p. 448):

1. Goal: *reduce pain, discomfort.*

a. Narcotics—morphine, possibly meperidine HCl (Demerol) or hydromorphone (Dilaudid); note response. *Avoid* IM.

b. Humidified oxygen 2–4 L/min; mouth care—oxygen is drying.

c. *Position:* semi-Fowler's to improve ventilation.

2. Goal: *maintain adequate circulation,* stabilize heart rhythm.

a. Monitor vital signs and urine output; observe for cardiogenic shock.

b. Monitor ECG for arrhythmias.

c. Give medications as ordered: *antiarrhythmics*—lidocaine HCl, atropine, quinidine *HCl,* procainamide (Pronestyl), bretylium (Bretylol); propranolol (Inderal); verapamil; *anticoagulants*—heparin sodium, bishydroxycoumarin or dicoumarin; *thrombolytic agents*—streptokinase (tPA), APSAC/anistreplase (Eminase).

d. Recognize heart failure: edema, cyanosis, dyspnea, cough, crackles.

e. Check lab data—normal; serum enzymes (CK 20-220 IU/L depending on gender; CK-MB 0–12 IU/L; LDH < 115 IU/L; LDH$_1$ < LDH$_2$); blood gases (pH 7.35–7.45; P$_{CO_2}$ 35–45 mEq/L; P$_{O_2}$ 80–100 mm Hg; HCO$_3$ 22–26); electrolytes (K$^+$ 3.5–5.0 mEq/L); clotting time (aPTT 25–41 sec; PT 11–15 sec).

f. CVP—zero level at right atrium; fluctuates with respiration; normal range 5–15 cm H$_2$O; note trend; increases with heart failure.

g. ROM of lower extremities; TED hose/antiembolic stockings.

3. Goal: *decrease oxygen demand/promote oxygenation, reduce cardiac workload.*

a. O$_2$ as ordered.

b. Activity: bed rest (24–48 hr) with bedside commode; planned rest periods; control visitors.

c. *Position:* semi-Fowler's to facilitate lung expansion and decrease venous return.

d. Anticipate needs of patient: call light, water.

e. Assist with feeding, turning.

f. Environment: quiet, comfortable.

g. Reassurance; stay with anxious patient.

h. Give medications as ordered: cardiotonics, calcium channel blockers, vasodilators, vasopressors.

4. Goal: *maintain fluid electrolyte, nutritional status.*

a. IV (keep vein open); CVP; vital signs; urine output—30 mL/hr.

b. Lab data within normal limits (Na$^+$ 135–145 mEq/L; K$^+$ 3.5–5.0 mEq/L).

 c. Monitor ECG—*hyperkalemia:* peaked T wave; *hypokalemia:* depressed T wave.

d. *Diet:* progressive *low* calorie, *low* sodium, *low* cholesterol, *low* fat, without caffeine.

5. Goal: *facilitate fecal elimination.*

a. Medications: stool softeners to prevent Valsalva maneuver (straining); mouth breathing during bowel movement; recognize complications of Valsalva maneuver—chest pain, cyanosis, diaphoresis, arrhythmias.

b. Bedside commode if possible.

6. Goal: *provide emotional support.*

a. Recognize fear of dying: denial, anger, withdrawal.

b. Encourage expression of feelings, fears, concerns.

c. Discuss rehabilitation, lifestyle changes: prevent cardiac-invalid syndrome by promoting self-care activities, independence.

7. Goal: *promote sexual functioning.*
   a. Encourage discussion of concerns regarding activity, inadequacy, limitations, expectations—include partner (usually resume activity 5–8 wk after uncomplicated MI or when patient can climb two flights of stairs).
   b. Identify need for referral for sexual counseling.
8. Goal: *health teaching.*
   a. Diagnosis and treatment regimen.
   b. *Caution* about when to *avoid* sexual activity: after heavy meal, alcohol ingestion; when fatigued, tense, under stress; with unfamiliar partners; in extreme temperatures.
   c. Information about sexual activity: less fatiguing positions (side to side; noncardiac on top); vasodilators, if ordered, before intercourse; select comfortable, familiar environment.
   d. Available community resources for information, support groups (e.g., American Heart Association, Stop Smoking Clinics).
   e. Medications: administration, importance, untoward effects, pulse taking.
   f. Control risk factors: rest, diet, exercise, no smoking, weight control, stress-reduction techniques.
   g. Need for follow-up care for regulation of medications, evaluating risk factors.
   h. Prepare for angioplasty or coronary bypass if planned.

◆ **F. Evaluation/outcome criteria:**
1. No complications: stable vital signs; relief of pain.
2. Adheres to prescribed medication regimen, demonstrates knowledge about medications.
3. Activity tolerance is increased, participates in program of progressive activity.
4. Reduction or modification of risk factors. Plans to alter lifestyle (e.g., loses weight, quits smoking).

VII. Cardiac valvular defects: alteration in the structure of a valve; impede flow of blood or permit regurgitation.

A. Pathophysiology:
1. *Stenosis*—narrowing of valvular opening due to adherence, thickening, and rigidity of valve cusp from fibrosis, scarring, and calcification.
2. *Insufficiency* (incompetence)—incomplete closure of valve due to contraction of chordae tendineae, papillary muscles; or to calcification, scarring of leaflets. Results in regurgitation.
3. *Mitral stenosis:*
   a. Most common residual cardiac lesion of rheumatic fever.

   b. Affects women <45 yr more often than men.
   c. Narrowing of mitral valve.
   d. Interferes with filling of left ventricle.
   e. Produces pulmonary hypertension, right ventricular failure.
4. *Mitral insufficiency* (incompetence):
   a. Leaking/regurgitation of blood back into left atrium.
   b. Results from rheumatic fever, bacterial endocarditis; less common.
   c. Affects *men* more often.
   d. Produces pulmonary congestion, right ventricular failure.
5. *Aortic stenosis:*
   a. Fusion of valve flaps between left ventricle and aorta.
   b. Congenital or acquired from atherosclerosis or from rheumatic fever and bacterial endocarditis; seen in *men* more often; pulmonary circulation congested, cardiac output decreased.
6. *Aortic insufficiency:*
   a. Incomplete closure of valve between left ventricle and aorta (regurgitation).
   b. Left ventricular failure leading to right ventricular heart failure.

B. Risk factors:
1. Congenital abnormality.
2. History of rheumatic fever.
3. Atherosclerosis.

◆ **C. Assessment:** Table 7–6.

◆ **D. Analysis/nursing diagnosis:**
1. *Decreased cardiac output* related to inadequate ventricular filling.
2. *Fluid volume excess* related to compensatory response to decreased cardiac output.
3. *Impaired gas exchange* related to pulmonary congestion.
4. *Activity intolerance* related to impaired cardiac function.
5. *Fatigue* related to poor oxygenation.

◆ **E. Nursing care plan/implementation:**
1. Goal: *reduce cardiac workload.*
2. Goal: *promote physical comfort and psychological support.*
3. Goal: *prevent complications.*
4. Goal: *prepare for surgery* (commissurotomy, valvuloplasty [valvotomy], or valvular replacement, depending on defect and severity of condition).
5. See section on cardiac surgery, p. 452, for specific nursing actions.

◆ **F. Evaluation/outcome criteria:**
1. Relief of symptoms.
2. Increase in activity level.
3. No complications following surgery.

VIII. Cardiac catheterization: a diagnostic procedure to evaluate cardiac status. Introduces a catheter into the

Adult

Instructions:
Check boxes for items that apply
Draw a line through items that do not apply
Document variances on the opposite side

CRITICAL PATHWAYS, AKA
PATIENT CARE MANAGEMENT PLAN:
ACUTE CORONARY SYNDROME/ACUTE MI

DATE	/ /	/ /	/ /
	ED	**Day 1 ICU/Telemetry**	**Day 2**
1 Discharge Planning / Referrals	☐ Initiate Cardiology Consult	☐ Evaluation of home situation ☐ Code status _____	☐ SW referral as needed
2 Diagnostic Tests / Treatments	☐ H & P ☐ BUN ☐ EKG x2 CXR ☐ CBC ☐ Creatinine ☐ Lipid panel ☐ CK MB #1 ☐ Troponin ☐ PT/PTT ☐ Electrolytes	☐ EKG ☐ CK MB #2 at 8 hrs. ☐ CK MB #3 at 16 hrs. ☐ Troponin ☐ PTT per heparin protocol ☐ Platelet count	☐ Transfer to telemetry 24-48hrs after admission Consider cardiac cath or noninvasive test for ischemia prior to discharge
3 Nutrition / Diet	☐ NPO	☐ Cardiac prudent diet	☐ Cardiac prudent diet
4 Treatments and Medications	☐ Medical Therapy ☐ MSO$_4$ ☐ Primary PTCA ☐ ASA ☐ Thrombolytic Therapy ☐ Beta Blocker ☐ IV fluids / Saline lock ☐ Heparin ☐ O$_2$ OR ☐ Nitrates ☐ Enoxaparin	☐ IV Fluids / Saline lock ☐ ACE Inhibitor ☐ O$_2$ ☐ Heparin ☐ Nitrates or ☐ MSO$_4$ ☐ Enoxaparin ☐ ASA ☐ Stool ☐ Beta Blocker Softener	☐ IV to saline lock ☐ Heparin Drip ☐ O$_2$ DC'd if ☐ MSO$_4$ D/C'd indicated ☐ ASA ☐ ACE Inhibitor ☐ PO Beta Blockers ☐ Stool Softener ☐ IV Beta Blocker DC'd ☐ NTG drip D/C'd
5 Activity Cardiac Rehab	☐ Bedrest with commode	CR step 1: ☐ Bedrest with commode ☐ PT referral	CR step 2: ☐ Begin self care with assistance ☐ PT evaluation
6 Nursing Assessment/ Intervention ◆	VS per ED routine I & O O$_2$ sat. > 92% Cardiac Monitor Saline lock	D E N ☐ EKG monitor / Telemetry ☐ ☐ ☐ Wt _____ VS per unit routine ☐ ☐ ☐ I & O ☐ ☐ ☐ O$_2$ sat > 92% ☐ ☐ ☐ Saline lock ☐ ☐ ☐ AxO x3, speech clear, memory intact, swallow intact ☐ ☐ ☐ Abdomen soft nontender, bowel sounds present, tolerates diet ☐ ☐ ☐ Voiding adequate amounts, urine clear, yellow to amber ☐ ☐ ☐ Normal ROM and strength appropriate for patient ☐ ☐ ☐ Circulation and sensation intact ☐ ☐ ☐ Coping appropriately ☐ ☐ ☐ Communicates needs and concerns, behavior appropriate to age and situation ☐ ☐ ☐	D E N ☐ EKG monitor / Telemetry ☐ ☐ ☐ Wt _____ VS per unit routine ☐ ☐ ☐ I & O ☐ ☐ ☐ O$_2$ sat > 92% ☐ ☐ ☐ Saline lock ☐ ☐ ☐ AxO X3, speech clear, memory intact, swallow intact ☐ ☐ ☐ Abdomen soft nontender, bowel sounds present, tolerates diet ☐ ☐ ☐ Voiding adequate amounts, urine clear, yellow to amber ☐ ☐ ☐ Normal ROM and strength appropriate for patient ☐ ☐ ☐ Circulation and sensation intact ☐ ☐ ☐ Coping appropriately ☐ ☐ ☐ Communicates needs and concerns, behavior appropriate to age and situation ☐ ☐ ☐
7 Alteration in Comfort: Pain	☐ Instruct patient on pain scale and need to call RN for pain Initial pain level _____	☐ Instruct patient or pain scale and need to call RN for pain	☐ Assess for pain
8 Anxiety	Anxiety level identified Low ☐ Med ☐ High ☐ ☐ Appropriate actions taken (see nursing notes for med/high)	☐ Cooperates with care	☐ Receives information about activities ☐ Participates in care ☐ Verbalizes fears and concerns.
9 Knowledge Deficit	☐ Inform patient of plan of care ☐ Teach patient how to use pain scale	☐ Reinforce use of pain scale ☐ "Recovery After Your Heart Attack" booklet given to patient	☐ Pt. knows he/she had an MI and what it means ☐ Cardiovascular disease risk factors reviewed ☐ Medication teaching started
SIGNATURE BOX	A/D: E: P/N:	A/D: E: P/N:	A/D: E: P/N:

Admitting diagnosis _____

Discharge diagnosis _____

/ /	/ /	/ /	/ /
Day 3	**Day 4**	**Day 5 / Discharge**	**Discharge Outcomes**
☐ Outpatient Cardiac Rehab Referral made	☐ Home care referral as needed	☐ Refer family to CPR class	☐ CPR class referral made ☐ Outpt. Cardiac Rehab referral made ☐ Home situation adequate / no help ☐ Home care referral completed ☐ Appt. made for f/u MD visit
☐ Nutrition consult			☐ Cardiac evaluation complete
☐ Cardiac prudent diet	☐ Cardiac prudent diet	☐ Cardiac prudent diet	☐ Patient / family able to identify elements of cardiac prudent diet ☐ Written materials given
☐ DO O$_2$ ☐ ASA ☐ PO Beta Blockers ☐ ACE Inhibitors ☐ Stool Softener	☐ Evaluate women for HRT ☐ ASA ☐ PO Beta Blockers ☐ ACE Inhibitors ☐ Stool Softener	☐ ASA ☐ PO Beta Blockers ☐ ACE Inhibitors ☐ Lipid lowering agent	☐ Discharge meds Rx given ☐ Pt. verbalizes understanding how to take d/c medications ☐ Medication teaching sheet completed and signed by patient and nurse
CR step 3: Ambulate x 3 without significant change in VS ☐ ☐ Teach Pt. methods to evaluate exertion ☐	CR step 4: Ambulate 5 x day Independent self care ☐ ☐ ☐ ☐ ☐ Stair climbing if appropriate ☐	☐ Verbalizes activity limits	☐ Inpatient Cardiac Rehab. complete ☐ ADLs with stable VS
D E N ☐ EKG monitor / Telemetry ☐ ☐ ☐ Wt _____ VS per unit routine ☐ ☐ ☐ I & O ☐ ☐ ☐ O$_2$ sat > 92% ☐ ☐ ☐ Saline lock ☐ ☐ ☐ AxO X3 speech clear, memory intact, swallow intact ☐ ☐ ☐ Abdomen soft nontender, bowel sounds present, tolerates diet ☐ ☐ ☐ Voiding adequate amounts, urine clear, yellow to amber ☐ ☐ ☐ Normal ROM and strength appropriate for patient ☐ ☐ ☐ Circulation and sensation intact ☐ ☐ ☐ Coping appropriately ☐ ☐ ☐ Communicates needs and concerns, behavior appropriate to age and situation ☐ ☐ ☐	D E N ☐ EKG monitor / Telemetry ☐ ☐ ☐ Wt _____ VS per unit routine ☐ ☐ ☐ I & O ☐ ☐ ☐ O$_2$ sat > 92% ☐ ☐ ☐ Saline lock ☐ ☐ ☐ AxO X3, speech clear, memory intact, swallow intact ☐ ☐ ☐ Abdomen soft nontender, bowel sounds present, tolerates diet ☐ ☐ ☐ Voiding adequate amounts, urine clear, yellow to amber ☐ ☐ ☐ Normal ROM and strength appropriate for patient ☐ ☐ ☐ Circulation and sensation intact ☐ ☐ ☐ Coping appropriately ☐ ☐ ☐ Communicates needs and concerns, behavior appropriate to age and situation ☐ ☐ ☐	D E N ☐ EKG monitor / Telemetry ☐ ☐ ☐ Wt _____ VS per unit routine ☐ ☐ ☐ I & O ☐ ☐ ☐ O$_2$ sat > 92% ☐ ☐ ☐ Saline lock ☐ ☐ ☐ AxO X3, speech clear, memory intact, swallow intact ☐ ☐ ☐ Abdomen soft nontender, bowel sounds present, tolerates diet ☐ ☐ ☐ Voiding adequate amounts, urine clear, yellow to amber ☐ ☐ ☐ Normal ROM and strength appropriate for patient ☐ ☐ ☐ Circulation and sensation intact ☐ ☐ ☐ Coping appropriately ☐ ☐ ☐ Communicates needs and concerns, behavior appropriate to age and situation ☐ ☐ ☐	☐ Referral to smoking cessation program made ☐ Referral to stress reduction program made ☐ D/C instructions given to patient, pt. verbalizes understanding
☐ Assess for pain	☐ Assess for pain		☐ Patient is pain free ☐ Verbalizes appropriate actions to take if chest pain recurs ☐ Verbalizes appropriate use of EMC system
☐ Receives information about activities ☐ Participates in care ☐ Verbalizes fears and concerns	☐ Retains information ☐ Participates in care	☐ Retains information ☐ Participates in care ☐ Verbalizes understanding of appropriate life style changes	☐ Verbalizes ability to manage at home ☐ Continuing care arrangements made if appropriate
☐ "Recovery After Your Heart Attack" booklet reviewed. ☐ Patient is able to identify risk factors ☐ Teach pulse taking	☐ Instruct patient and family on risk factors reduction ☐ Review "Recovery After Your Heart Attack" booklet ☐ Give D/C instructions	☐ Complete D/C instruction sheet ☐ RN and Pt. sign forms ☐ Patient/family member demonstrates pulse taking ☐ Review D/C instructions	☐ MI teaching record complete ☐ DC summary complete
A/D:	A/D:	A/D:	A/D:
E:	E:	E:	E:
P/N:	P/N:	P/N:	P/N:

Source: UCSF Healthcare, San Francisco, Calif. With permission from Jane E. Hirsch, RN, MS, Vice President, Nursing and Patient Care Services.

TABLE 7–6 Comparison of Symptomatoloy for Valvular Defects

◆ Assessment	Mitral Stenosis	Mitral Insufficiency	Aortic Stenosis	Aortic Insufficiency
Subjective Data				
Fatigue	✓	✓	✓	✓
Shortness of breath	✓			
Orthopnea	✓		✓	✓
Paroxysmal nocturnal dyspnea	✓		✓	✓
Cough	✓	✓		
Dyspnea on exertion		✓	✓	✓
Palpitations		✓	✓	
Syncope on exertion			✓	
Angina			✓	✓
Weight loss		✓		
Objective Data				
Vital signs				
Blood pressure:				
Low or normal	✓	✓		
Normal or elevated			✓	✓
Pulse:				
Weak, irregular	✓	✓		
Rapid, "waterhammer"				✓
Respirations:				
Increased, shallow	✓			
Cyanosis	✓			
Jugular vein distention	✓			
Enlarged liver	✓		✓	
Dependent edema	✓		✓	
Murmur	✓	✓	✓	✓

heart, blood vessels; analyzes blood samples for oxygen content, cardiac output, pulmonary artery blood flow; done before heart surgery; frequently combined with angiography to visualize coronary arteries; also provides access for specialized cardiac techniques (e.g., internal pacing and coronary angioplasty).

A. Approaches

1. *Right-heart* catheterization—venous approach (antecubital or femoral) → right atrium → right ventricle → pulmonary artery.
2. *Left-heart* catheterization—retrograde approach: right brachial artery or percutaneous puncture of femoral artery → ascending aorta → left ventricle.
   a. Transseptal: femoral vein → right atrium → septum → left atrium → left ventricle.
   b. Angiography/arteriography: done during left-heart catheterization.

B. Precatheterization

◆ 1. **Assessment:**
   a. *Subjective data*
      (1) Allergies: iodine, seafood.
      (2) Anxiety.
   b. *Objective data*
      (1) Vital signs: baseline data.
      (2) Distal pulses: mark for reference after catheterization.

◆ 2. **Analysis/nursing diagnosis:**
   a. *Anxiety* related to fear of unknown.

   b. *Knowledge deficit* (learning need) related to limited exposure to information or sudden need for procedure.

◆ 3. **Nursing care plan/implementation:**
   a. Goal: *provide for safety, comfort.*
      (1) Signed informed consent.
      (2) NPO (except for medications 6–8 hr before).
      (3) Have patient urinate before going to lab.
      (4) Give sedatives, as ordered, 30 min before procedure (e.g., midazolam HCl [Versed] IV, diazepam [Valium] PO).
   b. Goal: *health teaching.*
      (1) Procedure: length (1–3 hr).
      (2) Expectations (strapped to table for safety, must lie still, awake but mildly sedated).
      (3) Sensations (hot, flushed feeling in head with dye injection; thudding in chest from premature beats during catheter manipulation; desire to cough, particularly with right-heart angiography and contrast-medium injection).
      (4) Alert physician to unusual sensations (coolness, numbness, paresthesia).

C. Postcatheterization

◆ 1. **Assessment** (potential complications):
   a. *Subjective data*

◆ 4. **Evaluation/outcome criteria:**

   a. Displays moderate anxiety level.

   b. Verbalizes/demonstrates postoperative expectations.

   c. Quits smoking before surgery.

B. Postoperative

◆ 1. **Assessment:**

   a. *Subjective data*

     (1) Pain.

     (2) Fatigue—sleep deprivation.

   b. *Objective data*

     (1) Neurological: level of consciousness; pupillary reactions; movement of limbs (purposeful, spontaneous).

     (2) Respiratory: rate changes (increases occur with obstruction, pain; decreases occur with CO_2 retention); depth (shallow with pain, atelectasis); symmetry; skin *color;* patency/ *drainage* from chest tubes, *sputum* (amount, color); endotracheal tube placement (bilateral breath sounds).

     (3) Cardiovascular:

       (a) BP—*hypotension* may indicate heart failure, tamponade, hemorrhage, arrhythmias, or thrombosis; *hypertension* may indicate anxiety, hypervolemia.

       (b) Pulse: radial, apical, pedal; rate (>100 may indicate shock, fever, hypoxia, arrhythmias); rhythm, quality.

       (c) CVP or Swan-Ganz (*elevated* in cardiac failure); temperature (normal postop: 98.6°–101.6°F oral).

     (4) GI: nausea, vomiting, distention.

     (5) Renal: urine—minimum output (30 mL/hr); color; specific gravity (<1.010 occurs with *overhydration,* renal tubular damage; >1.020 present with *dehydration,* oliguria, blood in urine).

◆ 2. **Analysis/nursing diagnosis:**

   a. *Decreased cardiac output* related to decreased myocardial contractility or postoperative hypothermia.

   b. *Pain* (acute) related to incision.

   c. *Ineffective airway clearance* related to effects of general anesthesia.

   d. *Altered tissue perfusion* related to postoperative bleeding or thromboemboli.

   e. *Fluid volume deficit* related to blood loss.

   f. *Risk for infection* related to wound contamination.

   g. *Altered thought processes* related to anesthesia or stress.

   h. *Altered role performance* related to uncertainty about future.

◆ 3. **Nursing care plan/implementation:**

   a. Goal: *provide constant monitoring to prevent complications.*

     (1) Respiratory:

       (a) Observe for respiratory distress: restlessness, nasal flaring, *Cheyne-Stokes* respiration, dusky/cyanotic skin; assisted or controlled ventilation via endotracheal tube common 6–24 hr; supplemental O_2 after extubation.

      ▶ (b) Suctioning; cough, deep breathe.

      ◪ (c) Elevate *head of bed.*

       (d) Position chest tube to facilitate drainage; mediastinal sump tube maintains patency—"milking" not necessary. See also chest tube care in Table 11–7.

     (2) *Cardiovascular:*

      ◪ (a) Vital signs: BP >80–90 mm Hg systolic; *CVP:* range 5–15 cm H_2O unless otherwise ordered; pulmonary artery line (Swan-Ganz): mean pressure 4–12 mm Hg; I&O: report <30 mL/hr of urine from indwelling urinary catheter.

       (b) ECG; PVCs occur most frequently following aortic valve replacement and bypass surgery.

       (c) Peripheral pulses if leg veins used for grafting.

       (d) Activity: turn q2h; ROM; progressive, early ambulation.

     (3) Inspect dressing for bleeding.

     (4) Medications according to therapeutic directives—*cardiotonics* (digoxin); *coronary vasodilators* (nitrates); *antibiotics* (penicillin); *analgesics; anticoagulants* (with valve replacements); *antiarrhythmics* (quinidine, procainamide HCl [Pronestyl]).

   b. Goal: *promote comfort, pain relief.*

     (1) Medicate: Demerol or morphine sulfate—severe pain lasts 2–3 days.

     (2) Splint incision when moving or coughing.

     (3) Mouth care: keep lips moist.

     ◪ (4) *Position:* use pillows to prevent tension on chest tubes, incision.

   c. Goal: *maintain fluid, electrolyte, nutritional balance.*

     (1) I&O; urine specific gravity.

     (2) Measure chest drainage—should *not* exceed 200 mL/hr for first 4–6 hr.

     (3) Give fluids as ordered; maintain IV patency.

     (4) *Diet:* clear fluids → solid food if no nausea, GI distention; sodium intake *restricted,* low fat.

   d. Goal: *promote emotional adjustment.*

     (1) Anticipate behavior disturbances (depression, disorientation often occur

Adult

3 days postop) related to medications, fear, sleep deprivation.
(2) Calm, oriented, supportive environment, as personalized as possible.
(3) Encourage verbalization of feelings (family and patient).
(4) Encourage independence to avoid cardiac-cripple role.
e. Goal: *health teaching.*
(1) Alterations in lifestyle; activity, diet, work; resumption of sexual activity usually when patient can climb two flights of stairs.
(2) Available community resources for cardiac rehabilitation (e.g., American Heart Association, Mended Hearts).
(3) Drug regimen: purpose, side effects.
(4) Potential complications: dyspnea, pain, palpitations common postoperatively.

◆ 4. **Evaluation/outcome criteria:**
a. No complications; incision heals.
b. Activity level increases—no signs of overexertion (e.g., fatigue, dyspnea, pain).
c. Relief of symptoms.
d. Returns for follow-up medical care.
e. Takes prescribed medications; knows purposes and side effects.

XI. Minimally invasive direct coronary artery bypass (MIDCAB): a variation of CABG for patients in whom sternotomy and cardiopulmonary bypass is contraindicated or unnecessary. The left internal mammary is anastomosed to the left anterior descending coronary artery through a thoracic incision without bypass.

XII. Heart failure (HF): inability of the heart to meet the peripheral circulatory demands of the body; cardiac decompensation; combined right and left ventricular heart failure.
A. Pathophysiology: increased cardiac workload or decreased effective myocardial contractility → decreased cardiac output (forward effects). Left ventricular failure → pulmonary congestion; right atrial and right ventricular failure → systemic congestion → peripheral edema (backward effects). Compensatory mechanisms in HF include tachycardia, ventricular dilation, and hypertrophy of the myocardium; develops in 50–60% of heart disease patients.
B. Risk factors:
1. Decreased myocardial contractility:
a. Myocarditis.
b. MI.
c. Tachyarrhythmias.
d. Bacterial endocarditis.
e. Acute rheumatic fever.
2. Increased cardiac workload:
a. Elevated temperature.

b. Physical/emotional stress.
c. Anemia.
d. Hyperthyroidism (thyrotoxicosis).
e. Valvular defects.
◆ **C. Assessment:**
1. *Subjective data*
a. Shortness of breath.
(1) Orthopnea (sleeps on two or more pillows).
(2) Paroxysmal nocturnal dyspnea (sudden breathlessness during sleep).
(3) Dyspnea on exertion (climbing stairs).
b. Apprehension; anxiety; irritability.
c. Fatigue; weakness.
d. Reported weight gain; feeling of puffiness.
2. *Objective data* (Table 7–7)
a. Vital signs:
(1) BP: decreasing systolic; narrowing pulse pressure.
(2) Pulse: pulsus alternans (alternating strong-weak-strong cardiac contraction), increased.
(3) Respirations: crackles, *Cheyne-Stokes.*
b. Edema: dependent, pitting (1+ to 4+ mm).
c. Liver: enlarged, tender.
d. Neck veins: distended.
e. Chest x-ray:
(1) Cardiac enlargement.
(2) Dilated pulmonary vessels.
(3) Diffuse interstitial lung edema.
◆ **D. Analysis/nursing diagnosis:**
1. *Decreased cardiac output* related to decreased myocardial contractility.
2. *Activity intolerance* related to generalized weakness and inadequate oxygenation.
3. *Fatigue* related to edema and poor oxygenation.
4. *Altered tissue perfusion* related to peripheral edema and inadequate blood flow.
5. *Fluid volume excess* related to compensatory mechanisms.
6. *Impaired gas exchange* related to pulmonary congestion.
7. *Anxiety* related to shortness of breath.
8. *Sleep pattern disturbance* related to paroxysmal nocturnal dyspnea.

TABLE 7–7   Left Ventricular Compared with Right Ventricular Heart Failure

Left Ventricular Failure	Right Ventricular Failure
Pulmonary crackles	Jugular venous distention
Tachypnea	Peripheral edema
S₃ gallop	Perioral and peripheral cyanosis
Cardiac murmurs	Congestive hepatomegaly
Paradoxical splitting of S₂	Ascites
	Hepatojugular reflux

◆ **E. Nursing care plan/implementation** (see **Clinical Pathway for Congestive Heart Failure**):

1. Goal: *provide physical rest/reduce emotional stimuli.*

   ✎ a. *Position: sitting* or *semi*-Fowler's until tachycardia, dyspnea, edema resolved; change position frequently; pillows for support.

   b. Rest: planned periods; limit visitors, activity, noise. Chair and commode privileges.

   ⬭ c. Support: stay with anxious patient; have supportive family member present; administer sedatives/tranquilizers as ordered.

   d. Warm fluids if appropriate.

2. Goal: *provide for relief of respiratory distress; reduce cardiac workload.*

   ▶ a. Oxygen: low flow rate; encourage deep breathing (5–10 min q2h); auscultate breath sounds for congestion, pulmonary edema.

   ✎ b. *Position:* elevating head of bed 20–25 cm (8–10 in) alleviates pulmonary congestion.

   ⬭ c. Medications as ordered:

      (1) *Digitalis* preparations.

      (2) *ACE inhibitors*—captopril, enalapril.

      (3) *Inotropic agent*—dobutamine, dopamine.

      (4) *Diuretics*—thiazides, furosemide, metolazone.

      (5) *Tranquilizers*—phenobarbital, diazepam (Valium), chlordiazepoxide (Librium) HCl.

      (6) *Vasodilators*—hydrolazine, isosorbide.

3. Goal: *provide for special safety needs.*

   ▶ a. Skin care:

      (1) Inspect, massage, lubricate bony prominences.

      (2) Use foot cradle, heel protectors; sheepskin.

   b. Side rails up if hypoxic (disoriented).

   c. Vital signs: monitor for signs of fatigue, pulmonary emboli.

   d. ROM: active, passive; elastic stockings.

4. Goal: *maintain fluid and electrolyte balance, nutritional status.*

   ▯ a. Urine output: 30 mL/hr minimum; estimate insensible loss in diaphoretic patient. Monitor BUN, serum creatinine, and electrolytes.

   b. Daily weight; same time, clothes, scale.

   c. IV: use microdrip to avoid circulatory overloading.

   ▮●▯ d. *Diet:*

      (1) *Low* sodium as ordered.

      (2) Small, frequent feedings.

      (3) Discuss food preferences with patient.

5. Goal: *health teaching.*

   a. Diet restrictions; meal preparation.

   b. Activity restrictions, if any; planned rest periods.

   c. Medications: schedule (e.g., diuretic in early morning to limit interruption of sleep) purpose, dosage, side effects (importance of daily pulse taking, daily weights, intake of *potassium*-containing foods).

   d. Available *community resources* for dietary assistance, weight reduction, exercise program.

◆ **F. Evaluation/outcome criteria:**

1. Increase in activity level tolerance—fatigue decreased.

2. No complications—pulmonary edema, respiratory distress.

3. Reduction in dependent edema.

XIII. Pulmonary edema: sudden transudation of fluid from pulmonary capillaries into alveoli. **Life-threatening condition.**

A. **Pathophysiology:** increased pulmonary capillary permeability; increased hydrostatic pressure (pulmonary hypertension); decreased blood colloidal osmotic pressure; fluid accumulation in alveoli → decreased compliance → decreased diffusion of gas → hypoxia, hypercapnea.

B. **Risk factors:**

1. Left ventricular failure.

2. Pulmonary embolism.

3. Drug overdose.

4. Smoke inhalation.

5. CNS damage.

6. Fluid overload.

◆ C. **Assessment:**

1. *Subjective data*

   a. Anxiety.

   b. Restlessness at onset progressing to agitation.

   c. Stark fear.

   d. Intense dyspnea, orthopnea, fatigue.

2. *Objective data*

   a. Vital signs:

      (1) Pulse: tachycardia; gallop rhythm.

      (2) Respiration: tachypnea, moist, bubbling, wheezing, labored.

      (3) Temperature: normal to subnormal.

   b. Skin: pale, cool, diaphoretic, cyanotic.

   c. Auscultation: crackles, wheezes.

   d. Cough: productive of large quantities of pink, frothy sputum.

   e. Right ventricular heart failure: distended (bulging) neck veins, peripheral edema, hepatomegaly, ascites.

   f. Mental status: restless, confused, stuporous.

   ▯ g. Arterial blood gases: hypoxia; pulse oximetry: decreased O_2 saturation.

   h. Chest x-ray: haziness of lung fields, cardiomegaly.

Instructions:
Circle variances and document
on opposite side

UCSF Health Care
UCSF/Mount Zion Medical Center
PATIENT CARE MANAGEMENT PLAN: Congestive Heart Failure

DATE	/ /	/ /	/ /
	ED	**Day 1**	**Day 2**
1 **Discharge Planning / Referrals**	Consider Cardiology Consult	☐ Evaluated home situation Identify if patient is seen by home care ☐ Yes ☐ No ☐ Code status _____ Advanced directives ☐ Yes ☐ No	☐ SW referral made ☐ Define discharge needs ☐ Notify home care if patient was seen by home care before admission
2 **Diagnostic Tests / Treatments**	☐ H & P ☐ BUN/Cr ☐ EKG x2 ☐ Electrolytes ☐ CXR ☐ UA ☐ CBC ☐ PT/INR Consider CK MB and Troponin Consider TSH	☐ Telemetry ☐ BUN/ Cr ☐ Electrolytes ☐ ECHO (if not recent or if LV function and valve status are not known) ☐ Fasting lipid panel	☐ Telemetry ☐ BUN/ Cr ☐ Electrolytes ☐ Eval. for ischemia completed EF _____ NYHA baseline I II III IV (circle)
3 **Nutrition / Diet**	☐ NPO	☐ Cardiac prudent diet ☐ Other _____	☐ Cardiac prudent diet ☐ Other _____ ☐ Nutrition consult
4 **Treatments and Medications**	☐ IV fluids / Saline lock ☐ O₂ ☐ Nitrates ☐ MSO₄ ☐ Furosemide IV/PO	☐ IV fluids / Saline lock ☐ O₂ at _____ L/min. ☐ Nitrates ☐ MSO₄ ☐ ASA ☐ Digoxin ☐ ACE Inhibitor/ARBs ☐ Stool Softener ☐ Furosemide IV/PO ☐ K supplements IV/PO ☐ Hydralizine ☐ Beta Blocker	☐ IV to saline lock ☐ O₂ at _____ L/min. ☐ ASA ☐ ACE Inhibitor/ARBs ☐ Beta Blocker ☐ Nitrates ☐ Furosemide ☐ K supplements ☐ Stool softener ☐ Digoxin
5 **Activity Cardiac Rehab**	☐ Bedrest with commode	☐ Bedrest with commode ☐ PT referral	Begin self care with assistance O₂ pre. ambulation _____ O₂ post. ambulation _____ Pt. evaluation

| **6** **Nursing Assessment/ Intervention** ◆ | ☐ VS per ED routine
☐ I & O
☐ O₂ sat. > 92%
☐ Cardiac Monitor
☐ Saline lock
Wt. _____ | | | A E P | Ht _____
Wt _____
Target Wt. (see MD order) _____
VS per unit routine
I&O
O₂ sat > 92%
Saline lock
AxO x 3, speech clear, memory
  intact, swallow intact
Abdomen soft nontender, bowel
  sounds present, tolerates diet
Voiding adequate amounts, urine
  clear, yellow to amber
Foley cath. draining clear yellow to
  amber urine
Normal ROM and strength
  appropriate for patient
Circulation & sensation intact | | | A E P | Wt _____
VS per unit routine
I&O
O₂ sat > 92%
Saline lock
AxO x 3, speech clear, memory
  intact, swallow intact
Abdomen soft nontender, bowel
  sounds present, tolerates diet
Voiding adequate amounts, urine
  clear, yellow to amber
Foley cath. draining clear yellow to
  amber urine
Normal ROM and strength
  appropriate for patient
Circulation & sensation intact |

7 **Anxiety**	Anxiety level identified Low ☐ Med ☐ High ☐ ☐ Appropriate actions taken (see nursing notes)	☐ Cooperates with care	☐ Receives information about activities ☐ Participates in care ☐ Verbalizes fears and concerns
8 **Knowledge Deficit**	☐ Inform patient of plan of care	☐ CHF patient portion of pathway given to patient/family ☐ CHF booklet (Krames) given to patient ☐ Exacerbation factors identified: _____ _____ _____	☐ Show CHF video ☐ Medication teaching started ☐ Patient verbalizes exacerbation factors
Signature	A	A	A
	P	P	P
	N	N	N

EF NYHA class   I   II   III   IV   (circle)   **Admitting diagnosis** _____

Type of dysfunction_____   **Discharge diagnosis** _____

/ / **Day 3**	/ / **Day 4 / Discharge**	/ / **Discharge Outcomes**
☐ Home care referral as needed Room air O₂ _____ Home O₂ at _____		☐ CPR class referral made ☐ Outpt. Cardiac Rehab referral made if pt. has knowledge CAD ☐ Home situation adequate / no help ☐ Home care referral completed ☐ Appt. made for f/u MD visit
☐ D/c Telemetry		☐ Cardiac evaluation complete EF _____ Type of cardiac dysfunction _____ NYHA class _____ ☐ Lipid status known
☐ Cardiac prudent diet ☐ Other _____	☐ Cardiac prudent diet ☐ Other _____	☐ Patient / family able to identify elements of cardiac prudent diet ☐ Written materials given

☐ O₂ at _____ L/min.
☐ ASA
☐ Beta Blocker
☐ ACE Inhibitor
☐ Nitrates
☐ Furosemide
☐ K supplements
☐ Stool softener
☐ Digoxin
	☐ Home O₂ at _____ L/min.
	☐ ASA
	☐ Beta Blocker
	☐ ACE Inhibitor / ARBs
	☐ Nitrates
	☐ Furosemide
	☐ K supplements
	☐ Stool softener
	☐ Digoxin
		☐ D/C meds Rx given
		☐ Pt. verbalized understanding how to
		  take D/C medications
		☐ Medication teaching sheet completed
		  and signed by patient and nurse
		☐ Pt. identified who will pick up Rx.
		☐ Financial considerations addressed
		☐ Home O₂ arranged if needed

Ambulate x3 without significant change in VS ☐ ☐ ☐ Pt. evaluation Teach Pt. methods to evaluate exertion	Ambulate 5 x day ☐ ☐ ☐ ☐ ☐ Independent self care Stair climbing if appropriate ☐ Verbalizes activity limits	☐ Inpatient Cardiac Rehab. Complete ☐ ADLs with stable VS

A E P
Wt _____
VS per unit routine   ☐ ☐ ☐
I&O   ☐ ☐ ☐
O₂ sat > 92%   ☐ ☐ ☐
Saline lock   ☐ ☐ ☐
AxO x 3, speech clear, memory
  intact, swallow intact ☐ ☐ ☐
Abdomen soft nontender, bowel
  sounds present, tolerates diet ☐ ☐ ☐
Voiding adequate amounts, urine
  clear, yellow to amber ☐ ☐ ☐
Foley cath. dc'd, voiding without
  difficulty   ☐ ☐ ☐
Normal ROM and strength
  appropriate for patient ☐ ☐ ☐
Circulation & sensation intact ☐ ☐ ☐
	A E P
	Wt _____
	VS per unit routine ☐ ☐ ☐
	I&O ☐ ☐ ☐
	O₂ sat > 92% ☐ ☐ ☐
	Saline lock ☐ ☐ ☐
	AxO x 3, speech clear, memory
	  intact, swallow intact ☐ ☐ ☐
	Abdomen soft nontender, bowel
	  sounds present, tolerates diet ☐ ☐ ☐
	Voiding adequate amounts, urine
	  clear, yellow to amber ☐ ☐ ☐
	Normal ROM and strength
	  appropriate for patient ☐ ☐ ☐
	Circulation & sensation intact ☐ ☐ ☐
		☐ D/C instructions given to patient, patient
		  verbalizes understanding.
		☐ Patient at target weight (if known)

☐ Receives information about activities
☐ Participates in care
☐ Verbalizes fears and concerns
	☐ Retains information
	☐ Participates in care
	☐ Verbalizes understanding of proper life
	  style changes
		☐ Coping skills adequate
		☐ Continuing care arrangements made if
		  appropriate

Symptom management plan: _____ _____ _____ _____ ☐ Medication teaching reviewed ☐ Give D/C instructions	☐ Medication teaching reviewed ☐ Review D/C instructions ☐ Complete D/C instruction sheet ☐ RN and PT sign forms	☐ D/C summary complete ☐ Patient verbalizes diagnosis and management plan
A	A	A
P	P	P
N	N	N

Adult

◆ **D. Analysis/nursing diagnosis:**

1. *Decreased cardiac output* related to decreased myocardial contractility.
2. *Impaired gas exchange* related to pulmonary congestion.
3. *Altered tissue perfusion* related to inadequate blood flow.
4. *Anxiety,* severe, related to difficulty breathing.
5. *Fear* related to life-threatening situation.

◆ **E. Nursing care plan/implementation:**

1. Goal: *promote physical, psychological relaxation measures to relieve anxiety.*
   a. Slow respirations: morphine sulfate 3–10 mg IV/SC/IM, as ordered, to reduce respiratory rate, sedate, and produce vasodilation.
   b. Remain with patient.
   c. Encourage slow, deep breathing; assist with coughing.
   d. Work calmly, confidently, unhurriedly.
   e. Frequent rest periods.
2. Goal: *improve cardiac function, reduce venous return, relieve hypoxia.*
   a. O₂: 100%, preferably by demand valve to slow respiratory rate, provide uniform ventilation, reduce venous return, and inhibit "leaky capillary" syndrome. Possibly PEEP.
   b. IV: D₅W.
   c. Give aminophylline, as ordered, to lower venous pressure and increase cardiac output.
   d. *Position:* high Fowler's, extremities in dependent position, to reduce venous return and facilitate breathing.
   e. Medications as ordered: digitalis; *diuretics*—furosemide (Lasix); *inotropic agents*—dobutamine (Dobutrex), dopamine; nitroglycerin, nitroprusside.
   f. Vital signs; auscultate breath sounds.
   g. *Diet:* low sodium; fluid *restriction* as ordered.
3. Goal: *health teaching* (include family or significant other).
   a. Medications.
      (1) Side effects.
      (2) Potassium supplements if indicated.
      (3) Pulse taking.
   b. Exercise; rest.
   c. *Diet:* low sodium.
   d. Signs of complications: edema; weight gain of 2–3 lb (0.9–1.4 kg) in a few days; dyspnea.

◆ **F. Evaluation/outcome criteria:**

1. No complications; vital signs stable; clear breath sounds.
2. No weight gain; weight loss if indicated.
3. Alert, oriented, calm.

XIV. Shock: a critically severe deficiency in nutrients, oxygen, and electrolytes delivered to body tissues, plus deficiency in removal of cellular wastes; results from cardiac failure, insufficient blood volume, or increased vascular bed size.

A. Types, pathophysiology, and risk factors:

1. *Hypovolemic* (hemorrhagic, hematogenic)—markedly decreased **volume** of blood (hemorrhage or plasma loss from intestinal obstruction, burns, physical trauma, or dehydration) → decreased venous return, cardiac output → decreased tissue perfusion.
2. *Cardiogenic*—failure of cardiac muscle **pump** (myocardial infarction) → generally decreased cardiac output → pulmonary congestion, hypoxia → inadequate circulation; high mortality rate.
3. *Distributive:*
   a. *Neurogenic*—massive **vasodilation** from reduced vasomotor, vasoconstrictor tone (e.g., spinal shock, head injuries, anesthesia, pain); interruption of sympathetic nervous system; blood volume is normal but inadequate for vessels → decreased venous return → tissue hypoxia.
   b. *Vasogenic* (anaphylactic, septic, endotoxic)—severe reaction to foreign protein (insect bites, drugs, toxic substances, aerobic, gram-negative organisms) → histamine release → **vasodilation,** venous stasis → diminished venous return.

◆ **B. Assessment:** varies, depending on degree of shock (Table 7–8).

1. *Subjective data*
   a. Anxiety; restlessness.
   b. Dizziness; fainting.
   c. Thirst.
   d. Nausea.
2. *Objective data*
   a. Vital signs:

      (1) *BP*—hypotension (postural changes in early shock; systolic <70 mm Hg in late shock).

TABLE 7–8   Signs of Hypovolemic Shock

Blood Loss (% of Total)	◆ Assessment Data
800–1500 mL (15–30%)	Restlessness Pulse >100 Systolic pressure unchanged Diastolic pressure ↑ Urine output ↓
2000 mL (30–40%)	Mental status ↓ Pulse >120 Respirations >30 Systolic pressure ↓
>2500 mL (>40%)	Cold, clammy skin Pulse > 120 Respirations >30 Narrow pulse pressure (= systolic − diastolic)

(2) *Pulse*—tachycardia, thready; irregular (cardiogenic shock); could be slow if conduction system of heart damaged.

(3) *Respirations*—increased depth, rate; wheezing (anaphylactic shock).

(4) *Temperature*—decreased (elevated in septic shock).

  b. Skin:
    (1) Pale (or mottled), cool, clammy (warm to touch in septic shock).
    (2) Urticaria (anaphylactic shock).

  c. Level of consciousness: alert, oriented → unresponsive.

  d. CVP:

(handwritten: 5-15 norm.)

    (1) *Below 5* cm H_2O with hypovolemic shock.
    (2) *Above 15* cm H_2O with cardiogenic, possibly septic shock.

  e. Urine output: decreased ($<$30 mL/hr).

  f. Capillary refill: slowed; normally nailbed "pinks up" within 2 sec after blanching (nailbed pressure).

C. Analysis/nursing diagnosis:
1. *Altered tissue perfusion* related to vasoconstriction or decreased myocardial contractility.
2. *Impaired gas exchange* related to ventilation-perfusion imbalance.
3. *Decreased cardiac output* related to loss of circulating blood volume or diminished cardiac contractility.
4. *Altered urinary elimination* related to decreased renal perfusion.
5. *Fluid volume deficit* related to blood loss.
6. *Anxiety* related to severity of condition.
7. *Risk for injury* related to death.

◆ **D. Nursing care plan/implementation:** Goal: *promote venous return, circulatory perfusion.*

1. *Position:* foot of bed *elevated* 20 degrees (12–16 inches), knees straight, trunk horizontal, head slightly elevated; *avoid* Trendelenburg position.
2. Ventilation: monitor respiratory effort, loosen restrictive clothing; O_2 as ordered.
3. Fluids: maintain IV infusions; give blood, plasma expanders as ordered (exception— **stop** **blood** **immediately** in anaphylactic shock).
4. Vital signs:
  a. CVP (decreased with hypovolemia) arterial line, Swan-Ganz (increased pulmonary artery wedge pressue indicating cardiac failure).
  b. Urine output (insert catheter for hourly output).
  c. Monitor ECG (increased rate, dysrhythmias).
5. Medications (depending on type of shock) as ordered:

  a. *Antihypotensives*—epinephrine (Adrenalin), norepinephrine (Levophed), isoproterenol (Isuprel), dopamine (Intropin).
  b. *Antiarrhythmics.*
  c. *Cardiac glycosides.*
  d. *Adrenocorticoids.*
  e. *Antibiotics.*
  f. *Vasodilators* (nitroprusside).
  g. *Beta-adrenergics* (dobutamine).

6. Mechanical support: military (or medical) antishock trousers (MAST) or pneumatic antishock garment (PASG); used to promote internal autotransfusion of blood from legs and abdomen to central circulation; at lower pressures may control bleeding and promote hemostasis; do *not* remove (deflate) suddenly to examine underlying areas or BP will drop precipitously; *compartment syndrome* may result with prolonged use and high pressure; controversial.

◆ **E. Evaluation/outcome criteria:**
1. Vital signs stable, within normal limits.
2. Alert, oriented.
3. Urine output $>$30 mL/hr.

XV. Disseminated intravascular coagulation (DIC): diffuse or widespread coagulation initially within arterioles and capillaries leading to hemorrhage.

A. Pathophysiology: activation of coagulation system from tissue injury → fibrin microthrombi form in brain, kidneys, lungs → microinfarcts, tissue necrosis → red blood cells, platelets, prothrombin, other clotting factors trapped, destroyed in process → excessive clotting → release of fibrin split products → inhibition of platelet clotting → profuse bleeding.

B. Risk factors:
1. Obstetric complications.
2. Neoplastic disease.
3. Low perfusion states (e.g., burns, hypothermia).
4. Infections.

◆ **C. Assessment**—*objective data:*
1. Skin, mucous membranes: petechiae, ecchymosis.
2. Extremities (fingers, toes): cyanosis.
3. Bleeding: venipuncture sites, wound, oral, rectal, vaginal.
4. Urine output: oliguria → anuria.
5. Level of consciousness: convulsions, coma.
6. Lab data: *prolonged*—prothrombin time (PT) $>$15 sec; *decreased*—platelets, fibrinogen level.

◆ **D. Analysis/nursing diagnosis:**
1. *Altered tissue perfusion* related to peripheral microthrombi.
2. *Risk for injury* (death) related to bleeding.
3. *Risk for impaired skin integrity* related to ischemia.

4. *Altered urinary elimination* related to renal tubular necrosis.

◆ **E. Nursing care plan/implementation:** goal—*prevent and detect further bleeding.*

1. Carry out nursing measures designed to alleviate underlying problem (e.g., shock, birth of fetus, surgery/irradiation for cancer, antibiotics for infection).

2. Medications: heparin sodium IV, 1000 U/hr, if ordered, to reverse abnormal clotting (controversial).

3. IVs: blood to lessen shock; platelets, cryoprecipitate, fresh plasma to restore clotting factors, fibrinogen.

4. Observe: vital signs, CVP (normal 5–15 mm Hg), PAP (normal 20–30 systolic and 8–12 diastolic), and intake and output for signs of shock or fluid overload from frequent infusions; specimens for occult blood (urine, stool).

5. *Precautions: avoid* IM injections if possible; pressure 5 min to venipuncture sites; *no* rectal temperatures.

◆ **F. Evaluation/outcome criteria:**

1. Clotting mechanism restored (increased platelets, normal PT).

2. Renal function restored (urine output >30 mL/hr).

3. Circulation to fingers, toes; no cyanosis.

4. No irreversible damage from renal, cerebral, cardiac, or adrenal hemorrhage.

XVI. Pericarditis: inflammation of parietal or visceral pericardium or both; acute or chronic condition; may occur with or without effusion. Cardiac tamponade may result.

A. Pathophysiology: fibrosis or accumulation of fluid in pericardium → compression of cardiac pumping → decreased cardiac output → increased systemic, pulmonic venous pressure.

B. Risk factors:

1. Bacterial, viral, fungal infections.

2. Tuberculosis.

3. Collagen diseases.

4. Uremia.

5. Transmural MI.

6. Trauma.

◆ **C. Assessment:**

1. *Subjective data*

a. Pain:

(1) *Type*—sharp, moderate to severe.

(2) *Location*—wide area of pericardium, may radiate: right arm, jaw/teeth.

(3) *Precipitating factors*—movement, deep inspiration, swallowing.

b. Chills; sweating.

c. Apprehension; anxiety.

d. Fatigue.

e. Abdominal pain.

f. Shortness of breath.

2. *Objective data*

a. Vital signs:

(1) BP: decreased pulse pressure; pulsus paradoxus—abnormal drop in systolic BP of >8–10 mm Hg during inspiration.

(2) Pulse: tachycardia.

(3) Temperature: elevated; erratic course; low grade.

b. Pericardial friction rub.

c. Increased CVP; distended neck veins; dependent pitting edema; liver engorgement.

d. Restlessness.

e. Lab data: *elevated* AST (SGOT), WBC; CT or MRI—pericardial thickening

f. Serial ECGs: increased ST segment; echocardiogram: pericardial fluid.

◆ **D. Analysis/nursing diagnosis:**

1. *Decreased cardiac output* related to impaired cardiac muscle contraction.

2. *Pain* related to pericardial inflammation.

3. *Anxiety* related to unknown outcome.

4. *Fatigue* related to inadequate oxygenation.

◆ **E. Nursing care plan/implementation:**

1. Goal: *promote physical and emotional comfort.*

a. *Position:* semi-Fowler's (upright or sitting); bed rest.

b. Vital signs: q2–4h and prn; apical and radial pulse; notify physician if heart sounds decrease in amplitude or if pulse pressure *narrows*, indicating cardiac tamponade; cooling measures as indicated.

c. O₂ as ordered.

d. Medications as ordered:

(1) *Analgesics*—aspirin, morphine sulfate, meperidine or codeine.

(2) *Nonsteroidal anti-inflammatory agents*—indomethacin.

(3) *Antimicrobial.*

(4) *Digitalis and diuretics,* if heart failure present.

e. Assist with aspiration of pericardial sac (pericardiocentesis) if needed: medicate as ordered; *elevate* head 60 degrees; monitor ECG; have defibrillator and pacemaker available.

f. Prepare for pericardiectomy (excision of constricting pericardium) as ordered.

g. Continual emotional support.

h. Enhance effects of analgesics: positioning; turning; warm drinks.

i. Monitor for **signs of cardiac tamponade:** tachycardia; tachypnea; hypotension; pallor; narrowed pulse pressure; pulsus paradoxus; distended neck veins.

2. Goal: *maintain fluid, electrolyte balance.*

a. Parenteral fluids as ordered; strict I&O.

b. Assist with feedings; *low-sodium* diet may be ordered.

◆ **F. Evaluation/outcome criteria:**

1. Relief of pain, dyspnea.
2. No complications (e.g., cardiac tamponade).
3. Return of normal cardiac functioning.

XVII. Chronic arterial occlusive disease: arteriosclerosis obliterans most common occlusive disorder of the arterial system (aorta, large and medium-size arteries); frequently involves the femoral, iliac, and popliteal arteries.

A. Pathophysiology: fatty deposits in intimal, medial layer of arterial walls; plaque formation → narrowed arterial lumens; decreased distensibility → decreased blood flow; ischemic changes in tissues.

B. Risk factors:

1. Age (>50).
2. Sex (men).
3. Diabetes mellitus.
4. Hyperlipidemia—obesity.
5. Cigarette smoking.
6. Hypertension.
7. Family history.

◆ **C. Assessment:**

1. *Subjective data*
   a. Pain:
      (1) *Type*—cramplike.
      (2) *Location*—foot, calf, thigh, buttocks.
      (3) *Duration*—variable, may be relieved by rest.
      (4) *Precipitating causes*—exercise (intermittent claudication), but occasionally may occur when at rest.
   b. Tingling, numbness in toes, feet.
   c. Persistent coldness of one or both lower extremities.
2. *Objective data*
   a. Lower extremities:
      (1) Pedal pulses—absent or diminished.
      (2) Skin—shiny, glossy; dry, cold, chalky white, decreased/absent hair, ulcers, gangrene.
   b. Lab data: *increased* serum cholesterol, triglycerides, CBC, platelets
   c. Arteriography—indicates location, nature of occlusion. Noninvasive: ultrasound, segmental limb pressure, exercise testing.

◆ **D. Analysis/nursing diagnosis:**

1. *Altered tissue perfusion* related to peripheral vascular disease.
2. *Risk for activity intolerance* related to pain and sensory changes.
3. *Pain* related to ischemia.
4. *Risk for impaired skin integrity* related to poor circulation.
5. *Risk for injury* related to numbness of extremities.

◆ **E. Nursing care plan/implementation:**

1. Goal: *promote circulation; decrease discomfort.*
   a. *Position:* elevate head of bed on blocks (3–6 inches), because gravity aids perfusion to thighs, legs; elevating legs increases pain.
   b. Comfort: keep warm: *avoid* chilling or use of heating pads, which may burn skin; apply bed socks.
   c. Circulation: check pedal pulses, skin color, temperature qid.
   d. Medications:
      (1) *Vasodilators.*
      (2) *Antiplatelet*—ASA, ticlopidine, dipyridamole.
      (3) *Dihydropyridines*—nifedipine, amlodipine.
      (4) *Xanthine derivatives*—pentoxifylline.
2. Goal: *prevent infection, injury.*
   a. Skin care: use bed cradle, sheepskin, heel pads; mild soap; dry thoroughly; lotion; do *not* massage, to prevent release of thrombus.
   b. Foot care: wear properly fitting shoes, slippers when out of bed; inspect for injury or pressure areas; nail care by podiatrist.
3. Goal: *health teaching.*
   a. Skin care; inspect daily.
   b. Activity: balance exercise, rest to increase collateral circulation; walk only until painful.
   c. Exercises: walking, Buerger-Allen exercises (gravity alternately fills and empties blood vessels).
   d. *Diet:* low-fat, heart-healthy diet to slow disease progression.
   e. Lifestyle choices: *avoid* smoking.
   f. Recognizes and reports signs of occlusion (e.g., pain, cramping, numbness in extremities, color changes—white or blue, temperature changes—cool to cold).

◆ **F. Evaluation/outcome criteria:**

1. Decreased pain.
2. Skin integrity preserved; no loss of limb.
3. Quits smoking.
4. Does exercises to increase collateral circulation.

XVIII. Aneurysms (thoracic or abdominal aortic): localized or diffuse dilations/outpouching of a vessel wall, usually an artery; exerts pressure on adjacent structures; affects primarily men over age 60; >6 cm diameter, 50% will rupture; resected surgically, reconstructed with synthetic or vascular graft.

A. Risk factors:

1. Atherosclerosis.
2. Trauma.
3. Syphilis.
4. Congenital weakness.
5. Local infection.
6. Cigarette smoking.

◆ **B. Assessment:**
1. *Subjective data*
   a. Pain:
      (1) Constant, boring, neuralgic, inter-mittent—low back, abdominal.
      (2) Angina—sudden onset may mean rupture or dissection, which are **emergency** conditions.
   b. Dyspnea; orthopnea—pressure on tra-chea or bronchus.
2. *Objective data*
   a. Vital signs:
      (1) Radial pulses differ.
      (2) Tachycardia.
      (3) Hypotension following rupture lead-ing to shock.
   b. Pulsating mass: abdominal, chest wall pulsation; edema of chest wall (thoracic aneurysm); periumbilical (abdominal aneurysm); audible bruit over aorta.
   c. Cyanosis, mottled below level of aneurysm.
   d. Veins: dilated, superficial—neck, chest, arms.
   e. Cough: paroxysmal, brassy.
   f. Diaphoresis, pallor, fainting following rupture.
   g. Peripheral pulses:
      (1) Femoral present.
      (2) Pedal weak or absent.
   h. Stool bloody from irritation.
◆ **C. Analysis/nursing diagnosis:**
1. *Risk for injury* related to possible aneurysm rupture.
2. *Pain* related to pressure on lumbar nerves.
3. *Anxiety* related to risk of rupture.
◆ **D. Nursing care plan/implementation:**
1. Goal: *provide emergency care before surgery for dissection or rupture.*
   a. Vital signs: frequent, depending on sever-ity (systolic BP <100 mm Hg and pulse >100 with rupture).
   b. IVs: may have 2–4 sites; lactated Ringer's may be ordered.
   c. Urine output: monitored every 15–30 min.
   d. O$_2$: usually via nasal prongs.
   e. Medications as ordered: antihyperten-sives to prevent extension of dissection.
   f. Transport to operating room quickly.
   g. See **The Perioperative Experience,** p. 500, for general preoperative care.
2. Goal: *prevent complications postoperatively.*
   a. *Position:* initially flat in bed; *avoid* sharp flexion of hip and knee, which places pressure on femoral and popliteal arte-ries; turn gently side to side; note ery-thema on back from pooled blood.
   b. Vital signs: CVP; hourly peripheral pulses distal to graft site, including neurovascu-

lar check of lower extremities; absent pulses for 6–12 hr indicates occlusion; check with Doppler blood flow detector.
   c. Urine output: hourly from indwelling catheter.
      (1) Immediately report anuria or olig-uria (<30 mL/hr).
      (2) Check color for hematuria.
      (3) Monitor daily blood urea nitrogen (BUN) and creatinine.
   d. Observe *for signs of atheroembolization* (patchy areas of ischemia); report change in color, motor ability, or sensation of lower extremities.
   e. Observe for *signs of bowel ischemia* (de-creased/absent bowel sounds, pain, guaiac-positive diarrhea, abdominal distention); may have nasogastric tube.
   f. Measure abdominal girth; increase seen with graft leakage.
3. Goal: *promote comfort.*
   a. *Position:* alignment, comfort; prevent heel ulcers.
   b. Medication: narcotics.
4. Goal: *health teaching.*
   a. Minimize recurrence: *avoid* trauma, in-fection, smoking, high-cholesterol diet, obesity.
   b. Regular medical supervision.
◆ **E. Evaluation/outcome criteria:**
1. Surgical intervention before rupture.
2. No loss of renal function.

XIX. Varicose veins: abnormally lengthened, tortuous, di-lated superficial veins (saphenous); result of incom-petent valves, especially in lower extremities; process is irreversible.
   A. Pathophysiology: dilated vein → venous stasis → edema, fibrotic changes, pigmentation of skin, lowered resistance to trauma.
   B. Risk factors:
   1. Heredity.
   2. Obesity.
   3. Pregnancy.
   4. Chronic disease (heart, liver).
   5. Occupations requiring long periods of stand-ing.
◆ **C. Assessment:**
   1. *Subjective data*
      a. Dull aches; heaviness in legs.
      b. Pain; muscle cramping.
      c. Fatigue in lower extremities, increased with hot weather, high altitude, history of risk factors.
   2. *Objective data*
      a. Nodular protrusions along veins.
      b. Edema.
      c. *Diagnostic tests:* Trendelenburg test; phle-bography; Doppler flowmeter.
◆ **D. Analysis/nursing diagnosis:**

1. *Altered tissue perfusion* related to venous valve incompetence.
2. *Pain* related to edema and muscle cramping.
3. *Risk for activity intolerance* related to leg discomfort.
4. *Body image disturbance* related to disfigurement of leg.

◆ **E. Nursing care plan/implementation:**
1. Goal: *promote venous return from lower extremities.*
   a. Activity: walk every hour.
   b. Discourage prolonged sitting, standing, sitting with crossed legs.
   ◢ c. *Position:* elevate legs q2–3h; elastic stockings or Ace wraps.
2. Goal: *provide for safety.*
   a. Assist with early ambulation.
   b. *Surgical asepsis* with wounds, leg ulcers.
   c. Observe for hemorrhage—if occurs: *ele-*◢*vate* leg, apply pressure, notify physician.
   ◖◗ d. Observe for allergic reactions if sclerosing drugs used; have antihistamine available.
3. Goal: *health teaching.*
   a. Weight-reducing techniques, dietary approaches if indicated.
   b. Preventive measures: leg elevation; *avoiding* prolonged standing, sitting, high chairs, tight girdles, constrictive clothing; wear support hose.
   ▯ c. Expectations for *Trendelenburg test:*

   > (1) While patient is lying down, *elevate* leg 65 degrees for approximately 1 min to empty veins.
   > (2) Apply tourniquet high on upper thigh (do *not* constrict deep veins).
   > (3) Patient stands with tourniquet in place.
   > (4) Filling of veins is observed.
   > (5) Normal response is slow filling from below in 20–30 sec, with no change in rate when tourniquet is removed.
   > (6) Incompetent veins distend very quickly with back flow.

   d. Prepare for sclerotherapy or vein ligation and stripping.

◆ **F. Evaluation/outcome criteria:**
1. Relief or control of symptoms.
2. Activity without pain.

XX. **Vein ligation and stripping:** surgical intervention for advancing varicosities, stasis ulcerations, and cosmetic needs of patient. Procedure involves ligation of the saphenous vein at the groin, where it joins the femoral vein; saphenous stripping from the groin to the ankle; legs are wrapped with a pressure bandage. Frequently done as outpatient surgery.

◆ **A.** See preceding section on varicose veins for assessment data and nursing diagnosis of the patient requiring surgery.

◆ **B. Nursing care plan/implementation:**
1. Goal: *prevent complications* after discharge.
   ◢ a. *Position:* elevate legs as instructed.
   b. Activity:
   (1) *No* chair sitting to prevent venous pooling, thrombus formation. *Avoid* standing in one place.
   c. Bleeding: report to MD
2. Goal: *health teaching* to prevent recurrence.
   a. Weight reduction.
   b. *Avoid* constricting garments.
   c. Change positions frequently.
   d. Wear support hose/stockings to enhance venous return.
   e. *No* crossing legs at knees.

◆ **C. Evaluation/outcome criteria:**
1. No complications—hemorrhage, infection, nerve damage, deep-vein thrombosis.
2. No recurrence of varicosities.
3. Adequate circulation to legs: strong pedal pulses.
4. Resume daily activities; free of pain.

XXI. **Thrombophlebitis:** formation of a blood clot in an inflamed vein, secondary to phlebitis or partial obstruction; may lead to venous insufficiency and pulmonary embolism. Deep vein thrombosis is most serious form.

A. Pathophysiology: endothelial inflammation → formation of platelet plug (blood clot) → slowing of blood flow → increase in procoagulants in local area → initiation of clotting mechanisms.

B. Risk factors:
1. Immobility/stasis—prolonged sitting, bed rest, obesity, pregnancy.
2. Venous disease.
3. Age—increased incidence in elderly.
4. Gender—more often women.
5. Hypercoagulability of blood.
6. Intimal damage—IVs, drug abuse.
7. Fractures.
8. Oral contraceptives (related to estrogen content).

◆ **C. Assessment:**
1. *Subjective data*
   a. Calf stiffness, soreness.
   b. Severe pain: walking, dorsiflexion of foot (*Homan's sign*—may be unreliable).
2. *Objective data*
   a. Vein: redness, heat, hardness, threadiness.
   b. Limb: swollen, pale, cold.
   c. Vital signs: low-grade fever.
   ▯ d. *Diagnostic tests:* venogram, impedance plethysmography (electrical resistance to blood flow), ultrasonography.

◆ **D. Analysis/nursing diagnosis:**
1. *Altered peripheral tissue perfusion* related to venous stasis.
2. *Pain* related to inflammation.

Adult

3. *Activity intolerance* related to leg pain.
4. *Risk for injury* related to potential pulmonary emboli.

◆ **E. Nursing care plan/implementation:**
 1. Goal: *provide rest, comfort, and relief from pain.*
  a. Bed rest until therapeutic level of heparin reached (5–7 days with traditional heparin; after 24 hr with low-molecular-weight heparin).
  b. *Position:* as ordered; usually extremity *elevated;* watch for pressure points.
  ▶ c. Apply warm, moist heat to affected area as prescribed (cold may also be ordered).
  d. Assess progress of affected area: swelling, pain, soreness, temperature, color.
  e. Administer analgesics as ordered.
 2. Goal: *prevent complications.*
  a. Observe for signs of embolism (pain at site of embolism); allergic reaction (anaphylactic shock) with streptokinase.
  b. *Precautions: no* rubbing or massage of limb.
  c. Medications: anticoagulants (sodium heparin, enoxaparin, Coumadin); streptokinase (Varidase), tissue plasminogen activator (Table 7–9).
  d. Bleeding: hematuria, epistaxis, ecchymosis.
  e. Skin care, to relieve increased redness/maceration from hot or cold applications.
  f. ROM: unaffected limb.
 3. Goal: *health teaching.*
  a. *Precautions:* tight garters, girdles; sitting with legs crossed; oral contraceptives.
  b. *Preventive* measures: walking daily, swimming several times weekly if possible, wading, rest periods with legs *elevated,* elastic stockings (may remove at bedtime).
  c. Medication side effects: anticoagulants—pink toothbrush, hematuria, easily bruised.

  (1) Carry Medic Alert card/bracelet.
  (2) **Contraindicated** drugs—aspirin, glutethimide (Doriden), chloramphenicol (Chloromycetin), neomycin, phenylbutazone (Butazolidin), barbiturates.
  d. Prepare for surgery (thrombectomy, vein ligation).

◆ **F. Evaluation/outcome criteria:**
 1. No complications (e.g., embolism).
 2. No recurrence of symptoms.
 3. Free of pain—ambulates without discomfort.

XXII. Peripheral embolism: fragments of thrombi, globules of fat, clumps of tissue, calcified plaques, or air moves in the circulation and lodges in vessel, obstructing blood flow; thrombic emboli most common; may be venous or arterial.

Conditions Affecting Tissue Perfusion

I. Iron deficiency anemia (hypochromic microcytic anemia): inadequate production of red blood cells due to lack of heme (iron); common in infants, pregnant women, and premenopausal women.
 A. Pathophysiology: decreased dietary intake, impaired absorption, or increased utilization of iron decreases the amount of iron bound to plasma transferrin and transported to bone marrow for hemoglobin synthesis; decreased hemoglobin in erythrocytes decreases amount of oxygen delivered to tissues.
 B. Risk factors:
 1. *Excessive menstruation.*
 2. *Gastrointestinal bleeding*—peptic ulcer, hookworm, tumors.
 3. *Inadequate diet*—anorexia, fad diets, cultural practices.

TABLE 7–9 Nursing Responsibilities with Anticoagulant Therapy

	Heparin	Warfarin (Coumadin)	Low-Molecular-Weight Heparin (LMWH)
Monitor	PTT (25–38 sec) (2–3 times baseline)	PT (11–15 sec) (1½–2½ times baseline)	Antifactor Xa, CBC, platelets
Inspect	Ecchymosis, bleeding gums, petechiae, hematuria	Bleeding, ecchymosis	Bleeding, hemorrhage, unusual bruising
Administer	With an infusion pump; **never** mix with other drugs; **never** aspirate; **avoid** massaging site	Same time every day; PO	Subcutaneous bid
Avoid	Salicylates and other anticoagulants, e.g., antacids, corticosteroids, penicillin, phenytoin	Same as heparin	Warfarin, platelet aggregation inhibitors (e.g., ASA, NSAIDs, dextran)
Antidote	Protamine sulfate	Vitamin K	Protamine sulfate

4. *Poor absorption*—stomach, small intestine disease.

◆ **C. Assessment:**

1. *Subjective data*
   a. Fatigue: increasing.
   b. Headache.
   c. Change in appetite; difficulty swallowing due to pharyngeal edema/ulceration; heartburn.
   d. Shortness of breath on exercise.
   e. Extremities: numb, tingling.
   f. Flatulence.
   g. Menorrhagia.

2. *Objective data*
   a. Vital signs:
      (1) *BP*—increased systolic, widened pulse pressure.
      (2) *Pulse*—tachycardia.
      (3) *Respirations*—tachypnea.
      (4) *Temperature*—normal or subnormal.
   b. Skin/mucous membranes: pale, dry; tongue—smooth, shiny, bright red; cheilosis (cracked, painful corners of mouth).
   c. Sclera: pearly white.
   d. Nails: brittle, spoon shaped, flattened.
   e. Lab data: *decreased*—hemoglobin (<10 g/dL blood), serum iron (<65 μg/dL blood); *increased* total iron-binding capacity.

◆ **D. Analysis/nursing diagnosis:**

1. *Altered nutrition, less than body requirements,* related to inadequate iron absorption.
2. *Altered tissue perfusion* related to reduction in red cells.
3. *Risk for activity intolerance* related to profound weakness.
4. *Impaired gas exchange* related to decreased oxygen-carrying capacity.

◆ **E. Nursing care plan/implementation:**

1. Goal: *promote physical and mental equilibrium.*
   a. *Position:* optimal for respiratory excursion; deep breathing; turn frequently to prevent skin breakdown.
   b. Rest: balance with activity, as tolerated; assist with ambulation.
   c. Medication (hematinics):
      (1) Oral iron therapy (ferrous sulfate)—give *with* meals.
      (2) Intramuscular therapy (iron dextran)—use second needle for injection after withdrawal from ampule; use *Z-track method;* inject 0.5 mL of air before withdrawing needle, to prevent tissue necrosis; use 2- to 3-inch needle; rotate sites; do *not* rub site or allow wearing of constricting garments after injection.

d. Keep warm: *no* hot water bottles, heating pads, due to decreased sensitivity.
e. *Diet: high* in protein, iron, vitamins (see **Unit 9**); assistance with feeding, if needed; nonirritating foods with mouth or tongue soreness.

2. Goal: *health teaching.*
   a. Dietary regimen.
   b. Iron therapy: explain purpose, dosage, side effects (black or green stools, constipation, diarrhea); take with meals.
   c. Activity: exercise to tolerance, with planned rest periods.

◆ **F. Evaluation/outcome criteria:**

1. Hemoglobin and hematocrit level return to normal range.
2. Tolerates activity without fatigue.
3. Selects foods appropriate for dietary regimen.

II. Hemolytic anemia (normocytic normochromic anemia): premature destruction (hemolysis) of erythrocytes; occurs extravascularly (autoimmune) or intravascularly (dialysis, heart valves).

A. Risk factors—autoimmune hemolytic anemia:

1. *Warm reacting* (idiopathic): women, lupus, rheumatoid arthritis, myeloma.
2. *Cold reacting* (e.g., Raynaud's): older women, Epstein-Barr virus.
3. *Drug induced:* methyldopa, penicillin, quinine.

◆ **B. Assessment:**

1. *Subjective data*
   a. Fatigue; physical weakness.
   b. Dizziness.
   c. Shortness of breath.
   d. Diaphoresis on slight exertion.

2. *Objective data*
   a. Skin: pallor, jaundice.
   b. Posture: drooping.
   c. Lab data:
      (1) *Decreased* hematocrit.
      (2) *Increased* reticulocyte count; bilirubin.
      (3) Direct Coombs' test *positive.*

◆ **C.** See section on **iron deficiency anemia** for analysis, nursing care plan/implementation, and evaluation/outcome criteria.

III. Pernicious anemia (megaloblastic macrocytic anemia): lack of intrinsic factor found in gastric mucosa, which is necessary for vitamin B_{12} (extrinsic factor) absorption; slow developing, usually after age 50; may be an autoimmune disorder.

A. Pathophysiology: atrophy or surgical removal of glandular mucosa in fundus of stomach → degenerative changes in brain, spinal cord, and peripheral nerves from lack of vitamin B_{12}.

B. Risk factors:

1. Partial or complete gastric resection.

Adult

2. Prolonged iron deficiency; veganism.
3. Heredity.
◆ **C. Assessment:**
1. *Subjective data*
   a. Hands, feet: tingling, numbness.
   b. Weakness, fatigue.
   c. Sore tongue, anorexia.
   d. Difficulties with memory, balance.
   e. Irritability, mild depression.
   f. Shortness of breath.
   g. Palpitations.
2. *Objective data*
   a. Skin: pale, flabby, jaundiced.
   b. Sclera: icterus (yellow).
   c. Tongue: smooth, glossy, red, swollen.
   d. Vital signs:
      (1) *BP*—normal or elevated.
      (2) *Pulse*—tachycardia.
   e. Nervous system:
      (1) Decreased vibratory sense in lower extremities.
      (2) Loss of coordination.
      (3) *Babinski* present (flaring of toes with stimulation of sole of foot).
      (4) Positive *Romberg* (loses balance when eyes closed).
      (5) Increased or diminished reflexes.
   f. Lab data: *decreased* hemoglobin, RBCs, platelets, gastric secretions (achlorhydria), *Schilling test* (radioactive vitamin B$_{12}$ urine test).

◆ **D. Analysis/nursing diagnosis:**
1. *Altered nutrition, less than body requirements,* related to B$_{12}$ deficiency.
2. *Impaired physical mobility* related to numbness of extremities.
3. *Fatigue* related to decreased oxygen-carrying capacity.
4. *Altered oral mucous membrane* related to changes in gastric mucosa.
5. *Altered thought processes* related to progressive neurological degeneration.

E. Nursing care plan/implementation:
1. *Goal: promote physical and emotional comfort.*
   a. Activity: bed rest or activity as tolerated—restrictions depend on neurological or cardiac involvement.
   b. Comfort: keep extremities warm—light blankets, loose-fitting socks.
   c. Medication: vitamin B$_{12}$ therapy as ordered.
   d. *Diet:*
      (1) Six small feedings.
      (2) Soft or pureed.
      (3) Organ meats, fish, eggs.
   e. Mouth care: before and after meals, to increase appetite and relieve mouth discomfort.
2. Goal: *health teaching.*

a. Medication:
   (1) Lifelong therapy.
   (2) Injection techniques; rotation of sites.
b. Diet.
c. Rest; exercise to tolerance.
◆ **F. Evaluation/outcome criteria:**
1. No irreversible neurological or cardiac complications.
2. Takes vitamin B$_{12}$ for the rest of life—uses safe injection technique.
3. Returns for follow-up care.

IV. Polycythemia vera: abnormal increase in circulating red blood cells (myeloproliferative disorder); considered to be a form of malignancy; occurs more frequently among middle-aged Jewish men.
   A. Pathophysiology: unknown causes → massive increases of erythrocytes, myelocytes (bone marrow leukocytes), and thrombocytes → increased blood viscosity/volume and tissue/organ congestion; increased peripheral vascular resistance; intravascular thrombosis usually develops in middle age, particularly in Jewish men; in contrast, *secondary* polycythemia occurs as a compensatory response to tissue hypoxia associated with prolonged exposure to high altitude, chronic lung disease, and heart disease.
◆ **B. Assessment:**
1. *Subjective data*
   a. Headache; dizziness; ringing in ears.
   b. Weakness; loss of interest.
   c. Feelings of abdominal fullness.
   d. Shortness of breath; orthopnea.
   e. Pruritus, especially after bathing.
   f. Pain: gouty-arthritic.
2. *Objective data*
   a. Skin: mucosal erythema, ruddy complexion (reddish purple).
   b. Ecchymosis; gingival (gum) bleeding.
   c. Enlarged liver, spleen.
   d. Hypertension.
   e. Lab data:
      (1) *Increased*—hemoglobin, hematocrit, RBCs, leukocytes, platelets, uric acid.
      (2) *Decreased* bone marrow iron.

◆ **C. Analysis/nursing diagnosis:**
1. *Altered tissue perfusion* related to capillary congestion.
2. *Risk for injury* related to dizziness, weakness.
3. *Fluid volume excess* related to mass production of red blood cells.
4. *Risk for impaired skin integrity* related to pruritus.
5. *Ineffective breathing pattern* related to shortness of breath, orthopnea.
◆ **D. Nursing care plan/implementation:**
1. Goal: *promote comfort and prevent complications.*

a. Observe for signs of bleeding, thrombosis—stools, urine, gums, skin, ecchymosis.

b. Reduce occurrence: *avoid* prolonged sitting, knee gatch.

c. Assist with ambulation.

d. *Position:* elevate head of bed.

e. Skin care: cool-water baths to decrease pruritus; may add bicarbonate of soda to water.

f. Fluids: *force,* to reduce blood viscosity and promote urine excretion; 1500–2500 mL/24 hr.

g. *Diet: avoid* foods high in iron, to reduce RBC production.

h. Assist with venesection (phlebotomy), as ordered; 350–500 mL blood every other day until Hct low normal.

2. Goal: *health teaching.*

a. *Diet:* foods to *avoid* (e.g., liver, egg yolks); fluids to be increased.

b. Signs/symptoms of complications: infections, hemorrhage.

c. *Avoid:* falls, bumps; hot baths/showers (worsens pruritus).

d. Drugs: myelosuppressive agents (busulfan [Myleran], cyclophosphamide [Cytoxan], chlorambucil, radioactive phosphorus); purpose; side effects.

e. Procedures: venesection (phlebotomy) if ordered.

◆ **E. Evaluation/outcome criteria:**

1. Acceptance of chronic disease.

2. Reports at prescribed intervals for follow-up.

3. Remission: reduction of bone marrow activity, blood volume and viscosity (RBC <6,500,000/μL; Hgb <18 g/dL; Hct <45%; WBC <10,000/μL).

4. No complications (e.g., thrombi, hemorrhage, gout, CHF, leukemia).

V. Leukemia (acute and chronic): a neoplastic disease involving the leukopoietic tissue in either the bone marrow or lymphoid areas; acute leukemia occurs in children, young adults; chronic forms occur in later adult life.

A. Types:

1. Acute nonlymphocytic (ANLL)—also known as acute myelogenous leukemia (AML); seen generally in older age (>60 yr).

2. Acute lymphoblastic (ALL)—common in children 2–10 yr.

3. Chronic lymphocytic (CLL)—generally affects the elderly.

4. Chronic myelogenous (CML)—also known as chronic granulocytie leukemia (CGL); more likely to occur between 25 and 60 yr.

B. Pathophysiology: displacement of normal marrow cells by proliferating leukemic cells (abnormal, immature leukocytes) → normochromic anemia, thrombocytopenia.

C. Risk factors:

1. Viruses.

2. Genetic abnormalities.

3. Exposure to chemicals.

4. Radiation.

5. Treatment for other types of cancer (e.g., alkylating agents).

◆ **D. Assessment:**

1. *Subjective data*

a. Fatigue, weakness.

b. Anorexia, nausea.

c. Pain: joints, bones (acute leukemia).

d. Night sweats, weight loss, malaise.

2. *Objective data*

a. Skin: pallor due to anemia; jaundice.

b. Fever: frequent infections; mouth ulcers.

c. Bleeding: petechiae, purpura, ecchymosis, epistaxis, gingiva.

d. Organ enlargement: spleen, liver.

e. Enlarged lymph nodes; tenderness.

f. Bone marrow aspiration: increased presence of blasts.

g. Lab data:
(1) WBC—15,000–>100,000/μL
(2) RBC—normal to severely *decreased.*
(3) Hgb—low or normal.
(4) Platelets—low to *elevated.*

◆ **E. Analysis/nursing diagnosis:**

1. *Risk for infection* related to immature or abnormal leukocytes.

2. *Activity intolerance* related to hypoxia and weakness.

3. *Fatigue* related to anemia.

4. *Altered tissue perfusion* related to anemia.

5. *Anxiety* related to diagnosis and treatment.

6. *Altered oral mucous membrane* related to susceptibility to infection.

7. *Fear* related to diagnosis.

8. *Ineffective individual or family coping* related to potentially fatal disease.

◆ **F. Nursing care plan/implementation:**

1. Goal: *prevent, control, and treat infection.*

a. *Protective isolation* if indicated.

b. Observe for early signs of infection:
(1) Inflammation at injection sites.
(2) Vital-sign changes.
(3) Cough.
(4) Obtain cultures.

c. Give antibiotics as ordered.

d. Mouth care: clean q2h, examine for new lesions, *avoid* trauma.

2. Goal: *assess and control bleeding, anemia.*

a. Activity: *restrict* to prevent trauma.

b. Observe for hemorrhage: vital signs; body orifices, stool, urine.

c. Control localized bleeding: ice, pressure at least 3–4 min after needle sticks, positioning.

d. Use soft-bristle or foam-rubber toothbrush to prevent gingival bleeding.

e. Give blood/blood components as ordered; observe for transfusion reactions.
3. Goal: *provide rest, comfort, nutrition.*
   a. Activity: 8 hr sleep or rest; daily nap.
   b. Comfort measures: flotation mattress, bed cradle, sheepskin.
   c. Analgesics: without delay.
      (1) Mild pain (acetaminophen [Tylenol], propoxyphene HCl [Darvon] without aspirin).
      (2) Severe pain (codeine, meperidine HCl [Demerol]).
   d. *Diet:* bland.
      (1) *High* in protein, minerals, vitamins.
      (2) *Low* roughage.
      (3) Small, frequent feedings.
      (4) Favorite foods.
   e. Fluids: 3000–4000 mL/day.
4. Goal: *reduce side effects from therapeutic regimen.*
   a. Nausea: antiemetics, usually half-hour *before* chemotherapy.
   b. Increased uric acid level: force fluids.
   c. Stomatitis: antiseptic anesthetic mouthwashes.
   d. Rectal irritation: meticulous toileting, sitz baths, topical relief (e.g., Tucks).
5. Goal: *provide emotional/spiritual support.*
   a. Contact clergy if patient desires.
   b. Allow, encourage patient-initiated discussion of death (developmentally appropriate).
   c. Allow family to be involved in care.
   d. If death occurs, provide privacy, listening, sharing of grief for family.
6. Goal: *health teaching.*
   a. Prevent infection.
   b. Limit activity.
   c. Control bleeding.
   d. Reduce nausea.
   e. Mouth care.
   f. Chemotherapy: regimen; side effects.

◆ **G. Evaluation/outcome criteria:**
1. Alleviate symptoms; obtain remission.
2. Prevent complications (e.g., infection).
3. Ventilates emotions—accepts and deals with anger.
4. Experiences peaceful death (e.g., pain free).

VI. Idiopathic thrombocytopenic purpura (ITP): potentially fatal disorder characterized by spontaneous increase in platelet destruction; possible autoimmune response; seen predominantly in 2- to 4-year-olds and girls/women ≥10 years old. Remissions occur spontaneously or following splenectomy; in contrast, *secondary thrombocytopenia* (STP) is caused by viral infections, drug hypersensitivity (i.e., *quinidine, sulfonamides*), lupus, or bone marrow failure; treat cause.

◆ **A. Assessment:**
1. *Subjective data*
   a. Spontaneous skin hemorrhages—lower extremities.
   b. Menorrhagia.
   c. Epistaxis.
2. *Objective data*
   a. Bleeding: GI, urinary, nasal; following minor trauma, dental extractions.
   b. Petechiae; ecchymosis.
   c. *Tourniquet test*—positive, demonstrating increased capillary fragility.
   d. Lab data:
      (1) *Decreased* platelets (<100,000/μL).
      (2) *Increased* bleeding time.

◆ **B. Analysis/nursing diagnosis:**
1. *Risk for injury* related to hemorrhage.
2. *Altered tissue perfusion* related to fragile capillaries.
3. *Impaired skin integrity* related to skin hemorrhages.

◆ **C. Nursing care plan/implementation:**
1. Goal: *prevent complications from bleeding tendencies.*
   a. *Precautions:*
      (1) Injections—use small-bore needles; rotate sites; apply direct pressure.
      (2) *Avoid* bumping, trauma.
      (3) Use swabs for mouth care.
   b. Observe for signs of bleeding, petechiae following blood pressure reading, ecchymosis, purpura.
   c. Administer steroids (e.g., prednisone) with ITP to increase platelet count; give platelets for count below 20,000–30,000/μL with STP; high-dose immunoglobulins.
2. Goal: *health teaching.*
   a. *Avoid* traumatic activities:
      (1) Contact sports.
      (2) Violent sneezing, coughing, nose blowing.
      (3) Straining at stool.
      (4) Heavy lifting.
   b. *Signs of decreased platelets*—petechiae, ecchymosis, gingival bleeding, hematuria, menorrhagia.
   c. Use Medic Alert tag/card.
   d. *Precautions:* self-medication; particularly *avoid* aspirin-containing drugs.
   e. Prepare for splenectomy if drug therapy unsuccessful (prednisone, cyclophosphamide, azathioprine [Imuran]).

◆ **D. Evaluation/outcome criteria:**
1. Returns for follow-up.
2. No complications (e.g., intracranial hemorrhage).
3. Platelet count >200,000/μL.

4. Skin remains intact.
5. Resumes self-care activities.

VII. Splenectomy: removal of spleen following rupture due to acquired hemolytic anemia, trauma, tumor, or idiopathic thrombocytopenic purpura.

◆ **A. Analysis/nursing diagnosis:**
1. *Risk for fluid volume deficit* related to hemorrhage.
2. *Risk for infection* related to impaired immune response.
3. *Pain* related to abdominal distention.
4. *Ineffective breathing pattern* related to high abdominal incision.

◆ **B. Nursing care plan/implementation:**
▶ 1. Goal: *prepare for surgery.*
   a. Give whole blood, as ordered.
   b. Insert nasogastric tube to decrease postoperative abdominal distention, as ordered.
2. Goal: *prevent postoperative complications.*
   a. Observe for:
      (1) *Hemorrhage*—bleeding tendency with thrombocytopenia due to decreased platelet count.
      (2) *Gastrointestinal distention*—removal of enlarged spleen may result in distended stomach and intestines, to fill void.
   b. Recognize 101°F temp as normal for 10 days.
   c. Incision: splint when coughing, to prevent high incidence of atelectasis (common complication), pneumonia with upper-abdominal incision.
3. Goal: *health teaching.*
   a. Increased risk of infection postsplenectomy.
   b. Report signs of infection immediately.

◆ **C. Evaluation/outcome criteria:**
1. No complications (e.g., respiratory, subphrenic abscess or hematoma, thromboemboli, infection).
2. Complete and permanent remission—occurs in 60–80% of patients.

Fluid and Electrolyte Imbalances

Imbalances in fluid and electrolytes may be due to changes in the total quantity of either substance (deficit or excess), protein deficiencies, or extracellular fluid volume shifts. Older patients and very young patients are particularly susceptible.

I. Fluid volume deficit (dehydration): mechanism that influences fluid balance and sodium levels; decreased quantities of fluid and electrolytes may be caused by *deficient intake* (poor dietary habits, anorexia, and nausea), *excessive output* (vomiting, nasogastric suction, and prolonged diarrhea), or *failure of regulatory mechanism* that influences fluid balance and sodium levels.

A. Pathophysiology: water moves out of the cells to replace a significant water loss; cells eventually become unable to compensate for the lost fluid, and cellular dehydration begins, leading to circulatory collapse.

B. Risk factors:
1. No fluids available.
2. Available fluids not drinkable.
3. Inability to take fluids independently.
4. No response to thirst; does not recognize the need for fluids.
5. Inability to communicate need; does not speak same language.
6. Aphasia.
7. Weakness, comatose.
8. Inability to swallow.
9. Psychological alterations.
10. Overuse of diuretics.
11. Increased vomiting.
12. Fever.
13. Wounds, burns.
14. Blood loss.

◆ **C. Assessment:**
1. *Subjective data*
   a. Thirst.
   b. Behavioral changes: apprehension, apathy, lethargy, confusion, restlessness.
   c. Dizziness.
   d. Numbness and tingling of hands and feet.
   e. Anorexia and nausea.
   f. Abdominal cramps.
2. *Objective data*
   a. Sudden weight loss of 5%.
   b. Vital signs:
      (1) *Decreased* BP; postural changes.
      (2) *Increased* temperature.
      (3) Irregular, weak, rapid pulse.
      (4) *Increased* rate and depth of respirations.
   c. Skin: cool and pale in absence of infection; decreased turgor.
   d. Urine: oliguria to anuria, high specific gravity.
   e. Eyes: soft, sunken.
   f. Tongue: furrows.
   g. Lab data:
      (1) Blood—*increased* hematocrit and BUN.
      (2) Urine—*decreased* 17-ketosteroids.

◆ **D. Analysis/nursing diagnosis:**
1. *Fluid volume deficit* related to inadequate fluid intake.

◆ **E. Nursing care plan/implementation:**
1. Goal: *restore fluid and electrolyte balance*—increase fluid intake to hydrate client.

a. IVs as ordered; small, frequent drinks by mouth.

b. Daily weights (same time of day) to monitor progress of fluid replacement.

c. I&O, hourly outputs (when in acute state).

d. *Avoid* hypertonic solutions (may cause fluid shift when compensatory mechanisms begin to function).

2. Goal: *promote comfort.*

a. Frequent skin care (lack of hydration causes dry skin, which may increase risk for skin breakdown).

b. *Position:* change every hour to relieve pressure.

c. Medications as ordered: antiemetics, antidiarrheal.

3. Goal: *prevent physical injury.*

a. Frequent mouth care (mucous membrane dries due to dehydration; therefore, patient is at risk for breaks in mucous membrane, halitosis).

b. Monitor IV flow rate—observe for circulatory overload, pulmonary edema related to potential fluid shift when compensatory mechanisms begin or patient is unable to tolerate rate of fluid replacement.

c. Monitor vitals, including level of consciousness (decreasing BP and level of consciousness indicate continuation of fluid loss).

d. Prepare for surgery if hemorrhage present (internal bleeding can only be relieved by surgical intervention).

◆ **F. Evaluation/outcome criteria:**

1. Mentally alert.
2. Moist, intact mucous membranes.
3. Urinary output approximately equal to intake.
4. No further weight loss.
5. Gradual weight gain.

II. **Fluid volume excess** (fluid overload): most common cause is an increase in sodium; excessive quantities of fluid and electrolytes may be due to *increased ingestion,* tube feedings, intravenous infusions, multiple tap-water enemas, or a *failure of regulatory systems,* resulting in inability to excrete excesses.

A. **Pathophysiology:** hypo-osmolar water excess in extracellular compartment leads to intracellular water excess because the concentration of solutes in the intracellular fluid is greater than that in the extracellular fluid. Water moves to equalize concentration, causing swelling of the cells. The most common cause is an increase in sodium.

B. **Risk factors:**

1. Excessive intake of electrolyte-free fluids.
2. Increased secretion of ADH in response to stress, drugs, anesthetics.

3. Decreased or inadequate output of urine.
4. Psychogenic polydipsia.
5. Certain medical conditions: tuberculosis; encephalitis; meningitis; endocrine disturbances; tumors of lung, pancreas, duodenum, heart failure.
6. Inadequate kidney function or kidney failure.

◆ **C. Assessment:**

1. *Subjective data*

a. Behavioral changes: irritability, apathy, confusion, disorientation.
b. Headache.
c. Anorexia, nausea, cramping.
d. Fatigue.
e. Dyspnea.

2. *Objective data*

a. Vital signs: elevated blood pressure.
b. Skin: warm, moist; edema—eyelids, facial, dependent, pitting.
c. Sudden weight gain of 5 lbs.
d. Pink, frothy sputum; productive.
e. Constant, irritating cough.
f. Crackles in lungs.
g. Pulse, bounding.
h. Engorgement of neck veins in sitting position.
i. Urine: polyuria, nocturia.
j. Lab data:
   (1) Blood—*decreasing* hematocrit, BUN.
   (2) Urine—*decreasing* specific gravity.

D. **Analysis/nursing diagnosis:**

1. *Fluid volume excess* related to excessive fluid intake or decreased fluid output.

E. **Nursing care plan/implementation:**

1. Goal: *maintain oxygen to all cells.*

a. *Position:* semi-Fowler's or Fowler's to facilitate improved gas exchange.
b. Vital signs: q4h.
c. Fluid restriction.
d. Possible rotating tourniquets as needed (especially for interstitial-to-plasma shift).

2. Goal: *promote excretion of excess fluid.*

a. Medications as ordered: diuretics.
b. If in kidney failure: may need dialysis; explain procedure.
c. Assist patient during paracentesis, thoracentesis, phlebotomy.
   (1) Monitor vital signs to detect shock.
   (2) Prevent injury by monitoring sterile technique.
   (3) Prevent falling by stabilizing appropriate position during procedure.
   (4) Support patient psychologically.

3. Goal: *obtain/maintain fluid balance.*

a. Daily weights; 1 kg = 1000 mL fluid.
b. Measure: all edematous parts, abdominal girth, I&O.
c. *Limit:* fluids by mouth, IVs, sodium.
d. Strict monitoring of IV fluids.

4. Goal: *prevent tissue injury.*
   a. Skin and mouth care as needed.
   b. Evaluate feet for edema and discoloration when patient is out of bed.
   c. Observe suture line on surgical patients (potential for evisceration due to excess fluid retention).
   d. IV route preferred for parenteral medications; *Z track* if medications are to be given IM (otherwise injected liquid will escape through injection site).
5. Goal: *health teaching.*
   a. Improve nutritional status with low-sodium diet.
   b. Identify cause that put patient at risk for imbalance, methods to avoid this situation in the future.
   c. Desired and side effects of diuretics and other prescribed medications.
   d. Monitor urinary output, ankle edema; report to health care manager when fluid retention is noticed.
   e. Limit fluid intake when kidney/cardiac function impaired.

◆ F. **Evaluation/outcome criteria:**
   1. Fluid balance obtained.
   2. No respiratory, cardiac complications.
   3. Vital signs within normal limits.
   4. Urinary output improved, no evidence of edema.

III. **Common electrolyte imbalances:** electrolytes are taken into the body in foods and fluids; normally lost through sweat and urine. May also be lost through hemorrhage, vomiting, and diarrhea. Electrolytes have major influences on: body water regulation and osmolality, acid-base regulation, enzyme reactions, and neuromuscular activity. Clinically important electrolytes are:

A. **Sodium** (Na$^+$): normal 135–145 mEq/L. Most prevalent cation in extracellular fluid. Controls osmotic pressure; essential for neuromuscular functioning and intracellular chemical reactions. Aids in maintenance of acid-base balance. Necessary for glucose to be transported into cells.
   1. *Hyponatremia*—sodium deficit, resulting from either a sodium loss or water excess. Serum-sodium level below 135 mEq/L; symptoms usually do not occur until below 120 mEq/L unless rapid drop.
   2. *Hypernatremia*—excess sodium in the blood, resulting from either high sodium intake, water loss, or low water intake. Serum-sodium level above 145 mEq/L.

B. **Potassium** (K$^+$): normal 3.5–5.0 mEq/L. Direct effect on excitability of nerves and muscles. Contributes to intracellular osmotic pressure and influences acid-base balance. Major cation of the cell. Required for storage of nitrogen as muscle protein.
   1. *Hypokalemia*—potassium deficit related to dehydration, starvation, vomiting, diarrhea, diuretics. Serum-potassium level below 3.5 mEq/L; symptoms may not occur until below 2.5 mEq/L.
   2. *Hyperkalemia*—potassium excess related to severe tissue damage, renal disease, excess administration of oral or IV potassium. Serum-potassium level above 5 mEq/L; symptoms usually occur when above 6.5 mEq/L.

C. **Calcium** (Ca^{2+}): normal 4.5–5.5 mEq/L. Essential to muscle metabolism, cardiac function, and bone health. Controlled by parathyroid hormone; reciprocal relationship between calcium and phosphorus.
   1. *Hypocalcemia*—loss of calcium related to inadequate intake, vitamin D deficiency, hypoparathyroidism, damage to the parathyroid gland, decreased absorption in the GI tract, excess loss through kidneys. Serum-calcium level below 4.5 mEq/L.
   2. *Hypercalcemia*—calcium excess related to hyperparathyroidism, immobility, bone tumors, renal failure, excess intake of Ca^{2+} or vitamin D. Serum-calcium level above 5.5 mEq/L.

D. **Magnesium** (Mg^{2+}): normal 1.5–2.5 mEq/L. Essential to cellular metabolism of carbohydrates and proteins.
   1. *Hypomagnesemia*—magnesium deficit related to impaired absorption from GI tract, excessive loss through kidneys, and prolonged periods of poor nutritional intake. Hypomagnesemia leads to neuromuscular irritability. Serum-magnesium level below 1.5 mEq/L.
   2. *Hypermagnesemia*—magnesium excess related to renal insufficiency, overdose during replacement therapy, severe dehydration, repeated enemas with Mg^{2+} sulfate (epsom salts). Serum-magnesium level above 2.5 mEq/L.

◆ E. Table 7–10 provides assessment, analysis, nursing care plan/implementation, and evaluation/outcome criteria of the various electrolyte imbalances.

IV. **Acid-base balance:** concentration of hydrogen ions in extracellular fluid is determined by the ratio of bicarbonate to carbonic acid. The normal ratio is 20:1. Even when arterial blood gases are abnormal, if the ratio remains at 20:1, no imbalance will occur. Table 7–11 shows blood gas variations with acid-base imbalances.
   A. **Causes of blood gas abnormalities:** Table 7–12.
   B. **Types of acid-base imbalance:**
      1. *Acidosis:* hydrogen ion concentration increases and pH decreases.

TABLE 7–10 Electrolyte Imbalances

Disorder and Related Condition	Assessment — Subjective Data	Objective Data	◆ Analysis/Nursing Diagnosis	◆ Nursing Care Plan/Implementation	◆ Evaluation/Outcome Criteria
Hyponatremia Addison's disease Starvation GI suction Thiazide diuretics Excess water intake, enemas Fever Fluid shifts Ascites Burns Small-bowel obstruction Profuse perspiration	Apathy, apprehension, mental confusion, delirium Fatigue Vertigo, headache Anorexia, nausea Abdominal and muscle cramps	*Pulse:* rapid and weak *BP:* postural hypotension Shock, coma *GI:* weight loss, diarrhea, loss through NG tubes Muscle weakness	*Diarrhea* *Fluid volume excess* *Altered nutrition, less than body requirements* *Sensory-perceptual alteration (kinesthetic)*	*Obtain normal sodium level:* identify cause of deficit, *increase sodium intake* PO (salty foods), IVs—hypertonic solutions *Prevent further sodium loss:* irrigate NG tubes with saline; hourly I&O to monitor kidney output *Prevent injury* related to shock, dizziness, decreased sensorium; dangle before ambulation Skin care	Na⁺ 135–145 mEq/L No complications of shock present Return of muscle strength Alert, oriented Limits intake of plain water
Hypernatremia High sodium intake Low water intake Diarrhea High fever with rapid respirations Impaired renal functions Acute tracheobronchitis	Lethargy Restlessness, agitation Confusion	*BP and temperature:* elevated *Neuromuscular:* diminished reflexes *Skin:* flushed; firm turgor *GI:* mucous membrane dry, sticky *GU:* decreased output	*Fluid volume deficit* *Fluid volume excess* *Altered nutrition, less than body requirements* *Sensory-perceptual alteration (kinesthetic)*	*Obtain normal sodium level:* decrease sodium intake I&O to recognize signs and symptoms of complications, e.g., heart failure, pulmonary edema	Na⁺ 135–145 mEq/L No complaint of thirst Alert, oriented Relaxed in appearance Identifies high-sodium foods to avoid
Hypokalemia *Decreased intake:* Poor potassium food intake Excessive dieting Nausea Alcoholism IV fluids without added potassium *Increased loss:* GI suctioning, vomiting, diarrhea Ulcerative colitis Drainage: ostomy, fistulas Medications: potassium-losing diuretics, digoxin, cathartics Increased aldosterone production Renal disorders	Apathy, lethargy, fatigue, weakness Irritability, mental confusion Anorexia, nausea Leg cramps	*Muscles:* weakness, paralysis, paresthesia, hyporeflexia *Respirations:* shallow to respiratory arrest *Cardiac:* decreased BP; elevated, weak, irregular pulse; arrhythmias ECG: low, flat T waves; prolonged ST segment: elevated U wave; potential arrest *GI:* vomiting, flatulence, constipation; decreased motility → distention → paralytic ileus *GU:* urine not concentrated; polyuria, nocturia; kidney damage *Speech:* slow	*Decreased cardiac output* *Fatigue* *Altered cardiopulmonary tissue perfusion* *Ineffective breathing patterns* *Constipation* *Bathing/hygiene self-care deficit* *Impaired home maintenance management* *Sensory-perceptual alteration (gustatory)*	*Replace lost potassium: increase potassium in diet* (see Unit 9); liquid PO potassium medications—dilute in juice to aid taste; give potassium only if kidneys functioning *Prevent injury to tissues:* prevent infiltration, pain, tissue damage *Prevent potassium loss:* irrigate NG tubes with saline, not water	K⁺ 3.5–5.0 mEq/L Identifies cause of imbalance Lists foods to include in diet Lists signs and symptoms of imbalance Return of muscle strength No cardiac arrhythmias

Condition / Causes	Signs and Symptoms	Physical Assessment	Nursing Diagnoses	Interventions	Outcomes
Hyperkalemia Burns Crushing injuries Kidney disease Excessive infusion or ingestion of K^+ Adrenal insufficiency Mercurial poisoning	Irritability Weakness, muscle cramps Nausea, intestinal cramps	*Muscles:* paresthesia, flaccid muscle paralysis (later) *Cardiac:* irregular pulse; arrhythmias; bradycardia → asystole *ECG:* high T waves; depressed ST segment; widened QRS complex; diminished or absent P waves; ventricular fibrillation *GI:* explosive diarrhea; hyperactive bowel sounds *Kidney:* scanty to no urine	*Decreased cardiac output Altered urinary elimination Activity intolerance Ineffective breathing patterns Diarrhea Impaired home maintenance management*	*Decrease amount of potassium in body;* identify and treat cause of imbalance; give *foods low in K^+*; *avoid drugs or IV fluids containing K^+* If kidney failure present, may need to prepare for dialysis	**K^+ 3.5–5.0 mEq/L** No complications (e.g., arrhythmias, acidosis, respiratory failure)
Hypocalcemia Acute pancreatitis Diarrhea Peritonitis Damage to parathyroid during thyroidectomy Hypothyroidism Burns Pregnancy and lactation Low vitamin D intake Multiple blood transfusions Renal disorders Massive infection	Fatigue Tingling/numbness; fingers and circumoral Abdominal cramps Palpitations Dyspnea	*Muscle spasms:* tonic muscles, carpopedal, laryngeal *Neuromuscular:* grimacing; hyperirritable facial nerves Tetany → convulsions *Orthopedic:* osteoporosis → fractures *Cardiac:* arrhythmias → arrest *GI:* diarrhea	*Pain Diarrhea Altered nutrition, less than body requirements Risk for injury Sensory-perceptual alteration (gustatory)*	*Prevent tetany* (**medical emergency**): calcium gluconate IV, 2.5–5.0 mL 10% solution; repeated q10min to maximum dose of 30 mL *Prevent tissue injury due to hypoxia and sloughing;* administer slowly; *avoid infiltration* *Prevent injury related to medication administration. Caution:* drug interaction with carbonate, phosphate, digitalis; *avoid hypercalcemia* *In less acute condition:* increase calcium intake—calcium gluconate or lactate	**Ca^{2+} 4.5–5.5 mEq/L** No signs of tetany Absent *Trousseau's* and *Chvostek's* signs Lists foods high in vitamin D and calcium
Hypercalcemia Parathyroid glands: overactive; tumor Increased immobility Decreased renal function Bone cancer Increased vitamin D and calcium intake Milk-alkali syndrome—self-administration of antacids; increased milk in diet to relieve GI symptoms	*Pain:* flank, deep bone, shin splints Muscle weakness, fatigue Anorexia, nausea Headache Thirst → polyuria	*Muscles:* relaxed *GU:* kidney stones *GI:* increased milk intake, constipation, dehydration *Neurological:* stupor → coma	*Decreased cardiac output Constipation Activity intolerance Altered urinary elimination Pain*	*Reduce calcium intake:* decrease foods high in *calcium*; identify cause of imbalance; give steroids, diuretics as ordered; isotonic saline IV *Prevent injury:* prevent pathological fractures (e.g., advanced cancer); prevent renal calculi by *increasing fluid intake*	**Ca^{2+} 4.5–5.5 mEq/L** No pain reported No fractures/calculi seen on x-ray exam

Continued

Adult

Adult

TABLE 7–10 Electrolyte Imbalances—cont'd

Disorder and Related Condition	◆ Assessment		◆ Analysis/Nursing Diagnosis	◆ Nursing Care Plan/Implementation	◆ Evaluation/Outcome Criteria
	Subjective Data	Objective Data			
Hypomagnesemia Impaired GI absorption Prolonged malnutrition or starvation Alcoholism Excess loss of magnesium through kidneys, related to increased aldosterone production Prolonged diarrhea Draining GI fistulas	Agitation Depression Confusion Paresthesia	*Muscles:* irritable, tremors, spasticity, tetany → convulsions *Cardiac:* arrhythmias, tachycardia	*Risk for injury related to seizure activity* *Decreased cardiac output*	*Provide safety:* prevent injury to disoriented patient; administer magnesium salts PO or IV *Health teaching:* prevention; diet—*high-magnesium* foods: fruits, green vegetables, whole grain cereals, milk, meats, nuts	Mg^{2+} 1.5–2.5 mEq/L
Hypermagnesemia Renal failure Diabetic ketoacidosis Severe dehydration Antacid therapy	Drowsiness, lethargy	*Neuromuscular:* loss of deep-tendon reflexes *Respiratory:* depression *Cardiac:* arrest, hypotension	*Ineffective breathing pattern* *Decreased cardiac output* *Fluid volume deficit* *Fluid volume excess* *Altered cardiopulmonary tissue perfusion*	*Obtain normal magnesium level:* IV calcium; fluids; possible dialysis	Mg^{2+} 1.5–2.5 mEq/L No complications (e.g., respiratory depression, arrhythmias) Identifies magnesium-based antacids (e.g., Gelusil) Deep-tendon reflexes 2+

TABLE 7–11   Blood Gas Variations with Acid-Base Imbalances

Blood Gas Feature	Normal Value	Respiratory Acidosis	Respiratory Alkalosis	Metabolic Acidosis	Metabolic Alkalosis
		Value with:			
HCO_3 (bicarbonate)	22–26 mm Hg	Normal or ↑	Normal or ↓	↓	↑
P_{CO_2}	35–45 mm Hg	↑	↓	Normal or ↓	Normal or ↑
(Carbonic acid*)	(1.05–1.35)	↑	↓	Normal or ↓	Normal or ↑
pH (hydrogen-ion concentration)	7.35–7.45	↓	↑	↓	↑

↑ = increased; ↓ = decreased.
*To obtain carbonic acid level, multiply P_{CO_2} value by 0.03.

2. *Alkalosis:* hydrogen ion concentration decreases and pH increases.
3. *Metabolic imbalances:* bicarbonate is the problem. In primary conditions, the level of bicarbonate is directly *proportional* to pH.
   a. *Metabolic acidosis:* excessive acid is produced or added to the body, bicarbonate is lost, or acid is retained due to poorly functioning kidneys. Deficit of bicarbonate.
   b. *Metabolic alkalosis:* excessive acid is lost or bicarbonate or alkali is retained. Excess of bicarbonate.
   c. As compensatory mechanism, P_{CO_2} will be *low in metabolic acidosis,* as the body attempts to eliminate excess carbonic acid and elevate pH. P_{CO_2} will become *elevated in metabolic alkalosis.*
4. *Respiratory imbalances:* carbonic acid is the problem. In primary conditions, P_{CO_2} is inversely proportional to the pH.
   a. *Respiratory acidosis:* pulmonary ventilation decreases, causing an elevation in the level of carbon dioxide or carbonic acid. Excess of P_{CO_2}.
   b. *Respiratory alkalosis:* pulmonary ventilation increases, causing a decrease in the level of carbon dioxide or carbonic acid. Deficit of P_{CO_2}.
   c. As a compensatory mechanism, the level of bicarbonate will *increase in respiratory acidosis* and *decrease in respiratory alkalosis.*
◆ **C. Assessment:** Table 7–13.
◆ **D. Analysis/nursing diagnosis:**
1. *Impaired gas exchange* related to hyperventilation.
2. *Ineffective breathing pattern* related to decreased thoracic movements.
3. *Ineffective airway clearance* related to retained secretions.
4. *Risk for injury* related to poorly functioning kidneys.
5. *Altered renal tissue perfusion* related to dehydration.

TABLE 7–12   Blood Gas Abnormalities: Causes

Decreased P_{O_2}

Collapsed alveoli (atelectasis)
1. Airway obstruction
   a. By the tongue
   b. By a foreign body
2. Failure to take deep breaths
   a. Pain (rib fracture, pleurisy)
   b. Paralysis of respiratory muscles (spinal cord injury, polio)
   c. Depression of the respiratory center (head injury, drug overdose)
3. Collapse of the whole lung (pneumothorax)
Fluid in the alveoli
1. Pulmonary edema
2. Pneumonia
3. Near-drowning
4. Chest trauma
Other gases in the alveoli
1. Smoke inhalation
2. Inhalation of toxic chemicals
3. Carbon monoxide poisoning
Respiratory arrest

Elevated P_{CO_2}

Decreased CO_2 elimination (hypoventilation)
1. Decreased tidal volume
   a. Pain (rib fractures, pleurisy)
   b. Weakness (myasthenia gravis)
   c. Paralysis (spinal cord injury, polio)
2. Decreased respiratory rate
   a. Head injury
   b. Depressant drugs
   c. Stroke
Increased CO_2 production
1. Fever
2. Muscular exertion
3. Anaerobic metabolism

6. *Altered urinary elimination,* related to renal failure.
7. *Fluid volume excess* related to altered kidney function.
8. *Fluid volume deficit* related to diarrhea or dehydration.
9. *Knowledge deficit* related to self-administration of antacid medications.
◆ **E. Nursing care plan/implementation:** see Table 7–13.
◆ **F. Evaluation/outcome criteria:** see Table 7–13.

TABLE 7–13 **Acid-Base Imbalances**

Disorder and Related Conditions	◆Assessment		◆Nursing Care Plan/ Implementation	◆Evaluation/ Outcome Criteria
	Subjective Data	**Objective Data**		
Respiratory Acidosis Acute bronchitis Emphysema Respiratory obstruction Atelectasis Damage to respiratory center Pneumonia Asthmatic attack Drug overdose	Headache Irritability Disorientation Weakness Dyspnea on exertion Nausea	Increased respirations Cyanosis Tachycardia Diaphoresis Dehydration Coma (CO_2 narcosis) Hyperventilation to *compensate* if no pulmonary pathology present ──────────── HCO$_3$ normal, PaCO_2 elevated, pH <7.35	*Assist with normal breathing:* encourage coughing; ▶ suction airway; postural drainage; pursed-lip ◢ breathing; raise HOB *Protect from injury:* oxygen at 2 L; encourage fluids; *avoid* sedation; medica- ◖▷ tions as ordered—bicarbonates, antibiotics, bronchial dilators, detergent *Health teaching:* identify cause, prevent future episodes; increase awareness regarding risk factors and early signs of impending imbalance; encourage compliance	Normal acid-base balance obtained Respiratory rate slows, <30 No signs of pulmonary infection (e.g., sputum colorless, breath sounds clear) Demonstrates breathing exercises (e.g., diaphragmatic breathing)
Metabolic Acidosis Diabetic ketoacidosis Hyperthyroidism Severe infections Lactic acidosis in shock Renal failure → uremia Prolonged starvation diet; low-protein diet Diarrhea, dehydration Hepatitis Burns	Headache Restlessness Apathy, weakness Disorientation Thirst Nausea, abdominal pain	Kussmaul's respirations: deep, rapid air hunger; ↑temperature Vomiting, diarrhea Dehydration Stupor → convulsions → coma ──────────── HCO$_3$ below normal PaCO_2 normal, K$^+$ >5, pH <7.35	*Restore normal metabolism:* correct underlying prob- ◖▷ lem; sodium bicarbonate PO/IV; sodium lactate; fluid replacement, Ringer's solution; *diet:* ◖▮ high calorie *Prevent complications: regu-* ◖▷ *lar* insulin for ketoacidosis; hourly outputs; prepare for dialysis if in kidney failure *Health teaching:* identify signs and symptoms of primary illness; prevent complications, cardiac arrest; diet instructions	Normal acid-base balance obtained No rebound respiratory alkalosis following therapy No tetany following return of normal pH Alert, oriented No signs of K$^+$ excess
Respiratory Alkalosis Hyperventilation—CO_2 loss Fever Metabolic acidosis Increased ICP, encephalitis Salicylate poisoning After intensive exercise Hypoxia, high altitudes	Circumoral paresthesia Weakness Apprehension	Increased respirations Increased neuromuscular irritability; hypereflexia, muscle twitching, tetany, positive *Chvostek's* sign Convulsions Unconsciousness Hypokalemia ──────────── HCO$_3$ normal, PaCO_2 decreased, pH >7.45	*Increase carbon dioxide level:* rebreathing into a paper bag; adjusting respirator for CO_2 retention and oxygen inspired *Prevent injury:* safety measures for those who are unconscious; hypothermia for elevated temperature *Health teaching:* recognize stressful events; counseling if problem is hysteria	Normal acid-base balance obtained Recognizes psychological and environmental factors causing condition Respiratory rate returns to normal limits No cardiac arrhythmias Alert, oriented

Adult

TABLE 7–13   Acid-Base Imbalances—cont'd

Disorder and Related Conditions	◆Assessment		◆ Nursing Care Plan/ Implementation	◆ Evaluation/ Outcome Criteria
	Subjective Data	Objective Data		
Metabolic Alkalosis Potassium deficiencies Vomiting GI suctioning Intestinal fistulas Inadequate electrolyte replacement Increased use of antacids Diuretic therapy, steroids Increased ingestion/ injection of bicarbonates	Lethargy Irritability Disorientation Nausea	*Respirations:* shallow; apnea, decreased thoracic movement; cyanosis *Pulse:* irregular → cardiac arrest *Muscles:* twitching → tetany, convulsions *G.I.:* vomiting, diarrhea, paralytic ileus HCO_3 elevated above 26, $Paco_2$ normal, K^+ <3.5, pH >7.45	*Obtain, maintain acid-base balance:* irrigate NG ▶ tubes with saline; monitor I&O; IV saline, potassium added; isotonic solutions PO; monitor vital signs *Prevent physical injury:* monitor for potassium loss, side effects of medications *Health teaching:* increase sodium when loss expected; instructions regarding self-administration of medications (e.g., baking soda)	Normal acid-base balance obtained No signs of potassium deficit Respiratory rate 16–20 No arrhythmias— pulse regular Lists food sources high in potassium

Conditions Affecting Gas Transport

I. **Pneumonia:** acute inflammation of lungs with exudate accumulation in alveoli and other respiratory passages that interferes with ventilation process.

A. **Types:**
1. *Typical/classic pneumonia: pneumococcal;* related to diminished defense mechanisms, immunocompromised, critically ill, history of smoking, general anesthesia/abdominal surgery, exposure to airborne pathogens, hospitalization, recent respiratory tract infection, viral influenza, increased age, and chronic obstructive pulmonary disease (COPD).
   a. *Lobar pneumonia*—occurs abruptly when an acute bacterial infection affects a large portion of a lobe; causes pleuritic pain, heavy sputum production.
   b. *Bronchopneumonia*—involves patchy infiltration over a general area.
   c. *Alveolar pneumonia*—caused by virus; diffuse bilateral infection without patchy infiltrates.
2. *Atypical pneumonia:* related to contact with specific organisms.
   a. *Mycoplasma pneumoniae* or *Legionella pneumophila,* if untreated, can lead to serious complications such as disseminated intravascular coagulation (DIC), thrombocytopenic purpura, renal failure, inflammation of the heart, neurological disorders, or possible death.

   b. *Pneumocystis carinii* in conjunction with AIDS.
3. *Aspiration pneumonia:*
   a. *Noninfectious:* aspiration of fluids (gastric secretions, foods, liquids, tube feedings) into the airways.
   b. *Bacterial aspiration pneumonia:* related to poor cough mechanisms due to anesthesia, coma (mixed flora of upper respiratory tract cause pneumonia).
4. *Hematogenous pneumonia bacterial infections:* related to spread of bacteria from the bloodstream.

B. **Pathophysiology:** caused by infectious or noninfectious agents, clotting of an exudate rich in fibrogen, consolidated lung tissue.

◆ C. **Assessment:**
1. *Subjective data*
   a. Pain location: chest (affected side), referred to abdomen, shoulder, flank.
   b. Irritability, restlessness.
   c. Apprehensiveness.
   d. Nausea, anorexia.
   e. History of exposure.
2. *Objective data*
   a. Cough
      (1) Productive, rust (blood) or yellowish sputum (greenish with atypical pneumonia).
      (2) Splinting of affected side when coughing.
   b. Sudden increased fever, chills.
   c. Nasal flaring, circumoral cyanosis.
   d. Respiratory distress: tachypnea.
   e. Auscultation:

(1) Decreased breath sounds on *affected* side.

(2) Exaggerated breath sounds on *unaffected* side.

(3) Crackles, bronchial breath sounds.

(4) Dullness on percussion over consolidated area.

(5) Possible pleural friction rub.

f. Chest retraction (air hunger in infants).

g. Vomiting.

h. Facial herpes simplex.

i. *Diagnostic studies:*

(1) Chest x-ray: haziness to consolidation.

(2) Sputum culture: Gram stain and culture; specific organisms, usually pneumococcus.

(3) Bronchoscopy if sputum results are inconclusive.

j. Lab data:

(1) Blood culture: organism specific except when viral.

(2) WBC: leukocytosis.

(3) Sedimentation rate: *elevated.*

◆ **D. Analysis/nursing diagnosis:**

1. *Ineffective airway clearance* related to retained secretions.

2. *Activity intolerance* related to inflammatory process.

3. *Pain* related to continued coughing.

4. *Knowledge deficit* related to proper management of symptoms.

5. *Risk for fluid volume deficit* related to tachypnea.

◆ **E. Nursing care plan/implementation:**

1. Goal: *promote adequate ventilation.*

a. Deep breathe, cough.

b. Remove respiratory secretions, suction prn.

c. High humidity with or without oxygen therapy.

▶ d. Intermittent positive-pressure breathing (IPPB); incentive spirometry, chest physiotherapy, as ordered and needed to loosen secretions.

e. Use of expectorants as ordered.

f. Change position frequently.

▶ g. Percussion with postural drainage.

2. Goal: *control infection.*

a. Monitor vital signs; hypothermia for elevated temperature.

b. Administer antibiotics as ordered to control infection—cephalexin (Keflex), cephalothin (Keflin), erythromycin, gentamicin sulfate (Garamycin), penicillin G. *Note:* need cultures before starting on antibiotics.

3. Goal: *provide rest and comfort.*

a. Planned rest periods.

b. Adequate hydration by mouth, I&O; IVs as needed.

c. *Diet:* high carbohydrate, high protein to meet energy demands and assist in the healing process.

d. Mild analgesics for pain—*no* opioids.

4. Goal: *prevent potential complications.*

a. Cross infection: use good hand-washing technique.

b. Hyperthermia: tepid baths, hypothermia blanket.

c. Respiratory insufficiency and acidosis: clear airway, promote expectoration of secretions.

d. Assess cardiac and respiratory function.

e. Remain ambulatory whenever possible.

5. Goal: *health teaching.*

a. Proper disposal of tissues, cover mouth when coughing.

b. Expected side effects of prescribed medications.

c. Need for rest, limited interactions, increased caloric intake.

d. Need to avoid future respiratory infections. *Immunization:* influenza each year for those at risk. Vaccine for pneumococcal pneumonia every 5 years.

e. Correct dosage of antibiotics and the importance of taking entire prescription at prescribed times (times evenly distributed throughout the 24 hr period to maintain blood level of antibiotic) for increased effectiveness.

◆ **F. Evaluation/outcome criteria:**

1. Adheres to medication regimen.

2. Has improved gas exchange as shown by improved pulmonary function tests.

3. No acid-base or fluid imbalance: normal pH.

4. Energy level increased.

5. Sputum production decreased, normal color.

6. Vital signs stable.

7. Breath sounds clear.

8. Cultures negative.

9. Reports comfort level increased.

II. Atelectasis: collapsed alveoli in part or all of the lung.

A. Pathophysiology: due to compression (tumor), airway obstruction, decreased surfactant production, or progressive regional hypoventilation.

B. Risk factors:

1. Shallow breathing due to pain, abdominal distention, narcotics, or sedatives.

2. Decreased ciliary action due to anesthesia, smoking.

3. Thickened secretions due to immobility, dehydration.

4. Aspiration of foreign substances.

5. Bronchospasms.

◆ C. **Assessment:**
1. *Subjective data*
   a. Restlessness.
   b. Pain.
2. *Objective data*
   a. Tachypnea.
   b. Tachycardia.
   c. Dullness on percussion.
   d. Absent bronchial breathing.
   e. Tactile fremitus in affected area.
   f. X-ray:
      (1) Patches of consolidation.
      (2) Elevated diaphragm.
      (3) Mediastinal shift.

◆ D. **Analysis/nursing diagnosis:**
1. *Impaired gas exchange* related to shallow breathing.
2. *Pain,* acute, related to collapse of lung.
3. *Fear* related to altered respiratory status.

◆ E. **Nursing care plan/implementation:**
1. Goal: *relieve hypoxia.*
   a. Frequent respiratory assessment.
   b. Respiratory hygiene measures, cough, deep breathe.
   c. Oxygen as ordered.
   d. Monitor effects of respiratory therapy, ventilators, breathing assistance measures to ensure proper gas exchange.
   e. *Position:* on unaffected side to allow for lung expansion.
2. Goal: *prevent complications.*
   a. Antibiotics as ordered.
   b. *Sterile technique* when tracheal bronchial suctioning to reduce risk of possible infection.
   c. Turn, cough, and deep breathe.
   d. *Increase fluid* intake to liquefy secretions.
3. Goal: *health teaching.*
   a. Need to report signs and symptoms listed in assessment data for early recognition of problem.
   b. Importance of coughing and deep breathing to improve present condition and prevent further problems.

◆ F. **Evaluation/outcome criteria:**
1. Lung expanded on x-ray.
2. Acid-base balance obtained and maintained.
3. No pain on respiration.
4. Activity level increased.

III. **Pulmonary embolism:** undissolved mass that travels in bloodstream and occludes a blood vessel; can be thromboemboli, fat, air, or catheter. Constitutes a **critical medical emergency.**
   A. **Pathophysiology:** obstructs blood flow to lung → increased pressure on pulmonary artery and reflex constriction of pulmonary blood vessels → poor pulmonary circulation → pulmonary infarction.
   B. **Risk factors:**
   1. Thrombophlebitis.
   2. Recent surgery.
   3. Invasive procedures.
   4. Immobility.
   5. Obesity
   6. Myocardial infarction, heart failure.
   7. Smoking.
   8. Varicose veins.
   9. Hormone replacement therapy.

◆ C. **Assessment:**
1. *Subjective data*
   a. Chest pain: substernal, localized; type—crushing, sharp, stabbing with respirations.
   b. Sudden onset of profound dyspnea.
   c. Restless, irritable, anxious.
   d. Sense of impending doom.
2. *Objective data*
   a. Respirations: either rapid, shallow or deep, gasping.
   b. Elevated temperature.
   c. Auscultation: friction rub, crackles; diminished breath sounds.
   d. Shock:
      (1) Tachycardia.
      (2) Hypotension.
      (3) Skin: cold, clammy.
   e. Cough: hemoptysis.
   f. X-ray: area of density.
   g. ECG changes that reflect right-sided failure.
   h. Echocardiogram shows increased pulmonary dynamics.
   i. Lung scan.
   j. Lab data:
      (1) *Decreased* $PaCO_2$.
      (2) *Elevated* WBC.

◆ D. **Analysis/nursing diagnosis:**
1. *Ineffective breathing pattern* related to shallow respirations.
2. *Impaired gas exchange* related to dyspnea.
3. *Pain* related to decreased tissue perfusion.
4. *Altered peripheral tissue perfusion* related to occlusion of blood vessel.
5. *Fear* related to emergency condition.
6. *Anxiety* related to sense of impending doom.

◆ E. **Nursing care plan/implementation:**
1. Goal: *monitor for signs of respiratory distress.*
   a. Auscultate lungs for areas of decreased/absent breath sounds.
   b. *Elevate head of bed.*
   c. Monitor ABGs.
   d. Monitor pulse oximetry; administer oxygen, supplemental humidification as indicated.
   e. Monitor blood coagulation studies, e.g., aPTT.

f. Administer *anticoagulation* therapy, *thrombolytic* agents, morphine for pain, vasopressor medications.

g. Fluids: IV/PO as indicated.

h. Monitor signs: Homans', acidosis.

i. Ambulate as tolerated/indicated; change position.

j. Prepare for surgery if peripheral embolectomy is indicated.

2. Goal: *health teaching.*

a. Prevent further occurrence; importance of antiembolism stockings, intermittent pneumatic compression devices.

b. Decrease stasis.

c. If history of thrombophlebitis, *avoid* birth control pills.

d. Need to continue medication.

e. Follow-up care.

◆ **F. Evaluation/outcome criteria:**

1. No complications; no further incidence of emboli.

2. Respiratory rate returns to normal.

3. Coagulation studies within normal limits (aPTT 25–41 sec, ABGs within normal limits).

4. Reports comfort achieved.

IV. Histoplasmosis: infection found mostly in central United States. *Not transmitted from human to human but from dust and contaminated soil.* Progressive histoplasmosis, seen most frequently in middle-aged white males who have COPD, is characterized by cavity formation, fibrosis, and emphysema.

A. Pathophysiology: spores of *Histoplasma capsulatum* (from droppings of infected birds and bats) are inhaled, multiply, and cause fungal infections of respiratory tract. Leads to necrosis and healing by encapsulation.

◆ **B. Assessment:**

1. *Subjective data*

a. Malaise.

b. Chest pain, dyspnea.

2. *Objective data*

a. Weight loss.

b. Nonproductive cough.

c. Fever.

d. Positive skin test for histoplasmosis.

e. Benign acute pneumonitis.

f. Chest x-ray: nodular infiltrate.

g. Sputum culture shows *Histoplasma capsulatum.*

h. Hepatomegaly, splenomegaly.

◆ **C. Analysis/nursing diagnosis:**

1. *Ineffective airway clearance* related to pneumonitis.

2. *Ineffective breathing pattern* related to dyspnea.

3. *Pain,* acute, related to infectious process.

4. *Risk for infection* related to repeated exposure to fungal spores.

5. *Impaired gas exchange* related to chronic pulmonary disease.

6. *Knowledge deficit* related to prevention of disease and potential side effects of medications.

◆ **D. Nursing care plan/implementation:**

1. Goal: *relieve symptoms of the disease:*

a. Administer medications as ordered.

(1) Amphotericin B (IV) and ketoconazole.

(a) Monitor for drug side effects: local phlebitis, renal toxicity, hypokalemia, anemia, anaphylaxis, bone marrow depression.

(b) *Azotemia* (presence of nitrogen-containing compounds in blood) is monitored by biweekly BUN or creatinine levels.

BUN >40 mg/dL or creatinine >3.0 mg/dL necessitates stopping amphotericin B until values return to within normal limits.

(2) Aspirin, diphenhydramine HCl (Benadryl), promethazine HCl (Phenergan), prochlorperazine (Compazine): used *to decrease systemic toxicity* of chills, fever, aching, nausea, and vomiting.

2. Goal: *health teaching:*

a. Desired effects and side effects of prescribed medications; importance of taking medications for entire course of therapy (usually from 2 wk to 3 mo).

b. Importance of follow-up laboratory tests to monitor toxic effects of drug.

c. Identify source of contamination if possible and *avoid* future contact if possible.

d. Importance of deep breathing, pursed-lip breathing, coughing (see **VI. Emphysema,** p. 482, for specific care).

e. Signs and symptoms of chronic histoplasmosis, COPD, drug toxicity, and drug side effects, as in (1)(a), above.

◆ **E. Evaluation/outcome criteria:**

1. Complies with treatment plan.

2. Respiratory complications avoided.

3. Symptoms of illness decreased.

4. No further spread of disease.

5. Source of contamination identified and removed.

V. Tuberculosis: inflammatory, communicable disease that commonly attacks the lungs, although may occur in other body parts.

A. Pathophysiology: exposure to causative organism *(Mycobacterium tuberculosis)* in the alveoli in susceptible individual leads to inflammation. Infection spreads by lymphatics to hilus; antibodies are released, leading to fibrosis, calcification, or inflammation. Exudate formation leads to caseous necrosis, then liquefication of caseous material leads to cavitation.

B. Risk factors:
1. Persons who have inhaled the tubercle bacillus infectious particles called droplet nuclei.
2. Persons who have diseases or therapies known to suppress the immune system.
3. Immigrants from Latin America, Africa, Asia, and Oceania living in the United States for less than 1 year.
4. Americans living in those regions for a prolonged time.
5. Residents of U.S. metropolitan cities such as New York, Miami; those who live in poverty and are in overcrowded, poorly ventilated living conditions.
6. Men >65 yr.
7. Women between ages 26–44 yr and >65 yr.
8. Children <5 yr.

◆ **C. Assessment:**
1. *Subjective data*
   a. Loss of appetite, weight loss.
   b. Weakness, loss of energy.
   c. Pain: knifelike, chest.
   d. Though patient may be symptom free, the disease is found on screening.
2. *Objective data*
   a. Night sweats, chills.
   b. Fever: low grade, late afternoon.
   c. Pulse: increased.
   d. Respiratory assessment:
      (1) Productive persistent cough, hemoptysis.
      (2) Respirations: normal, increased depth.
      (3) Asymmetrical lung expansion.
      (4) Increased tactile fremitus.
      (5) Dullness to percussion.
      (6) Crackles following short cough.
   e. Hoarseness.
   f. Unexplained weight loss.
   g. *Diagnostic tests:*
      (1) *Positive tuberculin test (Mantoux)*—reaction to test begins approximately 12 hr after administration with area of redness and a central area of induration. The peak time is 48 hr. Determination of positive or negative is made. A reaction is positive when it measures 10 mm. Contacts reacting from 5–10 mm may need to be treated prophylactically. This test is referred to as purified protein derivative (PPD) or intradermal skin test.
      (2) *Sputum:* three specimens tested positive for acid fast (smear and culture). Positive equals greater than 10 AFB per field.
      (3) *X-ray:* infiltration cavitation.

h. Lab data: blood—*decreased* RBC, *increased* sedimentation rate.

i. Classification of tuberculosis:

Class	Description
0	No TB exposure, not infected.
1	TB exposure, no evidence of infection.
2	TB infection, no disease.
3	TB: current disease (persons with completed diagnostic evidence of TB—both a significant reaction to tuberculin skin test and clinical or x-ray evidence of disease).
4	TB: no current disease (persons with previous history of TB or with abnormal x-ray films but no significant tuberculin skin test reaction or clinical evidence).
5	TB: suspected (diagnosis pending) (used during diagnostic testing period of suspected persons, for no longer than 3 mo).

◆ **D. Analysis/nursing diagnosis:**
1. *Ineffective airway clearance* related to productive cough.
2. *Impaired gas exchange* related to asymmetrical lung expansion.
3. *Pain* related to unresolved disease process.
4. *Body image disturbance* related to feelings about tuberculosis.
5. *Social isolation* related to fear of spreading infection.
6. *Knowledge deficit* related to medication regimen.

◆ **E. Nursing care plan/implementation:**
1. Goal: *reduce spread of disease.*
   a. Administer medications: isoniazid (INH), rifampin, pyrazinamide, ethambutol, or streptomycin; or drug combinations such as Rifadin or Rifamate. Patient will be treated as an outpatient; may need to go to clinic for directly observed therapy (DOT) to ensure compliance of this long-term medication regimen.
   b. The following may need to take 300 mg of INH daily for 1 yr as *prophylactic* measure: positive skin test reactors, including contacts; persons who have diseases or are receiving therapies that affect the immune system; persons who have leukemia, lymphoma, or uncontrolled diabetes or who have had a gastrectomy.
   c. *Avoid direct contact with sputum.*
      (1) Use good hand-washing technique after contact with patient, personal articles.
      (2) Have patient cover mouth and nose when coughing and sneezing, and use disposable tissues to collect sputum.

Adult

d. *Provide good circulation of fresh air.* (Changes of air dilute the number of organisms. This plus chemotherapy provide protection needed to prevent spread of disease.)

▶ e. Implement airborne or droplet precautions (Table 7–14).

2. Goal: *promote nutrition.*
   a. *Increased protein, calories* to aid in tissue repair and healing.
   b. Small, frequent feedings.
   c. *Increased fluids,* to liquefy secretions so they can be expectorated.

3. Goal: *promote increased self-esteem.*
   a. Encourage patient and family to express concerns regarding long-term illness and treatment protocol.
   b. Explain methods of disease prevention, and encourage contacts to be tested and treated if necessary.
   c. Encourage patient to maintain role in family while home treatment is ongoing and to return to work and social contacts as soon as it is determined safe for progress of treatment plan.

4. Goal: *health teaching.*
   a. Desired effects and side effects of medications:
      (1) *INH* may affect memory and ability to concentrate. May result in peripheral neuritis, hepatitis, rash, or fever.
      (2) *Streptomycin* may cause eighth cranial nerve damage and vestibular ototoxity, causing hearing loss; may cause labyrinth damage, manifested by vertigo and staggering; also may cause skin rashes, itching, and fever.
      (3) Important for patient to know that medication regimen must be adhered to for entire course of treatment.
      (4) Discontinuation of therapy may allow organism to flourish and make the disease more difficult to treat.

TABLE 7–14 Airborne and Droplet Precautions ↺

When Used

For infectious diseases that are transmitted through inhalation of airborne particles (e.g., tuberculosis) or infected microorganisms in droplets (e.g., *Haemophilus influenzae,* pertussis)

Precautions

Isolate in private room (patients infected with same disease can be placed in same room)
Patient should wear mask if out of room for testing, etc.
Masks to be worn by personnel when working within 3 ft of patient
Gowns *not* necessary
Contaminated articles need to be labeled before being sent for decontamination
Provide adequate ventilation in patient's room
Careful hand washing

b. Need for follow-up, long-term care, and contact identification.
c. Importance of nutritious diet, rest, avoidance of respiratory infections.
d. Identify community agencies for support and follow-up.
e. Inform that this communicable disease must be reported.

◆ **F. Evaluation/outcome criteria:**
1. Complies with medication regimen.
2. Lists desired effects and side effects of medications prescribed.
3. Gains weight, eats food high in protein and carbohydrates.
4. Sputum culture becomes negative.
5. Retains role in family.
6. No complications (i.e., no hemorrhage, bacillus not spread to others).

VI. **Emphysema:** chronic disease with excessive inflation of the air spaces distal to the terminal bronchioles, alveolar ducts, and alveoli; characterized by increased airway resistance and decreased diffusing capacity. Emphysema, asthma, and chronic bronchitis together constitute chronic obstructive pulmonary disease (COPD).

A. **Pathophysiology:** imbalance between proteases, which break down lung tissue, and α_1-antitrypsin, which inhibits the breakdown. Increased airway resistance during expiration results in air trapping and hyperinflation → increased residual volumes. Increased dead space → unequal ventilation → perfusion of poorly ventilated alveoli → hypoxia and carbon dioxide retention (hypercapnia). Chronic hypercapnia reduces sensitivity of respiratory center; chemoreception in aortic arch and carotid sinus become principal regulators of respiratory drive (respond to hypoxia).

B. **Risk factors:**
1. Smoking.
2. Air pollution: long-term exposure to environmental irritants, fumes, dust.
3. Antienzymes and α_1-antitrypsin deficiencies.
4. Destruction of lung parenchyma.
5. Family history and increased age.

◆ **C. Assessment:**
1. *Subjective data*
   a. Weakness, lethargy.
   b. History of repeated respiratory infections, shortness of breath.
   c. Long-term smoking.
   d. Irritability.
   e. Inability to accept medical diagnosis and treatment plan.
   f. Refusal to stop smoking.
   g. Dyspnea on exertion, dyspnea at rest.
2. *Objective data*
   a. Increased BP.
   b. Increased pulse

c. Nostrils: flaring.

d. Cough: chronic, productive.

e. Episodes of wheezing, crackles.

f. Increased anterior-posterior diameter of chest (barrel chest).

g. Use of accessory respiratory muscles, abdominal and neck.

h. Asymmetrical thoracic movements, decreased diaphragmatic excursion.

i. *Position:* sits up, leans forward to compress abdomen and push up diaphragm, increasing intrathoracic pressure, producing more efficient expiration.

j. Pursed lips for greater expiratory breathing phase (*pink puffer*).

k. Weight loss due to hypoxia.

l. Skin: ruddy color, nail clubbing; when combined with bronchitis: cyanosis (*blue bloater*).

m. Respiratory: *early* disease—alkalosis; *late* disease—acidosis, respiratory failure.

n. Spontaneous pneumothorax.

o. Cor pulmonale (**emergency cardiac condition** involving right ventricular failure due to increased pressure within pulmonary artery).

p. X-ray: hyperinflation of lung, flattened diaphragm; lung scan differentiates between ventilation and perfusion.

q. Pulmonary function tests:
  (1) Prolonged rapid, forced exhalation.
  (2) *Decreased:* vital capacity (<4000 mL); forced expiratory volume.
  (3) *Increased:* residual volume (may be 200%); total lung capacity.

r. Lab data:
  (1) PaO_2 <80 mm Hg, pH <7.35.
  (2) $PaCO_2$ >45 mm Hg.

  Note: In patients whose compensatory mechanisms are functioning, lab values may be out of the normal range, but if a 20:1 ratio of bicarbonate to carbonic acid is maintained, then appropriate acid-base balance also will be maintained. (Carbonic acid value can be obtained by multiplying the PCO_2 value by 0.003.)

◆ **D. Analysis/nursing diagnosis:**

1. *Impaired gas exchange* related to thick pulmonary secretions.

2. *Ineffective breathing pattern* related to hyperinflated alveoli.

3. *Ineffective airway clearance* related to pulmonary secretions.

4. *Altered nutrition, less than body requirements,* related to weight loss due to hypoxia.

5. *Infection* related to chronic disease process and decreased ciliary action.

6. *Activity intolerance* related to increased energy demands used for breathing.

7. *Sleep pattern disturbance* related to changes in body positions necessary for breathing.

8. *Anxiety* related to disease progression.

9. *Knowledge deficit* related to disease, treatment, and self-care needs.

◆ **E. Nursing care plan/implementation:**

1. Goal: *promote optimal ventilation.*

  a. Institute measures designed to decrease airway resistance and enhance gas exchange.

  b. *Position:* Fowler's or leaning forward to encourage expiratory phase.

  c. Oxygen with humidification, as ordered—no more than 2 L/min to prevent depression of hypoxic respiratory drive (see Oxygen Therapy in **Unit 11,** p. 762). May need long-term oxygen therapy as disease progresses, to improve quality of life and reduce risk of complications.

  d. Intermittent positive-pressure breathing (IPPB) with nebulization as ordered.

  e. Assisted ventilation.

  f. Postural drainage, chest physiotherapy.

  g. Medications, as ordered:
    (1) *Bronchodilators* to increase airflow through bronchial tree: inhaled: β_2-adrenergic agonists (albuterol, metaproterenol); anticholinergic agent: ipratropium (Atrovent); aminophylline, theophylline, terbutaline, isoproterenol (Isuprel).
    (2) *Antimicrobials* to treat infection (determined by sputum cultures and sensitivity): trimethoprim and sulfamethoxazole (Bactrim, Septra); doxycycline, erythromycin, amoxicillin, cephalosporins, and macrolides (condition deteriorates with respiratory infections).
    (3) *Corticosteroids* to decrease inflammation, mucosal edema, improve pulmonary function during exacerbation; systemic: prednisone, methylprednisolone sodium succinate (Solu-Medrol); inhaled: trimcinolone acetonide (Azmacort), beclomethasone (Beclovent, Vanceril), flunisolide (AeroBid).
    (4) *Expectorants* (increase water intake to achieve desired effect): glyceryl guaiacolate (Robitussin).
    (5) *Bronchial detergents*/liquefying agents (Mucomyst).

  h. Immunotherapy: helps ward off life-threatening influenza and pneumonia. Flu vaccination every October or November. Pneumococcal vaccination routinely one dose; revaccinate 5 years later if high risk.

2. Goal: *employ comfort measures and support other body systems.*

a. Oral hygiene prn; frequently patient is mouth breather.

b. Skin care: waterbed, air mattress, foam pads to prevent skin breakdown.

▶ c. Active and passive ROM exercises to prevent thrombus formation; antiembolic stocking or woven elastic (Ace) bandages may be applied.

d. Increase activities to tolerance.

e. Adequate rest and sleep periods to prevent mental disturbances due to sleep deprivation and to reduce metabolic rate.

3. Goal: *improve nutritional intake.*

a. *High-protein, high-calorie diet* to prevent negative nitrogen balance.

b. Give small, frequent meals.

c. Supplement diet with high-calorie drinks.

d. *Push fluids* to 3000 mL/day, unless contraindicated—helps moisten secretions.

4. Goal: *provide emotional support for patient and family.*

a. Identify factors that increase anxiety:

(1) Fears related to mechanical equipment.

(2) Loss of body image.

(3) Fear of dying.

b. Assist family coping:

(1) Do *not* reinforce denial or encourage overconcern.

(2) Give accurate, up-to-date information on patient's condition.

(3) Be open to questioning.

(4) Encourage patient-family communication.

(5) Provide appropriate diversional activities.

5. Goal: *health teaching.*

a. Breathing exercises, such as pursed-lip breathing and diaphragmatic breathing.

b. Stress-management techniques.

c. Methods to stop smoking.

d. Importance of avoiding respiratory infections.

e. Desired effects and side effects of prescribed medications, possible interactions with over-the-counter drugs.

f. Purposes and techniques for effective bronchial hygiene therapy.

g. Rest/activity schedule that increases with ability.

h. Food selection for high-protein, high-calorie diet.

i. Importance of taking 2500–3000 mL fluid per day (unless contraindicated by another medical problem).

j. Importance of medical follow-up.

◆ F. Evaluation/outcome criteria:

1. Takes prescribed medication.

2. Participates in rest/activity schedule.

3. Improves nutritional intake, gains appropriate weight for body size.

4. No complications of respiratory failure, cor pulmonale.

5. No respiratory infections.

6. Acid-base balance maintained through compensatory mechanisms, acidosis prevented.

VII. **Asthma:** sometimes called reactive airway disease (RAD) or reversible obstructive airway disease (ROAD); a complex inflammatory process that causes increased airway resistance and, over time, airway tissue damage. Characterized by airway inflammation and hyperresponsiveness to a variety of stimuli such as allergens, cold air, dust, smoke, exercise, medications (e.g., aspirin), some food additives, and viral infections. *Immunologic* asthma occurs in childhood and follows other allergic disease. *Nonimmunologic* asthma occurs in adulthood and is associated with a history of recurrent respiratory tract infections.

A. **Pathophysiology:** triggers initiate the release of inflammatory mediators such as histamine, which produce airway obstruction through smooth muscle constriction, microvascular leakage, mucous plugging, and swelling. This process involves *six sequential steps:* (1) triggering—the allergic or antigenic stimuli activate the inflammatory (mast) cells; (2) these mast cells signal the systemic immune system to release proinflammatory substances; (3) migration of circulating inflammatory cells to regions of inflammation in the respiratory tract; (4) migrating cells are activated by the proinflammatory mediators; (5) this results in tissue damage; and (6) resolution. The airways of many asthma patients are chronically inflamed.

1. *Immunologic,* or allergic asthma in persons who are atopic (hypersensitivity state that is subject to hereditary influences); immunoglobulin E (IgE) usually elevated.

2. *Nonimmunologic,* or nonallergic asthma in persons who have a history of repeated respiratory tract infections; age usually >35 yr.

3. *Mixed,* combined immunologic and nonimmunologic; any age, allergen or nonspecific stimuli.

B. **Risk factors:**

1. History of allergies to identified or unidentified irritants; seasonal and environmental inhalants.

2. Recurrent respiratory infection.

◆ C. **Assessment:**

1. *Subjective data*

a. History: URI, rhinitis, allergies, family history of asthma.

b. Increasing tightness of the chest → dyspnea.

c. Anxiety, restlessness.

d. Attack history:

(1) *Immunologic:* contact with allergen to which person is sensitive; seen most often in children and young adults.

(2) *Nonimmunologic:* develops in adults >35 yr; aggravated by infections of the sinuses and respiratory tract.

2. *Objective data*
   a. Peak flowmeter level drops.
   b. Respiratory assessment: increased rate, audible expiratory wheeze (also inspiratory when severe) on auscultation, hyperresonance on percussion, rib retractions, use of accessory muscles on inspiration.
   c. Tachycardia, tachypnea.
   d. Cough: dry, hacking, persistent.
   e. General appearance: pallor, cyanosis, diaphoresis, chronic barrel chest, elevated shoulders, flattened molar bones, narrow nose, prominent upper teeth, dark circles under eyes, distended neck veins, orthopnea.
   f. Expectoration of tenacious mucoid sputum.
   g. *Diagnostic tests:*
      (1) Forced vital capacity (FVC): *decreased.*
      (2) Forced expiratory volume in 1 second (FEV$_1$): *decreased.*
      (3) Peak expiratory flow rate: *decreased.*
      (4) Residual volume: *increased.*
   h. Lab data: Blood gases—*elevated* PCO_2; *decreased* PO_2, pH.

   Emergency note: Persons severely affected may develop *status asthmaticus,* a **life-threatening** asthmatic attack in which symptoms of asthma continue and do not respond to usual treatment. Could lead to respiratory failure and hypoxemia.

◆ **D. Analysis/nursing diagnosis:**
   1. *Ineffective airway clearance* related to tachypnea.
   2. *Impaired gas exchange* related to constricted bronchioles.
   3. *Anxiety* related to breathlessness.
   4. *Activity intolerance* related to persistent cough.
   5. *Knowledge deficit* related to causal factors and self-care measures.

◆ **E. Nursing care plan/implementation:**
   1. Goal: *promote pulmonary ventilation.*
   a. *Position:* high Fowler's for comfort.
   b. Medications as ordered:
      (1) *Rescue* medications: corticosteroids, e.g., prednisone, methylprednisolone (Medrol); beta-adrenergic agonists, such as albuterol (Proventil, Ventolin), metaproterenol (Alupent, Metaprel).
      (2) *Maintenance* medications: nonsteroidal anti-inflammatory drugs: cromolyn (Intal), nedocromil (Tilade); corticosteroids: beclomethasone (Vanceril), trimcinolone (Azmacort); leukotriene inhibitors/receptor antagonists: zafir-

lukast (Accolate), zileuton (Zyflo); theophylline (Theo-Dur, Slo-Bid, Uni-Dur, theophylline ethylenediamino [Aminophylline]); anticholinergic: ipratropium (Atrovent); β$_2$-agonists: salmeterol (Serevent).
      (3) *Antibiotics* to control infection.
   c. Oxygen therapy with increased humidity as ordered.
   d. Frequent monitoring for respiratory distress.
   e. Rest periods and gradual increase in activity.
   2. Goal: *facilitate expectoration.*
   a. High humidity.
   b. *Increase fluid* intake.
   c. Monitor for dehydration.
   d. Respiratory therapy: IPPB.
   3. Goal: *health teaching to prevent further attacks:*
   a. Identify and avoid all asthma triggers.
   b. Teach importance of peak flow meter readings.
   c. Medications—when to use, how to use, side effects, withdrawals.
   d. Methods to facilitate expectoration—increase humidity, postural drainage when appropriate, percussion techniques.
   e. Breathing techniques to increase expiratory phase.
   f. Stress-management techniques.
   g. Importance of recognizing early signs of asthma attack and beginning treatment immediately.
   h. Steps to take during an attack.

◆ **F. Evaluation/outcome criteria:**
   1. No complications.
   2. Has fewer attacks.
   3. Takes prescribed medications, avoids infections.
   4. Adjusts lifestyle.
   5. Pulmonary function tests return to normal.

VIII. Bronchitis: acute or chronic inflammation of bronchus resulting as a complication from colds and flu. *Acute bronchitis* is caused by an extension of upper-respiratory infection, such as a cold, and can be given to others. It can also result from an irritation from physical or chemical agents. *Chronic bronchitis* is characterized by hypersecretion of mucus and chronic cough for 3 months per year for 2 consecutive years.
   A. Pathophysiology: bronchial walls are infiltrated with lymphocytes and macrophages; lumen becomes obstructed due to decreased ciliary action and repeated bronchospasms. Hyperventilation of alveolar sacs occurs. Long-term condition results in respiratory acidosis, recurrent pneumonitis, emphysema, or cor pulmonale.
   B. Risk factors:
   1. Smoking.

2. Repeated respiratory infections.
3. History of living in area where there is much air pollution.

◆ **C. Assessment:**

1. *Subjective data*
   a. History: recurrent, chronic cough, especially when arising in the morning.
   b. Anorexia.
2. *Objective data*
   a. Respiratory:
      (1) Shortness of breath.
      (2) Use of accessory muscles.
      (3) Cyanosis, dusky complexion "blue bloater."
      (4) Sputum: excessive, nonpurulent.
      (5) Vesicular and bronchovesicular breath sounds; wheezing.
   b. Weight loss.
   c. Fever.
   d. Pulmonary function tests:
      (1) *Decreased* forced expiratory volume.
      (2) PaO_2 <90 mm Hg; $PaCO_2$ >40 mm Hg.
   e. Lab data:
      (1) RBC: *elevated* to compensate for hypoxia (polycythemia).
      (2) WBC: *elevated* to fight infection.

◆ **D. Analysis/nursing diagnosis:**

1. *Ineffective airway clearance* related to excessive sputum.
2. *Ineffective breathing pattern* related to need to use accessory muscles for breathing.
3. *Impaired gas exchange* related to shortness of breath.
4. *Activity intolerance* related to increased energy used for breathing.

◆ **E. Nursing care plan/implementation:**

1. Goal: *assist in optimal respirations.*
   a. *Increase* fluid intake.
   ▶ b. IPPB, chest physiotherapy.
   c. Administer medications as ordered:
      (1) Bronchodilators.
      (2) Antibiotics.
      (3) Bronchial detergents, liquefying agents.
2. Goal: *minimize bronchial irritation.*
   a. *Avoid* respiratory irritants (e.g., smoke, dust, cold air, allergens).
   b. Environment: air-conditioned, increased humidity.
   c. Encourage nostril breathing rather than mouth breathing.
3. Goal: *improve nutritional status.*
   a. Diet: soft, *high* calorie.
   b. Small, frequent feedings.
4. Goal: *prevent secondary infections.*
   a. Administer antibiotics as ordered.
   b. *Avoid* exposure to infections, crowds.
5. Goal: *health teaching.*

a. *Avoid* respiratory infections.
b. Medications: desired effects and side effects.
c. Methods to stop smoking.
d. Rest and activity balance.
e. Stress management.

◆ **F. Evaluation/outcome criteria:**

1. Stops smoking.
2. Acid-base balance maintained.
3. Respiratory infections less frequent.

IX. Acute adult respiratory distress syndrome (ARDS) (formerly called by other names, including *shock lung*): noncardiogenic pulmonary infiltrations resulting in stiff, wet lungs and refractory hypoxemia in previously healthy adult. Acute hypoxemic respiratory failure without hypercapnea.

A. Pathophysiology: damage to alveolar capillary membrane, increased vascular permeability to pulmonary edema, and impaired gas exchange; decreased surfactant production and potential atelectasis; severe hypoxia → death.

B. Risk factors:

1. Primary:
   a. Shock, multiple trauma.
   b. Infections.
   c. Aspiration, inhalation of chemical toxins.
   d. Drug overdose.
   e. Disseminated intravascular coagulation (DIC).
   f. Emboli, especially fat emboli.
2. Secondary:
   a. Overaggressive fluid administration.
   b. Oxygen toxicity.

◆ **C. Assessment:**

1. *Subjective data*
   a. Restlessness, anxiety.
   b. History of risk factors.
   c. Severe dyspnea (Table 7–15).
2. *Objective data*
   a. Cyanosis.
   b. Tachycardia.
   c. Hypotension.
   d. Hypoxemia, acidosis.
   e. Crackles.
   f. Death if untreated.

◆ **D. Analysis/nursing diagnosis:**

1. *Anxiety* related to serious physical condition.
2. *Ineffective breathing pattern* related to severe dyspnea.
3. *Impaired gas exchange* related to alveolar damage.
4. *Altered tissue perfusion* related to hypoxia.

◆ **E. Nursing care plan/implementation:**

1. Goal: *assist in respirations.*
   ▶ a. May require mechanical ventilatory support to maintain respirations.
   b. May need to be transferred to ICU.
   ▶ c. May need oxygen to combat hypoxia.
   d. Suction prn.

TABLE 7–15   Differentiating Between Causes of Dyspnea

	Asthma	Chronic Obstructive Pulmonary Disease	Pneumothorax	Pulmonary Edema	Pulmonary Emboli
Characteristics	Episodic, acute History of allergies Recent cold or flu	History of emphysema, bronchitis Heavy smoker Recent cold or respiratory infection	Chest pain: sudden, sharp *Sudden* onset; associated with coughing, air travel, strenuous exertion	History of myocardial infarction Rapid weight gain Cough Taking diuretics Increasing need for pillows for sleep	Sudden dyspnea Sharp chest pain Recent immobilization, surgery, or fracture of lower extremeties History of thrombophlebitis, use of birth control pills, sickle cell anemia
Assessment Findings	Wheezing Hyperresonance Chest may be silent with bronchospasms	Use of pursed-lip breathing Wheezing, crackles "Barrel" chest Uses accessory muscles to breathe	Tracheal deviation Asymmetrical chest motion Diminished breath sounds	Crackles Pink, frothy sputum Gallop (S_3) Air hunger	Tachycardia Hypotension Tachypnea Pleural rub

e. Monitor blood gas results to detect early signs of acidosis/alkalosis.

f. If not on ventilator, assess vital signs and respiratory status every 15 min.

g. Cough, deep breathe every hour.

h. May need:
  ► (1) Chest percussion, vibration.
  ► (2) Postural drainage, suction.
  ◗ (3) Bronchodilator medications.

2. Goal: *prevent complications.*

a. Decrease anxiety and provide psychological care:
  (1) Maintain a calm atmosphere.
  (2) Encourage rest to conserve energy.
  (3) Emotional support.

b. Obtain fluid balance:
  (1) Slow IV flow rate.
  ◗ (2) Diuretics: rapid acting, low dose.

► c. Monitor:
  (1) Pulmonary artery and capillary wedge pressure.
  (2) Central venous pressure (CVP), cardiac output, peripheral perfusion.
  (3) I&O.
  (4) Assess for bleeding tendencies, potential for disseminated intravascular coagulation.

d. Protect from infection:
  ► (1) *Strict aseptic* technique.
  ◗ (2) Antibiotic therapy.

e. Provide physiological support:
  (1) Maintain nutrition.
  (2) Skin care.

3. Goal: *health teaching.*

a. Briefly explain procedures as they are happening (emergency situation can frighten patient).

b. Give rationale for follow-up care.

c. Identify risk factors as appropriate for prevention of recurrence.

◆ **F. Evaluation/outcome criteria:**
1. Patient survives and is alert.
2. Skin warm to touch.
3. Respiratory rate within normal limits.
4. Lab values and pressures within normal limits.
5. Urinary output >30 mL/hr.

X. Pneumothorax: presence of air within the pleural cavity; occurs spontaneously or as a result of trauma (Figure 7–6).

A. Types:
1. *Closed* (spontaneous): rupture of a subpleural bulla, tuberculous focus, carcinoma, lung abscess, pulmonary infarction, severe coughing attack, or blunt trauma.
2. *Open* (traumatic): communication between atmosphere and pleural space because of opening in chest wall.
3. *Tension:* one-way leak; may occur during mechanical ventilation or CPR, or as a complication of any type of spontaneous or traumatic pneumothorax. Positive pressure within chest cavity resulting from accumulated air that cannot escape during expiration. Leads to collapse of lung, mediastinal shift, and compression of the heart and great vessels.

B. Pathophysiology: pressure builds up in the pleural space, lung on the affected side collapses, and the heart and mediastinum shift toward the unaffected lung.

◆ **C. Assessment:**
1. *Subjective data*
  a. Pain

Adult

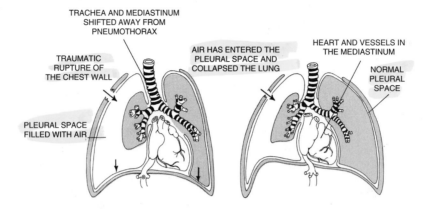

PNEUMOTHORAX
(OPEN —THE CHEST WALL INJURY PERMITS
AIR TO FLOW IN AND OUT OF THE PLEURAL
SPACE ON THE AFFECTED SIDE)

TRACHEA AND MEDIASTINUM
SHIFTED AWAY FROM
PNEUMOTHORAX

TRAUMATIC
RUPTURE OF
THE CHEST WALL

AIR HAS ENTERED THE
PLEURAL SPACE AND
COLLAPSED THE LUNG

HEART AND VESSELS IN
THE MEDIASTINUM

NORMAL
PLEURAL
SPACE

PLEURAL SPACE
FILLED WITH AIR

INHALATION: AIR ENTERS THE INJURED
SIDE, CAUSING COLLAPSE OF THE LUNG
AND SHIFT OF THE MEDIASTINUM AND
HEART TOWARD THE UNAFFECTED SIDE

EXHALATION: THE AIR IS PARTIALLY
FORCED FROM THE AFFECTED SIDE
PLEURAL SPACE AND THE MEDIASTINUM
SHIFTS TOWARD THE AFFECTED SIDE

(1) Sharp, aggravated by activity.
(2) Location—chest; may be referred to shoulder, arm on affected side.
  b. Restlessness, anxiety.
  c. Dyspnea.
2. *Objective data*
  a. Cough.
  b. Cessation of normal movements on affected side.
  c. Absence of breath sounds on affected side.
  d. Pallor, cyanosis.
  e. Shock.
  f. Tracheal deviation to unaffected side.
  g. X-ray; air in pleural space.

◆ **D. Analysis/nursing diagnosis:**
  1. *Ineffective breathing pattern* related to collapse of lung.
  2. *Impaired gas exchange* related to abnormal thoracic movement.
  3. *Pain* related to trauma to chest area.
  4. *Fear* related to emergency situation.

◆ **E. Nursing care plan/implementation:**
  1. Goal: *prevent damage until medical intervention available:*
    a. Place sterile occlusive gauze dressing over wound.
    b. Tape dressing on three sides to allow air to escape during expiration.
    c. Place patient on *affected side* to diminish possibility of tension pneumothorax.
  2. Goal: *protect against injury during thoracentesis.*
    a. Provide sterile equipment.
    b. Explain procedure.

  c. Monitor vital signs for shock.
  d. Monitor for respiratory distress, mediastinal shift.
3. Goal: *promote respirations.*
  a. *Position:* Fowler's.
  ▶ b. Oxygen therapy as ordered.
  c. Encourage slow breathing to improve gas exchange.
  d. Careful administration of narcotics to prevent respiratory depression (*avoid morphine*).
▶ 4. Goal: *prepare patient for closed chest drainage, physically and psychologically.*
  a. Explain purpose of the procedure—to provide means for evacuation of air and fluid from pleural cavity; to reestablish negative pressure in pleural space; to promote lung reexpansion.
  b. Explain procedure and apparatus (see Chest tubes in Table 11–7).
  c. Cleanse skin at tube insertion site; place patient in *sitting position,* ensuring safety by having locked over-bed table for patient to lean on, or have a nurse stay with patient so appropriate position is maintained throughout the procedure.
5. Goal: *prevent complications with chest tubes.*
  a. Observe for and immediately report crepitations (air under skin, also called *subcutaneous emphysema*), labored or shallow breathing, tachypnea, cyanosis, tracheal deviation, or signs of hemorrhage.
  b. Monitor for signs of infection.
  c. Ensure that tubing stays intact.

► d. *Monitor proper tube function.* Attach chest tube to a water-sealed drainage apparatus and use wall suction for negative pressure. Monitor amount and color of tube drainage every 2 hr. Notify MD if bloody drainage exceeds 100 mL/hr. Chest drainage system should be at least 1 ft (30 cm) below the chest tube insertion site. Change dressing at tube insertion site every 48 hr. Air bubbles will continue in the water-seal chamber for 24–48 hr after insertion. Persistent air bubbles indicate an air leak between alveoli and pleural space. Fluctuation of fluid level is expected (when suction is off) because respiration changes the pleural pressure. If a clot forms in the tube, gently squeeze the tube, without occluding it, to move the clot, or follow specific orders as written. Make sure tube is free of kinks. When moving patient, do *not* clamp tube; disconnect it from the wall suction. See key points for nursing intervention with chest tubes.

   e. *Change position* every 1–2 hr.
   f. Arm and shoulder ROM.
6. Goal: *health teaching.*
   a. How to prevent recurrence by avoiding overexertion; *avoid* holding breath.
   b. Signs and symptoms of condition.
   c. Methods to stop smoking.
   d. Encourage follow-up care.

◆ **F. Evaluation/outcome criteria:**
   1. No complications noted.
   2. Closed system remains intact until chest tubes are removed.
   3. Lung reexpands, breath sounds heard, pain diminished, symmetrical thoracic movements.

XI. Hemothorax: *presence of blood* in pleural cavity related to trauma or ruptured aortic aneurysm. See **X. Pneumothorax,** p. 487, for assessment, analysis/nursing diagnosis, nursing care plan/implementation, and evaluation/outcome criteria. Table 7–16 compares pneumothorax and hemothorax.

XII. Chest trauma

Flail chest: multiple rib fractures resulting in instability of the chest wall, with subsequent paradoxical breathing (portion of lung under injured chest wall moves in on inspiration while remaining lung expands; on expiration the injured portion of the chest wall expands while unaffected lung tissue contracts). **Sucking chest wound:** penetrating wound of chest wall with hemothorax and pneumothorax, resulting in lung collapse and mediastinal shift toward unaffected lung.

◆ **A. Assessment:**
   1. *Subjective data*
      a. Severe, sudden, sharp pain.
      b. Dyspnea.

   c. Anxiety, restlessness, fear, weakness.
   2. *Objective data*
      a. Vital signs:
         (1) Pulse: tachycardia, weak.
         (2) BP: hypotension.
         (3) Respirations: shallow, decreased expiratory force, tachypnea, stridor, accessory muscle breathing.
      b. Skin color: cyanosis, pallor.
      c. Chest:
         (1) Asymmetrical chest expansion (*paradoxical movement*).
         (2) Chest wound, rush of air through trauma site.
         (3) Crepitus over trauma site (from air escaping into surrounding tissues).
         (4) Lateral deviation of trachea, mediastinal shift.
      d. Pneumothorax: documented by absence of breath sounds, x-ray examination.
      e. Hemothorax: documented by needle aspiration by physician, x-ray examination.
      f. Shock; blood and fluid loss.
      g. Hemoptysis.
      h. Distended neck veins.

◆ **B. Analysis/nursing diagnosis:**
   1. *Ineffective airway clearance* related to shallow respirations.
   2. *Impaired gas exchange* related to asymmetrical chest expansion.
   3. *Pain* related to chest trauma.
   4. *Fear* related to emergency situation.

TABLE 7–16   Comparison of Pneumothorax and Hemothorax

	Pneumothorax (Free Air Between Visceral and Parietal Pleurae)	Hemothorax (Blood in Pleural Space)
Cause	*Spontaneous*—air enters without trauma; rupture of bleb (vesicle) on pleura; non–life threatening *Traumatic*—open chest wound: life threatening; closed chest wound—usually non–life threatening unless untreated *Tension*—air cannot escape via route of entry; causes atelectasis	Blunt trauma (assaults, falls) Penetrating trauma (knives, gunshot wounds)
◆ Assessment Findings	Minimal to sudden onset; sharp chest pain; dyspnea; cough; hypotension; tachypnea; tachycardia; mediastinal shift (tracheal deviation)	Asymptomatic or pleuritic pain and dyspnea; decreased or absent breath sounds; often discovered during chest x-ray; in severe cases: shock

5. *Risk for trauma* related to fractured ribs.
6. *Risk for infection* related to open chest wound.

◆ **C. Nursing care plan/implementation:**
   1. Goal: *restore adequate ventilation and prevent further air from entering pleural cavity:* **MEDICAL EMERGENCY.**
      ▶ a. In emergency situation: place air-occlusive dressing or hand over open wound as patient exhales forcefully against glottis (*Valsalva maneuver* helps expand collapsed lung by creating positive intrapulmonary pressures); or place patient's weight onto *affected* side. Administer oxygen.
      b. Assist with endotracheal tube insertion; patient will be placed on volume-controlled ventilator. (See discussion of ventilators under Oxygen Therapy, **Unit 11.**)
      ▶ c. Assist with thoracentesis and insertion of chest tubes with connection to water-seal drainage as ordered. (See Chest tubes section in Table 11–7.)
      d. Monitor vital signs to determine early shock.
      e. Monitor blood gases to determine early acid-base imbalances.
      ◖▮ f. Pain medications given with caution, so as not to depress respiratory center.

◆ **D. Evaluation/outcome criteria:**
   1. Respiratory status stabilizes, lung reexpands.
   2. Shock and hemorrhage are prevented.
   3. No further damage done to surrounding tissues.
   4. Pain is controlled.

XIII. Thoracic surgery: used for bronchogenic and lung carcinomas, lung abscesses, tuberculosis, bronchiectasis, emphysematous blebs, and benign tumors.
   A. Types:
   1. *Thoracotomy*—incision in the chest wall, pleura is entered, lung tissue examined, biopsy secured. *Chest tube is needed postoperatively.*
   2. *Lobectomy*—removal of a lobe of the lung. *Chest tube is needed postoperatively.*
   3. *Pneumonectomy*—removal of an entire lung. *No chest tube is needed postoperatively.*

◆ **B. Analysis/nursing diagnosis:**
   1. *Risk for injury* related to chest wound.
   2. *Impaired gas exchange* related to pain from surgical procedure.
   3. *Ineffective airway clearance* related to decreased willingness to cough due to pain.
   4. *Pain* related to surgical incision.
   5. *Impaired physical mobility* related to large surgical incision and chest tube drainage apparatus.
   6. *Knowledge deficit* related to importance of coughing and deep breathing to prevent complications.

◆ **C. Nursing care plan/implementation:**
   1. *Preoperative care.*
      a. Goal: *minimize pulmonary secretions.*

      (1) Humidify air to moisten secretions.
      (2) Use IPPB, as ordered, to improve ventilation.
      ◖▮ (3) Administer bronchodilators, expectorants, and antibiotics as ordered.
      ▶ (4) Use postural drainage, cupping, and vibration to mobilize secretions.
      b. Goal: *preoperative teaching.*
      (1) Teach patient to cough against a closed glottis to increase intrapulmonary pressure for improved expiratory phase.
      (2) Instruct in diaphragmatic breathing and coughing.
      (3) Encourage to stop smoking.
      (4) Instruct and supervise practice of postoperative arm exercises—flexion, abduction, and rotation of shoulder—to prevent ankylosis.
      (5) Explain postoperative use of chest tubes, IV, and oxygen therapy.
   2. *Postoperative care.*
      a. Goal: *maintain patent airway.*
      ▶ (1) Auscultate chest for breath sounds; report diminished or absent breath sounds on unaffected side (indicates decreased ventilation → respiratory embarrassment).
      (2) Turn, cough, and deep breathe, every 15 min to 1 hr first 24 hr and prn according to pulmonary congestion heard on auscultation.
      b. Goal: *promote gas exchange.*
      (1) Splint chest during coughing—support incision to help *cough up sputum (most important activity postoperatively).*
      ◪ (2) *Position:* high Fowler's.
         (a) Turn patient who has had a *pneumonectomy* to *operative* side (*avoid* extreme lateral positioning and mediastinal shift) to allow unaffected lung expansion and drainage of secretions; can also be turned onto back.
         (b) Patient who has had a *lobectomy* or *thoracotomy* can be turned on *either* side or back because chest tubes will be in place.
      c. Goal: *reduce incisional stress and discomfort*—pad area around chest tube when turning on operative side to maintain tube patency and promote comfort.
      d. Goal: *prevent complications related to respiratory function.*
      ▶ (1) Maintain chest tubes to water-seal drainage system.
      (2) See Chest tubes section in Table 11–7.
      (3) Observe for *mediastinal shift* (trachea should always be midline; movement toward either side indicates shift).

■ (a) Move patient onto back or toward opposite side.

(b) **MEDICAL EMERGENCY:** *Notify physician immediately.*

e. Goal: *maintain fluid and electrolyte balance.*

▶ (1) Administer parenteral infusion *slowly* (risk of pulmonary edema due to decrease in pulmonary vasculature with removal of lung lobe or whole lung).

f. Goal: *postoperative teaching.*

▶ (1) Prevent ankylosis of shoulder—teach passive and active ROM exercises of operative arm.

(2) Importance of early ambulation, as condition permits.

(3) Importance of stopping smoking.

(4) Dietary instructions—nutritious diet to aid in healing process.

(5) Importance of deep breathing, coughing exercises, to prevent stasis of respiratory secretions.

(6) Importance of *increased fluids* in diet to liquefy secretions.

(7) Desired and side effects of prescribed medications.

(8) Importance of rest, *avoidance* of heavy lifting and work during healing process.

(9) Importance of follow-up care; give names of referral agencies where patient and family can obtain assistance.

(10) Signs and symptoms of complications.

◆ **D. Evaluation/outcome criteria:**

1. Patient or significant other or both will be able to:

a. Give rationale for activity restriction and demonstrate prescribed exercises.

b. Identify name, dosage, side effects, and schedule of prescribed medications.

c. State plans for necessary modifications in lifestyle, home.

d. Identify support systems.

2. Wound heals without complications.

3. Obtains ROM in affected shoulder.

4. No complications of thoracotomy:

a. *Respiratory*—pulmonary insufficiency, respiratory acidosis, pneumonitis, atelectasis, pulmonary edema.

b. *Circulatory*—hemorrhage, hypovolemia, shock, myocardial infarction.

c. *Mediastinal shift.*

d. *Renal failure.*

e. *Gastric distention.*

XIV. Tracheostomy: opening into trachea, temporary or permanent. *Rationale:* airway obstruction due to foreign body, edema, tumor, excessive tracheobronchial secretions, respiratory depression, decreased gaseous diffusion at alveolar membrane, or

increased dead space (e.g., severe emphysema).

◆ **A. Analysis/nursing diagnosis:**

1. *Ineffective airway clearance* related to increased secretions and decreased ability to cough effectively.

2. *Ineffective breathing pattern* related to physical condition that necessitated tracheostomy.

3. *Impaired verbal communication* related to inability to speak when tracheostomy tube cuff inflated.

4. *Fear* related to need for specialized equipment to breathe.

◆ **B. Nursing care plan/implementation:**

1. *Preoperative care:*

a. Goal: *relieve anxiety and fear.*

(1) Explain purpose of procedure and equipment.

(2) Demonstrate suctioning procedure.

(3) Establish means of postoperative communication, e.g., paper and pencil, "magic slate," picture cards, and call bell. Specialized tubes such as a fenestrated tracheostomy tube or a tracheostomy button allow the individual to talk when the external opening is plugged.

(4) Remain with patient as much as possible.

2. *Postoperative care:*

a. Goal: *maintain patent airway* (Table 7–17).

TABLE 7–17 ▶Tracheostomy Suctioning Procedure

1. Suction as necessary to facilitate respirations. Explain to patient what to expect.

■2. *Position:* semi-Fowler's to prevent forward flexion of neck, to facilitate respiration, to promote drainage, and to minimize edema.

3. Administer *mist* to tracheostomy because natural humidifying of oropharynx pathways has been eliminated.

4. Auscultate for moist, noisy respirations because nonproductive coughing may indicate need for suctioning.

5. Prevent hypoxia by administering *100% oxygen before suctioning* (unless contraindicated).

6. Use *strict aseptic technique* and sterile suctioning catheters with each aspiration; use sterile saline to clear catheter of secretions. Keep dominant hand gloved with sterile glove, nondominant hand with nonsterile glove to control thumb control of suction. Suction tracheostomy before nose or mouth.

7. *Do not apply suction when inserting* suction catheter to prevent injury to respiratory tract and prevent loss of oxygen. Insert catheter about 5 in (12.5 cm).

8. If patient coughs during suctioning, gently remove catheter to permit ejection and suction of mucus.

9. Apply suction intermittently for *no longer* than 5–10 sec because prolonged suction decreases arterial oxygen concentrations. Allow 2–3 min between attempts.

10. Cuff deflation: if high-volume, low-pressure cuffed tube is used, deflation not necessary. If other tracheostomy cuffed tube is used, deflate for 5 min every hour to prevent damage to trachea.

11. Use caution not to dislodge tube when changing dressing or ties that secure tube.

Adult

b. Goal: *alleviate apprehension.*
  (1) Remain with patient as much as possible.
  (2) Encourage patient to communicate feelings using preestablished communication system.
c. Goal: *improve nutritional status.*
  (1) Provide nutritious foods/liquids the patient can swallow.
  (2) Give supplemental drinks to maintain necessary calories.
d. Goal: *health teaching.*
  (1) Explain all procedures.
  (2) Teach alternative methods of communication (best if done before the tracheostomy if it is not an emergency situation).
  (3) Teach self-care of tracheostomy as soon as possible.

◆ **C. Evaluation/outcome criteria:**
  1. Airway patent.
  2. Acid-base balance maintained.
  3. No respiratory infection/obstruction.

PROTECTIVE FUNCTIONS

I. Burns: wounds caused by exposure to excessive heat, chemicals, fire, steam, radiation, or electricity; most often related to carelessness or ignorance; 10,000–12,000 deaths annually; survival best at ages 15–30 yr and in burns covering less than 20% of total body surface.

   A. Pathophysiology:
   1. *Emergent phase* (injury to 72 hr): shock due to pain, fright, or terror → fatigue, failure of vasoconstrictor mechanisms → hypotension. Capillary dilation, increased permeability → plasma loss to blisters, edema → hemoconcentration → hypovolemia → hypotension → decreased renal perfusion → potential shut-down.
   2. *Acute phase* (3–5 days): interstitial to plasma fluid shift → hemodilution → hypervolemia → diuresis.

◆ **B. Assessment:**
   1. *Subjective data:* how the burn occurred.
   2. *Objective data:*
      a. Extent of body surface involved: *"rule of nines"*—head and both upper extremities, 9% each; front and back of trunk, 18% each; lower extremities, 18% each; and perineum, 1%. Requires adjustment for variation in size of head and lower extremities according to age.
      b. *Location*—facial, perineal, and hand and foot burns have potentially more complications because of poor vascularization.
      c. *Depth* of burn (Table 7–18):
         (1) *First degree (superficial)*—epidermal tissue only; not serious unless large areas involved.
         (2) *Second degree (shallow or deep partial thickness)*—epidermal and dermal tissue, hospitalization required if more than 10% of body surface involved (major burn).
         (3) *Third degree (full thickness)*—destruction of all skin layers; requires immediate hospitalization; involvement of 10% of body surface considered major burn.
         (4) *Fourth degree (deep penetrating)*—muscles (fascia), bone.
      d. Indications of airway burns, e.g., singed nasal hair, progressive hoarseness, sooty expectoration; edema may occur in 1 hr; increased mortality rate.
      e. Poorer prognosis—*infants*, due to immature immune system and effects of fluid loss; *elderly*, due to degenerative diseases and poor healing.
      f. Medical history—presence of hypertension, diabetes, alcohol abuse, or chronic obstructive pulmonary disease increases complication rate.

◆ **C. Analysis/nursing diagnosis:**
   1. *Impaired skin integrity* related to thermal injury.
   2. *Pain* (depending on type of burn) related to exposure of sensory receptors.
   3. *Fluid volume excess or deficit* related to hemodynamic changes.
   4. *Risk for infection* related to destruction of protective skin.
   5. *Impaired gas exchange* related to airway injury.
   6. *Body image disturbance* related to scarring, disfigurement.
   7. *Ineffective individual or family* coping related to traumatic experience.

◆ **D. Nursing care plan/implementation:**
   1. Goal: *alleviate pain, relieve shock, and maintain fluid and electrolyte balance.*
      a. Medications: give opioid analgesic and anxiolytics incrementally.

TABLE 7–18   Burn Characteristics According to Depth of Injury

Classification	Tissue Damage	Appearance	Pain	Clinical Course
Superficial (first degree)	Epidermis	Mild to fiery red erythema; no blisters	Very painful	Ordinarily heals in 3–7 days
Partial thickness; superficial or deep (second degree)	Epidermis and dermis	*Superficial:* mottled, moist, pink or red; may or may not blanch with pressure; usually blisters *Deep:* dry-white or deep red	*Superficial:* extreme pain and hypersensitivity to touch *Deep:* may or may not be painful	Healing takes 10–18 days; if infection develops in deep burn, it converts to full-thickness burn *Deep:* often grafted
Full thickness (third degree)	All layers of skin and subcutaneous tissue	Charred, leathery or pale and dry	Usually absent	Heals only with grafting or scarring
*Fourth degree	All layers of skin, subcutaneous tissue, muscle, and bone	Black	Same as full thickness	Same as full thickness

*Used in some classification systems. May require several days after a severe burn to determine fourth degree.

b. *Fluids:* IV therapy (see **Unit 11**); colloids, crystalloids, or 5% dextrose according to burn formula.

c. Monitor hydration status:

▶ (1) Insert indwelling catheter.

(2) Note color, odor, and amount of urine hourly.

(3) *Strict* intake and output; hourly for 36 hr with large burns.

(4) Check hematocrit (normal: men >40%; women >37%). Increased Hct with intravascular fluid depletion.

(5) Weigh daily.

2. Goal: *prevent physical complications.*

▶ a. Vital signs: hourly; central venous pressure (CVP) for signs of shock or fluid overload with at-risk patients.

b. Assess respiratory function (particularly with head, neck burns); patent airway; breath sounds.

c. Give medications as ordered—*tetanus booster; antibiotics* to treat documented infection; *sedatives* and *analgesics; antipyretics*—**avoid** aspirin; H$_2$ blockers.

d. *Isolation:* protective; contact isolation (hand washing, protective clothing).

e. *Positioning:* turn q2h; prevent contractures.

(1) Head and neck burns—use pillows under shoulders only for hyperextension of neck.

(2) Hand burns—splints.

(3) Arm and hand burns—keep arms at 90-degree angle from body and slightly above shoulders.

(4) Ankle and foot burns—splints; elevate to prevent edema.

(5) Splints to maintain functional positions.

(6) ROM exercises according to therapy guidelines; usually several times per day; active exercises most beneficial.

f. *Diet:* begin oral fluids at once; food as tolerated—*high* protein, *high* calorie for energy and tissue repair (promote positive nitrogen balance); enteral feedings if protein and calorie goals not met.

g. Observe for: constriction (circumferential or chest wall burns); check peak inspiratory pressure in intubated patient—report increased pressure; check pulses in burned extremities every 1–2 hr for 24 hr—report loss of pulses.

3. Goal: *promote emotional adjustment and provide supportive therapy.*

a. Care by same personnel as much as possible, to develop rapport and trust.

b. Involve patient in care plans.

c. Answer questions clearly, accurately.

d. Encourage family involvement and participation.

e. Provide diversional activities and change furnishings or room adornments when possible, to prevent perceptual deprivation related to immobility.

f. Point out signs of progress (e.g., decreased edema, healing) because patient and family tend to become discouraged and cannot see progress.

g. Encourage self-care to highest level tolerated.

h. Anticipate psychological changes:

(1) *Acute period*—severe anxiety: medicate with *anxiolytics* as ordered; maintain eye contact; explain procedures.

(2) *Intermediate period*—reactions associated with pain, dependency, depression, anger; give medications to decrease pain; explain procedures; have open, nonjudgmental attitude; use consistent approaches to care; contract with patient regarding division of responsibilities; encourage self-care.

(3) *Recuperative period*—grief process reactivated. Anxiety, depression, anger, bargaining, as patient tries to cope with altered body image, leaving security of hospital, finances. Encourage verbalization; refer to support group to assist adaptation.

4. Goal: *promote wound healing*—wound care:

a. *Open method*—exposure of burns to air; useful in burns of face; thin layer (2–4 mm) topical antimicrobial ointment applied.

b. *Closed method*—dressings applied to burned areas, changed 1–3 times/day; give PO pain medication 30 min before change; IV pain medication during dressing change; tubbing facilitates removal.

c. *Multiple dressing change*—common approach; dressings changed bid to q4h depending on wound condition.

d. *Topical antimicrobial therapies* (Table 7–19).

e. *Tubbing and debridement.*

(1) Hydrotherapy—body temperature bath water; loosens dressings so some float off; soak 20–30 min; encourage limb exercises; do *not* leave unattended; loss of body heat may occur, with chilling and poor perfusion resulting.

(2) Removal of eschar *(debridement)*—done with forceps and curved scissors; medicate for pain before; use *sterile technique;* only loose eschar removed, to prevent bleeding; examine wound for infection, color change, decreased granulation—report changes immediately. Chemical debridement also done; agent digests necrotic tissue.

TABLE 7–19   Topical Antimicrobials Used in Burn Care ⬤⬤

Agent	Advantages	Disadvantages	▶ Nursing Implications
Silver sulfadiazine 1% (Silvadene)	Broad-spectrum antimicrobial Antifungal Nonstaining Relatively painless No systemic metabolic abnormalities	Less eschar penetration than mafenide acetate (Sulfamylon) Decreased granulocyte formation; transient leukopenia Macular rash	Check for allergy to sulfa
Mafenide acetate (Sulfamylon) cream or solution	Eschar penetration Effective with *Pseudomonas* Topical of choice for electrical burns Suitable for open or closed method of treatment (cream) Used for gram-negative organisms	Severe pain and burning sensation (lasts 30 min) Metabolic acidosis Carbonic anhydrase inhibitor Ineffective against fungi May cause hypersensitivity rash	⬤⬤ Administer pretreatment analgesic Monitor for metabolic acidosis and hyperventilation Check for allergy to sulfa; observe for rash
Silver nitrate	Low cost Broad spectrum Effective with *Candida*	Continuous wet soaks Superficial penetration Black staining of sheets Stinging Electrolyte imbalances (low sodium, low chloride, low calcium, low potassium), alkalosis	Check serum electrolytes daily Rewet dressing to keep moist
Petroleum and mineral oil–based (e.g., Bacitracin, Neosporin, Polysporin)	Bactericidal, gram-positive and gram-negative organisms Painless Prevents drying of wound	Limited ability to penetrate eschar	Apply in thin layer (1 mm) Reapply as needed.

TABLE 7–20   Wound Coverings

Example	Advantages	Disadvantages	▶ Nursing Implications
Biological Xenograph	Promotes healing of clean wound; relieves pain; readily available; reduces water and heat loss	Easily digested by wound collagenase; allergic reactions	Overlap edges slightly; trim away when skin underneath has healed
Homograft-cadaver skin	Reduces water and heat loss; relieves pain; used with antimicrobial mesh; may be left in place until rejection occurs	May harbor disease	Observe for signs of infection
Amnion	Relieves pain; reduces water and heat loss; has bacteriostatic properties	Limited shelf life; requires special preparation for use; may harbor diseases	Change cover dressing q48h; leave on wound until it sloughs
Biosynthetic (Temporary) Biobrane	Protects from microbial penetration; decreases pain; promotes healing in partial-thickness burn	Not effective for preparing a granulation bed	Must be secured to skin with sutures, closure straps, tape, or staples; wrap with gauze; after 48 hr, check for adherence; once adherence has occurred, may be left open to air; check for signs of infection
Biosynthetic (Semipermanent) Integra Artificial Skin	Postexcisional treatment of life-threatening full or deep partial-thickness burns when autograft not available	Infection rate lower than autograft	Maintain integrity of covering; 18–20 days before thin autograft applied. *Avoid* hydrotherapy; observe for infection.

f. Wound coverage, to decrease chances of infection:
  (1) Temporary and semipermanent wound coverings (Table 7–20).
  (2) *Autograft*—patient donates skin for wound coverage

  (a) Types—free grafts (unattached to donor site) and pedicle grafts (attached to donor site).
  (b) Procedure—general anesthesia; donor sites shaved and prepared; graft applied to granulation bed;

face, hands, and arms grafted first.

(c) *Post–skin-graft care:*

▶ (i) Sheet grafts: roll cotton-tipped applicator over graft to remove excess exudate; maintain dressings; *aseptic technique;* mesh grafts: irrigate as ordered.

(ii) Third to fifth day—graft takes on pink appearance if it has taken.

(iii) Padding, then splints applied to immobilize grafted extremities.

(iv) Pressure garments worn up to 18 months to decrease hypertrophic scarring.

5. Goal: *health teaching.*

a. Mobility needs: exercise; physical therapy; splints, braces.

b. Community resources: mental health practitioner or psychotherapist if needed for problems with self-image or sexual role; referrals as needed.

c. Techniques to camouflage appearance: slacks, turtlenecks, long sleeves, wigs, makeup.

◆ E. **Evaluation/outcome criteria:**

1. Return of vital signs to preburn levels.

2. Minimal to no hypertrophic scarring.

3. Free of infection; demonstrates wound care.

4. Maintains functional mobility of limbs; no contractures.

5. Adjusts to changes in body image; no depression.

6. Regains independence; returns to work, social activities.

II. **Lyme disease:** a spirochetal illness (syndrome); most common tick-borne infectious disease in United States; prevalent Northeast, upper Midwest, and coastal northern California. Reporting is **mandatory.** With *early* treatment, recovery is usually quick and complete.

A. **Stages:**

1. *Stage I.* Rash (erythema migrans) at site of tick bite; bull's-eye or target pattern; may appear as hives or cellulitis; common in moist areas (groin, armpit, behind knees). Flulike symptoms may occur (joint pain, chills, fever).

2. *Stage II.* If untreated, may progress to cardiac problems (10% of patients) or neurological disturbances—Bell's palsy (10% of patients); occasionally meningitis, encephalitis, and eye damage may result.

3. *Stage III.* From 4 wk to 1 yr after the tick bite, "arthritis," primarily large joint, develops in half the patients. If untreated, chronic neurological problems may develop.

◆ B. **Assessment** (depends on stage): History is important—where do they live or work? Recent travel? Outdoor activities (gardening, hiking, camping, clearing brush)? Knowledge of tick bite and how removed? Pets?

1. *Subjective data:*

a. Malaise (stage I).

b. Headache (stage I).

c. Joint, neck, or back pain (stages I and III).

d. Weakness (stages II and III).

e. Chest pain (stage II).

f. Light-headedness (stage II).

g. Numbness, pain in arms or legs (stage III).

2. *Objective data:*

a. Rash—erythema migrans (stage I); at least 5 cm/lesion.

b. Dysrhythmias; heart block (stage II).

c. Facial paralysis (stage II).

d. Conjunctivitis, iritis, optic neuritis (stage II).

e. Lab data: Lyme titer—*elevated* (stages II and III). Often inconclusive.

f. *Diagnostic tests:* isolation of *Borrelia burgdorferi* in tissue or body fluid; diagnostic levels of IgM or IgG antibodies in serum or CSF.

◆ C. **Analysis/nursing diagnosis:**

1. *Anxiety* related to diagnosis.

2. *Pain* related to joint inflammation.

3. *Fatigue* related to viral illness.

4. *Impaired physical mobility* related to joint pain.

5. *Altered thought processes* related to neurological deficit.

6. *Decreased cardiac output* related to dysrhythmias.

7. *Knowledge deficit* (learning need) related to treatment and course of disease.

◆ D. **Nursing care plan/implementation:**

1. Goal: *minimize irreversible tissue damage and complications.*

a. Medications according to presenting symptoms: *stage I*—oral antibiotics for 21 days (doxycycline, amoxicillin, cefotaxime); *stages II and III*—oral (see stage I) or intravenous antibiotics for 21–28 days (ceftriaxone).

b. If hospitalized, monitor vital signs q4h for increased temperature, signs of heart failure; check level of consciousness and cranial nerve functioning.

c. Note treatment response: worsening of symptoms during first 24 hr; redder rash, higher fever, greater pain (*Jarisch-Herxheimer reaction*).

2. Goal: *alleviate pain, promote comfort.*

a. Medications: salicylates, nonsteroidal anti-inflammatory agents, or other analgesic, as ordered; observe for side effects (GI irritation).

Adult

b. Rest: give instructions on relaxation techniques; create a quiet environment.

3. Goal: *maintain physical and psychological well-being.*

   a. Activity: ROM at regular intervals; *medicate for pain* before exercise; encourage proper posture to reduce joint stress; rest periods between activities and treatments.

   b. Referral: occupational or physical therapy as appropriate.

   c. Reassurance: give psychological support; encourage discussion of feelings.

4. Goal: *health teaching.*

   a. Information on disease. Transmission from tick not likely if removed before 48 hours of attachment.

   b. Instructions for home IV antibiotics with heparin lock, if ordered.

   c. Side effects of antibiotics (drug specific); importance of completing therapy.

   d. Signs of disease recurrence (later stages of disease: less severe attacks).

   e. Preventing subsequent infections: wear proper clothing and tick repellent on clothing (20–30% DEET); conduct "tick checks" of self, children, and pets; proper tick removal (use tweezers, steady, gentle traction).

   f. Start vaccination series (LYMErix); three injections at 0, 1, and 12 months.

◆ **E. Evaluation/outcome criteria:**

1. Achieves reasonable comfort.

2. Regains normal physiological and psychological functioning—no irreversible complications; vital signs within normal limits.

3. Resumes previous activity level; returns to work.

4. Adheres to follow-up care recommendations.

5. Knows ways to minimize risk of reinfection.

III. Rheumatoid arthritis: chronic, systemic, collagen, inflammatory disease; etiology unknown; may be autoimmune, viral, or genetic; affects primarily women age 20–40 yr; present in 2–3% of total population; follows a course of exacerbations and remissions.

  A. Pathophysiology: synovitis with edema → proliferation of various blood material (formation of pannus) → destruction and fibrosis of cartilage (fibrous ankylosis); calcification of fibrous tissue (osseous ankylosis). See Figure 7–7.

◆ **B. Assessment:**

1. *Subjective data:*

   a. Joints: pain; morning stiffness; swelling.

   b. Easily fatigues; malaise.

   c. Anorexia; weight loss.

2. *Objective data:*

   a. Subcutaneous nodules over bony prominences.

   b. Bilateral symmetrical involvement of joints: crepitation, creaking, grating.

   c. Deformities: contractures, muscle atrophy.

   d. Lab data: blood: *decreased*—hemoglobin/hematocrit; RBCs; *increased*—WBCs (12,000–15,000), sedimentation rate (>20 mm/hr), rheumatoid factor.

◆ **C. Analysis/nursing diagnosis:**

1. *Pain* related to joint destruction.

2. *Impaired physical mobility* related to joint contractures.

FIGURE 7–7 Rheumatoid arthritis. (From Thomas, CL [ed]: Taber's Cyclopedic Medical Dictionary, ed 18. FA Davis, Philadelphia, 1997, p 153.)

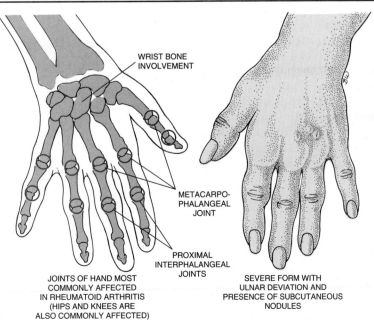

WRIST BONE INVOLVEMENT

METACARPO-PHALANGEAL JOINT

PROXIMAL INTERPHALANGEAL JOINTS

JOINTS OF HAND MOST COMMONLY AFFECTED IN RHEUMATOID ARTHRITIS (HIPS AND KNEES ARE ALSO COMMONLY AFFECTED)

SEVERE FORM WITH ULNAR DEVIATION AND PRESENCE OF SUBCUTANEOUS NODULES

3. *Risk for injury* related to the inflammatory process.
4. *Body image disturbance* related to joint deformity.
5. *Self-care deficit* related to musculoskeletal impairment.
6. *Risk for activity intolerance* related to fatigue and stiffness.
7. *Altered nutrition, less than body requirements,* related to anorexia and weight loss.
8. *Self-esteem disturbance* related to chronic illness.

◆ **D. Nursing care plan/implementation:**
1. Goal: *prevent or correct deformities.*
  a. Activity:
    (1) Bed rest during exacerbations.
  ▶ (2) Daily ROM—active and passive exercises *even* in acute phase 5–10 min periods; *avoid* fatigue and persistent pain.
    (3) Heat or pain medication before exercise.
  b. Medications: *aspirin* (high dosages); *nonsteroidals; steroids; antacids* given for possible GI upset with ASA, steroids; *disease-modifying antirheumatics* (methotrexate, hydroxychloroquine, sulfasalazine).
  c. *Fluids:* at least 1500 mL liquid daily to avoid renal calculi; milk for GI upset.
2. Goal: *health teaching.*
  a. Side effects of medications: tarry stools (GI bleeding); tinnitus (ASA).
  b. Psychosocial aspects: possible need for early retirement; financial hardship; loss of libido; unsatisfactory sexual relations.
  c. Prepare for joint repair or replacement if indicated.

◆ **E. Evaluation/outcome criteria:**
1. Remains as active as possible; limited loss of mobility; performs self-care activities.
2. No side effects from drug therapy (e.g., GI bleeding).
3. Copes with necessary lifestyle changes; complies with treatment regimen.

IV. Lupus erythematosus: chronic inflammatory disease of connective tissue; may affect or involve any organ; vague etiology, but genetic factors, viruses, hormones, and drugs are being investigated; occurs primarily in women ages 18–35 yr. Two forms: discoid lupus erythematosus (DLE) affects skin only, and systemic lupus erythematosus (SLE) affects multiple organs.

A. Pathophysiology: possible toxic effects from immune complexes deposited in tissue (antibody-antigen trapping in organ capillaries)—fibrinoid necrosis of collagen in connective issue, small arterial walls (kidneys and heart particularly) → cellular death, obstructed blood flow.

◆ **B. Assessment:**
1. *Subjective data:*

  a. Pain: joints.
  b. Anorexia; weight loss.
  c. Photophobia; sensitivity to sun.
  d. Weakness.
  e. Nausea, vomiting.
2. *Objective data:*
  a. Fever.
  b. Rash: butterfly distribution across nose, cheeks.
  c. Lesions: raised, red, scaling plaques—coinlike (discoid).
  d. Ulceration: oral or nasopharyngeal.
  e. Lab data:
    (1) Blood: *increased* LE cells; *decreased*—RBCs, WBCs, thrombocytes.
    (2) *Urine*—hematuria, proteinuria (nephritis).

◆ **C. Analysis/nursing diagnosis:**
1. *Risk for injury* related to possible autoimmune disorder.
2. *Pain* related to joint inflammation.
3. *Risk for activity intolerance* related to extreme fatigue, anemia.
4. *Body image disturbance* related to chronic skin eruptions.
5. *Altered nutrition, less than body requirements,* related to anorexia, nausea, vomiting.
6. *Altered oral mucous membrane* related to ulcerations.

◆ **D. Nursing care plan/implementation:**
1. Goal: *minimize or limit immune response and complications.*
  a. Activity: rest; 8–10 hr sleep; unhurried environment; assist with stressful activities; ROM to prevent joint immobility and stiffness.
  b. Skin care: hygiene; topical steroid cream as ordered for inflammation, pruritus, scaling.
  c. Mouth care: several times daily if stomatitis present; *soft, bland, or liquid diet* to prevent irritation.
  d. *Diet: low* sodium if edematous; *low* protein with renal involvement.
  e. Observe for signs of complications:
    (1) Cardiac/respiratory (tachycardia, tachypnea, dyspnea, orthopnea).
    (2) GI (diarrhea, abdominal pain, distention).
    (3) *Renal* (increased weight, oliguria, decreased specific gravity).
    (4) *Neurological* (ptosis, ataxia).
    (5) *Hematological* (malaise, weakness, chills, epistaxis); **report immediately.**
  f. Medications, as ordered:
    (1) *Analgesics.*
    (2) *Anti-inflammatory* agents (aspirin, prednisone) and *immunosuppressive drugs* (azathioprine [Imuran], cy-

clophosphamide [Cytoxan]) to control inflammation.

    (3) *Antimalarials* for skin and joint manifestations.

  2. Goal: *health teaching.*

    a. Disease process: diagnosis, prognosis, effects of treatment.

    b. *Avoid* precipitating factors:

      (1) Sun (aggravates skin lesions; thus, cover body as much as possible).

      (2) Altering dosage of medications.

      (3) Pregnancy requires medical clearance.

      (4) Fatigue, stress.

      (5) Infections.

    c. Medications: side effects of immunosuppressives and corticosteroids.

    d. Regular exercise: walking, swimming; but *avoid* fatigue.

    e. Wear Medic Alert bracelet.

◆ **E. Evaluation/outcome criteria:**

  1. Attains a state of remission.

  2. No organ involvement (e.g., cardiac, renal complications).

  3. Keeps active within limitations.

  4. Continues follow-up medical care—recognizes symptoms requiring immediate attention.

V. Acquired immunodeficiency syndrome (AIDS): the terminal stage of the disease continuum caused by human immunodeficiency virus (HIV), a retrovirus; typically progresses from asymptomatic seronegative status to asymptomatic seropositive status to subclinical immune deficiency to lymphadenopathy (early AIDS) to AIDS-related complex (middle stage with combination of symptoms) to AIDS; hallmarks of HIV infection include opportunistic infections: *Pneumocystis carinii* pneumonia (PCP); cytomegalovirus (CMV); *Mycobacterium tuberculosis;* hepatitis B; herpes simplex or zoster; candidiasis; may take 7–10 yr before signs and symptoms occur.

  A. High-risk populations:

    1. Men, homosexual or bisexual (71%).

    2. Injection drug users (IDU)/heterosexual (10%).

    3. IDU/homosexual (9%).

    4. Hemophiliacs and multiple transfusion recipients (1%).

    5. Heterosexual (5%).

    6. Undetermined/other (4%).

  B. Pathophysiology: abnormal response to foreign antigen stimulation (acquired immunity) → deficiency in cell-mediated immunity—T lymphocytes, specifically helper cells (T4 cells) and hyperactivity of the humoral system (B cells).

◆ **C. Assessment:**

  1. *Subjective data:*

    a. Fatigue: prolonged; associated with headache or light-headedness.

    b. Unexplained weight loss: >10%.

  2. *Objective data:*

    a. Fever: prolonged or night sweats >2 wk.

    b. Lymphadenopathy.

    c. Skin or mucous membrane lesions: purplish-red, nodules (*Kaposi's sarcoma*).

    d. Cough: persistent, heavy, dry.

    e. Diarrhea: persistent.

    f. Tongue/mouth "thrush"; oral hairy leukoplakia.

    g. *Diagnostic tests* (with permission of patient): enzyme-linked immunosorbent assay (ELISA); Western blot test.

    h. Lab data: *decreased*—CD4 (T4) lymphocytes, hematocrit, WBC, platelets. *Seropositive*—syphilis, hepatitis B; ELISA—*positive*; Western blot test—*positive* (mean time for seroconversion is 6 wk after infection).

◆ **D. Analysis/nursing diagnosis:**

  1. *Risk for infection* related to immunocompromised state.

  2. *Fatigue* related to anemia.

  3. *Altered nutrition, less than body requirements,* related to anorexia.

  4. *Impaired skin integrity* related to nonhealing viral lesions, Kaposi's sarcoma.

  5. *Diarrhea* related to infection or parasites.

  6. *Risk for activity* intolerance related to shortness of breath.

  7. *Ineffective airway clearance* related to pneumonia.

  8. *Visual sensory/perception alteration* related to retinitis.

  9. *Risk for altered body temperature* (fever) related to opportunistic infections.

  10. *Social isolation* related to stigma attached to AIDS.

  11. *Powerlessness* related to inability to control disease progression.

  12. *Altered thought processes* related to dementia.

  13. *Ineffective individual coping* related to poor prognosis.

  14. *Risk for violence, self-directed,* related to anger, panic, or depression.

◆ **E. Nursing care plan/implementation:**

  1. Goal: *reduce risk of infection; slow disease progression.*

    a. Observe signs of opportunistic infections: weight loss, diarrhea, skin lesions, sore throat.

    b. Monitor vital signs (including temperature).

    c. Note secretions and excretions: changes in color, consistency, or odor indicating infection.

    d. *Diet:* monitor fluid and electrolytes; strict measurement; encourage adequate dietary intake (*high* calorie, *high* protein, *low* bulk); 5–10 times RDA for water-soluble vitamins (B complex, C); favorite foods from home; enteral feedings. Six small meals/day.

e. *Protective isolation*, if indicated, for severe immunocompromise.

f. Antiviral medications, as ordered: nucleoside reverse transcriptase inhibitors, e.g., zidovudine (Retrovir); nonnucleoside reverse transcriptase inhibitors, e.g., nevirapine (Viramune); protease inhibitors, e.g., indinavir sulfate (Crixivan); drug toxicity and numerous side effects likely (rash, GI upset); large number of pills and tight administration schedule; costly; potential for drug resistance.

2. Goal: *prevent the spread of disease.*
   a. Frequent hand washing, even after wearing gloves.
   b. *Avoid* exposure to blood, body fluids of patient; wear gloves, gowns; proper disposal of needles, IV catheters (Table 7–21).

3. Goal: *provide physical and psychological support.*
   a. Oral care: frequent.
   b. Cooling bath: 1:10 concentration of isopropyl alcohol in tepid water; *avoid* plastic-backed pads with night sweats.
   c. Encourage verbalization of fears, concerns without condemnation; may suffer loss of job, lifestyle, significant other.
   d. Determine status of support network: arrange contact with support group.
   e. Observe for severe emotional symptoms (suicidal tendencies).
   f. Address issues surrounding death to ensure quality of life: advance directive prepared and on file; code blue status; reassurance of comfort and pain control.

4. Goal: *health teaching.*
   a. Avoidance of environmental sources of infection (kitty litter, bird cages, tub bathing).
   b. Precautions following discharge: risk-reducing behaviors; condoms (latex), limit number of sexual partners, *avoid* exposure to blood or semen during intercourse.
   c. Family counseling; availability of community resources.
   d. Information on disease progression and life span.
   e. Stress-reduction techniques: visualization, guided imagery, meditation.
   f. Expected side effects with drug therapy; importance of compliance.

◆ **F. Evaluation/outcome criteria:**
   1. Relief of symptoms (e.g., afebrile, gains weight).
   2. Resumes self-care activities; returns to work; improved quality of life.
   3. Accepts diagnosis; participates in support group.
   4. Progression of disease slows; improved survival probability.
   5. Retains autonomy, self-worth.
   6. Permitted to die with dignity.

TABLE 7–21   Standard Precautions

- **Wash your hands** and any other skin surfaces immediately and thoroughly if they become contaminated with blood or other body fluids. Use lots of soap and hot water.

- **Wear clean gloves** whenever there is potential exposure to blood or other body fluids except sweat. Wear surgical gloves for performing venipunctures, for touching mucous membranes or nonintact skin, or whenever there is a possibility of exposure to blood or body fluids. **Remove gloves** after contact with each patient. **Discard used gloves** immediately after use in an appropriate receptacle (e.g., a plastic bag with a "biohazard" label). **Wash your hands** immediately after removing gloves.

- Use *mask, protective eyewear, face shield, gown* during any procedure that is likely to generate splashes of blood or other body fluids.

- Handle all **needles, intravenous equipment,** and **sharp instruments** with extreme care:
  1. *Never* recap, remove, bend, or break needles after use or manipulate them in any other way by hand.
  2. Dispose of syringes, needles, scalpel blades, and other sharp items in a puncture-resistant container kept within easy reach.

The Perioperative Experience

I. Preoperative preparation
◆ **A. Assessment:**
   1. *Subjective data:*
      a. Understanding of proposed surgery—site, type, extent of hospitalization.
      b. Previous experiences with hospitalization.
      c. Age-related factors.
      d. Allergies—iodine, latex, adhesive tape, cleansing solutions, medications.
      e. Medication/substance use—prescribed, OTC, smoking, alcohol, recreational drugs.
      f. Cultural and religious background.
      g. Concerns or feelings about surgery:
         (1) Exaggerated ideas of surgical risk, e.g., fear of colostomy when none is being considered.
         (2) Nature of anesthesia, e.g., fears of going to sleep and not waking up, saying or revealing things of a personal nature.

(3) Degree of pain, i.e., may be incapacitating.

(4) Misunderstandings regarding prognosis.

h. Identification of significant others as a source of patient support or care responsibilities postdischarge.

2. *Objective data:*

a. Speech patterns indicating anxiety—repetition, changing topics, avoiding talking about feelings.

b. Interactions with others—withdrawn or involved.

c. Physical signs of anxiety, i.e., increased pulse, respirations; clammy palms, restlessness.

d. Baseline physiological status: vital signs; breath sounds; peripheral circulation; weight; hydration status (hematocrit, skin turgor, urine output); degree of mobility; muscle strength.

◆ **B. Analysis/nursing diagnosis:**

1. *Anxiety* related to proposed surgery.

2. *Knowledge deficit* (learning need) related to incomplete teaching or lack of understanding.

3. *Fear* related to threat of death or disfigurement.

4. *Risk for injury* related to surgical complications.

5. *Ineffective individual coping* related to anticipatory stress.

◆ **C. Nursing care plan/implementation:**

1. Goal: *reduce preoperative and intraoperative anxiety and prevent postoperative complications.*

a. *Preoperative teaching:*

(1) Provide information about hospital nursing routines and preoperative procedures to reduce fear of unknown.

(2) Explain purpose of diagnostic procedures to enhance ability to cooperate and tolerate procedure.

(3) What will occur and what will be expected in the postoperative period:

(a) Will return to room, postanesthesia care unit, or intensive care unit.

(b) Special equipment—monitors, tubes, suction equipment.

(c) Pain control methods.

b. *Management of latex allergy if present.* Three forms: *immediate reaction* (most serious, life threatening)—flushing, diaphoresis, pruritus, nausea, vomiting, cramping, hypotension, dyspnea; *delayed response* (most common, discomfort)—localized symptoms 18–24 hr after contact; and *contact dermatitis.* Exposure to latex through skin, mucous membranes, inhalation, internal tissue, and intravascular; sources include: anesthesia masks, tourniquets, ECG electrodes, adhesive tape, warming blankets, elastic bandages, gloves, tubes/catheters, irrigation syringes. **Nursing goal:** provide latex-free environment.

2. Goal: *instruct in exercises to reduce complications.*

a. *Diaphragmatic breathing*—refers to flattening of diaphragm during inspiration, which results in enlargement of upper abdomen; during expiration the abdominal muscles are contracted, along with the diaphragm.

(1) The patient should be in a *flat, semi-Fowler's,* or *side position,* with knees flexed and hands on the midabdomen.

(2) Have the patient take a deep breath through nose and mouth, letting the abdomen rise. Hold breath 3–5 seconds.

(3) Have patient exhale through nose and mouth, squeezing out all air by contracting the abdominal muscles.

(4) Repeat 10–15 times, with a short rest after each five to prevent hyperventilation.

(5) Inform patient that this exercise will be repeated 5–10 times every hour postoperatively.

b. *Coughing*—helps clear chest of secretions and, although uncomfortable, will not harm incision site.

(1) Have patient lean forward slightly from a sitting position, and place patient's hands over incisional site; this acts as a splint during coughing.

(2) Have patient inhale and exhale slowly several times.

(3) Have patient inhale deeply, hold breath 3 seconds, and cough sharply three times while exhaling—patient's mouth should be slightly open.

(4) Tell patient to inhale again and to cough deeply once or twice. If unable to cough deeply, patient should "huff" cough to stimulate cough.

c. *Turning and leg exercises*—help prevent circulatory stasis, which may lead to thrombus formation, and postoperative flatus or "gas pains," as well as respiratory problems.

(1) Tell patient to turn on one side with uppermost leg flexed; use side rails to facilitate the movement.

(2) In a supine position, have patient do five repetitions every hour of: ankle

pumps, quad sets, gluteal tightenings, and straight-leg raises.

▶ (3) Apply intermittent pulsatile compression device or sequential compression device to promote venous return.

3. Goal: *reduce the number of bacteria on the skin to eliminate incision contamination.* **Skin preparation:**

a. Prepare area of skin wider and longer than proposed incision in case a larger incision is necessary.

b. Gently scrub with an antimicrobial agent.
   (1) Note possibility of allergy to iodine.
   (2) Hexachlorophene should be left on the skin for 5–10 min.
   (3) If benzalkonium Cl (Zephiran) solution is ordered, do *not* soap skin before use; soap reduces effectiveness of benzalkonium by causing it to precipitate.

c. Hair should remain *unless* it interferes with surgical procedure.
   (1) Note any nicks, cuts, or irritations, potential infection sites.
   (2) Depilatory creams or clipping of hair is preferred to shaving with a razor; nick may result in cancellation of surgery.
   (3) Skin prep may be done in surgery.

4. Goal: *reduce the risk of vomiting and aspiration during anesthesia; prevent contamination of abdominal operative sites by fecal material.* **Gastrointestinal tract preparation:**

a. *No* food or fluid at least 6–8 hr before surgery.

b. Remove food and water from bedside.

c. Place NPO signs on bed or door.

d. Inform kitchen and oncoming nursing staff that patient is NPO for surgery.

e. Give IV infusions up to time of surgery if dehydrated or malnourished.

▶ f. Enemas: two or three may be given the evening before surgery with intestinal, colon, or pelvic surgeries; 3 days of cleansing with large-intestine procedures.

g. Possible antibiotic therapy to reduce colonic flora with large-bowel surgery.

▶ h. Gastric or intestinal intubation may be inserted the evening before major abdominal surgery.
   (1) Types of tubes:
      (a) *Levin:* single lumen; sufficient to remove fluids and gas from stomach; suction may damage mucosa.
      (b) *Salem-sump:* large lumen; prevents tissue-wall adherence.
      (c) *Miller-Abbott:* long single or double lumen; required to remove the contents of jejunum or ileum.

   (2) Pressures: *low* setting with Levin and intestinal tubes; *high* setting with Salem-sump; excessive pressures will result in injury to mucosal lining of intestine or stomach.

5. Goal: *promote rest and facilitate reduction of apprehension.*

a. Medications as ordered: on evening before surgery may give barbiturate—pentobarbital (Nembutal), secobarbital (Seconal).

b. Quiet environment: eliminate noises, distractions.

c. *Position:* reduce muscle tension.

d. Back rub.

6. Goal: *protect from injury; ensure final preparation for surgery.* Day of surgery:

a. Operative permit signed and on chart; physician responsible for obtaining informed consent.

b. Shower or bathe.
   (1) Dress: hospital pajamas.
   (2) Remove: hair pins (cover hair); nail polish, to facilitate observation of peripheral circulation; jewelry (tape wedding bands securely); pierced earrings; contact lenses; dentures (store and give mouth care); give valuable personal items to family; chart disposition of items.

c. Proper identification—check band for secureness and legibility.

d. Vital signs—baseline data.

e. Void, to prevent distention and possible injury to bladder.

f. Give preoperative medication to ensure smooth induction and maintenance of anesthesia—*antianxiety* (e.g., midazolam, diazepam, lorazepam); *narcotics* (e.g., meperidine, morphine, fentanyl); *anticholinergics* (e.g., atropine, glycopyrrolate).
   (1) Administered 45–75 min before anesthetic induction.
   (2) Side rails up (client will begin to feel drowsy and light-headed).
   (3) Expect complaint of dry mouth if anticholinergics given.
   (4) Observe for side effects—narcotics may cause nausea and vomiting, hypotension, arrhythmias, and/or respiratory depression.
   (5) Quiet environment until transported to operating room.

g. Note completeness of chart:
   (1) Surgical checklist completed.
   (2) Vital signs recorded.
   (3) Routine laboratory reports present.
   (4) Preoperative medications given.
   (5) Significant patient observations.

h. Assist patient's family in finding proper waiting room.

(1) Inform family members that the surgeon will contact them after the procedure is over.

(2) Explain length of time patient is expected to be in recovery room.

(3) Prepare family for any special equipment or devices that may be needed to care for patient postoperatively (e.g., oxygen, monitoring equipment, ventilator, blood transfusions).

II. Intraoperative preparation—anesthesia: blocks transmission of nerve impulses, suppresses reflexes, promotes muscle relaxation, and in some instances achieves reversible unconsciousness.

A. Intravenous conscious sedation—produces sedation and amnesia in ambulatory procedures, short surgical or diagnostic procedures. Allays fear and anxiety, elevates pain threshold, maintains consciousness and protective reflexes, and returns patient quickly to normal activities. Commonly used agents are benzodiazepines (midazolam, diazepam) and narcotics (fentanyl, meperidine, morphine).

B. Regional anesthesia—purpose is to block pain reception and transmission in a specified area. Commonly used drugs are lidocaine HCl, tetracaine HCl, cocaine HCl, and procaine HCl. Types of regional anesthetics:

1. *Topical*—applied to mucous membranes or skin; drug anesthetizes the nerves immediately *below* the area. May be used for bronchoscopic or laryngoscopic examinations. *Side effects:* rare anaphylaxis.

2. *Local infiltration*—used for minor procedures; anesthetic drug is injected directly into the area to be incised, manipulated, or sutured. *Side effects:* rare anaphylaxis.

3. *Peripheral nerve block*—regional anesthesia is achieved by injecting drug into or around a nerve after it passes from vertebral column; procedure is named for nerve involved, such as brachial-plexus block. Requires a high degree of anatomical knowledge. *Side effects:* may be absorbed into bloodstream. Observe for signs of excitability, twitching, changes in vital signs, or respiratory difficulties.

4. *Field block*—a group of nerves is injected with anesthetic as the nerves branch from a major or main nerve trunk. May be used for dental procedures, plastic surgery. *Side effects:* rare.

5. *Epidural anesthesia*—anesthetizing drug is injected into the epidural space of vertebral canal; produces a bandlike anesthesia around body. Frequently used in obstetrics. Rare complications. Slower onset than spinal anesthesia, not dependent on patient position for level of anesthesia, no postoperative headaches.

6. *Spinal anesthesia*—anesthetizing drug is injected into the subarachnoid space and mixes with spinal fluid; drug acts on the nerves as they emerge from the spinal cord, thereby inhibiting conduction in the autonomic, sensory, and motor systems.

a. *Advantages:* rapid onset; produces excellent muscle relaxation.

b. Utilization: surgery on lower limbs, inguinal region, perineum, and lower abdomen.

c. *Disadvantages:*

(1) Loss of sensation below point of injection for 2–8 hr—watch for signs of *bladder distention;* prevent injuries by maintaining alignment, keeping bedclothes straightened.

(2) Patient awake during surgical procedure—*avoid* light or upsetting conversations.

(3) Leakage of spinal fluid from puncture site—keep flat in bed for 24–48 hr to prevent headache. Keep well hydrated to aid in spinal-fluid replacement.

(4) Depression of vasomotor responses—frequent checks of vital signs.

7. *Intravenous regional anesthesia*—used in an extremity whose circulation has been interrupted by a tourniquet; the anesthetic is injected into vein, and blockage is presumed to be achieved from extravascular leakage of anesthetic near a major nerve trunk. Precautions as for peripheral nerve block.

C. General anesthesia—a reversible state in which the patient loses consciousness due to the inhibition of neuronal impulses in the brain by a variety of chemical agents; may be given intravenously, by inhalation, or rectally.

1. *Side effects:*

a. Respiratory depression.

b. Nausea, vomiting.

c. Excitement.

d. Restlessness.

e. Laryngospasm.

f. Hypotension.

♦ 2. **Nursing care plan/implementation**—Goal: *prevent hazardous drug interactions.*

a. *Notify anesthesiologist* if patient is taking any of the following drugs:

(1) *Antidepressants,* such as Prozac—long half-life; monitor renal and liver function.

(2) *Antihypertensives,* such as reserpine, hydralazine, and methyldopa—*potentiate* the hypotensive effects of anesthetic agents.

(3) *Anticoagulants,* such as heparin, warfarin (Coumadin)—increase bleeding times, which may result in excessive *blood loss* or hemorrhage.

(4) *Aspirin and NSAIDs*—decrease platelet aggregation and may result in increased *bleeding.*

(5) *Steroids,* such as cortisone—anti-inflammatory effect may *delay* wound healing.

b. *Stages of inhalation anesthesia and nursing goals:*

(1) Stage I—extends from beginning of induction to loss of consciousness. **Nursing goal:** *reduce external stimuli,* because all movement and noises are exaggerated for the patient and can be highly distressing.

(2) Stage II—extends from loss of consciousness to relaxation; stage of delirium and excitement. **Nursing goal:** *prevent injury* by assisting anesthesiologist to restrain patient if necessary; maintain a quiet, nonstimulating environment.

(3) Stage III—extends from loss of lid reflex to cessation of voluntary respirations. **Nursing goal:** *reduce risk of untoward effects* by preparing the operative site, assisting with procedures, and observing for signs of complications.

(4) Stage IV—indicates overdose and consists of respiratory arrest and vasomotor collapse due to medullary paralysis. **Nursing goal:** *promote restoration of ventilation and vasomotor tone* by assisting with cardiac arrest procedures and by administering cardiac stimulants or narcotic antagonists as ordered.

D. Intravenous agents—rapid and pleasant induction of anesthesia. Three categories: *barbiturates* (thiopental), *narcotics,* and *neuromuscular blocking agents* (succinylcholine, curare, pancuronium). Ketamine also used—may produce *emergence delirium.* IV drugs require liver metabolism and renal excretion.

E. Hypothermia—a specialized procedure in which the patient's body temperature is lowered to 28°–30°C (82°–86°F).

1. Reduces tissue metabolism and oxygen requirements.

2. Used in heart surgery, brain surgery, and surgery on major blood vessels.

◆ 3. **Nursing care plan/implementation:**

a. Goal: *prevent complications:*

(1) Monitor vital signs for shock.

(2) Note level of consciousness.

(3) Record intake and output accurately.

(4) Maintain good body alignment; reposition to prevent edema, pressure, or discoloration of skin.

(5) Maintain patent IV.

b. Goal: *promote comfort.*

(1) Apply blankets to rewarm and prevent shivering.

(2) Mouth care.

c. Goal: observe for indications of **malignant hyperthermia**—common during induction; may occur 24–72 hr postoperatively. Genetic defect of muscle metabolism; early sign is unexplained ventricular dysrhythmia, tachypnea, cyanosis, skin mottling; elevated temperature is not reliable indicator.

▶ (1) Administer 100% O_2.

▶ (2) Cool with ice packs or cooling blankets.

(3) Give dantrolene (muscle relaxant) per order.

◆ **F. Evaluation/outcome criteria:** complete reversal of anesthetic effects (e.g., spontaneous respirations, pupils react to light). No indication of intraoperative complications—cardiac arrest, laryngospasm, aspiration, hypotension, malignant hyperthermia.

III. Postoperative experience

◆ **A. Assessment:**

1. *Subjective data:*

a. Pain: location, onset, intensity.

b. Nausea.

2. *Objective data:*

a. Operative summary:

(1) Type of operation performed.

(2) Pathological findings if known.

(3) Anesthesia and medications received.

(4) Problems during surgery that will affect recovery, e.g., arrhythmias, bleeding (estimated blood loss).

(5) Fluids received: type, amount.

(6) Need for drainage or suction apparatus.

b. Observations:

(1) Patency of airway.

(2) Vital signs.

(3) Skin color and dryness.

(4) Level of consciousness.

(5) Status of reflexes.

(6) Dressings.

(7) Type and rate of IV infusion and blood transfusion.

(8) Tubes/drains: urinary, chest, Penrose, Hemovac; note color and amount of drainage.

◆ **B. Analysis/nursing diagnosis:**

1. *Ineffective breathing pattern* related to general anesthesia.

2. *Ineffective airway clearance* related to absent or weak cough.

3. *Risk for aspiration* related to vomiting.

4. *Pain* related to surgical incision.

5. *Altered tissue perfusion* related to shock.

6. *Risk for fluid volume deficit* related to blood loss.
7. *Risk for injury* related to disorientation.
8. *Risk for infection* related to disruption of skin integrity.
9. *Urinary retention* related to anesthetic effects.
10. *Constipation* related to decreased peristalsis.

◆ C. **Nursing care plan/implementation**—*immediate postanesthesia nursing care:* refers to time following surgery that is usually spent in the recovery room (1–2 hr).

1. Goal: *promote a safe, quiet, nonstressful environment.*
   a. Side rails up at all times.
   b. Nurse in constant attendance.
2. Goal: *promote lung expansion and gas exchange.*
3. Goal: *Prevent aspiration and atelectasis.*
   ◪ a. *Position:* side or back, with head turned to side to prevent obstruction of airway by tongue; allows for drainage from mouth.
   b. Airway: leave the oropharyngeal or nasopharyngeal airway in place until patient awakens and begins to eject; gagging and vomiting may occur if not removed before pharyngeal reflex returns.
   ◪ c. After removal of airway: turn on side in a *lateral position;* support upper arm with pillow.
   ▶ d. Suction: remove excessive secretions from mouth and pharynx.
   e. Encourage coughing and deep breathing: aids in upward movement of secretions.
   ▶ f. Give humidified oxygen as necessary: reduces respiratory irritation and keeps bronchotracheal secretions soft and moist.
   ▶ g. Mechanical ventilation: respirators if needed (see Ventilators in **Unit II,** p. 763).
4. Goal: *promote and maintain cardiovascular function.*
   a. Vital signs, as ordered: usually q15min until stable.
      (1) Compare with preoperative vital signs.
      (2) | **Immediately report:** systolic blood pressure that *drops 20* mm Hg or more, a pressure *below 80* mm Hg, or a pressure that continually drops 5–10 mm Hg over several readings; pulse rates *under 60 or over 110* beats/min, or irregularities; respirations *over 30*/min; becoming shallow, quiet, slow; use of neck and diaphragm muscles (symptoms of *respiratory depression*).
   b. Observe for other alterations in circulatory function—pallor; thready pulse; cold, moist skin; decreased urine output, restlessness.
      (1) Immediately report to physician.
      ▶ (2) Initiate oxygen therapy.

◪ (3) Place patient in shock position unless contraindicated—feet elevated, legs straight, head *slightly* elevated to increase venous return.
   c. Intravenous infusions: time, rate, orders for added medications.
   ▶ d. Monitor *blood transfusions* if ordered: observe for signs of *reaction* (chills, elevated temperature, urticaria, laryngeal edema, and wheezing). Table 7–22 illustrates the nursing care plan/implementation.
   e. If reaction occurs, immediately stop transfusion and notify physician. Send stat urine to lab.
5. Goal: *promote psychological equilibrium.*
   a. Reassure on awakening—orient frequently.
   b. Explain procedures even though patient does not appear alert.
   c. Answer patient's questions briefly and accurately.
   d. Maintain quiet, restful environment.
   e. Comfort measures:
      (1) Good body alignment.
      (2) Support dependent extremities to *avoid* pressure areas and possible nerve damage.
      (3) Check for constriction: dressings, clothing, bedding.
      (4) Check IV sites frequently for patency and signs of infiltration (swelling, blanching, cool to touch).
6. Goal: *maintain proper function of tubes and apparatus* (see Table 11–7).

D. **General postoperative nursing care:** refers to period of time from admission to the general nursing unit until anticipated recovery and discharge from the hospital. See Table 7–22 for a review of postoperative complications.

1. Goal: *promote lung expansion, gaseous exchange, and elimination of bronchotracheal secretions.*
   a. Turn, cough, and deep breathe q2h.
   ▶ b. Use incentive spirometer as ordered to enable patient to observe depth of ventilation.
   c. Administer nebulization as ordered to help mobilize secretions.
   d. Encourage hydration to thin mucous secretions.
   e. Assist in ambulation as soon as allowed.
2. Goal: *provide relief of pain.*
   a. Assess type, location, intensity, and duration; possible causative factors, such as poor body alignment or restrictive bandages.
   b. Observe and evaluate reaction to discomfort.
   c. Use comfort measures, such as back rubs and proper ventilation, staying with patient and encouraging verbalization.

Adult

TABLE 7–22   Postoperative Complications

Condition and Etiology	◆ Assessment: Signs and Symptoms	◆ Nursing Care Plan/Implementation
Respiratory Complications —Most Common Are Atelectasis, Pneumonias (Lobar, Bronchial, and Hypostatic), and Pleuritis; Other Complications Are Hemothorax and Pneumothorax		
Atelectasis—undetected preoperative upper respiratory infections, aspiration of vomitus: irritation of the tracheobronchial tree with increased secretions of mucus due to intubation and inhalation anesthesia, a history of heavy smoking, or chronic obstructive pulmonary disease; severe postoperative pain or high abdominal or thoracic surgery, which inhibits deep breathing; and debilitation or old age, which lowers the patient's resistance	Dyspnea; ↑ temperature; absent or diminished breath sounds over affected area, asymmetrical chest expansion, ↑ respirations and pulse rate; tracheal shift to affected side when severe; anxiety and restlessness	1. *Position:* unaffected side 2. Turn, cough, and deep breathe ▶ 3. *Postural drainage* ▶ 4. Nebulization 5. *Force* fluids if not contraindicated
Pneumonia—see *Atelectasis* for etiology	Rapid, shallow, painful respirations; crackles; diminished or absent breath sounds; asymmetrical lung expansion; chills and fever, productive cough, rust-colored sputum; and circumoral and nailbed cyanosis	1. *Position of comfort*—semi-Fowler's to high Fowler's 2. *Force* fluids to 3000 mL/day ▶ 3. Provide humidification of air and oxygen therapy ▶ 4. Oropharyngeal suction prn 5. Assist during coughing 6. Administer antibiotics and analgesics as ordered 7. *Diet:* high calorie, as tolerated 8. Cautious disposal of secretions; proper oral hygiene
Pleuritis—see *Atelectasis* for etiology	Knifelike chest pain on inspiration; intercostal tenderness; splinting of chest by patient; rapid, shallow respirations; pleural friction rub; ↑ temperature; malaise	1. *Position: affected* side to splint the chest ▶ 2. Manually splint patient's chest during cough ▶ 3. Apply binder or adhesive strapping as ordered 4. Administer analgesics as ordered
Hemothorax—chest surgery, gunshot or knife wounds, and multiple fractures of chest wall	Chest pain; increased respiratory rate; dyspnea, decreased or absent breath sounds; decreased blood pressure; tachycardia, and mediastinal shift may occur (heart, trachea, and esophagus great vessels are pushed toward unaffected side)	1. Observe vital signs closely for signs of shock and respiratory distress 2. Assist with thoracentesis (needle aspiration of fluid) 3. Assist with insertion of thoracotomy ▶ tube to closed-chest drainage (see care of water-sealed drainage system)
Pneumothorax, closed or tension— thoracentesis (needle nicks the lung), rupture of alveoli or bronchi due to accidental injury, and chronic obstructive lung disease	Marked dyspnea, sudden sharp chest pain, subcutaneous emphysema (air in chest wall tissue); cyanosis; tracheal shift to unaffected side; hyperresonance on percussion, decreased or absent breath sounds; increased respiratory rate, tachycardia; asymmetrical chest expansion, feeling of pressure within chest; *mediastinal shift*—severe dyspnea and cyanosis, deviation of larynx and trachea toward unaffected side, deviation either medially or laterally of apex of heart, decreased blood pressure; distended neck veins; increased pulse and respirations	1. Remain with patient—keep as calm and quiet as possible 2. *Position:* high Fowler's (sitting) 3. Notify physician through another nurse, and have thoracentesis equipment brought to bedside ▶ 4. Administer oxygen as necessary 5. Take vital signs to evaluate respiratory and cardiac function 6. Assist with thoracentesis ▶ 7. Assist with initiation and maintenance of closed-chest drainage

TABLE 7–22   Postoperative Complications—cont'd

Condition and Etiology	◆ Assessment: Signs and Symptoms	◆ Nursing Care Plan/Implementation

Circulatory Complications—Shock, Thrombophlebitis, Pulmonary Embolism, and Disseminated Intravascular Coagulation (DIC)

Condition and Etiology	Assessment: Signs and Symptoms	Nursing Care Plan/Implementation
Shock—hemorrhage, sepsis, decreased cardiac contractility (myocardial infarction, cardiac failure, tamponade), drug sensitivities, transfusion reactions, pulmonary embolism, and emotional reaction to pain or deep fear	Dizziness; fainting; restlessness; anxiety *BP:* ↓ or falling *Pulse:* weak, thready *Respirations:* ↑, shallow *Skin:* pale, cool, clammy, cyanotic ↓ temperature; oliguria; CVP <5 cm H$_2$O; thirst	1. *Position:* foot of bed raised 20 degrees, knees straight, trunk horizontal, head slightly elevated; *avoid* Trendelenburg's position 2. Administer blood transfusions, plasma expanders, and intravenous infusions as ordered; medications specific to type of shock 3. Check: vital signs, CVP, temperature 4. Insert urinary catheter to monitor hourly urine output 5. Administer oxygen as ordered
Thrombophlebitis—injury to vein wall by tight leg straps or leg holders during gynecological surgery; hemoconcentration due to dehydration or fluid loss; stasis of blood in extremities due to postoperative circulatory depression	Calf pain or cramping, redness and swelling (the left leg is affected more frequently than the right); slight fever, chills; *Homans'* sign and tenderness over the anteromedian surface of thigh	1. Maintain complete bed rest, *avoiding positions* that restrict venous return 2. Apply elastic stockings to prevent swelling and pooling of venous blood 3. Apply warm, moist soaks to area as ordered 4. Administer anticoagulants as ordered 5. Use bed cradle over affected limb 6. Provide active and passive ROM exercises in unaffected limb
Pulmonary embolism—obstruction of a pulmonary artery by a foreign body in bloodstream, usually a blood clot that has been dislodged from its original site	*Sudden,* severe stabbing chest pain; *severe* dyspnea; cyanosis; *rapid* pulse; anxiety and apprehension; pupillary dilation: *profuse* diaphoresis; *loss of* consciousness	1. Administer oxygen and inhalants while patient *is sitting upright* 2. Maintain bed rest and frequent reassurance 3. Administer heparin sodium, as ordered 4. Administer analgesics, such as morphine SO$_4$, to reduce pain and apprehension

Disseminated Intravascular Coagulation (DIC) (see p. 459).

Wound Complications—Infection, Dehiscence, and Evisceration

Condition and Etiology	Assessment: Signs and Symptoms	Nursing Care Plan/Implementation
Wound infection—*obesity or undernutrition,* particularly protein and vitamin deficiencies; *decreased* antibody production in aged; *decreased* phagocytosis in newborn; metabolic disorder, such as diabetes mellitus, Cushing's syndrome, malignancies, and shock; breakdown in aseptic technique	Redness, tenderness, and heat in area of incision; wound drainage; ↑ temperature; ↑ pulse rate.	1. Assist in cleansing and irrigation of wound and insertion of a drain 2. Give antibiotics as ordered; observe responses
Wound dehiscence and evisceration—obesity and undernutrition, particularly protein and vitamin C deficiencies; immunosuppression; metabolic disorders; cancer; liver disease; common site is midline abdominal incision, frequently about 7 days postoperatively; precipitating factors include: abdominal distention, vomiting, coughing, hiccups, and uncontrolled motor activity	Slow parting of wound edges with a gush of pinkish serous drainage; or rapid parting with coils of intestines escaping onto the abdominal wall: the latter accompanied by pain and often by vomiting. Patient reports "giving" sensation.	1. *Position:* bed rest, low Fowler's or horizontal position 2. Notify physician stat 3. Cover exposed coils of intestines with sterile towels or dressing and keep moist with sterile normal saline 4. Monitor vital signs frequently 5. Remain with patient; reassure that physician is coming 6. Prepare for physician's arrival; set up IV, suction equipment, and nasogastric tube; obtain sterile gown, mask, gloves, towels, and warmed normal saline 7. Notify surgery that patient will be returning to operating room

Continued

TABLE 7–22 Postoperative Complications—cont'd

Condition and Etiology	◆ Assessment: Signs and Symptoms	◆ Nursing Care Plan/Implementation
Urinary Complications—Retention and Infections		
Urinary retention—obstruction in bladder or urethra; neurological disease; mechanical trauma as in childbirth or gynecological surgery; psychological conditioning that inhibits voiding in bed; prolonged bed rest; pain with lower abdominal surgery	Inability to void within 8 hr postsurgery, despite adequate fluid replacement; palpable bladder, frequent voiding of small amounts of urine or dribbling; suprapubic pain	1. Assist patient to stand, or use bedside commode if not contraindicated 2. Provide privacy 3. Reduce tension, provide support 4. Use warm bedpan 5. Run tap water 6. Place patient's feet in warm water 7. Pour warm water over perineum ▶ 8. Catheterize if conservative measures fail
Urinary tract infections—urinary retention, bladder distention, repeated or prolonged catheterization	*Urinary:* burning and frequency *Pain:* low back or flank Pyuria, hematuria; ↑ temperature, chills; anorexia; positive urine culture	1. *Push fluids* to 3000 mL daily, unless contraindicated 2. *Avoid* stimulants such as caffeine 3. Give antibiotics, sulfonamides, or acidifying agents as ordered ▶ 4. Give perianal care after each bowel movement
Gastrointestinal Complications—Gastric Distention, Paralytic Ileus, and Intestinal Obstruction		
Gastric distention—depressed gastric motility due to sympathoadrenal stress response; idiosyncrasy to drugs: emotions, pain, shock; fluid and electrolyte imbalances	Feeling of fullness, hiccups, overflow vomiting of dark, foul-smelling liquid; severe retention leads to decreased blood pressure (due to pressure on vagus nerve) and other symptoms of shock syndrome	1. Report signs to physician *immediately* 2. Insert or assist in insertion of NG tube; attach to intermittent suction ▶ 3. Irrigate NG tube with *saline* (water will deplete electrolytes and result in metabolic alkalosis) 4. Administer IV infusions with electrolytes as ordered
Paralytic ileus—see *Gastric distention*	Greatly decreased or absent bowel sounds, failure of either gas or feces to be passed by rectum; nausea and vomiting; abdominal tenderness and distention; fever; dehydration	1. Notify physician ▶ 2. Insert or assist with insertion of NG tube; attach to low, intermittent suction ▶ 3. Insert rectal tube 4. Administer IV infusion with electrolytes as ordered 5. Irrigate nasogastric tube with saline ▶ 6. Assist with insertion of Miller-Abbott tube if indicated 7. Administer medications to increase peristalsis as ordered
Intestinal obstruction—due to poorly functioning anastomosis, hernia, adhesions, fecal impaction	Severe, colicky abdominal pains, mild to severe abdominal distention, nausea and vomiting, anorexia and malaise; fever; lack of bowel movement; electrolyte imbalance; high-pitched tinkling bowel sounds	▶ 1. Assist with insertion of nasoenteric tube and attach to intermittent suction 2. Maintain IV infusions with electrolytes 3. Encourage nasal breathing to *avoid* air swallowing ▶ 4. Check abdomen for distention and bowel sounds every 2 hr 5. Encourage verbalization 6. Plan rest periods for patient 7. Administer oral hygiene frequently
Transfusion Reactions—Allergic, Febrile, and Hemolytic		
Allergic and febrile reactions—unidentified antigen or antigens in donor blood or transfusion equipment; previous reaction to transfusions; small thrombi; bacteria; lysed red blood cells	Fever to 103°F, may have *sudden* onset; chills; itching; erythema; urticaria; nausea; vomiting; dyspnea and wheezing, occasionally	1. *Stop* transfusion and notify physician 2. Administer *antihistamines,* as ordered 3. Send stat urine to lab for analysis ▶ 4. Institute *cooling* measures if indicated 5. Maintain *strict* input and output records 6. Send remaining blood to lab for analysis, and order recipient blood sample for analysis

TABLE 7–22   Postoperative Complications—cont'd

Condition and Etiology	◆ Assessment: Signs and Symptoms	◆ Nursing Care Plan/Implementation
Transfusion Reactions—Allergic, Febrile, and Hemolytic *(Continued)*		
Hemolytic reaction—infusion of incompatible blood (less common, more serious)	*Early:* chills and fever; throbbing headache, feeling of burning in face; hypotension; tachycardia; chest, back, or flank pain; nausea, vomiting; feeling of doom; *later:* spontaneous and diffuse bleeding; icterus; oliguria; anuria; hemoglobinuria	1. *Stop* infusion immediately; take vital signs and notify physician 2. Send patient blood sample and unused blood to lab for analysis 3. Send stat urine to lab 4. Save *all* urine for observation of discoloration 5. Administer parenteral infusions to combat shock, as ordered 6. Administer medications as ordered—*diuretics, sodium bicarbonate, hydrocortisone,* and *vasopressors*
Emotional Complications		
Emotional disturbances—grief associated with loss of body part or loss of body image; previous emotional problems; decreased sensory and perceptual input; sensory overload; fear and pain; decreased resistance to stress as a result of age, exhaustion, or debilitation	Restlessness, insomnia, depression, hallucinations, delusions, agitation, suicidal thoughts	1. Report symptoms to physician 2. Encourage verbalization of feelings; give realistic assurance 3. Orient to time and place as necessary 4. Provide safety measures, such as side rails 5. Keep room lit, to reduce incidence of visual hallucinations 6. Administer tranquilizers as ordered. 7. Use restraints as a *last* resort

d. Reduce incidence of pain: change position frequently; support dependent extremities with pillows, sandbags, and footboards; keep bedding dry and straight.

e. Give analgesics or tranquilizers as ordered; assure patient that they will help.

f. Observe for desired and untoward effects of medication.

3. Goal: *promote adequate nutrition and fluid and electrolyte balance.*

   a. Parenteral fluids, as ordered.

   b. Monitor blood pressure, I&O to assess adequate, deficient, or excessive extracellular fluid volume.

   c. *Diet:* liquid when nausea and vomiting stop and bowel sounds are established, progress as ordered.

4. Goal: *assist patient with elimination.*

   a. Encourage voiding within 8–10 hr after surgery.

      (1) Allow patient to stand or use commode, if not contraindicated.

      (2) Run tap water or soak feet in warm water to promote micturition.

      (3) Catheterization if bladder is distended and conservative treatments have failed.

   b. Maintain accurate I&O records.

   c. Expect bowel function to return in 2–3 days.

5. Goal: *facilitate wound healing and prevent infection.*

   a. Incision care: *avoid* pressure to enhance venous drainage and prevent edema.

   b. Elevate injured extremities to reduce swelling and promote venous return.

   c. Support or splint incision when coughing.

   d. Check dressings q2h for drainage.

   e. Change dressings on draining wounds prn; *aseptic technique;* protective ointments to reduce skin irritation may be ordered.

   f. Carefully observe wound suction (e.g., *Jackson-Pratt*), if applied, for kinking or twisting of the tubes.

6. Goal: *promote comfort and rest.*

   a. Recognize factors that may cause restlessness—fear, anxiety, pain, oxygen lack, wet dressings.

   b. Comfort measures: analgesics or barbiturates; apply oxygen as indicated; change positions; encourage deep breathing; massage back to reduce restlessness.

   c. Allow rest periods between care—group activities.

   d. Give antiemetic for relief of nausea and vomiting, as ordered.

   e. Vigorous oral hygiene (brushing) to prevent "surgical mumps" or parotitis from preop atropine or general anesthesia.

7. Goal: *encourage early movement and ambulation to prevent complications of immobilization.*
   a. Turn or reposition q2h.
   ▶ b. ROM: passive and active exercises.
   c. Encourage leg exercises.
   ▶ d. Use preventive treatments—antiembolic stockings, graduated compression stockings, or external pneumatic compression sleeves:
      (1) With compression stockings, highest pressure (100%) at ankles, lowest pressure (40%) at midthigh.
      (2) Compression sleeves, three chambers sequentially inflated-deflated to stimulate venous return.
   e. Assist with standing or use of commode if allowed.
   f. Encourage resumption of personal care as soon as possible.
   g. Assist with ambulation in room as soon as allowed. *Avoid* chair sitting because it enhances venous pooling and may predispose to thrombophlebitis.

◆ E. **Evaluation/outcome criteria:**
   1. Incision heals without infection.
   2. No complications, e.g., atelectasis, pneumonia, thrombophlebitis.
   3. Normal bowel and bladder functions resume.
   4. Carries out activities of daily living, self-care.
   5. Accepts possible limitations: dietary, activity, body image (e.g., no depression, complies with treatment regimen).

NUTRITION

I. General nutritional deficiencies
◆ **A. Assessment:**
1. *Subjective data:*
   a. Mental irritability or confusion.
   b. History of poor dietary intake.
   c. History of lack of adequate resources to provide adequate nutrition.
   d. Lack of knowledge about proper diet, food selection, or preparation.
   e. History of eating disorders.
   f. Paresthesia (burning and tingling): hands and feet.
2. *Objective data:*
   a. *Appearance:* listless; *posture:* sagging shoulders, sunken chest, poor gait.
   b. *Muscle:* weakness, fatigue, wasted appearance.
   c. *GI:* indigestion, vomiting, enlarged liver, spleen.
   d. *Cardiovascular:* tachycardia on minimal exertion; bradycardia at rest; enlarged heart, elevated BP.
   e. *Hair:* brittle, dry, thin, sparse; lack of natural shine; color changes; can be easily plucked out.
   f. *Skin:* dryness (xerosis), scaly, dyspigmentation, petechiae, lack of fat under skin.
   g. *Mouth:*
      (1) *Teeth:* missing, abnormally placed, caries.
      (2) *Gums:* bleed easily, receding.
      (3) *Tongue:* swollen, sore.
      (4) *Lips:* red, swollen, angular fissures at corners.
   h. *Eyes:* pale conjunctiva, corneal changes.
   i. *Nails:* brittle, ridged.
   j. *Nervous system:* abnormal reflexes.
   k. Lab data: blood: *decreased* albumin, iron-binding capacity, lymphocyte, hemoglobin, and hematocrit.
   l. Anthropometric measurements document nutritional deficiencies.

◆ **B. Analysis/nursing diagnosis:**
1. *Altered nutrition, less than body requirements,* related to poor dietary intake.
2. *Knowledge deficit* related to nutritional requirements.
3. *Altered health maintenance* related to inability to provide own nutritional care.
4. *Ineffective individual coping* related to eating disorders.
5. *Ineffective family coping, disabling,* related to inadequate resources or knowledge to provide appropriate family nutrition.

◆ **C. Nursing care plan/implementation:**
1. Goal: *prevent complications of specific deficiency.*
   a. Identify etiology of nutritional deficiency.
   b. Recognize signs of nutritional deficiencies (Table 7–23).

TABLE 7–23   Essential Nutrients and Potential Deficiencies

Nutrient	Function	Deficiency Leads to
Calcium	Aids in formation and maintenance of bones and teeth; permits healthy nerve functioning and normal blood clotting	↑ neuromuscular irritability, impaired blood clotting
Phosphorus	Bone building	Rickets
Magnesium	Cellular metabolism of carbohydrates and protein	↓ cellular metabolism of carbohydrates and protein; tetany
Sodium	Fluid and electrolyte balance; acid-base balance; electrochemical impulses of nerves and muscles	Fluid and electrolyte imbalance; ↓ muscle contraction
Potassium	Osmotic pressure and water balance	Fluid and electrolyte imbalance; ↓ cardiac and skeletal muscular contractility
Chloride	Fluid and electrolyte balance; acid-base balance; digestion	Fluid imbalances; alkalosis
Iron	Hemoglobin formation; cellular oxidation	Anemia; ↑ risk of infection
Iodine	Synthesis of thyroid hormone; overall body metabolism	Goiter
Zinc	Constituent of cell enzyme system; CO_2 carrier in RBC	↓ metabolism of protein and carbohydrates; delayed wound healing; ↑ risk of infection
Vitamin A	Collagen synthesis	Poor healing; scaly skin
Vitamin C	Capillary integrity	Poor healing; bruising
Vitamin K	Coagulation	Bruising and hemorrhage
Pyridoxine and thiamine	Antibody, RBC, and WBC formation	↑ risk of infection; anemia
Protein	Wound repair; clotting; WBC production; phagocytosis	Poor healing; edema
Fats	Cellular energy; cell membrane integrity	Impaired tissue repair
Carbohydrates	Cellular energy; spare protein	Interference with healing

Adult

c. Identify foods high in deficient nutrient (see **Unit 9**).

d. Evaluate economic resources to purchase appropriate foods.

e. Identify community resources for assistance.

f. Monitor progress for potential additional illnesses.

2. Goal: *health teaching*.

a. Effects of nutritional deficiencies on health.

b. Foods to include in diet to avoid deficits.

◆ **D. Evaluation/outcome criteria:**

1. Complications do not occur.

2. Patient gains weight.

3. Patient selects appropriate foods to alleviate deficiency.

II. Celiac disease (gluten enteropathy, nontropical sprue): immune to gluten, causing impaired absorption and digestion of nutrients through the small bowel. Affects adults and children and is characterized by inability to digest and use sugars, starches, and fats.

A. Pathophysiology: intolerance to the gliadin fraction of grains causing degeneration of the epithelial surface of the intestine, atrophy of the intestinal villi, and impaired absorption of essential nutrients.

B. Risk factors:

1. Possible genetic or familial factors.

2. Hypersensitivity response.

3. History of childhood celiac disease.

◆ **C. Assessment:**

1. *Subjective data:* family history.

2. *Objective data:*

a. Loss: weight, fat deposits, musculature.

b. Anemia.

c. Vitamin deficiencies.

d. Abdomen distended with flatus.

e. Stools: diarrhea, foul smelling, bulky, fatty, float in commode.

f. Skin condition known as dermatitis herpetiformis.

g. History of acute attacks of fluid and electrolyte imbalances.

h. *Diagnostic tests:* stool for fat; barium enema; antibody tests, including endomyosial (EMA); blood studies of iron, folate, proteins, minerals, and clotting factors; small bowel biopsy.

i. *Gluten-free diet* leads to remission of symptoms.

◆ **D. Analysis/nursing diagnosis:**

1. *Altered nutrition, less than body requirements,* related to inability to digest and use sugars, starches, and fats.

2. *Diarrhea* related to intestinal response to gluten in diet.

3. *Fluid volume deficit* related to loss through excessive diarrhea.

4. *Knowledge deficit* related to dietary restrictions to control symptoms.

◆ **E. Nursing care plan/implementation:**

1. Goal: *prevent weight loss.*

a. *Diet: high* in calories, protein, vitamins, and minerals, and gluten free.

(1) *Avoid* wheat, rye, oats, barley.

(2) All other foods permitted.

b. Daily weights to monitor weight changes.

2. Goal: *health teaching.*

a. Nature of disease.

b. Dietary restrictions and allowances.

c. Complications of noncompliance.

◆ **F. Evaluation/outcome criteria:**

1. No further weight loss.

2. Normal stools.

3. Fluid/electrolyte balance obtained and maintained.

III. Hepatitis: inflammation of the liver.

A. Pathophysiology:

1. Infection with either *hepatitis A* (formerly called infectious hepatitis), *hepatitis B* (formerly called serum hepatitis), *hepatitis C* (single-stranded RNV virus of the *Flaviviridae* family; usually asymptomatic), *delta hepatitis* (infection caused by a defective RNA virus that requires HBV to multiply), or *hepatitis E* (major etiological agent of the enterically transmitted non-A, non-B hepatitis worldwide) → inflammation, necrosis, and regeneration of liver parenchyma. Hepatocellular injury impairs clearance of urobilinogen → elevated urinary urobilinogen; and, as injury increases → conjugated bilirubin not reaching the intestines → decreased urine and fecal urobilinogen → increased serum bilirubin → jaundice.

2. Failure of liver to detoxify products → increased toxic products of protein metabolism → gastritis and duodenitis.

B. Risk factors:

1. Exposure to virus.

2. Exposure to carriers of virus.

3. Exposure to hepatotoxins such as dry-cleaning agents.

4. Nonimmunized.

◆ **C. Assessment:**

1. *Subjective data:*

a. Anorexia, nausea.

b. Malaise, dull ache in right upper quadrant, abdominal pain.

c. Repugnance to food, cigarette smoke, strong odors, alcohol.

d. Headache.

2. *Objective data:*

a. Fever.

b. Liver: enlarged (hepatomegaly), tender, smooth.

c. Skin: icterus in sclera of eyes, jaundice; rash; pruritus; petechiae, bruises.

TABLE 7–24 Etiology, Incidence, Epidemiological, and Clinical Comparison of Hepatitis A, Hepatitis B, Hepatitis C, and Delta Hepatitis

	Hepatitis A	Hepatitis B	Hepatitis C	Delta Hepatitis
Incubation	2–6 wk	4 wk–6 mo	Variable: 14–160 days; average, 50 days	Same as hepatitis B
Communicable	Until 7–9 days after jaundice occurs	Several months—as long as virus present in blood	As long as virus present in blood	As long as virus present in blood
Transmission	Fecal-oral; blood; sexual	Parenteral; sexual; perinatal	Percutaneous, via contaminated blood, parenteral drug abuse; some fecal-oral forms; sexual, perinatal	Parenteral; blood
Sources	Crowding; contaminated food, milk, or water	Contaminated needles, syringes, surgical instruments	Persons who have received 15 or more blood transfusions; IV drug users; persons traveling to contaminated areas	Contaminated needles, syringes
Portal of entry	GI tract; asymptomatic carriers	Integumentary: blood plasma or transfusions	Blood	Integumentary: blood
HB antigen	Not present	Present	Not present	Present as with hepatitis B
Incidence	Sporadic epidemics; increased in children <15	Increased in ages 15–29, particularly in heroin addiction; occupational hazard for laboratory workers, nurses, physicians	All ages groups; higher in adults because of exposure to risk factors	Same as hepatitis B
Immunity	*Preexposure:* immune globulin, 0.02 mL/kg *Postexposure:* within 2 wk of exposure, as above	*Preexposure:* hepatitis B vaccine *Postexposure:* immune globulin with high amounts of anti-HBs (HBIG); hepatitis B vaccine	None; immune globulin may be given	None
Prevention	Hand washing, use of gloves; hepatitis A vaccine	Care when handling products contaminated by blood, use of gloves; Hepatitis B vaccine	Same as hepatitis B	Same as hepatitis B
Severity	Mild	Mild to moderate	Mild to moderate	Moderate to severe
Fever	Common	Uncommon	Uncommon	Uncommon
Nausea/vomiting	Common	Common	Common	Common

d. Urine: normal, dark.
e. Stool: normal, clay colored, loose.
f. Vomiting, weight loss.
g. Lymph nodes: enlarged.
h. Lab data:
  (1) Blood—leukocytosis.
  (2) *Increased* AST (SGOT), ALT (SGPT), and bilirubin levels, alkaline phosphatase.
  (3) Urine—*increased* urobilinogen.
i. See Table 7–24.

◆ **D. Analysis/nursing diagnosis:**
1. *Pain* related to inflammation of liver.
2. *Impaired skin integrity* related to pruritus.
3. *Activity intolerance* related to fatigue.
4. *Risk for infection* to others related to incubation/infectious period.
5. *Altered nutrition, less than body requirements,* related to repugnance of food.

TABLE 7–25 Contact Precautions

1. Private room if the patient's hygiene is poor. In general, patients with the same infection *may share* a room.
2. Masks are *not* indicated.
3. Gowns are indicated if soiling is likely.
4. Gloves are indicated for touching infective material.
5. Hands must be washed before and after touching the patient or potentially contaminated articles.
6. Contaminated articles should be discarded or bagged and labeled.

6. *Social isolation* related to isolation precautions.

◆ **E. Nursing care plan/implementation:**
  1. Goal: *prevent spread of infection to others.*
    a. Isolation according to type
      (1) *Hepatitis A:*
        (a) Contact precautions (Table 7–25).
        (b) Private room preferred.

(c) Gown/gloves for direct contact with feces.
(d) Hand washing when in direct contact with feces.
(2) *Hepatitis B:* blood and body fluid precautions.
  (a) Needle/dressing precautions.
  (b) Private room not necessary.
  (c) Gown: only if enteric precautions also necessary.
  (d) Hand washing: use gloves when in direct contact with blood.
(3) *Hepatitis C:* blood and body fluid precautions.
  (a) Same as hepatitis B, except when in countries with fecal-oral form, then use hepatitis A precautions also.
(4) *Delta:*
  (a) Same as hepatitis B.
b. Passive immunity for contacts.
(1) *Hepatitis A:* hepatitis A vaccine (Havrix, VAQTA), immune serum globulin (ISG), administered before and after exposure.
(2) *Hepatitis B:* hepatitis B immune globulin (HBIG) (Recombivax HB, Energix-B) or ISG.
(3) *Hepatitis C:* prophylaxis not as effective; IG may be given.
(4) *Delta:* same as for hepatitis B.
c. Goal: *promote healing.*
(1) *Diet* as tolerated:
  (a) NPO with parenteral infusions, when in acute stage.
  (b) *High* protein, *high* carbohydrate, *low* fat, offered in frequent small meals.
  (c) Push fluids, if not contraindicated; I&O.
(2) Medications:
  (a) Antiviral for patients with persistently elevated ALT levels.
  (b) Interferon for initial treatment of hepatitis C.
d. Goal: *monitor for worsening of disease process, failure to respond to prescribed treatment.*
(1) Observe urine—dark due to presence of bile and stool, clay colored.
(2) Observe sclera, lab tests for increasing jaundice.
(3) Mental confusion, unusual somnolence may indicate decreased liver function.
(4) Weigh daily—increase indicates fluid retention and possible ascites.
e. Goal: *health teaching.*
(1) Diet and fluid intake to promote liver regeneration.

(2) Importance of rest and limited activity to reduce metabolic workload of liver.
(3) Personal hygiene practices to prevent contamination.
(4) *Avoid:* alcohol, blood donations, and contact with communicable infections.
(5) Follow-up case referral; may take 6 mo for full recovery.
(6) Teach contacts about available immunizations.
2. Goal: *promote comfort.*
a. Bed rest to combat fatigue and reduce metabolic needs until hepatomegaly subsides; *semi-Fowler's* or *supine* positioning.
b. Oral hygiene q1–2h to decrease nausea.
c. ROM exercises to maintain muscle strength.
d. *Measures to reduce pruritus:*
(1) Mild, oil-based lotion to reduce itching.
(2) Nails cut short, cotton gloves, long-sleeved clothing to prevent skin injury from scratching.
(3) Environment: cool and dry.
(4) Cool wet soaks to skin.
(5) Diversional activities.
(6) Medications as ordered:
  (a) *Emollients* to relieve dry skin.
  (b) *Topical corticosteroids* to reduce inflammation.
  (c) *Antihistamines* to reduce itch.
  (d) *Tranquilizers and sedatives* to allow rest and prevent exhaustion.
◆ **F. Evaluation/outcome criteria:**
1. Tolerates food; nausea and vomiting decreased.
2. Signs of infection/inflammation absent.
3. No complications, hemorrhage, liver damage, ascites.
4. No jaundice noted.

IV. **Pancreatitis:** inflammatory disease of the pancreas that may result in autodigestion of the pancreas by its own enzymes.
  A. Pathophysiology: proteolytic enzymes within the pancreas are activated by endotoxins, exotoxins, ischemia, anoxia, or trauma. Pancreatic enzymes begin process of autodigestion of pancreas and surrounding tissues; also activate other enzymes that digest cellular membranes. Autodigestion leads to edema, hemorrhage, vascular damage, coagulation necrosis, and fat necrosis.
  B. Risk factors:
1. Obesity.
2. Alcoholism, alcohol consumption.
3. Biliary tract disease.
4. Abdominal trauma.
5. Surgery.

6. Drugs.
7. Metabolic disease.
8. Intestinal disease.
9. Obstruction of the pancreatic ducts.
10. Infections.
11. Carcinoma.
12. Adenoma.
13. Hypercalcemia.

◆ **C. Assessment:**

1. *Subjective data:*

   a. Pain:

      (1) Sudden onset; severe, widespread, constant, and incapacitating.

      (2) Location—epigastrium, right upper quadrant (RUQ) and left upper quadrant (LUQ) of abdomen; radiates to back, flanks, and substernal area.

   b. Nausea.

   c. History of risk factors.

   d. Dyspnea.

2. *Objective data:*

   a. *Elevated:* temperature, pulse, respirations, BP (unless in shock).

   b. *Decreased* breath sounds related to atelectasis/pleural effusion.

   c. *Increased* crackles, cyanosis.

   d. Hemorrhage, shock.

   e. Vomiting.

   f. Fluid and electrolyte imbalances, dehydration.

   g. *Decreased* bowel sounds; abdominal tenderness with guarding.

   h. *Stools:* bulky, pale, foul smelling, steatorrhea (excessive fat in stools).

   i. *Skin:* pale, moist, cold; may be jaundiced.

   j. Muscle rigidity.

   k. Supine position leads to increased pain.

   l. Fluid accumulation in the abdomen.

   m. Lab data:

      (1) *Elevated:*

         (a) Amylase, serum, and urine.

         (b) Serum lipase, AST (SGOT).

         (c) Alkaline phosphatase.

         (d) Bilirubin, glucose; serum and urine.

         (e) Urine protein, WBC.

         (f) Leukocytes.

         (g) BUN.

         (h) LDH (liver function, lactate dehydrogenase).

      (2) *Decreased:*

         (a) Serum calcium.

         (b) Protein.

   n. Ultrasound for gallstones, CAT scan.

◆ **D. Analysis/nursing diagnosis:**

1. *Altered nutrition, less than body requirements,* related to nausea and vomiting.

2. *Pain* related to inflammatory and autodigestive processes of pancreas.

3. *Fluid volume deficit* related to inflammation, decreased intake, and vomiting.

4. *Ineffective breathing pattern* related to pain and pleural effusion.

5. *Knowledge deficit* related to risk factors and disease management.

◆ **E. Nursing care plan/implementation:**

1. Goal: *control pain.*

   a. Medications: analgesics—meperidine (*not* morphine or codeine due to spasmodic effect).

   b. *Position:* sitting with knees flexed.

2. Goal: *rest injured pancreas.*

   a. NPO.

   b. NG tube to low suction.

   c. Medications:

      (1) *Antiulcers.*

      (2) *Antibiotics.*

      (3) *Antiemetics.*

      (4) *Antispasmodics.*

      (5) *Anticholinergics.*

      (6) *Histamine-2 receptors* (cimetidine).

3. Goal: *prevent fluid and electrolyte imbalance.*

   a. Monitor: vitals, CVP.

   b. IVs, fluids, blood, albumin, plasma.

4. Goal: *prevent respiratory and metabolic complications.*

   a. Cough, deep breathe, change position.

   b. Monitor: blood sugar as ordered.

   c. Monitor calcium levels: *Chvostek's* and *Trousseau's sign* positive when calcium deficit exists (see **XVI. Thyroidectomy,** p. 599, for description of tests).

5. Goal: *provide adequate nutrition.*

   a. *Low-fat diet.*

   b. Bland, small, frequent meals.

   c. Vitamin supplements.

   d. *Avoid* alcohol.

6. Goal: *prevent complications.*

   a. Monitor for signs of:

      (1) Peritonitis.

      (2) Perforation.

      (3) Respiratory complications.

      (4) Hypotension, shock.

      (5) DIC.

      (6) Hemorrhage from ulcers, varices.

      (7) Anemia.

      (8) Encephalopathy.

7. Goal: *health teaching.*

   a. Food selections for low-fat, bland diet.

   b. Necessity of vitamin therapy.

   c. Importance of avoiding alcohol.

   d. Signs and symptoms of recurrence.

   e. Importance of rest, to prevent relapse.

   f. Desired effects and side effects of prescribed medications:

      (1) Narcotics for pain.

      (2) Antiemetics for nausea and vomiting.

      (3) Pancreatic hormone and enzymes to replace enzymes not reaching duodenum.

◆ **F. Evaluation/outcome criteria:**
1. Pain is relieved.
2. No complications, e.g., peritonitis, respiratory.
3. States dietary allowances and restrictions.
4. Takes medications as ordered; states purposes, side effects.

V. **Cirrhosis:** chronic inflammation and fibrosis (irreversible scarring) of the liver in which some liver cells (hepatocytes) undergo necrosis and others undergo proliferative regeneration.

   A. Pathophysiology: progressive destruction of hepatic cells → loss of normal metabolic function of the liver and formation of scar tissue. Regeneration and proliferation of fibrous tissue → obstruction of the portal vein → increased portal hypertension, ascites, liver failure, and eventual death.

   B. Risk factors:
   1. Alcohol abuse most common cause.
   2. Nutritional deficiency with decreased protein intake.
   3. Hepatotoxins.
   4. Virus.
   5. Hepatitis B and C.

◆ **C. Assessment:**
   1. *Subjective data:*
      a. Chronic feeling of malaise.
      b. Anorexia, nausea.
      c. Abdominal pain.
      d. Pruritus.
   2. *Objective data:*
      a. GI:
         (1) Malnutrition, weight loss.
         (2) Vomiting.
         (3) Flatulence.
         (4) Ascites.
         (5) Enlarged liver and spleen.
         (6) Glossitis.
         (7) Fetid breath (sweet, musty odor).
      b. Blood—coagulation defects, possible esophageal varices, portal hypertension, bleeding from gums and injection sites.
      c. Skin and hair—edema, jaundice, spider angioma (telangiectasias); palmar erythema, decreased pubic and axillary hair.
      d. Reproductive—menstrual abnormalities, gynecomastia, testicular atrophy, impotence.
      e. Neurological deficits, including memory loss, hepatic coma, decreased level of consciousness: flapping tremor, grimacing.
      f. Lab data:
         (1) *Decreased:* albumin, potassium, magnesium, blood urea nitrogen (BUN).
         (2) *Elevated:* prothrombin time, globulins, ammonia, AST (SGOT), Bromsulphalein (BSP), alkaline phosphate, uric acid, blood sugar.
      g. *Diagnostic tests*
         (1) Celiac angiography, hepatoportography
         (2) Liver biopsy
         (3) Paracentesis

◆ **D. Analysis/nursing diagnosis:**
   1. *Altered nutrition, less than body requirements,* related to decreased intake, nausea, and vomiting.
   2. *Risk for injury* related to decreased prothrombin production.
   3. *Activity intolerance* related to fatigue.
   4. *Fatigue* related to anorexia and nutritional deficiencies.
   5. *Self-esteem disturbance* related to physical body changes.
   6. *Risk for impaired skin integrity* related to pruritus.

◆ **E. Nursing care plan/implementation:**
   1. Goal: *provide for special safety needs.*
      a. Monitor vitals (including neurological) frequently for hemorrhage from esophageal varices (may have *Sengstaken-Blakemore* or *Linton* tube inserted).
      b. Prepare patient for *LeVeen shunt* surgery for portal hypertension as needed.
      c. Assist with *paracentesis* performed for ascites; monitor vitals to prevent shock during procedure.
   2. Goal: *relieve discomfort caused by complications.*
      a. *Position: semi-Fowler's* or *Fowler's* to decrease pressure on diaphragm due to ascites.
      b. Deep breathing q2h to prevent respiratory complications.
      c. Skin care, topical medications to relieve pruritus; nail care to decrease possibility of further skin injury.
      d. Frequent oral hygiene related to nausea, vomiting, and fetid breath.
   3. Goal: *improve fluid and electrolyte balance.*
      a. IV fluids and vitamins.
      b. I&O, hourly urines during acute attacks.
      c. Daily: girths, weights to monitor fluid balance.
      d. Diuretics as ordered to decrease edema.
      e. May receive serum albumin to promote adequate vascular volume, prevent azotemia and encephalopathy, and promote diuresis (observe carefully, because albumin could escape quickly through cell walls and cause increase in ascites).
   4. Goal: *promote optimum nutrition within dietary restrictions.*
      a. NPO during acute episodes.
      b. Small, frequent meals when able to eat.
      c. *Low protein* (to decrease the amount of nitrogenous materials in the intestines) and *sodium* (to decrease fluid retention).

d. *Moderate carbohydrate* (to meet energy demands) and *fat* (to make diet more palatable to anorexic patients).
5. Goal: *provide emotional support.*
   a. Quiet environment during acute episodes to decrease external stimuli.
   b. Identify *community agencies* for assistance far patient, e.g., Alcoholics Anonymous; for family, Al-Anon/Alateen.
6. Goal: *health teaching.*
   a. *Avoid* alcohol, exposure to infections.
   b. Dietary allowances, restrictions (see **Unit 9,** Sodium-restricted diet, p. 682, and Purine-restricted diet, p. 682).
   c. Drugs: names, purposes.
   d. Signs, symptoms of disease; complications.
   e. Stress-management techniques.

◆ **F. Evaluation/outcome criteria:**
1. No complications.
2. Nutritional status improves; lists dietary restrictions.
3. No alcohol consumption.
4. Lists signs and symptoms of progression of disease and complications.
5. Complies with discharge plan, becomes involved with an alcohol treatment program.

VI. Esophageal varices: life-threatening hemorrhage from tortuous dilated, thin-walled veins in submucosa of lower esophagus. May rupture when chemically or mechanically irritated or when pressure is increased because of sneezing, coughing, use of the Valsalva maneuver, or excessive exercise.

A. Pathophysiology: portal hypertension related to cirrhosis of the liver → distended branches of the azygos vein and inferior vena cava where they join the smaller vessels of the esophagus.

B. Risk factors for hemorrhage:
1. Exertion that increases abdominal pressure.
2. Trauma from ingestion of coarse foods.
3. Acid pepsin erosion.

◆ **C. Assessment:**
1. *Subjective data:*
   a. Fear.
   b. Dysphagia.
   c. History: alcohol ingestion, liver dysfunction.
2. *Objective data:*
   a. Hematemesis.
   b. Hemorrhage: sudden, often fatal.
   c. Decreased BP; increased pulse, respirations.
   d. Melena (occult blood in stool).

◆ **D. Analysis/nursing diagnosis:**
1. *Fluid volume deficit* related to blood loss.
2. *Risk for injury* related to hemorrhage.
3. *Fear* related to massive blood loss.
4. *Ineffective individual coping* related to complications of cirrhosis.

◆ **E. Nursing care plan/implementation:**
1. Goal: *provide safety measures related to hemorrhage.*
   a. Recognize signs of shock; vitals q15min.
   b. Assist with insertion of *Sengstaken-Blakemore* (or Minnesota) or *Linton tube* (tube is large and uncomfortable for patient during insertion); explain procedure briefly to decrease fear and attempt to gain patient's cooperation.
   c. While tube is in place, observe for respiratory distress; if present, *deflate the balloon by releasing pressure; do not cut the tube.*
   d. Deflate the balloon as ordered to prevent necrosis.
   ► e. NG tube to low gastric suction; monitor for amount of bright-red blood; irrigate only as ordered using tepid, *not* iced, solutions.
   f. Vitamin K as ordered to control bleeding.
2. Goal: *promote fluid balance.*
   a. IV fluids, expanders, blood.
   b. Fresh blood as ordered to avoid increased ammonia; aids in coagulation.
3. Goal: *prevent complications of hepatic coma.*
   a. Saline cathartics as ordered to remove old blood from GI tract.
   b. Antibiotics as ordered to prevent infection.
   c. Reduce portal hypertension; give propranolol (Inderal), vasopressin (Pitressin).
4. Goal: *provide emotional support.*
   a. Stay with patient.
   b. Calm atmosphere.
5. Goal: *health teaching.*
   a. Explain use of tube to patient and family.
   b. Bland diet instructions.
   c. Recognize signs of bleeding.
   d. *Avoid* straining at stool.
   e. *Avoid* aspirin because of increased bleeding tendency.

◆ **F. Evaluation/outcome criteria:**
1. Survives acute bleeding episode.
2. Further episodes prevented by avoiding irritants, especially alcohol.
3. Improves nutritional status.
4. Recognizes symptoms of complications, e.g., bleeding.
5. Demonstrates knowledge of medications by avoiding aspirin.

VII. Diaphragmatic (hiatal) hernia: protrusion of part of stomach through diaphragm and into thoracic cavity (Figure 7–8). *Types:* sliding (most common); paraesophageal "rolling."

A. Pathophysiology: weakening of the musculature of the diaphragm, aggravated by increased intra-abdominal pressure → protrusion of the abdominal organs through the esophageal hiatus → reflux of gastric contents → esophagitis.

FIGURE 7–8 Hiatal hernia. (From Thomas, CL [ed]: Taber's Cyclopedic Medical Dictionary, ed 18. FA Davis, Philadelphia, 1997, p 890.)

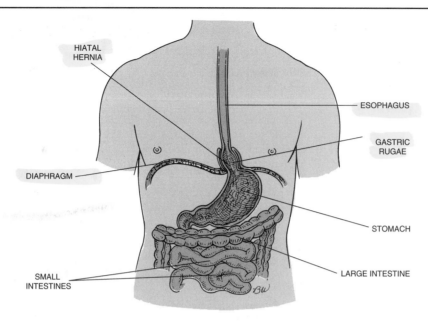

B. Risk factors:
1. Congenital abnormality.
2. Penetrating wound.
3. Age (middle-aged or elderly).
4. Women more than men.
5. Obesity.
6. Ascites.
7. Pregnancy.
8. History of constipation.

◆ **C. Assessment:**
1. *Subjective data:*
   a. Pressure: substernal.
   b. Pain: epigastric, burning.
   c. Eructation, heartburn after eating.
   d. Dysphagia.
   e. Symptoms aggravated when recumbent.
2. *Objective data:*
   a. Cough, dyspnea.
   b. Tachycardia, palpitations.
   c. Bleeding: hematemesis, melena, signs of anemia due to gastroesophageal irritation, ulceration, and bleeding.
   d. *Diagnostic tests:*
      (1) Chest x-rays, showing protrusion of abdominal organs into thoracic cavity.
      (2) Barium swallow (upper GI series) to show presence of hernia.
      (3) Endoscopy
   e. Symptoms parallel those of gastroesophageal reflux disease (GERD).

◆ **D. Analysis/nursing diagnosis:**
1. *Pain* related to irritation of lining of GI tract.
2. *Altered nutrition, less than body requirements,* related to dysphagia.

3. *Sleep pattern disturbance* related to increase in symptoms when recumbent.
4. *Risk for aspiration* related to reflux of gastric contents.
5. *Activity intolerance* related to dyspnea.
6. *Anxiety* related to palpitations.

◆ **E. Nursing care plan/implementation:**
1. *Presurgical:*
   a. Goal: *promote relief of symptoms.*
      (1) *Diet:*
         (a) Small, frequent feedings of soft, bland foods, to reduce abdominal pressure and reflux.
         (b) Fluid when swallowing solids may push food into stomach; hot fluid may work best.
         (c) *Avoid* eating 2 hr before bedtime.
         (d) *High*-protein, *low*-fat foods to decrease heartburn.
      (2) *Positioning: head elevated* to increase movement of food into stomach. Symptoms may decrease if head of bed at home is elevated on 8-inch blocks.
      (3) Weight reduction to decrease abdominal pressure.
      (4) Medications as ordered:
         (a) 30 mL antacid 1 hr *after* meals and at bedtime.
         (b) *Avoid* anticholinergic drugs, which decrease gastric emptying.
2. *Postsurgical:*
   a. Goal: *provide for postoperative safety needs.*
      (1) Respiratory: deep breathing, coughing, splint incision area.

▶ (2) *Nasogastric (NG) tube:* check patency.
    (a) Drainage: should be small amount.
    (b) Color: dark brown 6–12 hr after surgery, changing to greenish yellow.
    (c) Do *not* disturb tube placement to avoid traction on suture line.

▟ (3) *Position:* initially head of bed elevated slightly, then *semi-Fowler's;* turn side to side frequently, to prevent pressure on diaphragm.

▶ (4) Maintain closed chest drainage if indicated (see Table 11–7).

    (5) Check for return of bowel sounds.

b. Goal: *promote comfort and maintain nutrition.*
    (1) IVs for hydration and electrolytes.

▶ (2) Initiate feeding through *gastrostomy* tube if present.

> (a) Usually attached to intermittent, low suction after surgery.
> (b) Aspirate gastric contents before feeding—delay if 75 mL or more is present; report these findings to physician.
> ▟ (c) Feed in *high Fowler's* or sitting position; keep head elevated for 30 min after eating.
> (d) Warm feeding to room temperature; dilute with H_2O if too thick.
> (e) Give 50 mL H_2O before feeding; 200–500 mL feeding by gravity over 10–15 min; follow with 50 mL H_2O.
> (f) Give frequent mouth care.

c. Goal: *health teaching.*
    (1) *Avoid* constricting clothing and activities that increase intra-abdominal pressure, e.g., lifting, bending, straining at stool.
    (2) Weight reduction.
    (3) Dietary needs: small, frequent, soft, bland meals; chew thoroughly; upright position for at least 1 hr after meals.

◆ **F. Evaluation/outcome criteria:**
1. Relief from symptoms, comfortable.
2. Receiving adequate, balanced nutrition.
3. Describes dietary changes, recommended positioning, and activity limitations to prevent recurrence.

VIII. Gastroesophageal reflux disease (GERD): inappropriate relaxation of the lower esophageal sphincter (LES) in response to unknown stimulus.

    A. Pathophysiology: gastric volume or intra-abdominal pressure elevated, or LES tone decreased → frequent episodes of acid reflux →

breakdown of mucosal barrier → esophageal inflammation, hyperemia, and erosion → fibrotic tissue formation → esophageal stricture → impaired swallowing.

B. Risk factors:
1. Hiatal hernia.
2. Diet—foods that lower pressure of LES (fatty foods, chocolate, cola, coffee, tea).
3. Smoking.
4. Drugs (calcium channel blockers, NSAIDs, theophylline).
5. Elevated intra-abdominal pressure (obesity, pregnancy, heavy lifting).

◆ **C. Assessment:**
1. *Subjective data:*
    a. Heartburn (pyrosis)—substernal or retrosternal; may mimic angina; 20 min to 2 hr after eating.
    b. Regurgitation—sour or bitter taste not associated with belching or nausea.
    c. Dysphagia or odynophagia (difficult or painful swallowing)—severe cases.
    d. Belching, feeling bloated.
    e. Nocturnal cough.
2. *Objective data:*
    a. Hoarseness, wheezing.
    b. *Diagnostic tests:* 24 hr pH monitoring; barium swallow with fluoroscopy; endoscopy.

◆ **D. Analysis/nursing diagnosis:**
1. *Pain* related to acid reflux and esophageal inflammation.
2. *Knowledge deficit* (learning need) related to modifications needed to control reflux.

◆ **E. Nursing care plan/implementation:**
1. Goal: *promote comfort and reduce reflux episodes.*
    a. Medications as ordered:
      (1) *Antacids* to neutralize gastric acid.
      (2) *Histamine (H_2) receptor antagonists* (cimetidine, ranitidine, famotidine) to reduce gastric acid secretion and support tissue healing.
      (3) *Proton pump inhibitor* (omeprazole [Prilosec]) to inhibit gastric enzymes and suppress gastric acid secretion.
    b. *Diet: avoid* strong stimulants of acid secretion (caffeine, alcohol); *avoid* foods that reduce LES competence (fatty foods, onions, tomato-based foods); *increase* protein; *restrict* spicy, acidic foods until healing occurs.
    c. Activity: *avoid* heavy lifting, straining, constrictive clothing, bending over.
    ▟ d. *Position:* elevate head of bed 6–12 inches for sleeping. Reflux more likely on right side.
2. Goal: *health teaching.*
    a. Weight reduction if indicated.
    b. Smoking cessation.

Adult

c. Diet modification: avoid overeating—eat 4–6 small meals.

d. Medication administration.

e. Potential complications if uncontrolled (hemorrhage, aspiration).

◆ **F. Evaluation/outcome criteria:**

1. No heartburn reported.

2. Changes diet as instructed.

3. No complications of continued reflux.

IX. Peptic ulcer disease: circumscribed loss of mucosa, submucosa, or muscle layer of the gastrointestinal tract caused by a decreased resistance of gastric mucosa to acid-pepsin injury. *Peptic ulcer disease* is a chronic disease and may occur in the distal esophagus, stomach, upper duodenum, or jejunum. *Gastric ulcers,* located on the lesser curvature of the stomach, are larger and deeper than duodenal ulcers and tend to become *malignant. Duodenal ulcers* are located on the first part of the duodenum and are more common than gastric ulcers. *Esophageal ulcers* occur in the esophagus. *Stress ulcers,* an acute problem, occur after a major insult to the body.

A. Pathology: failure of the body to regenerate mucous epithelium at a sufficient rate to counterbalance the damage to tissue during the breakdown of protein; decrease in the quantity and quality of the mucus; poor local mucosal blood flow, along with individual susceptibility to ulceration. A *peptic ulcer* is a hole in the lining of the stomach, duodenum, or esophagus. This hole occurs when the lining of these organs is corroded by the acidic digestive juices secreted by the stomach cells. Excess acid is still considered to be significant in ulcer formation. The leading cause of ulcer disease is currently believed to be infection of the stomach by *Helicobacter pylori (H. pylori).* Another major cause of ulcers is chronic use of nonsteroidal anti-inflammatory drugs (NSAIDs). Cigarette smoking is also an important cause of ulcers.

B. Risk factors:

1. *Gastric ulcers.*

a. Infection with *H. pylori.*

b. Decreased resistance to acid-pepsin injury.

c. Increased histamine release → inflammatory reaction.

d. Ulcerogenic drugs (aggravate pre-existing conditions).

e. Cigarette smoking.

f. Increased alcohol and caffeine use (aggravates pre-existing conditions).

g. Gastric ulcer is thought to be a risk for gastric cancer.

h. Difficulty coping with stressful situations.

2. *Duodenal ulcers.*

a. Infection with *H. pylori.*

b. Elevated gastric acid secretory rate.

c. Elevated gastric acid levels postprandially (after eating).

d. Increased rate of gastric emptying → increased amount of acid in duodenum → irritation and breakdown of duodenal mucosa.

e. Ulcerogenic medication use (aggravates pre-existing conditions).

f. Cigarette smoking.

g. Alcohol and caffeine use (aggravates pre-existing condition).

h. Difficulty coping with stressful situations.

3. *Stress ulcers.*

a. Severe trauma or major illness.

b. Severe burns *(Curling's ulcer);* develop in 72 hr with majority of persons with burns over more than 35% of the body surface.

c. Head injuries or intracranial disease *(Cushing's ulcer).*

d. Medications in large doses: corticosteroids, salicylates, ibuprofen, indomethacin, phenylbutazone (Butazolidin).

e. Shock.

f. Sepsis.

◆ **C. Assessment:**

1. *Subjective data:*

a. *Gastric ulcers.*

(1) Pain.

(a) Type: gnawing, aching, burning.

(b) Location: epigastric, left of midline, localized.

(c) Occurrence: periodic pain, often 2 hr after eating.

(d) Relief: antacids; may be aggravated, *not* relieved, by food.

(e) Some patients report no discomfort at all.

(2) Weakness.

(3) History of risk factors as above.

b. *Duodenal ulcers.*

(1) Pain.

(a) Type: gnawing, aching, burning, hungerlike, boring.

(b) Location: right epigastric, localized; steady pain near midline of back may indicate perforation.

(c) Occurrence: 1–3 hr after eating, worse at end of day or during the night; initial attack occurs spring or fall; history of remissions and exacerbations.

(d) Relief: food, antacids, or both.

(e) Some patients report no discomfort at all.

(2) Nausea.

(3) History of risk factors (see **IX. B.,** on this page).

c. *Stress ulcers.*

(1) Pain: often painless until serious complication (hemorrhage, perforation) occurs.

(2) History of risk factors as above.

2. *Objective data.*

a. *Gastric ulcer.*
  (1) Vomiting blood (hematemesis).
  (2) Melena (tarry stools).
  (3) Weight loss.
  (4) X-ray (upper GI series) confirms "crater" (punched-out appearance, clean base).
  (5) Endoscopy confirms presence of ulcer; biopsy for cytology.
  (6) Monitor for blood loss: CBC, stool for occult blood.
  (7) Orthostatic hypotension.
  (8) *Lab data:* positive for *H. pylori.*
b. *Duodenal ulcer.*
  (1) Eructation.
  (2) Vomiting blood (hematemesis).
  (3) Regurgitation of sour liquid into back of mouth.
  (4) Constipation.
  (5) X-ray (upper GI series) confirms ulcer craters and niches, as well as outlet deformities: round or oval funnel-like lesion extending into musculature.
  (6) Endoscopy for direct visualization.
  (7) Monitor for blood loss: CBC, stool for occult blood.
  (8) Orthostatic hypotension.
  (9) *Lab data:* positive for *H. pylori.*
c. *Stress ulcer.*
  (1) GI bleeding.
  (2) Multiple, superficial erosions affecting large area of gastric mucosa.

◆ **D. Analysis/nursing diagnosis** (all types):
  1. *Pain* related to erosion of gastric lining.
  2. *Ineffective individual coping* related to inability to change lifestyle.
  3. *Altered nutrition, less than body requirements,* related to inadequate intake.
  4. *Knowledge deficit* regarding preventive measures.
  5. *Risk for injury* related to possible hemorrhage or perforation.

◆ **E. Nursing care plan/implementation** (all types):
  1. Goal: *promote comfort.*
    a. Medications as ordered to decrease pain (see 4. Goal: *health teaching*); sedatives to decrease anxiety.
    b. Prepare for *diagnostic tests.*
      (1) X-rays; upper GI series (barium swallow); lower GI (barium enema).
      (2) Endoscopy.
      (3) Gastric analysis, to determine amount of hydrochloric acid in GI tract.
  2. Goal: *prevent/recognize signs of complications.*
    a. Monitor vitals for shock.
    b. Check stool for occult blood/hemorrhage.
    c. Palpate abdomen for perforation (rigid,

boardlike); arterial bleeding.
  3. Goal: *provide emotional support.*
    a. Stress-management techniques.
    b. Restful environment.
    c. Prepare for surgery, if necessary.
  4. Goal: *health teaching.*
    a. Medications:
      (1) *Antibiotics.* Sometimes antibiotics work best if given in combination with Prilosec, H$_2$ blockers, or Pepto-Bismol. *Caution:* use of antibiotic treatment can cause allergic reactions, diarrhea, and severe antibiotic-induced colitis.
        (a) Tetracycline.
        (b) Amoxicillin.
        (c) Metronidazole (Flagyl).
        (d) Clarithromycin (Biaxin).
      (2) *Histamine antagonists: given with meals/bedtime* to block the action of histamine-stimulated gastric secretions (basal and stimulated); inhibit pepsin secretion and reduce the volume of gastric secretions.
        (a) Cimetidine (Tagamet) inhibits gastrin release; can be given PO, IV, or IM; *cannot* be given within 1 hr of antacid therapy.
        (b) Ranitidine (Zantac) has greater reduction of acid secretion, longer duration, less frequent administration (bid vs. qid), and fewer side effects than cimetidine.
        (c) Nizatidine (Axid).
        (d) Famotidine (Pepcid).
      (3) *Proton pump inhibitors* (gastric acid inhibitors): superior in treating esophageal ulcers; equal to other H$_2$ receptors for gastric and duodenal ulcers.
        (a) Omeprazole (Prilosec).
        (b) Lansoprazole (Prevacid).
        (c) Pantoprazole.
      (4) *Antiulcers: give 1–3 hr after meals and at bedtime* to decrease pain by lowering acidity; monitor for:
        (a) Diarrhea (seen most often with magnesium carbonate and magnesium oxide [Maalox, Mylanta]).
        (b) Constipation (seen most often with calcium carbonate [Tums] or aluminum hydroxide [Amphojel]).
        (c) Electrolyte imbalance (seen with systemic antacid, soda bicarbonate).
        (d) Best 1–3 hr *after meals.*
        (e) Liquids more effective than tablets; if taking tablets, chew slowly.

(5) *Sucralfate* (Carafate) and misoprostol (Cytotec): *given 1 hr before meals and at bedtime.*
  (a) Locally active topical agent that forms a protective coat on mucosa, prevents further digestive action of both acid and pepsin.
  (b) Must *not* be given within 30 min of antacids.
(6) *Anticholinergic*—when used, given before meals to decrease gastric acid secretion and delay gastric emptying.
(7) *Cisapride,* a serotonin-4 receptor agonist used to treat ulcers, gastric reflux, dyspepsia, gastroparesis, and chronic constipation.
(8) Important: *avoid aspirin* (could increase bleeding possibility).

b. *Diet:*
  (1) Change diet only to relieve symptoms; diet may not influence ulcer formation.
  (2) *Avoid* foods that increase acidity—caffeine and alcohol in moderation.
  (3) *Plan:*
    (a) Small, frequent meals (to prevent exacerbations of symptoms related to an empty stomach).
    (b) Weight control.

c. Complications—signs and symptoms:
  (1) Gastric ulcers may be premalignant.
  (2) Perforation.
  (3) Hemorrhage.
  (4) Obstruction.

d. *Lifestyle changes:*
  (1) Decrease:
    (a) Smoking.
    (b) Noise.
    (c) Rush.
    (d) Confusion.
  (2) Increase:
    (a) Communication.
    (b) Mental/physical rest.
    (c) Compliance with medical regimen.

◆ **F. Evaluation/outcome criteria:**
1. *Avoids* foods/liquids that cause irritation.
2. Takes prescribed medications.
3. Pain decreases.
4. No complications.
5. States signs and symptoms of complications.
6. Participates in stress-reduction activities.
7. Stops smoking.

X. Gastric surgery: peformed when ulcer medical regimen is unsuccessful, ulcer is determined to be precancerous, or complications are present.
  A. Types:
  1. *Subtotal gastrectomy:* removal of a portion of the stomach.

2. *Total gastrectomy:* removal of the entire stomach.
3. *Antrectomy:* removal of entire antrum (lower) portion of the stomach.
4. *Pyloroplasty:* repair of the pyloric opening of the stomach.
5. *Vagotomy:* interruption of the impulses carried by the vagus nerve, which results in reduction of gastric secretions and decreased physical activity of the stomach (being done less often).
6. Combination of vagotomy and gastrectomy.

◆ **B. Analysis/nursing diagnosis:**
1. *Pain* related to surgical incision.
2. *Ineffective breathing pattern* related to high surgical incision.
3. *Risk for trauma* related to possible complications postgastrectomy.
4. *Knowledge deficit* regarding medication regimen and factors that aggravate condition.
5. *Fear* related to possible precancerous lesion.
6. *Ineffective individual coping* related to adjustments in lifestyle needed to lessen symptoms.

◆ **C. Nursing care plan/implementation:**
1. Goal: *promote comfort in the postoperative period.*
  a. Analgesics: to relieve pain and allow patient to cough, deep breathe to prevent pulmonary complications.
  b. *Position: semi-Fowler's* to aid in breathing.
2. Goal: *promote wound healing.*
  a. Keep dressings dry.
  b. NG tube to low intermittent suction (Levin) or low continuous suction (Salem-sump).
    (1) Check drainage from NG tube; normally bloody first 2–3 hr postsurgery, then brown to dark green.
    (2) Excessive bright-red blood drainage: take vital signs; report vital signs, color and volume of drainage to MD **immediately.**
    (3) Irrigate gently with saline in amount ordered; do *not* irrigate against resistance; may not be done in early postoperative period.
    (4) Tape securely to face, but prevent obstructed vision.
    (5) Frequent mouth and nostril care.
3. Goal: *promote adequate nutrition and hydration.*
  a. Administer parenteral fluids as ordered.
  b. Accurate I&O.
  c. Check bowel sounds, at least q4h; NPO 1–3 days; bowel sounds normally return 21–36 hr; oral fluids as ordered when bowel sounds present—usually 30 mL, then small feedings, then bland liquids to soft diet.

d. Observe for nausea and vomiting due to suture line edema, food intake (too much, too fast).

4. Goal: *prevent complications.*
    a. Check dressing q4h for bleeding.
    b. *Vitamin B₁₂* and iron replacement as indicated to avoid pernicious anemia and iron deficiency anemia.
    c. *Avoid* dumping syndrome.

◆ **D. Evaluation/outcome criteria:**
1. Hemorrhage, dumping syndrome avoided.
2. Healing begins.
3. Adjust lifestyle to prevent recurrence/marginal ulcer.

XI. Dumping syndrome: hypoglycemic-type episode; occurs postoperativly after gastric resection (may also occur after vagotomy, antrectomy, or gastroenterostomy), when food and fluids that are more hyperosmolar than the jejunal secretions pass *quickly* into jejunum, producing fluid shifts from bloodstream to jejunum. This is a mild problem for about 20% of patients and will disappear in a few months to a year. Symptoms cause serious problem for about 7% of patients. This discomfort may occur during a meal or up to 30 min after the meal and last from 20–60 min. The reaction is greatest after the ingestion of sugar.

◆ **A. Assessment:**
1. *Subjective data:*
    a. Feeling of fullness, weakness, faintness.
    b. Palpitations.
    c. Nausea.
    d. Discomfort during or after eating.
2. *Objective data:*
    a. Diaphoresis.
    b. Diarrhea.
    c. Fainting.
    d. Symptoms of hypoglycemia.

◆ **B. Analysis/nursing diagnosis:**
1. *Altered nutrition, more than body requirements,* related to body's inability to properly digest high-carbohydrate, high-sodium foods.
2. *Diarrhea* related to food passing into jejunum too quickly.
3. *Risk for injury* related to hypoglycemia.
4. *Knowledge deficit* related to dietary restrictions.

◆ **C. Nursing care plan/implementation:**
1. Goal: *health teaching.*
    a. *Include:*
        (1) *Increased fat, protein* to delay emptying.
        (2) Rest after meals.
        (3) Small, frequent meals.
        (4) Fluids *between* meals.
    b. *Avoid:*
        (1) Foods high in *salt, carbohydrate.*
        (2) Large meals.

        (3) Stress at mealtime.
        (4) Fluids at mealtime.

◆ **D. Evaluation/outcome criteria:**
1. No complications.
2. Patient heals.
3. No further ulcers.
4. Incorporates health teaching into lifestyle and prevents syndrome.

XII. Total parenteral nutrition: provide nutrition through a central venous line to patients who are in a catabolic state; are malnourished and cannot tolerate food by mouth; are in negative nitrogen balance; or have conditions that interfere with protein ingestion, digestion, and absorption, e.g., Crohn's disease, major burns, and side effects of radiation therapy of abdomen.

A. Types of solutions:
1. Hydrolyzed proteins (Hyprotein, Amigen).
2. Synthetic amino acids (Freamine).
3. Usual components:
    a. 3–8% amino acid.
    b. 10–25% glucose.
    c. Multivitamins.
    d. Electrolytes.
    e. Fats (lipid or fat emulsions). Lipid emulsions are *contraindicated* if patient has allergy to eggs.
4. Supplements that can be added:
    a. Fructose.
    b. Alcohol.
    c. Minerals: iron, copper, calcium.
    d. Trace elements: iodine, zinc, magnesium.
    e. Vitamins: A, B, C.
    f. Androgen hormone therapy.
    g. Insulin.
    h. Heparin.

B. Administration:
1. Dosage varies with clinical condition; 1 L q5–8h; rate of flow must be constant.
2. Solution prepared under laminar flow hood (usually in pharmacy); solution must be *refrigerated;* when refrigerated, expires in 24 hr; once removed from refrigerator, expires in 12 hr.
3. Incompatible with many antibiotics; check with pharmacy.
4. Route: catheter inserted in a large vein (e.g., subclavian) by physician; placement confirmed by x-ray before beginning infusion (Figure 7–9).
5. *Side effects:*
    a. Hyperosmolar coma.
    b. Hyperglycemia >130 mg/dL.
    c. Septicemia.
    d. Thrombosis/sclerosis of vein.
    e. Air embolus.
    f. Pneumothorax.
6. Prolonged use: >10 days, fat needed; intralipids piggybacked close to insertion site;

Adult

FIGURE 7–9 Hyperalimentation. Patient with subclavian hyperalimentation line.

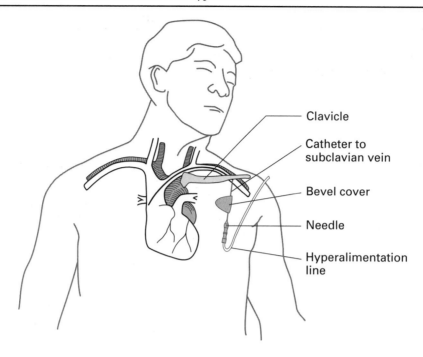

do *not* give through filter; observe for hypersensitivity (e.g., tachypnea, tachycardia, nausea, urticaria).

◆ **C. Analysis/nursing diagnosis:**
  1. *Fluid volume excess, potential,* related to inability to tolerate amount and consistency of solution.
  2. *Fluid volume deficit* related to state of malnutrition.
  3. *Risk for injury* related to possible complications.
  4. *Altered nutrition, more or less than body requirements,* related to ability to tolerate parenteral nutrition.

◆ **D. Nursing care plan/implementation:**
  1. Goal: *prevent infection.*
    ▶ a. Dressing change:
      (1) Strict *aseptic* technique.
      (2) Nurse and patient wear mask during dressing change.
      (3) Cleanse skin with solution as ordered:
        (a) Acetone to defat the skin, destroy the bacterial wall.
        (b) Iodine 1% solution as antiseptic agent.
      (4) Dressing changed q48–72h; transparent polyurethane dressings may be changed weekly.
      (5) Mark with nurse's initials, date and time of change.
      (6) Air occlusive dressing.
    b. Attach final filter on tubing setup, to prevent air embolism.
    c. Solution: change q12h to prevent infec-

tion.
    d. Culture wound and catheter tip if signs of infection appear.
    e. Monitor temperature q4h.
    f. Use lumen line for feeding *only* (not for CVP or medications).
  2. Goal: *prevent fluid and electrolyte imbalance.*
    a. Daily weights.
    b. I&O.
    c. Blood glucose q4h using glucometer; may need insulin coverage.
    d. Specific gravity q8h to determine hydration status; normal serum osmolality 275–295 mOsm, TPN 600–1400 mOsm.
    e. Infusion pump to maintain constant infusion rate.
  3. Goal: *prevent complications.*
    a. Warm TPN solution to room temperature to prevent chills.
    b. Monitor for signs of complications (Table 7–26).
      (1) Infiltration.
      (2) Thrombophlebitis.
      (3) Fever.
      (4) Hyperglycemia.
      (5) Fluid imbalance.
    c. Have patient perform *Valsalva maneuver* or apply a plastic-coated clamp when changing tubing to prevent air embolism.
    d. Tape tubings together to prevent accidental separation.

◆ **E. Evaluation/outcome criteria:**
  1. No signs of infection.
  2. Blood sugar <130 mg/dL.
  3. Specific gravity between 1.010 and 1.020.

TABLE 7–26   Complications Associated with Total Parenteral Nutrition

Problem	◆ Nursing Interventions
Infection Local infection (pain, redness, edema) Generalized, systemic infection (elevated temperature, WBC)	Sterile dressings; administer antibiotics as ordered; general comfort measures
Arterial Puncture Artery is punctured instead of vein Physician aspirates bright-red blood that is pulsating strongly	Needle is withdrawn and pressure is applied
Air Embolus Air enters venous system during catheter insertion or tubing changes; or catheter/tubing pull apart Chest pain, dizziness, cyanosis, confusion	Stat ABGs, chest x-ray, ECG Connect catheter to sterile syringes, and aspirate air Clean catheter tip, connect to new tubing *Place patient on left side with head lowered* (left Trendelenburg prevents air from going into pulmonary artery) *Prevention: have patient perform Valsalva maneuver or use plastic-coated clamp on catheter at insertion or tubing changes*
Catheter Embolus Catheter must be checked for placement by x-ray and observed when removed to be sure it is intact	Careful observation of catheter Monitor for signs of distress
Pneumothorax If needle punctures pleura, patient reports dyspnea, chest pain	May seal off or may need chest tubes

4. Wounds begin to heal.
5. Weight: no further loss, begins to gain.

XIII. **Diabetes:** heterogeneous group of diseases involving the disruption of the metabolism of carbohydrates, fats, and protein. If uncontrolled, serious vascular and neurological changes occur.
   A. **Types:**
      1. *Type 1:* formerly called *insulin-dependent diabetes mellitus (IDDM);* and also formerly called "juvenile-onset diabetes." Insulin needed to prevent ketosis; onset usually in youth but may occur in adulthood; prone to ketosis, unstable diabetes.
      2. *Type 2:* formerly called *non–insulin-dependent diabetes mellitus (NIDDM);* and also *formerly* called "maturity-onset diabetes" or "adult-onset diabetes." May be controlled with diet and oral hypoglycemics or insulin; patient less apt to have ketosis, except in presence of infection. May be further classified as *obese type 2* or *nonobese type 2.*
      3. *Type 3: gestational diabetes mellitus (GDM):* glucose intolerance during pregnancy in women who were not known to have diabetes before pregnancy; will be reclassified after birth; may need to be treated or may return to prepregnancy state and need no treatment.
      4. *Type 4:* diabetes secondary to another condition, such as pancreatic disease, other hormonal imbalances, or drug therapy such as receiving glucocorticoids.
   B. **Pathophysiology:**
      1. Type 1—absolute deficiency of insulin due to destruction of pancreatic beta cells by the interaction of genetic, immunological, hereditary, or environmental factors.
      2. Type 2—relative deficiency of insulin due to:
         a. An islet cell defect resulting in a slowed or delayed response in the release of insulin to a glucose load; or
         b. Reduction in the number of insulin receptors from continuously elevated insulin levels; or
         c. A postreceptor defect; or
         d. A major peripheral resistance to insulin induced by hyperglycemia. These factors lead to deprivation of insulin-dependent cells → a marked decrease in the cellular rate of glucose uptake, and therefore elevated blood glucose.
   C. **Risk factors:**
      1. Obesity.
      2. Family history of diabetes.
      3. Age 45 or older.
      4. Women whose babies at birth weighed more than 9 lb.
      5. History of autoimmune disease.
      6. Members of high-risk ethnic group (African-American, Latino, or Native American).
      7. History of gestational diabetes mellitus.
      8. Hypertension.
      9. Elevated HDL.
   ◆ D. **Assessment:**
      1. *Subjective data:*
         a. *Eyes:* blurry vision.
         b. *Skin:* pruritus vulvae.
         c. *Neuromuscular:* paresthesia, peripheral neuropathy, lethargy, weakness, fatigue, increased irritability.

Adult

d. *GI:* polydipsia (increased thirst).

e. *Reproductive:* impotence.

2. *Objective data:*

a. *Genitourinary:* polyuria, glycosuria, nocturia (nocturnal enuresis in children).

b. *Vital signs:*

(1) Pulse and temperature normal or elevated.

(2) BP normal or decreased, unless complications present.

(3) Respirations, increased rate and depth (*Kussmaul's* respirations).

c. *GI:*

(1) Polyphagia, dehydration.

(2) Weight loss, failure to gain weight.

(3) Acetone breath.

d. *Skin:* cuts heal slowly; frequent infections, foot ulcers, vaginitis.

e. *Neuromuscular:* loss of strength, peripheral neuropathy.

f. Lab data:

(1) *Elevated:*

(a) Blood sugar >126 mg/dL fasting or 200 mg/dL 1–2 hr after eating.

(b) Glucose tolerance test.

(c) Glycosuria (>170 mg/100 mL).

(d) Potassium (>5) and chloride (>145).

(e) Hemoglobin A_{1c} >7%.

(2) *Decreased:*

(a) pH (<7.4).

(b) $PaCO_2$ (<32).

g. Long-term pathological considerations:

(1) *Cataract formation and retinopathy:* thickened capillary basement membrane, changes in vascularization and hemorrhage, due to chronic hyperglycemia.

(2) *Nephropathy:* due to glomerulosclerosis, arteriosclerosis of renal artery and pyelonephritis, progressive uremia.

(3) *Neuropathy:* due to reduced tissue perfusion; affecting motor, sensory, voluntary, and autonomic functions.

(4) *Arteriosclerosis:* due to lesions of the intimal wall.

(5) *Cardiac:* angina, coronary insufficiency, myocardial infarction.

(6) *Vascular changes:* occlusions, intermittent claudication, loss of peripheral pulses, arteriosclerosis.

◆ **E. Analysis/nursing diagnosis:**

1. *Altered nutrition, less than body requirements,* related to inability to metabolize nutrients and weight loss.

2. *Altered nutrition, more than body requirements,* related to excessive glucose intake.

3. *Risk for injury* related to complications of uncontrolled diabetes.

4. *Body image disturbance* related to long-term illness.

5. *Knowledge deficit* related to management of long-term illness and potential complications.

6. *Ineffective individual coping* related to inability to follow diet/medication regimen.

7. *Sexual dysfunction* related to impotence from diabetes and treatment.

◆ **F. Nursing care plan/implementation:**

1. Goal: *obtain and maintain normal sugar balance.*

a. Monitor: vital signs; blood glucose before meals, at bedtime, and as symptoms demand (urine testing for glucose levels is not as accurate as capillary blood testing).

b. Medications:

(1) *Oral hypoglycemics:*

(a) Sulfonylureas; tolbutamide (Orinase), chlorpropamide (Diabenese), tolazamide (Tolinase), acetohexamide (Dymelor), glimepiride (Amaryl), glyburide (DiaBeta and Micronase), and glipizide (Glucocotrol).

(b) Others: metformin (Glucophage) increases body's sensitivity to insulin. Acarbose (Precose) inhibits cells of the small intestine from absorbing complex carbohydrates.

(2) *Insulin* (available as pork, beef, or human synthetic insulin):

(a) Lispro, a rapid-acting analogue of human insulin.

(b) Short acting (crystalline, regular) (Humulin R).

(c) Intermediate acting (Lente and NPH).

(d) Slow acting (protamine zinc).

(e) Long, extended acting (Ultralente, Ultratard).

(3) Methods of administration:

(a) Subcutaneous injection.

(b) Prefilled injectable insulin pens (Novopen and Novolin).

(c) Continuous subcutaneous insulin infusion therapy (insulin pumps).

c. *Diet,* as ordered.

(1) Carbohydrate, 50–60%; protein, 20%; fats, 30% (saturated fats limited to 10%, unsaturated fats, 90%).

(2) Calorie reduction in obese adults; enough calories to promote normal growth and development for children or nonobese adults.

(3) Limit refined sugars.

(4) Add vitamins, minerals as needed for well-balanced diet.

d. Monitor for signs of acute (hypoglycemia, ketoacidosis) or chronic (circulatory compromise, neuropathy, nephropathy, retinopathy) complications.

2. Goal: *health teaching:*

a. *Diet:* foods allowed, restricted, substitutions.

b. Medications: administration techniques, importance of using room-temperature insulin and rotating injection sites to prevent tissue damage.

c. Desired and side effects of prescribed insulin type; onset, peak, and duration of action of prescribed insulin.

d. Blood glucose testing techniques.

e. Signs of complications (Table 7–27).

f. Importance of health maintenance:

(1) Infection prevention, especially foot and nail care.

(2) Routine checkups.

(3) Maintain stable balance of glucose by carefully monitoring glucose level and making necessary adjustments in diet and activity level; seeking medical attention when unable to maintain balance; regular exercise program.

◆ **G. Evaluation/outcome criteria:**

1. Optimal blood-glucose levels achieved.

2. Ideal weight maintained.

3. Adequate hydration.

4. Carries out self-care activities: blood or urine testing, foot care, exchange diets, medication administration, exercise.

5. Recognizes and treats hyperglycemic or hypoglycemic reactions.

6. Seeks medical assistance appropriately.

XIV. Nonketotic hyperglycemic hyperosmolar coma (NKHHC): profound hyperglycemia and dehydration without ketosis or ketoacidosis; seen in non–insulin-dependent diabetes; brought on by infection or illness. This condition may lead to impaired consciousness and seizures. The patient is *critically ill.* Mortality rate is over 50%.

A. Pathophysiology: hyperglycemia greater than 1000 mg/dL causes osmotic diuresis, depletion of extracellular fluid, and hyperosmolarity related to infection or another stressor as the precipitating factor. Patient unable to replace fluid deficits with oral intake.

B. Risk factors:

1. Old age.

2. History of non–insulin-dependent diabetes.

3. Infections: pneumonia, pyelonephritis, pancreatitis, gram-negative infections.

4. Kidney failure: uremia and peritoneal dialysis or hemodialysis.

5. Shock:

a. Lactic acidosis related to bicarbonate deficit.

b. Myocardial infarction.

6. Hemorrhage:

a. GI.

b. Subdural.

c. Arterial thrombosis.

7. Medications:

a. Diuretics.

b. Glucocorticoids.

8. Tube feedings.

◆ **C. Assessment:**

1. *Subjective data:*

a. Confusion.

b. Lethargy.

2. *Objective data:*

a. Nystagmus.

b. Dehydration.

c. Aphasia.

d. Nuchal rigidity.

e. Hyperreflexia.

f. Lab data:

(1) Blood-glucose level 1000 mg/dL.

(2) Serum sodium and chloride—normal to *elevated.*

(3) BUN >60 mg/dL (higher than in ketoacidosis because of more severe gluconeogenesis and dehydration).

(4) Arterial pH—slightly *depressed.*

◆ **D. Analysis/nursing diagnosis:**

1. *Risk for injury* related to hyperglycemia.

2. *Altered renal peripheral tissue perfusion* related to vascular collapse.

3. *Ineffective airway clearance* related to coma.

◆ **E. Nursing care plan/implementation:**

1. Goal: *promote fluid and electrolyte balance.*

a. IVs: fluids and electrolytes, sodium chloride solution used initially to combat dehydration. Rate of infusion will be determined by BP assessment, cardiovascular status, balance between fluid input and output, and lab values.

b. Monitor I&O because of the high volume of fluid replaced in the critical stage of this condition.

c. Administer nursing care for the problem that precipitated this serious condition.

d. Food by mouth when client is able.

2. Goal: *prevent complications.*

a. Administer *regular* insulin (initial dose usually 5–15 U) and food, as ordered.

b. Uncontrolled condition leads to cardiovascular disease, renal failure, blindness, and diabetic gangrene.

◆ **F. Evaluation/outcome criteria:**

1. Blood sugar returns to normal level of 80–120 mg/dL.

2. Patient is alert to time, place, and person.

3. Primary medical problem resolved.

4. Patient recognizes and reports signs of imbalance.

Adult

TABLE 7–27   Comparison of Diabetic Complications

	Hypoglycemia	Ketoacidosis
Pathophysiology	Major metabolic complication when too little food or too large dose of insulin or hypoglycemic agents administered; interferes with oxygen consumption of nervous tissue	Major metabolic complication in which there is insufficient insulin for metabolism of carbohydrates, fats, and proteins; seen most frequently with patients who are insulin dependent; precipitated in the known diabetic by stressors (such as infection, trauma, major illness) that increase insulin needs
Risk factors	Too little food Emotional or added stress Vomiting or diarrhea Added exercise	Insufficient insulin or oral hypoglycemics Noncompliance with dietary instructions Major illness/infections Therapy with steroid administration Trauma, surgery Elevated blood sugar: >200 mg/dL
◆ Assessment	**Behavioral change:** *Subjective data*—nervous, irritable, anxious, confused, disoriented *Objective data*—abrupt mood changes, psychosis **Visual:** *Subjective data*—blurred vision, diplopia *Objective data*—dilated pupils **Skin:** *Objective data*—diaphoresis, **pale,** cool, clammy, goose bumps (piloerection), tenting **Vitals:** *Objective data*—tachycardia; palpitations, thready **Gastrointestinal:** *Subjective data*—hunger, nausea *Objective data*—diarrhea, vomiting **Neurological:** *Subjective data*—headache; lips/tongue: tingling, numbness *Objective data*—fainting, yawning; speech: incoherent; convulsions; coma **Musculoskeletal:** *Subjective data*—weak, fatigue *Objective data*—trembling Blood sugar: <80 mg/dL	**Behavioral change:** *Subjective data*—irritable, confused *Objective data*—drowsy **Visual:** *Objective data*—eyeballs: soft, sunken **Skin:** *Objective data*—loss of turgor, **flushed face,** pruritus vulvae **Vitals:** *Objective data*—respirations: *Kussmaul's;* breath: fruity; BP: hypovolemic shock **Gastrointestinal:** *Subjective data*—increased thirst and hunger, abdominal pain, nausea *Objective data*—vomiting, diarrhea, dry mucous membrane; lips, tongue: red, parched **Neurological:** *Subjective data*—headache; irritability; confusion; lethargy, weakness **Musculoskeletal:** *Subjective data*—fatigue; general malaise **Renal:** *Objective data*—polyuria Blood sugar: >130 mg/dL
◆ Analysis/nursing diagnosis	*Risk for injury* related to deficit of needed glucose *Knowledge deficit* related to proper dietary intake or proper insulin dosage *Altered nutrition, less than body requirements,* related to glucose deficiency	*Risk for injury* related to glucose imbalance *Knowledge deficit* related to proper balance of diet and insulin dosage
◆ Nursing care plan/implementation	Goal: *provide adequate glucose to reverse hypoglycemia:* administer simple sugar stat, PO or IV, glucose paste absorbed in mucous membrane; monitor blood sugar levels; identify events leading to complication Goal: *health teaching:* how to prevent further episodes (see Diabetes, Health teaching, p. 527); importance of careful monitoring of balance between glucose levels and insulin dosage	Goal: *promote normal balance of food and insulin:* **regular** insulin as ordered; IV saline, as ordered; bicarbonate and electrolyte replacements, as ordered; potassium replacements once therapy begins and urine output is adequate Goal: *health teaching:* diet instructions; desired effects and side effects of prescribed insulin or hypoglycemic agent (onset, peak, and duration of action); importance of recognizing signs of imbalance
◆ Evaluation/outcome criteria	Adheres to diet and correct insulin dosage Adjusts dosage when activity is increased Glucose level 80–120 mg/dL	Serious complications avoided Accepts prescribed diet Takes medication (correct dose and time) Glucose level 80–120 mg/dL

XV. **Cholecystitis/cholelithiasis:** inflammation of gall-bladder due to bacterial infection, presence of cholelithiasis (stones, cholesterol, calcium, or bile in the gallbladder), or choledocholithiasis (stone in the common bile duct) and/or obstruction. Acute cholecystitis is abrupt in onset, but the patient usually has a history of several attacks of fatty-food intolerance. Patient with chronic cholecystitis has a history of several attacks of moderate severity and has usually learned to avoid fatty foods to decrease symptoms.

A. **Pathophysiology:** calculi from increased concentration of bile salts, pigments, or cholesterol due to metabolic or hemolytic disorders, biliary stasis → precipitation of salts into stones, or inflammation causing bile constituents to become altered.

B. **Risk factors:**
1. Womanhood.
2. Obesity.
3. Pregnancy or previous pregnancies.
4. Use of birth control pills or hormone replacement therapy.
5. High-fat, low-fiber diets.
6. Rapid weight loss.
7. History of Crohn's disease.
8. Genetics.
9. Age: increased risk over 40.
10. Certain drugs to lower lipids; clofibrate (Atromid-S).
11. Other diseases: cirrhosis of liver.

◆ C. **Assessment:**
1. *Subjective data:*
   a. Pain:
      (1) Type—severe colic, radiating to the back under the scapula and to the right shoulder.
      (2) Positive *Murphy's sign*—a sign of gallbladder disease consisting of pain on taking a deep breath when pressure is placed over the location of the gallbladder.
      (3) Location—right upper quadrant, epigastric area, flank (Figure 7–10).
      (4) Duration—spasm of duct attempting to dislodge stone lasts until dislodged or relieved by medication, or sometimes by vomiting.
   b. GI—anorexia, nausea, feeling of fullness, indigestion, intolerance of fatty foods.
2. *Objective data:*
   a. GI—belching, vomiting, clay-colored stools.
   b. Vital signs—increased pulse, fever.
   c. Skin—chills, jaundice.
   d. Urine—dark amber.
   e. Lab data—*elevated:*
      (1) WBC.
      (2) Alkaline phosphatase.
      (3) Serum amylase, lipase.
      (4) AST (SGOT).
      (5) Bilirubin.
   f. *Diagnostic studies:*
      (1) Ultrasound.
      (2) Cholangiography.
      (3) Computed tomography (CT) scan.
      (4) Endoscopic retrograde cholangiopancreatography (ERCP).

◆ D. **Analysis/nursing diagnosis:**
1. *Pain* related to obstruction of bile duct due to cholelithiasis.
2. *Altered nutrition, more than body requirements,* related to ingestion of fatty foods.
3. *Altered nutrition, less than body requirements,* related to hesitancy to eat due to anorexia and nausea.
4. *Risk for fluid volume deficit* related to episodes of vomiting.
5. *Knowledge deficit* related to dietary restrictions.

◆ E. **Nursing care plan/implementation:**
1. Nonsurgical interventions:
   a. Goal: *promote comfort.*
      (1) Medications as ordered: meperidine, *antibiotics, antispasmodics, electrolytes.*
      (2) *Avoid* morphine due to spasmodic effect.
      (3) NG tube to low suction.
      (4) *Diet:* fat free when able to tolerate food.
      (5) Lithotripsy: gallstones fragmented by shock waves
      (6) Oral dissolution therapy: ursodeoxycholic acid (ursodiol [Actigall]).
   b. Goal: *health teaching:*
      (1) Signs, symptoms, and complications of disease.
      (2) Fat-free diet.
      (3) Desired effects and side effects of prescribed medications.
      (4) Prepare for possible removal of gallbladder (cholecystectomy) if conservative treatment unsuccessful.
2. Surgical interventions:
   a. *Preoperative*—Goal: *prevent injury:* see **I. Preoperative preparation,** p. 500.
   b. *Postoperative*—Goal: *promote comfort* (see also **III. Postoperative experience,** p. 504).
      (1) Laparoscopic laser cholecystectomy—tiny incisions/puncture wounds; gallbladder is removed using a video-guided system with a camera; patient is discharged that day or next day, able to resume normal diet and work activities in a few days.
      (2) Endoscopic retrograde cholangiopancreatography (ERCP) with papillotomy—removes stones from bile duct. No incision; done under sedation, not anesthesia.

FIGURE 7–10 Abdominal pain by location. (Modified from Caroline, NL: Emergency Care in the Streets, ed 5. Boston, Little, Brown, 1995, p 641; and from Thomas, CL, [ed]: Taber's Cyclopedic Medical Dictionary, ed 18. FA Davis, Philadelphia, 1997, p 3.)

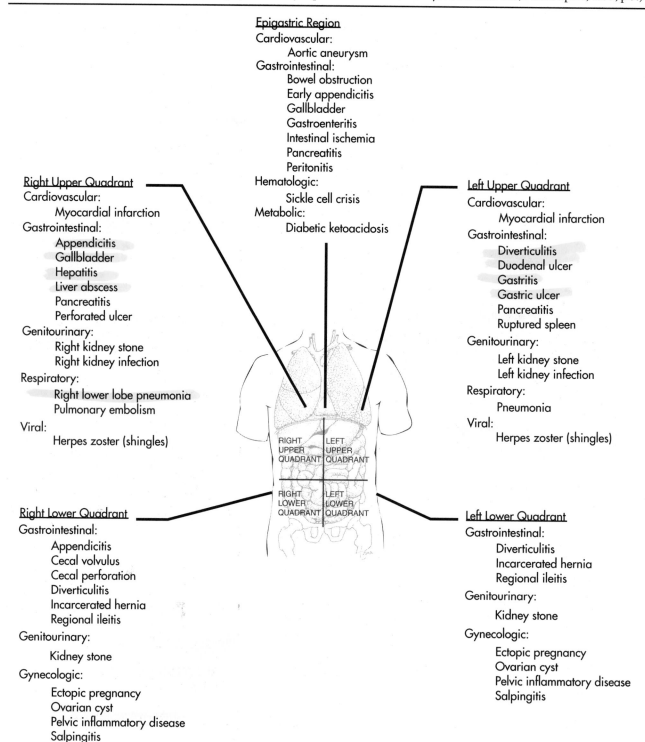

Epigastric Region
Cardiovascular:
  Aortic aneurysm
Gastrointestinal:
  Bowel obstruction
  Early appendicitis
  Gallbladder
  Gastroenteritis
  Intestinal ischemia
  Pancreatitis
  Peritonitis
Hematologic:
  Sickle cell crisis
Metabolic:
  Diabetic ketoacidosis

Right Upper Quadrant
Cardiovascular:
  Myocardial infarction
Gastrointestinal:
  Appendicitis
  Gallbladder
  Hepatitis
  Liver abscess
  Pancreatitis
  Perforated ulcer
Genitourinary:
  Right kidney stone
  Right kidney infection
Respiratory:
  Right lower lobe pneumonia
  Pulmonary embolism
Viral:
  Herpes zoster (shingles)

Left Upper Quadrant
Cardiovascular:
  Myocardial infarction
Gastrointestinal:
  Diverticulitis
  Duodenal ulcer
  Gastritis
  Gastric ulcer
  Pancreatitis
  Ruptured spleen
Genitourinary:
  Left kidney stone
  Left kidney infection
Respiratory:
  Pneumonia
Viral:
  Herpes zoster (shingles)

Right Lower Quadrant
Gastrointestinal:
  Appendicitis
  Cecal volvulus
  Cecal perforation
  Diverticulitis
  Incarcerated hernia
  Regional ileitis
Genitourinary:
  Kidney stone
Gynecologic:
  Ectopic pregnancy
  Ovarian cyst
  Pelvic inflammatory disease
  Salpingitis

Left Lower Quadrant
Gastrointestinal:
  Diverticulitis
  Incarcerated hernia
  Regional ileitis
Genitourinary:
  Kidney stone
Gynecologic:
  Ectopic pregnancy
  Ovarian cyst
  Pelvic inflammatory disease
  Salpingitis

RIGHT UPPER QUADRANT | LEFT UPPER QUADRANT
RIGHT LOWER QUADRANT | LEFT LOWER QUADRANT

(3) Open-incision cholecystectomy.

▶ (a) Promote tube drainage:

> (i) NG tube to low suction.
> (ii) *T-tube* to closed-gravity drainage, to preserve patency of edematous common duct and ensure bile drainage; usual amount 500–1000 mL/24 hr; dark brown drainage.
> (iii) Provide enough tubing to allow turning without tension.
> (iv) Empty and record bile drainage q8h.

◢ (b) *Position: low Fowler's* to *semi-Fowler's* to facilitate T-tube drainage.

(c) Dressing: dry to protect skin (because bile excoriates skin).

(d) Clamp T-tube as ordered.
   (i) Observe for abdominal distention, pain, nausea, chills, or fever.
   (ii) Unclamp tube and notify MD if symptoms appear.

c. Goal: *prevent complications.*
   (1) IV fluids with vitamins.
   (2) Cough, turn, and deep breathe with open incision, particularly with removal of gall bladder (prone to respiratory complication because of high incision).
   (3) Early ambulation to prevent vascular complications and aid in expelling flatus.
   (4) Monitor for jaundice: skin, sclera, urine, stools.
   (5) Monitor for signs of hemorrhage, infection.

d. Goal: *health teaching.*
   (1) *Diet:* fat free for 6 wk.
   (2) Signs of complications of food intolerance, pain, infection, hemorrhage.

▶ **F. Evaluation/outcome criteria:**
   1. No complications.
   2. Able to tolerate food.
   3. Plans follow-up care.
   4. Possible weight reduction.

Adult

ELIMINATION

Conditions Affecting Bowel Elimination

I. Appendicitis: obstruction of appendiceal lumen and subsequent bacterial invasion of appendiceal wall; acute emergency.

  A. Pathophysiology: when obstruction is partial or mild, inflammation begins in mucosa with slight appendiceal swelling, accompanied by periumbilical pain. As the inflammatory process escalates and/or obstruction becomes more complete, the appendix becomes more swollen, the lumen fills with pus, and mucosal ulceration begins. When inflammation extends to the peritoneal surface, pain is referred to the right lower abdominal quadrant. *Danger:* rigidity over the entire abdomen is usually indicative of ruptured appendix; the patient is then prone to peritonitis.

  B. Risk factors:
   1. Men more than women.
   2. Most frequently seen between age 10 and 30 yr.

  ◆ **C. Assessment:**
   1. *Subjective data:*
      a. Pain: generalized, then right lower quadrant at McBurney's point, with rebound tenderness.
      b. Anorexia, nausea.
   2. *Objective data:*
      a. Vital signs: elevated temperature, shallow respirations.
      b. Either diarrhea or constipation.
      c. Vomiting, fetid breath odor.
      d. Splinting of abdominal muscles, flexion of knees onto abdomen.
      e. Lab data:
         (1) WBC *elevated* (>10,000).
         (2) Neutrophil count *elevated* (>75%).
      f. *Diagnostic studies:*
         (1) Ultrasound.
         (2) CT scan.

  ◆ **D. Analysis/nursing diagnosis:**
   1. *Pain* related to inflammation of appendix.
   2. *Risk for trauma* related to ruptured appendix.
   3. *Knowledge deficit* related to possible surgery.

  ◆ **E. Nursing care plan/implementation:**
   1. Goal: *promote comfort.*
      a. *Preoperative:*
         (1) Explain procedures.
         (2) Assist with diagnostic workup.
      b. *Postoperative:*
         (1) Relieve pain related to surgical incision.
         (2) Prevent infection: wound care, dressing technique.
         (3) Prevent dehydration: IVs, I&O, fluids to solids by mouth as tolerated.
         (4) Promote ambulation to prevent postoperative complications.

  ◆ **F. Evaluation/outcome criteria:**
   1. No infection.
   2. Tolerates fluid; bowel sounds return.
   3. Heals with no complications.

II. Hernia: protrusion of the intestine through a weak portion of the abdominal wall.

  A. Types:
   1. *Reducible:* visceral contents return to their normal position, either spontaneously or by manipulation.
   2. *Irreducible, or incarcerated:* contents cannot be returned to normal position.
   3. *Strangulated:* blood supply to the structure within the hernia sac becomes occluded (usually a loop of bowel).
   4. Most common hernias: umbilical, femoral, inguinal, incisional, and hiatal.

  B. Pathophysiology: weakness in the wall may be either congenital or acquired. Herniation occurs when there is an increase in intraabdominal pressure from coughing, lifting, crying, straining, obesity, or pregnancy.

  ◆ **C. Assessment:**
   1. *Subjective data:*
      a. Pain, discomfort.
      b. History of feeling a lump.
   2. *Objective data:*
      a. Soft lump, especially when straining or coughing.
      b. Sometimes alteration in normal bowel pattern.
      c. Swelling.

  ◆ **D. Analysis/nursing diagnosis:**
   1. *Activity intolerance* related to pain and discomfort.
   2. *Risk for trauma* related to lack of circulation to affected area of bowel.
   3. *Pain* related to protrusion of intestine into hernia sac.

  ◆ **E. Nursing care plan/implementation:**
   1. Goal: *prevent postoperative complications.*
      a. Monitor bowel sounds.
      b. Prevent postoperative scrotal swelling with inguinal hernia by applying ice and support to scrotum.
   2. Goal: *health teaching.*
      a. Prevent recurrence with correct body mechanics.
      b. Gradual increase in exercise.

  ◆ **F. Evaluation/outcome criteria:** healing occurs with no further hernia recurrence.

III. Diverticulosis: a *diverticulum* is a small pouch or sac composed of mucous membrane that has protruded through the muscular wall of the intestine. The presence of several of these is called *diverticulosis.* Inflammation of the diverticula is called *diverticulitis.*

A. Pathophysiology: weakening in a localized area of muscular wall of the colon (especially the sigmoid colon), accompanied by increased intraluminal pressure.

B. Risk factors:
1. Diverticulosis:
   a. Age: seldom before 35 yr; 60% incidence in older adults.
   b. History of constipation.
   c. Diet history: low in vegetable fiber, high in carbohydrate.
2. Diverticulitis: highest incidence between ages 50 and 60 yr.

◆ **C. Assessment:**
1. *Subjective data:* pain: cramplike; left lower quadrant of abdomen.
2. *Objective data:*
   a. Constipation or diarrhea, flatulence.
   b. Fever.
   c. Rectal bleeding.
   d. *Diagnostic procedures:*
      (1) Palpation reveals tender colonic mass.
      (2) Barium enema (done only in absence of inflammation) reveals presence of diverticula.
      (3) Sigmoidoscopy/colonoscopy.

◆ **D. Analysis/nursing diagnosis:**
1. *Constipation* related to dietary intake.
2. *Pain* related to inflammatory process of intestines.
3. *Risk for fluid volume deficit* related to episodes of diarrhea or bleeding.
4. *Risk for injury* related to bleeding.
5. *Knowledge deficit* related to prevention of constipation.

◆ **E. Nursing care plan/implementation:**
1. Goal: *bowel rest during acute episodes.*
   a. *Diet:* soft, liquid.
   b. Fluids, IVs if oral intake not adequate.
   c. Medications:
      (1) *Antibiotics:* ciprofloxacin (Cipro), metronidazole (Flagyl), cephalexin (Keflex), doxycycline (Vibramycin).
      (2) *Antispasmodics:* chlordiazepoxide (Librax), dicyclomine (Bentyl), Donnatal, hyoscyamine (Levsin).
   d. Monitor stools for signs of bleeding.
2. Goal: *promote normal bowel elimination.*
   a. *Diet:* bland, *high* in vegetable fiber if no inflammation.
      (1) *Include:* fruits, vegetables, whole-grain cereal, unprocessed bran.
      (2) *Avoid:* foods difficult to digest (corn, nuts).
   b. Bulk-forming agents as ordered: methylcellulose, psyllium.
   c. Monitor: abdominal distention, acute bowel symptoms.

3. Goal: *health teaching.*
   a. Methods to avoid constipation.
   b. Foods to include/avoid in diet.
   c. Relaxation techniques.
   d. Signs and symptoms of complications of chronic inflammation: abscess, obstruction, fistulas, perforation, or hemorrhage.

◆ **F. Evaluation/outcome criteria:**
1. Inflammation decreases.
2. Bowel movements return to normal.
3. Pain decreases.
4. No perforation, fistulas, or abscesses noted.

IV. Ulcerative colitis: inflammation of mucosa and submucosa of the large intestine. Inflammation leads to ulceration with bleeding. Involved areas are continuous. Disease is characterized by remissions and exacerbations.

A. Pathophysiology: Currently believed to be an autoimmune disease. The body's immune system is called on to attack the inner lining of the large intestine, causing inflammation and ulceration. Edema and hyperemia of colonic mucous membrane → superficial bleeding with increased peristalsis, shallow ulcerations, abscesses; bowel wall thins and shortens and becomes at risk for perforation. Increased rate of flow of liquid ileal contents → decreased water absorption and diarrhea.

B. Risk factors:
1. Highest occurrence in young adults (age 20–40 yr).
2. Genetic predisposition: higher in caucasians, Jews.
3. Autoimmune response.
4. Infections.
5. More common in urban areas (upper-middle incomes and higher educational levels).
6. Nonsmokers/ex-smokers.
7. Genetic, inherited, or familial tendencies.
8. Chronic ulcerative colitis is a risk factor for colon cancer.

◆ **C. Assessment:**
1. *Subjective data:*
   a. Urgency to defecate, particularly when standing.
   b. Loss of appetite, nausea.
   c. Colic-like abdominal pain.
   d. History of intolerance to dairy products.
   e. Emotional depression.
2. *Objective data:*
   a. *Diarrhea:* 10–20 stools/day; can be chronic or intermittent, episodic or continual; stools contain blood, mucus, and pus.
   b. Weight loss and malnutrition, dehydration.
   c. Fever.
   d. Rectal bleeding.
   e. Lab data: *decreased:* RBC, potassium, sodium, calcium, bicarbonate related to excessive diarrhea.

f. Lymphadenitis.

g. *Diagnostic tests:*
  (1) Sigmoidoscopy/colonoscopy for visualization of lesions.
  (2) Barium enema.

◆ **D. Analysis/nursing diagnosis:**

1. *Diarrhea* related to increased flow rate of ileal contents.
2. *Self-esteem disturbance* related to progression of disease and increased number and odor of stools.
3. *Pain* (acute) related to inflammatory process.
4. *Fluid volume deficit* related to frequent episodes of diarrhea.
5. *Knowledge deficit* related to methods to control symptoms.
6. *Social isolation* related to continual diarrhea episodes.

◆ **E. Nursing care plan/implementation:**

1. Goal: *prevent disease progression and complications.*
  a. Administer medications:
    (1) *Salicylates:* sulfasalazine (Azulfidine), olsalazine (Dipentum), mesalamine (Asacol, Pentasa). All given PO in high doses. Mesalamine (Rowasa) is given in enema or suppository form.
    (2) *Corticosteroids:* prednisone, PO or IV. Hydrocortisone (Cortenema) is given by enema.
    (3) *Immunosuppressants:* azathioprine (Imuran), and 6-mercaptopurone (Purinethol), cyclosporine (Sandimmune), and methotrexate (Rheumatrex).
    (4) *Nicotine.*
    (5) *Sedatives and tranquilizers to produce rest and comfort.*
    (6) *Absorbents:* kaolin/pectin (Koapectate).
    (7) *Anticholinergics* and *antispasmotics to relieve cramping and diarrhea:* atropine sulfate, phenobarbital, diphenoxylate/atropine sulfate (Lomotil).
    (8) *Anti-infective* agents *to relieve bacterial overgrowth in bowel* and *limit secondary infections:* metronidazole (Flagyl).
    (9) *Potassium supplements to relieve deficiencies* related to excessive diarrhea.
    (10) Calcium folate and vitamin B_{12} when malabsorption is present.

2. Goal: *reduce psychological stress.*
  a. Provide quiet environment.
  b. Encourage verbalization of concerns.

3. Goal: *health teaching.*
  a. *Diet:*
    (1) *Avoid:* coarse-residue, high-fiber foods, e.g., raw fruits and vegetables, whole milk, cold beverages (because of inflammation).
    (2) *Include:* bland, *high*-protein, *high*-vitamin, *high*-mineral, *high*-calorie foods.
    (3) Parenteral hyperalimentation for severely ill.
    (4) Force fluids by mouth.
  b. Monitor for colon cancer, especially 8–10 years after incidence.

4. Goal: *prepare for surgery if medical regimen unsuccessful.*
  a. Possible surgical procedures:
    (1) Permanent ileostomy.
    (2) Continent ileostomy *(Kock pouch).*
    (3) Total colectomy, anastomosis with rectum.
    (4) Total colectomy, anastomosis with anal sphincter.

◆ **F. Evaluation/outcome criteria:**

1. Fluid balance is obtained and maintained.
2. Alterations in lifestyle are managed.
3. Stress-management techniques are successful.
4. Complications such as fistulas, obstruction, perforation, and peritonitis are avoided.
5. Patient is prepared for surgery if medical regimen is unsuccessful or complications develop.

V. Crohn's disease: a chronic inflammatory disease causing ulcerations in the small and large intestines. The immune system seems to react to a variety of substances and/or bacteria in the intestines, causing inflammation, ulceration, and bowel injury. Called Crohn's *colitis* when only large intestine is involved; Crohn's *enteritis* when only small intestine is involved; *terminal ileitis* when lowest part of small intestine is involved; Crohn's *enterocolitis* or *ileocolitis* when both small and large intestines are involved.

A. Pathophysiology: *one of two conditions called "inflammatory bowel disease"* (ulcerative colitis is the other) that affects all layers of the ileum, the colon, or both, causing patchy, shallow, longitudinal mucosal ulcers; possible correlation with autoimmune disease and adenocarcinoma of the bowel. Small, scattered shallow crater-like areas cause scarring and stiffness of the bowel → bowel becomes narrow → obstruction, then pain, nausea, and vomiting.

B. Risk factors:

1. Age: 15–20, 55–60 yr.
2. Caucasian, especially Jewish.
3. Familial predisposition.
4. Possible virus involvement.
5. Possible psychosomatic involvement.
6. Possible hormonal or dietary influences.

◆ **C. Assessment** (See IV. Ulcerative colitis, p. 533, for analysis/nursing diagnosis, nursing care plan/implementation, and evaluation/outcome criteria):

1. *Subjective data:*

a. Abdominal pain.
b. Anorexia.
c. Nausea.
d. Malaise.
e. History of isolated, intermittent, or recurrent attacks.

2. *Objective data:*
   a. Diarrhea.
   b. Weight loss, vomiting.
   c. Fever, signs of infection.
   d. Fluid/electrolyte imbalances.
   e. Malnutrition, malabsorption.
   f. Occult blood in feces.

VI. Intestinal obstruction: blockage in movement of intestinal contents through small or large intestine.

  A. Pathophysiology:

1. *Mechanical causes*—physical impediments to passage of intestinal contents, e.g., adhesions, hernias, neoplasms, inflammatory bowel disease, foreign bodies, fecal impactions, congenital or radiational strictures, intussusception, or volvulus.

2. *Paralytic causes*—passageway remains open, but peristalsis ceases, e.g., after abdominal surgery, abdominal trauma, hypokalemia, myocardial infarction, pneumonia, spinal injuries, peritonitis, or vascular insufficiency.

  ◆ **B. Assessment:**

1. *Subjective data:* pain related to
   a. *Proximal loop obstruction:* upper abdominal, sharp, cramping, intermittent pain.
   b. *Distal loop obstruction:* poorly localized, cramping pain.

2. *Objective data:*
   a. Bowel sounds: initially loud, high pitched; then when smooth muscle atony occurs, bowel sound absent.
   b. Increased peristalsis above level of obstruction in attempt to move intestinal contents through the obstructed area.
   c. Obstipation (no passage of gas or stool through obstructed portion of bowel; no reabsorption of fluids).
   d. Distention.
   e. Vomiting:
      (1) *Proximal loop obstruction:* profuse nonfecal vomiting.
      (2) *Distal loop obstruction:* less frequent fecal-type vomiting.
   f. Urinary output: decreased.
   g. Temperature: elevated; tachycardia; hypotension → shock if untreated.
   h. Dehydration, hemoconcentration, hypovolemia.
   i. Lab data:
      (1) Leukocytosis.
      (2) *Decreased:* sodium (<138), potassium (<3.5).

(3) *Increased:* bicarbonate (>26 mEq/L), BUN (>18 mg/dL).
(4) *pH:* If obstruction is at gastric outlet, pH will be *elevated,* indicating *metabolic alkalosis;* if obstruction is distal duodenal or proximal jejunal, the pH will *drop* and *metabolic acidosis* occurs.

◆ **C. Analysis/nursing diagnosis:**

1. *Fluid volume deficit* related to vomiting.
2. *Pain* related to increased peristalsis above the level of obstruction.
3. *Altered nutrition, less than body requirements,* related to vomiting.
4. *Risk for trauma* related to potential perforation.

◆ **D. Nursing care plan/implementation:**

1. Goal: *obtain and maintain fluid balance.*
   ▶ a. Nursing care of patient with nasogastric tube (see Table 11–7, p. 768).
      (1) *Miller-Abbott tube:* dual lumen, balloon inflated with air after insertion. *Caution:* do *not* tape tube to face until tube reaches point of obstruction.
      (2) *Cantor tube:* has mercury in distal sac, which helps move tube to point of obstruction. *Caution:* do *not* tape tube to face until tube reaches point of obstruction.
   b. Nothing by mouth, IV therapy, strict I&O.
   ▶ c. Take daily weights (early morning), monitor CVP for hydration status.
   ▶ d. Monitor abdominal girth for signs of distention and urinary output for signs of retention or shock.

2. Goal: *relieve pain and nausea.*
   a. Medications as ordered:
      (1) *Analgesics, antiemetics.*
      (2) If problem is paralytic: medical treatment includes neostigmine *to stimulate peristalsis.*
   b. Observe for bowel sounds, flatus (tape intestinal tube to face once peristalsis begins).
   c. Skin and frequent mouth care.

3. Goal: *prevent respiratory complications.*
   a. Encourage coughing and deep breathing.
   b. *Semi-Fowler's* or position of comfort.

4. Goal: *postoperative nursing care* (if treated surgically): see **Postoperative experience,** p. 504.

◆ **E. Evaluation/outcome criteria:**

1. Fluid balance obtained and maintained.
2. Shock prevented.
3. Obstruction resolved.
4. Pain decreased.
5. Fluids tolerated by mouth.
6. Complications such as perforation and peritonitis avoided.

VII. Fecal diversion—*stomas:* performed because of disease or trauma; may be temporary or permanent.

A. Types (Table 7–28).

1. *Temporary*—fecal stream rerouted to allow GI tract to heal or to provide outlet for stool when obstructed.
2. *Permanent*—intestine cannot be reconnected. Rectum and anal sphincter removed (abdominal perineal resection). Often performed for cancer of the colon and/or rectum.
3. *Continent ileostomy*—pouch is created inside the wall of the intestine. The pouch serves as a reservoir similar to a rectum. The pouch is emptied on a regular basis with a small tube.
4. *Ileoanal anastomosis*—the large intestine is removed and the small intestine is inserted into the rectum and attached just above the anus. The muscles of the rectum remain intact and the normal route of stool elimination is maintained.

◆ **B. Analysis/nursing diagnosis:**

1. *Bowel incontinence* related to lack of sphincter in newly formed stoma.
2. *Altered health maintenance* related to knowledge of ostomy care.
3. *Body image disturbance* related to stoma.
4. *Fear* related to medical condition requiring stoma.
5. *Fluid volume deficit* related to increased output through stoma.

◆ **C. Nursing care plan/implementation:**

1. *Preoperative period:*
   a. Goal: *prepare bowel for surgery.*
   (1) Administer neomycin as ordered to reduce colonic bacteria.
   (2) Administer cathartics, enemas as ordered to cleanse the bowel of feces.
   (3) Administer *low-residue* or *liquid diet* as ordered.
   b. Goal: *relieve anxiety and assist in adjustment to surgery.*
   (1) Provide accurate, brief, and reassuring explanations of procedures; allow time for questions.
   (2) Have enterostomal nurse visit to discuss ostomy management and placement of stoma appliance.
   (3) Offer opportunity for a visit with an Ostomy Association Visitor.
   c. Goal: *health teaching.*
   (1) Determine knowledge of surgery and potential impact.
   (2) Begin teaching regarding ostomy.
2. *Postoperative period:*
   a. Goal: *maintain fluid balance.*
   (1) Monitor I&O because large volume of fluid is lost through stoma.
   (2) Administer IV fluids as ordered.
   (3) Monitor losses through NG tube.
   b. Goal: *prevent other postoperative complications.*
   (1) Monitor for signs of intestinal obstruction.
   (2) Maintain sterility when changing dressings; *avoid* fecal contamination of incision.
   (3) Observe appearance of stoma: rosy pink, raised (Figure 7–11).
   c. Goal: *initiate ostomy care.*

TABLE 7–28   Comparison of Ileostomy and Colostomy

	Ileostomy	Colostomy
Procedure	Surgical formation of a fistula, or stoma, between the abdominal wall and *ileum;* continent ileostomy (*Kock* pouch) may be constructed	Surgical formation of an artificial opening between the surface of the abdominal wall and *colon* *Single barrel*—only one loop of bowel is opened to the abdominal surface *Double barrel*—two loops of bowel, a proximal and distal portion, are open to the abdominal wall; feces will be expelled from the proximal loop, mucus will be expelled from the distal loop; patient may expel some excreta from rectum as well
Reasons performed	Unresponsive ulcerative colitis: complications of ulcerative colitis, e.g., hemorrhage, carcinoma (suspected)	*Single barrel:* colon or rectal cancer *Double barrel:* relieve obstruction
Results	Permanent stoma	*Single barrel:* permanent stoma *Double barrel:* temporary stoma
Discharge	Green liquid, nonodorous	Consistency of feces dependent on diet and portion of the bowel used as the stoma; from brown odorous liquid to normal stool consistency
Nursing care	See **VII. Fecal diversion,** above	See **Tables 11–8, Emptying Colostomy Appliance,** and **11–9, Changing Colostomy Appliance,** pp. 771, 537

FIGURE 7–11 Colostomy sites. (From Thomas, CL [ed]: Taber's Cyclopedic Medical Dictionary, ed 18. FA Davis, Philadelphia, 1997, p 416.)

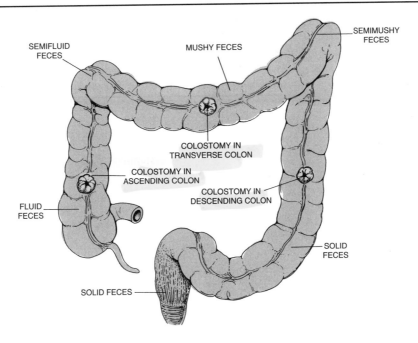

(1) Protect skin around stoma: use commercial preparation to toughen skin and use protective barrier wafer (Stomahesive) or paste (Karaya or substitute) to keep drainage (which can cause excoriation) off the skin.

(2) Keep skin around stoma clean and dry; empty appliance frequently. Check for drainage in appliance at least twice during each shift. If drainage present (diarrhea-type stool):

  (a) Unclip bottom of bag.

  (b) Drain into bedpan.

  (c) Use a squeeze-type bottle filled with warm water to rinse inside of appliance.

  (d) Clean clamp, if soiled.

  (e) Put a few drops of deodorant in appliance if not odorproof.

  (f) Fasten bottom of appliance securely (fold bag over clamp two or three times before closing).

  (g) Check for leakage under appliance every 2–4 hr.

(3) Change appliance when drainage leaks around seal, or approximately every 2–3 days. Initially, size of stoma will be large due to edema. Pouch opening should be slightly larger than stoma so it will not constrict. Stoma will need to be measured for each change until swelling subsides to ensure appropriate fit.

  (a) Gather equipment: gloves, skin prep packet, colostomy appliance measured to fit stoma properly (use stoma measuring guide), skin barrier, warm water and soap, face cloth/towel, plastic bag for disposal of old equipment.

  (b) Remove old appliance carefully, pulling from area with least drainage to area with most drainage.

  (c) Wash skin area (*not* stoma) with soap and water. Be careful *not to*: irritate skin, put soap on stoma, irritate stoma; do *not* put anything dry onto stoma. Remember: bowel is very fragile; working near bowel increases peristalsis so that feces and flatulence may be expelled.

  (d) Observe skin area for potential breakdown.

  (e) Use packet of skin prep on the skin around the stoma. Do *not* put this solution onto stoma, because it will cause irritation. Allow skin prep solution to dry on skin before applying colostomy appliance.

  (f) Apply skin barrier you have measured and cut to size.

  (g) Put appliance on so that bottom of appliance is easily accessible for emptying (e.g., if patient is *out* of bed most of the time, put the bottom facing the feet; if patient is *in* bed most of the time, have bottom face the side). Picture frame the adhesive portion of the appliance with 1-inch tape.

(h) Put a few drops of deodorant in appliance if not odorproof.

(i) Use clamp to fasten bottom of appliance.

(j) Talk to patient (or communicate in best way possible during and after procedure). *This is a very difficult alteration in body image.*

(k) Good hand-washing technique.

(4) Use deodorizing drops in appliance and provide adequate room ventilation to decrease odors. *Caution:* deodorizing drops must be safe for mucous membranes. *No* pinholes in pouch.

(5) If continent ileostomy, a *Kock pouch*, has been constructed, the patient does not have to wear an external pouch. The stool is stored intra-abdominally. The patient drains the pouch several times daily, when there is a feeling of fullness, using a catheter. The stoma is flat and on the right side of the abdomen.

    d. Goal: *promote psychological comfort.*

      (1) Support patient and family—accept feelings and behavior.

      (2) Recognize that such a procedure may initiate the grieving process.

    e. Goal: *health teaching.*

      (1) Self-care management skills related to ostomy appliance, skin care, and irrigation, if indicated (Table 7–29).

      (2) *Diet:* adjustments to control character of feces; *avoid* foods that increase flatulence.

TABLE 7–29 ▶**Colostomy Irrigation***

1. Assemble all equipment for irrigation and appliance change.
2. Remove and discard old pouch.
3. Clean the peristomal skin.
4. Apply the irrigating sleeve; place in toilet or bedpan.
5. Fill container with 500–1000 mL of warm water, *never* more than 1000 mL. Clear air from tubing. Insert lubricated tubing 2–4 inches into stoma. Do *not* force. Hold container about 18 inches above stoma. Infuse gently over 7–10 min.
6. Allow stool to empty into toilet. Evacuation usually occurs in 20–25 min.
7. If no return after irrigation, ambulate, gently massage abdomen, or give patient a warm drink.
8. Once complete, remove the sleeve, and follow guidelines for applying appliance.

*Colostomy irrigation is seldom used with newer colostomies.

      (3) Signs of complications of infection, obstruction, or electrolyte imbalance.

      (4) Community referral for follow-up care.

 ◆ **D. Evaluation/outcome criteria:**

    1. Demonstrates self-care skill for independent living.

    2. Makes dietary adjustments.

    3. Ostomy functions well.

    4. Adjusts to alteration in bowel elimination pattern.

VIII. Hemorrhoids: enlarged vein/veins in mucous membrane of rectum. Hemorrhoids can be internal or external. Bleeding internal hemorrhoids can be painful and are best treated by rubber band ligation, injection sclerotherapy, infrared coagulation, or surgery (scalpel, cautery, or laser). Laser surgery is usually done as an outpatient and causes minimal discomfort. High-fiber diets can minimize constipation and prevent hemorrhoids.

    A. Pathophysiology: venous congestion and interference with venous return from hemorrhoidal veins → increase in pelvic pressure, swelling, and distortion.

    B. Risk factors:

      1. Straining to expel constipated stool.

      2. Pregnancy.

      3. Intra-abdominal or pelvic masses.

      4. Interference with portal circulation.

      5. Prolonged standing or sitting.

      6. History of low-fiber, high-carbohydrate diet, which contributes to constipation.

      7. Family history of hemorrhoids.

      8. Enlarged prostate.

 ◆ **C. Assessment:**

    1. *Subjective data:* discomfort, anal pruritus, pain.

    2. *Objective data:*

      a. Bleeding, especially on defecation.

      b. Narrowing of stool.

      c. Grapelike clusters around anus (pink, red, or blue).

      d. *Diagnostic test:*

        (1) Visualization for external hemorrhoids.

        (2) Digital exam or proctoscopy for internal hemorrhoids.

 ◆ **D. Analysis/nursing diagnosis:**

    1. *Pain* related to defecation.

    2. *Constipation* related to dietary habits and pain at time of defecation.

    3. *Knowledge deficit* related to foods to prevent constipation.

 ◆ **E. Nursing care plan/implementation:**

    1. Goal: *reduce anal discomfort.*

      a. Sitz baths, as ordered; perineal care to prevent infection.

 ▶ b. Hot or cold compresses as ordered to reduce inflammation and pruritus.

c. Topical medications as ordered:
(1) *Anti-inflammatory:* hydrocortisone cream (Anusol).
(2) *Astringents:* witch hazel–impregnated pads.
(3) *Topical anesthetics:* pramoxine (Procto-Foam); dibucaine (Nupercainal).
d. *Bulk laxatives:* psyllium (Metamucil), Konsyl, polycarbophil (FiberCon).
2. Goal: *prevent complications related to surgery.*
a. Encourage postoperative ambulation.
b. Pain relief until packing removed.
c. Monitor for bleeding, infection, pulmonary emboli, phlebitis.
d. Facilitate bowel evacuation: stool softeners, laxatives, suppositories, oil enemas as ordered.
e. Monitor for syncope/vertigo during first postoperative bowel movement.
f. *Diet:*
(1) *Low* residue (postoperative)—until healing has begun.
(2) *High* fiber to prevent constipation after healing.
g. Increase fluid intake.
3. Goal: *health teaching*—methods to avoid constipation.

◆ **F. Evaluation/outcome criteria:**
1. No complications.
2. Patient has bowel movement.
3. Incorporates knowledge of correct foods into lifestyle.

Conditions Affecting Urinary Elimination

I. Pyelonephritis (PN): acute or chronic inflammation due to bacterial infection of the parenchyma and renal pelvis; 95% of cases caused by gram-negative enteric bacilli *(Escherichia coli)*; occurs more frequently in women.
A. Pathophysiology: inflammation of renal medulla or lining of the renal pelvis → nephron destruction; hypertrophy of nephrons needed to maintain urine output → impaired sodium reabsorption (salt wasting); inability to concentrate urine; progressive renal failure; hypertension (two-thirds of all cases).
B. Risk factors:
1. Urinary obstruction (tumors, prostate).
2. Cystitis.
3. Neurogenic bladder.
4. Pregnancy.
5. Catheterization, cystoscopy.
◆ **C. Assessment:**
1. *Subjective data:*

a. *Pain:* flank—one or both sides; back; dysuria; headache.
b. *Loss of appetite;* weight loss.
c. *Night sweats;* chills.
d. *Urination:* frequency, urgency.
2. *Objective data:*
a. Fever; shaking chills.
b. Lab data:
(1) *Blood*—polymorphonuclear leukocytosis >11,000/mm^3.
(2) *Urine*—leukocytosis, hematuria, white blood cell casts, proteinuria (<3 g in 24 hr), positive cultures; specific gravity—normal *or increased* with acute PN, *decreased* with chronic PN; cloudy; foul smelling.
c. Intravenous pyelogram (IVP)—may manifest structural changes.
◆ **D. Analysis/nursing diagnosis:**
1. *Altered urinary elimination* related to kidney disease.
2. *Pain* related to dysuria and kidney damage.
3. *Hyperthermia* related to inflammation.
4. *Risk for fluid volume excess* related to renal failure.
◆ **E. Nursing care plan/implementation:**
1. Goal: *combat infection, prevent recurrence, alleviate symptoms.*
a. Medications:
(1) *Antibiotics, urinary antiseptics,* and/or sulfonamides appropriate for causative organism; also reduce pain.
(2) *Analgesics* for pain—phenazopyridine (Pyridium); stronger if calculi present.
(3) *Antipyretics* for fever—acetaminophen (Tylenol).
b. *Fluids:* 1500–2000 mL/day to flush kidneys, relieve dysuria, reduce fever, prevent dehydration.
c. Observe hydration status: I&O (output minimum 1500 mL/24 hr); daily weight; urine—check each voiding for protein, blood, specific gravity; vital signs q4h to monitor for hypertension, tachycardia; skin turgor.
d. *Hygiene:* meticulous perineal care; cleanse with soap and water; antibiotic ointment may be used around urinary meatus with retention catheter.
▶ e. Cooling measures: tepid sponging.
f. *Diet:* sufficient calories and protein to prevent malnutrition; sodium supplement as ordered. Acid-ash to prevent renal calculus.
2. Goal: *promote physical and emotional rest.*
a. Activity: bed rest or as tolerated—depends on whether anemia or fever is present; encourage activities of daily living as tolerated.

b. Emotional support: encourage expression of fears (possible renal failure, dialysis); provide diversional activities; include family in care; answer questions.

3. Goal: *health teaching.*
   a. Medications: take regularly to maintain blood level; side effects.
   b. Personal care: perineal hygiene; avoid urethral contamination (wiping perineum front to back); *avoid* tub baths.
   c. Possible recurrence with pregnancy.
   d. Monitoring daily weight.

◆ **F. Evaluation/outcome criteria:**
   1. Normal renal function (minimum 1500 mL urine/24 hr).
   2. Blood pressure within normal range.
   3. No recurrence of symptoms.

II. Acute glomerulonephritis: see **Unit 5,** p. 249.

III. Acute renal failure: broadly defined as rapid onset of oliguria accompanied by a rising BUN and serum creatinine; usually reversible.

   A. Pathophysiology: acute renal ischemia → tubular necrosis → decreased urine output. *Oliguric phase* (<400 mL/24 hr)—waste products are retained → metabolic acidosis → water and electrolyte imbalances → anemia. *Recovery phase*— diuresis → dilute urine → rapid depletion of sodium, chloride, and water → dehydration.

   B. Types and risk factors:
   1. *Prerenal*—due to factors outside of kidney; usually circulatory collapse—cardiovascular disorders, hypovolemia, peripheral vasodilation, renovascular obstruction, severe vasoconstriction.
   2. *Intrarenal*—parenchymal disease from ischemia or nephrotoxic damage; nephrotoxic agents—poisons, such as lead (carbon tetrachloride); heavy metals (mercury); antibiotics (gentamicin); incompatible blood transfusion; alcohol myopathies; obstetric complications; acute renal disease—acute glomerulonephritis, acute pyelonephritis.
   3. *Postrenal*—obstruction in collecting system: renal or bladder calculi; tumors of bladder, prostate, or renal pelvis; gynecological or urological surgery in which ureters are accidentally ligated.

   ◆ **C. Assessment:**
   1. *Subjective data:*
      a. Sudden decrease or cessation of urine output   (<400 mL/24 hr).
      b. Anorexia, nausea, vomiting from azotemia.
      c. Sudden weight gain from fluid accumulation.
      d. Headache.
   2. *Objective data:*

   a. Vital signs (vary according to cause and severity):
      (1) *BP*—usually elevated.
      (2) *Pulse*—tachycardia, irregularities.
      (3) *Respirations*—increased rate, depth, crackles.
   b. Neurological: decreasing mentation, unresponsive to verbal or painful stimuli, psychoses, convulsions.
   c. Halitosis; cracked mucous membranes; uremic odor.
   d. Skin: dry, rashes, purpura, itchy, pale.
   e. Lab data:
      (1) Blood: *increased*—potassium, BUN, creatinine, WBC; *decreased*—pH, bicarbonate, hematocrit, hemoglobin.
      (2) Urine: *decreased*—volume, specific gravity (↓1.010); *increased*—protein, casts, red and white blood cells, sodium.

   ◆ **D. Analysis/nursing diagnosis:**
   1. *Altered urinary elimination* related to kidney malfunction.
   2. *Fluid volume excess* related to decreased urine output.
   3. *Altered nutrition, less than body requirements,* related to anorexia.
   4. *Altered oral mucous membrane* related to stomatitis.
   5. *Altered thought processes* related to uremia.

   ◆ **E. Nursing care plan/implementation:**
   1. Goal: *maintain fluid and electrolyte balance and nutrition.*
      a. Monitor: daily weight (should not vary more than ±1 lb); vital signs—include CVP;
         blood chemistries (BUN 6–20 mg/dL; creatinine 0.6–1.5 mg/dL).
      b. *Fluids:* IV as ordered; blood: plasma, packed cells, electrolyte solutions to replace losses; restricted to 400 mL/24 hr if hypertension present or during oliguric phase to prevent fluid overload.
      c. *Diet,* as tolerated: *high* carbohydrate, *low* protein, may be *low* potassium and *low* sodium; hypertonic glucose (TPN) if oral feedings not tolerated; intravenous L-amino acids and glucose.
      d. Control hyperkalemia: infusions of hypertonic glucose and insulin to force potassium into cells; calcium gluconate (IV) to reduce myocardial irritability from K⁺; sodium bicarbonate (IV) to correct acidosis; polystyrene sodium sulfonate (Kayexalate) or other exchange resins, orally or rectally (enema), to remove excess K⁺; continuous renal replacement therapy, peritoneal or hemodialysis.

e. Medications—*diuretics* (mannitol, furosemide [Lasix]) to increase renal blood flow and diuresis.

2. Goal: *use assessment and comfort measures to reduce occurrence of complications.*
   a. Respiratory: monitor rate, depth, breath sounds, arterial blood gases; encourage deep breathing, coughing, turning; use ▶ incentive spirometer or nebulizer as indicated.
   b. Frequent oral care to prevent stomatitis.
   c. Observe for signs of:
      (1) *Infection*—elevated temperature, localized redness, swelling, heat, or drainage.
      (2) *Bleeding*—stools, gums, venipuncture sites.

3. Goal: *maintain continual emotional support.*
   a. Same caregivers, consistency in procedures.
   b. Give opportunities to express concerns, fears.
   c. Allow family interactions.

4. Goal: *health teaching.*
   a. Preparation for dialysis (indications: uremia, uncontrolled hyperkalemia, or acidosis). **Continuous renal replacement therapy** (CRRT) may be used in ARF with fluid overload or rapidly developing azotemia and metabolic acidosis. Continuous ultrafiltration (8–24 hr) of extracellular fluid and uremic toxins. Patient's BP powers system. Arterial and venous access required.
   b. Dietary *restrictions:* low sodium, fluid restriction.
   c. Disease process; treatment regimen.

◆ F. **Evaluation/outcome criteria:**
1. Return of kidney function—normal creatinine level (<1.5 mg/dL), urine output.
2. Resumes normal life pattern (about 3 mo after onset).

IV. **Chronic renal failure:** as a result of progressive destruction of kidney tissue, the kidneys are no longer able to maintain their homeostatic functions; considered irreversible.

A. **Pathophysiology:** destruction of glomeruli → reduced glomerular filtration rate → retention of metabolic waste products; decreased urine output; severe fluid, electrolyte, acid-base imbalances → uremia. Clinical picture includes:
1. Ammonia in skin and alimentary tract by bacterial interaction with urea → inflammation of mucous membranes.
2. Retention of phosphate → decreased serum calcium → muscle spasms, tetany, and increased parathormone release → demineralization of bone.
3. Failure of tubular mechanisms to regulate blood bicarbonate → metabolic acidosis → hyperventilation.
4. Urea osmotic diuresis → flushing effect on tubules → decreased reabsorption of sodium → sodium depletion.
5. Waste product retention → depressed bone marrow function → decreased circulating RBCs → renal tissue hypoxia → decreased erythropoietin production → further depression of bone marrow → anemia.

B. **Risk factors:**
1. Diabetic retinopathy.
2. Chronic glomerulonephritis.
3. Chronic urinary obstruction, ureteral stricture, calculi, neoplasms.
4. Chronic pyelonephritis.
5. Hypertensive nephrosclerosis.
6. Congenital or acquired renal artery stenosis.
7. Systemic lupus erythematosus.

◆ C. **Assessment:**
1. *Subjective data:* excessive fatigue, weakness.
2. *Objective data:*
   a. Skin: bronze colored, uremic frost.
   b. Ammonia breath.
   c. Also see **III. Acute renal failure,** p. 540; symptoms gradual in onset.

◆ D. **Analysis/nursing diagnosis:**
1. In addition to the following, see **III. Acute renal failure,** p. 540.
2. *Fatigue* related to severe anemia.
3. *Risk for impaired skin integrity* related to pruritus.
4. *Ineffective individual coping* related to chronic illness.
5. *Body image disturbance* related to need for dialysis.
6. *Noncompliance* related to denial of illness.

◆ E. **Nursing care plan/implementation:**
1. Goal: *maintain fluid/electrolyte balance and nutrition.* (Also see **III. Acute renal failure,** p. 540.)
   a. *Diet: low* sodium; foods *high* in: calcium, vitamin B complex, vitamins C and D, and iron (to reduce edema, replace deficits, and promote absorption of nutrients).
   b. Medications: given to control BP, regulate electrolytes, control fluid volume; supplemental vitamins if deficient; electrolyte modifier (aluminum hydroxide [AluCap, Amphojel]), calcium carbonate to bind phosphate.
   c. I&O; intake should be equivalent to previous daily output to prevent fluid retention.

2. Goal: *employ comfort measures that reduce distress and support physical function.*
   a. Activity: bed rest; facilitate ventilation; turn, cough, deep breathe q2h; ROM—active and passive, to prevent thrombi.

b. Hygiene: mouth care to prevent stomatitis and reduce discomfort from mouth ulcers; perineal care.

c. Skin care: soothing lotions to reduce pruritus.

d. Encourage communication of concerns.

3. Goal: *health teaching.*

🔴📋a. *Dietary restrictions: no* added salt when cooking; change cooking water in vegetables during process to decrease potassium; read food labels to *avoid* Na$^+$ and K$^+$; protein restriction according to BUN/creatinine ratio (10:1).

b. Importance of daily weight: same scale, time, clothing.

c. Prepare for dialysis; transplantation.

F. **Evaluation/outcome criteria:**

1. Acceptance of chronic illness (no indication of indiscretions, destructive behavior, suicidal tendency).

2. Compliance with dietary restriction—no signs of protein excess (e.g., nausea, vomiting) or fluid/sodium excess (e.g., edema, weight gain).

V. **Dialysis:** diffusion of solute through a semipermeable membrane that separates two solutions; direction of diffusion depends on concentration of solute in each solution; rate and efficiency depend on concentration gradient, temperature of solution, pore size of membrane, and molecular size; two methods available (Table 7–30).

A. **Indications:** acute poisonings; acute or chronic renal failure; hepatic coma; metabolic acidosis; extensive burns with azotemia.

B. *Goals:*

1. *Reduce level of nitrogenous waste.*

2. *Correct acidosis, reverse electrolyte imbalances, remove excess fluid.*

C. *Hemodialysis:* circulation of patient's blood through a compartment formed of a semipermeable membrane (polysulfone, polyacrylonitrile) surrounded by dialysate fluid.

1. Types of venous access for hemodialysis:

a. External shunt (Figure 7–12).

(1) Cannula is placed in a large vein and a large artery that approximate each other.

(2) External shunts, which provide easy and painless access to bloodstream, are prone to infection and clotting and cause erosion of the skin around the insertion area.

(a) Daily cleansing and application of a sterile dressing.

(b) Prevention of physical trauma and avoidance of some activities, such as swimming.

b. Arteriovenous fistulas or graft (Figure 7–13).

(1) Large artery and vein are sewn together (anastomosed) below the surface of the skin (fistula) or subcutaneous graft using the saphenous vein, synthetic prosthesis, or bovine xenograft to connect artery and vein.

(2) Purpose is to create one blood vessel for withdrawing and returning blood.

(3) *Advantages:* greater activity range than AV shunt and no protective asepsis.

(4) *Disadvantage:* necessity of two venipunctures with each dialysis.

c. Vein catheterization.

TABLE 7–30 Comparison of Hemodialysis and Peritoneal Dialysis

	Hemodialysis	Peritoneal Dialysis
Process	Rapid—uses either external AV shunt (acute renal failure) or internal AV fistula (chronic renal failure); typical treatment is 3–4 hr, 3 days/wk; also used for barbiturate overdoses to remove toxic agent quickly	Intermittent—up to 36 hr for hospitalized patients; outpatients 4–8 hr, 5–6 times per week; dwell time 30–45 min for manual dialysis or 10–20 min for automatic cycler; either rigid stylet catheter or surgically inserted soft catheter; advantage for patients who cannot tolerate rapid fluid and electrolyte changes
		Continuous—two methods: (1) four cycles in 24 hr; dwell time is 4–5 hr during the day and 8–12 hr overnight; no need for machinery, electricity, or water source; surgically inserted soft catheter; closely resembles normal renal function; (2) automated cycler infuses and removes dialysate; generally done while patient sleeps; built-in alarms for patient safety.
Vascular access	Required	Not necessary; therefore suitable for patients with vascular problems
Heparinization	Required; systemic or regional	Little or no heparin necessary; therefore suitable for patients with bleeding problems
Complications (other than fluid and electrolyte imbalances, which are common to all)	Dialysis dysequilibrium syndrome (preventable) Mechanical dysfunctions of dialyzer	Peritonitis Hypoalbuminemia Bowel or bladder perforation Plugged or dislodged catheter

(1) Femoral or subclavian vein access is immediate.

(2) May be short- or long-term duration.

2. Complications during hemodialysis:

    a. *Dysequilibrium syndrome*—rapid removal of urea from blood → reverse osmosis, with water moving into brain cells → cerebral edema → possible headache, nausea, vomiting, confusion, and convulsions; usually occurs with initial dialysis treatments; shorter dialysis time and slower rate minimizes.

    b. *Hypotension*—results from excessive ultrafiltration or excessive antihypertensive medications.

    c. *Hypertension*—results from volume overload (water and/or sodium), causing *dysequilibrium syndrome* or anxiety.

    d. *Transfusion reactions* (see **Unit 11, Table 11–4**).

    e. *Arrhythmias*—due to hypotension, fluid overload, or rapid removal of potassium.

    f. *Psychological problems:*

        (1) Patients react in varying ways to dependence on hemodialysis.

        (2) Nurse needs to identify patient reactions and defense mechanisms and to employ supportive behaviors, e.g., include patient in care; continual repetition and reinforcement; do *not* interpret patient's behavior—for example, do *not* say, "You're being hostile" or "You're acting like a child"; answer questions honestly regarding quality and length of life with dialysis and/or transplantation; encourage independence as much as possible.

D. *Intermittent peritoneal dialysis:* involves introduction of a dialysate solution into the abdomen, where the peritoneum acts as the semipermeable membrane between the solution and blood in abdominal vessels. *Procedure:*

1. Area around umbilicus is prepared and anesthetized with local anesthetic, and a catheter is inserted into the peritoneal cavity through a trocar; the catheter is then sutured into place to prevent displacement.

2. Warmed dialysate is then allowed to flow into the peritoneal cavity. Inflow time: 5–10 min; 2 liters of solution are used in each cycle in the adult; solutions contain glucose, Na^+, Ca^{2+}, Mg^{2+}, K^+, Cl^-, and lactate or acetate.

3. When solution bottle is empty, dwell time (exchange time) begins. *Dwell time:* 10–20 min; processes of diffusion, osmosis, and filtration begin to move waste products from bloodstream into peritoneal cavity.

4. Draining of the dialysate begins with the unclamping of the outflow clamp. *Outflow time:* usually 10 min; returns less than 2 liters usually result from incomplete peritoneal emptying; turn side to side to increase return; multiple exchanges in 24 hr depending on patient need.

E. Continuous ambulatory peritoneal dialysis (CAPD): functions on the same principles as peritoneal dialysis, yet allows greater freedom and independence for dialysis patients. *Procedure:*

FIGURE 7–12 AV shunt (cannulae).

A. **On Dialyzer**

B. **Off Dialyzer (before bandaging)**

FIGURE 7–13 AV fistula.

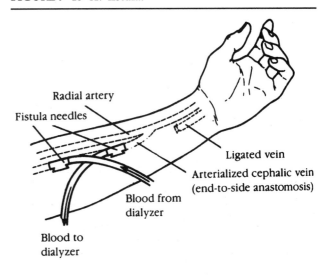

1. Dialysis solution is infused into peritoneum three times daily and once before bedtime.
2. *Dwell time*—≥4 hr for each daily exchange, and overnight for the fourth (8–12 hr).
3. Indwelling peritoneal catheter is connected to solution bag at all times—serves to fill and drain peritoneum; concealed in cloth pouch, strapped to the body during dwell time; patient can move about doing usual activities.

F. *Continuous cycling peritoneal dialysis* (CCPD): same principles as CAPD, except uses an automated system to infuse and remove dialysate; reduces nursing care needs with hospitalized patients. Cumbersome equipment inhibits nighttime mobility. *Procedure:*
1. Long exchanges without an automated cycler during the day and short exchanges with a cycler at night.
2. *Dwell time*—6–8 hr while sleeping.
3. Automatic alarms to prevent malfunction with home use.

VI. **Kidney transplantation:** placement of a donor kidney (from sibling, parent, cadaver) into the iliac fossa of a recipient and the anastomosis of its ureter to the bladder of the recipient; indicated in end-stage renal disease.

A. Criteria for recipient: irreversible kidney function; under 70 yr of age; patent and functional lower urinary tract; and good surgical risk, free of serious cardiovascular complications. *Contraindicated* in those with another life-threatening condition.

B. Donor selection:
1. Sibling or parent—survival rate of kidney is greater; preferred for transplantation.
2. Cadaver—greater rate of rejection following transplantation, although majority of transplantations are with cadaver kidneys.

C. Bilateral nephrectomy: necessary for patients with rapidly progressive glomerulonephritis, malignant hypertension, or chronic kidney infections; prevents complications in transplanted kidney (see **VII. Nephrectomy** for nursing care, p. 545).

◆ D. **Analysis/nursing diagnosis:**
1. *Altered urinary elimination* related to kidney failure.
2. *Fear* related to potential transplant rejection.
3. *Risk for infection* related to immunosuppression.
4. *Body image disturbance* related to immunosuppression.

◆ E. **Nursing care plan/implementation:**
1. *Preoperative:*
a. Goal: *promote physical and emotional adjustment.*
(1) Informed consent.
(2) Lab work completed—histocompatibility, CBC, urinalysis, blood type and crossmatch.

(3) Skin preparation.
b. Goal: *encourage expression of feelings:* origin of donor, fear of complications, rejection.
c. Goal: *minimize risk of organ rejection:* give medications: begin immunosuppression (azathioprine, corticosteroids, cyclosporine); antibiotics if ordered.
d. Goal: *health teaching.*
(1) Nature of surgery; placement of kidney.
(2) Postoperative expectations: deep breathing, coughing, turning, early ambulation; reverse isolation.
(3) Medications: *immunosuppressive* therapy: purpose, effect.

2. *Postoperative:*
a. Goal: *promote uncomplicated recovery of recipient.*
(1) Vital signs; CVP; I&O—urine output usually immediate with living donor; with cadaver kidney may not work for a week or more and dialysis will be needed within 24–48 hr. Report <100 mL/hr **immediately.**
▶ (2) *Isolation:* strict *reverse* isolation with immunosuppression; wear face mask when out of room.
▰ (3) *Position:* back to *nonoperative* side; *semi-Fowler's* to promote gas exchange.
▶ (4) Indwelling catheter care: *strict* asepsis; characteristics of urine—report gross hematuria, heavy sediment; clots; perineal care; bladder spasms may occur after removal of catheter.
(5) Activity: ambulate 24 hr after surgery; *avoid* prolonged sitting.
(6) Weigh daily.
(7) Medications: *immunosuppressives; analgesics* as ordered (pain decreases significantly after 24 hr).
(8) Drains: irrigate *only* on physician order; *meticulous* catheter care.
(9) *Diet:* regular after return of bowel sounds; liberal amounts of protein; *restrict* fluids, sodium, potassium *only if* oliguric.
b. Goal: *observe for signs of rejection*—most dangerous complication. Three classifications:

(1) Hyperacute—occurs within 5–10 min up to 48 hr after transplantation (rare).
(2) Acute—most common 7–14 days; varies depending on living (1 wk–6 mo) or cadaver (1 wk–2 yr) donor.
(3) Chronic—occurs several months to years.
◆ **Assessment:**
(a) *Subjective data:*

> (i) Lethargy, anorexia.
> (ii) Tenderness over graft site.
> (b) *Objective data:*
> (i) Lab data: Urine *decreased*—output, creatinine clearance, sodium; *increased*—protein. Blood: *increased*—BUN, creatinine.
> (ii) Rapid weight gain; more than 3 lb/day.
> (iii) Vital signs: BP, temperature—*elevated.*

c. Goal: *maintain immunosuppressive therapy.*

(1) Azathioprine *(Imuran)*—an antimetabolite that interferes with cellular division. *Side effects:*
  (a) Gastrointestinal bleeding (give PO form with food).
  (b) Bone marrow depression; leukopenia; anemia.
  (c) Development of malignant neoplasms.
  (d) Infection.
  (e) Liver damage.

(2) Prednisone—believed to affect lymphocyte production by inhibiting nucleic acid synthesis: anti-inflammatory action helps prevent tissue damage if rejection occurs. *Side effects:*
  (a) Stress ulcer with bleeding (give with food).
  (b) *Decreased* glucose tolerance (hyperglycemia).
  (c) Muscle weakness.
  (d) Osteoporosis.
  (e) Moon facies.
  (f) Acne and striae.
  (g) Depression and hallucinations.

(3) Cyclosporine (Neoral, Sandimmune)—polypeptide antibiotic used to prevent rejection of kidney, liver, or heart allografts; PO dose given with *room temperature chocolate milk or orange juice* in a glass dispenser. *Side effects:*
  (a) Nephrotoxicity (*increased* BUN, creatinine).
  (b) Hypertension.
  (c) Tremor.
  (d) Hirsutism, gingival hyperplasia.
  (e) *GI*—nausea, vomiting, anorexia, diarrhea, abdominal pain.
  (f) Infections—pneumonia, septicemia, abscesses, wound.

(4) Additional drugs may include cyclophosphamide (Cytoxan), antithymocyte (ATG), antilymphocyte globulin, muromonab-CD3 (OKT3),

tacrolimus (Prograf), and mycophenolate mofetil (CellCept).

d. Goal: *health teaching.*
  (1) Signs of rejection (see Goal b).
  (2) Drugs: side effects of immunosuppression (see Goal c).
  (3) Self-care activities: temperature, blood pressure, I&O, urine specimen collection.
  (4) Avoidance of infection.
  (5) See also goals of care, under **Postoperative experience,** p. 504.

◆ F. **Evaluation/outcome criteria:**
  1. No signs of rejection (e.g., no weight gain, oliguria).
  2. No depression.
  3. Patient resumes role responsibilities.

VII. Nephrectomy (radical or partial): removal of kidney through flank, retroperitoneal, abdominal, thoracic, or thoracic-abdominal approach; indicated with malignant tumors, severe trauma, or under certain conditions before renal transplantation (see **VI. Kidney transplantation,** p. 544).

◆ A. **Analysis/nursing diagnosis:**
  1. *Pain* related to surgical incision.
  2. *Risk for infection* related to wound contamination.
  3. *Risk for aspiration* related to vomiting.
  4. *Constipation* related to paralytic ileus.
  5. *Anxiety* related to possible loss of function in remaining kidney.
  6. *Dysfunctional grieving* related to perceived loss.

◆ B. **Nursing care plan/implementation:**
  1. *Preoperative:* Goal: *optimize physical and psychological functioning* (see **I. Preoperative preparation,** p. 500).
  2. *Postoperative:* Goal: *promote comfort and prevent complications.*
    a. Observe for signs of:
      (1) *Paralytic ileus*—abdominal distention, absent bowel sounds, vomiting (common complication following renal surgery).
      (2) *Hemorrhage.*
    b. Fluid balance: daily weight—maintain within 2% of preoperative level.

◆ C. **Evaluation/outcome criteria:**
  1. No complications (e.g., hemorrhage, paralytic ileus, wound infection).
  2. Acceptance of loss of kidney.

VIII. Renal calculi (urolithiasis): formation of calculi (stones) in renal calyces or pelvis that pass to lower regions of urinary tract—ureters, bladder, or urethra; occurs after age 30, with greatest incidence in *men,* particularly over age 50.
  A. **Pathophysiology:** organic crystals form (most consist of calcium salts or magnesium—ammonium phosphate (struvite) → obstruction, infection; increased backward pressure in kidney

→ hydronephrosis → atrophy, fibrosis of renal tubules.

B. Risk factors (in over 50% of cases, cause is idiopathic):
1. Urinary tract infection.
2. Urinary stasis—obstruction.
3. Metabolic factors—excessive intake of vitamin D or C, calcium carbonate.

◆ **C. Assessment** (depends on size, shape, location of stone):
1. *Subjective data:*
   a. Pain: occasional, dull, in loin or back when stones are in calyces or renal pelvis; *excruciating* in flank area (renal colic), radiating to groin when stones are ureteral.
   b. Nausea associated with pain.
2. *Objective data:*
   a. Pallor, sweating, syncope, shock, and vomiting due to pain.
   b. Palpable kidney mass with hydronephrosis.
   c. Fever and pyuria with infection.
   d. Lab data:
      (1) Urinalysis: abnormal—pH (acidic or alkaline); RBCs (injury); WBCs (infection); *increased*—specific gravity; casts; crystals; other organic substances, depending on type of stone (i.e., calcium, struvite, uric acid or cystine); *positive* culture.
      (2) Blood: *increased* calcium, phosphorus, total protein, alkaline phosphatase, creatinine, uric acid, BUN.
   e. *Diagnostic tests:*
      (1) IVP: reveals nonopaque stones, degree of obstruction.
      (2) X-ray; radiopaque stones seen.
      (3) Ultrasound may also be used.

◆ **D. Analysis/nursing diagnosis:**
1. *Pain* related to passage of stone.
2. *Altered urinary elimination* related to potential obstruction.
3. *Urinary retention* related to obstruction of urethra.

◆ **E. Nursing care plan/implementation:**
1. Goal: *reduce pain and prevent complications.*
   a. Medication: *narcotics, antiemetics, antibiotics.*
   b. Fluids: 3–4 L/day; IVs if nauseated, vomiting.
   c. Activity: ambulate to promote passage of stone, except bed rest during acute attack (colic).
   d. Reduce spasms: warm soaks to affected flank.
   e. Observe for signs of:
      (1) *Obstruction*—decreased urinary output, increased flank pain.
      (2) *Passage of stone* (90% will pass <5 mm size)—cessation of pain; filter urine with gauze.

   f. Monitor: hydration status—I&O, daily weight; vital signs—particularly temperature for sign of infection; urine—color, odor.
2. Goal: *health teaching.*
   a. Importance of fluids: minimum 3000 mL/day; 2 glasses during night.
   b. *Diet:* modify according to stone type.
      (1) *Calcium oxalate and calcium phosphate stones*—*low* calcium phosphorus and oxalate (e.g., *avoid* tea, cocoa, cola, beans, spinach, acidic fruits).
      (2) *Magnesium-ammonium phosphate*—*low* phosphorus.
      (3) *Uric acid stones*—*low* purine.
      (4) *Cystine stones*—*low* protein.
   c. *Acid-ash diet* with calcium oxalate and calcium phosphate stones, magnesium and ammonium phosphate (struvite) stones.
   d. *Alkaline-ash diet* with uric acid and cystine stones (see Common Therapeutic Diets in **Unit 9,** p. 683).
   e. Signs of urinary infection: dysuria, frequency, hematuria; seek immediate treatment.
   f. Prepare for removal if indicated; percutaneous or extracorporeal lithotripsy done for stones <1 cm; ureterolithotomy may also be ordered for larger stones; nephrectomy in *extreme* cases.

◆ **F. Evaluation/outcome criteria:**
1. Relief from pain.
2. No signs of urinary obstruction (e.g., increased flank pain, decreased urine output).
3. No recurrence of lithiasis (adheres to diet and fluid regimen).

IX. Lithotripsy. *Extracorporeal shock wave*—a noninvasive mechanical procedure used to break up renal calculi so they can pass spontaneously, in most cases. The trunk of the patient is submerged in distilled water. In addition to being strapped to a frame, the patient may also receive *sedation* and *analgesia* for pain from sound waves. The procedure takes 30–45 min, and remaining still is important. An underwater electrode generates shock waves that fragment the stone so it can be excreted in the urine a few days after the procedure. A degree of renal colic may occur, requiring *narcotics* for up to 3 days. *Nursing measures* should encourage ambulation and promote diuresis through *forcing* fluids. *Percutaneous lithotripsy*—nephrostomy tract above kidney region; nephroscope used to retrieve calculi. Urinary drainage from incision for 3–4 days is normal. May be required for large fragments remaining after extracorporeal lithotripsy. *Nursing measures* include: dressing changes to prevent infection and prevent skin breakdown, and administration of *antibiotics* and narcotics for pain.

X. **Benign prostatic hyperplasia** (BPH): bladder outlet obstruction resulting from an enlargement of the prostate gland.

    A. **Pathophysiology:** prostate enlarges, bulges upward, blocks flow of urine from bladder into urethra → obstruction → hydroureter, hydronephrosis.

    B. **Risk factors:**

        1. Changes in estrogen and androgen levels.

        2. Men >50.

◆ C. **Assessment:**

        1. *Subjective data—urination:*

          a. Difficulty starting stream.

          b. Smaller, less forceful.

          c. Dribbling.

          d. Frequency.

          e. Urgency.

          f. Nocturia.

          g. Retention (incomplete emptying).

          h. Inability to void after ingestion of alcohol or exposure to cold.

        2. *Objective data:*

          a. Catheterization for residual urine: 25–50 mL after voiding.

          b. Enlarged prostate on rectal exam.

          c. Lab data:

             (1) Urine—*increased* RBC, WBC.

             (2) Blood—*increased* creatinine, PSA.

◆ D. **Analysis/nursing diagnosis:**

        1. *Urinary retention* related to incomplete emptying.

        2. *Altered urinary elimination* related to obstruction.

        3. *Urinary incontinence* related to urgency, pressure.

        4. *Anxiety* related to potential surgery.

        5. *Body image disturbance* related to threat to male identity.

◆ E. **Nursing care plan/implementation:**

        1. Goal: *relieve urinary retention.*

          a. Catheterization: release maximum of 1000 mL initially; *avoid* bladder decompression, which results in hypotension, bladder spasms, ruptured blood vessels in bladder; empty 200 mL every 5 min.

▶   b. Patency: irrigate intermittently or continually, as ordered.

          c. Fluids: minimum 2000 mL/24 hr.

        2. Goal: *health teaching.*

          a. Preparation for surgery (cystostomy, prostatectomy):

             (1) Expectations—indwelling catheter (will feel urge to void).

             (2) *Avoid* pulling on catheter (this increases bleeding and clots).

             (3) Bladder spasms common 24–48 hr after surgery, particularly with transurethral resection and suprapubic approaches.

             (4) Threatening nature of procedure (possibility of impotence with perineal prostatectomy).

          b. See also **I. Preoperative preparation,** p. 500.

XI. **Prostatectomy:** surgical procedure to relieve urinary retention and frequency caused by benign prostatic hyperplasia or cancer of the prostate.

    A. Types

        1. *Transurethral resection (TUR)*—removal of obstructive prostatic tissue surrounding urethra by an electric wire (resectoscope) introduced through the urethra; hypertrophy may recur, and TUR repeated; little risk of impotence. Laser also being used.

        2. *Suprapubic*—low midline incision is made directly over the bladder; bladder is opened and large mass of prostatic tissue is removed through incision in urethral mucosa.

        3. *Retropubic*—removal of hypertrophied prostatic tissue high in pelvic area through a low abdominal incision; bladder is not opened; patient may remain potent.

        4. *Perineal*—removal of prostatic tissue low in pelvic area is accomplished through an incision made between the scrotum and the rectum; usually results in impotency and incontinence.

◆ B. **Nursing care plan/implementation:**

        1. *Preoperative:* see **X. Prostatic hyperplasia,** p. 547.

        2. *Postoperative:*

          a. Goal: *promote optimal bladder function and comfort.*

             (1) Urinary drainage: sterile closed-gravity system—maintain external traction as ordered.

             (2) Reinforce purposes, sensations to expect.

▶   (3) Bladder irrigation to control bleeding, keep clots from forming.

▶   (4) Suprapubic catheter care (suprapubic prostatectomy)—closed-gravity drainage system; observe character, amount, flow of drainage.

             (5) *After removal:*

               (a) Observe for urinary drainage q4h for 24 hr.

               (b) Skin care.

               (c) Report excessive drainage to physician.

             (6) Dressings: keep dry, clean; reinforce if necessary (may need to change suprapubic dressing if urinary drainage); notify physician of *excessive bleeding.*

             (7) Observe for signs of:

               (a) *Bladder distention*—distinct mound over pubis, slow drip in

Adult

collecting bottle; irrigate catheter as ordered.

(b) *Increased bleeding*—expect and report frank bleeding (if venous bleeding, increase traction on catheter); if bright red drainage, and clots (arterial bleeding), may need surgical control; cool, clammy, pale skin and increased pulse rate indicate shock.

b. Goal: *assist in rehabilitation.* Emotional support: *fears* of incontinence, loss of male identity, impotence.

c. Goal: *health teaching.*

(1) Expectations: mild incontinence, dribbling for a while (several months) after surgery; need to void as soon as urge is felt; *push fluids.*

(2) Exercises: perineal (Kegel) 1–2 days after surgery—buttocks are tightened for a count of ten, 20–50 times daily.

(3) *Avoid:*

(a) Long auto trips, vigorous exercise, heavy lifting (anything heavier than 10 lb), and sexual intercourse for about 3 wk or until medical permission, because they may increase tendency to bleed.

(b) Alcoholic beverages for 1 mo, because this may cause burning on urination; caffeine, because it causes diuresis.

(c) Tub baths, because they increase chance of infection.

(4) Medications: stool softeners or mild cathartics to decrease straining.

◆ **C. Evaluation/outcome criteria:**

1. Relief of symptoms.

2. No complications (e.g., hemorrhage, impotence).

XII. Urinary diversion. *Incontinent*—ileal conduit: anastomosis of ureters to a small portion of the ileum; stoma is called urostomy; urine flow is constant; requires external collection device. *Continent*—Kock pouch, Indiana pouch: segment of small bowel or colon is used to create a pouch; holds urine without leakage; requires self-catheterization.

A. Indications:

1. Congenital anomalies of bladder.

2. Neurogenic bladder.

3. Mechanical obstruction to urine flow (e.g., bladder cancer).

4. Chronic progressive pyelonephritis.

5. Trauma to lower urinary tract.

◆ **B. Analysis/nursing diagnosis:**

1. *Altered urinary elimination* related to surgical diversion.

2. *Risk for impaired skin integrity* related to leakage of urine.

3. *Risk for infection* related to contamination of stoma.

4. *Constipation* related to absence of peristalsis.

5. *Body image disturbance* related to stoma.

◆ **C. Nursing care plan/implementation:**

1. *Preoperative:* optimal bowel and stoma site preparation.

a. *Diet: low-*residue 2 days followed by clear liquids for 24 hr.

b. Medications:

(1) Neomycin (for bowel sterilization).

(2) Cathartics (GoLYTELY), enemas.

c. Site selection: appliance faceplate (incontinent diversion) must bond securely; *avoid* areas of pressure from clothing (waistline); usual site is right or left lower abdominal quadrant.

d. See also **I. Preoperative preparation,** p. 500.

2. *Postoperative:*

a. Goal: *prevent complications and promote comfort.*

(1) Observe for signs of:

(a) *Paralytic ileus* (common complication)—keep NG tube patent.

(b) *Stoma necrosis*—dusky or cyanotic color (**emergency** situation).

(2) Skin care: check for leakage around ostomy bag.

(3) Urinary drainage—stents or catheter in stoma; blood in urine in immediate postoperative period; mucus normal.

(4) See **III. Postoperative experience,** p. 504.

b. Goal: *health teaching.*

(1) Self-care activities:

(a) *Peristomal skin care*—prevent irritation, breakdown; proper cleansing—soap and water; adhesive remover, if needed.

(b) *Appliance application and emptying;* pouch opening 2–3 mm larger than stoma; do *not* remove each day; change appliance every 3–5 days or when leaking.

(c) *Odor control*—dilute urine, acidash diet, hygiene; *avoid* asparagus, tomatoes.

(d) *Use of night drainage system if necessary* for uninterrupted sleep.

(2) Signs *of complications:* change in urine color, clarity, quantity, smell; stomal color change (normal is bright pink or red).

◆ **D. Evaluation/outcome criteria:**

1. Acceptance of new body image.

2. Regains independence.

3. Demonstrates confidence in management of self-care activities.

SENSORY/PERCEPTUAL FUNCTIONS

I. Laryngectomy with radical neck dissection: removal of entire larynx, lymph nodes, submandibular salivary gland, sternomastoid muscle, spinal accessory nerves, and jugular vein for cancer of the larynx that extends beyond the vocal cords. Permanent tracheostomy; new methods of speech will have to be learned.

Partial laryngectomy: removal of lesion on larynx. Patient will be able to speak after operation, but quality of voice may be altered.

◆ **A. Assessment:**
1. *Subjective data:*
   a. Feeling of lump in throat.
   b. Pain: Adam's apple; may radiate to ear.
   c. Dysphagia.
2. *Objective data:*
   a. Hoarseness: persistent (longer than 2 weeks), progressive.
   b. Lymphadenopathy: cervical.
   c. Breath odor: foul.

◆ **B. Analysis/nursing diagnosis:**
1. *Impaired verbal communication* related to removal of larynx.
2. *Body image disturbance* related to radical neck dissection.
3. *Ineffective airway clearance* related to copious amounts of mucus.
4. *Fear* related to diagnosis of cancer.
5. *Impaired swallowing* related to edema.
6. *Impaired social interaction* related to altered speech.

◆ **C. Nursing care plan/implementation:**
1. *Preoperative care:*
   a. Goal: *provide emotional support and optimal physical preparation.*
      (1) Encourage verbalization of fears; answer all questions honestly, particularly about having no voice after surgery.
      (2) Visit from person with laryngectomy (contact New Voice Club, Lost Chord, or International Association of Laryngectomees).
   b. Goal: *health teaching.*
      (1) Prepare for tracheostomy.
      (2) Other means to speak (esophageal "burp" speech, tracheoesophageal prosthesis or electronic artificial larynx).
2. *Postoperative care:*
   a. Goal: *maintain patent airway and prevent aspiration.*
      ◪ (1) *Position:* semi-Fowler's (elevate 30–45 degrees), preventing forward flexion of neck to reduce edema and keep airway open.
      (2) Observe for hypoxia:
         (a) *Early signs:* increased respiratory and pulse rates, apprehension, restlessness.
         (b) *Late signs:* dyspnea, cyanosis; swallowing difficulties—patient should chew food well and swallow with water.

      (3) *Laryngectomy* tube care:
         (a) Observe for stridor (coarse, high-pitched inspiratory sound)—**report immediately.**
         (b) Have extra laryngectomy tube at bedside.
      ▶ (c) Suction with sterile equipment; 2–3 mL of sterile saline into stoma may be used to loosen secretions.

   b. Goal: *promote optimal physical and psychological function.*
      (1) Frequent mouth care.
      ▶ (2) *Wound:* exposed site; note color and amount of drainage.
      ▶ (3) *Tubes:* closed drainage system (*Hemovac, Jackson-Pratt*) (Figure 7–14); expect <100 up to 300 mL of serosanguineous drainage first postoperative day; drainage should decrease daily; observe patency.

FIGURE 7–14 Closed drainage system for constant suction. Suction is maintained by a plastic container. The container serves as both suction source and receptacle for blood. It is emptied as required, and drainage tubes are left in the neck for approximately 3 days. (From De Weese, DD: Saunders' Textbook of Otolaryngology. Mosby, St. Louis, 1987.)

Adult

◆ **A. Analysis/nursing diagnosis:**
1. *Sensory/perceptual alteration* related to edema and ear packing.
2. See The Perioperative Experience, p. 501, for diagnoses relating to surgery.

◆ **B. Nursing care plan/implementation:**
1. *Preoperative* health teaching.
   a. Important to keep head in position ordered by physician postoperatively.
   b. *Caution:* sneezing, blowing nose (keep mouth open), vomiting, coughing—all of which increase pressure in eustachian tubes (blow one side gently).
   c. Breathing exercises.
2. *Postoperative:*
   a. Goal: *promote physical and psychological equilibrium.*
      (1) *Position:* as ordered by physician—varies according to preference.
      (2) Activity: assist with ambulation; *avoid* rapid turning, which might increase vertigo.
      (3) Dressings: check frequently; may change cotton pledget in outer ear.
      (4) Give medications as ordered:
         (a) *Antiemetics.*
         (b) *Analgesics.*
         (c) *Antibiotics.*
      (5) Reassurance: reduction in hearing is normal; hearing may *not* immediately improve after surgery.
   b. Goal: *health teaching.*
      (1) Ear care: keep covered outdoors; keep outer ear plug clean, dry, and changed.
      (2) *Avoid:*
         (a) Water in ear for 6 wk:
            (i) Use barrier when washing hair.
            (ii) Use two pieces of cotton; saturate outer piece with petroleum jelly.
         (b) Pressure or vibration from loud noise, flying, or heavy lifting until advised by MD.

◆ **C. Evaluation/outcome criteria:**
1. Hearing improves—evaluate 1 mo postoperatively (may require hearing aid).
2. Returns to work (usually 2 wk after surgery).
3. Continues medical supervision.

VI. Deafness: (1) *Hard of hearing*—slight or moderate hearing loss that is serviceable for activities of daily living. (2) *Deaf*—hearing is nonfunctional for activities of daily living.

A. Risk factors:
1. *Conductive* hearing losses (transmission deafness):
   a. Impacted cerumen (wax).
   b. Foreign body in external auditory canal.
   c. Defects (thickening, scarring) of eardrum.
   d. Otosclerosis of ossicles.
2. *Sensorineural* hearing losses (perceptive or nerve deafness):
   a. Arteriosclerosis.
   b. Infectious diseases (mumps, measles, meningitis).
   c. Drug toxicities (quinine, streptomycin, neomycin SO_4).
   d. Tumors.
   e. Head traumas.
   f. High-intensity noises.
3. *Central* deafness:
   a. Tumors.
   b. Stroke (brain attack).
4. *Noise-induced or occupational noise* hearing loss:
   a. Blast injury.
   b. Firearms.
   c. Loud music.
5. *Aging* (presbycusis).

◆ **B. Assessment**—*objective data:*
1. Inattentive or strained facial expression.
2. Excessive loudness or softness of speech.
3. Frequent need to clarify content of conversation or inappropriate responses.
4. Tilting of head while listening.
5. Lack of response when others speak.

◆ **C. Analysis/nursing diagnosis:**
1. *Auditory/sensory/perceptual alteration* related to loss of hearing.
2. *Impaired social interaction* related to deafness.

◆ **D. Nursing care plan/implementation:**
1. Goal: *maximize hearing ability and provide emotional support.*
   a. Gain person's attention before speaking; *avoid* startling.
   b. Provide adequate lighting so person can see you when you are speaking.
   c. Look at the person when speaking.
   d. Use nonverbal cues to enhance communication, e.g., writing, hand gestures, pointing.
   e. Speak slowly, distinctly; do *not* shout (excessive loudness distorts voice).
   f. If person does not understand, use different words; write it down.
   g. Use alternative communication system:
      (1) Speech (lip) reading.
      (2) Sign language.
      (3) Hearing aid.
      (4) Paper and pencil.
      (5) Flash cards.
   h. Supportive, nonstressful environment; alert staff to patient's hearing impairment.
2. Goal: *health teaching.*
   a. Prepare for evaluative studies—audiogram.

b. Appropriate community resources: National Association of Hearing and Speech Agencies for *counseling services;* National Association for the Deaf to assist with *employment, education, legislation;* Alexander Graham Bell Association for the Deaf, Inc., serves as *information* center for those working with the deaf; American Hearing Society provides educational information, employment services, *social clubs.*

c. Use of hearing aid: care—(1) turn off aid when not using (open case at night to prevent draining battery); (2) keep extra battery available; (3) wash with mild soap and warm water; use pipe cleaner to remove wax; (4) do *not* wear aid in shower or with ear infection; (5) store same place every night and away from pets; (6) if aid does not work: check battery insertion, on-off switch, placement (if ear-molded aid), cleanliness.

d. Safety precautions: when crossing street, driving.

◆ **E. Evaluation/outcome criteria:**
  1. Method of communication established.
  2. Achieves independence (use of Dogs for Deaf, special telephones, visual signals).
  3. Copes with lifestyle changes (minimal depression, anger, hostility).

VII. Glaucoma (acute and chronic): increased intraocular pressure; second most common cause of blindness.

  A. Pathophysiology:
  1. *Acute (closed-angle)*—impaired passage of aqueous humor into the circular canal of Schlemm due to closure of the angle between the cornea and the iris. ***Medical emergency; requires surgery.***
  2. *Chronic (open-angle)*—degenerative changes in trabecular meshwork; local obstruction of aqueous humor between the anterior chamber and the canal. *Most common; treated with medication* (miotics, carbonic anhydrase inhibitors).
  3. *Secondary*—in some cases neovascularization (new vessels) may form; blocks passage of aqueous humor (uveitis, trauma, drugs, diabetes, retinal vein occlusion).
  4. Untreated: imbalance between rate of secretion of intraocular fluids and rate of absorption of aqueous humor → increased intraocular pressures → decreased peripheral vision → corneal edema → halos and blurring of vision → blindness.

  B. Risk factors—unknown, but associated with:
  1. Emotional disturbances.
  2. Hereditary factors.
  3. Allergies.
  4. Vasomotor disturbances.

◆ **C. Assessment:**
  1. *Subjective data:*
    a. *Acute* (closed-angle):
      (1) Pain: severe, in and around eyes.
      (2) Rainbow halos around lights.
      (3) Blurring of vision.
      (4) Nausea, vomiting.
    b. *Chronic* (open-angle):
      (1) Eyes tire easily.
      (2) Loss of peripheral vision.
      (3) Dull, morning headache.
  2. *Objective data:*
    a. Corneal edema.
    b. Decreased peripheral vision.
    c. Increased cupping of optic disc.
    d. Tonometry—pressures >22 mm Hg.
    e. Pupils: dilated.
    f. Redness of eye.

◆ **D. Analysis/nursing diagnosis:**
  1. *Visual sensory/perceptual alterations* related to increased intraocular pressure.
  2. *Pain* related to sudden increase in intraocular pressure.
  3. *Risk for injury* related to blindness.
  4. *Impaired physical mobility* related to impaired vision.

◆ **E. Nursing care plan/implementation:**
  1. Goal: *reduce intraocular pressure.*
    a. Activity: bed rest.
    b. *Position:* semi-Fowler's.
    c. Medications as ordered:
      (1) *Miotics* (pilocarpine, carbachol); may not be effective with intraocular pressure (IOP) >40 mm Hg.
      (2) *Carbonic anhydrase inhibitors* (acetazolamide [Diamox]).
      (3) *Anticholinesterase* (demecarium bromide [Humorsol]) to facilitate outflow of aqueous humor.
      (4) *Ophthalmic beta blockers* (timolol) to decrease IOP.
  2. Goal: *provide emotional support.*
    a. Place personal objects within field of vision.
    b. Assist with activities.
    c. Encourage verbalization of concerns, fears of blindness, loss of independence.
  3. Goal: *health teaching.*
    a. *Prevent* increased IOP by *avoiding:*
      (1) Anger, excitement, worry.
      (2) Constrictive clothing.
      (3) Heavy lifting.
      (4) Excessive *fluid* intake.
      (5) Atropine or other mydriatics that cause dilation.
      (6) Straining at stool.
      (7) Eye strain.
    b. Relaxation techniques; stress management if indicated.

c. Prepare for surgical intervention, if ordered: laser trabeculoplasty, trabeculectomy (filtering), laser peripheral iridotomy.

d. Medications: purpose, dosage, frequency;

> *eyedrop installation*—(1) wash hands; (2) head back, expose conjunctiva of lower lid, instill in center *without* touching eyelashes or eye; (3) close eyes gently, apply slight pressure to corner of eye to decrease systemic absorption; (4) wait at least 2 minutes before instilling a second eyedrop medication; have extra bottle in case of breakage or loss.

e. Activity: moderate exercise—walking.

f. Safety measures: eye protection (shield or glasses); Medic Alert band or tag; *avoid* driving 1–2 hr after instilling miotics.

g. Community resources as necessary.

◆ **F. Evaluation/outcome criteria:**

1. Eyesight preserved if possible.

2. Intraocular pressure lowered (<22 mm Hg).

3. Continues medical supervision for life—reports reappearance of symptoms immediately.

VIII. Cataract: developmental or degenerative opacification of the crystalline lens.

A. Risk factors:

1. Aging (most common).

2. Trauma (x-rays, infrared or possibly ultraviolet exposure).

3. Systemic disease (diabetes).

4. Congenital defect.

5. Drug effects (corticosteroids).

◆ **B. Assessment:**

1. *Subjective data*—vision: blurring, loss of acuity (see best in low-lit conditions); distortion; diplopia; photophobia.

2. *Objective data:*

    a. Blindness: unilateral or bilateral (particularly in congenital cataracts).

    b. Loss of red reflex; gray or cloudy white opacity of lens.

◆ **C. Analysis/nursing diagnosis:**

1. *Visual sensory/perceptual alterations* related to opacity of lens.

2. *Risk for injury* related to accidents.

3. *Social isolation* related to impaired vision.

IX. Cataract removal: removal of opacified lens because of loss of vision; extracapsular cataract extraction followed by intraocular lens (IOL) insertion is procedure of choice.

◆ **A. Nursing care plan/implementation:**

1. *Preoperative:*

    a. Goal: *prepare for surgery* (ambulatory center). Antibiotic drops or ointment, mydriatic eyedrops as ordered; note dilation of

pupils; *avoid* glaring lights; usually done under local anesthetic with sedation.

b. Goal: *health teaching.* Postoperative expectations: do *not* rub, touch, or squeeze eyes shut after surgery; eye patches will be on; assistance will be given for needs; overnight hospitalization not required unless complications occur; mild iritis usually occurs.

2. *Postoperative:*

a. Goal: *reduce stress on the sutures and prevent hemorrhage.*

    (1) Activity: ambulate as ordered, usually soon after surgery; generally discharged few hours after surgery.

    (2) *Position: flat* or *low Fowler's;* on *back* or turn to *nonoperative* side 3–4 wk, because turning to operative side increases pressure.

    (3) *Avoid* activities that increase IOP: straining at stool, vomiting, coughing, brushing teeth, brushing hair, shaving, lifting objects over 20 lb, *bending,* or *stooping;* wear glasses or shaded lens during day, eyeshield at night.

    (4) Provide mouthwash, hair care, personal items within easy reach, "step-in" slippers to *avoid* bending over.

b. Goal: *promote psychological well-being.* With elderly, frequent contacts to prevent sensory deprivation.

c. Goal: *health teaching.*

    (1) If intraocular lens not inserted, prescriptive glasses may be used (cataract glasses); explain about magnification, perceptual distortion, blind areas in peripheral vision; guide through activities with glasses; need to look through central portion of lens and turn head to side when looking to the side to decrease distortion.

    (2) Eye care: instillation of eyedrops (mydriatics and carbonic anhydrase inhibitors) to prevent glaucoma and adhesions if IOL not inserted; with IOL, steroid-antibiotic use—see Glaucoma, E.3.d., p. 554, for correct technique; eye shield at night to prevent injury for 1 mo.

    (3) Signs/symptoms of *infection* (redness, pain, edema, drainage); iris *prolapse* (bulging or pear-shaped pupil); *hemorrhage* (sharp eye pain, half-moon of blood).

    (4) *Avoid:* heavy lifting; potential eye trauma.

◆ **B. Evaluation/outcome criteria:**

1. Vision restored.

2. No complications (e.g., severe eye pain, hemorrhage).

3. Performs self-care activities (e.g., instills eye-drops).
4. Returns for follow-up ophthalmology care—recognizes symptoms requiring immediate attention.

X. Retinal detachment: separation of neural retina from underlying retinal pigment epithelium.

   A. Risk factors:
   1. Trauma.
   2. Degeneration.

◆ **B. Assessment:**
   1. *Subjective data:*
      a. Flashes of light before eyes.
      b. Vision: blurred, sooty (sudden onset); sensation of floating particles; blank areas of vision.
   2. *Objective data*—ophthalmic exam: retina is grayish in area of tear; bright red, horseshoe-shaped tear; B-scan ultrasonography.

◆ **C. Analysis/nursing diagnosis:**
   1. *Visual sensory/perceptual alteration* related to blurred vision.
   2. *Anxiety* related to potential loss of vision.
   3. *Risk for injury* related to blindness.

◆ **D. Nursing care plan/implementation:**
   1. *Preoperative:*
      a. Goal: *reduce anxiety and prevent further detachment.*
         (1) Encourage verbalization of feelings; answer all questions; reinforce physician's explanation of surgical procedures.
         (2) Activity: *bed rest;* eyes usually covered to promote rest and maintain normal position of retina; side rails up.
         (3) *Position:* according to location of retinal tear; involved area of eye should be in a dependent position.
         (4) Give medications as ordered: *cycloplegic* or *mydriatics* to dilate pupils widely and decrease intraocular movement.
         (5) Relaxing diversion: conversation, music.
      b. Goal: *health teaching.* Prepare for surgical intervention (often combination used):
         (1) *Cryopexy* or *cryotherapy*—supercooled probe is applied to the sclera, causing a scar, which pulls the choroid and retina together.
         (2) *Laser photocoagulation*—a beam of intense light from a carbon arc is directed through the dilated pupil onto the retina; seals hole if retina not detached.
         (3) *Scleral buckling*—the sclera is resected or shortened to enhance the contact between the choroid and retina; frequently combined with cryopexy.

         (4) *Banding or encirclement*—silicone band or strap is placed under the extraocular muscles around the globe.
         (5) *Pneumatic retinopexy*—instillation of expandable gas or oil to tamponade tear.
   2. *Postoperative:*
      a. Goal: *reduce intraocular stress and prevent hemorrhage.*
         (1) *Position: flat* or *low Fowler's;* sandbags may be used to position head; turn to nonoperative side if allowed, retinal tear dependent; special positions may be prone, side-lying, or sitting with face down on table if gas or oil bubble injected; position may be restricted 4–8 days.
         (2) Activity: bed rest; decrease intraocular pressure by *not* stooping or bending and *avoiding* prone position.
         (3) Give medications as ordered:
            (a) *Cycloplegics* (atropine).
            (b) *Antibiotics.*
            (c) *Corticosteroids* to reduce eye movements and inflammation and prevent infection.
         (4) ROM—isometric, passive; elastic stockings to avoid thrombus related to immobility.
      b. Goal: *support coping mechanisms.*
         (1) Plan all care with patient.
         (2) Encourage verbalization of feelings, fears.
         (3) Encourage family interaction.
         (4) Diversional activities.
      c. Goal: *health teaching.*
         (1) Eye care: eye patch or shield at night for about 2 wk to prevent touching eye while asleep; dark glasses; *avoid* rubbing, squeezing eyes.
         (2) Limitations: no reading, needlework for 3 wk, *no* physical exertion for 6 wk; OK to watch TV, walk, except with bubble restrictions.
         (3) Medications: dosage, frequency, purpose, side effects: avoid nonprescription medications.
         (4) *Signs of redetachment:* flashes of light, increase in "floaters," blurred vision, acute eye pain.

◆ **E. Evaluation/outcome criteria:**
   1. Vision restored.
   2. No further detachment—recognizes signs and symptoms.
   3. No injury occurs—accepts limitations.

XI. Blindness: legally defined as vision less than 20/200 with the use of corrective lenses, or a visual field of no greater than 20 degrees; greatest incidence after 65 yr.

A. Risk factors:
1. Glaucoma.
2. Cataracts.
3. Macular degeneration.
4. Diabetic retinopathy.
5. Atherosclerosis.
6. Trauma.

◆ **B. Analysis/nursing diagnosis:**
1. *Visual sensory/perceptual alteration* related to blindness.
2. *Impaired social interaction* related to loss of sight.
3. *Risk for injury* related to visual impairment.
4. *Self-care deficit* related to visual loss.

◆ **C. Nursing care plan/implementation:**
1. Goal: *promote independence and provide emotional support.*
   a. Familiarize with surroundings; encourage use of touch.
   b. Establish communication lines; answer questions.
   c. Deal with feelings of loss, overprotectiveness by family members.
   d. Provide diversional activities: radio, CDs, talking books, tapes.
   e. Encourage self-care activities; allow voicing of frustrations when activity is not done to satisfaction (spilling or misplacing something), to decrease anger and discouragement.
2. Goal: *facilitate activities of daily living.*
   a. *Eating:*
      (1) Establish routine placement for tableware, e.g., plate, glass.
      (2) Help person mentally visualize the plate as a clock or compass (e.g., "3 o'clock" or "east").
      (3) Take person's hand and guide the fingertips to establish spatial relationship.
   b. *Walking:*
      (1) Have person hold your forearm: walk a half step in front.
      (2) Tell the person when approaching stairs, curb, incline.
   c. *Talking:*
      (1) Speak when approaching person; tell them before you touch them.
      (2) Tell them who you are and what you will be doing.
      (3) *Do not avoid* words such as "see" or discussing the appearance of things.
3. Goal: *health teaching.*
   a. Accident prevention in the home.
   b. *Community resources:*
      (1) Voluntary agencies:
         (a) American Foundation for the Blind—provides catalogs of devices for visually handicapped.
         (b) National Society for the Preven-

tion of Blindness—comprehensive educational programs and research.
         (c) Recording for the Blind, Inc.—provides recorded educational books on free loan.
         (d) Lion's Club.
         (e) Catholic charities.
         (f) Salvation Army.
      (2) Government agencies:
         (a) Social and Rehabilitation Service—counseling and placement services.
         (b) Veterans Administration—screening and pensions.
         (c) State Welfare Department, Division for the Blind—vocational.

◆ **D. Evaluation/outcome criteria:**
1. Acceptance of disability—participates in self-care activities, remains socially involved.
2. Regains independence with rehabilitation.

XII. Traumatic injuries to the brain
A. Primary trauma:
1. *Concussion*—transient disorder due to injury in which there is brief loss of consciousness due to paralysis of neuronal function; recovery is usually total.
2. *Contusion*—structural alteration of brain tissue characterized by extravasation of blood cells (bruising); injury may occur on side of impact or on opposite side (when cranial contents shift forcibly within the skull with impact).
3. *Laceration*—tearing of brain tissue or blood vessels due to a sharp bone fragment or object or tearing force.
4. *Fracture*—linear (may result in epidural bleed); comminuted or depressed (may tear dura and result in CSF leak); basilar (most serious). Basilar skull fracture may result in meningitis or brain abscess; bleeding from nose or ears; CSF present in drainage; bruising over mastoid process (*Battle's sign*) and periorbital ecchymosis (raccoon eyes).

B. Secondary trauma (response to primary trauma):
1. *Hematomas:*
   a. *Subdural*—blood from ruptured or torn vein collects between arachnoid and dura; may be acute, subacute, or chronic.
   b. *Extradural* (epidural)—blood clot located between dura mater and inner surface of skull; most often from tearing of middle meningeal artery; **emergency** condition.
2. *Increased intracranial pressure* (see **XIII. Increased intracranial pressure,** p. 558).

C. Mechanisms of injury:
1. Deformation (blow to the head).
2. Acceleration-deceleration (coup-contracoup)—forward and rebounding motion.

3. Rotation (tension, stretching, shearing force).
   D. **Pathophysiology** of impaired CNS functioning:
   1. Depressed neuronal activity in reticular activating system → depressed *consciousness* (Table 7–31).
   2. Depressed neuronal functioning in lower brain stem and spinal cord → depression of reflex activity → decreased eye movements, unequal pupils → decreased response to light stimuli → widely dilated and fixed *pupils.*
   3. Depression of respiratory center → altered respiratory pattern → decreased rate → *respiratory arrest.*

◆ E. **Risk factors:** accidents—automobile, industrial and home, motorcycle, military.

◆ F. **Assessment:**
   1. *Objective data:*
      a. Headache.
      b. Dizziness, loss of balance.
      c. Double vision.
      d. Nausea.
   2. *Objective data:*
      a. Laceration or abrasion around face or head; profuse bleeding from scalp (highly vascular, poor vasoconstrictive abilities).
      b. Drainage from ears or nose (serosanguineous).
      c. Projectile vomiting, hematemesis.
      d. Vital signs indicating increased intracranial pressure (see **XIII. Increased intracranial pressure,** p. 558.)
      e. Neurological exam:
         (1) *Altered level of consciousness;* a numerical assessment, such as the Glasgow Coma Scale (Table 7–32), may be used. The lower the score, the poorer the prognosis, generally.
         (2) Pupils—equal, round, react to light; *or* unequal, dilated, unresponsive to light.
         (3) Extremities—paresis or paralysis.

(4) Reflexes—hypotonia or hypertonia; *Babinski* present (flaring of great toe when sole is stroked).

◆ G. **Analysis/nursing diagnosis:**
   1. *Altered thought processes* related to brain trauma.
   2. *Sensory/perceptual alteration* related to depressed neuronal activity.
   3. *Risk for injury* related to impaired CNS functioning.
   4. *Risk for aspiration* related to respiratory depression.
   5. *Self-care deficit* related to altered level of consciousness.
   6. *Ineffective breathing pattern* related to CNS trauma.

◆ H. **Nursing care plan/implementation:**
   1. Goal: *sustain vital functions and minimize or prevent complications.*
      ▶ a. Patent airway: endotracheal tube or tracheostomy may be ordered.
      ▶ b. Oxygen: as ordered (hypoxia increases cerebral edema).
      ◪ c. *Position: semiprone* or *prone* (coma position) with head level to prevent aspiration *(keep off back);* turn side to side to prevent stasis in lungs.
      d. Vital signs as ordered.
      e. Neurological check: pupils, level of consciousness, muscle strength; report changes.
      ▶ f. Seizure precautions: padded side rails.
      ◖ g. Medications as ordered:
         (1) *Steroids* (dexamethasone [Decadron]).
         (2) *Anticonvulsants* (phenytoin [Dilantin], phenobarbital).
         (3) *Analgesics* (**morphine contraindicated**).
      ▶ h. Cooling measures or hypothermia to reduce elevated temperature.

TABLE 7–31 Levels of Consciousness

Stage	Characteristics
Alertness	Aware of time and place
Automatism	Aware of time and place but demonstrates abnormality of mood (euphoria to irritability)
Confusion	Inability to think and speak in coherent manner; responds to verbal requests but is unaware of time and place
Delirium	Restlessness and violent activity; may not comply with verbal instructions
Stupor	Quiet and uncommunicative; may appear conscious—sits or lies with glazed look; unable to respond to verbal instructions; bladder and rectal incontinence may occur
Semicoma	Unresponsive to verbal instructions but responds to vigorous or painful stimuli
Coma	Unresponsive to vigorous or painful stimuli

TABLE 7–32 Glasgow Coma Scale

Best eye-opening response	Purposeful and spontaneous: To voice; To pain; No response; Untestable
Best verbal response	Oriented; Disoriented; Inappropriate words; Incomprehensible sounds; No response; Untestable
Best motor response	Obeys commands; Localizes pain; Withdraws to pain; Flexion to pain; Extension to pain; No response; Untestable

Adult

i. Assist with *diagnostic tests:*
(1) Lumbar puncture (**contraindicated** with increased intracranial pressure).
(2) Electroencephalogram (EEG).
j. *Diet:* NPO for 24 hr, progressing to clear liquids if awake.
k. Fluids: IVs; nasogastric *tube feedings;* I&O.
l. Monitor blood chemistries: sodium imbalance common with head injuries.
2. Goal: *provide emotional support and use comfort measures.*
a. Comfort: skin care, oral hygiene; sheepskins; wrinkle-free linen.
b. Eyes: lubricate q4h with artificial tears if periocular edema present.
c. ROM—passive, active; physical therapy as tolerated.
d. *Avoid* restraints.
e. Encourage verbalization of concerns about changes in body image, limitations.
f. Encourage family communication.

◆ **I. Evaluation/outcome criteria:**
1. Alert, oriented—no residual effects (e.g., cognitive processes intact).
2. No signs of increased intracranial pressure (e.g., decreased respirations, increased systolic pressure with widening pulse pressure, bradycardia).
3. No paralysis—regains motor/sensory function.
4. Resumes self-care activities.

XIII. Increased intracranial pressure (ICP): intracranial hypertension associated with altered states of consciousness.
A. Pathophysiology: increases in intracranial blood volume, cerebrospinal fluid, or brain tissue mass → increased intracranial pressure → impaired neural impulse transmission → cellular anoxia, atrophy.
B. Risk factors:
1. Congenital anomalies (hydrocephalus).
2. Space-occupying lesions (abscesses or tumors).
3. Trauma (hematomas or skull fractures).
4. Circulatory problems (aneurysms, emboli).
5. Inflammation (meningitis, encephalitis).
◆ **C. Assessment:**
1. *Subjective data:*
a. Headache (early, but nonspecific symptom).
b. Nausea.
c. Visual disturbance (diplopia).
2. *Objective data:*
a. Changes in level of consciousness (*early* sign).
b. Pupillary changes—unequal, dilated, and unresponsive to light (*late* sign).
c. Vital signs—changes are variable.
(1) Blood pressure—gradual or rapid elevation, widened pulse pressure.

(2) Pulse—bradycardia, tachycardia; significant sign is *slowing of pulse as blood pressure rises.*
(3) Respirations—pattern changes (*Cheyne-Stokes,* apneusis, *Biot's*), deep and sonorous; hiccups.
(4) Temperature—moderate elevation.
d. Projectile vomiting (more common in children).
e. *Diagnostic test:* Head CT—structural changes.
◆ **D. Analysis/nursing diagnosis:**
1. *Altered cerebral tissue perfusion* related to increased intracranial pressure.
2. *Altered thought processes* related to cerebral anoxia.
3. *Ineffective breathing pattern* related to compression of respiratory center.
4. *Risk for aspiration* related to unconsciousness.
5. *Self-care deficit* related to altered level of consciousness.
6. *Impaired physical mobility* related to abnormal motor responses.
◆ **E. Nursing care plan/implementation:** *promote adequate oxygenation and limit further impairment.*
1. Vital signs: report changes **immediately.**
2. Patent airway; keep alkalotic, to prevent increased intracranial pressure from elevated CO_2; hyperventilate if necessary.
3. Give medications as ordered:
a. *Hyperosmolar diuretics* (mannitol, urea) to reduce brain swelling.
b. *Steroids* (dexamethasone [Decadron]) for anti-inflammatory action.
c. *Antacids* or H_2 antagonist to prevent stress ulcer.
4. *Position:* head of bed *elevated* 30 degrees.
5. Fluids: *restrict;* strict I&O.
6. Cooling measures to reduce temperature, because fever increases ICP.
7. Prepare for surgical intervention (see **XIV.** Craniotomy, following).
◆ **F. Evaluation/outcome criteria:**
1. No irreversible brain damage—regains consciousness.
2. Resumes self-care activities.

XIV. Craniotomy: excision of a part of the skull (burr hole to several centimeters) for exploratory purpose and biopsy; to remove neoplasms, evacuate hematomas or excess fluid, control hemorrhage, repair skull fractures, remove scar tissue, repair or excise aneurysms, and drain abscesses; produces minimal neurological deficit.
◆ **A. Analysis/nursing diagnosis:**
1. *Altered cerebral tissue perfusion* related to edema.
2. *Altered thought processes* related to disorientation.
3. *Self-care deficit* related to continued neurological impairment.

4. Also see nursing diagnosis for **XII.** Traumatic injuries to the brain, **XIII.** Increased intracranial pressure, and The Perioperative Experience, p. 500.

◆ **B. Nursing care plan/implementation:**
   1. *Preoperative:*
      a. Goal: *obtain baseline measures.*
         (1) Vital signs.
         (2) Level of consciousness.
         (3) Mental, emotional status.
         (4) Pupillary reactions.
         (5) Motor strength and functioning.
      b. Goal: *provide psychological support:* listen; give accurate, brief explanations.
      c. Goal: *prepare for surgery.*
         (1) Cut hair; shave scalp (usually done in surgery); save hair if patient/family desire.
         (2) Cover scalp with clean towel.
         ▶ (3) Insert indwelling Foley catheter as ordered.
   2. *Postoperative:*
      a. Goal: *prevent complications and limit further impairment.*
         (1) Vital signs (*indications of complications*):
            (a) Decreased blood pressure—*shock.*
            (b) Widened pulse pressure—*increased ICP.*
            (c) Respiratory failure—*compression* of medullary *respiratory* centers.
            (d) Hyperthermia—disturbance of heat-regulating mechanism; *infection.*
         (2) Neurological:
            (a) Pupils—ipsilateral dilation (*increased ICP*), visual disturbances.
            (b) Altered level of consciousness.
            (c) Altered cognitive or emotional status—disorientation common.
            (d) Motor function and strength—hypertonia, hypotonia, seizures.
         (3) Blood gases, to monitor adequacy of ventilation.
         (4) Dressings: check frequently; *aseptic* technique; reinforce as necessary.
         (5) Observe for:
            (a) CSF leakage (glucose-positive drainage from nose, mouth, ears)—*report immediately.*
            (b) Periorbital edema—apply light ice compresses as necessary—remove crusts from eyelids.
         (6) Check integrity of seventh cranial nerve (facial)—incomplete closure of eyelids.
         ◢ (7) *Position:*
            (a) *Supratentorial surgery* (cerebrum)—*semi-Fowler's* (30-degree elevation); may *not* lie on operative side.

            (b) *Infratentorial* (brain stem, cerebellum)—*flat* in bed (prone); may turn to either side but *not* onto back.
         (8) Fluids: NPO until bowel sounds return, alert, and intact gag, swallow, and cough reflexes present.
         ◖▣ (9) Medications as ordered:
            (a) *Osmotic diuretics* (mannitol).
            (b) *Corticosteroids* (dexamethasone [Decadron]).
            (c) *Mild analgesics* (do not mask neurological or respiratory depression).
            (d) *Stool softeners* to prevent constipation and straining.
         (10) Orient frequently to person, time, place—to reduce restlessness, confusion.
         (11) Side rails up for safety.
         (12) *Avoid* restraints (may increase agitation and ICP).
         (13) Ice bags to head to reduce headache.
         (14) Activity: assist with ambulation.
      b. Goal: *provide optimal supportive care.*
         (1) Cover scalp once dressings are removed (scarves, wigs).
         (2) Deal realistically with neurological deficits—facilitate acceptance, adjustment, independence.
      c. Goal: *health teaching.*
         (1) Prepare for physical, occupational, or speech therapy, as needed.
         (2) Activities of daily living.

◆ **C. Evaluation/outcome criteria:**
   1. Regains consciousness—is alert, oriented.
   2. Resumes self-care activities within limits of neurological deficits.

XV. Epilepsy: seizure disorder characterized by sudden transient aberration of brain function; associated with motor, sensory, autonomic, or psychic disturbances.
   A. Seizure: involuntary muscular contraction and disturbances of consciousness from abnormal electrical activity.
   B. Risk factors:
      1. Brain injury.
      2. Infection (meningitis, encephalitis).
      3. Water and electrolyte disturbances.
      4. Hypoglycemia.
      5. Tumors.
      6. Vascular disorders (hypoxia or hypocapnia).
   C. Generalized seizures:
      1. *Tonic-clonic* (grand mal) seizures:
         a. **Pathophysiology:** increased excitability of a neuron → possible activation of adjacent neurons → synchronous discharge of impulses → vigorous involuntary sustained muscle spasms (*tonic* contractions). Onset of neuronal fatigue →

intermittent muscle spasms (*clonic con-tractions*) → cessation of muscle spasms → fatigue.

◆ b. **Assessment:**
(1) *Subjective data*—aura: flash of light; peculiar smell, sound; feelings of fear; euphoria.
(2) *Objective data:*
(a) *Convulsive stage*—tonic and clonic muscle spasms, loss of conscious-ness, breath holding, frothing at mouth, biting of tongue, urinary or fecal incontinence; lasts 2–5 min.
(b) *Postconvulsion*—headache, fatigue (postictal sleep), malaise, vomit-ing, sore muscles, choking on se-cretions, aspiration.

2. *Absence* (petit mal) seizures:
a. **Pathophysiology:** unknown etiology, mo-mentary loss of consciousness (10–20 sec); usually no recollection of seizure; re-sumes previously performed action.
◆ b. **Assessment**—*objective data:*
(1) Fixation of gaze; blank facial expres-sion.
(2) Flickering of eyelids.
(3) Jerking of facial muscle or arm.

3. *Minor motor* seizures:
a. *Myoclonic*—involuntary "lightning-like" jerking contraction of major muscles; may throw person to the floor; no loss of consciousness.
b. *Atonic*—brief, total loss of muscle tone; person falls to the floor; loss of conscious-ness (common in children).

D. **Partial (focal) seizures:**
1. *Partial motor:* arises from region in motor cortex (posterior frontal lobe); most com-monly begins in upper extremities, spreading to face and lower extremity (*jacksonian march*); noting progression is important in identifying area of cortex involved.
2. *Partial sensory:* sensory symptoms occur with partial seizure activity; varies with region in brain; transient.
3. *Partial complex* (psychomotor): arises out of anterior temporal lobe; frequently begins with an aura; characteristic feature is automa-tism (lip smacking, chewing, patting body, picking at clothes); lasts from 2–3 min to 15 min; do *not* restrain.

◆ E. **Analysis/nursing diagnosis:**
1. *Risk for injury* related to convulsive disorder.
2. *Anxiety* related to sudden loss of conscious-ness.
3. *Self-esteem disturbance* related to chronic ill-ness.
4. *Impaired social interaction* related to self-consciousness.

◆ F. **Nursing care plan/implementation** (general-ized seizures):
1. Goal: *prevent injury during seizure.*
a. Do *not* force jaws open during convul-sion.
b. Do *not* restrict limbs—protect from in-jury; place something soft under head (towel, jacket, hands).
c. Loosen constrictive clothing.
d. Note time, level of consciousness, type and duration of seizure.
▶ 2. Goal: *postseizure care:*
a. *Turn on side* to drain saliva and facilitate breathing.
b. Suction as necessary.
c. Orient to time and place.
d. Oral hygiene if tongue or cheek injured.
e. Check vital signs, pupils, level of con-sciousness.
3. Goal: *prevent or reduce recurrences of seizure activity.*
a. Encourage patient to identify precipitat-ing factors.
b. Moderation in diet and exercise.
c. Medications as ordered: phenytoin (Di-lantin); phenobarbital; carbamazepine (Tegretol); primidone (Mysoline); val-proate (Depacon).
4. Goal: *health teaching.*
a. Medications:
(1) Actions, side effects (apathy, ataxia, hyperplasia of gums).
(2) Complications with sudden with-drawal (*status epilepticus*—continu-ous seizure activity; give diazepam per order, O_2).
b. Attitude toward life and treatment; ad-here to medication program.
c. Clarify misconceptions, fears—especially about insanity, bad genes.
d. Maintain activities, interests—expect no driving until seizure free for period of time specified by state Department of Motor Vehicles.
e. *Avoid:* stress; lack of sleep; emotional up-set; alcohol.
f. Relaxation techniques; stress-manage-ment techniques.
g. Use Medic Alert band or tag.
h. Appropriate community resources.

◆ G. **Evaluation/outcome criteria:**
1. Avoids precipitating stimuli—achieves seizure control.
2. Complies with medication regimen.
3. Retains independence.

XVI. Transient ischemic attacks (TIAs): temporary, com-plete, or relatively complete cessation of cerebral blood flow to a localized area of brain, producing

symptoms (2–30 min) ranging from weakness ("drop attacks") and numbness to monocular blindness; an important precursor to stroke. Surgical intervention includes *carotid endarterectomy;* most common postoperative cranial nerve damage causes vocal cord paralysis or difficulty managing saliva and tongue deviation (cranial nerves VII, X, XI, XII); usually temporary; stroke may also occur.

XVII. **Ischemic stroke** (CVA, brain attack): brain lesion resulting from damage to blood vessels supplying brain (middle cerebral artery most common).

A. **Pathophysiology:** reduced or interrupted blood flow → interruption of nerve impulses down corticospinal tract → decreased or absent voluntary movement on one side of the body (fine movements are more affected than coarse movements); later, autonomous reflex activity → spasticity and rigidity of muscles.

B. **Risk factors:**
1. Cerebral thrombosis (most common), embolism, hemorrhage.
2. Prior ischemic episodes (TIAs).
3. Hypertension.
4. Oral contraceptives.
5. Emotional stress.
6. Family history.
7. Age.
8. Diabetes mellitus.

◆ C. **Assessment:**
1. *Subjective data:*
   a. Weakness: sudden or gradual loss of movement of extremities on one side.
   b. Difficulty forming words.
   c. Difficulty swallowing (dysphagia).
   d. Nausea, vomiting.
   e. History of TIAs.
2. *Objective data:*
   a. Vital signs:
      (1) BP—elevated; widened pulse pressure.
      (2) Temperature—elevated.
      (3) Pulse—normal, slow.
      (4) Respirations—tachypnea, altered pattern; deep; sonorous.
   b. Neurological:
      (1) Altered level of consciousness.
      (2) Pupils—unequal; vision—homonymous hemianopia.
      (3) Ptosis of eyelid, drooping mouth.
      (4) Paresis or paralysis (hemiplegia).
      (5) Loss of sensation and reflexes.
      (6) Incontinence of urine or feces.
      (7) Aphasia (see p. 550).

◆ D. **Analysis/nursing diagnosis:**
1. *Impaired physical mobility* related to hemiplegia.
2. *Impaired swallowing* related to paralysis.
3. *Impaired verbal communication* related to aphasia.

4. *Risk for aspiration* related to unconsciousness.
5. *Sensory/perceptual alterations* related to altered cerebral blood flow, visual field blindness.
6. *Altered thought processes* related to cerebral edema.
7. *Self-care deficit* related to paresis or paralysis.
8. *Body image disturbance* related to hemiplegia.
9. *Total incontinence* related to interruption of normal nerve transmission.
10. *Impaired social interaction* related to aphasia or neurological deficit.
11. *Risk for impaired skin integrity* related to immobility.
12. *Unilateral neglect* related to cerebral damage.

◆ E. **Nursing care plan/implementation** (see **Clinical Pathway for Stroke,** p. 562):
1. Goal: *reduce cerebral anoxia.*
   a. Patent airway:
      ▶ (1) Oxygen therapy as ordered; suctioning to prevent aspiration.
      (2) Turn, cough, deep breathe q2h due to high incidence of aspiration pneumonia.
   b. Activity: bed rest, progressing to out of bed as tolerated.
   ◪ c. *Position:*
      (1) Maximize ventilation.
      (2) Support with pillows when on side; use hand rolls and arm slings as ordered.
2. Goal: *promote cardiovascular function and maintain cerebral perfusion.*
   a. Vital signs; neurological checks.
   b. Medications as ordered:
      (1) *Antiplatelet aggregation inhibitors* (ASA, ticlopidine, dipyridamole [Persantine]).
      (2) *Antihypertensives* to prevent rupture.
      (3) *Anticoagulants* to prevent thrombus.
   c. *Fluids:* IVs to prevent hemoconcentration; I&O; weigh daily.
   d. ROM exercises to prevent contractures, muscle atrophy, phlebitis.
   e. Skin care and position changes to prevent decubiti.
3. Goal: *provide for emotional relaxation.*
   a. Identify grief reaction to changes in body image.
   b. Encourage expression of feelings, concerns.
4. Goal: *patient safety.*
   a. Identify existence of *homonymous hemianopia* (visual field blindness) and *agnosia* (disturbance in sensory information).
   b. Use side rails and assist as needed.
   c. Remind to walk slowly, take adequate rest periods, ensure good lighting, look where patient is going.

Modified Rankin Scale Bonita and Beaglehole, Stroke 1988; 10:1487-1500
Grade I – No deficit
Grade II – Functionally insignificant impairments of movements,
　　　　but with control movements through full range
Grade III – Presence of muscle contraction and movement against gravity or resistance,
　　　　but limited range and not controlled
Grace IV – Little or no active movements

UCSF / Health Care
UCSF / Mount Zion Medical Center
STROKE CLINICAL PATHWAY

DATE	/ /	/ /	/ /
	ED	**Day 1**	**Day 2**
Discharge Planning		☐ Evaluation of home situation ☐ Contact SW (social work)	☐ Discharge planning started ☐ SW evaluation
Consultations/ Referrals	☐ Evaluate for tPA ☐ Neurology consult ☐ PMD / House staff notified ☐ tPA consent ☐ Neurosurgery consult	☐ Neurology consult ☐ Dietary screen ☐ PT eval ☐ OT eval ☐ Speech/swallow eval	Complete day one evals: ☐ PT ☐ OT ☐ Speech/swallow ☐ Dietary eval
Diagnostic Tests/ Screening	☐ PT, INR　☐ CxR ☐ PTT　　☐ CT scan ☐ Electrolytes ☐ BUN ☐ CBC　　☐ Creatinine ☐ EKG　　☐ Dip Stick UA ☐ Type and ☐ Glucose 　 screen	☐ PT, INR ☐ PTT ☐ CBC ☐ Carotid ultrasound ☐ Echocardiogram+/- bubbles ☐ Hypercoag. Panel ☐ MRI/A	☐ PT, INR ☐ PTT
Treatments/ Medications	☐ Suction ☐ IV fluids _____ ☐ O₂ ☐ tPA ☐ Blood pressure control medications ☐ Heparin IV/SQ ☐ LMWH SQ ☐ Aspirin/Antiplatelets	☐ Suction ☐ Respiratory therapy ☐ IV fluids _____ ☐ Warfarin ☐ Heparin IV/SQ ☐ LMWH SQ ☐ Aspirin/Antiplatelets ☐ Stool softener ☐ Other	☐ Suction ☐ Respiratory therapy ☐ IV to saline lock ☐ Warfarin ☐ Heparin IV/SQ ☐ LMWH SQ ☐ Aspirin/Antiplatelets ☐ Stool softener ☐ Other
Diet / Nutrition	☐ NPO	Diet (check one): ☐ NPO ☐ Other _____ Feeding (check one): ☐ Oral self ☐ Feeding tube ☐ Oral assisted feed ☐ Supplements	Diet (check one): ☐ NPO ☐ Other _____ Feeding (check one): ☐ Oral self ☐ Feeding tube ☐ Oral assisted feed ☐ Supplements
Activity	☐ Bed rest	☐ Bed rest ☐ Other _____	☐ Physical therapy ☐ Speech therapy ☐ Occupational therapy
Nursing Assessment/ Intervention ◆	☐ VS as per ED routine ☐ I & O ☐ Baseline neuro exam ☐ Glasgow coma score ☐ Cardiac monitor ☐ Weight _____	A E P VS as per unit routine ☐☐☐ I&O ☐☐☐ O₂ sat above 92% ☐☐☐ Cardiac monitor ☐☐☐ Saline lock ☐☐☐ Neuro assessment q___hrs ☐☐☐ TEDs, SCD ☐☐☐ Bleeding precautions ☐☐☐ Aspirations precautions ☐☐☐ Falls precautions ☐☐☐ Regular apical pulse, peripheral 　pulses palpable and equal ☐☐☐ Abdomen soft nontender, bowel 　sounds present ☐☐☐ Voiding adequate amounts, urine 　clear yellow to amber ☐☐☐ Foley draining adequate 　amounts, clear urine ☐☐☐ Weight _____	A E P VS as per unit routine ☐☐☐ I&O ☐☐☐ O₂ sat above 92% ☐☐☐ Cardiac monitor ☐☐☐ Saline lock ☐☐☐ Neuro assessment q___hrs ☐☐☐ TEDs, SCD ☐☐☐ Bleeding precautions ☐☐☐ Aspirations precautions ☐☐☐ Falls precautions ☐☐☐ Regular apical pulse, peripheral 　pulses palpable and equal ☐☐☐ Abdomen soft nontender, bowel 　sounds present ☐☐☐ Voiding adequate amounts, urine 　clear yellow to amber, 　consider PVR ☐☐☐ Foley draining adequate 　amounts, clear urine ☐☐☐ Weight _____
Knowledge Deficit Patient/Family Teaching	☐ Patient/Family teaching regarding 　current status, immediate plan ☐ Give patient/family your health 　matter copy of patient pathway 　portion ☐ Pastoral support	☐ Include patient/family in 　plan of care ☐ Begin assessment of patient/family 　knowledge of stroke ☐ Stroke risk factors discussed	☐ Update plan of care ☐ PT/OT to start teaching 　patient/family: ☐ Mobility ☐ Safety ☐ Transfers ☐ Assistive devices ☐ Discharge goals ☐ SW to discuss D/C options ☐ Patient/Family able to identify risk 　factors

Adult

Type of Stroke _____ Location _____

Admission Rankin _____ Discharge Rankin _____

/ /	/ /	/ /
Day 3	**Day 4 / Discharge**	**Discharge Outcomes**
☐ D/C plan identified ☐ Transportation needs identified	☐ D/C plan in place ☐ Transportation arranged	☐ D/C Home ☐ D/C SNF ☐ D/C Rehab.
☐ Interdisciplinary form for SNF or Rehab. initiated ☐ Home care liaison referral	☐ Complete referral for SNF or Rehab. ☐ Home care arranged	F/U MD appointment made F/U with appropriate home care services arranged ☐ Refer to stroke support group
☐ PT, INR ☐ PTT ☐ If Foley d/c'd UA with micro ☐ BUN ☐ Creatinine	☐ If Foley d/c'd UA with micro ☐ PT, INR ☐ PTT ☐ BUN ☐ Creatinine	
☐ Suction ☐ Respiratory therapy ☐ Saline lock ☐ Warfarin ☐ Aspirin / Antiplatelets ☐ Stool softener ☐ LMWH SQ ☐ Laxative ☐ Other	☐ Suction ☐ Respiratory therapy ☐ Saline lock ☐ Warfarin ☐ Aspirin / Antiplatelets ☐ Stool softener ☐ LMWH SQ ☐ Laxative ☐ Other	☐ INR therapeutic ☐ D/C medications teaching complete ☐ LMWH administration teaching complete with patient or family ☐ Coumadin teaching complete ☐ FU with primary care MD arranged ☐ Next blood draw for INR arranged ☐ D/C Rx given to patient/family
Diet (check one): advance as tol: ☐ NPO ☐ Other _____ Feeding (check one): ☐ Oral self ☐ Feeding tube ☐ Oral assisted feed ☐ Supplements	Diet (check one): advance as tol: ☐ NPO ☐ Other _____ Feeding (check one): ☐ Oral self ☐ Feeding tube ☐ Oral assisted feed ☐ Supplements ☐ Feeding plan for home identified	☐ Nutritional needs met at home ☐ Patient tolerates self feeds or ☐ Family able to assist with feeds ☐ Feeding tube in place ☐ Home referral complete ☐ Feeding/nutrition teaching complete
☐ Physical therapy: advance as tol. ☐ Speech therapy ☐ Occupational therapy: advance as tol.	☐ Physical therapy: advance as tol. ☐ Speech therapy ☐ Occupational therapy: advance as tol.	☐ Assistive devices equipment given ☐ Delivery arranged ☐ Told where to obtain ☐ Home safety addressed ☐ Mobility, ADL, and communications needs addressed
A E P VS as per unit routine ☐ ☐ ☐ I&O ☐ ☐ ☐ O₂ sat above 92% ☐ ☐ ☐ Cardiac monitor ☐ ☐ ☐ Saline lock ☐ ☐ ☐ Neuro assessment q___hrs ☐ ☐ ☐ TEDs, SCD ☐ ☐ ☐ Bleeding precautions ☐ ☐ ☐ Aspirations precautions ☐ ☐ ☐ Falls precautions ☐ ☐ ☐ Regular apical pulse, peripheral pulses palpable and equal ☐ ☐ ☐ Abdomen soft nontender, bowel sounds present ☐ ☐ ☐ Voiding adequate amounts, urine clear yellow to amber, consider PVR ☐ ☐ ☐ Foley draining adequate amounts, clear urine ☐ ☐ ☐ Weight _____	A E P VS as per unit routine ☐ ☐ ☐ I&O ☐ ☐ ☐ O₂ sat above 92% ☐ ☐ ☐ Cardiac monitor ☐ ☐ ☐ Saline lock ☐ ☐ ☐ Neuro assessment q___hrs ☐ ☐ ☐ TEDs, SCD ☐ ☐ ☐ Bleeding precautions ☐ ☐ ☐ Aspirations precautions ☐ ☐ ☐ Falls precautions ☐ ☐ ☐ Regular apical pulse, peripheral pulses palpable and equal ☐ ☐ ☐ Abdomen soft nontender, bowel sounds present ☐ ☐ ☐ Voiding adequate amounts, urine clear yellow to amber, consider PVR ☐ ☐ ☐ Foley draining adequate amounts, clear urine ☐ ☐ ☐ Weight _____	☐ Negative for DVT ☐ Skin intact/alterations addressed ☐ BM within last 24 hrs ☐ Afebrile ☐ Neurologically stable
☐ Update plan of care ☐ Warfarin teaching started, appropriate teaching material given ☐ Feeding/nutrition teaching initiated ☐ PT teaching ☐ OT teaching ☐ Patient/family states ways to modify risk factors	☐ Update plan of care ☐ Warfarin teaching started, appropriate teaching material given ☐ Feeding/nutrition teaching ☐ PT teaching ☐ OT teaching ☐ Patient/family states ways to modify risk factors	Patient/family able to verbalize instructions on: ☐ D/C ☐ D/C medications ☐ Precautions ☐ Activity ☐ F/U services ☐ MD appointment

Adult

5. Goal: *health teaching.*
    a. Exercise routines.
    b. Diet: self-feeding, but assist as needed.
    c. Resumption of self-care activities.
    d. Use of supportive devices; transfer techniques.

◆ **F. Evaluation/outcome criteria:**
  1. No complications (e.g., pneumonia).
  2. Regains functional independence—resumes self-care activities.
  3. Return of control over body functions (e.g., bowel, bladder, speech).

XVIII. Bacterial meningitis (see **Unit 5,** p. 253).

XIX. Encephalitis (also includes aseptic meningitis): inflammation of the brain and its coverings due to direct viral invasion, which usually results in a lengthy coma.

  A. Pathophysiology: brain tissue injury → release of enzymes that increase vascular dilation, capillary permeability → edema formation → increased intracranial pressure → depression of CNS function.

  B. Risk factors:
    1. Arboviruses.
    2. Enteroviruses (poliovirus, echovirus).
    3. Herpesvirus.
    4. Varicella-zoster (chickenpox).
    5. Postinfection complication (measles, mumps, smallpox).

◆ **C. Assessment:**
  1. *Subjective data:*
    a. Headache—severe.
    b. Fever—sudden.
    c. Nausea, vomiting.
    d. Sensitivity to light (photophobia).
    e. Difficulty concentrating.
  2. *Objective data:*
    a. Altered level of consciousness.
    b. Nuchal rigidity.
    c. Tremors; facial weakness.
    d. Nystagmus.
    e. Elevated temperature.
    f. *Diagnostic test:* lumbar puncture—fluid cloudy; *increased* neutrophils, protein.
    g. Lab data: blood—slight to moderate leukocytosis (about 14,000).

◆ **D. Analysis/nursing diagnosis:**
  1. *Self-care deficit* related to altered level of consciousness.
  2. *Risk for injury* related to coma.
  3. *Sensory/perceptual alteration* related to brain tissue injury.
  4. *Altered thought processes* related to increased intracranial pressure.

◆ **E. Nursing care plan/implementation:**
  1. Goal: *support physical and emotional relaxation.*
    a. Vital signs; neurological signs as ordered.
    b. Seizure precautions.
    c. *Position:* to maintain patent airway; prevent contractures; ROM.
    d. Medications as ordered:
      (1) *Analgesics* for headache and neck pain.
      (2) *Antipyretics* for fever.
      (3) *Antivirals.*
      (4) *Anticonvulsants* for seizures.
      (5) *Antibiotics* for infection in aseptic meningitis.
      (6) *Osmotic diuretics* (mannitol) to reduce cerebral edema.
      (7) *Corticosteroids* for inflammation.
    e. No isolation.
  2. Goal: *health teaching:* self-care activities with residual motor and speech deficits; physical therapy.

◆ **F. Evaluation/outcome criteria:**
  1. Regains consciousness; is alert, oriented.
  2. Performs self-care activities with minimal assistance.

COMFORT, REST, ACTIVITY, AND MOBILITY

I. **Pain**—the "fifth vital sign" in the care of patients; a complex subjective sensation; unpleasant sensory and emotional experience associated with real or potential tissue damage. *Pain is considered to be whatever the person experiencing it says it is, existing whenever he or she says it does.*

 A. **Classifications:**
   1. *Acute pain:* lasts typically less than 1 mo; characterized by tachycardia, tachypnea, increased BP, diaphoresis, dilated pupils.
   2. *Chronic pain:* persists or is recurring for longer than 3 mo; often characterized by lassitude, sleep disturbance, decreased appetite, weight loss, diminished libido, constipation, depression.
   3. *Somatogenic* (organic/physiological):
     a. *Nociceptive:* somatic or visceral pain—sensations, normal pain transmission, such as aching or pressure (e.g., cancer pain, chronic joint and bone pain).
     b. *Neuropathic:* aberrant processes in peripheral and/or central nervous system; part of a defined neurological problem; sensations such as sharp, burning, shooting pain (e.g., nerve compression, polyneuropathy, central pain of stroke, phantom pain after amputation).
   4. *Psychogenic* (without organic pathology sufficient to explain pain).

 B. **Components of pain experience**—pain related to:
   1. *Stimuli*—sources: chemical, ischemic, mechanical trauma, extremes of heat/cold.
   2. *Perception*—viewed with fear by children, can be altered by level of consciousness, interpreted and influenced by previous and current experience, is more severe when alone at night or immobilized.
   3. *Response*—variations in physiological, cultural, and learned responses; anxiety is created; pain seen as justified punishment; pain used as means for attention-getting.

 ◆ C. **Assessment:**
   1. *Subjective data* (see Table 7–33):
     a. *Site*—medial, lateral, proximal, distal.
     b. *Strength:*
       (1) Certain tissues are more sensitive.
       (2) Change in intensity.
       (3) Based on expectations.
       (4) Affected by distraction or concentration, state of consciousness.
       (5) Described as slight, medium, severe, excruciating.
     c. *Quality*—aching, burning, crushing, dull, piercing, shifting, throbbing, tingling.
     d. *Antecedent factors*—physical exertion, eating, extreme temperatures, physical and emotional stressors (e.g., fear).
     e. *Previous experience*—influences reaction to pain.
     f. *Behavioral clues*—demanding, worried, irritable, restless, difficult to distract, sleepless.
   2. *Objective data:*
     a. *Verbal clues*—moaning, groaning, crying.
     b. *Nonverbal clues*—clenching teeth, grimacing, splinting of body parts, body position, knees drawn up, involuntary reflex movements, tossing/turning, rhythmic rubbing movements, voice pitch and speed, eyes shut.
     c. *Physical clues*—breathing irregularities, abdominal distention, skin color changes, skin temperature changes, excessive salivation, perspiration.
     d. *Time/duration*—onset duration, recurrence, interval, last occurrence.

 ◆ D. **Analysis/nursing diagnosis:**
   1. *Pain,* acute or chronic, related to specific patient condition.
   2. *Activity intolerance* related to discomfort.
   3. *Sleep pattern disturbance* related to pain.
   4. *Fatigue* related to state of discomfort or emotional stress.
   5. *Ineffective individual coping* related to chronic pain.

TABLE 7–33   Required Pain Assessment on Admission for Hospitalized Patients

Do you have pain now? Have you had pain in the recent past? If "yes" to either question, the following data are obtained:

- Pain intensity (use a scale appropriate for the patient population)
- Location (ask patient to mark on diagram or point to the site)
- Quality, patterns of radiation, character (use patient's own words)
- Onset, duration, variations, and patterns
- Alleviating and aggravating factors
- Present pain management regimen and effectiveness
- Pain management history (medication history, barriers to reporting pain and using analgesics, manner of expressing pain)
- Effects of pain (impact on daily life, function, sleep, appetite, relationships with others, emotions, concentration)
- Patient's pain goal (pain intensity and goals related to function, activities, quality of life)
- Physical examination/observation of site(s) of pain

Source: Joint Commission on Accreditation of Healthcare Organizations, Oakbrook Terrace, Ill., 1999. (www.jcaho.org)

Adult

◆ **E. Nursing care plan/implementation:**
1. Goal: *provide relief of pain.*
   a. Assess level of pain; ask patient to rate on scale of 0 to 10 (0 = no pain; 10 = worst pain) or smile/sad faces. Use age-, condition-, and language-appropriate scale (Table 7–34).
   b. Determine cause and try nursing *comfort* measures *before* giving drugs:
      (1) *Environmental factors:* noise, light, odors, motion.
      (2) *Physiological needs:* elimination, hunger, thirst, fatigue, circulatory impairment, muscle tension, ventilation, pressure on nerves.
      (3) *Emotional:* fear of unknown, helplessness, loneliness (especially at night).
   c. *Relieve:* anger, anxiety, boredom, loneliness.
   d. Report **sudden, severe, new** pain; pain **not** relieved by medications or comfort measures; pain associated with **casts** or **traction.**
   e. *Remove pain stimulus:*
      (1) Administer pain medication—*nonopioids:* NSAIDs—ketorolac (Toradol); *opioids:* first-line analgesics include morphine, hydromorphone, fentanyl, oxycodone, hydrocodone (see Table 10–9); *adjuvants:* local anesthetics, sedatives, muscle relaxants; give at appropriate time intervals; do *not* withhold due to overestimated danger of addiction.
      (2) *Avoid* cold (to reduce immediate tissue reaction to trauma).
      (3) *Apply* heat (to relieve ischemia).
      (4) Change activity (e.g., restrict activity in cardiac pain).
      (5) Change, loosen dressing.
      (6) Comfort (e.g., smooth wrinkled sheets, change wet dressing).
      (7) Give food (e.g., for ulcer).
   f. *Reduce pain-receptor reaction.*
      (1) Ointment (use as coating).

   g. Assist with medical/surgical interventions to *block pain-impulse transmission:*
      (2) Local anesthetics.
      (3) Padding (of bony prominences).
      (1) Injection of local anesthetic into nerve (e.g., dental).
      (2) Cordotomy—sever anterolateral spinal cord nerve tracts.
      (3) Electrical stimulation—transcutaneous (skin surface), percutaneous (peripheral nerve).
      (4) Peripheral nerve implant—electrode to major sensory nerve.
      (5) Dorsal column stimulator—electrode to dorsal column.
   h. *Minimize barriers to effective pain management:*
      (1) Achieve "balanced analgesia"; around-the-clock administration of NSAIDs or acetaminophen if possible, continuous infusion, patient-controlled analgesia (PCA); combination therapy (opioids, nonopioids, adjuvants).
      (2) Accept patient and family report of pain.
      (3) Discuss fear of addiction with patient/family (incidence <1% when opioids taken for pain relief).
      (4) Discuss fear of respiratory depression with staff; preventable; related to sedation.
   i. *Document response to pain-relief measures.*
2. Goal: *use nonpharmacological methods to reduce pain.*
   a. *Distraction,* e.g., TV (cerebral cortical activity blocks impulses from thalamus).
   b. *Aromatherapy*—assists in relaxation.
   c. *Hypnosis*—assess appropriateness for use for psychogenic pain and for anesthesia; needs to be open to suggestion.
   d. *Acupuncture*—assess emotional readiness and belief in it.
3. Goal: *alter interpretation and response to pain.*
   a. Administer *narcotics*—result: no longer sees pain as disturbing.
   b. Administer *hypnotics*—result: changes perception and decreases reaction.
   c. Help patient obtain interpersonal satisfaction from ways other than attention received when in pain.
4. Goal: *promote patient control of pain and analgesia: patient-controlled analgesia* (PCA), an analgesia administration system designed to maintain optimal serum analgesia levels; safely delivers intermittent bolus doses of a narcotic analgesic; preset to maximum hourly dose.
   a. *Advantages:* decreased patient anxiety; improved pulmonary function; fewer side effects.

TABLE 7–34   Format for Assessing Pain 💡

FIRST, assess the pain:

Frequency	Is it intermittent or constant?
Intensity	What is the quality of the pain? Sharp or dull? Throbbing? Squeezing?
Radiation	Does the pain move to other parts of the body?
Severity	On a scale of 1 to 10, how bad is the pain?
Timing	When did the pain begin? How long does it last? Does anything make it worse or take the pain away? What precedes the pain?

b. *Limitations:* requires an indwelling intravenous line; analgesia targets central pain, may not relieve peripheral discomfort; cost of PCA unit.

5. Goal: *health teaching.*
   a. Explain causes of pain and how to describe pain.
   b. Explain that it is acceptable to admit existence of pain.
   c. Relaxation exercises.
   d. Biofeedback methods of pain perception and control.
   e. Proper medication administration (PCA, continuous around-the-clock dosing), when necessary, for self-care.

◆ **F. Evaluation/outcome criteria:**
   1. Verbalizes comfort; awareness of pain decreased.
   2. Knows source of pain; how to reduce stimulus and perception.
   3. Uses alternative measures for pain relief.
   4. Able to cope with pain, e.g., remains active, relaxed appearance; verbal and nonverbal clues of pain absent.

II. Immobility: impaired physical mobility or limitation of physical movement may be accompanied by a number of complications that can involve any or all of the major systems of the body. Regardless of the cause of immobilization, there are a number of conditions that arise primarily as a complication of immobility. These are discussed in Table 7–35.

   A. Types of immobility:
      1. *Physical*—physical restriction due to limitation in movement or physiological processes (e.g., breathing).
      2. *Intellectual*—lack of action due to lack of knowledge (e.g., mental retardation, brain damage).
      3. *Emotional*—immobilized when highly stressed (e.g., after loss of loved person or diagnosis of terminal illness).
      4. *Social*—decreased social interaction due to separation from family when hospitalized or when alone, as in old age.

   B. Risk factors:
      1. Pain, trauma, injury.
      2. Loss of body function or body part.
      3. Chronic disease.
      4. Emotional, mental illness; neglect.
      5. Malnutrition.
      6. Bed rest, traction, surgery, medications.

   ◆ **C. Assessment:**
      1. *Subjective data: psychological/social effects* of immobility:
         a. Decreased motivation to learn; decreased retention.
         b. Decreased problem-solving abilities.
         c. Diminished drives; decreased hunger.

         d. Changes in body image, self-concept.
         e. Exaggerated emotional reactions, inappropriate to situation or person; aggression, apathy, withdrawal.
         f. Deterioration of time perception.
         g. Fear, anxiety, feelings of worthlessness related to change in role activities, e.g., when no longer employed.
      2. *Objective data: physical effects* of immobility:
         a. Cardiovascular.
            (1) Orthostatic hypotension.
            (2) Increased cardiac load.
            (3) Thrombus formation.
         b. Gastrointestinal.
            (1) Anorexia.
            (2) Diarrhea.
            (3) Constipation.
         c. Metabolic.
            (1) Tissue atrophy and protein catabolism.
            (2) BMR reduced.
            (3) Fluid/electrolyte imbalances.
         d. Musculoskeletal.
            (1) Demineralization (osteoporosis).
            (2) Contractures and atrophy.
            (3) Skin breakdown.
         e. Respiratory.
            (1) Decreased respiratory movement.
            (2) Accumulation of secretions in respiratory tract.
            (3) O_2/CO_2 level imbalance.
         f. Urinary.
            (1) Calculi.
            (2) Bladder distention, stasis.
            (3) Infection.
            (4) Frequency.

   ◆ **D. Analysis/nursing diagnosis:**
      1. *Impaired physical mobility* related to specific patient condition.
      2. *Impaired skin integrity* related to physical immobilization.
      3. *Urinary retention* related to incomplete emptying of bladder.
      4. *Constipation* related to inactivity.
      5. *Risk for disuse syndrome* related to lack of range of motion.
      6. *Bathing/hygiene self-care deficit* related to musculoskeletal impairment.
      7. *Sensory/perceptual alteration* related to complications of immobility.
      8. *Body image disturbance* related to physical limitations.

   ◆ **E. Nursing care plan/implementation:**
      1. Goal: *prevent physical, psychological hazards.*
         a. Apply nursing measures to promote venous flow, muscle strength, endurance, joint mobility, skin integrity.
         b. Assess and counteract *psychological* impact of immobility (e.g., feelings of helplessness, hopelessness, powerlessness).

TABLE 7–35 **Complications of Immobilization**

◆ Disorder	Pathophysiology	◆ Assessment	◆ Analysis/Nursing Diagnosis	◆ Nursing Care Plan/Implementation	◆ Evaluation/Outcome Criteria
Orthostatic hypotension	A decrease in BP >30/15 caused by failure of vasomotor responses to compensate for change from a recumbent to an upright position	*Subjective data:* weakness; dizziness. *Objective data:* decreased BP >30/15 measured 2 min after moving from a supine to a sitting or standing position; loss of muscle tone and strength; patient may faint	*Decreased cardiac output* related to orthostatic hypotension. *Risk for injury* related to vertigo. *Activity intolerance* related to dizziness	*Prevent trauma resulting from sudden decrease in BP* 1. Change position gradually 2. Elastic stockings 3. Leg exercises 4. Dangle before getting up 5. Tilt table 6. Sitting and lying BP 7. Monitor side effects of drugs *Health teaching* 1. Explains signs and symptoms to patient 2. Encourage patient to dangle before standing 3. Encourage slow movement from sitting to standing 4. Exercises to maintain muscle tone	Patient tolerates increased activity. No trauma occurs. BP remains within normal limits
Cardiac overload	When the body is recumbent, some of the total blood volume that would be in the legs as a result of gravity is redistributed to other parts of the body, thereby increasing the circulating volume and increasing the workload of the heart; heart rate, which is decreased because blood is prevented from entering the thoracic vessels by pressure from the Valsalva maneuver, increases when normal breathing resumes	*Subjective data:* fear; apprehension. *Objective data:* Valsalva maneuver (pressure against the closed glottis when breath is held) 10–20 times/hr, when trying to move in bed; tachycardia; decreased exercise tolerance	*Risk for injury* related to increased workload of heart. *Activity intolerance* related to increased workload of heart. *Fear* related to tachycardia	*Prevent injury and further ischemic damage to cardiac tissue by decreasing workload of heart* 1. Out of bed in chair when possible 2. *Semirecumbent* position when in bed; pillows between legs when side-lying 3. Exercises: passive and active ROM, isometric 4. Encourage participation in self-care 5. Turn every 2 hr, dangle 6. *Avoid* Valsalva, fatigue 7. Minimize constipation 8. Encourage slow, deep breathing when moving in bed *Health teaching* 1. Exhale while turning; do *not* hold breath 2. Measures to conserve energy	No complications noted. Patient tolerates increased activity. Heart rate within normal limit
Thrombus formation	Mass of blood constituents formed in the heart or blood vessels due to pooling of blood from lack of activity;	*Subjective data:* discomfort over involved vessel. *Objective data:* increased RBC; venous stasis; hypercoagulability	*Altered peripheral tissue perfusion* related to obstructed vessel. *Risk for injury* related to emboli	*Prevent injury by reducing risk factors and venous stasis* 1. *Position:* change q1–2h 2. *Do not* gatch bed (causes pressure against leg vessels) 3. Increase fluid intake	No thromboemboli. *Note:* If *Homans'* sign present (discomfort behind knee on forced dorsiflexion of the foot), see nursing

Assessment / Problem	Analysis	Subjective/Objective data	Nursing diagnosis	Nursing plan/implementation	Evaluation/outcome criteria
Thrombus formation—cont'd	increased viscosity related to dehydration or possible external pressure			4. Monitor coagulation lab values 💊 5. *Medications:* anticoagulation therapy, as prescribed for patients at risk (immobilized, trauma, low pelvic surgery) 6. Ambulate as soon as possible *Health teaching* 1. How to recognize signs of thrombophlebitis/thromboemboli 2. Leg exercise program to strengthen muscles for improved tone, to prevent pooling of blood in vessels 3. Precautions necessary when on anticoagulation therapy 4. Side effects of anticoagulation therapy (bleeding from gums, body fluids, obvious bleeding)	care for patient with thromboemboli, p. 463
Respiratory congestion related to decreased respiratory movements	Decreased thoracic movement due to restriction against bed or chair, lack of position change, restrictive clothing or binders/bandages, or abdominal distention	*Subjective data:* dyspnea; pain *Objective data:* trauma; immobilization of thorax or abdomen, due to position in bed; inability to cough or deep breathe; abdominal distention	*Ineffective breathing pattern* related to splinting to reduce pain *Ineffective airway clearance* related to retained secretions *Impaired physical mobility* related to trauma	*Prevent complications related to respiratory status* ▲ 1. Maintain a clear airway, assist with ventilation prn 2. Remove or minimize causes of dyspnea 3. Conserve patient's energy (periods of rest and activity—patient able to cough more effectively when rested) ▲ 4. Incentive spirometry *Promote comfort* 1. Maintain hydration and nutrition ▣ 2. *Position:* change q2h; out of bed in chair when possible (chest expansion greater when sitting in chair) *Health teaching* 1. Methods to allay anxieties precipitated by dyspnea 2. Effective breathing and coughing exercises	No respiratory complications or excess secretions noted
Respiratory congestion related to pooled secretions	Inability of cilia to move normal secretions out of bronchial tree due to ineffective coughing, lack of thoracic expansion, or effects of medications	*Subjective data:* dyspnea; pain *Objective data:* dehydration; 💊 drugs—anticholinergic, CNS depressants, anesthesia; inadequate coughing; stationary position	*Ineffective airway clearance* related to pooled secretions *Impaired gas exchange* related to ineffective coughing	*Prevent atelectasis, infection, stasis of air and secretions in lungs* ▲ 1. Maintain patent airway; cough; suction; change position 2. See nursing care plan for Respiratory congestion related to decreased respiratory movements (see above) *Health teaching* 1. Effective coughing techniques 2. Importance of adequate hydration	No respiratory complications Patient coughs and removes secretions

Continued

Adult

Adult

TABLE 7–35   Complications of Immobilization—cont'd

Disorder	Pathophysiology	◆ Assessment	◆ Analysis/Nursing Diagnosis	◆ Nursing Care Plan/Implementation	◆ Evaluation/Outcome Criteria
Oxygen–carbon dioxide imbalance	Imbalance in oxygen and carbon dioxide levels related to pulmonary congestion, ineffective breathing patterns, trauma, or effects of medications	*Subjective data:* confusion, irritable, restless, dyspnea *Objective data:* hypoxia, hypercapnia, cyanosis	*Impaired gas exchange* related to immobilization	*Promote improved respirations* 1. Change position frequently 2. Increase humidification 3. Monitor side effects of administered medication, especially narcotics, barbiturates 4. See nursing care plan for Respiratory congestion related to decreased respiratory movements (see p. 569)	No respiratory complications Respiratory rate and depth are adequate for maintaining balance of oxygen and carbon dioxide
Malnutrition of immobilized adult	Lack of adequate dietary intake to maintain healthy tissue related to lack of food; lack of knowledge about food; problems with ingestion, digestion, or absorption; or psychosocial factors that influence patient's motivation to eat	*Subjective data:* anorexia, nausea; diet history validating lack of adequate nutritional intake; mental irritability *Objective data:* 1. Recent weight loss of >10% 2. Decreased: healing ability, GI motility, absorption, secretion of digestive enzymes 3. *Appearance:* listlessness, muscle weakness; posture—sagging shoulders, sunken chest 4. Anthropometric data (measurement of size, weight, and body proportions): <85% of standard 5. *Cardiovascular:* tachycardia (>100 beats/min) on minimal exertion; bradycardia at rest 6. *Hair:* brittle, dry, thin 7. *Skin:* dry, scaly 8. Lack of financial resources: sociocultural influences 9. *Decreased* blood values: serum albumin, ironbinding capacity, lymphocyte levels, hematocrit, and hemoglobin	*Altered nutrition, less than body requirements,* related to decreased appetite *Knowledge deficit* related to nutrition requirements	*Improved nutritional intake* to maintain basal metabolism requirements and replace losses from catabolism 1. Provide balanced or prescribed diet, soft or ground food if cannot chew or is edentulous 2. *Increase* fluid intake 3. Attain/maintain normal weight 4. Feed, assist with feeding, or place foods within patient's reach *Promote comfort* ▲ 1. Mouth care: to facilitate mastication of food → improved digestion and absorption 2. Relieve constipation (see nursing care plan for constipation, p. 571) 3. Observe for stomatitis, bleeding, changes in skin texture, color 4. Medications: monitor nausea and vomiting side effects of prescribed medications; administer *antiemetics* as ordered to control nausea and vomiting 5. Ambulate to alleviate flatulence and distention 6. Alleviate pain and discomfort by distractions, increased social interactions, pleasant environment, backrubs, and administration of prn pain medications, as ordered *Health teaching* 1. Diet and elimination 2. See Unit 9 for foods *high in protein and carbohydrate*	No complications Patient obtains/maintains normal weight No tissue breakdown

Constipation	Waste material in the bowel is too hard to pass easily; or bowel movements are so infrequent that patient has discomfort	*Subjective data:* discomfort, pain, distress, and pressure in the rectum; reported decrease in normal elimination pattern *Objective data:* immobilization; hard-formed stool, possible palpable impaction; decreased bowel sounds; bowel elimination less frequent than usual	*Constipation* related to decreased water and fiber intake *Knowledge deficit* related to dietary and exercise requirements to prevent constipation	*Promote normal pattern of bowel elimination* 1. Administer: *stool softeners* or *bulk cathartics* as ordered; oil retention, soap suds enemas as ordered 2. Encourage change of position and activity as tolerated 3. Provide *high-bulk diet* 4. *Increase fluid* intake 5. Provide for privacy 6. Encourage regular time for evacuation *Health teaching* 1. Dietary instructions regarding *increased fiber* 2. Exercise program as tolerated 3. *Increase fluids*	Patient has normal bowel elimination pattern No impactions Increases fluid and fiber in diet
Osteoporosis	Metabolic bone disorder in which there is a generalized loss of bone density due to an imbalance between formation and bone resorption; immobilization can cause calcium losses of 200–300 mg/day *Risk factors:* women, family history; postmenopause, thin and/or small frame, anorexia or bulimia, diet low in calcium; use of corticosteroids and anticonvulsants; inactive lifestyle; cigarette smoking, excessive use of alcohol	*Subjective data:* backache *Objective data:* demineralization of bone seen on x-ray; kyphosis; spontaneous fracture of bone (hip, spine, wrist); collapsed vertebrae; loss of height; stooped posture	*Pain* related to bone fractures or body structural changes	*Prevent injury related to decreased bone strength* 1. *Position:* correct body alignment, firm mattress 2. Encourage self-care activities: plan maximum activity allowed by physical condition; muscle exercises against resistance as tolerated 3. Rest/activity pattern: encourage ROM exercise; *avoid fatigue* 4. *Weight-bearing* positions, tilt table 5. *Diet:* high protein, high vitamin D, calcium rich 6. *Increase fluids* to prevent renal calculi (calcium from bones could cause kidney stones) *Health teaching* 1. Dietary instructions: foods to include for high-protein, high-vitamin D, high-calcium diet 2. Exercise program 3. Signs and symptoms of renal calculi 4. *Avoid smoking, alcohol*	No fractures No renal calculi Incorporates dietary improvements in daily menu selection Participates in exercise program on a regular basis Regular bone density tests (1–2 years for ages 40–65+)
Contractures	Abnormal shortening of muscle tissue, rendering the muscle highly resistant to stretching; related to lack of active or passive ROM, or	*Subjective data:* pain *Objective data:* muscles—fixed, shortened, decreased tone; resistance of muscles to stretch; decreased ROM in affected limb	*Impaired physical mobility* related to muscle weakness and contractures *Pain* related to injury *Self-care deficit* related to immobility	*Prevent deformities* 1. Active or passive ROM 2. *Positioning:* functional, correct alignment 3. Footboard to prevent footdrop 4. *Avoid knee gatch*	ROM maintained No deformities noted

Continued

Adult

Adult

TABLE 7–35 **Complications of Immobilization—cont'd**

Disorder	Pathophysiology	◆ Assessment	◆ Analysis/Nursing Diagnosis	◆ Nursing Care Plan/Implementation	◆ Evaluation/Outcome Criteria
Contractures—cont'd	improper support and positioning of joints affected by arthritis or injury			*Health teaching* 1. Importance of ROM exercises 2. Correct anatomical positions	No skin breakdown
Skin breakdown	Presence of risk factors that could lead to skin breakdown, such as immobility, inadequate nutrition, lack of position changes	*Subjective data:* fatigue; pain; inability to turn on own *Objective data:* interruption of skin integrity, especially over ears, occiput, heels, sacrum, scrotum, elbows, trochanter, ischium, scapula; immobilization; malnutrition	*Impaired skin integrity* related to lack of frequent position change	*Prevent skin breakdown* 1. Change position q1–2h and prn, out of bed when possible 2. Protect from infection 3. Increase *dietary* intake: protein, carbohydrates 4. Increase *fluids* Assess for/reduce *contributing factors known to cause decubitus ulcers:* incontinence, stationary position, malnutrition, obesity, sensory deficits, emotional disturbances, paralysis *Promote healing* 1. Wash gently, pat dry—*to avoid skin abrasion* 2. Clean, dry, wrinkle-free bed linens and pads 3. Massage skin with lotion that does *not contain alcohol* (alcohol dries skin) 4. Protect with wafer barrier, alternating mattress, sheepskin pads, protectors, flotation devices 5. *No* "doughnuts" or rubber rings (interfere with circulation of tissue within center of ring)	
Urinary stasis	Immobility leads to inability to completely empty the bladder, which increases risk for urinary tract infection and renal calculi	*Subjective data:* pain, due to infection or renal calculi *Objective data:* difficulty in urinating due to position or lack of privacy; infection related to catheter insertion or stasis of urine; hematuria	*Altered urinary elimination* related to inability to empty bladder	*Prevent urinary infections, stasis, and renal calculi* 1. Increase activity as allowed 2. Check for distended bladder 3. Increase *fluids,* I&O 4. *Diet:* acid ash to increase acidity, thereby preventing infection 5. *Avoid* catheterization; use intermittent catheterization instead of Foley whenever possible or *Credé maneuver* to empty bladder (manual exertion of pressure on the bladder to force urine out) 6. Bladder training	No urinary infections or evidence of renal calculi; bladder emptied, no urinary stasis

c. Help maintain accurate sensory processing to prevent and lessen *sensory disturbances.*

d. Help adapt to *altered body image* due to increased dependency, sensory deprivation, and changes in status and power that accompany immobility.

e. Offer counseling when sexual expression is impaired.

2. Goal: *health teaching:* how to prevent physical problems related to immobility (e.g., anticonstipation diet, range of motion, skin care); teach activities while immobile that encourage independence and provide sensory stimulation.

◆ **F. Evaluation/outcome criteria:**

1. Minimal contractures, skin breakdown, muscle atrophy or loss of strength.

2. Interest in self and environment; positive self-image.

3. Returns to optimal level of physical activity.

III. Fractures: disruptions in the continuity of bone as the result of trauma or various disease processes, such as *Cushing's* syndrome or osteoporosis, that weaken the bone structure.

A. Types (Figure 7–15):

1. *Open or compound*—fractured bone extends *through skin* and mucous membranes; increased potential for infection.

2. *Closed or simple*—fractured bone *does not* protrude through skin.

3. *Complete*—fracture extends through *entire bone,* disrupting the periosteum on both sides of the bone, producing two or more fragments.

4. *Incomplete*—fracture extends *only part way* through bone; bone continuity is not totally interrupted.

5. *Greenstick* or *willow-hickory stick*—fracture of *one side of bone; other side merely bends;* usually seen only in children.

6. *Impacted or telescoped*—fracture in which bone fragments are *forcibly driven into* other or adjacent bone structures.

7. *Comminuted*—fracture having *more than one* fracture line and with bone fragment broken into *several pieces.*

8. *Depressed*—fracture in which bone or bone fragments are driven *inward,* as in skull or facial fractures.

9. See also **VI,** Total hip replacement, p. 583.

B. Methods used to reduce/immobilize fractures: reduction or setting of the bone—restores bone alignment as nearly as possible.

1. *Closed reduction*—manual traction or manipulation. Usually done under anesthesia to reduce pain and muscle spasm. Maintenance of reduction and immobilization is accomplished by casting (fiberglass or plaster of Paris).

2. *Open reduction*—operative procedure utilized to achieve bone alignment; pins, wire, nails, or rods may be used to secure bone fragments in position; prosthetic implants may also be used.

3. *Traction reduction*—force is applied in two directions: to obtain alignment, and to reduce or eliminate muscle spasm. Used for fractures of long bones. May be:

a. Continuous—used with fractures or dislocations of bones or joints.

b. Intermittent—used to reduce flexion contractures or lessen pain and muscle spasm.

c. Applied as follows:

(1) *Skin*—traction applied to skin by using a commercial foam-rubber *Buck's* traction splint or by using adhesive, plastic, or a moleskin strip bound to the extremity by elastic bandage; exerts indirect traction on bone or muscles (e.g., *Bryant's, Buck's* extension, head, pelvic, *Russell's*) (Figure 7–16, parts *A* through *E*).

(2) *Skeletal*—direct traction applied to bone using pins *(Steinman),* wires *(Kirschner).* Pin is inserted through the bone in or close to the involved area and usually protrudes through skin on both sides of the extremity. Skeletal traction for fractured vertebrae accomplished with tongs (e.g., *Crutchfield* tongs, *Gardner-Wells* tongs) (Figure 7–16, parts *F* through *H*).

d. Specific types of traction:

(1) *Cervical*—direct traction applied to cervical vertebrae using a head halter or *Crutchfield, Gardner-Wells,* or *Vinke* tongs that are inserted into the skull (see Figure 7–16, parts *C* and *G*). Traction is increased with weights until vertebrae move into position and alignment is regained. After reduction is obtained, weights are decreased to the amount needed to maintain reduction. *Weight amount is prescribed by physician.*

(2) *Balanced suspension*—countertraction produced by a force other than patient's body weight; extremity is suspended in a traction apparatus that maintains the line of traction despite changes in the patient's position (e.g., *Russell's* leg traction, *Thomas'* splint with *Pearson's* attachment). See Figure 7–16, parts *E* and *F.*

(3) *Running*—traction that exerts a pull in one plane; countertraction is supplied by the weight of the patient's body or can be increased through use

FIGURE 7–15 Types of fractures and terminology. (From Thomas, CL [ed]: Taber's Cyclopedic Medical Dictionary, ed 18. FA Davis, Philadelphia, 1997, p 754.)

FRAGMENTS UNDISPLACED

FRAGMENTS SEPARATED DUE TO BREAK FROM WITHIN (COMPOUND FRACTURE)

FRAGMENTS SEPARATED BY EXTERNAL FORCE SUCH AS BULLET (COMPOUND FRACTURE)

PROXIMAL PORTION OF BONE

MIDDLE PORTION OF BONE

DISTAL PORTION OF BONE

GREENSTICK   DISPLACED   INCOMPLETE   COMPLETE

COMMINUTED   SEGMENTAL   BUTTERFLY   SPIRAL   HAIR-LINE

TYPES OF FRACTURES AND TERMINOLOGY

of weights and pulleys in the opposite direction (e.g., *Buck's* extension, *Russell's* traction). See Figure 7–16, parts *A* through *C*.

(4) *Halo*—an apparatus that employs both a plastic and metal frame; molded frame extends from the axilla to iliac crest and houses a metal frame. The struts of the frame extend to skull and attach to round metal (halo) device. The halo is attached to skull by four pins—two located an-

terolaterally and two located posterolaterally. They are inserted into external cortex of the cranium (see Figure 7–16, part *H*). Used to immobilize the cervical spine following spinal fusion, give some correction to scoliosis before spinal fusion, and immobilize nondisplaced fracture of spine.

4. *Immobilization*—maintains reduction and promotes healing of bone fragments. Achieved by:

   a. *External fixation:*

FIGURE 7–16 Types of skin and skeletal traction.

Skin

A. Bryant's traction

B. Buck's traction

C. Head halter traction

D. Pelvic traction

E. Russell's traction

Skeletal

F. Balanced suspension traction

G. Crutchfield tongs

H. Halo vest

Adult

(1) Casts—types:
  (a) *Spica*—applied to immobilize hip or shoulder joints.
  (b) Body cast—applied to trunk.
  (c) Arm or leg cast—joints above and below site included in cast.
(2) Splints, continuous traction.
(3) External fixation devices (Charnley)—multiple pins/rods through limb above and below fracture site, attached to external metal supports. Patient able to become ambulatory.

b. *Internal fixation*—pins, wires, nails, rods. See Total hip replacement, p. 583, and Total knee replacement, p. 585.

◆ **C. Assessment:**

1. *Subjective data:*
   a. Pain, tenderness.
   b. Tingling, numbness.
   c. Nausea.
   d. History of traumatic event.
   e. Muscle spasm.

2. *Objective data:*
   a. Function: abnormal or lost.
   b. Deformities.
   c. Ecchymosis, increased heat over injured part.
   d. Localized edema.
   e. Crepitation (grating sensations heard or felt as bone fragments rub against each other).
   f. Signs of shock.
   g. Indicators of anxiety.
   h. X-ray: *fracture*—positive interruption of bone; *dislocation*—abnormal position of bone.

◆ **D. Analysis/nursing diagnosis:**

1. *Pain* related to interruption in bone.
2. *Impaired physical mobility* related to fracture/treatment modality.
3. *Risk for injury* related to complications of fractures.
4. *Knowledge deficit* regarding cast care, crutch walking, traction.
5. *Constipation* related to immobilization.
6. *Risk for impaired skin integrity* related to immobility or friction from materials used to immobilize the fracture during healing.

◆ **E. Nursing care plan/implementation:**

1. Goal: *promote healing and prevent complications of fractures* (Table 7–36).
   a. *Diet: high* protein, iron, vitamins, to improve tissue repair; *moderate* carbohydrates to prevent weight gain; no increase in calcium, to prevent kidney stones (decalcification and demineralization occur when patient is immobilized).
   (1) Encourage *increased fluid intake,* to prevent kidney stones.
   (2) Prevent or correct constipation through *increasing bulk foods, fruits, and fruit juices,* or using prescribed stool softeners, laxatives, or cathartics as necessary.
   b. Provide activities to reduce perceptual deprivation—reading, handcrafts, music, special interests/hobbies that can be done while maintaining correct position for healing.

2. Goal: *prevent injury or trauma in relation to:*
   ▶ a. *Fracture care:*
      (1) Maintain affected part in optimum alignment.
      (2) Maintain skin integrity; check all bony prominences for evidence of pressure q4h and prn, depending on amount of pressure.
      (3) Monitor: circulation in, sensation of, and motion of (CSM) affected part q15min for first 4 hr; q1h until 24 hr; q4h and prn, depending on amount of edema (Table 7–37).
      (4) Maintain mobility in unaffected limb and unaffected joints of affected limb by active and passive ROM; prevent footdrop by using ankle-top sneakers.
   ▶ b. *Skin traction:*
      (1) Maintain correct alignment:
         (a) If tape or moleskin is used, shave extremity and apply benzoin to improve adherence of strip and reduce itching.
         (b) Check apparatus for slippage, bunching; replace prn.
      (2) Prevent tissue injury:
         (a) Check all bony prominences for evidence of pressure: q15min for first 4 hr; q1h until 24 hr, q4h and prn, depending on amount of edema.
         (b) Nonadhesive traction may be removed q8h to check skin (e.g., *Bryant's*).
   ▶ c. *Skeletal traction:*
      (1) Maintain affected part in optimum alignment:
         (a) Ropes on pulleys.
         (b) Weights hang free.
         (c) *Elevate* head of bed as prescribed.
         (d) Check knots routinely.
      (2) Maintain skin integrity:
         (a) Frequent skin care.
         (b) Keep bed linens free of crumbs and wrinkles.
      (3) Prevent infection: special skin care to pin insertion site tid. Keep area around pins clean and dry. Use prescribed solution for cleansing.

TABLE 7–36 Complications of Fractures

Complication	◆ Assessment	◆ Analysis/Nursing Diagnosis	◆ Nursing Care Plan/Implementation	◆ Evaluation/Outcome Criteria
Shock (see p. 507)				
Thrombophlebitis (see p. 507)				
Fat emboli: serious, potentially life-threatening complication in which pressure changes in interior of fracture force molecules of fat from marrow into systemic circulation; may cause problems in respiratory or nervous system; seen most frequently on third day after multiple fractures, fractures of long bones, or comminuted fracture	*Subjective data:* dyspnea, severe chest pain; confusion, agitation; decrease in level of consciousness; numbness; feeling faint; history of diabetes, obesity *Objective data:* cyanosis; pupillary changes; muscle twitching; petechiae—chest, buccal cavity, axilla, conjunctiva, soft palate; extremities—pallor; cold; shock; vomiting	*Risk for injury* related to fat emboli *Altered tissue perfusion* related to fat emboli	1. *Position:* high Fowler's to relieve respiratory symptoms 2. Administer oxygen stat, to relieve anoxia and reduce surface tension of fat globules 3. Institute respiratory support measures, as ordered—IPPB, respiratory assistive devices: **be prepared for CPR** in event of respiratory failure 4. Monitor vital signs, cardiac monitor, q15min during acute episode and prn (shock/cardiac failure possible) 5. Obtain baseline data and monitor level of consciousness, neurological signs q15min during acute episode and prn (neurological involvement possible) 6. Administer parenteral fluids, as ordered: IV alcohol, blood and fluid replacements 7. Administer medications as ordered: corticosteroids; digitalis; aminophylline; heparin sodium 8. **DO NOT RUB ANY LEG CRAMPS, BUT REPORT IMMEDIATELY**	Patient alert Pain relieved Respiratory, cardiac, and neurological systems have no permanent damage
Nerve compression: pressure on nerve in affected area from edema, dislocation of bone, or immobilization apparatus; if pressure not relieved, permanent paralysis can result	*Subjective data:* discomfort, pain, referred pain; burning, tingling, "stinging sensation"; numbness, altered sensation, inability to distinguish touch *Objective data:* limited movement; muscle weakness; paralysis; reflexes—diminished, irritable, or absent; color changes related to impaired circulation	*Pain* related to pressure on nerve *Potential for physical injury* related to pressure on nerve *Impaired tissue perfusion* related to impaired circulation *Impaired physical mobility* related to joint contracture, numbness	1. Monitor for potential signs q1h for first 48 hr; neurovascular assessment q12h and prn as condition indicates (circulation, sensation, and motion [CSM]) 2. *Elevate* affected limb; flex hand or foot of affected extremity; passive and active ROM exercises 3. **Be prepared to cut cast or remove constrictions if signs of impairment exist** 4. Begin active ROM exercises to unaffected extremities 5. Use footboard to prevent footdrop 6. Encourage use of trapeze if applicable 7. Isometric exercises, as ordered 8. Ambulation, weight bearing as ordered, support casts	Sensation, motor function are normal No complications noted

Continued

TABLE 7–36 **Complications of Fractures—cont'd**

Complication	◆ Assessment	◆ Analysis/Nursing Diagnosis	◆ Nursing Care Plan/Implementation	◆ Evaluation/Outcome Criteria
Avascular necrosis/circulatory impairment: interference with normal circulation to affected area due to interruption of blood vessel, pressure on the vessel from dislocation, edema, or immobilization devices; results of impaired circulation lead to discomfort and, if not corrected, necrosis of tissue and bone due to lack of oxygen supply	*Subjective data:* tenderness; pain, especially on passive motion *Objective data:* edema, swelling in affected area; decreased color, temperature, mobility; bleeding from wound	*Risk for altered peripheral tissue perfusion* related to vessel damage	1. Monitor for potential signs q1h for first 48 hr; blanching, coolness, edema; palpate pulse above and below injury; report absent pulse or major discrepancies stat 2. *Elevate* affected limb to decrease edema 3. Report to physician if signs persist 4. Be prepared to assist with bivalving of casts, or cut cast to relieve pressure 5. Monitor size of drainage stains on casts; measure accurately and report if size increases	Circulation adequate to limb, to prevent tissue damage
Infection	*Subjective data:* pain *Objective data:* elevated temperature and pulse: erythema—discoloration of surrounding skin; edema—sudden, local induration; drainage—thin, watery, foul-smelling exudate; crepitus (may be indicative of gas gangrene); with cast—warm area, foul smell	*Risk for injury* related to tissue destruction *Altered peripheral tissue perfusion* related to swelling	1. Monitor vital signs, drainage 2. Ensure patient has had prophylactic tetanus toxoid 3. May have prophylactic antibiotics ordered if wound was contaminated at time of injury 4. Instruct patient *not* to touch open wound or pin sites or put anything inside cast (could interrupt skin integrity and become potential source of infection)	No infection or heals with no serious complications
Delayed union/nonunion: failure of bone to heal within normal time related to lack of use, inadequate circulation, other complicating medical conditions such as diabetes or poor nutrition	*Subjective data:* pain *Objective data:* lack of callus formation on x-ray: poor alignment	*Risk for injury* related to poor healing of bone fracture *Impaired physical mobility* related to lower-limb fractures *Dressing/grooming, bathing/hygiene, self-care deficit* related to upper-limb fracture	1. Maintain immobilization and alignment of affected limb 2. Maintain adequate nutrition 3. *Avoid* trauma to affected limb 4. Monitor for circulatory or infection complication 5. Dietary instructions regarding foods containing *calcium* and *protein* necessary for bone healing	Bone heals No complications noted Pain decreased Ambulation and self-care return to preinjury status
Skin breakdown (related to cast)	*Subjective data:* pain *Objective data:* temperature and pulse elevated; erythema; edema—cast edges, exposed distal portion of limb, limb area within cast; drainage and foul odor from break in skin (may be under cast and stain through or exit at ends of cast); crepitus (crackling sound could indicate gas gangrene); hyperactive reflexes	*Impaired skin integrity* related to cast trauma	1. If open wound: verify tetanus administration; monitor site through cast window, change dressing daily and prn 2. Apply lotion or cornstarch to exposed skin (*no powder*) 3. Petal tape edges of cast to reduce irritation 4. Inspect skin for irritation, edema, odor, drainage—q2h initially, then q3h 5. Instruct patient *not* to place any object under the cast because skin abrasions may lead to decubitus ulcers	No skin breakdown

Duodenal distress (with spica cast): spica cast incorporates the trunk and affected limb and can cause respiratory or abdominal distress when edema is present under the cast or cast is too tight to allow for normal body functions

Subjective data: anorexia, nausea, abdominal pain
Objective data: duodenal distress, vomiting, distention, cast too tight

Ineffective breathing related to pressure from cast
Pain related to abdominal distress from pressure
Fear related to cast constriction

6. Promote drying of cast by leaving it uncovered and exposed to air for 48 hr; use *no plastic*
7. Prevent indenting casts with fingertips or hard surface; place on pillows; use palms of hands when positioning affected limb
8. *Avoid* excessive padding of Thomas splint in groin area—padding traps moisture, may lead to skin breakdown

1. Place on firm mattress; use bed boards if necessary to reduce muscle spasm
2. Maintain warmth by covering uncasted areas
3. *Avoid* turning for first 8 hr; when turning: use enough personnel to logroll; do *not* use bar between legs as turning device; support chest with pillows
4. Monitor for signs of respiratory distress: increased respirations, apprehension
5. Monitor for signs of duodenal distress: vomiting, distention; *if these signs occur:* place in *prone* position; have cast bivalved; may need NG tube; monitor for fluid imbalance
6. Protect cast with nonabsorbent material during elimination

Complications avoided or detected early enough to prevent serious damage

Adult

TABLE 7–37 ♥ **Assessing Injured Limb: CSM**

C Circulation
Is it warm to touch?
Are both limbs equal in size?
Are peripheral pulses present?
Is there adequate capillary refill?

S Sensation
Does the patient feel pain?
Can the patient distinguish different sensations, e.g., painful stimuli vs. soft touch?
Is the patient aware of the position of the limb?

M Motion
Can the patient move extremities that are not immobilized?
Can the patient do this independently?
Can the patient do this on command?

(4) Monitor circulation in, sensation of, and motion of affected part (see E.2.a. Fracture care, p. 576).
(5) Maintain mobility in unaffected limb and unaffected joints; prevent foot-drop of affected limb.

▶ d. *Running traction:*
(1) Keep well centered in bed.
▧ (2) *Elevate head of bed only* to point of countertraction.
(3) *No* turning from side to side—will cause rubbing of bony fragments.
(4) Check distal circulation frequently.
(5) Frequent back care to prevent skin breakdown.
(6) Fracture bed pan for toileting.
(7) *Avoid* excessive padding of splints in groin area to prevent tissue trauma.

▧ ▶ e. *Balanced suspension traction:*
(1) Maintain alignment and countertraction:
(a) Ropes on pulleys.
(b) Weights hang free.
(c) *Elevate* head of bed as prescribed.
(d) Check knots routinely.
(2) May move patient, but turn only slightly (no more than 30 degrees to *unaffected* side).
(3) Heel of affected leg must remain free of the bed.
(4) *20-degree angle* between thigh and bed.
(5) Check for pressure from sling to popliteal area.
(6) Provide foot support to prevent foot-drop.
(7) Maintain *abduction* of extremity.
(8) Check for signs of infection at pin insertion sites; cleanse tid as ordered.
(9) If tape or moleskin is used, shave extremity and apply benzoin to improve adherence of strip and reduce itching.

▶ f. *Cervical traction:*
(1) May be placed on specialized bed, e.g., *Stryker frame.*
▧ (2) *Position:* maintain body alignment.
(3) Keep tongs free from bed, and keep weights hanging freely to allow traction to function properly.

▶ g. *Halo traction:*
(1) Several times a day, check screws to the head and screws that hold the upper portion of the frame, to determine correct position.
◖▭ (2) Pin sites cleansed tid with bacteriostatic solution to prevent infection.
(3) Monitor for signs of infection.
▧ (4) *Position* as any other patient in body cast, except *no* pressure to rest on halo—pillows may be placed under abdomen and chest when patient is prone.
(5) Institute ROM exercises to prevent contractures.
(6) Turn frequently to prevent development of pressure areas.
(7) Allow patient to verbalize about having screws placed in skull.
(8) Postapplication nursing care same as pin insertion for other traction.

▶ h. *External fixation devices:*
(1) Pin care same as for skeletal traction.
(2) Teach clothing adjustment.
(3) Teach to adjust for size of apparatus.

i. *Internal fixation devices:*
(1) Monitor for signs of infection/allergic reaction to materials used for maintenance of reduction (drainage, pain, increased temperature).
(2) Position as ordered to prevent dislocation.

▶ j. *Casts:*
(1) Support drying cast on firm pillow; *avoid* finger imprints on cast.
▧ (2) *Elevate* limb to reduce edema.
(3) Prevent complications of fractures as listed.
(4) Closely monitor *circulation* (blanching, swelling, decreased temperature); *sensation* (absence of feeling; pain or burning); and *motion* (inability to move digits of affected limb).
(5) **Be prepared to notify MD or cut cast if circulatory impairment occurs.**
(6) Protect skin integrity: *avoid* pressure of edges of cast; petal prn.
(7) Monitor for signs of infection if skin integrity impaired.

3. Goal: *provide care related to ambulation with crutches.*
▶ a. See Table 7–38.
b. Measure crutches correctly (Table 7–39).

TABLE 7–38 Teaching Crutch Walking

A. When only *one* leg can bear weight:
1. *Swing-to-gait:* crutches forward; swing body to crutches.
   a. Move both crutches forward.
   b. Move both legs to meet the crutches.
   c. Continue pattern.
2. *Swing-through gait:* crutches forward; swing body through crutches.
   a. Move both crutches forward.
   b. Move both legs farther ahead than crutches.
   c. Continue pattern.
3. *Three-point gait:* crutches and affected extremity forward; swing forward, placing nonaffected foot ahead of or between crutches.
   a. Both crutches and affected limb move at same time.
   b. Move both crutches and affected leg (e.g., left) ahead 6 inches.
   c. Move unaffected leg (e.g., right) to same place as left and crutches.
   d. Continue pattern.
B. When *both* legs can move separately and bear some weight:
1. *Four-point gait:* right crutch forward, left foot forward; swing weight to right side while bringing left crutch forward, then right foot forward; gait simulates normal walking.
   a. Move right crutch forward 4–6 inches.
   b. Move left foot forward same distance as right crutch.
   c. Move left crutch forward ahead of left foot.
   d. Move right foot forward to meet right crutch.
   e. Continue pattern.
2. *Two-point gait:* same as four-point gait but faster; one crutch and opposite leg moving forward at same time.
   a. Opposite crutch and limb move together.
   b. Move right crutch and left leg ahead 6 inches.
   c. Move left crutch and right leg ahead.
   d. Continue pattern.
C. When patient is *unable* to walk: *tripod gait:* crutches forward at a wide distance; drag legs to point just behind crutches, balance, and repeat.

---

(1) Subtract 16 inches from total height; top of crutch should be 2 inches below the axilla.
(2) Complete extension of the elbows should be possible *without* pressure of axilla bar into the axilla.
(3) Handgrip should be adjusted so that complete wrist extension is possible.
(4) Instruct in correct body alignment:
   (a) Head erect.
   (b) Back straight.
   (c) Chest forward.
   (d) Feet 6–8 inches apart, wide base for support.

4. Goal: *provide safety measures related to possible complications following fracture* (see Table 7–36).
5. Goal: *health teaching.*
   a. Explain and show apparatus before application, if possible.
   b. Pin care at least once daily to prevent granulation and cellulitis.

TABLE 7–39 ▶Measuring Crutches Correctly

1. Have patient lie on a flat surface. Measure from anterior fold of axilla to 4 inches lateral to heel.
2. Have patient stand. Measure from 1–2 inches below axilla to 2 inches in front of and 6 inches to the side of the foot.
3. Hand placement on bar of crutch: have patient stand upright, support body weight with hand on bar (*not* putting weight on axilla). Elbow flexion should be 30 degrees.
4. Slightly pad the shoulder rests of the crutches for general comfort.
5. Make sure there are nonskid rubber tips on the crutches.

---

   c. Correct position for rest/sleep and prevention of injury with halo traction—*no* pressure on halo.
   d. Purpose of cast: to immobilize, to support body tissues, to prevent or correct deformities.
   e. Teach signs and symptoms of complications to report related to cast care (i.e., numbness, odor, crack/break in cast; extremity cold, bluish).
   f. Isometric exercises for use with affected joint.
▶ g. *Safety measures with crutches:*
   (1) Weight bearing on hands, *not* axilla.
   (2) Position crutches 4 inches to side and 4 inches to front.
   (3) Use short strides, looking ahead, not at feet.
   (4) Prevent injury: if patient begins to fall, throw crutches to side to prevent falling on them; body should be relaxed.
   (5) Check for environmental hazards: rugs, water spills.
◆ **F. Evaluation/outcome criteria:**
1. No injury or complications related to apparatus or immobilization (e.g., infection, tissue injury, altered circulation/sensation, dislocation).
2. Bone remains in correct alignment and begins to heal.
3. Demonstrates elevated limb position to relieve edema with casted extremity.
4. Lists complications related to circulation or neurological impairment and infection.
5. Begins to use affected part.
6. Demonstrates correct technique for ambulation with crutches—no pressure on axilla, uses strength of arms and wrists.
7. No falls while using crutches.

IV. Compartment syndrome: an accumulation of fluid in the muscle compartment, resulting in an increase in pressure that reduces blood flow to the tissues. Can lead to neuromuscular deficit, amputation, and death.

A. **Pathophysiology:** inability of the fascia surrounding the muscle group to expand to accommodate the increased volume of fluid → compartment pressure increases → venous flow impaired → arterial flow continues, increasing capillary pressure → fluid pushed into the extravascular space → intracompartment pressure further increased → prolonged or severe ischemia → muscle and nerve cells destroyed, contracture, loss of function, necrotic tissue, infection, release of potassium, hydrogen, and myoglobin into bloodstream.

B. **Risk factors:**
   1. Fractures.
   2. Burns.
   3. Crushing injuries.
   4. Restrictive bandages.
   5. Cast.
   6. Prolonged lithotomy positioning.

◆ C. **Assessment:**
   1. *Subjective data:*
      a. Severe, unrelenting pain, unrelieved by narcotics and associated with passive stretching of muscle.
      b. Paresthesias.
   2. *Objective data:*
      a. Edema; tense skin over limb.
      b. Paralysis.
      c. Decreased or absent peripheral pulses.
      d. Poor capillary refill.
      e. Limb temperature change (colder).
      f. Ankle-arm pressure index (API) decreased; 0.4 indicates ischemia (see **Unit II,** Doppler ultrasonography, p. 749).
      g. Urine output—decreased (developing acute tubular necrosis); reddish-brown color.

◆ D. **Analysis/nursing diagnosis:**
   1. *Pain* related to tissue swelling and ischemia.
   2. *Risk for injury* related to neuromuscular deficits.
   3. *Impaired physical mobility* related to contracture and loss of function.
   4. *Risk for infection* related to tissue necrosis.
   5. *Altered urinary elimination* related to acute tubular necrosis from myoglobin accumulation.
   6. *Body image disturbance* related to limb disfigurement.

◆ E. **Nursing care plan/implementation:**
   1. Goal: *recognizes early indications of ischemia.*
      a. Assess neurovascular status frequently (q1h): skin temperature, capillary refill, peripheral pulses, mobility, and sensation.
      b. Listen to patient complaints; report suspected complications.
      c. Report nonrelief of pain with narcotics.
      d. Recognize unrelenting pain with passive muscle stretching.

   2. Goal: *prevent complications.*
      a. *Elevate* injured extremity initially; if ischemia suspected, keep extremity at *heart level* to prevent compensatory increase in blood flow.
      b. *Avoid* tight bandages, splints, or casts.
      c. Monitor intravenous infusion for signs of infiltration.
      d. Prepare patient for fasciotomy (incision of skin and fascia to release tight compartment).

◆ F. **Evaluation/outcome criteria:**
   1. Relief from pain; normal perfusion restored.
   2. Neurovascular status within normal limits.
   3. Retains function of limb; no contractures or infection.
   4. Compartment pressure returns to normal (<20 mm Hg.).
   5. No systemic complications (e.g., normal cardiac and renal function, acid-base balance within normal limits).

V. **Osteoarthritis:** joint disorder characterized by degeneration of articular cartilage and formation of bony outgrowths at edges of weight-bearing joints.

   A. **Pathophysiology:** excessive friction combined with risk factors → thinning of articular cartilage, narrowing of joint space, and loss of joint stability; cartilage erodes, producing shallow pits on articular surface and exposing bone in joint space. Bone responds by becoming denser and harder.

   B. **Risk factors:**
      1. Aging (>50).
      2. Rheumatoid arthritis.
      3. Arteriosclerosis.
      4. Obesity.
      5. Trauma.
      6. Family history.

◆ C. **Assessment:**
   1. *Subjective data:*
      a. Pain; tender joints.
      b. Fatigability, malaise.
      c. Anorexia.
      d. Cold intolerance.
      e. Extremities: numb, tingling.
   2. *Objective data:*
      a. Joints:
         (1) Enlarged.
         (2) Stiff, limited movement.
         (3) Swelling, redness, and heat around affected joint.
         (4) Shiny stretched skin over and around joint.
         (5) Subcutaneous nodules.
      b. Weight loss.
      c. Fever.
      d. Crepitation (creaking or grating of joints).

e. Deformities, contractures.

f. Cold, clammy extremities.

g. Lab data: *decreased* Hgb, *elevated* WBC.

h. *Diagnostic tests:* x-ray, thermography, arthroscopy.

◆ **D. Analysis/nursing diagnosis:**

1. *Pain* related to friction of bones in joints.

2. *Bathing/hygiene self-care deficit* related to decreased mobility of involved joints.

3. *Risk for injury* related to fatigability.

4. *Impaired physical mobility* related to stiff, limited movement.

5. *Impaired home maintenance management* related to contractures.

◆ **E. Nursing care plan/implementation:**

1. Goal: *promote comfort: reduce pain, spasms, inflammation, swelling.*

a. Medications as prescribed.

(1) *Nonsteroidal anti-inflammatory agents:* aspirin (Ecotrin), acetaminophen (Tylenol), ibuprofen (Motrin), indomethacin (Indocin), corticosteroids, nabumetone (Relafen), naproxen (Naprosyn).

(2) *Antimalarials:* chloroquine (Aralen), hydroxychloroquine (Plaquenil), to relieve symptoms.

b. Heat to reduce muscle spasms, stiffness.

c. Cold to reduce swelling and pain.

d. Prevent contractures:

(1) Exercise.

(2) Bed rest on firm mattress during attacks.

(3) Splints to maintain proper alignment.

e. *Elevate* extremity to reduce swelling.

f. Rest.

g. Assistive devices to decrease weight bearing of affected joints (canes, walkers).

2. Goal: *health teaching to promote independence.*

a. Encourage self-care with assistive devices for activities of daily living (ADL).

b. Activity, as tolerated, with ambulation-assistive devices.

c. Scheduled rest periods.

d. Correct body posture and body mechanics.

3. Goal: *provide for emotional needs.*

a. Accept feelings of frustration regarding long-term debilitating disorder.

b. Provide diversional activities appropriate for age and physical condition to promote comfort and satisfaction.

◆ **F. Evaluation/outcome criteria:**

1. Remains independent as long as possible.

2. No contractures.

3. States comfort has improved.

4. Uses methods that are successful in pain control.

VI. **Total hip replacement:** femoral head and acetabulum are replaced by a prosthesis, which is cemented into the bone with plastic cement. Performed to replace a joint with limited and painful function due to bony alkalosis and deformity, caused by degenerative joint disease or when vascular supply to femoral head is compromised from a fracture. Goal of the surgery: restore or improve mobilization of hip joint and prevent complications of extended immobilization.

A. **Risk factors:**

1. Rheumatoid arthritis.

2. Osteoarthritis.

3. Complications of femoral neck fractures—avascular necrosis and malunion (Table 7–40).

4. Congenital hip disease.

TABLE 7–40   Fractures of the Hip

Risk Factors	Types	◆Assessment	Surgical Intervention
Osteoporosis Age >60 Women Caucasian Postmenopausal Immobility/sedentary lifestyle	Intracapsular (femoral neck; within hip joint and capsule)	Slight trauma Pain, groin and hip Lateral rotation, shortening of leg, minimal deformity	Total hip replacement
	Extracapsular (outside hip joint; also called intertrochanteric)	Direct trauma Severe pain External rotation, shortening of leg, obvious deformity	Internal fixation with nail (open reduction) Possible total hip replacement
	Subtrochanteric (below lesser trochanter)	Direct trauma Leg pain near fracture site External rotation, shortening of leg, deformity Presence of hematoma	Internal fixation with nail (open reduction) Closed reduction

◆ **B. Analysis/nursing diagnosis:**
1. *Risk for injury* related to implant surgery.
2. *Knowledge deficit* regarding joint replacement surgery.
3. *Impaired physical mobility* related to major hip surgery.
4. *Pain* related to surgical incision.
5. *Risk for impaired skin integrity* related to immobility.

◆ **C. Nursing care plan/implementation** (see **Clinical Pathway for Primary Hip Arthroplasty**):
1. *Preoperative:*
    a. Goal: *prevent thrombophlebitis or pulmonary emboli.*
        (1) Antiembolic stockings.
        (2) *Increase* fluid intake.
    b. Goal: *prevent infection:* antibiotics as ordered, given prophylactically.
    c. Goal: *health teaching.*
        (1) *Isometric exercises*—gluteal, abdominal, and quadricep setting; dorsiflexion and plantarflexion of the feet.
        (2) Use of trapeze.
        (3) Explain position of operative leg and hip postoperatively to prevent *adduction* and flexion.
        (4) Transfer techniques—bed to chair and chair to crutches; dangle at bedside first time out of bed.
        (5) Assist patient with skin scrubs with antibacterial soap.
2. *Postoperative:*
    a. Goal: *prevent respiratory complications.*
        (1) Turn, cough, and deep breathe.
        (2) Incentive spirometry.
    b. Goal: *prevent complications of shock or infection.*
        ▶ (1) Check dressings for drainage q1h for first 4 hr; then q4h and prn; may have Hemovac or other drainage tubes inserted in wound to keep dressing dry.
        (2) Monitor I&O and vital signs hourly for 4 hr, then q4h and prn.
    c. Goal: *prevent contractures, muscle atrophy:* initiate exercises as soon as allowed: isometric quadriceps, dorsiflexion and plantarflexion of foot, and flexion and extension of the ankle.
    d. Goal: *promote early ambulation and movement.*
        (1) Use trapeze.
        (2) Transfer technique (pivot on unaffected leg); crutches/walker.
        (3) Initiate progressive ambulation as ordered; ensure *maximum extension* of leg when walking.
        (4) Administer anticoagulation therapy as ordered prophylactically to prevent thromboemboli.
        (5) Recognize early side effects of medications and report appropriately.

e. Goal: *prevent constipation.*
    (1) *Increase* fluid intake.
    (2) Use fracture bed pan.
f. Goal: *prevent dislocation of prosthesis.*
    ◨ (1) Maintain *abduction* of the affected joint (prevent external rotation); *elevate* head of bed, turn according to physician's order. When turning to unaffected side, turn with abduction pillow between legs to maintain abduction.
    ▶ (2) *Buck's extension* or *Russell's traction* may be applied (temporary skin traction).
    (3) Plaster booties with an abduction bar may be used.
    ◨ (4) Wedge Charnley (triangle-shaped) pillow to *maintain abduction* between knees and lower legs.
    ◨ (5) Provide periods throughout day when patient lies flat in bed to *prevent hip flexion* and strengthen hip muscles.
    (6) Report signs of dislocation: *anteriorly*—knee flexes, leg turns outward, leg looks longer than other, femur head may be felt in groin area; *posteriorly*—leg turns inward, appears shorter than other, greater trochanter elevated.
g. Goal: *promote comfort.*
    (1) Initiate skin care; monitor pressure points for redness; back care q2h.
    (2) Alternating pressure mattress; sheepskin when sitting in chair.
h. Goal: *health teaching.*
    (1) Exercise program with written list of activity restrictions.
    (2) Methods to *prevent* hip adduction.
    (3) *Avoid* sitting for more than 1 hr: stand, stretch, and walk frequently to *prevent* hip flexion contractures.
    ◨ (4) Advise *not to exceed 90 degrees of hip flexion* (dislocation can occur, particularly with posterior incisions); *avoid* low chairs.
    (5) Teach alternative methods of usual self-care activities to prevent hip dislocation—e.g., *avoid:* bending from waist to tie shoes, sitting up straight in a low chair, using a low toilet seat.
    (6) *Avoid* crossing legs, driving a car for 6 wk.
    (7) Wear support hose for 6 wk to enhance venous return and avoid thrombus formation.

◆ **D. Evaluation/outcome criteria:**
1. Participates in postoperative nursing care plan to prevent complications.
2. Reports pain has decreased.
3. Ambulates with assistive devices.

4. Complications of immobility avoided.
5. Able to resume self-care activities.

VII. Total knee replacement: both sides of the joint are replaced by metal or plastic implants.
◆ **A. Analysis:** see Total hip replacement, p. 583.
◆ **B. Nursing plan/implementation:**
　1. See **VI.** Total hip replacement, p. 583.
　2. Goal: *achieve active flexion beyond 70 degrees.*
　▶ a. *Immediately postop:* may have continuous passive motion (CPM) device for flexion/extension of affected knee. Maximum flexion 110 degrees.
　▶ b. Monitor drainage in *Hemovac* (q15 min for first 4 hr, q1h until 24 hr; q4h and prn while Hemovac in place).
　 c. Analgesics as ordered for pain.
　 d. While dressings are still on: quadriceps-setting exercises for approximately 5 days (consult with physical therapist for specific instructions).
　 e. After dressings removed: active flexion exercises.
　 f. *Avoid* pressure on heel.
◆ **C. Evaluation/outcome criteria:**
　1. No complications of infection, hemorrhage noted.
　2. ROM of knee increases with exercises.

VIII. Amputation: surgical removal of a limb as a result of trauma or circulatory impairment (gangrene). The amount of tissue amputated is determined by the severity of disease or trauma and the ability of the remaining tissue to heal.
　A. Risk factors:
　1. Atherosclerosis obliterans.
　2. Uncontrolled diabetes mellitus.
　3. Malignancy.
　4. Extensive and intractable infection.
　5. Result of severe trauma.
◆ **B. Assessment** *(preoperative):*
　1. *Subjective data:* pain in affected part.
　2. *Objective data:*
　　a. Soft-tissue damage.
　　b. Partial or complete severance of a body part.
　　c. Lack of peripheral pulses.
　　d. Skin color changes, pallor → cyanosis → gangrene.
　　e. Infection, hemorrhage, or shock.
◆ **C. Analysis/nursing diagnosis:**
　1. *Impaired physical mobility* related to lower-limb amputation.
　2. *Body image disturbance* related to loss of body part.
　3. *Pain* related to interruption of nerve pathways.
　4. *Anxiety* related to potential change in lifestyle.
　5. *Knowledge deficit* related to rehabilitation goals.

◆ **D. Nursing care plan/implementation:**
　1. Goal: *prepare for surgery, physically and emotionally.*
　　a. Validate that patient and family are aware that amputation of body part is planned.
　　b. Validate that informed consent is signed.
　　c. Allow time for grieving.
　　d. If time allows, prepare patient for postoperative phase, e.g., teach arm-strengthening exercises if lower limb is to be amputated; teach alternative methods of ambulation.
　　e. Provide time to discuss feelings.
　　f. Prepare surgical site to decrease possibility of infection (e.g., shave, scrub as ordered).
　　g. Discuss postoperative expectations.
　2. Goal: *promote healing postoperatively.*
　▶ a. Monitor respiratory status q1–4h and prn: rate, depth of respiration; auscultate for signs of congestion; and question patient about chest pain (pulmonary emboli common complication).
　　b. Monitor for hemorrhage; keep tourniquet at bedside.
　 c. Medicate for pain as ordered—patient may have phantom limb pain.
　　d. Support stump on pillow for first 24 hr; **remove pillow** after 24 hr to prevent contracture.
　▰ e. *Position: turn patient on to stomach* to prevent hip contracture.
　　f. ROM exercises for joint above amputation to prevent joint immobilization; strengthening exercises for arms, nonaffected limbs, abdominal muscles.

　▶ g. | *Stump care:*
(1) Early postoperative dressings changed prn.
(2) As incision heals, bandage is applied in cone shape to prepare stump for prosthesis.
(3) Inspect for blisters, redness, abrasions.
(4) Remove stump sock daily and prn.

　　h. Assist in rehabilitation program.
◆ **E. Evaluation/outcome criteria:**
　1. Begins rehabilitation program.
　2. No hemorrhage, infection.
　3. Adjusts to altered body image.

IX. Gout: disorder of purine metabolism; genetic disease believed to be transmitted by a dominant gene, characterized by recurrent attacks of acute pain and swelling of one joint (usually the great toe).
　A. Pathophysiology: urate crystals and infiltrating leukocytes appear to damage the intracellular phagolysosomes, resulting in leakage of lysomal enzymes into the synovial fluid, causing tissue damage and joint inflammation.

Adult

PCA -	Patient Controlled Analgesia
SCDs -	Sequential Compression Device
AES -	Antiembolism Stockings
MSW -	Medical Social Worker
D/C-	Discontinue
Y-	Yes
N-	No

Circle items not completed, and document exceptions.
Review circled items daily. Date circled items when
completed. Items with boxes are for non-Nursing discipline.

	DOS Date: / / THA	Day 1 / /	Day 2
• Milestones		• **Patient dangles and stands first time with physical therapy** **Y N**	
1. Discharge Planning	Admission nursing assessment completed		☐ MSW interview and collaborates with Home Care Liaison Interdisciplinary Team collaborates with MSW regarding discharge goal ☐ MSW assess services, equipment, transportation and possible placement
2. MD Consult/Activity			☐ D/C wound drains ☐ Dressing changed to light dressing
3. Diagnostic Tests ⬚		CBC P.T. (if on Warfarin)	CBC P.T. (if on Warfarin)
4. Treatments Instrumentation	Balanced Suspension/abduction pillow Foley AES, SCDs Wound Drains O_2 via nasal prongs I&O	Balanced Suspension/abduction pillow Foley AES, SCDs Wound Drains O_2 via nasal prongs I&O	D/C Balanced Suspension Abduction pillow D/C Foley AES, SCDs D/C O_2 I&O
5. Diet and Nutrition	Diet as tolerated	Diet as tolerated	Diet as tolerated
6. Medications 🔵 a. Antibiotics b. Pain Management c. Anticoagulation d. Bowel Regimen e. IV	IV Antibiotics PCA with Basal or Parenteral Analgesics Anticoagulation IV continuous	IV Antibiotics PCA with Basal or Parenteral Analgesics Anticoagulation IV continuous	D/C Antibiotics D/C Basal, continue self-dose PCA or parenteral analgesics and begin oral analgesics ATC x24 Anticoagulation Bowel intervention IV continuous
7. Activity	Bed rest with operated leg in balanced suspension/abduction pillow Reposition as needed Adjust balanced suspension/abduction pillow prn	☐ PT: evaluation instruction isometrics, precautions, PT program • **Dangle (stand if pt tolerates)** Complete bath/partial bath Adjust balanced suspension/abduction pillow prn	☐ PT: advances activity as tol. incl. transfers ADLs and gait ☐ PT: Adv. exercises as tol. Partial Bath, OOB to chair, toilet Adjust abduction pillow prn
8. Nursing Assessment ♦ CSM= circulation, sensation, movement	VS every 4 hrs with O_2 sats CSM every 4 hrs Systems assessment every 8 hrs	VS every 4 hrs with O_2 sats CSM every 4 hrs Systems assessment every 8 hrs	VS every 8 hrs CSM every 4 hrs Systems assessment every 8 hrs
9. Patient Teaching	Orientation to room, call light and nursing care Begin teaching to include: 1. PCA/analgesic instruction 2. Positioning, THA precautions 3. Protocol for advancing diet 4. Purpose of anticoagulation, AES, SCDs 5. ICS, C + DB 6. Pain scale, 0-10	Reinforce teaching for: 1. PCA 2. Positioning, THA precautions, ROM 3. Advancing diet 4. Anticoagulation, AES, SCDs 5. ICS, C + DB 6. Reinforce pain scale ☐ PT: Post-op exercise instruction	Teach ATC PO pain management Teach sx hip dislocation Balance diet to include iron & fiber 🍽 Reinforce teaching for: 1. THA precautions 2. Advancing diet 3. Anticoagulation, AES, SCDs 4. ICS, C + DB

HEALTH CARE ACTIVITIES/PHYSICIAN ORDER REQUIRED

Adult

PRIMARY HIP ARTHROPLASTY (THA) CLINICAL PATHWAY

Day 3 / /	Day 4 / /	Day 5 / /	Discharge Outcomes
• **Final post discharge destination made and transportation initiated** Y N		• **Patient is discharged Y N** • **Patient independent in and out of bed Y N**	
• **Initiate Home Care Referral Form or Interfacility Transfer Form**	☐ MSW confirm Transportation ☐ Home Care Referral Made by Home Care Liaison	Give clinic appointment Prescriptions for discharge meds • **Discharge patient**	Patient/caregiver receives discharge resources: 1. supplies 2. equipment 3. home care or other d/c arrangements
		☐ Dressing change	
P.T. (if on Warfarin)	Duplex scan D/C hip x-rays P.T. (if on Warfarin) Platelet Count (Enoxaparin)	P.T. (if on Warfarin)	Correct prosthetic placement by x-ray confirmation Urine clear
Abduction pillow AES, D/C SCDs Monitor drsg for drainage, change prn D/C I&O	Abduction pillow AES Monitor drsg for drainage, change prn	Abduction pillow AES	Wound healing with minimum redness or drainage
Diet as tolerated	Diet as tolerated	Diet as tolerated	Tolerates normal diet
D/C PCA or parenteral analgesics Continue Oral Analgesics ATC x24 Anticoagulation	Discharge planning for: Analgesics Anticoagulation Oral analgesics prn Anticoagulation Bowel intervention	Discharged on: Oral Analgesics prn Appropriate anticoagulation Oral analgesics prn Anticoagulation	Pain under control by self report on oral analgesics Normal circulation to extremities Abdomen soft, reports GI comfort
HL IV	HL IV	D/C HL	
☐ PT: advances activity as tol. incl. transfers, ADLs and gait ☐ PT: Adv. exercises as tol. ☐ PT: Assess and order equip.	☐ PT: advances activity as tol. incl. transfers, ADLs and gait ☐ PT: Adv. exercises as tol. ☐ PT: Stair climbing	• **In/out of bed independently** ☐ PT: advances activity as tol. incl. transfers, ADLs and gait ☐ PT: Adv. exercises as tol. ☐ PT: Stair climbing	Follows THA precautions and uses assistive devices correctly Independent in/out of bed
Self bath with help Adjust abduction pillow prn Assist with progressive gait	Self bath with help Adjust abduction pillow prn Assist with progressive gait	Self bath with help Adjust abduction pillow prn Assist with progressive gait	
VS every 8 hrs CSM every 4 hrs· Systems assessment every 8 hrs	VS every 8 hrs CSM every 4 hrs Systems assessment every 8 hrs	VS every 8 hrs CSM every 4 hrs Systems assessment every 8 hrs	Temp < 38 for 24 hours prior to D/C CSM status same as prior to surgery or improved All systems returned to baseline
Bacteremia teaching, "Protecting Your Joint From Infection" given. Review S+S of infection Reinforce teaching for: 1 THA precaution 2. Anticoagulation, AES Teach ATC vs prn pain management	Anticoagulation teaching S+S thrombophlebitis. Watch ADL videotape Reinforce teaching for: 1. THA precautions 2. Anticoagulation, AES 3. Prn pain medication management	Review staple/wound care Give "Care of your wound" handout Reinforce teaching for: 1. THA precautions 2. Anticoagulation, AES Discharge medication teaching	Able to verbalize S+S: wound infection, thrombophlebitis, bacteremia, hip and wound precautions, diet high in *iron* and *fiber*, indications and side effects of discharge medications

Adult

Adult

PRIMARY HIP ARTHROPLASTY (THA) CLINICAL PATHWAY

	DOS THA Date: / /	Day 1 / /	Day 2 / /
10. Comfort	Verbalizes acceptable level of pain at _____ and able to cooperate with activities Uses PCA/analgesic appropriately	Verbalizes acceptable level of pain at _____ and able to cooperate with activities Uses PCA/analgesic appropriately	Verbalizes acceptable level of pain at _____ and able to cooperate with activities Uses PCA appropriately without basal rate and takes po pain meds appropriately
11. Physical Mobility	Uses overhead trapeze appropriately Maintains operated leg in balanced suspension with THA precautions/abduction pillow in place Tolerates balanced suspension/abduction pillow Follows THA positioning guidelines	Uses overhead trapeze appropriately Dangles with assist, stands if tol Tolerates balanced suspension/abduction pillow Follows THA precautions	Up to chair 30 min BID and amb in room Stands with PT assist and progress ambulation Uses walker or crutches approp. Maintains THA precautions with abduction pillow
12. Bowel and Bladder Function	Urine output > 30 cc/hour Bowel sounds present Abdomen soft, non-distended Tolerates diet.	Urine output > 30 cc/hour Bowel sounds present Abdomen soft, non-distended Tolerates diet.	Urine output > 30 cc/hour Bowel sounds present + flatus Abdomen soft, non distended. Has bowel movement
13. Self Care Ability		Verbalizes understanding of care needs Assists staff as able Uses bedpan with max assist	Washes face, arms, and chest with set up Uses bedpan with moderate assist
14. Skin Integrity	Skin intact Dressing dry and intact PURV _____	Skin intact Dressing dry and intact	Skin intact Dressing dry and intact
15. Safety Falls Assessment * If score ≥ 6 follow orthopaedic standardized NCP or individualize "intervention Guideline" for PT at risk for fall.		65 or older .... 1 Mental status limitations ...... 5 History of falls .... 5 Mobility limitations .... 4 Elimination problems .... 2 Medications .... 1 TOTAL SCORE .... _____ *	65 or older .... 1 Mental status limitations ...... 5 History of falls .... 5 Mobility limitations .... 4 Elimination problems .... 2 Medications .... 1 TOTAL SCORE .... _____ *

B. Risk factors:
1. Men.
2. Age (>50).
3. Genetic/familial tendency.
4. Prolonged hyperuricemia (elevated serum uric acid).
5. Obesity.
6. Moderate to heavy alcohol intake.
7. Hypertension.
8. Abnormal kidney function.

◆ **C. Assessment:**
1. *Subjective data:*
    a. Pain: excruciating.
    b. Fatigue.
    c. Anorexia.
2. *Objective data:*
    a. Joint: erythema (redness), hot, swollen, difficult to move; skin stretched and shiny over joint.
    b. Subcutaneous nodules, tophi (deposits of urate) on hands and feet.
    c. Weight loss.
    d. Fever.
    e. Sensory changes, with cold intolerance.

f. Lab data:
  (1) Serum uric acid: *increased significantly* (6.5/100 mL in women, 7.5/100 mL in men) in chronic gout; only *slightly increased* in acute gout.
  (2) WBC: 12,000–15,000/μL.
  (3) Erythrocyte sedimentation rate: >20 mm.
  (4) 24 hr urinary uric acid: slightly *elevated.*
  (5) Proteinuria (chronic gout).
  (6) Azotemia (presence of nitrogen-containing compounds in blood) in chronic gout.

g. *Diagnostic tests:* arthrocentesis, x-rays.

◆ **D. Analysis/nursing diagnosis:**
1. *Pain* related to inflammation and swelling of affected joint.
2. *Impaired physical mobility* related to pain.
3. *Knowledge deficit* related to diet restrictions and increased fluid needs.
4. *Altered urinary elimination* related to kidney damage.

Day 3	Day 4	Day 5	Discharge Outcomes
Verbalizes acceptable level of pain at_____ and able to cooperate with activities Reports pain relief with non-pharmacologic methods (i.e. turning, positioning, relaxation, etc. Tolerates ATC po pain meds	Verbalizes acceptable level of pain at_____ and able to cooperate with activities Requests po prn pain meds approp.	Verbalizes acceptable level of pain at_____ and able to cooperate with activities Able to verbalize understanding of indications and side effects of D/C meds Requests prn po pain meds approp.	Pain controlled by self report on oral analgesics.
Ambulates with PT assistance in hall Tolerates 30 min in chair TID Able to get in and out of bed with moderate assist Uses walker or crutches approp. Maintains THA precautions	Increases walking distance with PT or Nsg Assist in hall Uses walker or crutches approp. Able to get in and out of bed with minimal assist Maintains THA precautions	Increases walking distance with PT or Nsg Assist in hall Uses walker or crutches approp. Able to get in and out of bed with minimal assist Maintains THA precautions	Independent/min assist in and out of bed Verbalizes understanding of hip precautions No dislocation of prosthesis
Voids spontaneously Bowel sounds present + flatus Abdomen soft, non-distended	Voids spontaneously Bowel sounds present + flatus Has bowel movement.	Voids spontaneously Bowel pattern same as pre op status	Voids spontaneously Bowel pattern normal
Washes areas in reach Uses bedpan with minimal assist Uses bathroom with mod assist	Washes areas in reach Uses bathroom with minimal assist	Bathes self Independent/min assist to bathroom with assistive devices	Able to bathe self/bathe with set-up Independent/min assist to bathroom with assistive devices
Skin intact Dressing dry and intact PURV _____	Skin intact Dressing dry and intact	Skin intact Dressing dry and intact PURV _____	Skin intact Incision well approximated without redness or drainage
65 or older .... 1 Mental status limitations ...... 5 History of falls .... 5 Mobility limitations .... 4 Elimination problems .... 2 Medications .... 1 TOTAL SCORE .... _____ *	65 or older .... 1 Mental status limitations ...... 5 History of falls .... 5 Mobility limitations .... 4 Elimination problems .... 2 Medications .... 1 TOTAL SCORE .... _____ *	65 or older .... 1 Mental status limitations ...... 5 History of falls .... 5 Mobility limitations .... 4 Elimination problems .... 2 Medications .... 1 TOTAL SCORE .... _____ *	

Source: UCSF Healthcare, San Francisco, Calif. With permission from Jane E. Hirsch, RN, MS, Vice President, Nursing and Patient Care Services.

Adult

◆ **E. Nursing care plan/implementation:**
1. Goal: *decrease discomfort.*
   a. Administer antigout medications as ordered:
      (1) Treatment of *acute* attacks: colchicine, phenylbutazone (Butazolidin), indomethacin (Indocin), allopurinol (Zyloprim), naproxen (Naprosyn), corticosteroids (prednisone).
      (2) *Preventive therapy:* probenecid (Benemid), sulfinpyrazone (Anturane). These drugs are not used during acute attacks.
   b. Absolute rest of affected joint → gradual increase in activities, to prevent complications of immobilization; at the same time, rest for comfort.
2. Goal: *prevent kidney damage.*
   a. *Increase* fluid intake to 2000–3000 mL/day.
   b. Monitor urinary output.
3. Goal: *health teaching.*
   a. Need for *low-purine diet* during acute attack (see VII. Purine-restricted diet, Common Therapeutic Diets, **Unit 9,** p. 682.

b. Importance of *increased fluid in diet.*
c. Signs and symptoms of increased progression of disease.
d. Dosage and side effects of prescribed medications.

◆ **F. Evaluation/outcome criteria:**
1. Swelling decreased.
2. Discomfort alleviated.
3. Mobility returned to status before attack.
4. Lab values return to normal.

X. Herniated/ruptured disk (ruptured nucleus pulposus): strain or injury to a weakened cartilage between vertebrae can result in herniation of the nucleus, causing pressure on nerve roots in spinal canal, pain, and disability.

   A. Pathophysiology: pulpy substance of disk interior (nucleus pulposus) bulges or ruptures through the outer annulus fibrosus → irritation and pressure on nerve endings in the spinal ligaments → muscle spasm and distortion of the joints of vertebral arches.

   B. Risk factors:
   1. Strain as result of poor body mechanics.
   2. Trauma.

3. History of back injuries.
4. Degenerative disc (Spondylosis).

◆ **C. Assessment:**
1. *Lumbar injuries* (90% of herniations):
   a. *Subjective data:*
      (1) Pain: low back, radiating to buttocks, posterior thigh, and calf; relieved by recumbency; aggravated by sneezing, coughing, and flexion; sciatic pain continues even when back pain subsides.
      (2) Numbness, tingling.
   b. *Objective data:*
      (1) Muscle weakness—leg and foot.
      (2) Inability to flex leg.
      (3) Sensory loss, leg and foot.
      (4) Alterations in posture: leans to side, unable to stand up straight.
      (5) Edema: leg and foot.
      (6) Positive *Lasègue's sign:* straight leg raising with hip flexed and knee extended will produce sciatic pain.
2. *Cervical injuries* (10% of herniations):
   a. *Subjective data:*
      (1) Pain—upper extremities, radiating to hands and fingers; aggravated by coughing, sneezing, and straining.
      (2) Tingling, burning sensation in upper extremities and back of neck.
   b. *Objective data:*
      (1) Upper extremities: weakness and atrophy.
      (2) Neck: restricted movement.
      (3) *Diagnostic tests* for both lumbar and cervical injuries.
         (a) Spine x-rays.
         (b) CT scan.
         (c) MRI.
         (d) Myelography (less preferred than CAT scan or MRI).
         (e) Electromyography.
         (f) Neurological exam: special attention to sensory status, including pain, touch, and temperature identification, and to motor status, including strength, gait, and reflexes.

◆ **D. Analysis/nursing diagnosis:**
1. *Pain* related to pressure on nerve roots.
2. *Fear* related to disease progression and/or potential surgery.
3. *Knowledge deficit* related to correct body mechanics.
4. *Impaired physical mobility* related to continued pain.
5. *Sleep pattern disturbance* related to difficulty finding comfortable position.

◆ **E. Nursing care plan/implementation:**
1. Goal: *relieve pain and promote comfort.*
   a. Bed rest with bedboard.
   b. *Position*—avoid twisting.
      (1) *Lumbar disk: William's* (head elevated 30 degrees, knee gatch elevated to flatten the lumbosacral curve). Can be duplicated at home with pillow placement.
      (2) *Cervical: low Fowler's.*
   c. Medications as ordered:
      (1) *Analgesics.*
      (2) *Muscle relaxants.*
      (3) *Anti-inflammatory.*
      (4) *Stool softeners.*
   d. Moist heat.
   e. Fracture bedpan.
   f. Gradual increase in activity.
   g. Brace application for support.
   h. Traction application prn for comfort.
   i. Prepare for surgery if medical regimen unsuccessful.
2. Goal: *health teaching.*
   a. Correct body mechanics, keep back straight.
   b. Exercise program as symptoms decrease.

◆ **F. Evaluation/outcome criteria:**
1. Reports pain decreased.
2. Mobility increased, normal body posture attained.

XI. **Laminectomy:** excision of dorsal arch of vertebrae with or without spinal fusion of two or more vertebrae with a bone graft from iliac crest, to stabilize spine. See **Clinical Pathway for Posterior Spinal Fusion,** p. 592.

◆ **A. Analysis/nursing diagnosis:**
1. *Pain* related to edema of surgical procedure.
2. *Impaired physical mobility* related to pain and discomfort resulting from surgery.

◆ **B. Nursing care plan/implementation:**
1. Goal: *relieve anxiety.*
   a. Answer questions, explain routines.
   b. See The Perioperative Experience, p. 500.
2. Goal: *prevent injury postoperatively.*
   a. Monitor vital signs:
      (1) Neurological signs, e.g., check sensation and motor strength of limbs.
      (2) Respiratory status (risk for respiratory depression with cervical laminectomy).
   b. Monitor I&O (urinary retention common, especially with cervical laminectomy); may need catheterization. Encourage fluids.
   c. Monitor bowel sounds (paralytic ileus common with lumbar laminectomy).
   d. Monitor dressing for possible bleeding.
   e. Bed *position* as ordered:
      (1) *For lumbar laminectomy: head of bed flat;* supine with slight flexion of legs; with pillow between knees for turning and side-lying position.

(2) *For cervical laminectomy: head of bed elevated,* neck immobilized with collar or sandbags.

  f. Encourage deep breathing to prevent respiratory complications.

  g. Prevent strain or flexion at surgical site: log-rolling with spinal fusion.

  h. Some surgical interventions that require small incisions (microsurgery) have no specific postoperative positions.

3. Goal: *promote comfort.*

  a. Administer analgesics if sciatic-type pain continues after lumbar surgery (arm pain after cervical surgery), due to edema from trauma of surgery.

4. Goal: *prepare for early discharge.*

  a. Patients having microsurgery for repair of herniated disk will usually be discharged from the hospital 1 day postoperative; teaching regarding allowed and restricted activities must be done early.

5. Goal: *health teaching.*

  a. How to *turn and move* from side to side in one motion, *sit up,* and *get out of bed without twisting spine;* to get out of bed: raise head of bed while in side-lying position, then put feet over edge of bed, and stand.

  b. Proper positioning and *ambulation* techniques.

  c. Correct posture, *body mechanics,* activities to prevent further injury; increase activities according to tolerance.

  d. Physiotherapy; encourage compliance for full rehabilitation.

◆ **C. Evaluation/outcome criteria:**

1. No respiratory, bowel, or bladder complications noted.

  a. Lung sounds clear.

  b. Bowel sounds present; able to pass gas and feces.

  c. Urinary output adequate.

2. Regains mobility.

3. Comfort level increases: reports leg and back pain decreased.

4. Demonstrates protective positioning and ambulation techniques.

XII. Spinal cord injuries: trauma from hyperextension, hyperflexion, axial compression, lateral flexion, or shearing of the spine.

  A. Types:

1. *C-1 and C-2 injury level*—resulting deficit:

  a. Phrenic nerve involvement.

  b. Diaphragmatic paralysis.

  c. Respiratory difficulties (require permanent ventilatory support).

  d. Possible quadriplegia.

  e. Possible death.

2. *C-4 through T-1 injury level*—resulting deficit: possible quadriplegia.

3. *Thoracic-lumbar injury level*—resulting deficit: possible paraplegia.

  B. Pathophysiology: trauma → vertebral dislocation or fractures → cord trauma, compression, or severance of the cord.

  C. Risk factors:

1. Motor vehicle accidents.

2. Diving, surfing, contact sports.

3. Falls.

4. Gunshot wounds.

◆ **D. Assessment:**

1. *Subjective data:*

  a. Pain at the level of injury.

  b. Numbness/weakness, loss of sensation below level of injury.

  c. Psychological distress related to severity of injury and its effects.

2. *Objective data:*

  a. Symptoms depend on extent of injury to spinal cord/spinal nerves.

  b. Paralysis: motor, sphincter.

    (1) Initially a period of *flaccid paralysis* and loss of reflexes, called *spinal* or *neural shock.*

    (2) *Incomplete injuries* may lead to loss of voluntary movement and sensory deficits below injury level (symptoms vary depending on injury).

    (3) *Complete injury* leads to loss of function and all voluntary movement below level of injury.

  c. Respiratory distress.

  d. Alterations in temperature control.

  e. Alterations in bowel and bladder function.

  f. Involved muscles become spastic and hyperreflexic within days or weeks.

◆ **E. Analysis/nursing diagnosis:**

1. *Ineffective breathing pattern* related to high-level injury.

2. *Impaired physical mobility* related to injuries affecting lower limbs.

3. *Fear* related to uncertain future health status.

4. *Anxiety* related to loss of control over own activities of daily living.

5. *Bathing/hygiene self-care deficit* related to injuries above T-1.

6. *Impaired home maintenance management* related to possible quadriplegia and paraplegia.

7. *Risk for altered body temperature* related to absence of sweating below level of injury.

8. *Risk for injury* related to equipment necessary for daily activities.

9. *Tactile sensory/perceptual alterations* related to injury level.

10. *Body image disturbance* related to permanent change in physical status.

◆ **F. Nursing care plan/implementation:**

1. Goal: *maintain patent airway.*

Circle items not completed or not within normal limits, and document exceptions. Review circled items daily.
Date circled items when completed. Items with boxes are for non-Nursing discipline charting.

Name:_____

		Pre Admit	Day of Surgery	/ / Day 1	/ / Day 2
PCA-	Patient Controlled Analgesia				
SCDs-	Sequential Compression Device				
AES-	Antiembolism Stockings				
MSW -	Medical Social Worker				
D/C -	Discontinue				
Y-	Yes				
N-	No				

HEALTH CARE TEAM ACTIVITIES - PHYSICIAN ORDER REQUIRED

	Pre Admit	Day of Surgery	Day 1	Day 2
Milestones				• **Stands 5 minutes Y N**
1. Discharge Planning	Spine Service Nurse/Case Manager assesses home situation and collaborates with MSW			☐ MSW interview and collaborates with Home Care Liaison Interdisciplinary Team collaborates with MSW regarding discharge goal ☐ MSW assess services, equipment, transportation and possible placement
2. MD/Consult/ Activity	Pain management consult as indicated	☐ PT requisition	☐ Pain management Pharmacy consult	☐ D/C drain
3. Diagnostic Tests			CBC	CBC

4. Treatments/ Instrumentation ▶		Intake + Output
		AES, SCDs
		Foley
		O$_2$ via nasal prongs
		Assess wound
		Wound drain
		  Type _____
		  Site _____
		Describe drainage _____
			Intake + Output
			AES, SCDs
			Foley
			O$_2$ via nasal prongs
			Assess wound
			Wound drain
			  Type _____
			  Site _____
			Describe drainage _____
				Intake + Output
				AES, SCDs
				Foley
				O$_2$ via nasal prongs
				Assess wound
				Wound drain
				  Type _____
				  Site _____
				Describe drainage _____

5. Diet/Nutrition	NPO after midnight day before surgery	NPO	NPO	Ice chips, 30 cc/hr if bowel sounds
6. Medications a) Routine b) Pain Management c) Bowel Regimen d) IV (intravenous) HL (saline lock)	Discontinue non-steroidal anti-inflammatory drugs 2 weeks before surgery Continue analgesics as ordered and evaluate analgesic use Fleets enema evening before surgery	IV Antibiotic PCA with Basal IV continuous	IV Antibiotic PCA with Basal IV continuous	D/C IV Antibiotic (48˚ post surgery) PCA with Basal Bowel intervention Suppository IV continuous
7. Activity / Mobility		Bedrest Logroll q 2 hours	Bedrest Logroll q 2 hours	Bedrest Logroll q 2 hours Dangle 2-3 times • **Stands 5 minutes** Notify orthotist if able to stand
8. Physical Therapy (PT) Occupational Therapy (OT)	Physical therapy instructions Occupational therapy instructions		☐ PT evaluation Instruction supine exercises Dangle if ordered	☐ PT advance exercises as tolerated. Dangle, stand if tolerated. Instruct body mechanics self care mobilization exercises ☐ OT Evaluation as needed
9. Assessment ◆ **VS=T, R, P, BP** **CSM= Circulation Sensation Movement** **GI=Bowel sounds** **Pulmonary=Auscultate lung fields**	VS Q 4˚	VS Q 4˚ CSM q 4 hours GI/GU q 4 hours Pulmonary q 4 hours O$_2$ sat q 4 hours Neurological assess Q shift Cardiovascular Q shift Musculoskeletal Q shift Skin assessment Q shift Psychosocial/Behavioral Assessment Q shift	VS q 4 hours CSM q 4 hours GI/GU q 4 hours Pulmonary q 4 hours O$_2$ sat q 4 hours Neurological Q shift Cardiovascular Q shift Musculoskeletal Q shift Skin assessment Q shift Psychosocial/Behavioral Assessment Q shift	VS QID CSM QID GI/GU q 8 hours Pulmonary q 4 hours O$_2$ sat q 4 hours Neurological Q shift Cardiovascular Q shift Musculoskeletal Q shift Skin assessment Q shift Psychosocial/Behavioral Assessment Q shift
10. IV Access IV WNL: No erythema, drainage, tenderness or swelling. Document time for IV assessment / interventions		DOS TYPE SITE TYPE SITE TYPE SITE	DAY 1 TYPE SITE TYPE SITE TYPE SITE	DAY 2 TYPE SITE TYPE SITE TYPE SITE
11. Patient Teaching ICS-Incentive Spirometer TCDB-turn, cough, deep breathe	Pt teaching re: D/C options, post hospitalization destination options, purpose of invasive lines/tubes, ICU stay, PCA use, diet advancement Give pt clinical pathway patient version	Teach PCA and ICS, logroll, positioning, T,C,DB Confirm pt has received pt version of clinical pathway	Review PCA, ICS, logroll, positioning, T,C,DB Reinforce PT bed exercises and activity progress Review pt version of clinical pathway	Explain brace molding procedure Review dangling Teach anxiety reduction strategies Evaluate pt for *Bridge to Home* protocol Give *Bridge to Home* pamphlet of appropriate Review pt version of clinical pathway

For IV Access columns: insert date, WNL, erythema, tenderness, drainage, swelling, tubing change, site care, line D/C

Clinical Pathway: Posterior Spinal Fusion (PSF)

Day 3	Day 4 / /	Day 5 / /	Day 6 / /	Day 7 / /	Discharge Outcomes Date _____
	• **Brace molded Y N**			• **Discharge Y N**	
	☐ Home Care Liaison assesses equipment and transport needs Start Home Care referral	☐ Home Care Liaison starts Home Care Referral Continue Home Care Referral/ insurance info	☐ Home Care Liaison confirms transport and equipment needs	Give clinic appointment and prescriptions for discharge meds • **Discharge patient**	Patient is discharged
☐ Change dressing Apply light dressing or steri strips open to air	☐ Brace molded by orthotist	☐ Brace returned and fitted	☐ Brace adjusted if needed	☐ Dressing change ☐ PDP completed ☐ Prescriptions written	Brace fits properly
CBC, UA, C + S, if fever or urine cloudy			Full spine x-ray (in brace if ordered)		Spine alignment confirmed per x-ray
Intake + Output AES, SCDs D/C Foley D/C O₂ Assess wound	D/C Intake + Output AES, SCDs Assess wound	AES, discontinue SCDs when ambulating independently Assess wound	Wears AES Assess wound	Discontinue AES on discharge	
Clear liquids, if flatus passed	Advance diet Type of diet ____ % taken B __ L __ D __	Advance diet Type of diet ____ % taken B __ L __ D __	Advance diet Type of diet ____ % taken B __ L __ D __	Advance diet Type of diet ____ % taken B __ L __ D __	Patient tolerates diet
Begin PO medications + FESO₄, MVI, DOSS PCA, no Basal Begin PO medications around the clock for 24 hours Bowel intervention IV continuous	PO medications Discontinue PCA PO pain medications, prn Bowel intervention HL IV	PO medications PO pain medications, prn Bowel intervention DC IV	PO medications PO pain medications, prn Bowel intervention	PO medications PO pain medications, prn Bowel intervention	Pain under control by self report on oral analgesics Abdomen soft Reports GI comfort
Dangle 2-3 times. Logroll • **Stand in AM 8-10 minutes for brace mold** Chair 30 minutes maximum	Stand, sit in chair for meals Progress activity per MD order	Sit in chair for meals Progress activity Wear brace as ordered	Sit in chair for meals Progress to independence or goal Wear brace as ordered	Progress to independence or goal Wear brace as ordered	Independent in/out of bed and ambulates with/without assistive device
☐ PT advance activity as tolerated including transfers and gait ☐ OT: Increase independent lower extremities with bed mobility, standing tolerance and precautions.	☐ PT advance activity as tolerated including transfers, gait and home exercise program. ☐ OT: Independent in lower extremities self care. Independent with caregiver transfer training.	☐ PT advance to stairs ☐ OT Don/Doff brace with assistance Independent in transfer activities (car, toilet, chair, shower chair)	☐ PT/OT: Order equipment as needed. Review progression of activity after discharge		Patient meets physical therapy D/C criteria
VS BID CSM BID GI/GU BID Pulmonary BID Discontinue O₂ sat Neurological Q shift Cardiovascular Q shift Musculoskeletal Q shift Skin assessment Q shift Psychosocial/Behavioral Assessment Q shift	VS BID CSM BID GI/GU BID Pulmonary BID Neurological Q shift Cardiovascular Q shift Musculoskeletal Q shift Skin assessment Q shift Psychosocial/Behavioral Assessment Q shift	VS BID CSM BID GI/GU BID Pulmonary BID Neurological Q shift Cardiovascular Q shift Musculoskeletal Q shift Skin assessment Q shift Psychosocial/Behavioral Assessment Q shift	VS BID CSM BID GI/GU BID Pulmonary BID Neurological Q shift Cardiovascular Q shift Musculoskeletal Q shift Skin assessment Q shift Psychosocial/Behavioral Assessment Q shift	VS BID CSM BID GI/GU BID Pulmonary BID Neurological Q shift Cardiovascular Q shift Musculoskeletal Q shift Skin assessment Q shift Psychosocial/Behavioral Assessment Q shift	Temp < 38 for 24 hours prior to D/C; CSM status same as prior to surgery or improved; All system returned to baseline Coping appropriately; communicates needs and concerns
DAY 3 TYPE / SITE / TYPE / SITE / TYPE / SITE	DAY 4 TYPE / SITE / TYPE / SITE / TYPE / SITE	DAY 5 TYPE / SITE / TYPE / SITE / TYPE / SITE	DAY 6 TYPE / SITE / TYPE / SITE / TYPE / SITE	DAY 7 TYPE / SITE / TYPE / SITE / TYPE / SITE	
Give "After Spine Surgery" booklet. Reinforce anxiety reduction strategies Start *Bridge to Home* program Review pt version of clinical pathway	Reinforce PT body mechanics Review brace molding *Bridge to Home* Program Review pt version of clinical pathway	Review "After Spine Surgery" booklet with patient and family Reinforce relaxation techniques and deep breathing Reinforce brace Don/Doff Technique *Bridge to Home* Program Review pt version of clinical pathway	Reinforce PT instructions Review pt version of clinical pathway *Bridge to Home* Program	Instruct discharge medications / follow-up appointments and give prescriptions Review pt version of clinical pathway Give certificate for completion of *Bridge to Home* Program	Able to verbalize S+S of wound infection, brace and skin care, activity progression, limitations, medications, when to call physician

Adult

Name: _____

	Pre Admit	Day of Surgery\ PSF	/ / Day 1	/ / Day 2
12. Pain Relief		Verbalize acceptable level of pain at_____ Uses PCA appropriately	Verbalizes acceptable level of pain at _____ and able to cooperate with activities Uses PCA appropriately	Verbalizes acceptable level of pain at _____ and able to cooperate with activities Uses PCA appropriately
13. Physical Mobility		Logrolls and repositions with maximal assistance	Logrolls with moderate-maximal assistance Participates in P.T. exercises and activity progression	Logrolls with mod - max assist Dangles 2 times, maximal assistance Stands 5 minutes
14. Tissue Perfusion		CSM status at baseline	CSM status at baseline	CSM status at baseline
15. Respiratory Function		Uses ICS. O$_2$ sat > 94% Cooperates with C,T, & DB Respiratory system WNL	C,T, & DB Uses ICS q 1 hour volume_____ O$_2$ sat > 94% Respiratory system WNL	C,T, & DB Uses ICS q 2 hours volume_____ O$_2$ sat > 94% Respiratory system WNL
16. Skin Integrity		WNL: skin warm, dry and intact. Normal color and turgor. PURV_____	WNL: skin warm, dry and intact. Normal color and turgor.	WNL: skin warm, dry and intact. Normal color and turgor.
17. Anxiety		Receives information about post-op care	Receives information about post-op activities and procedures Participates in care Exhibits mild to severe anxiety	Receives information about activities Participates in care Begins to use functional coping mechanisms Verbalizes fears and concerns
18. Bowel and Bladder Function		Urine output > 30 cc/hour Bowel sounds minimal or absent Abdomen soft, non-tender	Urine output > 30 cc/hour Bowel sounds minimal or absent Abdomen soft, non-tender	Urine output > 30 cc/hour Bowel sounds present Abdomen soft, non-tender Passing flatus or has a bowel movement
19. Musculoskeletal Neurological Cardiovascular Sysems Function		Systems WNL	Systems WNL	Systems WNL
20. Self Care Ability			Verbalizes understanding of care needs, assists staff as able	Washes face, arms and chest
21. Safety Falls Assessment *Follow orthopaedic standardized NCP.		65 or older ....1 Mental status limitations ..5 History of falls ....5 Mobility limitations...........4 Elimination problems ....2 Medications ....1 TOTAL SCORE................._____ *	65 or older ....1 Mental status limitations ..5 History of falls ....5 Mobility limitations...........4 Elimination problems ....2 Medications ....1 TOTAL SCORE................._____ *	65 or older ....1 Mental status limitations ..5 History of falls ....5 Mobility limitations...........4 Elimination problems ....2 Medications ....1 TOTAL SCORE................._____ *

Y = Yes
N = No

PATIENT OUTCOMES

▶ a. Suction, cough, tracheostomy care, prn.
▶ b. Oxygen, ventilator care.
c. Monitor blood gas levels.
2. Goal: *prevent further damage.*
  a. Immobilize spine.
  b. Firm mattress, *Stryker frame, Foster frame, CircO-electric* bed, traction, braces (see **III. Fractures,** p. 580).
  c. Skeletal traction via tongs: *Crutchfield, Gardner-Wells* (see **III. Fractures,** p. 573).
  d. Halo traction (see **III. Fractures,** pp. 574, 580).
3. Goal: *relieve edema:* anti-inflammatory medications, corticosteroids.
4. Goal: *relieve discomfort:* analgesics, sedatives, muscle relaxants.
5. Goal: *promote comfort:*
  a. Maintain fluid intake: PO/IV, I&O.
  b. Increase nutritional intake.
  c. Prevent contractures and decubiti.
  d. Assist patient to deal with psychosocial issues, e.g., role changes.

e. Begin rehabilitation plan.
6. Goal: *prevent complications.*
  a. Monitor for spinal shock during initial phase of injury (see **XIII. Spinal shock,** p. 595).
  b. Monitor for hyperreflexia with severed spinal cord injuries (see **XIV. Autonomic hyperreflexia,** p. 596).
7. Goal: *health teaching.*
  a. Self-care techniques for highest level of independence; include significant others in teaching.
  b. How to use ambulation assistive devices (battery-operated wheelchair controlled by mouthpiece or hand controls, depending on level of paralysis).
  c. Identify community resources for follow-up care and career counseling.
  d. Signs and symptoms of autonomic hyperreflexia (see **XIV.** p. 596).
  e. Methods to prevent skin breakdown, infections of respiratory, urinary tract.

Clinical Pathway: Posterior Spinal Fusion (PSF)

/ /	/ /	/ /	/ /	/ /	Discharge Outcomes
Day 3	**Day 4**	**Day 5**	**Day 6**	**Day 7**	**Date** _____
Verbalizes pain at acceptable level Uses PCA appropriately w/o basal + takes po pain medication around the clock	Verbalizes pain at acceptable level; on PO prn pain medication	Pain at acceptable level with PO medication prn	Pain at acceptable level with PO medication prn	Pain at acceptable level with PO medication prn	Pain at acceptable level with PO medication prn
Logrolls, minimal-moderate assistance Dangles 2 times, moderate assistance Stands 8-10 minutes for brace mold	Gets in/out of bed, moderate assistance Sits in chair for meals 1-2 times Walks in room, moderate-maximal	Gets in/out of bed, minimal assistance Sits in chair 2-3 times Walks to hall, moderate assistance 3x Wearing brace as ordered Reports need for adjustment of brace	Gets in/out of bed Sits in chair 2-3 times Walks in hall minimal assistance times 3	Gets in/out of bed independently Sits in chair 2-3 times Walks, independently 3 times Reports brace correctly fitting	Independent in/out of bed Walking on level and up/ down stairs or reached goal Patient/family demonstrate on/off brace technique
CSM status at baseline	CSM status at baseline	CSM status at baseline	CSM status at baseline	CSM status at baseline	CSM status at baseline
C, T, & DB Uses ICS q 2" volume_____ O₂ sat >94% on room air Respiratory system WNL	Uses ICS independently volume____ Respiratory system WNL	Uses ICS independently volume____ Respiratory system WNL	Uses ICS independently volume____ Respiratory system WNL	Respiratory system WNL	Respiratory system WNL
WNL: skin warm, dry and intact. Normal color and turgor. PURV	WNL: skin warm, dry and intact. Normal color and turgor.	WNL: skin warm, dry and intact. Normal color and turgor.	WNL: skin warm, dry and intact. Normal color and turgor. PURV	WNL: skin warm, dry and intact. Normal color and turgor.	Skin clean, dry, and intact; wound well-approximated without redness/swelling
Receives and verbalizes understanding of information booklet Participates in care Anxiety reduction strategies Able to group requests Exhibits decreased anxiety	Verbalizes understanding of information Participates in care Able to use anxiety reduction strategies	Verbalizes understanding of information Participates in care Able to make decisions	Participates in care Discusses plans for going home Makes decisions	Participates in care Verbalizes ability to manage at home Makes decisions	Verbalizes ability to manage at home and/or with continuing care arrangements
Voiding without difficulty Bowel sounds present Abdomen non-tender Passing flatus or has a bowel movement	Voiding without difficulty Bowel sounds present Abdomen non-tender Passing flatus, or has a bowel movement	Voiding Bowel sounds present Abdomen non-tender Passing flatus, or has a bowel movement	Voiding Bowel sounds present Abdomen non-tender Passing flatus, and has a bowel movement	Voiding Bowel sounds present Abdomen non-tender Passing flatus, or has a bowel movement	Voiding Had BM during hospitalization
Systems WNL	Systems WNL	Systems WNL	Systems WNL	Systems WNL	Systems WNL
Washes areas in reach Feeds self	Washes areas in reach Feeds self	Bathes self with minimal assistance	Bathes and toilets self with minimal assistance	Independent in self care or reaches goal	Independent in self care or reaches goal
65 or older ....1 Mental status limitations .5 History of falls ....5 Mobility limitations..........4 Elimination problems ....2 Medications ....1 TOTAL SCORE..............____*	65 or older ....1 Mental status limitations .5 History of falls ....5 Mobility limitations..........4 Elimination problems ....2 Medications ....1 TOTAL SCORE..............____*	65 or older ....1 Mental status limitations .5 History of falls ....5 Mobility limitations..........4 Elimination problems ....2 Medications ....1 TOTAL SCORE..............____*	65 or older ....1 Mental status limitations .5 History of falls ....5 Mobility limitations..........4 Elimination problems ....2 Medications ....1 TOTAL SCORE..............____*	65 or older ....1 Mental status limitations .5 History of falls ....5 Mobility limitations..........4 Elimination problems ....2 Medications ....1 TOTAL SCORE..............____*	No falls

Adult

Source: UCSF Healthcare, San Francisco, Calif. With permission from Jane E. Hirsch, RN, MS, Vice President, Nursing and Patient Care Services.

f. Bowel, bladder program.

◆ **G. Evaluation/outcome criteria:**
 1. Complications avoided.
 2. Accomplishes self-care to greatest level for injury.
 3. Participates in rehabilitation plan.
 4. Grieves over loss and begins to integrate self into society.

XIII. Spinal shock: temporary flaccid paralysis and areflexia following a severe injury to the spinal cord.
 A. Pathophysiology: squeezing or shearing of the spinal cord due to fractures or dislocation of vertebrae; interruption of sensory tracts; loss of conscious sensation; interruption of motor tracts; loss of voluntary movement; loss of facilitation; loss of reflex activity; loss of muscle tone; loss of stretch reflexes, leading to bowel and bladder retention. If injury between T-1 and L-2, leads to loss of sympathetic tone and decrease in blood pressure. Afferent impulses are unable to ascend from below the injured site to the brain,

and efferent impulses are unable to descend to points below the site.
 B. Risk factors:
 1. Automobile/motorcycle accidents.
 2. Athletic accidents, e.g., diving in shallow water.
 3. Gunshot wounds.
◆ **C. Assessment:**
 1. *Subjective data:*
  a. Loss of sensation below level of injury.
  b. Inability to move extremities.
  c. Pain at level of injury.
 2. *Objective data:*
  a. Neurological exam:
   (1) *Absent:* pinprick, pressure, and vibratory sensations below level of injury; reflexes below level of injury.
   (2) Muscles: flaccid.
  b. Vital signs:
   (1) BP decreased (loss of vasomotor tone below level of injury).
   (2) Bradycardia.

(3) Elevated temperature.

(4) Respirations: may be depressed; possible respiratory failure if diaphragm involved.

c. Absence of sweating below level of injury.

d. Urinary retention.

e. Abdominal distention: retention of feces, paralytic ileus.

f. Skin: cold, clammy.

◆ **D. Analysis/nursing diagnosis:**

1. *Decreased cardiac output* related to loss of vasomotor tone below level of injury.

2. *Ineffective breathing pattern* related to injuries involving diaphragm.

3. *Improved physical mobility* related to loss of voluntary movement of limbs.

4. *Urinary retention* related to loss of stretch reflexes.

5. *Fear* related to serious physical condition.

6. *Risk for injury* related to potential organ damage if shock continues.

◆ **E. Nursing care plan/implementation:**

1. Goal: *prevent injury related to shock.*

▶ a. Maintain patent airway: intubation and mechanical ventilation may be necessary with cervical spinal injuries due to involvement of diaphragm.

b. Monitor vital signs; *profound hypotension* and *bradycardia* are most dangerous aspects of spinal shock.

c. Administer blood/IV fluids as ordered.

d. Nutrition and hydration:

(1) NPO in acute stage: maintain nutrition by IV infusions as ordered.

(2) When allowed to eat: *high-protein, high-calorie, high-vitamin diet.*

e. Maintain proper *position* to prevent further injury.

(1) Backboard is necessary to transport from place of injury.

(2) Support head in neutral alignment and prevent flexion.

(3) Skeletal traction will be applied once diagnosis is made.

f. Monitor urinary output q1h; may have Foley catheter while in shock; later intermittent catheterization will be used as needed.

▶ g. Relieve bowel distention; use lubricant containing anesthetic, as necessary, when checking for or removing impaction.

◆ **F. Evaluation/outcome criteria:**

1. Complications are avoided.

2. Body functions are maintained.

XIV. Autonomic dysreflexia (autonomic hyperreflexia): a group of symptoms in which many spinal cord autonomic responses are activated simultaneously. This may occur when cord lesions are *above the sixth thoracic* vertebra; it is *most commonly* seen with cervical

and high thoracic cord injuries; may occur up to 6 yr after injury.

A. Pathophysiology: pathological reflex condition, which is an acute **medical emergency** characterized by extreme hypertension and exaggerated autonomic responses to stimuli.

B. Risk factors:

1. Distention of bladder or rectum.

2. Stimulation of skin, e.g., decubitus ulcers, wrinkled clothing.

3. Stimulation of pain receptors.

◆ **C. Assessment:**

1. *Subjective data:*

a. Severe, pounding headache.

b. Blurred vision; sees spots in front of eyes.

c. Nausea.

d. Restlessness.

e. Feels flushed.

2. *Objective data:*

a. Severe hypertension (systolic BP may reach 300 mm Hg).

b. Bradycardia (30–40/min); fever.

c. Profuse diaphoresis, above level of injury.

d. Flushing of skin above level of injury.

e. Pale skin below level of injury.

f. Pilomotor spasm (goose flesh); chills.

g. Nasal congestion.

h. Distended bladder, bowel.

i. Skin breakdown.

j. Seizures.

◆ **D. Analysis/nursing diagnosis:**

1. *Dysreflexia* related to high spinal cord injury.

2. *Risk for injury* related to complications of hypertension, CVA.

3. *Visual sensory/perceptual alteration* related to blurred vision.

4. *Urinary retention* related to inability to empty bladder due to spinal injury.

5. *Constipation* related to inability to establish successful bowel training program.

6. *Impaired skin integrity* related to immobility.

◆ **E. Nursing plan/implementation:**

1. Goal: *decrease symptoms to prevent serious side effects.*

a. *Elevate head of bed;* this lowers BP in persons with high spinal cord injuries.

b. Identify and correct source of stimulation if possible; notify physician.

c. Monitor vital signs (BP) q15min and prn; uncontrolled hypertension can lead to stroke, blindness, death.

d. Give medications as ordered: nitrates, nifedipine (Procardia), or hydralazine (Apresoline).

▶ 2. Goal: *maintain patency of catheter.*

a. Monitor output; palpate for distended bladder.

b. Check for tubing kinks; irrigate catheter prn.

c. Insert new catheter *immediately* if blocked. Do *not* Credé (see Table 7–35, p. 572) or tap the bladder; it could exacerbate the response.

d. Culture if infection suspected.

3. Goal: *promote regular bowel elimination.*

▶ a. Bowel training program.

b. Administer suppository/enemas/laxatives as ordered and prn.

c. When checking for and removing impaction, first use *anesthetic ointment* (e.g., dibucaine [Nupercainal] ointment) to decrease irritation.

4. Goal: *prevent decubitus ulcers.*

a. Meticulous skin care.

b. *Position change q1–2h.*

c. Flotation pads, alternating pressure mattress on bed and wheelchair.

5. Goal: *health teaching.*

a. How to recognize risk factors that could initiate this condition.

b. Methods to prevent situations that increase risk, e.g., bowel program, bladder program, skin care, position change schedule.

◆ **F. Evaluation/outcome criteria:**

1. BP remains within normal limits.

2. No complications occur.

XV. Hyperthyroidism (also called *thyrotoxicosis; Graves' disease):* spectrum of symptoms of accelerated metabolism caused by excessive amounts of circulating thyroid hormone. *Graves' disease* is most common cause of hyperthyroidism. The three components of *Graves' disease* are *hyperthyroidism, ophthalmopathy* (protrusion of the eyes), and *skin lesions* (dermopathy). *Graves' disease* is triggered by: stress, smoking, radiation of the neck, some medications (interleukin-2), and infections. *Treatment* of hyperthyroidism is accomplished by antithyroid medications, radioactive iodine administration (capsule given once), or surgery. Patients may need to take supplemental thyroid hormone (levothyroxine) after treatment.

A. Pathophysiology: diffuse hyperplasia of thyroid gland → overproduction of thyroid hormone and increased blood serum levels. Hormone stimulates mitochondria to increase energy for cellular activities and heat production. As metabolic rate increases, fat reserves are utilized, despite increased appetite and food intake. Cardiac output is increased to meet increased tissue metabolic needs, and peripheral vasodilation occurs in response to increased heat production. Neuromuscular hyperactivity → accentuation of reflexes, anxiety, and increased alimentary tract mobility. *Graves' disease* is caused by stimulation of the gland by immunoglobulins of the IgG class.

B. Risk factors:

1. Possible autoimmune response resulting in increase of a gamma globulin called *long-acting thyroid stimulator* (LATS).

2. Occurs in third and fourth decade.

3. Affects women more than men.

4. Emotional trauma, infection, increased stress.

5. Overdose of medications used to treat hypothyroidism.

6. Use of certain weight-loss products.

◆ **C. Assessment:**

1. *Subjective data:*

a. Nervousness, mood swings.

b. Palpitations.

c. Heat intolerance.

d. Dyspnea.

e. Weakness.

2. *Objective data:*

a. Eyes: exophthalmos, characteristic stare, lid lag.

b. Skin:

(1) Warm, moist, velvety.

(2) Increased sweating; increased melanin pigmentation.

(3) Pretibial edema with thickened skin and hyperpigmentation.

c. Weight loss *despite* increased appetite.

d. Muscle: weakness, tremors, hyperkinesia.

e. Vital signs: BP—increased systolic pressure, widened pulse pressure; tachycardia.

f. Goiter: thyroid gland noticeable and palpable.

g. Gynecological: abnormal menstruation.

h. GI: frequent bowel movements.

i. Activity pattern: overactivity leads to fatigue, which leads to depression, which stimulates patient into overactivity, and pattern continues. *Danger:* total exhaustion.

j. Lab data:

(1) *Elevated:* serum T_4 (>11 μg/100 mL), free T_4 or free T_4 index, T_3 level (>35%) and free T_3 level.

(2) *Elevated:* thyroid uptake of radioiodine (RAIU).

(3) *Elevated:* metabolic rate (BMR).

(4) *Decreased:* WBC caused by *decreased* granulocytosis (<4500).

◆ **D. Analysis/nursing diagnosis:**

1. *Altered nutrition, less than body requirements,* related to elevated basal metabolic rate.

2. *Risk for injury* related to exophthalmos and tremors.

3. *Activity intolerance* related to fatigue from overactivity.

4. *Fatigue* related to overactivity.

5. *Anxiety* related to tachycardia.

6. *Sleep pattern disturbance* related to excessive amounts of circulating thyroid hormone.

Adult

◆ **E. Nursing care plan/implementation:**
1. Goal: *protect from stress:* private room, restrict visitors, quiet environment.
2. Goal: *promote physical and emotional equilibrium.*
   a. Environment: quiet, cool, well ventilated.
   b. Eye care:
      (1) Sunglasses to protect from photophobia, dust, wind.
      (2) Protective drops (methylcellulose) to soothe exposed cornea.
   c. *Diet:*
      (1) *High:* calorie, protein, vitamin B.
      (2) 6 meals/day, as needed.
      (3) Weigh daily.
      (4) *Avoid* stimulants (coffee, tea, colas, tobacco).
3. Goal: *prevent complications.*
   a. Medications as ordered:
      (1) Propylthiouracil to block thyroid synthesis; hyperthyroidism returns when therapy is stopped.
      (2) Methimazole (Tapazole) to inhibit synthesis of thyroid hormone.
      (3) Iodine preparations: used in combination with other medications when hyperthyroidism not well controlled; saturated solution of potassium iodide (SSKI) or *Lugol's* solution; more palatable if diluted with water, milk, or juice; give through a *straw* to prevent staining teeth. Takes 2–4 wk before results are evident.
      (4) Propranolol (Inderal), atenolol (Tenormin), metoprolol (Lopressor) given to counteract the increased metabolic effect of thyroid hormones, but do not alter their levels. Relieve the symptoms of tachycardia, tremors, and anxiety.
   b. Monitor for *thyroid storm (crisis)*—**medical emergency:** acute episode of thyroid overactivity caused when increased amounts of thyroid hormone are released into the bloodstream and metabolism is markedly increased.

   (1) **Risk factors** for thyroid storm: patient with uncontrolled hyperthyroidism (usually *Graves' disease*) who undergoes severe sudden stress, such as:
      (a) Infection.
      (b) Surgery.
      (c) Beginning labor to give birth.
      (d) Taking inadequate antithyroid medications before thyroidectomy.
   ◆ (2) **Assessment:**
      (a) *Subjective data*—thyroid storm:
         (i) Apprehension.
         (ii) Restlessness.
      (b) *Objective data*—thyroid storm:
         (i) Vital signs: elevated temperature (106°F), hypotension, extreme tachycardia.
         (ii) Marked respiratory distress, pulmonary edema.
         (iii) Weakness and delirium.
         (iv) **If untreated, patient could die of heart failure.**
   (3) Medications—thyroid storm:
      (a) Propylthiouracil or methimazole (Tapazole) *to decrease synthesis of thyroid hormone.*
      (b) Sodium iodide IV; Lugol's solution orally *to facilitate thyroid hormone synthesis.*
      (c) Propranolol (Inderal) *to slow heart rate.*
      (d) Aspirin *to decrease temperature.*
      (e) Steroids *to combat crisis.*
      (f) Diuretics, digitalis *to treat heart failure.*
4. Goal: *health teaching.*
   a. Stress-reduction techniques.
   b. Importance of medications, their desired effects and side effects.
   c. Methods to protect eyes from environmental damage.
   d. Signs and symptoms of thyroid storm (see E. 3. b., p. 598).
5. Goal: *prepare for additional treatment as needed.*
   a. *Radioactive iodine therapy:* 131I, a radioactive isotope of iodine to decrease thyroid activity.
      (1) 131I dissolved in water and given by mouth.
      (2) Hospitalization necessary only when large dose is administered.
      (3) Minimal precautions needed for usual dose.
         (a) Sleep alone for several nights.
         (b) Flush toilet several times after use.
      (4) Effectiveness of therapy seen in 2–3 wk; single dose controls 90% of patients.
      (5) Monitor for signs of hypothyroidism.
   b. Surgery: see **XVI.** Thyroidectomy, following.
◆ **F. Evaluation/outcome criteria:**
1. Complications avoided.
2. Compliance with medical regimen.
3. No further weight loss.
4. Able to obtain adequate sleep.

XVI. Thyroidectomy: partial removal of thyroid gland (for hyperthyroidism) or total removal (for malignancy of thyroid).

A. **Risk factor:** unsuccessful medical treatment of hyperthyroidism.

◆ B. **Analysis/nursing diagnosis:**
1. *Risk for injury* related to possible trauma to parathyroid gland during surgery.
2. *Ineffective breathing pattern* related to neck incision.
3. *Pain* related to surgical incision.
4. *Altered nutrition, less than body requirements,* related to difficulty in swallowing because of neck incision.
5. *Impaired verbal communication* related to possible trauma to nerve during surgery.
6. *Risk for altered body temperature* related to thyroid storm.

◆ C. **Nursing care plan/implementation:** *Prepare for surgery* (see **I.** Preoperative preparation, p. 500). *Postoperative:*
1. Goal: *promote physical and emotional equilibrium.*
   a. *Position:* semi-Fowler's to reduce edema.
   b. Immobilize head with pillows/sandbags.
   c. Support head during position changes to *avoid* stress on sutures, prevent flexion or hyperextension of neck.
2. Goal: *prevent complications of hypocalcemia and tetany,* due to accidental trauma to parathyroid gland during surgery; signs of tetany indicate necessity of *calcium gluconate IV.*
   a. Check *Chvostek's sign*—tapping face in front of ear produces spasm of facial muscles.
   b. Check *Trousseau's sign*—compression of upper arm (usually with BP cuff) elicits carpal (wrist) spasm.
   c. Monitor for *respiratory distress* (due to laryngeal nerve injury, edema, bleeding); keep tracheostomy set/suction equipment at bedside.
   d. Monitor for elevated temperature, indicative of *thyroid storm* (see objective assessment data for thyroid storm).
   e. Monitor vital signs, check dressing and beneath head, shoulders for bleeding q1h and prn for 24 hr; *hemorrhage* is possible complication; if swallowing is difficult, loosen dressing. If patient still complains of tightness when dressing is loosened, look for further signs of hemorrhage.
   f. Check voice postoperatively as soon as responsive after anesthesia and every hour (assess for possible *laryngeal nerve damage*); crowing voice sound indicates laryngeal nerves on both sides have been injured; *respiratory distress possible from swelling.*
      (1) *Avoid* unnecessary talking to lessen hoarseness.
      (2) Provide alternative means of communication.
3. Goal: *promote comfort measures.*
   a. Narcotics as ordered.
   b. Offer iced fluids.
   c. Ambulation and *soft diet,* as tolerated.
4. Goal: *health teaching.*
   a. How to support neck to prevent pressure on suture line: place both hands behind neck when moving head or coughing.
   b. Signs of hypothyroidism; needs supplemental thyroid hormone if total thyroidectomy.
   c. Signs and symptoms of hemorrhage and respiratory distress.
   d. Importance of adequate rest and nutritious diet.
   e. Importance of voice rest in early recuperative period.

◆ D. **Evaluation/outcome criteria:**
1. No respiratory distress, hemorrhage, laryngeal damage, tetany.
2. Preoperative symptoms relieved.
3. Normal range of neck motion obtained.
4. States signs and symptoms of possible complications.

XVII. Hypothyroidism (myxedema): deficiency of circulating thyroid hormone; often a final consequence of *Hashimoto's thyroiditis* and *Graves' disease.*

A. **Pathophysiology:** atrophy, destruction of gland by endogenous antibodies or inadequate pituitary thyrotropin production → insidious slowing of body processes, personality changes, and generalized, interstitial nonpitting (mucinous) edema—myxedema; pronounced involvement in systems with high protein turnover (e.g., cardiac, GI, reproductive, hematopoietic).

B. **Risk factors:**
1. Total thyroidectomy; inadequate replacement therapy.
2. Inherited autosomal recessive gene coding for disorder.
3. Hypophyseal failure.
4. Dietary iodine deficiencies.
5. Irradiation of thyroid gland.
6. Overtreatment of hyperthyroidism.
7. Chronic lymphocytic thyroiditis.
8. Postpartum thyroiditis.
9. Viral thyroiditis.
10. Medications, such as amiodarone HCl (Cordarone), used to treat abnormal heart rhythms.

◆ C. **Assessment:**
1. *Subjective data:*
   a. Weakness, fatigue, lethargy.
   b. Headache.
   c. Slow memory, psychotic behavior.
   d. Loss of interest in sexual activity.
2. *Objective data:*
   a. Depressed basal metabolism rate (BMR).

b. Cardiomegaly, bradycardia, hypotension, anemia.
c. Menorrhagia, amenorrhea, infertility.
d. Dry skin, brittle nails, coarse hair, hair loss.
e. Slow speech, hoarseness, thickened tongue.
f. Weight gain: edema, generalized interstitial; peripheral nonpitting; periorbital puffiness.
g. Intolerance to cold.
h. Hypersensitive to narcotics and barbiturates.
i. *Lab data:*
> (a) *Elevated:* thyroid-releasing hormone (TRH), thyroid-stimulating hormone (TSH), cholesterol (>220 mg/dL), lipids (>850 mg/dL), protein (>8g/dL).
> (b) *Normal-low:* serum thyroxine (T_4), serum triiodothyrinine (T_3).
> (c) *Decreased:* radioactive iodine uptake (RAIU).

◆ **D. Analysis/nursing diagnosis:**
1. *Risk for injury* related to hypersensitivity to drugs.
2. *Altered nutrition, more than body requirements,* related to decreased BMR.
3. *Activity intolerance* related to fatigue.
4. *Constipation* related to decreased peristalsis.
5. *Decreased cardiac output* related to hypotension and bradycardia.
6. *Risk for impaired skin integrity* related to dry skin and edema.
7. *Social isolation* related to lethargy.

◆ **E. Nursing care plan/implementation:**
1. Goal: *provide for comfort and safety.*
   a. Monitor for infection or trauma; may precipitate *myxedema coma,* which is manifested by: unresponsiveness, bradycardia, hypoventilation, hypothermia, and hypotension.
   b. Provide warmth; prevent heat loss and vascular collapse.
   c. Administer thyroid medications as ordered: levothyroxine (Synthroid)—most common drug used; liothyronine sodium (Cytomel); dosage adjusted according to symptoms.
2. Goal: *health teaching.*
   a. *Diet: low* calorie, *high* protein.
   b. Signs and symptoms of hypothyroidism and hyperthyrodism.
   c. Lifelong medications, dosage, desired effects and side effects.
   d. Medication dosage adjustment: take one-third to one-half the usual dose of narcotics and barbiturates.
   e. Stress-management techniques.
   f. Exercise program.

◆ **F. Evaluation/outcome criteria:**
1. No complications noted. Most common complications: atherosclerotic coronary heart disease, acute organic psychosis, and myxedema coma.
2. Dietary instructions followed.
3. Medication regimen followed.
4. Thyroid hormone balance obtained and maintained.

XVIII. Cushing's disease: an endogenous overproduction of adrenocorticotropic hormone (ACTH) that can be caused by pituitary-dependent adenomas. **Cushing's syndrome:** condition marked by chronic excessive circulating cortisol with or without pituitary involvement. One of the most common causes of Cushing's syndrome is the administration of cortisone-like medications for treatment of a variety of conditions.

A. Pathophysiology:
1. Excess glucocorticoid production, leading to:
   a. *Increased* gluconeogenesis → raised serum-glucose levels → glucose in urine, increased fat deposits in face and trunk.
   b. *Decreased* amino acids → protein deficiencies, muscle wasting, poor antibody response, and lack of collagen.

B. Risk factors:
1. Adrenal hyperplasia.
2. Excessive hypothalamic stimulation.
3. Tumors: adrenal, hypophyseal, pituitary, bronchogenic, or gallbladder.
4. Excessive steroid therapy.

◆ **C. Assessment:**
1. *Subjective data:*
   a. Headache, backache.
   b. Weakness, decreased work capacity.
   c. Mood swings.
2. *Objective data:*
   a. Hypertension, weight gain, pitting edema.
   b. Characteristic fat deposits, truncal and cervical obesity (buffalo hump).
   c. Pendulous abdomen, purple striae, easy bruising.
   d. Moon face, acne.
   e. Hyperpigmentation.
   f. Impotence.
   g. Virilization in women: hirsutism, breast atrophy, and amenorrhea.
   h. Pathological fractures, reduced height.
   i. Slow wound healing.
   j. Lab data:
   > (1) Urine: *elevated* 17-ketosteroids (>12 mg/24 hr) and glucose (>120 mg/dL).
   > (2) Plasma: *elevated* 17-hydroxycorticosteroids, cortisol (>10 >μg/dL). Cortisol *does not decrease during the day* as it should.
   > (3) Serum: *elevated*—glucose, RBC, WBC; *diminished*—potassium, chlorides, eosinophils, lymphocytes.

k. X-rays and scans to determine tumors/metastasis.

◆ **D. Analysis/nursing diagnosis:**

1. *Body image disturbance* related to changes in physical appearance.
2. *Activity intolerance* related to backache and weakness.
3. *Risk for injury* related to infection and bleeding.
4. *Knowledge deficit* related to management of disease.
5. *Pain* related to headache.

◆ **E. Nursing care plan/implementation.**

1. Goal: *promote comfort.*
   a. Assist with preparation of diagnostic workup.
   b. Explain procedures.
   c. Protect from trauma.
2. Goal: *prevent complications;* monitor for:
   a. Fluid balance—I&O, daily weights.
   b. Glucose metabolism—blood, urine for sugar and acetone.
   c. Hypertension—vital signs.
   d. Infection—skin care, urinary tract; check temperature.
   e. Mood swings—observe behavior.
3. Goal: *health teaching.*
   a. Diet: *increased* protein, potassium; *decreased* calories, sodium.
   b. Medications:
      (1) Cytotoxic agents: aminoglutethimide (Cytadren), trilostane (Modrastane), mitotane (Lysodren)—decrease cortisol production.
      (2) Replacement hormones as needed.
   c. Signs and symptoms of progression of disease as noted in assessment.
   d. Preparation for adrenalectomy if medical regimen unsuccessful.

◆ **F. Evaluation/outcome criteria:**

1. Symptoms controlled by medication.
2. No complications—adrenal steroids within normal limits.
3. If adrenalectomy necessary, see following section.

XIX. **Adrenalectomy:** surgical removal of adrenal glands because of tumors or uncontrolled overactivity; also bilateral adrenalectomy may be performed to control metastatic breast or prostate cancer.

A. **Risk factors:**
   1. Pheochromocytoma.
   2. Adrenal hyperplasia.
   3. Cushing's syndrome.
   4. Metastasis of prostate or breast cancer.
   5. Adrenal cortex or medulla tumors.

◆ B. **Assessment:**
   1. *Objective data:* validated evidence of:
      a. Benign lesion (unilateral adrenalectomy) or malignant tumor (bilateral adrenalectomy).

b. Adrenal hyperfunction that cannot be managed medically.
c. Bilateral excision for metastasis of breast and sometimes metastasis of prostate cancer.

◆ **C. Analysis/nursing diagnosis:**

1. *Knowledge deficit* related to planned surgery.
2. *Risk for physical injury* related to hormone imbalance.
3. *Risk for decreased cardiac output* related to possible hypotensive state resulting from surgery.
4. *Risk for infection* related to decreased normal resistance.
5. *Altered health maintenance* related to need for self-administration of steroid medications, orally or by injection.

◆ **D. Nursing care plan/implementation:**

1. Goal: *preoperative: reduce risk of postoperative complications.*
   a. Prescribed steroid therapy, given 1 wk before surgery, is gradually decreased; will be given again postoperatively.
   b. Antihypertensive drugs are discontinued because surgery may result in severe hypotension.
   c. Sedation as ordered.
   d. General preoperative measures (see p. 500).
2. Goal: *postoperative: promote hormonal balance.*
   a. Administer hydrocortisone parenteral therapy as ordered; rate indicated by fluid and electrolyte balance, blood sugar, and blood pressure.
   b. Monitor for signs of *Addisonian (adrenal) Crisis* (see p. 602).
3. Goal: *prevent postoperative complications.*
   a. Monitor vital signs until stability is regained; if on *vasopressor* drugs such as metaraminol (Aramine):
      (1) Maintain flow rate as ordered.
      (2) Monitor BP q5–15 min, notify physician of significant elevations in BP (dose needs to be decreased) or drop in BP (dose needs to be increased). *Note:* readings that are normotensive for some may be hypotensive for patients who have been hypertensive.
   ▶ b. NPO—attach *nasogastric tube* to intermittent suction; abdominal distention is common side effect of this surgery.
   c. Respiratory care:
      (1) Turn, cough, and deep breathe.
      (2) Splint flank incision when coughing.
      (3) Administer narcotics to reduce pain and allow patient to cough; flank incision is close to diaphragm, making coughing very painful.
   ▶ (4) Auscultate breath sounds q2h; decreased or absent sounds could indicate pneumothorax.

(5) Sudden chest pain and dyspnea should be reported *immediately* (spontaneous pneumothorax).

☑ d. *Position: flat* or *semi*-Fowler's.

e. Mouth care.

f. Monitor dressings for bleeding; reinforce prn.

g. Ambulation, as ordered.
(1) Check BP q15min when ambulation is first attempted.
(2) Place elastic stockings on lower extremities to enhance stability of vascular system.

h. *Diet*—once NG tube removed, diet as tolerated.

4. Goal: *health teaching.*

a. *Signs and symptoms of adrenal crisis:*
(1) Pulse: rapid, weak, or thready.
(2) Temperature: elevated.
(3) Severe weakness and hypotension.
(4) Headache.
(5) Convulsions, coma.

b. Importance of maintaining steroid therapy schedule to ensure therapeutic serum level.

c. Weigh daily.

d. Monitor blood-glucose levels daily.

e. Report undesirable side effects of steroid therapy or adrenal crisis to physician.

f. *Avoid* persons with infections, due to decreased resistance.

g. Daily schedule: include adequate rest, moderate exercise, good nutrition.

◆ **E. Evaluation/outcome criteria:**

1. Adrenal crisis avoided.
a. Vitals within normal limits.
b. No neurological deficits noted.

2. Healing progresses: no signs of infection or wound complications.

3. Adjusts to alterations in physical status.
a. Complies with medication regimen.
b. Avoids infections.
c. Incorporates good nutrition, periods of rest and activity into daily schedule.

XX. Addison's disease: chronic primary adrenal corticotropic insufficiency. A hormonal (endocrine) disorder involving destruction of the adrenal glands, which then are unable to produce sufficient adrenal hormones (cortisol) necessary for the normal body functions.

A. Pathophysiology:

1. Atrophy of adrenal gland is most common cause of adrenal insufficiency; manifested by *decreased* adrenal cortical secretions.

a. Deficiency in mineralocorticoid secretion *(aldosterone)* → increased sodium excretion → dehydration → hypotension → decreased cardiac output and resulting decrease in heart size.

b. Deficiency in glucocorticoid secretion *(cortisol)* → decrease in gluconeogenesis → hypoglycemia and liver glycogen deficiency, emotional disturbances, diminished resistance to stress. Cortisol deficiency → failure to inhibit anterior pituitary secretion of ACTH and melanocyte-stimulating hormone → increased levels of ACTH and hyperpigmentation.

c. Deficiency in androgen hormone → less axillary and pubic hair in women (testes supply adequate sex hormone in men, so no symptoms are produced).

B. Risk factors:

1. Autoimmune processes.
2. Infection.
3. Malignancy.
4. Vascular obstruction.
5. Bleeding.
6. Environmental hazards.
7. Congenital defects.
8. Bilateral adrenalectomy.
9. Tuberculosis.

◆ **C. Assessment:**

1. *Subjective data:*
a. Muscle weakness, fatigue, lethargy.
b. Dizziness, fainting.
c. Nausea, food idiosyncrasies, anorexia.
d. Abdominal pain/cramps.

2. *Objective data:*
a. Vital signs: decreased BP, orthostatic hypotension, widened pulse pressure.
b. Pulse—increased, collapsing, irregular.
c. Temperature—subnormal.
d. Vomiting, diarrhea, and weight loss.
e. Tremors.
f. Skin: poor turgor, excessive pigmentation (bronze tone).
g. Lab data:
(1) Blood:
(a) *Decreased:* sodium (<135 mEq/L); glucose (<60 mg/dL), chloride (<98 mEq/L), bicarbonate (<23 mEq/L).
(b) *Increased:* hematocrit, potassium (>5 mEq/L).
(2) Urine: *decreased* (or absent) 17-ketosteroids, 17-hydroxycorticosteroids (<5 mg/24 hr).
h. *Diagnostic tests:*
(1) CT scan, MRI.
(2) ACTH stimulation test (cortisol levels are measured *before* and *after* administration of synthetic ACTH).

◆ **D. Analysis/nursing diagnosis:**

1. *Fluid volume deficit* related to decreased sodium.

2. *Altered renal tissue perfusion* related to hypotension.

3. *Decreased cardiac output* related to aldosterone deficiency.

4. *Risk for infection* related to cortisol deficiency.

5. *Activity intolerance* related to muscle weakness and fatigue.

6. *Altered nutrition, less than body requirements,* related to nausea, anorexia, and vomiting.

◆ **E. Nursing care plan/implementation:**

1. Goal: *decrease stress.*
   a. Environment: quiet, nondemanding schedule.
   b. Anticipate events for which extra resources will be necessary.

2. Goal: *promote adequate nutrition.*
   a. *Diet: acute phase—high* sodium, *low* potassium; *nonacute phase—increase* carbohydrates and protein.
   b. *Fluids:* force, to balance fluid losses; monitor I&O, daily weights.
   c. Administer lifelong exogenous replacement therapy as ordered:
      (1) *Glucocorticoids*—prednisone, hydrocortisone.
      (2) *Mineralocorticoids*—fludrocortisone (Florinef).

3. Goal: *health teaching.*
   a. Take medications *with* food or milk.
   b. May need antacid therapy to prevent GI disturbances.
   c. Side effects of steroid therapy.
   d. *Avoid* stress; may need adjustment in medication dosage when stress is increased.
   e. Signs and symptoms of *addisonian (adrenal) crisis:* very serious condition characterized by severe hypotension, shock, coma, and vasomotor collapse related to strenuous activity, infection, stress, omission of prescribed medications. **If untreated, could quickly lead to death.**

4. Goal: *prevent serious complications if Addisonian Crisis evident.*
   a. Complete bed rest; *avoid* stimuli.
   b. High dose of hydrocortisone IV or cortisone IM.
   c. Treat shock—IV saline.
   d. I&O, vital signs q15min to 1 hr or prn until crisis passes.

◆ **F. Evaluation/outcome criteria:**

1. No complications occur.
2. Medication regimen followed, is adequate for patient's needs.
3. Adequate nutrition and fluid balance obtained.

XXI. Multiple sclerosis: progressive neurological disease, common in northern climates, characterized by demyelination of brain and spinal cord leading to degenerative neurological function; chronic remitting and relapsing disease; cause unknown. Visual problems are often the first indication of multiple sclerosis. Classifications of multiple sclerosis: relapsing-remitting, primary-progressive, secondary-progressive, and progressive-relapsing. Exacerbations aggravated by fatigue, chilling, and emotional distress.

A. Pathophysiology: multiple foci (patches) of nerve degeneration throughout brain, spinal cord, optic nerve, and cerebrum cause nerve impulses to be interrupted (blocked) or distorted (slowed). Researchers suggest that in genetically susceptible people, the disease results from an abnormal autoimmune response to some agent, perhaps a virus or environmental trigger.

B. Risk factors:

1. Northern climate.
2. Onset age: 20–40 yr.
3. Two to three times more common in women than men.

◆ **C. Assessment:**

1. *Subjective data:*
   a. Extremities: weak, numb, decreased sensation.
   b. Emotional instability, apathy, irritability, mood swings, fatigue.
   c. Eyes: diplopia (double vision), spots before eyes (scotomas), potential blindness.
   d. Difficulty in swallowing.
   e. Pain.

2. *Objective data:*
   a. Nystagmus (involuntary rhythmic movements of eyeball) and decreased visual acuity.
   b. Inappropriate outbursts of laughing or crying (sometimes related to ingestion of hot food).
   c. Disorders of speech.
   d. Susceptible to infections.
   e. Tremors to severe muscle spasms and contractures.
   f. Changes in muscular coordination; *gait:* ataxic, spastic.
   g. Changes in bowel habits, e.g., constipation.
   h. Urinary frequency and urgency.
   i. Incontinence (urine and feces).
   j. Sexual dysfunction.
   k. Cognitive changes/depression.
   l. *Lab tests:* cerebrospinal fluid has presence of gamma globulin IgG.
   m. *Diagnostic tests:*
      (1) Neurological examination.
      (2) Positive *Lhermitte's* sign (electric shock–like sensation along spine on flexion of the head).
      (3) Positive Babinski reflex.
      (4) MRI detects plaques.

◆ **D. Analysis/nursing diagnosis:**

1. *Impaired physical mobility* related to changes in muscular coordination.

2. *Self-esteem disturbance* related to chronic, debilitating disease.
3. *Altered health maintenance* related to spasms and contractures.
4. *Risk for impaired skin integrity* related to contractures.
5. *Constipation* related to immobility.
6. *Impaired swallowing* related to tremors.
7. *Visual sensory/perceptual alteration* related to nystagmus and decreased visual acuity.

◆ **E. Nursing care plan/implementation:**
1. Goal: *maintain normal routine as long as possible.*
   a. Maintain mobility—encourage walking as tolerated; active and passive ROM; splints to decrease spasticity.
   b. *Avoid* fatigue, infections.
   c. Frequent position changes to prevent skin breakdown and contractures; *position at night: prone* to minimize flexor spasms of knees and hips.
   d. Bowel/bladder training program to minimize incontinence.
   e. *Avoid* stressful situations.
2. Goal: *decrease symptoms*—medications as ordered:
   a. Methylprednisolone (high dose, IV) plus sodium succinate, followed by gradual tapering of steroids to treat at initial diagnosis.
   b. Methylprednisolone (Solu-Medrol), prednisone (Deltasone), and dexamethasone (Decadron) used to treat acute relapses.
   c. Methotrexate (Rheumatrex) (low dose) used to delay progression of impairment.
   d. Interferon β-1b (Betaseron) reduces number of lesions and frequency of relapses.
   e. Glatiramer (Copaxone) to reduce number of relapses.
   f. Baclofen (Lioresal) for alleviating spasticity 5 mg three times daily, increased by 5 mg every three days; not to exceed 80 mg/day (20 mg four times daily). Optimal effect between 40 and 80 mg; sudden withdrawal of medication may cause *hallucinations* and *rebound spasticity.*
   g. Diazepam (Valium), dantrolene (Dantrium) to relieve *muscle spasm.*
   h. Carbamazepine (Tegretol) or amitriptyline HCl (Elavil) for dysesthesias or neuralgia.
   i. Ciprofloxacin (Cipro) to treat bladder dysfunction.
   j. Psyllium hydrophilic mucilloid (Metamucil) to treat bowel dysfunction.
   k. Phenytoin (Dilantin) to treat sensory symptoms.
   l. Analgesics to treat pain.
3. Goal: *health teaching to prevent complications.*

   a. Signs and symptoms of disease; measures to prevent exacerbations.
   b. Teach to monitor respiratory status to prevent infections.
   c. Importance of physical therapy to prevent contractures.
   d. Possible counseling or community support group for assistance in accepting long-term condition.
   e. Teach special skin care to prevent decubitus ulcers.
   f. Teach use of assistive devices to maintain independence.
4. Goal: *provide psychosocial support.*
   a. Answer questions of patient and family members.
   b. Provide referrals to appropriate agencies.
   c. Monitor for signs of suicide (higher incidence of suicide in patients with MS than the general population).
   d. Encourage communication.

◆ **F. Evaluation/outcome criteria:**
1. Establishes daily routine; adjusts to altered lifestyle.
2. Injuries prevented; no falls.
3. Urinary and bowel routines established; incontinence decreased.
4. Infections avoided.
5. Symptoms minimized by medications.

XXII. **Myasthenia gravis:** Chronic neuromuscular disease characterized by weakness and easy fatigability of facial, oculomotor, pharyngeal, and respiratory muscles. The muscle weakness increases during periods of activity and improves after periods of rest.
   A. Pathophysiology: inadequate acetylcholine or excessive or altered cholinesterase, leading to impaired transmission of nerve impulses to muscles at myoneural junction.
   B. Risk factors:
   1. Possible autoimmune reaction.
   2. Thymus tumor.
   3. Young women and older men, but can occur at any age.
   ◆ **C. Assessment:**
   1. *Subjective data:*
      a. Diplopia (double vision).
      b. Severe generalized fatigue.
   2. *Objective data:*
      a. Muscle weakness: hands and arms affected first.
      b. Ptosis (drooping of eyelids), expressionless facies.
      c. Hypersensitivity to narcotics, barbiturates, tranquilizers.
      d. Abnormal speech pattern, with high-pitched nasal voice.
      e. Difficulty chewing/swallowing food.
      f. Decreased ability to cough and deep breathe, vital capacity.

g. Positive Tensilon test (administration of edrophonium chloride, 10 mg IV, produces relief of symptoms within 30 sec).

h. Positive Prostigmin test (1.5 mg subcutaneous neostigmine methylsulfate, produces relief of symptoms within 15 min; increased muscle strength within 30 min).

◆ **D. Analysis/nursing diagnosis:**
1. *Ineffective breathing pattern* related to weakness.
2. *Risk for injury* related to muscle weakness.
3. *Activity intolerance* related to severe fatigue.
4. *Bathing/dressing self-care deficit* related to progressive disease.
5. *Impaired physical mobility* related to decrease in strength.
6. *Anxiety* related to physical symptoms and disease progression.
7. *Knowledge deficit* related to medication administration and expected effectiveness.

◆ **E. Nursing care plan/implementation:**
1. Goal: *promote comfort.*
   a. Passive and active ROM, as tolerated, to increase strength.
   b. Mouth care: before and after meals.
   c. *Diet:* as tolerated, soft, pureed, or tube feedings.
   d. Skin care to prevent decubiti.
   e. Eye care: remove crusts; patch affected eye prn.
   f. Monitor respiratory status—suction airway prn.
2. Goal: *decrease symptoms.*
   a. Administer medications as ordered:
      (1) Anticholinesterase (neostigmine [Prostigmin], pyridostigmine [Mestinon]) to elevate concentration of acetylcholine at myoneural junction.
      (2) Give *before* meals to aid in chewing, *with* milk or food to decrease GI symptoms; may be given parenterally.
3. Goal: *prevent complications.*
   a. Respiratory assistance if breathing pattern not adequate.
   b. Monitor for choking/increased oral secretion.
   c. **Avoid:** narcotics, barbiturates, tranquilizers.
4. Goal: *promote increased self-concept.*
   a. Encourage independence when appropriate.
   b. Encourage communication; provide alternative methods when speech pattern impaired.
5. Goal: *health teaching.*
   a. Medication information:
      (1) Adjust dosage to maintain muscle strength.
      (2) Medication must be taken at prescribed time to avoid:

(a) *Myasthenic crisis* (too little medication).
(b) *Cholinergic crisis* (too much medication).
   b. *Signs and symptoms of crisis:* dyspnea, severe muscle weakness, respiratory distress, difficulty in swallowing.
   c. Importance of *avoiding upper respiratory infections.*
   d. Determine methods to conserve energy, to maintain independence as long as possible, while avoiding overexertion.
   e. *Refer* to Myasthenia Gravis Foundation and other *community agencies* for assistance in reintegration into the community and plans for follow-up care.

◆ **F. Evaluation/outcome criteria:**
1. Independence maintained as long as possible.
2. Respiratory arrest avoided.
3. Infection avoided.
4. Medication regimen followed and crisis avoided.

XXIII. Parkinson's disease: progressive disease of the brain occurring generally in later life; characterized by stiffness of muscles and by tremors.

A. Pathophysiology: depigmentation of the substantia nigra of basal ganglia → decreased dopamine (neurotransmitter necessary for proper muscle movement) → decreased and slowed voluntary movement, masklike facies, and difficulty initiating ambulation. Decreased inhibitions of alpha-motoneurons → increased muscle tone → rigidity of both flexor and extensor muscles and tremors at rest.

B. Risk factors:
1. Age >40; most often 50–60 yr.
2. Affects men and women equally.
3. Cause unknown; possibly connected to arteriosclerosis or viral infection.
4. Drug-induced parkinsonian syndromes have been linked to:
   a. Phenothiazines.
   b. Reserpine (Serpasil).
   c. Butyrophenones (haloperidol).

◆ **C. Assessment:**
1. *Subjective data:*
   a. Insomnia.
   b. Depression.
   c. Defects in judgment related to emotional instability; dementia (memory loss).
2. *Objective data:*
   a. Limbs, shoulders: stiff, offer resistance to passive ROM.
   b. Loss of coordination, muscular weakness with rigidity.
   c. Shuffling gait: difficulty in initiating, then propulsive, trunk bent forward.
   d. Tremors: pill-rolling of fingers, to-and-fro head movements.

e. Loss of postural reflexes.

f. Weight loss, constipation.

g. Difficulty in maintaining social interactions because of impaired speech, lack of facial affect, drooling.

h. Facies: wide-eyed, decreased eye blinking, decreased facial expression.

i. Akinesia (abnormal absence of movement).

j. Excessive salivation, drooling.

k. Speech: slowed, slurred.

l. Judgment defective (e.g., poor decision making); intelligence intact.

m. Heat intolerance.

◆ **D. Analysis/nursing diagnosis:**

1. *Impaired physical mobility* related to loss of coordination.

2. *Altered health maintenance* related to defective judgment.

3. *Risk for injury* related to altered gait.

4. *Dressing/grooming self-care deficit* related to muscular rigidity.

5. *Sleep pattern disturbance* related to insomnia.

6. *Body image disturbance* related to tremors and drooling.

7. *Social isolation* related to altered physical appearance.

8. *Altered nutrition, less than body requirements,* related to lack of appetite.

9. *Impaired swallowing* related to excessive drooling.

10. *Constipation* related to dietary changes.

◆ **E. Nursing care plan/implementation:**

1. Goal: *promote maintenance of daily activities.*

a. ROM exercises, skin care, physical therapy.

b. Encourage ambulation; discourage sitting for long periods.

c. Assist with meals—*high protein, high calorie; soft diet;* small, frequent feedings; encourage increased fluids.

d. Encourage compliance with medication regimen:

(1) *Dopamine agonists:*

(a) Levodopa: given in increasing doses until symptoms are relieved; given *with food* to decrease GI symptoms. *Side effects:* nausea, vomiting, anorexia, postural hypotension, mental changes, cardiac arrhythmias. Levodopa (L-Dopa) helps restore dopamine deficiency in striated muscles: 500–1000 mg/day in divided doses; increase by 100–750 mg/day every 3–7 days until response reached; usual maintenance dose should not exceed 18 g/day.

(b) Carbidopa-levodopa (Sinemet): 25/250 mg/day in 3–4 divided doses. Limits the metabolism of levodopa peripherally and provides more levodopa for the brain.

(2) *Anticholinergics:* effective in lessening muscle rigidity.

(a) Benztropine mesylate (Cogentin): 0.5–6 mg/day in 1–2 divided doses.

(b) Biperiden (Akineton): 2 mg 3–4 times daily, not to exceed 16 mg/day.

(c) Trihexyphenidyl (Artane): 1–2 mg/day; increased by 2 mg every 3–5 days; usual maintenance dose 5–15 mg/day in 3–4 divided doses.

(3) *Antihistamines:* have mild central anticholinergic properties.

2. Goal: *protect from injury.*

a. Monitor BP, side effects of medications, e.g., orthostatic hypotension.

b. Monitor for GI disturbances.

c. *Avoid* pyridoxine (vitamin B_6): cancels effect of levodopa.

d. Levodopa *contraindicated* with:

(1) Glaucoma (causes increased intraocular pressure).

(2) Monoamine oxidase (MAO) inhibitors (causes possible hypertensive crisis).

3. Goal: *health teaching.*

a. Teach patient and family about medications: dosage range, side effects, not discontinuing medications abruptly.

b. Exercise program to maintain ROM and normal body posture; also to get adequate rest to prevent fatigue.

c. *Dietary adjustment and precautions* regarding cutting food in small pieces to prevent choking, taking fluid with food for easier swallowing.

d. Importance of adding *roughage* to *diet* to prevent constipation.

e. Assist patient and family to adjust to this chronic debilitating illness.

◆ **F. Evaluation/outcome criteria:**

1. Activity level maintained.

2. Symptoms relieved by medications; no drug interactions.

3. Complications avoided.

XXIV. Amyotrophic lateral sclerosis (ALS; Lou Gehrig's disease): progressive degeneration of motor neurons within the brain, spinal cord, or both, leading to death within 2–7 years, usually from infection (pneumonia) or consequences of respiratory or bulbar paralysis. There are three types of ALS: classic sporadic, familial, and Mariana Islands (Guam).

A. Pathophysiology: myelin sheaths destroyed, replaced by scar tissue; involves lateral tracts of spinal cord, eventually medulla and ventral tracts.

B. Risk factors:

1. Affects men more than women.
2. Usually in middle age.
3. Viral infection possible causal agent.
4. Possible familial or genetic component.

◆ **C. Assessment:**

1. *Subjective data:*
   a. Early symptoms: fatigue, awkwardness.
   b. Dysphagia, dysarthria.
   c. Alert, no sensory loss.
2. *Objective data:*
   a. Symptoms depend on which motor neurons affected.
   b. Decreased fine finger movement.
   c. Progressive muscular weakness, atrophy, especially lower limbs at onset of disease; later, arms, hands, and shoulders.
   d. Spasticity of flexor muscles; one side of body becomes more involved than other.
   e. Progressive respiratory difficulties → diaphragmatic paralysis.
   f. Progressive disability of upper and lower extremities.
   g. Fasciculations (muscle twitching visible under skin).
   h. *Diagnostic tests:*
      (1) Electromyography (EMG).
      (2) Nerve conduction velocities (NCV).

◆ **D. Analysis/nursing diagnosis:**

1. *Ineffective airway clearance* related to difficulty in coughing.
2. *Ineffective breathing pattern* related to progressive respiratory difficulties and eventually respiratory paralysis.
3. *Altered health maintenance* related to inability to perform self-care activities.
4. *Impaired physical mobility* related to progressive muscular weakness.
5. *Self-care deficits: bathing/hygiene and dressing/grooming*

6. *Powerlessness* related to lifestyle of progressive physical helplessness.
7. *Impaired swallowing* related to disease progression.

◆ **E. Nursing care plan/implementation:**

1. Goal: *maintain independence as long as possible.*
   a. Assistance with ADL; splints, prosthetic devices to support weak limbs and maintain mobility.
   b. Skin care to prevent decubiti.
   c. *Soft/liquid diet* to aid in swallowing, prevent choking; suction prn; *head of bed elevated* when eating.
   d. Respiratory assistance as needed; ventilators as disease progresses and diaphragm becomes involved.
   e. Arrange long-term care arrangements if home maintenance no longer feasible.
   f. Emotional support, when patient is alert; continue involving patient in decisions regarding care.
   g. Medications: riluzolet (Rilutek); has some effect in reducing disease progression; other drugs offer temporary relief of symptoms.
2. Goal: *health teaching.*
   a. Skin care to prevent decubitus ulcer.
   b. Explain ramifications of disease so patient and family can make decisions regarding future care, whether patient will remain at home as disease progresses or enter a long-term care facility.
   c. How to use suction apparatus to clear airway.
   d. Care of nasogastric or gastrostomy feeding tube.

◆ **F. Evaluation/outcome criteria:**

1. Obtains physical and emotional support.
2. Complications avoided in early stage of disease.
3. Remains in control of ADL as long as possible.
4. Skin breakdown avoided.
5. Peaceful death.

Adult

CANCER

I. The cancer patient: Cancer is a multisystem stressor. Regardless of the specific type of cancer, certain aspects of the disease and of nursing care are the same. The following principles apply universally and should be referred to when studying individual kinds of cancer.

A. Pathophysiology: result of altered cellular mechanisms. Several theories about causation, but current thinking is multiple causation. Alterations result in a progressive, uncontrolled multiplication of cells, with selective ability to invade and metastasize.

B. Risk factors:
1. Heredity, e.g., retinoblastoma.
2. Familial susceptibility, e.g., breast.
3. Acquired diseases, e.g., ulcerative colitis.
4. Virus, e.g., Burkitt's tumor.
5. Environmental factors:
   a. Tobacco.
   b. Alcohol.
   c. Radiation.
   d. Occupational hazards.
   e. Drugs, e.g., immunosuppressive, cytotoxic.
   f. Asbestos.
6. Age.
7. Air pollution.
8. Diet, e.g., high animal protein.
9. Chronic irritation.
10. Precancerous lesions, e.g., gastric ulcers.
11. Stress.

◆ **C. Assessment:**
1. Specific symptoms depend on the anatomical and functional characteristics of the organ or structure involved.
2. *Mechanical effects:*
   a. *Pressure*—tumors growing in confined areas such as bone produce pain early, whereas tumors growing in expandable areas such as the abdomen may be undetected for some time.
   b. *Obstruction*—tumors that compress tubular structures such as the esophagus, bronchi, or lymph channels may cause symptoms such as swallowing difficulties, shortness of breath, edema. Symptoms depend on location of tumor and on the particular organ or structure receiving pressure.
   c. *Interruptions of blood supply*—compression of blood vessels or diversion of blood supply may cause necrosis or ulceration or may precipitate hemorrhage.
3. *Systemic effects:*
   a. Anorexia, weakness, weight loss.
   b. Metabolic disturbances—malabsorption syndrome.
   c. Fluid and electrolyte imbalances.
   d. Hormonal imbalances—increased antidiuretic hormone (ADH), adrenocorticotropic hormone (ACTH), thyrotropin (TSH), or parathyroid hormone (PTH).
   e. *Diagnostic tests:*
      (1) *Biopsy*—excision of part of tumor mass.
      (2) *Needle biopsy*—aspiration of cells from subcutaneous masses or organs such as liver.
      (3) *Exfoliative cytology*—scraping of any endothelium (cervix, mucous membranes, skin) and applying to slide.
      (4) *X-rays*—detect tumor growth in GI, respiratory, and renal systems.
      (5) *Endoscopy*—visualization of body cavity through endoscope.
      (6) *Computed tomography (CT)*—visualization of a body part whereby layers of tissue can be seen utilizing the very narrow beams of this type of x-ray equipment.
      (7) *Magnetic resonance imaging (MRI)*—a scanning device using a magnetic field for visualization.
   f. Lab data:
      (1) *Blood and urine tests*—refer to **Appendix A** for normal values.
      (2) *Alkaline phosphatase*—greatly *increased* in osteogenic carcinoma (>92 U/L).
      (3) *Calcium*—*elevated* in multiple myeloma bone metastases (>10.5 mg/dL).
      (4) *Sodium*—*decreased* in bronchogenic carcinoma (<135 mEq/L).
      (5) *Potassium*—*decreased* in extensive liver carcinoma (<3.5 mEq/L).
      (6) *Serum gastrin*—measures gastric secretions. *Decreased* in gastric carcinoma. Normal value 0–180 ng/L.
      (7) *Neutrophilic leukocytosis*—tumors.
      (8) *Eosinophilic leukocytosis*—brain tumors, Hodgkin's disease.
      (9) *Lymphocytosis*—chronic lymphocytic anemia.

◆ **D. Analysis/nursing diagnosis:**
1. *Pain* related to diagnostic procedures, pressure, obstruction, interruption of blood supply, or potential side effects of drugs.
2. *Anxiety* related to fear of diagnosis or disease progression, treatment, and its known or expected side effects.
3. *Altered nutrition, less than body requirements,* related to anorexia.
4. *Risk for injury* related to radioactive contamination of excreta.
5. *Body image disturbance* related to loss of body parts, change in appearance as a result of therapy.

6. *Powerlessness* related to diagnosis and own perception of its meaning.

7. *Self-esteem disturbance* related to impact of cancer diagnosis.

8. *Risk for infection* related to immunosuppression from radiation and chemotherapy.

9. *Altered urinary elimination* related to dehydration.

10. *Risk for injury* related to normal tissue damage from radiation source.

11. *Fluid volume deficit* related to nausea and vomiting.

12. *Diarrhea* related to radiation of bowel.

13. *Constipation* related to dehydration.

◆ **E. Nursing care plan/implementation**—general care of the cancer patient:

1. Goal: *promote psychosocial comfort.* (See also **Unit 6.**)

   a. Assist with diagnostic workup by providing psychological support and information about specific disease, diagnostic tests, diagnosis, and treatment options.

   b. Reduce anxiety by listening, making referrals for special problems (peer support groups, self-help groups such as Reach to Recovery), supplying information, or correcting misinformation, as appropriate.

   c. Stress-management techniques (see Orientation, **Unit 1**).

   d. Nursing management related to depressed patient (see **Unit 6**).

2. Goal: *minimize effects of complications.*

   a. Anorexia/anemia:

      (1) *Decrease anemia* by:

         (a) Providing well-balanced, *iron-rich, small, frequent* meals.

         (b) Administering supplemental vitamins and iron as ordered.

         ▶ (c) Administering packed red blood cells as ordered.

         ▶ (d) Maintaining hyperalimentation as ordered.

         (e) Monitoring red blood cell count.

      (2) *Enhance nutrition* by providing nutritional supplements and a *diet high in protein*; necessary because of increased metabolism related to metastatic process. *Consult* with dietitian for suggestions of best food for individual patient.

   b. Hemorrhage: monitor platelet count and maintain platelet infusions as ordered. Teach patient to monitor for any signs of bleeding.

   c. Infection: observe for signs of sepsis (changes in vital signs, temperature of skin, mentation, urinary output or pain); monitor laboratory values (WBCs); administer antibiotics as ordered.

   d. Pain and discomfort: alleviate by frequent position changes, diversions, conversations, guided imagery, relaxation, back rubs, and narcotics as ordered.

   e. Assist in adjusting to altered body image by encouraging expression of fears and concerns. Do *not* ignore patient's questions, and give honest answers: be available.

   f. Fatigue. Encourage periods of rest and a decrease in daily exertion.

3. Goal: *general health teaching.*

   a. Self-care skills to maintain independence; e.g., patient who has a colostomy should know how to manage the colostomy before going home.

   b. Importance of follow-up care and routine physical examinations to monitor for general health and possible signs of further disease.

   c. Dietary instructions, adjustments necessary to maintain nutrition during and after treatment.

   d. Health maintenance programs: teach hazards of the use of tobacco and alcohol. *Avoid* high-fat, low-roughage diet.

   e. Risk factors: family history, stress, age, diet, occupation, environment.

   f. Access to information: patients should have telephone numbers where questions can be answered and symptoms reported 24 hours a day.

F. General surgical intervention: surgery may be *diagnostic, curative* (when the lesion is localized or with minimal metastases to the lymph nodes), *palliative* (to decrease symptomatology), or *reconstructive.* (Also see The Perioperative Experience, p. 500, and specific types of cancer, following.)

◆ 1. **Nursing care plan/implementation**—*preoperative:*

   a. Goal: *prevent respiratory complications.*

      (1) Coughing and deep-breathing techniques.

      (2) *No* smoking for 1 wk before surgery.

   b. Goal: *counteract nutritional deficiencies.*

      (1) *Diet:*

         (a) *High* protein, *high* carbohydrate for tissue repair.

         (b) Vitamin and mineral supplements.

         (c) Hyperalimentation as ordered.

      (2) Blood transfusions may be needed if counts are low.

   c. Goal: *reduce apprehension.*

      (1) Clarify postoperative expectations.

      (2) Explain care of ostomies or tubes.

      (3) Answer patient's questions honestly.

2. *Postoperative:*

   a. Goal: *prevent complications.*

(1) Monitor respiratory status and hemodynamic status.

▶ (2) Wound care; active and passive exercises as allowed; respiratory hygiene; coughing, deep breathing, and turning; fluids (see **III. Postoperative experience,** p. •••).

b. Goal: *alleviate pain and discomfort.*

(1) Encourage early ambulation, depending on surgical procedure.

(2) Administer prescribed medications as needed.

(3) Administer stool softeners and enemas as ordered.

c. Goal: *health teaching.*

(1) Involve patient, significant others, and family members in rehabilitation program.

(2) Prepare for further therapies, such as radiation or chemotherapy.

(3) *Support groups,* as appropriate: Reach to Recovery, Ostomy Associates, Laryngectomy Association.

(4) Develop skills to deal with disease progression if cure not realistic or metastasis evident (see **J.** Palliative care, p. 614).

G. **Chemotherapy:** used as single treatment or in combination with surgery and radiation, for early or advanced diseases. Used to cure, increase survival time, or decrease specific life-threatening complications. Antineoplastic agents' primary mode of action involves interfering with the supply and utilization of building blocks of nucleic acids, as well as interfering with intact molecules of DNA or RNA, which are needed for replication and cell growth. Bone marrow, hair follicles, and the gastrointestinal tract are three areas of the body in which cells are actively dividing; this is why most side effects are related to these areas of the body. Most often antineoplastic agents are used in combination.

1. *Types: alkylating* agents, *antimetabolites, antitumor antibiotics, antimiotic* agents, *plant alkaloids, enzymes, hormones,* and *biotherapy.* (e.g., BCG, interferon) (see Table 10–8).

2. *Major problem:* lacks specificity, thus affecting normal as well as malignant cells.

3. *Major side effects:* bone marrow depression, stomatitis, nausea and vomiting, gastrointestinal ulcerations, diarrhea, and alopecia (Table 7–41).

4. *Routes of administration:* oral, intramuscular, intravenous (*Hickman or Groshong catheter*), subclavian lines, porta caths, peripheral, intra-arterial (may have infusion pump for continuous or intermittent flow rate), intracavity (e.g., bladder through cystoscopy). (See p. 611 for information about administration of IV chemotherapeutic agents.)

◆ 5. **Nursing care plan/implementation:**

a. Goal: *assist with treatment of specific side effects.*

(1) *Nausea and vomiting*—antiemetic drugs as ordered and scheduled; small, frequent, *high-calorie, high-potassium, high-protein* meals; chopped or blended foods for ease in swallowing; include milk and milk products when tolerated for *increased calcium;* carbonated drinks; frequent mouth care; *antacid* therapy as ordered; rest after meals; *avoid* food odors during preparation of meals; pleasant environment during meals; appropriate

▶ distractions; IV therapy; *nasogastric* tube for control of severe nausea or as route for *tube feeding* if unable to take food by mouth; *hyperalimentation.*

(2) *Diarrhea*—low-residue diet; *increased potassium;* increased fluids; atropine SO_4–diphenoxylate HCl (Lomotil) or kaolin-pectin (Kaopectate) as ordered; *avoid* hot or cold foods/liquids.

(3) *Stomatitis* (painful mouth)—soft toothbrushes or sponges (toothettes); mouth care q2–q4; viscous lidocaine HCl (Xylocaine) as ordered before meals. Oral salt and soda mouth rinses; *avoid* commercial mouthwashes that contain high level of alcohol, which could be very irritating to mucous membranes. *Avoid* hot foods/liquids; include *bland* foods at cool temperatures; remove dentures if sores are under dentures; moisten lips with lubricant.

(4) *Skin care*—monitor: wounds that do not heal, infections (patient receives frequent sticks for blood tests and therapy); *avoid* sunlight; use sunblock, especially if receiving doxorubicin (Adriamycin).

(5) *Alopecia*—be gentle when combing or lightly brushing hair; use wigs, night caps, scarves; provide frequent linen changes. Advise patient to have hair cut short before treatment with drugs known to cause alopecia (bleomycin, cyclosphosphamide, dactinomycin, daunorubicin hydrochloride, doxorubicin hydrochloride, 5-fluorouracil, ICRF-159, hydroxyurea, methotrexate, mitomycin, VP 16-213, vincristine). Other techniques may be used, depending on patient's age and protocol in clinical agency.

(6) *Extravasation*—infiltration of chemotherapeutic agents into surrounding tissues. Document and treat according to agency protocols for administered drug.

Adult

TABLE 7–41 Common Side Effects of Chemotherapeutic Agents

	Nausea and Vomiting	Mucositis	Diarrhea	Skin Reactions	Lung	Neurological
Alkylating Agents						
Busulfan	0	+	0	Hyperpigmentation	0	0
Carboplatin	+	0	0	0	0	0
Cisplatin	+	0	0	Alopecia	0	+
Chlorambucil	0	0	0	0	+	0
Cyclophosphamide	+	0	0	0	+	0
DTIC	+	0	0	0	0	0
Ifosfamide	+	0	0	Alopecia	0	Encephalopathy
Mechlorethamine	+	+	+	Alopecia, rash	0	0
Melphalan	0	0	0	0	0	0
Antimetabolites						
Cytosine arabinoside	0	0	+	0	+	0
Fludarabine	+	0	0	0	0	0
5-Fluorouracil	0	+	+	Phlebitis	0	Cerebellar
Hydroxyurea	0	0	0	Skin atrophy	0	0
Methotrexate	+	+	+	Dermatitis	+	0
with leucovorin	+	+	+	Dermatitis	+	0
2-Deoxycoformycin	+	0	0	Erythema	0	Lethargy, coma
6-Mercaptopurine	+	0	0	Rash	0	0
Thioguanine	+	+	0	0	0	0
2-Chlorodeoxyadenosine	+	0	0	0	0	0
Antitumor Antibiotics						
Bleomycin	0	0	0	Erythema	+	0
Dactinomycin	+	+	0	Alopecia, rash	0	0
Daunorubicin	+	+	+	Alopecia, vesicant	0	0
Doxorubicin	+	+	+	Alopecia, vesicant	0	0
Idarubicin	+	+	+	Alopecia, vesicant	0	0
Mitomycin C	+	+	0	Vesicant	+	0
Mitoxantrone	+	+	+	Alopecia, vesicant	0	0
Nitrosoureas						
Carmustine (BCNU)	+	0	0	0	+	0
Lomustine (CCNU)	+	0	0	0	0	0
Streptozocin	+	0	0	0	0	0
Thiotepa	+	+	+	Alopecia, rash	0	0
Plant Alkaloids						
Etoposide	0	0	0	0	0	0
Vinblastine	+	+	0	Alopecia, vesicant	0	+
Vincristine	0	0	0	Vesicant	0	+ Neuropathy
Taxol	+	0	0	Alopecia	0	Neuropathy

+, present; 0, absent.

Source: Adapted from Ewald G, McKenzie C: Manual of Medical Therapeutics. Little, Brown, Boston, 1995.

b. Goal: *health teaching.*

(1) Orient patient and family to purpose of proposed drug regimen and anticipated side effects.

(2) Advise that frequent checks on hematological status will be necessary (patient will receive frequent IV sticks, lab tests).

(3) Advise patient/family on increased risk for infection (*avoid* uncontrolled crowds and individuals with upper respiratory tract infections or childhood diseases).

(4) Monitor injection site for signs of extravasation (infiltration); site must be changed if leakage suspected, and guidelines to neutralize must be followed according to drug protocol.

◔ 6. **Nursing precautions with chemotherapy:**

a. Nurse should wear gloves and mask when preparing chemotherapy drugs for administration. Mixing of drug into IV bag done under laminar flow hood.

b. Drugs are toxic substances, and nurses must take every precaution to handle them with care.

c. When expelling air bubbles from syringes, care must be taken that the drugs are not sprayed into the atmosphere.

d. Contaminated needles and syringes should be disposed of intact (to prevent aerosol generation) in plastic-lined box according to environmental standards. Disposable equipment should be used whenever possible.

e. If skin becomes contaminated with a drug, wash under running water.

f. Nurses should know the half-life and excretion route of the drugs being administered and take the special precautions necessary. For example, while the drug is actively being excreted, use gloves when touching patient, stool, urine, dressings, vomitus, etc.

g. If the nurse is in the early phase of pregnancy, she should seek specific information about risks to her unborn child before caring for the patient receiving chemotherapeutic agents.

H. Radiation therapy: used in high doses to kill cancer cells, or palliatively for pain relief. *Side effects of radiation therapy* depend on site of therapy (side effects are variable in each individual): nausea, vomiting, stomatitis, esophagitis, dry mouth, diarrhea, depression of bone marrow, suppression of immune response, decreased life span, and sterility.

1. **External radiation:** cobalt or linear accelerator machine.

   a. *Procedure:* daily treatments, Monday through Friday, for prescribed number of times according to size and location of tumor (length of treatment schedule is usually 4–6 wk). Patient remains alone in room during treatment. (Nurse, therapist, family members cannot stay in room with patient due to radiation exposure during treatment.) Patient instructed to lie still so exactly same area irradiated each treatment. Marks (tattoos or via permanent-ink markers) are made on skin to delineate area of treatment; marks must *not* be removed during entire treatment course.

   ◆ b. **Nursing care plan/implementation:**

      (1) Goal: *prevent tissue breakdown.*

         (a) Do *not* wash off site-identification marks (tattoos cannot be removed); dosage area is carefully calculated and must be exact for each treatment.

         (b) Assess skin daily and teach patient to do same (most radiation therapy is done on outpatient basis, so patient needs skills to manage independently).

         (c) Keep skin dry; cornstarch usually the only topical application allowed:

         (d) *Contraindications:*

            (i) Talcum powders, due to potential radiation dosage alteration.

            (ii) Lotions, due to increased moistening of skin.

         (e) Reduce skin friction by *avoiding* constricting bedclothes or clothing and by using electric shaver.

         (f) Dress areas of skin breakdown with nonadherent dressing and paper tape.

      (2) Goal: *decrease side effects of therapy.*

         (a) Provide meticulous oral hygiene.

         (b) If diarrhea occurs, may need IV infusions, *antidiarrheal* medications; monitor bowel movements, possible adhesions from surgery and radiation treatments.

         (c) Monitor vital signs, particularly respiratory function, and BP (sloughing of tissue puts patient at risk for hemorrhage).

         (d) Monitor hematological status—bone marrow depression can cause fatal toxicosis and sepsis.

      ▶ (e) Institute *reverse isolation* as necessary to prevent infections (reverse isolation usually instituted if less than 50% neutrophils).

      (3) Goal: *health teaching.*

         (a) Instruct patient to *avoid:*

            (i) Strong sunlight; must wear sunblock lotion, protective clothing over radiation site.

            (ii) Extremes in temperature to the area (hot-water bottles, ice caps).

            (iii) Synthetic, nonporous clothes or tight constrictive clothing over area.

            (iv) Eating 2–3 hr before treatment and 2 hr after, to decrease nausea; give small, frequent meals *high* in protein and carbohydrates and *low* in residue.

            (v) Strong alcohol-base mouthwash; use daily salt and soda mouthwash.

            (vi) Fatigue, an overwhelming problem. Need to pace themselves, nap; may need someone to drive them to therapy; can continue with usual activities as tolerated.

            (vii) Crowds and persons with upper respiratory infections or any other infections.

         (b) Provide appropriate birth control information for patients of childbearing age.

2. **Internal radiation: sealed** (radium, iridium, cesium):

a. Used for localized masses, e.g., mouth, cervix, breast, testes. Due to exposure from radiation source, precautions must be taken while it is in place. Health care personnel and family must adhere to *principles of time, distance, and shielding to decrease exposure (shortest* amount of time possible, stay as *far away* as possible from the source of radiation, and wear *protective* lead apron, gloves). If source of radiation accidentally falls out, it should be picked up only with *forceps*. Radiation officer should be notified immediately. Patient should be notified immediately. Patient should be in private room, and bed should be in the center of the room, if possible, to protect others. Unless the walls are lead lined, radiation will penetrate them; placing the bed in *center of room* will decrease exposure. Once the source of radiation has been removed, there is no exposure from patient, excretions, or linens.

◆ b. **Nursing care plan/implementation:**

▶ (1) Goal: *assist with cervical radium implantation* (cervical radium is used here as the most common example of internal radiation source).

    (a) *Before insertion*—give douche, enema, perineal prep; insert Foley, as ordered.

    (b) *After implantation*—check position of applicator q24h.

       ◢ (i) Keep patient on bed rest in *flat position* to avoid displacing applicator (may turn to side for eating).

       (ii) Notify physician if temperature elevates, nausea and/or vomiting occur (indicates radiation reaction or infection).

       (iii) *After removal* of implant (48–144 hr)—bathe, douche, and remove catheter as ordered.

(2) Goal: *health teaching.*

    (a) Explain that nursing care will be limited to essential activities in postinsertion period.

    (b) Signs and symptoms of complications so patient can notify staff if something unusual happens (bleeding, radiation source falls out, fever, etc.).

◆ c. **Nursing precautions for sealed internal radiation:**

(1) **Never handle radium directly**—if applicators should accidentally be removed, pick up applicator by strings with long-handled forceps and **notify radiation officer.**

(2) Linen must remain in patient's room and *not* be sent to laundry until source of radiation has been accounted for and returned to its container.

(3) **Time, distance,** and **shielding** are factors that increase or decrease potential effects on personnel. Need to minimize exposure of nursing staff, patient's family, and other health professionals. Nurses who may be pregnant should *not* care for patients with radiation because of possible damage to the fetus from radiation exposure. Children under 16 should *not* be allowed to visit while internal radiation is in use.

3. **Internal radiation: unsealed** (radioisotope/radionuclide)

a. Source of radiation is given orally or intravenously or instilled into a cavity as a liquid.

◆ b. **Nursing care plan/implementation:** Goal: *reduce radiation exposure of others.*

(1) *Isolate* patient and tag room with radioactivity symbol.

(2) *Rotate* personnel to avoid overexposure *(principles of time, distance, and shielding).* Staff should use good handwashing technique. Patient should be in a room with running water. (Nurse who may be pregnant should *not* care for patient while radiation source still active.)

(3) Encourage family to maintain telephone contact or use intercom, to decrease exposure to others.

(4) Plan independent diversional activities.

◆ c. *Specific nursing precautions* (post in chart, on patient's door).

(1) *Radioactive iodine* (^{131}I): half-life 8.1 days; excreted in urine, saliva, perspiration, vomitus, feces.

    (a) Wear gloves and isolation gowns when handling patient, excreta, or dressings directly.

    (b) Collect paper plates, eating utensils, dressings, and linen in impermeable bags; label and dispose according to agency protocol.

    (c) Collect excreta in shielded container and send to lab daily to monitor excretion rate and disposal.

(2) *Radioactive phosphorus* (^{32}P): half-life 14 days; injected into cavity or given IV or orally.

Adult

■ (a) If injected into cavity, turn patient q10–15min for 2 hr to ensure distribution.

(b) No radiation hazard unless leakage from instillation site or from patient's excreta, which are collected in lead-lined containers and brought to the radioisotope laboratory for disposal. Linen is collected in container, marked *radioactive,* and brought to the radioisotope lab for special handling.

(c) Seepage will stain linens *blue;* wear gloves when handling contaminated linens, dressings. Excreta disposed of as in (b).

(3) *Radioactive gold* (^{198}Au): half-life 2.7 days; usually injected into pleural or abdominal cavity.

(a) May seep from instillation site or drainage tubes in cavity; stains *purple.*

■ (b) Turn patient q15min for 2 hr, as in (2)(a).

(c) Same precautions regarding handling excreta as in (1)(a) and (2)(b).

◆ **4. Precautions for nurses:**

a. Use *principles of time, distance,* and *shielding* when caring for patients who are having active radiation therapy treatments.

b. Nurses who may be pregnant should *not* accept an assignment caring for patients who have active radiation in place.

c. *Always* use gloves, gowns to protect skin and clothing.

d. Wear detection badge to determine exposure to energy source.

I. Immunotherapy: it has been hypothesized that clinical malignancy may occur as a result of failure of the immunological surveillance system of the body to fight off cancer cells as they develop. The goal of immunotherapy is to immunize patients against their own tumors.

1. *Nonspecific* immunotherapy—encourages a host-immune response by use of an unrelated agent. Bacille Calmette-Guérin (BCG) vaccine and *Corynebacterium parvum* are the two agents used for this type of immunotherapy.

2. *Specific* immunotherapy—uses substances that are antigenically related to the tumor that stimulate a specific host-immune response.

3. *Side effects*—malaise, chills, nausea, vomiting, diarrhea; local reaction at site of injection, such as pruritus, scabbing.

◆ **4. Nursing care plan/implementation:**

a. Goal: *decrease discomfort associated with side effects of therapy.*

(1) Identify measures to lessen symptoms of side effects (see E. Nursing care plan/implementation—general care of the cancer patient, p. 609).

(2) Know type of immunotherapy being used, adverse and desirable effects of therapy.

(3) Administer fluids, encourage rest.

(4) Administer acetaminophen as ordered to decrease flulike symptoms.

(5) Administer antiemetics as ordered for nausea.

(6) Monitor for respiratory distress.

(7) Administer analgesics as ordered for pain.

b. Goal: *health teaching.*

(1) Comfort measures to decrease side effects of therapy.

(2) Expected and side effects of therapy.

(3) Investigational nature of therapy.

(4) Care of site of administration.

(5) Answer questions honestly.

J. Palliative care: when treatment has been ineffective in control of the disease, the nurse must plan palliative, terminal care. Cure is not possible for such patients in an advanced phase of malignancy. Symptoms increase in severity; patients and family have many special problems.

1. General problems of terminal cancer patient:

a. *Cachexia:* progressive weakness, wasting, and weight loss.

b. *Anemia:* leukopenia, thrombocytopenia, hemorrhage.

c. *Gastrointestinal disturbances:* anorexia, constipation.

d. *Tissue breakdown* leading to decubiti, seeping wounds.

e. *Urine:* retention, incontinence, renal calculi, tumor obstruction of ureters.

f. *Hypercalcemia* occurs in 10–30% of patients.

g. *Pain* due to tumor growth, obstruction, vertebral compression, or secondarily to complications, e.g., decubiti, stiffened joints, stomatitis. Also neuropathy, due to prolonged use of neurotoxic chemotherapeutic agents such as vincristine.

h. *Fatigue:* major and debilitating problem.

◆ **2. Nursing care plan/implementation:**

a. Goal: *make patient as comfortable as possible;* involve nursing staff, family, support personnel, clergy, volunteers, support groups, hospice, etc.

(1) *Nutrition:* obtain nutritional consultation; *high-calorie, high-protein diet;* small, frequent meals; blenderized or strained; commercial nutritional supplements (Ensure, Vivonex, Sustacal).

(2) Prevent tissue breakdown and vascular complications: frequent turning,

massage, air mattress, active and passive ROM exercises.

(3) GI tract disturbances: observe for toxic reactions to therapy, particularly vomiting and diarrhea; administer medications: *antiemetics, antidiarrheal* agents as ordered.

(4) Relieve pain.

(a) Use supportive measures such as massage, relaxation techniques, guided imagery; and drugs for pain relief: administer codeine, fentanyl, aspirin–oxycodone HCl (Percodan), pentazocine (Talwin), morphine, methadone, as ordered.

(b) Methods of administration: oral, injected, rectal, analgesic patches, or pumps (IV or SC).

(c) Monitor for side effects of narcotics: depressed respiratory status, constipation, anorexia.

b. Goal: *assist patient to maintain self-esteem and identity.*

(1) Encourage self-care.

(2) Spend time with patient; isolation is a great fear for the dying patient.

c. Goal: *assist patient with psychological adjustment*—see nursing care for grieving patients, dying patients (see **Unit 6**).

◆ **K. Evaluation/outcome criteria:**

1. Tolerates treatment modality—complications of surgery are avoided or minimized; tolerates chemotherapy; completes radiation therapy.

2. Side effects of treatment are managed by effective nursing care and health teaching.

3. Maintains good nutritional status.

4. Uses effective coping mechanisms or seeks appropriate assistance to deal with psychosocial concerns.

5. Makes choices for follow-up care based on accurate information.

6. Finds methods to control pain and minimize discomfort.

7. Participates in decisions regarding continuation of therapy (living will, health care proxy, DNR decisions).

8. Dignity maintained until death and during dying.

II. Lung cancer

A. Pathophysiology: *squamous cell carcinoma:* undifferentiated, pleomorphic in appearance; accounts for 45–60% of all lung cancer; *small-cell (oat-cell) carcinoma:* small, dark cells located between cells of mucosal surfaces; characterized by early metastasis and poor prognosis; *large-cell (giant-cell) carcinoma:* located in the peripheral areas of the lung, has poor prognosis; *adenocarcinoma:* found in men and women; not necessarily related to smoking.

B. Risk factors:

1. Heavy cigarette smoking, 20 yr smoking history.

2. Exposure to certain industrial substances, such as asbestos.

3. Increased incidence in women during the last decade of life.

C. Annual incidence: 178,100 new cases; 160,400 estimated deaths.

◆ **D. Assessment:**

1. *Subjective data:*

a. Dyspnea.

b. Pain: on swallowing; dull and poorly localized chest pain, referred to shoulders.

c. Anorexia.

d. History of cigarette smoking over a period of years; recurrent respiratory infections with chills and fever, especially pneumonia or bronchitis.

2. *Objective data:*

a. Wheezing; dry to productive persistent cough; hemoptysis, hoarseness.

b. Weight loss.

c. Positive diagnosis: cytology report of cells from bronchoscopy.

d. Chest pain.

e. Signs of metastasis.

◆ **E. Analysis/nursing diagnosis:**

1. *Ineffective breathing pattern* related to pain.

2. *Impaired gas exchange* related to tumor growth.

3. *Pain* related to disease progression.

4. *Fear* related to uncertain future.

5. *Powerlessness* related to inability to control symptoms.

6. *Knowledge deficit* related to disease and treatment.

◆ **F. Nursing care plan/implementation:**

1. Goal: *make patient aware of diagnosis and treatment options.*

a. Allow time to talk and to discuss diagnosis.

b. Patient makes informed decision regarding treatment.

2. Goal: *prevent complications related to surgery* for patient who is diagnosed early and for whom surgery is an option: wedge or segmental resection, laser therapy, lobectomy, or pneumonectomy are usual procedures.

a. See Nursing care plan/implementation for the patient having thoracic surgery, p. 490.

b. Monitor vital signs, including accurate respiratory assessment for respiratory congestion, blood loss, infection.

c. Assist patient to deep breathe, cough, change position.

3. Goal: *assist patient to cope with alternative therapies* when surgery is deemed not possible.

Adult

a. *Radiation:* megavoltage x-ray, cobalt—usual form of radiation. (See Nursing care plan/implementation for the patient having radiation therapy, p. 612.)

b. *Chemotherapy:*
  (1) Cisplatin and VP-16 with irradiation has become standard form of induction chemotherapy. Cyclophosphamide (Cytoxan), doxorubicin (Adriamycin), CCNU, methotrexate, vincristine sulfate (Oncovin) are the other drugs given for lung cancer.
  (2) See Nursing care plan/implementation for the patient having chemotherapy, p. 610.

4. Goal: *health teaching.*
  a. Encourage patient to stop smoking to offer best possible air exchange.
  b. Encourage *high-protein, high-calorie diet* to counteract weight loss.
  c. *Force fluids,* to liquefy secretions so they can be expectorated.
  d. Encourage adequate rest and activity to prevent problems of immobility.
  e. Desired effects and side effects of medications prescribed for therapy and pain relief.
  f. Coping mechanisms for maximal comfort and advanced disease (see **J.** Palliative care, p. 614).

◆ **G. Evaluation/outcome criteria:**
  1. Copes with disease and treatment.
  2. Side effects of treatment are minimized by proper nursing management.
  3. Acid-base balance is maintained by careful management of respiratory problems.
  4. Patient is aware of the seriousness of the disease.

III. Colon and rectal cancer
  A. Risk factors:
  1. Men, middle age, personal or family history of colon and rectal cancer, personal or family history of polyps in the rectum or colon, ulcerative colitis.
  2. Diet high in beef and low in fiber.
  3. *Gardner's syndrome* (multiple colonic adenomatous polyps, osteomas of the mandible or skull, multiple epidermoid cysts, or soft-tissue tumors of the skin).

  B. Annual incidence: 131,200 new cases, 56,600 estimated deaths.

◆ **C. Assessment:**
  1. *Subjective data:*
    a. Change in bowel habits.
    b. Anorexia.
    c. Weakness.
    d. Abdominal cramping or vague discomfort with or without pain.

e. Chills.
2. *Objective data:*
  a. Diarrhea (pencil-like or ribbon-shaped feces) or constipation.
  b. Weight loss.
  c. Rectal bleeding; anemia.
  d. Fever.
  e. Digital exam reveals palpable mass if lesion is in ascending or descending colon.
  f. Signs of intestinal obstruction: constipation, distention, pain, vomiting, fecal oozing.
  g. *Diagnostic tests:*
    (1) Digital examination.
    (2) Slides of stool specimen, for occult blood.
    (3) Proctoscopy.
    (4) Sigmoidoscopy, colonoscopy.
    (5) Barium enema.
  h. Lab data: occult blood, blood serotonin *increased,* carcinoembryonic antigen (CEA); *positive* radioimmunoassay of serum or plasma indicates presence of carcinoma or adenocarcinoma of colon; positive result after resection indicates return of tumor.

◆ **D. Analysis/nursing diagnosis:**
  1. *Constipation or diarrhea* related to presence of mass.
  2. *Altered health maintenance* related to care of stoma.
  3. *Sexual dysfunction* related to possible nerve damage during radical surgery.
  4. *Body image disturbance* related to colostomy.

◆ **E. Nursing care plan/implementation** (see also **E.** Nursing care plan/implementation—general care of the cancer patient, p. 609):
  1. *Radiation:* to reduce tumor or for palliation.
  2. *Chemotherapy:* to reduce tumor mass and metastatic lesions.
    a. *Antitumor antibiotics*—mitomycin C, doxorubicin hydrochloride (Adriamycin).
    b. *Alkylating agents*—methyl-CCNU.
    c. *Antimetabolites*—5-fluorouracil (5-FU).
    d. *Steroids* and *analgesics* for symptomatic relief.
  3. Prepare patient for surgery (colostomy) if necessary.

◆ **F. Evaluation/outcome criteria:**
  1. Return of peristalsis and formed stool following resection and anastomosis.
  2. Adjusts to alteration in bowel elimination route following abdominoperineal resection (e.g., no depression, resumes lifestyle).
  3. Demonstrates self-care skills with colostomy.
  4. Makes dietary adjustments that affect elimination as indicated.
  5. Identifies alternative methods of expressing sexuality, if needed.

IV. **Breast cancer**
  A. **Risk factors:**
    1. Women > age 50.
    2. Family history of breast cancer.
    3. Never bore children, or bore first child after age 30.
    4. Had breast cancer in other breast.
    5. Menarche before age 11.
    6. Menopause after age 50.
    7. Exposure to endogenous estrogens.
    8. Exposure to ionizing radiation.
    9. High alcohol and fat intake may increase risk.
  B. **Annual incidence:** 181,600 new cases; 44,190 estimated deaths.
  ◆ C. **Assessment:**
    1. *Subjective data:*
      a. Burning, itching of nipple.
      b. Reported painless lump.
    2. *Objective data:*
      a. Firm, nontender lump or mass.
      b. Asymmetry of breast.
      c. Nipple—retraction, discharge.
      d. Alteration in breast skin—redness, dimpling, ulceration.
      e. Palpation reveals lump.
      f. *Diagnostic tests:* mammography, needle biopsy, core biopsy, excisional biopsy—level of estrogen-receptor protein predicts response to hormonal manipulation of metastatic disease and may represent a prognostic indicator for primary cancer; carcinoembryonic antigen (CEA) useful with metastatic disease of the breast.
  ◆ D. **Analysis/nursing diagnosis:**
    1. *Risk for injury* related to surgical intervention.
    2. *Body image disturbance* related to effects of surgery, radiation, or chemotherapy.
    3. *Altered sexuality patterns* related to loss of breast.
  ◆ E. **Nursing care plan/implementation** (see also **E.** Nursing care plan/implementation—general care of the cancer patient, p. 609):
    1. Goal: *assist through treatment protocol.*
      a. *Radiation*—primary treatment modality; adjunctive, external, or implantation to primary lesion site or nodes.
      b. *Chemotherapy* usually given in combinations.
        (1) *Cytotoxic* agents to destroy tumor and control metastasis.
        (2) *Alkylating* agents: cyclophosphamide (Cytoxan).
        (3) *Antitumor antibiotics:* doxorubicin (Adriamycin).
        (4) *Antimetabolites:* fluorouracil (5-FU); methotrexate (Amethopterine, MTX).
        (5) *Plant alkaloids:* vincristine sulfate (Oncovin).
        (6) *Hormones* to control metastasis, provide palliation: androgens, fluoxymesterone (Halotestin), testosterone (Teslac), diethylstilbesterol (estrogen).
        (7) *Antiestrogens:* tamoxifen (Nolvadex) may be used after initial treatment.
        (8) *Cortisols:* cortisone, prednisolone (Delta-Cortef), prednisolone acetate (Meticortelone), prednisone (Deltasone, Delta).
      c. *Surgery.*
        (1) *Preoperative:*
          (a) Goal: *prepare for surgery—types:*
            (i) *Lumpectomy* (with or without radiation)—used when lesion is small; section of breast is removed (often accompanied by radiation therapy and then radium interstitial implant).
            (ii) *Simple mastectomy*—breast removed, no alteration in nodes.
            (iii) *Modified radical mastectomy*—breast, some axillary nodes, subcutaneous tissue removed; pectoralis minor muscle removed.
            (iv) *Radical mastectomy*—breast, axillary nodes, and pectoralis major and minor muscles removed.
            (v) *Reconstructive surgery*—done at time of initial mastectomy or (most often) later, when other adjuvant therapy has been completed.
          (b) Goal: *promote comfort.*
            (i) Allow patient and family to express fears, feelings.
            (ii) Provide correct information about diagnostic tests, operative procedure, postoperative expectations.
            (iii) Patient may be hospitalized for 24 hours or less. Have telephone number available for questions. Make appropriate community referrals.
        (2) *Postoperative:*
          (a) Goal: *facilitate healing.*
            (i) Observe pressure dressings for bleeding; will appear under axilla and toward the back.
            (ii) Report if dressing becomes saturated; reinforce dressing as need; monitor drainage from Hemovac or suction pump.

(iii) *Position: semi-Fowler's* to facilitate venous and lymphatic drainage; use pillows to *elevate affected* arm *above right atrium,* to prevent edema if nodes removed.

(b) Goal: *prevent complications.*
   (i) Monitor vital signs for shock.
   (ii) Use gloves when emptying drainage.
   (iii) Maintain joint mobility—flexion and extension of fingers, elbow, shoulder.
   (iv) ROM as ordered to prevent ankylosis.

(v) If skin graft done, check donor site and limit exercises.

(c) Goal: *facilitate rehabilitation.*
   (i) Encourage patient, significant others, and family to look at incision.
   (ii) Involve patient in incisional care, as tolerated.
   (iii) *Refer* to Reach to Recovery program of the American Cancer Society
   (iv) Exercise program, hydrotherapy for postmastectomy patients, to reduce lymphedema.

FIGURE 7–17 Breast self-examination. *(A)* Examine breasts during bath or shower because flat fingers glide easily over wet skin. Use right hand to examine left breast and vice versa. *(B)* Sit or stand before a mirror. Inspect breasts with hands at sides, then raised overhead. Look for changes in contour or dimpling of skin. *(C)* Place hands on hips and press down firmly to flex chest muscles. *(D)* Lie down with one hand under head and pillow or folded towel under that scapula. *(E)* Palpate that breast with the other hand using concentric circle method. It usually takes three circles to cover all breast tissue. Include the tail of the breast and the axilla. Repeat with other breast. *(F)* End in a sitting position. Palpate the areola areas of both breasts, and inspect and squeeze nipples to check for discharge.

(d) Goal: *health teaching.*
   (i) How to avoid injury to affected area; how to prevent lymphedema.
   (ii) Exercises to gain full ROM.
   (iii) Availability of prosthesis, reconstructive surgery.
   (iv) Correct breast self-examination (BSE) technique (patient is at risk for breast cancer in remaining breast) (Figure 7–17). Best time for exam: *premenopausal* women, seventh day of cycle; *postmenopausal* women, same day each month.

◆ **F. Evaluation/outcome criteria:**
1. Identifies feelings regarding loss.
2. Demonstrates postmastectomy exercises.
3. Gives rationale for avoiding fatigue and avoiding constricting garments on affected arm; necessity for avoiding injury (cuts, bruises, burns) while carrying out activities of daily living.
4. Describes signs and symptoms of infection.
5. Demonstrates correct BSE technique.

V. **Uterine cancer** (endometrial): originates from epithelial tissues of the endometrium; second only to cervical cancer as cause of pelvic cancer. Slow growing; metastasizes late; responsive to therapy with early diagnosis; Pap test not as effective—more effective to have endometrial tissue sample (Tables 7–42 and 7–43). Table 7–44 discusses cervical cancer.

A. **Risk factors:**
1. History of infertility (nulliparity).
2. Failure of ovulation.
3. Prolonged estrogen therapy.
4. Obesity.
5. Menopause after age 52.
6. Diabetes.

B. **Annual incidence:** 37,400 new cases; 6400 estimated deaths.

◆ **C. Assessment:**
1. *Subjective data:*
   a. History of risk factor(s).
   b. Pain (late symptom).

2. *Objective data:*
   a. Obese.
   b. Abnormal cells obtained from aspiration of endocervix or endometrial washings.
   c. Postmenopausal uterine bleeding.
   d. Abnormal menses; intermenstrual or unusual discharge.

◆ **D. Analysis/nursing diagnosis:**
1. *Pain* related to surgery.
2. *Risk for injury* related to surgery.
3. *Body image disturbance* related to loss of uterus.

◆ **E. Nursing care plan/implementation** (see also care of the cancer patient, p. 609):
1. Goal: *assist patient through treatment protocol.*
   a. *Radiation*—external, internal, or both with poor surgical risk patient.
   b. *Chemotherapy*—to reduce tumors and produce remission of metastasis. Antineoplastic drugs: dacarbazine (DTIC), doxorubicin (Adriamycin), medroxyprogesterone acetate (Provera), megestrol acetate (Megace).
2. Goal: *prepare patient for surgery—types:*
   a. *Subtotal hysterectomy:* removal of the uterus; cervical stump remains.
   b. *Total hysterectomy:* removal of entire uterus, including cervix (abdominally [approximately 70%] or vaginally).
   c. *Total hysterectomy with bilateral salpingo-oophorectomy:* removal of entire uterus, fallopian tubes, and ovaries.
3. Goal: *reduce anxiety and depression:* allow for expression of feelings, concerns about feminity, role, relationships.
4. Goal: *prevent postoperative complications.*
   ▶ a. Catheter care—temporary bladder atony may be present as a result of edema or nerve trauma, especially when vaginal approach is used.

TABLE 7–42 Papanicolaou-Smear Classes

Class	Recommended Actions
I Normal	
II Atypical cells, nonmalignant	Treat vaginal infections; repeat Pap smears
III Suspicious cells	Biopsy; dilation and curettage
IV Abnormal cells; suspicious of malignancy	Biopsy; dilation and curettage; conization
V Malignant cells present	See Table 7–43

TABLE 7–43 Uterine Cancer: Recommended Treatment, by Stage of Invasion

Stage of Invasion		Recommended Treatment
0	(In situ) Atypical hyperplasia	Cryosurgery, conization
I	Uterus is of normal size	Hysterectomy
II	Uterus slightly enlarged, but tumor is undifferentiated	Radiation implant, x-ray; hysterectomy 4–6 wk postradiation
III	Uterus enlarged, tumor extends outside uterus	Radiation implant, total hysterectomy 4–6 wk postradiation
IV	Advanced metastatic disease	Radiation, chemotherapy; progestin therapy to reduce pulmonary lesions

Adult

TABLE 7–44   International System of Staging for Cervical Carcinoma

Stage	Location	Prognosis	Treatment
0	In situ	Highly curable	Conization
I	Cervix	Cure rate decreases as stage progresses	Radiation
II	Cervix to upper vagina		Radiation
III	Cervix to pelvic wall or lower third of vagina		Surgeries: 1. Panhysterectomy, wide vaginal excision with removal of lymph nodes; ileal conduit
IV	Cervix to true pelvis, bladder, or rectum		2. Pelvic exenteration: a. Anterior: removal of vagina and bladder; ileal conduit b. Posterior: removal of rectum and vagina; colostomy c. Total: both anterior and posterior 3. Chemotherapy

▶ b. Observe for abdominal distention and hemorrhage:
  (1) Auscultate for bowel sounds.
  (2) Measure abdominal girth.
  (3) Use rectal tube to decrease flatus.
  c. *Decrease pelvic congestion* and prevent venous stasis.
  ▰ (1) *Avoid* high Fowler's position.
  (2) Antiembolic stockings as ordered.
  ▶ (3) Institute passive leg exercises.
  (4) Apply abdominal support as ordered.
  (5) Encourage early ambulation.
5. Goal: *support coping mechanisms* to prevent psychosocial response of depression: allow for verbalization of feelings.
6. Goal: *health teaching* to prevent complication of hemorrhage, infection, thromboemboli.
  a. *Avoid:*
  (1) Douching or coitus until advised by physician.
  (2) Strenuous activity and work for 2 mo.
  (3) Sitting for long time and wearing constrictive clothing, which tend to increase pelvic congestion.
  b. Explain hormonal replacement if applicable; correct dosage, desired and side effects of prescribed medications.
  c. Explain:
  (1) Menstruation will no longer occur.
  (2) Importance of reporting symptoms, e.g., fever, increased or bloody vaginal discharge, and hot flashes.
◆ F. **Evaluation/outcome criteria:**
  1. Adjusts to altered body image.
  2. No complications—hemorrhage, shock, infection, thrombophlebitis.

VI. **Prostate cancer:** malignant neoplasm, usually adenocarcinoma; most common cause of cancer in men.
  A. **Risk factors:**
  1. Men > age 50.

2. Familial history.
3. Geographic distribution, environmental (e.g., industrial exposure to cadmium).
4. Hormonal factors (testosterone).
5. Diet (high fat).
B. **Annual incidence:** 185,000 new cases; 40,000 estimated deaths.
◆ C. **Assessment:**
  1. *Subjective data:*
  a. Difficulty in starting urinary stream (hesitancy); urgency.
  b. Pain due to metastasis in lower back, hip, legs; perianal or rectal discomfort.
  c. Symptoms of cystitis; frequency, urgency.
  2. *Objective data:*
  a. Urinary: smaller, less forceful stream; terminal dribbling; frequency, nocturia; *retention* (inability to void after ingestion of alcohol or exposure to cold).
  b. *Diagnostic tests:* digital rectal examination (DRE); transrectal ultrasonography (TRUS). Needle biopsy or tissue specimen reveals positive cancer cells.
  c. Lab data: *increased:*
  (1) Prostate-specific antigen (PSA)—over 4 ng/mL.
  (2) Urine RBCs (hematuria).
  (3) Gleason score for prostate cancer grading system (range: 2–10).
◆ D. **Analysis/nursing diagnosis:**
  1. *Altered urinary elimination* related to incontinence.
  2. *Altered sexuality pattern* related to nerve damage and erectile dysfunction.
  3. *Anxiety* related to diagnosis.
  4. *Pain* related to metastasis to bone.
◆ E. **Nursing care plan/implementation** (see also care of the cancer patient, p. 609):
  1. Goal: *assist patient through decisions about treatment protocol* (varies by stage: 0–IV).

a. *Radiation*—alone or in conjunction with surgery. Types: external beam radiation, 3-D conformal (focal), radioactive seed implants (brachytherapy).

b. *Surgery*—cryosurgery; radical retropubic prostatectomy (see p. 547).

c. Other options: hormones (*luteinizing hormone–releasing hormone agonists* [Lupron, Zoladex, Casodex, Nilandron]), *antiandrogen* (flutamide [Eulexin]); drugs in conjunction with orchiectomy, to limit production of androgens (*androgen deprivation therapy*).

d. **Watchful waiting**—recommended with small contained tumor; older men; where surgery is contraindicated for other serious health problems.

◆ **F. Evaluation/outcome criteria:** see Prostatectomy, pp. 547–548.

VII. Bladder cancer: bladder is most common site of urinary tract cancer.

A. Risk factors:
1. Contact with certain dyes.
2. Cigarette smoking.
3. Excessive coffee intake.
4. Prolonged use of analgesics with phenacetin.
5. Three times more common in men.

B. Annual incidence: 54,500 new cases; 12,100 estimated deaths.

◆ **C. Assessment:**
1. *Subjective data:*
   a. Frequency, urgency.
   b. Pain: flank, pelvic; dysuria.
2. *Objective data:*
   a. Painless hematuria (initially).
   b. *Diagnostic tests:*
      (1) Cystoscopy, intravenous pyelogram *(IVP)*—mass or obstruction.
      (2) Bladder biopsy, urine cytology—malignant cells.
   c. Lab data: urinalysis—*increased* RBC (>4.8/μL—men, >4.3/μL—women); erythrocytes (>30 mg/dL).

◆ **D. Analysis/nursing diagnosis:**
1. *Risk for injury* related to surgical intervention.
2. *Altered urinary elimination* related to surgery.

◆ **E. Nursing care plan/implementation** (see also care of the cancer patient, p. 609):
1. Goal: *assist patient through treatment protocol.*
   a. *Radiation:* cobalt, radioisotopes, radon seeds; often before surgery to slow tumor growth.
   b. *Chemotherapy:*
      (1) *Antitumor antibiotics:* doxorubicin hydrochloride (Adriamycin), mitomycin.
      (2) *Antimetabolites:* 5-fluorouracil (5-FU).
      (3) *Alkylating* agents: thiotepa.
      (4) *Sedatives, antispasmodics.*

2. Goal: *prepare patient for surgery*—types:
   a. *Transurethral fulguration or excision:* used for small tumors with minimal tissue involvement.
   b. *Segmental resection:* up to half the bladder may be resected.
   c. *Cystectomy with urinary diversion:* complete removal of the bladder; performed when disease appears curable.
3. Goal: *assist with acceptance of diagnosis and treatment.*
4. Goal: *prevent complication during postoperative period.*
   a. *Transurethral fulguration or excision:*
      (1) Monitor for clots, bleeding, spasms.
   ▶ (2) Maintain patency of Foley catheter.
   b. *Urinary diversion with stoma:*
      (1) Protect skin, ensure proper fit of appliance—because constantly wet with urine (see also Ileal conduit, p. 548, and ostomies and stoma care, pp. 537–538).
      (2) Prevent infection by increasing *acidity* of urine and increasing *fluid* intake.
      (3) *Health teaching.*
         (a) Self-care of stoma and appliance.
         (b) Expected and side effects of medications.
         (c) Importance of follow-up visits for early detection of metastasis.

◆ **F. Evaluation/outcome criteria:**
1. Accepts treatment plan.
2. Uses prescribed measures to decrease side effects of surgery, radiation, chemotherapy.
3. Plans follow-up visits for further evaluation.
4. Maintains dignity.

VIII. Laryngeal cancer
A. Risk factors:
1. Eight times more common in men.
2. Occurs most often after age 60.
3. Cigarette smoking.
4. Alcohol.
5. Chronic laryngitis, vocal abuse.
6. Family predisposition to cancer.

B. Annual incidence: 10,900 new cases; 4230 estimated deaths.

◆ **C. Assessment:**
1. *Subjective data:*
   a. Dysphagia—pain in areas of Adam's apple; radiates to ear.
   b. Dyspnea.
2. *Objective data:*
   a. Persistent hoarseness.
   b. Cough and hemoptysis.
   c. Enlarged cervical nodes.
   d. General debility and weight loss.
   e. Foul breath.
   f. Diagnosis made by history, laryngoscopy with biopsy and microscopic study of cells.

◆ **D. Analysis/nursing diagnosis:**
1. *Impaired verbal communication* related to removal of larynx.
2. *Body image disturbance* related to radical surgery.
3. *Ineffective airway clearance* related to increased secretions through tracheostomy.

◆ **E. Nursing care plan/implementation** (see also care of the cancer patient, p. 609): treatment primarily surgical (laryngectomy—see p. 549); radiation therapy may also be indicated.

◆ **F. Evaluation/outcome criteria:** see Laryngectomy, p. 549.

IX. Additional types of cancer—Table 7–45.

FIGURE 7–18 Testicular self-examination. (From Morton, PG: Health Assessment in Nursing. FA Davis, Philadelphia, 1993, p 451.)

Testicular self-examination

To help detect abnormalities early, every male should examine his testes once a month. Instruct the client to follow this procedure:

1 If possible, take a warm bath or shower before beginning; the scrotum, which tends to contract when cold, will be relaxed, making the testes easier to examine.

2 With one hand, lift the penis and check the scrotum (the sac containing the testes) for any change in shape, size, or color. The left side of the scrotum normally hangs slightly lower than the right.

3 Next, check the testes for lumps and masses. Locate the crescent-shaped structure at the back of each testis. This is the epididymis, which should feel soft.

4 Use the thumb and first two fingers of your left hand to squeeze the spermatic cord gently; it extends upward from the epididymis, above the left testis. Then repeat on the right side, using your right hand. Check for lumps and masses by palpating along the entire length of the cord.

5 Next, examine each testis. To do so, place the index and middle fingers on its underside and the thumb on top, then gently roll the testis between the thumb and fingers. A normal testis is egg-shaped, rubbery-firm, and movable within the scrotum; it should feel smooth, with no lumps. Both testes should be the same size.

6 Promptly report any lumps, masses, or changes to the physician.

TABLE 7–45   Selected Cancer Problems

| | ◆ Assessment | | | | |
	Subjective Data	Objective Data	Risk Factors	Annual Incidence	Specific Treatment
GASTROINTESTINAL TRACT					
Oral cancer	Difficulty chewing, swallowing, moving tongue or jaws; history of heavy smoking, alcohol use, or chewing tobacco	Sore that bleeds and does not heal; persistent red or white patch; diagnosis by biopsy; early detection: dental checks	Heavy smoking and drinking, user of chewing tobacco, men > age 40 (affects twice as many men as women)	30,750 new cases; 8440 estimated deaths	*Surgery*, with reconstructive surgery useful for cure and palliatively (see care of cancer patient having surgery, pp. 609–610) *Radiation* using simulated computer localization to avoid destruction of normal tissue (see care of patient having radiation therapy, pp. 612–614)
Esophageal cancer	Dysphagia—difficulty in swallowing; discomfort described as lump in throat, pressure in chest, pain; fatigue, lethargy, apathy, depression; anorexia	Weight loss; regurgitation, vomiting; diagnostic tests—*barium swallow, esophagoscopy, biopsy*	Over age 50, alcoholism, use of tobacco; increasing risk in nonwhite women, in people with achalasia (inability to relax lower esophagus with swallowing) or hiatal hernias	12,500 new cases; 12,200 estimated deaths	*Surgery*: resection with anastomosis, or removal with gastrostomy *Radiation*: best form of therapy ⬤ *Chemotherapy*: antineoplastic drugs ineffective; medications to reduce symptoms of pain, discomfort, and anxiety; see nursing care plan/implementation for patient with cancer (p. 609); having radiation therapy (pp. 612–614); having chemotherapy (pp. 611–612); having surgery (pp. 609–610)
Stomach cancer	Vague feeling of fullness, pressure, or epigastric pain following ingestion of food; anorexia, nausea, intolerance of meat; malaise	Eructation, regurgitation, vomiting; melena, hematemesis, anemia; jaundice, diarrhea, ascites; big belly, upper gastric area; often palpable mass	Men, lower socioeconomic classes, colder climates, early exposure to dietary carcinogens, blood group A, pernicious anemia, atrophic achlorhydric gastritis	22,400 new cases; 14,000 estimated deaths	*Surgery*: gastrectomy (see gastric surgery, p. 522, for nursing care). *Radiation*: not as useful because dosage needed would cause side effects unlikely to be tolerated by patient ⬤ *Chemotherapy* alone or in conjunction with surgery: antitumor antibiotics, antimetabolites, nitrosoureas, hematinics (see nursing care plan for patient having chemotherapy, pp. 611–612)
Pancreatic cancer	Anorexia, nausea; pain in upper abdomen, radiating to back; dyspnea	Jaundice, vomiting, weight loss; determination of solid mass in area of pancreas by *computed tomography* and *ultrasound*; tissue identification by thin-needle *percutaneous biopsy*	Excessive use of alcohol; exposure to dry-cleaning chemicals, gasoline; coffee and decaffeinated coffee; possibly diabetes and chronic pancreatitis	27,600 new cases; 28,100 estimated deaths	*Surgery*: removal (must then have supplemental pancreatic enzymes; some patients become insulin-dependent diabetics) or bypass to relieve obstruction (see nursing care plan/implementation for patient with diabetes, pp. 526–527) ⬤ *Chemotherapy*: pain relief, antiemetics, insulin, pancrelipase, 5-fluorouracil cyclophosphamide (5-FU), cytoxan, carmustine (BCNU), methotrexate, vincristine, mitomycin-C (see nursing care plan/implementation for patient having chemotherapy, pp. 611–612)

Continued

Adult

Adult

TABLE 7–45   Selected Cancer Problems—cont'd

	◆ Assessment				
	Subjective Data	Objective Data	Risk Factors	Annual Incidence	Specific Treatment
GASTROINTESTINAL TRACT—cont'd Pancreatic cancer—cont'd					*Radiation:* intraoperative high dose to pancreatic tumors with external high beam; palliative radiation therapy for pain (see nursing care plan/implementation for patient having radiation therapy, pp. 612–614; see nursing care plan/implementation for patient with cancer, p. 609)
SKIN Skin cancer: basal cell	Reported painless lesion	Scaly plaques, papules that ulcerate; pale, waxy, pearly nodule or red, sharply outlined patch; unusual skin condition, change in size or color, or other darkly pigmented growth or mole	Exposure to sun, coal tar, pitch, arsenic compounds, creosote, radium; fair complexion	900,000 new cases; 7300 estimated deaths; 44,200 of those are malignant melanoma	*Surgery:* electrodesiccation (dehydration of tissue by use of needle electrode); cryosurgery (destruction of tissue by application of extreme cold) (see care of cancer patient, p. 609) *Radiation therapy* (see care of patient having radiation therapy, pp. 612–614) *Prevention: avoid* sun from 10 A.M.–3 P.M.; use protective clothing, sunblock lotion
NERVOUS SYSTEM Brain	*Headache:* steady, intermittent, severe (may be intensified by physical activity); nausea; lethargy, easy fatigability; forgetfulness, disorientation, impaired judgment; visual disturbances; blackouts	Vomiting, may be projectile; sight loss, auditory changes; signs of increased intracranial pressure; seizures; paresthesia; behavior changes. *diagnostic studies*—CT scan, arteriography, cytology of cerebrospinal fluid	None known for primary tumors; brain is common site for metastasis	17,600 new cases (brain and spinal cord); 13,200 estimated deaths	*Surgery:* craniotomy with excision of lesion; ventricular shunt to allow for drainage of fluid (see nursing care plan/implementation for craniotomy, p. 559; see nursing care plan/implementation for patient with cancer, p. 609) *Radiation:* cobalt (local or entire CNS); total brain radiation causes alopecia, which may be permanent (see nursing care plan/implementation for patient having radiation therapy, pp. 612–614; could be used alone, with surgery, or with chemotherapy *Chemotherapy:* antineoplastic alkylating agents; nitrosoureas (cross blood-brain barrier to reduce tumor)—carmustine (BCNU), lomustine (CCNU); semustine (methyl-CCNU); cerebral diuretics to reduce edema; anticonvulsants; analgesics; sedatives (see nursing care plan/implementation for patient having chemotherapy, pp. 611–612)

ENDOCRINE

Thyroid cancer

Painless nodule; dysphagia; difficulty breathing

Radiation exposure in childhood

18,100 new cases; 1200 estimated deaths

Enlarged thyroid, thyroid nodule; palpable thyroid, lymph nodes; hoarseness; hypofunctional nodule seen on *isotopic imaging scanning; needle biopsy for cytology studies*

Surgery: total thyroidectomy, possible radical neck dissection (see Thyroidectomy, pp. 598–599)
Radiation: external, or with radioactive iodine (^{131}I) (see care of patient having radiation therapy, pp. 612–614)
Chemotherapy: chlorambucil, doxorubicin, vincristine (Leukeran, Adriamycin, Oncovin, respectively) (see care of patient having chemotherapy, pp. 611–612)

BLOOD AND LYMPH TISSUES

Hodgkin's disease

Fatigue; generalized pruritis; anorexia

For young adults from 15–35 yr old, not clearly defined, some relationship to socioeconomic status; men-women ratio is 1.5:1; increased frequency among caucasians

7500 new cases; 1300 estimated deaths

Painless enlargement of lymph nodes, especially in cervical area; fever, night sweats; hepatosplenomegaly; anemia; peak age of incidence, 15–35; *diagnostic tests*—biopsy shows presence of *Reed-Sternberg cells; x-rays, scans, laparotomy*

Staging and treatment:
Stage I—involvement of a single node or a single node region; excision of lesion, and total nodal radiation (see care of patient having radiation therapy, pp. 612–614).
Stage II—involvement of two or more lymph node regions on same side of diaphragm; excision of lesion and radiation (see care of patient having radiation therapy, pp. 612–614)
Stage III—involvement of lymph node regions on both sides of the diaphragm, which may include the spleen; combination of radiation and chemotherapy
Stage IV—involvement of one or more extralymphatic organs or tissues, with or without lymphatic involvement; treated with chemotherapy alone, radiation therapy alone, or both
Presence or absence of symptoms of night sweats, significant fever, and weight loss; treated with *chemotherapy,* MOPP protocol—Mustargen (mechlorethamine HCl, alkylating agent), Oncovin (vincristine, plant alkaloid), procarbazine (antineoplastic); prednisone (corticosteroid) (see care of patient having chemotherapy, pp. 611–612)

Continued

Adult

Adult

TABLE 7–45 Selected Cancer Problems—cont'd

	◆ Assessment				
	Subjective Data	**Objective Data**	**Risk Factors**	**Annual Incidence**	**Specific Treatment**
BLOOD AND LYMPH TISSUES—cont'd					
Non-Hodgkin's lymphoma	Night sweats	Nontender lymphadenopathy, enlarged liver and spleen, weight loss, fever	Age 50–60 yr	53,600 new cases; 23,800 estimated deaths	Stage I—rarely observed, but remission possible with radiation therapy Stage II—radiation therapy Stage III and IV—combination chemotherapy, with or without radiation therapy
Multiple myeloma	Weakness; history of frequent infections, especially pneumonias; severe bone pain on motion; neurological symptoms, paralysis	Fractures of long bones; deformity of: sternum, ribs, vertebrae, pelvis; hepatosplenomegaly; anemia and bleeding tendencies *Elevated* uric acid	Exposure to ionizing radiation; middle-aged or older women	13,200 new cases; 11,400 estimated deaths	*Surgery:* relieve spinal cord compression; orthopedic procedures to relieve or support bone problems (see nursing care plan/implementation for patients with internal fixation for fractures, pp. 576, 580; patient with spinal cord injuries when paralysis occurs, p. 591) *Radiation:* for some lesions (see nursing care plan/implementation for patients having radiation therapy, pp. 612–614) *Chemotherapy:* alkylating agents; antitumor antibiotics; plant alkaloids; hormones—melphalan and prednisone (see nursing care plan/implementation for patients having chemotherapy, pp. 611–612)
URINARY ORGANS					
Kidney cancer	Anorexia, nausea; fatigue; abdominal or flank pain	Painless, gross hematuria; firm, nontender, palpable kidney; vomiting and weight loss; *complications*—hypertension, nephrotic syndrome, lung metastasis *Lab and diagnostic tests:* IVP; urinalysis—presence of red cells and albumin; CBC—*decrease* in red cells and leukocytes, *reduction* in serum albumin, *elevation* of alpha globulin	More common among men than women, whites than blacks; radiation exposure, possible familial influence; common site of metastasis from lung, breast	30,000 new cases; 1900 estimated deaths	*Surgery:* nephrectomy (see pre/postoperative nursing care, p. 545) *Radiation:* local and irradiation of metastatic sites when tumor is radiosensitive (see nursing care plan/implementation for patient having radiation therapy, pp. 612–614) *Chemotherapy:* plant alkaloids—vincristine (Oncovin); antitumor antibiotics—dactinomycin (Actinomycin D), doxorubicin (Adriamycin); alkylating agents—cyclophosphamide (Cytoxan) (see nursing care plan/implementation for patient having chemotherapy, pp. 611–612)

	Signs/Symptoms	Risk Factors	Statistics	Treatment
GENITAL ORGANS Testicular cancer	Aching or dragging sensation in groin, usually painless	Second most common malignancy among men age 25–40 yr; possibly exposure to chemical carcinogens; trauma, orchitis; gonadal dysgenesis; cryptorchidism (undescended testicles)	7400 new cases; 300 estimated deaths; 95–100% 5 yr survival rate for early-detected nonmetastasized lesions	*Surgery:* orchiectomy (see nursing care plan/implementation for the preop and postop patient, pp. 501, 505, 509, 510) *Radiation:* see nursing care plan/implementation for patient having radiation therapy, pp. 612–614 ◉ *Chemotherapy:* cisplatin, Bleomycin, Etoposide, steroids (see nursing care plan/implementation for patient having chemotherapy, pp. 611–612)
Cervical cancer	Vague pelvic or low back discomfort, pressure, or pain Intermenstrual, postcoital, or postmenopausal bleeding; vaginal discharge—serosanguineous and malodorous hypermenorrhea; abdominal distention with urinary frequency; abnormal Pap test (see Table 7–42); recommended guidelines by American Cancer Society: *Pap test* annually; after three consecutive normal tests, MD may recommend less frequent testing; pelvic/uterine exam every 3 yr	Early age at first intercourse; multiple sex partners; low socioeconomic status; exposure to herpesvirus 2	14,500 new cases; 6400 estimated deaths	*Staging* (see Table 7–44) *Stage 0*—carcinoma in situ; no distinct tumor observable; stage may last for 8–10 yr; cure rate 100% following treatment of wedge or cone resection of cervix during childbearing years, or simple hysterectomy *Stage I*—malignant cells infiltrate cervical mucosa; lesion bleeds easily; cure rate 80% with treatment of hysterectomy *Stage II*—neoplasm spreads through cervical muscular layers, involves upper third of vaginal mucosa; cure rate 50% with treatment of radical hysterectomy *Stage III*—neoplasm involves lower third of vagina; cure rate 25% with pelvic exenteration *Stage IV*—involves metastasis to bladder, rectum, and surrounding tissues; considered incurable *Radiation:* external or internal or both, in conjunction with surgery or alone, depending on stage of disease or condition of patient (see nursing care plan/implementation for patient having radiation therapy, pp. 612–614) ◉ *Chemotherapy:* progestin, antineoplastics, megestrol (Megace), medroxyprogesterone (Curretab, Provera); alkylating agents—dacarbazine (DTIC)

EMERGENCY NURSING PROCEDURES

I. Purpose—to initiate assessment and intervention procedures that will speed total care of the patient toward a successful outcome.

II. Emergency nursing procedures for adults are detailed in Table 7–46.

III. Legal issues—see **Unit 3.**

TABLE 7–46   Nursing Care of the Adult in Medical and Surgical Emergencies

Condition	◆ Assessment: Signs and Symptoms	▶ Prehospitalization Nursing Care	▶ In-hospital Nursing Care
Cardiovascular Emergencies			
Myocardial infarction—ischemia and necrosis of cardiac muscle secondary to insufficient or obstructed coronary blood flow	*Prehospital:* *Chest pain:* viselike choking, unrelieved by rest or nitroglycerin *Skin:* ashen, cold, clammy *Vital signs:* pulse—rapid, weak, thready; increased rate and depth of respirations; dyspnea *Behavior:* restless, anxious *In hospital:* *C/V:* blood pressure and pulse pressure decreased *Heart sounds:* soft; S_3 may be present *Respirations:* fine basilar crackles *Lab:* ECG consistent with tissue necrosis (Q waves) and injury (ST-segment elevation); serum enzymes elevated	1. If coronary suspected, call physician, paramedic service, or emergency ambulance 2. Calm and reassure patient that help is coming 3. Place in *semi-Fowler's* position 4. Keep patient warm but not hot	1. Rapidly assess hemodynamic and respiratory status 2. Start IV as ordered—usually 5% D/W per microdrip to establish lifeline for emergency drug treatment 3. Draw blood for electrolytes, enzymes, as ordered 4. Place on cardiac monitor 5. Relieve pain—morphine SO_4 IV as needed 6. Take 12-lead ECG Once patient is stable, transfer to CCU
Cardiac arrest—cardiac standstill or ventricular fibrillation secondary to rapid administration or overdose of anesthetics or narcotic drugs, obstruction of the respiratory tract (mucus, vomitus, foreign body), acute anxiety, cardiac disease, dehydration, shock, electric shock, or emboli	Cyanosis, gasping *Respirations:* rapid, shallow, absent *Pulse:* weak, thready, >120 beats/min, absent Muscle twitching *Pupils:* dilated *Skin:* cold, clammy Loss of consciousness	*CPR* 1. *Position:* flat on back 2. Shake vigorously—establish unresponsiveness 3. Call for help 4. Tilt head back (chin lift) 5. Check for breathing—listen at mouth, look at chest, feel with cheek *No breathing:* 1. Kneel close to head; place hand on forehead, bringing lower jaw forward and opening airway 2. Pinch nostrils shut and blow two full breaths into patient's mouth 3. Lips must form airtight seal 4. Watch chest for adequate expansion; clear throat if indicated 5. Check pulse—if present, breathe into mouth every 5 sec	1. If monitored, note rhythm; call for help and note time 2. Countershock if rhythm is ventricular fibrillation or ventricular tachycardia 3. If countershock unsuccessful, begin CPR, as in prehospital care

TABLE 7–46   Nursing Care of the Adult in Medical and Surgical Emergencies—cont'd

Condition	◆ Assessment: Signs and Symptoms	▶ Prehospitalization Nursing Care	▶ In-hospital Nursing Care
		No heartbeat: *One- or two-person lay rescuers CPR:* 80 chest compressions per minute, with two rescue breaths between every 15 compressions (no difference in ratio for one or two persons); with EMS responders 5 compressions to one breath Check pulse at neck after 1 min and every few minutes thereafter Check pupils to determine effectiveness of CPR—should begin to constrict *Provide early defibrillation* with Automated External Defibrillator (AED) within 5 min of arrest if indicated	*Two-person rescue* *First person:* begins CPR as described in prehospital care *Second person:* 1. Pages arrest team 2. Brings defibrillator to bedside and countershocks, if indicated by rhythm; defibrillate within 3 min of arrest if indicated 3. Brings emergency cart to bedside 4. Suctions airway, if indicated due to vomitus or secretions 5. Bags patient with 100% O_2 6. Assists with intubation when arrest team arrives 7. Establishes intravenous line if one is not available
		If heartbeat returns: assist respiration and monitor pulse; continue CPR until help arrives	
Shock—cellular hypoxia and impairment of cellular function secondary to: trauma, hemorrhage, fright, dehydration, cardiac insufficiency, allergic reactions, septicemia, impairment of nervous system, poisons	**Early shock** *Sensorium:* conscious, apprehensive, and restless; some slurring of speech *Pupils:* dull but reactive to light *Pulse:* rate <140/min; amplitude full to mildy decreased *Blood pressure:* normal to slightly decreased *Neck veins:* normal to slightly flat in supine position; may be full in septic shock or grossly distended in cardiogenic shock *Skin:* cool, clammy, pale *Respirations:* rapid, shallow *GI:* nausea, vomiting, thirst *Renal:* urine output 20–40 mL/hr	1. Check breathing—clear airway if necessary; if no breathing, give artificial respirations; if breathing is irregular or labored, raise head and shoulders 2. Control bleeding by placing pressure on the wound or at pressure points (proximal artery) 3. Make comfortable and reassure 4. Cover lightly to prevent heat loss, but do *not* bundle up 5. If neck or spine injury is suspected—do *not* move, unless victim in danger of more injury	1. Check vital signs rapidly—pulse, pupils, respirations 2. Check airway; clear if necessary; PO_2 should be maintained above 60 mm Hg; elevated PCO_2 indicates need for intubation and ventilatory assistance 3. Control gross bleeding 4. Prepare for insertion of intravenous line and central lines—if abdominal injuries present 5. Peripheral line should be placed in upper extremity if fluids being lost in abdomen
		If patient unconscious or has wounds of the lower face and jaw—place on *side* to promote drainage of fluids; position patient on *back* unless otherwise indicated	1. Draw blood for specimens: Hgb, Hct, CBC, glucose, CO_2, sodium amylase, BUN, K^+; type and crossmatch, blood gases, enzymes, prothrombin times 2. Prepare infusion of 5% D/NS *unless* hypernatremia suspected; dextran if blood loss

Continued

TABLE 7–46   Nursing Care of the Adult in Medical and Surgical Emergencies—cont'd

Condition	◆ Assessment: Signs and Symptoms	▶ Prehospitalization Nursing Care	▶ In-hospital Nursing Care
	Severe or late shock *Sensorium:* confused, disoriented, apathetic, unresponsive; slow, slurred speech, often incoherent *Pupils:* dilating, dilated, slow or nonreactive to light *Pulse:* rate >150 beats/min, thready, weak *Blood pressure:* 80 mm Hg or unobtainable *Neck veins:* flat in a supine position—no filling; full to distended in septic *or* cardiogenic shock *Skin:* cold, clammy, mottled; circumoral cyanosis, dusky, cyanotic *Eyes:* sunken—vacant expression *Renal:* urine output <20 mL/hr	1. *Raise* feet 6–8 inches unless patient has head or chest injuries; if victim becomes less comfortable, lower feet 2. If patient complains of thirst, do *not* give fluids unless you are more than 6 hr away from professional medical help; under *no* conditions give water to patients who are unconscious, having seizures or vomiting, appearing to need general anesthetic, or with a stomach, chest, or skull injury 3. Be calm and confident; reassure patient help is on the way	1. Assess and intervene as for early shock; then obtain information as to onset and past history 2. Catheterize and monitor patient urine output as ordered 3. Take 12-lead ECG 4. Insert nasogastric tube and assess aspirate for volume, color, and blood; save specimen if poison or drug overdose suspected 5. *If CVP low*—infuse 200–300 mL over 5–10 min *If CVP rises* sharply, fluid restriction necessary; if remains low, hypovolemia present 6. *If patient febrile*—blood cultures and wound cultures will be ordered 7. *If urine output* scanty or absent—give mannitol as ordered
Respiratory Emergencies			
Choking—obstruction of airway secondary to aspiration of a foreign object	Gasping, wheezing; looks panicky, but can still breathe, talk, cough Cough: weak, ineffective; breathing sounds like high-pitched crowing; color—white, gray, blue Difficulty speaking; clutches throat	Do not interfere if coughing; do *not* slap on back; watch closely; call for assistance ▶ *Victim standing, sitting and conscious:* Perform *obstructive airway maneuver* (formally Heimlich maneuver), stand behind victim, wrap arms around waist, place fist against abdomen, and with your other hand, press it into the victim's abdomen with a quick upward thrust until the obstruction is relieved or the victim becomes unconscious *Victim lying down:* Roll the victim onto his or her back; straddle the victim's thighs; place heel of hand in the middle of abdomen; place other hand on top of the first; stiffen arms and deliver 6–10 abdominal thrusts	As in prehospital care As in prehospital care

TABLE 7–46   Nursing Care of the Adult in Medical and Surgical Emergencies—cont'd

Condition	◆ Assessment: Signs and Symptoms	▶ Prehospitalization Nursing Care	▶ In-hospital Nursing Care
		Unconscious victim: *Lay rescuers*—proceed to CPR. No abdominal thrusts or blind finger sweeps *EMS responders*—Try to ventilate; if unsuccessful, deliver abdominal thrusts using technique described for obstructive airway; probe mouth for foreign objects; keep repeating above procedure until ventilation occurs; as victim becomes more deprived of air, muscles will relax and maneuvers that were previously unsuccessful will begin to work; when successful in removing obstruction, give two breaths; check pulse; start CPR if indicated	As in prehospital care; when probing mouth for foreign object, turn *head to side,* unless patient has neck injury; ✒ in event of neck injury, *raise* the arm opposite you and roll the head and shoulders as a unit, so that head ends up supported on the arm
		On **obese or pregnant** victims—use chest thrusts instead of abdominal thrusts	
		You are victim and alone: Place your two fists for abdominal thrusts; bend over back of chair, sink, etc. and exert hard, repeated pressure on abdomen to force object up; push fingers down your throat to encourage regurgitation	
Acute respiratory failure—sudden onset of an abnormally low PaO$_2$ (<60 mm Hg) or high PCO$_2$ (>60 mm Hg) secondary to: lung disease or trauma, peripheral or central nervous system depression, cardiac failure, severe obesity, airway obstruction, environmental abnormality	*Hypoxia* *Sensorium:* acute apprehension *Respiration:* dyspnea; shallow, rapid respirations *Skin:* circumoral cyanosis; pale, dusky skin and nailbeds *C/V:* slight hypertension and tachycardia, or hypotension and bradycardia *Hypercapnia* *Sensorium:* decreasing mentation; headache *Skin:* flushed, warm, moist *C/V:* hypertension; tachycardia	If you suspect respiratory distress, call physician; calm and reassure patient; place in a chair or semisitting ✒ position; keep warm but not hot; phone for ambulance; *if respirations cease* or patient becomes unconscious, clear airway and commence respiratory resuscitation; check pulse: initiate CPR if necessary; continue resuscitation until help arrives	Check patient's ability to speak; maintain airway by placing in ✒ *high Fowler's position;* check vital signs: BP, pulse rate and rhythm, temperature, skin color, rate and depth of respirations *Prepare for intubation if:* 1. Patient has flail chest 2. Patient is comatose without gag reflex 3. Has respiratory arrest; maintain mouth to mouth until intubation 4. PaCO$_2$ > 55 mm Hg 5. PaO$_2$ < 60 mm Hg 6. F$_1$O$_2$ > 50% using nasal cannula, catheter, or mask 7. Respiratory rate > 36 *After intubation:* 1. Check bilateral lung sounds 2. Observe for symmetrical lung expansion 3. Maintain humidified oxygen at lowest F$_1$O$_2$ possible to achieve PaO$_2$ of 60 mm Hg

Continued

TABLE 7–46 **Nursing Care of the Adult in Medical and Surgical Emergencies—cont'd**

Condition	◆ Assessment: Signs and Symptoms	▶ Prehospitalization Nursing Care	▶ In-hospital Nursing Care
Abdominal injuries			1. Observe for rigidity 2. Check for hematuria 3. Auscultate for bowel sounds 4. Assist with paracentesis to confirm bleeding in abdominal cavity 5. Prepare for exploratory laparotomy 6. Insert nasogastric tube—to detect presence of upper GI bleeding 7. Monitor vital signs *If organs protruding:* 1. *Flex* patient's knees 2. Cover intestines with sterile towel soaked in saline 3. Do *not* attempt to replace organs
Fractures			1. Administer tetanus toxoid as ordered 2. Observe for pain, peripheral pulses, pallor, loss of sensation and/or movement 3. Assist with wound cleansing, casting, x-rays, reduction 4. Prepare for surgery if indicated 5. Monitor vital signs
Burns—tissue trauma secondary to scalding fluid or flame, chemicals, or electricity	*Superficial (first degree):* Erythema and tenderness Usually sunburn	Relieve pain by applying cold, wet towel or cold water (not iced)	1. Cleanse thoroughly with mild detergent and water 2. Apply gauze or sterile towel 3. Administer sedatives and narcotics as ordered 4. Arrange for follow-up care, or prepare for admission if burn ambulatory care impractical

	Partial thickness (second degree):
	Swelling, blisters; moisture due to escaping plasma
		1. Douse with cold water until pain relieved
		2. Blot skin dry and cover with clean towel
		3. Do *not:* break blisters, remove pieces of skin, or apply antiseptic ointments
		4. If arm or leg burned, keep *elevated*
		5. Seek medical attention if *second-degree* burns:
		  a. Cover 10% of body surface
		  b. Involve hands, feet, or face
			1. Check tetanus immunization status
			2. Administer sedatives or narcotics as ordered
			3. Assess respiratory and hemodynamic status; oxygen or ventilatory assist as indicated, intravenous infusions as ordered to combat shock
			4. Remove all clothing from burn area
			5. Using *aseptic technique,* cleanse burns as indicated.

TABLE 7–46   Nursing Care of the Adult in Medical and Surgical Emergencies—cont'd

Condition	◆ Assessment: Signs and Symptoms	▶ Prehospitalization Nursing Care	▶ In-hospital Nursing Care

	Full thickness (third degree): White, charred areas	1. Do *not* remove charred clothing
		2. Cover burned area with clean towel, sheet
		◩ 3. *Elevate* burned extremities
		4. Apply cold pack to hand, face, or feet
		◩ 5. Sit up patient with face or chest wound to assist respirations
		6. Maintain airway
		7. Observe for shock
		8. Do *not:*
		   a. Put ice water on burns or immerse wounds in ice water—may increase shock
		   b. Apply ointments
		9. Calm and reassure victim
		10. Get medical help promptly
		11. *If* patient conscious, not vomiting, and medical assistance is more than 6 hr away: may give sips of weak solution of salt, soda, and water
			1. Do *not* break blebs or attempt debridement
			2. Assist with application of dressings as ordered
			3. Maintain frequent checks of vital signs, urine output
			4. Provide psychological support—explain procedures, orient, etc.
			5. Assist with application of splints as ordered
			◖▭ 6. Administer tetanus immune globulin or toxoid as ordered
			7. Assist with transfer to hospital unit

	Fourth degree: Black	Same as full thickness.	
	Chemical burns	1. Flush with copious amounts of water 2. Get rid of clothing over burned area	1. Flush with copious amounts of water ◖▭ 2. Administer sedation or narcotics as ordered
	Burns of the eye: Acid	1. Flush eye with water for at least 15 min 2. Pour water from inside to outside of eye to *avoid contaminating unaffected eye* 3. Cover—seek medical attention at once	1. Irrigate with water; *never* use neutralizing solution ◖▭ 2. Instill 0.5% tetracaine as ordered 3. Apply patch
	Alkali (laundry detergent or cleaning solvent)	1. Do *not* allow a patient to rub eye 2. Flush eye with water for at least 30 min 3. Cover—seek medical attention at once	As above for acid
Abdominal Emergencies			
Aortic aneurysm—rupture or dissection	Primarily men > age 60 Sudden onset of excruciating pain: abdominal, lumbosacral, groin, or rectal Orthopnea, dyspnea Fainting, hypotension; if dissecting, marked hypertension may be present Palpable, tender, pulsating mass in umbilical area Femoral pulse present; dorsalis pedis—weak or absent	1. Notify physician ◩ 2. Lay patient flat, or raise head if in respiratory distress 3. Cover—keep warm but *not* hot 4. Institute shock measures as above 5. Calm; reassure that help is on the way.	1. Assess respiratory and hemodynamic status 2. Institute shock measures (see p. 459) if indicated 3. Evaluate and compare peripheral pulses 4. Assist with x-rays 5. Assist with emergency preoperative treatment

Continued

Adult

TABLE 7–46 **Nursing Care of the Adult in Medical and Surgical Emergencies—cont'd**

Condition	◆ Assessment: Signs and Symptoms	▶ Prehospitalization Nursing Care	▶ In-hospital Nursing Care

Blunt injuries—spleen	Left upper quadrant pain, tenderness and moderate rigidity; left shoulder pain *(Kehr's sign)*
	Hypotension; weak, thready pulse; increased respirations (shock)
		1. Lay patient *flat*
		2. Institute shock measures (see p. 459)
			1. Assess respiratory and hemo-dynamic status
			  a. Maintain airway and ventilation as indicated
			  b. Institute infusions of colloid or crystalloids as ordered
			  c. Insert both CVP and arterial monitoring lines
			  d. Insert *Foley* catheter
			2. Prepare for splenectomy

Eye and Ear Emergencies			
Chemical burns	See *Burns*	See *Burns*	See *Burns*
Blunt injuries secondary to flying missiles, e.g., balls, striking face against car dashboard	Decreased visual acuity, diplopia, blood in anterior chamber Pain, conjunctiva reddened, edema of eyelids	1. Prevent victim from rubbing eye 2. Cover with patch to protect eye 3. Seek medical help immediately	1. Test visual acuity of each eye using *Snellen* or *Jaeger* chart 2. Assist with *fluorescein* administration—to facilitate identifying breaks in cornea
Sharp ocular trauma—secondary to small or larger foreign bodies	Reports feeling as if something were hitting eye Pain, tearing, reddened conjunctiva Blurring of vision Foreign object may be visible	1. Keep victim from rubbing eye 2. Cover very lightly—do *not* apply pressure	1. Check visual acuity in both eyes 2. Check pupils 3. Instill 1% tetracaine HCl as ordered to relieve pain 4. Administer antibiotic drops or ointment as ordered 5. Apply eye patch 6. Provide instructions for subsequent care and follow-up

Foreign bodies in ears—beans, peas, candy, foxtails, insects	Decreased hearing; pulling, poking at ear and ear canal; buzzing, discomfort	1. Do *not* attempt to remove object
		2. Seek medical assistance
			1. Inspect ear canal
			2. Assist with sedating children—restraint may be necessary
			3. Assist with procedures to remove object:
			  a. Forceps or curved probe for *foxtails, irregularly shaped* objects
			  b. 10F or 12F catheter with tip cut squarely off and attached to suction to remove *round* object
			4. Irrigate external auditory canal to flush out *insects,* materials that do not absorb water; do *not* irrigate if danger of perforation

Questions

Select the one best answer for each question.

1. Nursing preparations for a gastroscopy procedure include:
   1. Holding the patient NPO for 24 hours before the procedure.
   2. Having an operative or procedure permit signed.
   3. Reassuring the patient that gastroscopy is not an uncomfortable procedure, though he or she will need to lie quietly.
   4. Removing dentures and administering pain medication before the procedure.

2. Which nursing action is the *first* priority during a generalized tonic-clonic seizure episode?
   1. Observe and record all events that occur before, during, and after the seizure.
   2. Maintain a patent airway by turning the head to the side.
   3. Protect the patient from injury.
   4. Monitor vital signs, with special attention directed to respiratory status.

3. Which nursing intervention would be the most beneficial in preparing the patient psychologically for ileostomy surgery?
   1. Include the patient's family in preoperative teaching sessions.
   2. Encourage the patient to express his or her concerns and to ask questions regarding the management of the ileostomy.
   3. Thorough, brief explanation of all preoperative and postoperative procedures.
   4. Have a member of an "ostomy club" visit the patient.

4. Which of the following indicates circulatory constriction in the patient with a newly applied long leg cast?
   1. Tingling and numbness of toes.
   2. Inability to move toes.
   3. Blanching or cyanosis of toes.
   4. Complaints of pressure or tightness of the cast.

5. Paralytic ileus is described by the nurse as:
   1. Edema of the intestinal mucosa.
   2. Acute dilation of the colon.
   3. Absent, diminished, or uncoordinated autonomic stimulation of peristalsis.
   4. High, tinkling bowel sounds over the area of obstruction.

6. The doctor has ordered ambulation on crutches, with no weight bearing on the affected limb. An appropriate crutch gait for the nurse to teach the patient would be:
   1. Two-point gait.
   2. Three-point gait.
   3. Four-point gait.
   4. Tripod gait.

7. Nursing preparation for an upper GI series includes:
   1. NPO for 24 hours before the procedure.
   2. Administering an enema or cathartic to enhance visualization.
   3. Discouraging the patient from smoking the morning of the procedure because smoking can stimulate gastric motility.
   4. Instructing the patient that the test involves insertion of a rubber gastroscopy tube.

8. Burns are classified according to the depth of tissue destruction. The nurse would recognize a deep partial-thickness burn because the burn:
   1. Involves the epidermis only.
   2. Extends to the dermis and is very painful.
   3. Extends to subcutaneous tissues and is rarely painful.
   4. Extends to muscle and bone and is very painful.

9. The nurse's best explanation of the basic emotional issue underlying or contributing to the development of ulcers would be:
   1. Anxiety neurosis.
   2. Dependence-independence conflict.
   3. Repressed anger and hostility.
   4. Compulsive time orientation.

10. Which patient problem relating to altered nutrition is a consequence of impaired physical mobility?
    1. Increased appetite.
    2. Decreased protein catabolism.
    3. Increased carbohydrate needs.
    4. Increased secretion of digestive enzymes.

11. The signs and symptoms of open-angle glaucoma are related to:
    1. An imbalance between the rate of secretion of intraocular fluids and the rate of absorption of aqueous humor.
    2. A degenerative disease characterized by narrowing of the arterioles of the retina and areas of ischemia.
    3. An infectious process that causes clouding and scarring of the cornea.
    4. A dysfunction of aging in which the retina of the eye buckles from inadequate fluid pressures.

12. Patients suffering from dumping syndrome should be advised by the nurse to:
    1. Drink liquids between meals.
    2. Drink liquids only with meals.
    3. Drink liquids any time they want.
    4. Restrict fluid intake to 1200 mL/day.

13. Urinary output is closely assessed after nephrectomy. Which assessment finding is an early indicator of fluid retention in the postoperative period?
    1. Increased specific gravity of urine.
    2. Daily weight gain of 2 lb or more.
    3. A urinary output of 50 mL/hr.
    4. Periorbital edema.

14. Which statement by the nurse accurately describes the Miller-Abbott tube?
    1. A double-lumen tube, with one lumen leading to the inflatable balloon and the other lumen used for aspiration.
    2. A plastic or rubber tube with holes near its tip facilitating withdrawal of fluids from the stomach.
    3. A single-lumen, saline-, air-, or water-weighted tube approximately 6 feet long.
    4. A 10-foot-long rubber tube with a saline, air, or water bag at its end.

15. The correct interpretation of the above arrhythmia is:
    1. Sinus rhythm with multifocal premature ventricular contractions (PVCs).
    2. Atrial fibrillation with unifocal PVCs.
    3. Sinus tachycardia with unifocal PVCs.
    4. Second-degree atrioventricular block with unifocal PVCs.

16. If treatment with thyroid hormone is effective, the nurse should expect:
    1. Diuresis, a decrease in pulse rate, and an increase in blood pressure.
    2. Diuresis, a widening pulse pressure, and an increase in both temperature and respiratory rate.
    3. Increased pulse rate, decreased respiratory rate, and decreased puffiness.
    4. Weight loss, increased diastolic blood pressure, and decreased pulse rate.

17. A patient was admitted to the hospital with deep partial-thickness burns of the left leg and thigh. The nurse would expect this patient's serum-sodium level to be within normal limits at the time of admission because:
    1. The pituitary has increased ADH release.
    2. Vascular fluid losses due to exudate and edema formation have resulted in hemoconcentration.
    3. Sodium has diffused from disrupted cells into the vascular compartment.
    4. Increased serum potassium has depressed aldosterone secretion by the adrenal cortex.

18. Nursing actions for patients with Addison's disease include:
    1. Providing a low-sodium diet.
    2. Restricting fluids to 1500 mL/day.
    3. Administering insulin-replacement therapy.
    4. Reducing physical and emotional stress.

19. The nurse explains to a patient that a vagotomy is done in conjunction with a subtotal gastrectomy because the vagus nerve:

    1. Stimulates increased gastric motility.
    2. Decreases gastric motility, thereby preventing the movement of HCl out of the stomach.
    3. Stimulates both increased gastric secretion and gastric motility.
    4. Stimulates decreased gastric secretion, thereby increasing nausea and vomiting.

20. In planning care for a patient with hyperkalemia, the nurse knows that the treatment of choice to reduce hyperkalemia is:
    1. Morphine sulfate.
    2. Sodium polystyrene sulfonate (Kayexalate).
    3. Insulin and 50% glucose solution.
    4. Synthetic aldosterone.

21. Understanding that prolonged immobilization could lead to decubitus ulcers, the nurse plans interventions to prevent alterations in skin integrity. Which would be the *least* appropriate intervention?
    1. Use of a bed cradle.
    2. Giving backrubs with alcohol.
    3. Encouraging a high-protein diet.
    4. Frequent assessment of the skin.

22. The nurse knows that the physiological response to the stress of extensive burns may result in the following complication in the postburn period:
    1. Curling's ulcer due to elevated serum cortisol.
    2. Positive nitrogen balance due to mobilization of body proteins.
    3. Decreased hematocrit due to red-blood-cell agglutination by epinephrine.
    4. Hypothermia and hyperthermia due to failure of hypothalamic temperature regulators.

23. The nurse knows that the arrhythmia shown above, if untreated, is most likely to:
    1. Progress to ventricular fibrillation.
    2. Increase the blood pressure suddenly.
    3. Intensify chest pain from a myocardial infarction (MI).
    4. Cause no observable change in the patient.

24. Several hours after a long leg cast has been applied, the nurse notices that the patient's toes have become edematous. The physician decides to bivalve the cast. The nurse explains to the patient that this procedure:
    1. Requires recasting after 24 hours.
    2. Includes splitting and spreading the cast down the middle to relieve constriction.
    3. Includes splitting and spreading the cast on each side and cutting the underlying padding.
    4. Should be followed by placing the patient's leg in a dependent position.

25. Which statement would the nurse include in teaching regarding nasogastric tubes?
    1. Nasogastric tubes should be irrigated with sterile water.
    2. Patient should be in a sitting position with head slightly flexed for tube insertion.
    3. When resistance is met while irrigating a nasogastric tube, pressure should be increased to complete that irrigation, and the physician should be notified at the completion.
    4. Ice chips can be taken as often as desired to promote comfort in the throat.

26. To correctly instill pilocarpine in a patient's eyes, the nurse should gently pull down the lower lid of the eye and instill the drops:
    1. Directly on the central surface of the cornea.
    2. On the inner canthus of the eye.
    3. Into the conjunctival sac.
    4. Directly on the dilated pupil.

27. The nurse anticipates that the backbone of treatment for patients with myasthenia gravis will be:
    1. Adrenergic drugs.
    2. Anticholinergic drugs.
    3. Anticholinesterase drugs.
    4. Cholinergic drugs.

28. A patient's burns were treated by the closed method. The burned left leg was cleaned and the left ankle debrided. Mafenide 1% (Sulfamylon) was applied, and the leg was wrapped in fine mesh gauze. Nursing measures when this approach is used include:
    1. Cleansing of the wound daily and maintenance of strict isolation to prevent air contamination.
    2. Cleansing of the wound daily, or more often if needed, and application of new dressings using clean technique.
    3. Cleansing the wound one or more times each day and application of new dressing using sterile technique.
    4. Cleansing of the wound daily and utilization of heat lamps to help maintain normal body temperature.

29. The nurse tells a postoperative gastrectomy patient that dumping syndrome is a significant problem for:
    1. 70–80% of patients having gastrectomies.
    2. 50% of patients having gastrectomies.
    3. 25% of patients having gastrectomies.
    4. 5–10% of patients having gastrectomies.

30. The nurse knows that, in contrast to patients with hypothyroidism, women with hyperthyroidism have:
    1. Increased serum cholesterol.
    2. Increased basal metabolic rate and serum T_3 and T_4.
    3. Increased serum thyroid-stimulating hormone (TSH).
    4. Increased menstrual volume.

31. Pilocarpine is the drug of choice in the treatment of open-angle glaucoma. The expected outcome following administration would be:
    1. Blocked action of cholinesterase at the cholinergic nerve endings, and therefore increased pupil size.

    2. Constricted pupil and therefore widened outflow channels and increased flow of aqueous fluid.
    3. Impaired vision from decreased aqueous humor production.
    4. Constriction of aqueous veins and therefore decreased venous pooling in the eye.

32. Hyponatremia may develop in patients with burns due to:
    1. Displacement of sodium in edema fluids and loss through denuded areas of skin.
    2. Increased aldosterone secretion.
    3. Inadequate fluid replacement.
    4. Metabolic acidosis.

33. A patient has had a partial gastrectomy, vagotomy, and gastrojejunostomy. Which complication would the nurse primarily anticipate in this patient's postoperative period?
    1. Thrombophlebitis from decreased mobility.
    2. Abdominal distention due to air swallowing.
    3. Atelectasis due to shallow breathing.
    4. Urinary retention due to prolonged use of anticholinergic medications.

34. The nurse tells a postoperative gastrectomy patient that the nasogastric tube will be removed:
    1. Standard only on the fourth postoperative day.
    2. When bowel sounds are established and the patient has passed flatus or stool.
    3. Thirty-six hours after the cessation of bloody drainage.
    4. After 2 days of alternate clamping and unclamping of the tube.

35. A patient with burns is to receive fluid replacement therapy. Besides assessing size and depth of the burn, which physical parameters are also important baseline data for fluid replacement therapy?
    1. Age, sex, and vital signs.
    2. Age, weight, vital signs, and skin turgor.
    3. Vital signs, level of mentation, and urine output.
    4. Vital signs and quantity and specific gravity of urine.

36. The nurse is to administer the drug of choice for long-term control of generalized tonic-clonic seizures. This drug is:
    1. Phenobarbital.
    2. Diazepam (Valium).
    3. Diphenylhydantoin (Dilantin) sodium.
    4. Trimethadione (Tridione).

37. An angiogram was performed using a catheter inserted into the left femoral artery. Which nursing action is the *first* priority following this procedure?
    1. Monitoring vital signs until stable.
    2. Frequently checking the puncture site for fresh bleeding, swelling, or increasing tenderness.
    3. Measuring the quantity and specific gravity of urinary output.
    4. Checking the peripheral pulses distal to the femoral puncture site.

38. Which replacement fluid will the nurse *least* often be expected to administer to a patient with burns within the first 24 hours postburn?
    1. Ringer's lactate.
    2. Whole blood.
    3. Dextran.
    4. Dextrose and water.

39. The nurse must observe for which imbalance to occur with prolonged nasogastric suctioning?
    1. Hypernatremia.
    2. Hyperkalemia.
    3. Metabolic alkalosis.
    4. Hypoproteinemia.

40. After left nephrectomy, a patient has a large flank incision. In order to facilitate deep breathing and coughing, the nurse should:
    1. Have the patient lie on the unaffected side.
    2. Coordinate breathing and coughing exercises with administration of analgesics.
    3. Maintain the patient in high Fowler's position.
    4. Push fluid administration to loosen respiratory secretions.

41. The postoperative nephrectomy patient should be closely observed by the nurse for:
    1. Hemorrhage.
    2. Hyperkalemia.
    3. Respiratory alkalosis and tetany.
    4. Polyuria.

42. Two days postoperatively, a patient who has had an ileostomy begins to refuse care and repeatedly says to the staff, "Leave me alone, I just want to sleep." What would be the first nursing action?
    1. Provide accurate, brief, and reassuring explanations of all procedures.
    2. Encourage ambulation in the hall with other patients.
    3. Invite a member of an "ostomy club" to visit the patient.
    4. Encourage the patient to verbalize his or her feelings, fears, and questions.

43. Before insertion of a Miller-Abbott tube, the balloon is tested for patency and capacity and then deflated. Which nursing measure will ease the insertion of the nasoenteric tube?
    1. Chilling the tube before insertion.
    2. Administering a sedative to reduce anxiety.
    3. Warming the tube before insertion.
    4. Positioning the patient in low Fowler's position.

44. Small, frequent feedings of which type of diet would the nurse recommend for patients experiencing dumping syndrome?
    1. Low-protein, high-fat, low-carbohydrate diet.
    2. High-protein, high-fat, high-carbohydrate diet.
    3. High-protein, high-fat, low-carbohydrate diet.
    4. Low-protein, low-fat, high-carbohydrate diet.

45. The nurse recognizes that myasthenia gravis is:
    1. An upper motor neuron lesion.
    2. A lower motor neuron lesion.
    3. A combined upper and lower motor neuron lesion.
    4. A genetic dysfunction.

46. The mouth care measure that should be used with caution by the nurse when a patient has a nasogastric tube is:
    1. Regularly brushing teeth and tongue with soft brush.
    2. Sucking on ice chips to relieve dryness.
    3. Occasionally rinsing mouth with a nonastringent substance and massaging gums.
    4. Application of lemon juice and glycerine swabs to the lips

47. The nurse can expect hyperkalemia to develop following burn damage because there is:
    1. Increased exudate formation at the burn site.
    2. Disruption of cell membrane integrity, allowing intracellular electrolytes to diffuse into the vascular compartment.
    3. Decreased aldosterone secretion, increasing sodium excretion, and retention of potassium.
    4. Hyperbilirubinemia secondary to red blood cell destruction.

48. Two days before discharge following a left nephrectomy, a patient expressed renewed concern over the ability to continue many activities with only one kidney. The nurse responds.
    1. "You seem depressed. Actually you are very lucky, since the pathology reports indicate your tumor was encapsulated."
    2. "Lots of people do quite well with only one kidney."
    3. "Would you like me to call the doctor so you two can discuss it?"
    4. "I can understand your concern, but your remaining kidney is sufficient to maintain normal renal functions."

49. A patient is admitted to the orthopedic unit with a long leg cast, used to immobilize a transverse fracture of the right tibia and fibula. The plaster of paris cast is damp, and the patient is complaining that it feels very hot. The nurse should:
    1. Explain to the patient that the cast will feel hot for several hours as the moisture evaporates and the cast hardens.
    2. Recognize that this is a sign of excessive pressure on the soft tissues and notify the physician.
    3. Tell the patient not to worry; this is a common complaint.
    4. Administer meperidine (Demerol), 50 mg IM, to relieve discomfort.

50. Diagnosis of myasthenia gravis is frequently based on the patient's response to an intravenous injection of edrophonium (Tensilon). If the patient responds positively to this drug, the nurse should expect:
    1. Exacerbation of symptomatology.
    2. Relief of ptosis but not of weakness in other facial muscles.

3. A prompt and dramatic increase in muscle strength.

4. A slight increase in muscle strength that is countered by an increase in muscle fatigability.

51. Assessment of the intraocular pressure as measured by tonometry would be normal if the value is in the range:
   1. 5–10 mm Hg.
   2. 12–22 mm Hg.
   3. 10–20 cm H_2O.
   4. 20–30 mm Hg.

52. On the morning of discharge, a patient who had an emergency abdominal hysterectomy is found sitting with her back to the door, staring out the window. She says that she no longer feels like a real woman. The nurse's response should be to:
   1. Ask her if she would like her diazepam (Valium).
   2. Notify the physician.
   3. Ask, "Can you tell me what makes you feel that way?"
   4. Reassure her that this is a common reaction.

53. Which behavior is *least* likely to be included in the nursing assessment of a patient with burns during the recovery period?
   1. Anxiety with mild confusion.
   2. Desperation and panic.
   3. Withdrawal and depression.
   4. Dependency and regression.

54. Forty-eight hours after a nephrectomy, a patient complains of increasing nausea and abdominal pressure. The nurse's *first* nursing action is to:
   1. Change the patient's position to relieve abdominal pressure.
   2. Auscultate bowel sounds.
   3. Insert a rectal tube to relieve flatus.
   4. Administer morphine SO_4, 6 mg, as ordered for the relief of discomfort.

55. Which instruction would be *inappropriate* when teaching a patient to use crutches?
   1. Use axilla to help carry weight.
   2. Use short strides to maintain maximum mobility.
   3. Keep feet 6–8 inches apart to provide a wide base for support.
   4. If the patient should begin to fall, throw crutches to the side to prevent falling on them.

56. The nurse explains that epileptic seizures or convulsions result from:
   1. Excessive exercise with lactic acid accumulation.
   2. Excessive, simultaneous, disordered neuronal discharge.
   3. Excessive cerebral metabolism, with local K^+ increased.
   4. Excessive circulating cerebrospinal fluid increasing cerebral pressures.

57. What nursing action best facilitates the passage of the nasoenteric tube from the stomach through the pylorus and into the duodenum?
   1. Gently advancing the tube 1–4 inches at regular time intervals.
   2. Positioning the patient on the right side for 2 hours after insertion.
   3. Maintaining strict bed rest and avoiding all unnecessary movement.
   4. Positioning the patient in a flat supine position.

58. During the initial stage of burns, a primary fluid imbalance occurs. The nurse knows that there has been a shift of fluids from:
   1. The cell to the interstitial space.
   2. The interstitial space into the cell.
   3. The interstitial space to the plasma.
   4. The plasma to the interstitial space.

59. Bed rest is ordered for a patient with chronic glaucoma during a period of acute distress, because activity tends to increase intraocular pressure. Which activity of daily living should this patient be instructed to avoid?
   1. Watching television.
   2. Brushing teeth and hair.
   3. Self-feeding.
   4. Passive range-of-motion exercises.

60. Nursing implications with diphenylhydantoin given during treatment of status epilepticus include giving the intravenous injection slowly and in small increments to prevent:
   1. Respiratory depression and/or arrest.
   2. Vasodepression and circulatory shock.
   3. Irritation and/or necrosis of the vein and surrounding tissue.
   4. Vasomotor stimulation, with a sudden, malignant increase in blood pressure.

61. The nurse would be alerted to a sudden increase in intraocular pressure if the patient with open-angle glaucoma complained of:
   1. Generalized decrease in peripheral vision over the past year.
   2. Difficulty with close vision.
   3. Increasing discomfort in the left eye with radiation to the forehead and left temple.
   4. Halos around lights.

62. The nurse will usually ambulate a patient postgastrectomy beginning:
   1. The day after surgery.
   2. 3–4 days after surgery.
   3. After 4 days of bed rest.
   4. Immediately after awakening from anesthesia.

63. If "cholinergic crisis" is demonstrated in a patient who has myasthenia gravis, all anticholinesterase drugs are withdrawn. To reduce symptoms, which of the following drugs should the nurse be prepared to give?
   1. Atropine.
   2. Ephedrine sulfate.
   3. Potassium chloride.
   4. Neostigmine bromide.

64. Equally important as the depth of tissue destruction in determining severity of burns is the total body surface involved. The nurse would anticipate potential fluid and electrolyte problems when burns are:
    1. Superficial partial thickness and cover 20% of the body surface.
    2. Deep partial thickness and cover 15% of the body surface.
    3. Full thickness and cover 10% of the body surface.
    4. Fourth degree and cover 5% of the body surface.

65. Patient teaching about glaucoma should include a comparison of the two types. Open-angle, or chronic glaucoma differs from closed-angle or acute glaucoma in that:
    1. Open-angle glaucoma occurs less frequently than closed-angle glaucoma.
    2. Open-angle glaucoma's symptomatology includes pain, severe headache, nausea, and vomiting; closed-angle glaucoma has a slow, silent, and generally painless onset.
    3. The obstruction to aqueous flow in open-angle glaucoma generally occurs somewhere in Schlemm's canal or aqueous veins. It does not narrow or close the angle of the anterior chamber, as in closed-angle glaucoma.
    4. Open-angle glaucoma rarely occurs in families; however, there is a hereditary predisposition for closed-angle glaucoma.

66. The adequacy of fluid volume replacement in the early postburn period is best reflected by:
    1. Blood pressure, pulse rates, and daily weights.
    2. Quantity of urinary output and vital signs.
    3. Hemoglobin and hematocrit levels.
    4. Serum-electrolyte levels and urinary output.

67. Which aspect of open-angle glaucoma and its medical treatment is the *most frequent* cause of patient non-compliance?
    1. Loss of mobility due to severe driving restrictions.
    2. The painful and insidious progression of this type of glaucoma.
    3. Decreased light and near-vision accommodation due to miotic effects of pilocarpine.
    4. The frequent nausea and vomiting accompanying use of miotic drugs.

68. Which would the nurse expect to see with the dumping syndrome?
    1. Feeling of hunger.
    2. Constipation.
    3. Increased strength.
    4. Diaphoresis.

69. The nurse observes a patient in the orthopedic clinic using a long pencil to scratch the skin under the cast. The nurse should:
    1. Ask the physician for an oral medication order to relieve itching.
    2. Explain to the patient that scratching under the cast should be avoided, because it may break the skin and cause an infection.

3. Assist the patient by gently rolling the casted leg in the palmar surfaces of the nurse's hands.
4. Take the pencil away from the patient.

70. The *best* explanation for the nurse to offer to a patient and family would be that myasthenia gravis is a:
    1. Degenerative dysfunction of the basal ganglia.
    2. Transmission dysfunction at the myoneural junction.
    3. Hypertrophic reaction in the anterior motor neurons of the spinal cord.
    4. Hereditary condition of cranial nerves VII, IX, and X.

71. Fifty-four hours after a patient sustained deep partial-thickness burns of the left leg and thigh, the patient's urine output increased from 1000 to 2300 mL/24 hr. Laboratory values were as follows: serum sodium, 136 mEq/L; serum potassium, 4 mEq/L; and hematocrit, 34%. The nurse knows that the changes in the patient's urinary output and lab studies indicate:
    1. Beginning of the interstitial-to-plasma fluid shift phase of burns.
    2. Kidney failure.
    3. Circulatory overload due to rapid IV infusion rate.
    4. Hyponatremia.

72. A nursing care plan includes observing for the most common patient problems arising from the use of pyridostigmine (Mestinon) and neostigmine bromide (Prostigmin), which include:
    1. Gastric distress—nausea, anorexia, diarrhea.
    2. Elimination problems—urinary retention.
    3. Central nervous system excitation—flushing, irritability.
    4. Cardiac arrhythmias—palpitations, PVCs.

73. Before discharge a postoperative gastrectomy patient asks the nurse pointedly, "How long will it be before I can eat three meals a day like the rest of my family?" The nurse responds:
    1. "Eating six meals a day can be a bother, can't it?"
    2. "Some patients can tolerate three meals a day by the time they leave the hospital. Maybe it will be a little longer for you."
    3. "You will probably have to eat six meals a day for the rest of your life."
    4. "It varies from patient to patient, but generally in 6–12 months most patients can return to their previous meal patterns."

74. The nurse would be correct in saying that two common causes of primary hypothyroidism are:
    1. Destruction of thyroid tissue by radioactive iodine during therapy for hyperthyroidism, and spontaneous atrophy due to autoimmune response.
    2. Spontaneous atrophy due to autoimmune response, and surgical removal of the thyroid gland.
    3. Surgical removal of the thyroid gland, and tumors of the pituitary gland that decrease the amount of circulating thyroxine.
    4. Tumors of the pituitary gland, and/or large doses of antithyroid drugs.

75. In order to take full advantage of the effects of pyridostigmine bromide and neostigmine bromide in reducing dysphagia related to myasthenia gravis, the nurse should plan to give the medications before meals. How long before?
    1. 2 hours.
    2. 45–60 minutes.
    3. 20–30 minutes.
    4. 10–15 minutes.

76. A patient recuperating from burns is withdrawn and depressed. The nurse can expect this patient to exhibit such psychological reactions during the recuperative stage because of:
    1. Pain and immobility.
    2. Changes in body image.
    3. Financial concerns.
    4. Anger.

77. Because medications have been increased for a patient with myasthenia gravis, it is important that the nurse observe for signs of "cholinergic crisis." These include:
    1. Dilated pupils, profuse diaphoresis, and trembling.
    2. Constricted pupils, hypersalivation, and hypotension.
    3. Dilated pupils, nausea, and tachycardia.
    4. Constricted pupils, dry mucous membranes, and bradycardia.

78. The nursing assessment of a patient recently diagnosed with hypothyroidism will likely reveal the most common clinical manifestations of hypothyroidism, which are:
    1. Increased body temperature, tachycardia, and fatigue.
    2. Decreased exercise tolerance and facial and pitting edema.
    3. Increased sluggishness, increased cold intolerance, and puffy eyelids, hands, and feet.
    4. Decreased facial expression, diarrhea, and weight gain.

79. In contrast to hypothyroidism, hyperthyroidism is due to excessive levels of thyroxine in the plasma. Clinical data gathered by the nurse indicating this endocrine dysfunction would include:
    1. Systolic hypertension and heat intolerance.
    2. Diastolic hypertension and widened pulse pressure.
    3. Heat intolerance and weight gain.
    4. Emotional hyperexcitability and anorexia.

80. Which statement by the nurse about myasthenia gravis is accurate?
    1. Thymectomies rarely produce remissions in myasthenia gravis.
    2. Myasthenia gravis is an acute illness that progresses rapidly.
    3. Myasthenia gravis has increased muscle strength as a major symptom.
    4. Myasthenia gravis may be an autoimmune disease.

81. Which nursing intervention would be included in the preoperative period for a patient who will have a partial gastrectomy, vagotomy, and gastrojejunostomy?

    1. Insertion of a nasogastric tube before surgery.
    2. Administration of diazepam (Valium), 4 mg, with 4 oz water 1 hour before surgery.
    3. Detailed description of the possible complications that could happen postoperatively.
    4. Instructions to avoid taking pain medication too frequently in the first 2 postoperative days to avoid drug dependency.

82. Both Cushing's syndrome and Addison's disease are due to dysfunction of the adrenal cortex. In order to plan for the care of a patient with Cushing's syndrome, the nurse should know that the primary pathology is:
    1. Increased cortisol secretion.
    2. Increased epinephrine secretion.
    3. Decreased aldosterone secretion.
    4. Decreased ACTH secretion.

83. Because cortisol is a glucocorticoid, the nurse caring for the patient with Cushing's syndrome should expect:
    1. Hypoglycemia due to increased insulin production.
    2. Skeletal-muscle wasting because glucocorticoids promote protein and fat mobilization.
    3. Dependent edema and severe hypokalemia due to abnormal aldosterone secretion.
    4. Discoloration or hyperpigmentation of the skin due to increased pituitary secretion of ACTH.

84. In Addison's disease, glucocorticoids, mineralocorticoids, and androgenic hormones are all reduced. Therefore, in contrast to Cushing's syndrome, the nurse should expect to find:
    1. Hypotension, weight loss, and physical and mental exhaustion.
    2. Hypertension, moon facies, and masculinization in women.
    3. Hypotension, hyperglycemia, and weight gain.
    4. Hypertension, male impotency, and menstrual disturbances.

85. Iron deficiency anemia is best described as:
    1. Hypochromic microcytic.
    2. Hyperchromic macrocytic.
    3. Hyperchromic microcytic.
    4. Hypochromic macrocytic.

86. The nurse should expect that a patient's emotional responses to acute rheumatoid arthritis would primarily depend on the patient's:
    1. Self-concept, body image, and usual effective coping strategies.
    2. Relationship with the patient's mother.
    3. Usual effective or palliative coping strategies only.
    4. Economic status and work history.

87. Because aldosterone is the major mineralocorticoid secreted by the adrenal cortex, which fluid and electrolyte imbalance should the nurse anticipate with decreased secretion of this hormone?
    1. Hyperkalemia.
    2. Hypernatremia.
    3. Hypervolemia.
    4. Hypercalcemia.

88. The care plan for a patient who is burned includes observing for side effects of mafenide 1% (Sulfamylon), such as:
    1. Severe electrolyte disturbances.
    2. Metabolic acidosis.
    3. Metabolic alkalosis.
    4. Staining of linen.

89. A patient complains of not having had a bowel movement since being admitted 2 days ago for multiple fractures of both lower legs. The patient is on bed rest and skeletal traction. Which intervention would be the *most* appropriate nursing action?
    1. Administer an enema.
    2. Put the patient on the bedpan every 2 hours.
    3. Ensure maximum fluid intake (3000 mL/day).
    4. Perform range-of-motion exercises to all extremities.

90. Which cardinal sign heralds the onset of thyroid storm?
    1. Fever.
    2. Tachycardia.
    3. Hypertension.
    4. Tremulousness.

91. The nurse would recognize drainage of blood from the nasogastric tube after gastrectomy surgery as abnormal if:
    1. It continued for 4–6 hours.
    2. It continued for a period longer than 12 hours.
    3. It turned greenish yellow in less than 24 hours.
    4. It was dark red in the immediate postoperative period.

92. Fluid therapy postburn may necessitate as much as 7 liters of fluid in 24 hours for a 70 kg individual. Using a 15 gtt/mL administration set, the drops per minute that the nurse would set to deliver this volume would be:
    1. 48 gtt/min.
    2. 75 gtt/min.
    3. 60 gtt/min.
    4. 90 gtt/min.

93. The nurse anticipates that osteoporosis may result from prolonged immobilization because of:
    1. Lack of weight bearing, which decreases osteoblastic activity.
    2. Decreased dietary calcium intake.
    3. Deposition of excess calcium phosphate salts.
    4. Lack of weight bearing, which increases bone formation.

94. The appropriate nursing response to the above arrhythmia would be to:
    1. Administer a bolus of lidocaine, 50 mg IV.
    2. Limit patient activity while the arrhythmia is present.

    3. Hold digoxin until atrioventricular node depression reverses.
    4. Do nothing, particularly with no symptoms.

95. The nurse knows that in a patient who has deep partial or full-thickness burns, the hematocrit is reduced due to:
    1. Lack of erythropoietin factor.
    2. Hemodilution and volume overload.
    3. Metabolic acidosis.
    4. Hypoalbuminemia.

96. Following gastrectomy surgery the nurse must observe for signs of pernicious anemia, which may be a problem after gastrectomy because:
    1. The extrinsic factor is produced in the stomach.
    2. The extrinsic factor is absorbed in the antral portion of the stomach.
    3. The intrinsic factor is produced in the stomach.
    4. Decreased hydrochloric acid production inhibits vitamin B_{12} reabsorption.

97. Which nursing intervention can aid in reducing the gastric side effects of pyridostigmine bromide (Mestinon) and neostigmine bromide (Prostigmin)?
    1. Give with milk, soda crackers, or antacids.
    2. Push fluids and encourage ambulation.
    3. Keep room cool and discourage visitors.
    4. Encourage food high in potassium.

98. The nurse would recognize a generalized tonic-clonic seizure if which of the following occurred?
    1. Brief, abrupt loss of consciousness lasting 10–20 seconds.
    2. Loss of consciousness for several minutes, with sustained and intermittent contractions of all motor muscle groups.
    3. Sustained and intermittent contractions of selected motor groups in a somewhat confined area.
    4. Twitching of facial muscles.

99. When testing the sensory response of a 75-year-old patient to dull or sharp objects, which finding would be considered normal? The patient is:
    1. Able to identify location of touch correctly but not the type of sensation.
    2. Able to identify type of sensation correctly but not the location.
    3. Able to identify both type and location correctly, but the response is slow.
    4. Unable to identify sensation in any area.

100. A patient is awaiting surgery for reduction of a fractured right femur. Skeletal traction has been applied. Which nursing diagnosis requires the nurse to function collaboratively to achieve the best outcome for the patient?
    1. Risk for impaired skin integrity.
    2. Pain (acute).
    3. Impaired physical mobility.
    4. Risk for fracture deformity.

101. Most adverse drug effects in the elderly occur because:
    1. The amount of body water is decreased.

2. Hormone activity is generally diminished.

3. The amount of body fat tends to increase with age.

4. CNS effects decrease in the elderly.

102. Which nursing diagnosis would be the priority in the care of a patient with acquired immunodeficiency syndrome (AIDS)?

1. Impaired skin integrity.

2. Anxiety (death).

3. Pain (acute).

4. Ineffective breathing pattern.

103. Which of the following is most important to include in teaching a patient about preventing heat cramps when working outside in hot weather?

1. Prior history of heat sensitivity.

2. Need to maintain sodium level in body.

3. Importance of drinking fluids to stay cool.

4. Risk of potassium and magnesium loss.

104. Which signs and symptoms indicate that the patient is experiencing hypovolemic shock?

1. Increased heart rate and decreased urine output.

2. Decreased urine output and pitting edema.

3. Fever and furrowed tongue.

4. Bounding pulse and crackles in the chest.

105. Which sign is the best indicator of early infection in a patient who is immunosuppressed?

1. Fever.

2. Sore throat.

3. Elevated sedimentation rate.

4. Decreased urine output.

106. The most important information to include when teaching a patient who is being discharged on continuous ambulatory peritoneal dialysis (CAPD) would be the need to:

1. Use sterile technique to prevent infection.

2. Increase protein in the diet.

3. Record blood pressure and weight daily.

4. Wear a medical identification bracelet.

107. A patient complaining of severe indigestion while walking in the hall, grabs his chest and falls to the floor. The first assessment to make would be to determine:

1. Unresponsiveness.

2. Breathing pattern.

3. Blood pressure.

4. Presence of a pulse.

108. A patient has hypotension, jugular venous distention, and muffled heart sounds on auscultation. The nurse would anticipate that the patient's treatment will be directed at:

1. Reversing cardiogenic shock.

2. Improving left ventricular function.

3. Reducing the degree of ventricular hypertrophy.

4. Managing pericardial effusion or tamponade.

109. On admission of a patient with status epilepticus who has been having a seizure for over 2 hours, the most important assessment data would be:

1. Total time unconscious.

2. Time of last meal.

3. Current arterial blood gases.

4. Time of last dose of anticonvulsant medication.

110. Which nursing assessment would identify the earliest indication of increasing intracranial pressure?

1. Temperature over 102°F.

2. Change in level of consciousness.

3. Widening pulse pressure.

4. Unequal pupils.

111. What is the most common reaction to an epidural narcotic for postoperative pain management that a nurse would observe?

1. Slowing of the respiratory rate.

2. Increase in the heart rate.

3. Increased urinary urgency.

4. Itching.

112. Which nursing diagnosis would be a postoperative priority for a patient being transferred from postanesthesia recovery to the surgical floor?

1. Decreased cardiac output related to blood loss.

2. Pain related to large abdominal incision.

3. Risk for infection related to surgical wound.

4. Risk for activity intolerance related to surgery.

113. Before administering oxygen therapy, the nurse would:

1. Review patient's history for indications of COPD.

2. Observe patient's respiratory pattern.

3. Draw arterial blood gases.

4. Auscultate bilateral breath sounds.

114. The priority nursing action for a patient admitted with a productive cough, weight loss, and a suspected diagnosis of tuberculosis is:

1. Instruction on preventing disease transmission.

2. Planning for frequent rest periods.

3. Recording accurate intake and output.

4. Reviewing current dietary patterns.

115. A patient who is suspected of experiencing respiratory distress from a left-sided pneumothorax should be positioned:

1. On the left side.

2. On the right side.

3. In semi-Fowler's position.

4. Prone.

116. The most important nursing diagnosis for a patient admitted with an intestinal obstruction is:

1. Risk for aspiration.

2. Risk for fluid volume deficit.

3. Altered nutrition, more than body requirements (hyperkalemia).

4. Nausea.

117. Following a myocardial infarction and the development of left ventricular failure, a decrease in which of the following laboratory values would be expected?

1. Alanine aminotransferase (ALT).

2. White blood cell count.

3. Creatine kinase isoenzyme.

4. Arterial pH.

Questions

118. The patient becomes pulseless with a monitored rhythm of sinus tachycardia following a motor vehicle accident and a fractured right femur. The nurse should prepare for:
    1. Mechanical ventilation and administration of sodium bicarbonate.
    2. CPR and epinephrine IV push.
    3. Atropine IV and intubation with mechanical ventilation.
    4. Isoproterenol (Isuprel) followed by CPR.

119. Which of the following symptoms experienced by a patient following an acute MI will most likely be relieved by oxygen administration?
    1. Metabolic alkalosis and an elevated CK-MB.
    2. Arrhythmias and related hypotension.
    3. Sweating and hyperoxemia.
    4. Hypertension and AV conduction problems.

120. The blood pressure of a patient, who is scheduled for a femoral-popliteal bypass of the right leg, is 168/120. The most appropriate nursing action would be to:
    1. Give the prescribed antihypertensive agent regardless of surgery.
    2. Check vital signs frequently to determine further changes in BP.
    3. Call the MD to see if surgery can be postponed.
    4. Administer an antianxiety agent IV per order.

121. A patient is scheduled for cardioversion to treat sustained atrial fibrillation. The nursing priority before the procedure would be to:
    1. Auscultate the heart sounds.
    2. Administer medication for sedation.
    3. Give the prescribed analgesic.
    4. Start an antibiotic IV per order.

122. The nurse determines that the expected normal urine output in 24 hours for a healthy adult is:
    1. 720 mL.
    2. 840 mL.
    3. 1500 mL.
    4. 3000 mL.

123. The patient's arterial blood gases are as follows: pH 7.43, Po_2 83; Pco_2 29; HCO_3 29. The nurse would instruct the patient to:
    1. Turn, cough, and deep breathe at least every 2 hours.
    2. Get up and walk at least three times a day to improve O_2 level.
    3. Try to breathe more slowly.
    4. Drink more fluids to flush the kidneys.

124. A person who is diabetic is brought into the emergency department by a friend who found him on the floor unconscious. The first nursing action would be to:
    1. Ask the friend what happened and how long the patient was unconscious.
    2. Assess the patient for signs of head trauma when he collapsed.
    3. Obtain a blood sugar level and start an IV infusion.

4. Contact the patient's immediate family to come to the hospital.

125. A patient with AIDS is afraid of getting toxoplasmosis. The most important precaution to take would be to:
    1. Wash all vegetables before cooking.
    2. Wear gloves when gardening.
    3. Wear a mask when traveling to foreign countries.
    4. Avoid contact with cats and birds.

126. Which information about recommended adult immunizations is accurate to include in health teaching?
    1. Tetanus and diphtheria booster is needed at least every 5 years.
    2. Pneumococcal pneumonia vaccine may be given once for lifetime protection.
    3. Influenza A and B vaccine are given one time, unless high risk.
    4. Measles and mumps vaccine are given to college-age students only.

127. The laboratory findings for a patient with polycythemia vera include major and minor criteria. Which of the following is the major or defining hematological finding?
    1. Leukocytosis >12,000/mm^3.
    2. Thrombocytosis >400,000/mm^3.
    3. RBC count >6 million/mm^3.
    4. Elevated leukocyte alkaline phosphatase.

128. Which patient, experiencing a change in cardiac rhythm after a myocardial infarction, would the nurse assess first?
    1. A conversion from normal sinus rhythm to atrial fibrillation.
    2. An increase in the PR interval to 0.26 seconds.
    3. Sinus tachycardia, rate of 110.
    4. One unifocal premature ventricular contraction in 1 minute.

129. Preoperative teaching for a patient scheduled for surgery to repair a detached retina will include the following information:
    1. Eye patches may be used postoperatively.
    2. No eye pain is expected postoperatively.
    3. Semi-Fowler's position will be used to reduce pressure in the eye.
    4. Return of normal vision is expected following surgery.

130. When ambulating a patient who is blind, the nurse should be positioned:
    1. Behind the patient, holding the patient's elbows.
    2. In front, with the patient holding the nurse's arm at elbow.
    3. On the patient's side, holding the dominant hand.
    4. On the patient's side, holding the nondominant hand.

131. The greatest reduction in falls and improved safety for the elderly patient with Parkinson's disease would occur with:
    1. Discouraging the patient from wearing slippers.

2. Buying shoes that fit snugly.

3. Raising the height of toilet seats.

4. Patient holding hands behind back when walking.

132. Assessment of a patient following a recent fracture of the left humerus revealed increasing pain with extension of the fingers of the left hand. Distal pulse is strong in the limb. Capillary refill is brisk, and there does not appear to be any restriction of the fingers from the cast. The most likely explanation of the pain is:

1. Possible development of compartment syndrome.

2. Disuse syndrome from immobility.

3. Normal response to sudden movement of fingers.

4. Compression of nerve at fracture site.

Answers/Rationale

1. (2) All permits must be signed before the procedure. Patients are NPO 6–8 hours, not 24 hours (**Answer 1**). Gastroscopy is an uncomfortable procedure; to mislead the patient by saying it is not uncomfortable (**Answer 3**) can only increase anxiety and discomfort during the procedure. This procedure involves the passage of a long tube into the stomach, with a lighted, mirrored lens that permits direct visualization of the stomach mucosa. The patient must lie quietly during insertion of the tube to prevent perforation of the esophagus. Usually *sedatives, not* pain medications (**Answer 4**), are given before the procedure.

> **Test-taking tip**—One answer is different from the others. Three of the choices deal with physical preparation.

IMP, 4, SECE, Management of Care

2. (3) The first priority is to protect the patient from injury. Do not restrain the patient's arms or legs, but make sure he or she does not hit anything. Protect the head with the nurse's hand, a towel, or a jacket. During the initial tonic phase, the patient usually stops breathing for up to a minute. There is no cause for alarm, as spontaneous breathing will, in most patients, return with no harm. In the absence of breathing, airway patency by this position change (**Answer 2**) is *not the first* priority. Muscle contraction will prevent "positioning" of the head. A padded tongue blade, once indicated during a seizure, is also no longer used. **Answers 1** and **4** are appropriate nursing actions *after* the seizure has ended.

> **Test-taking tip**—The correct choice is broadest, encompassing the other choices. Key word: *first* priority.

PL, 2, PhI, Physiological Adaptation

3. (2) Although all of these interventions are appropriate in the preoperative period, research indicates that the *best* postoperative outcomes are related to the patient's reduced preoperative anxiety levels. Patients who deny apprehension and refuse information, as well as those who are highly anxious and who are unable to ask questions or assimilate information, have the most difficult postsurgical course. Patients

who are able to express their concerns and who are given emotional support as well as accurate, brief explanations tend to have less pain and fewer postoperative complications. **Answers 1, 3,** and **4** do not address the patient's need to verbalize concerns.

> **Test-taking tip**—The correct answer is the only one that asks the patient what he or she would like to know.

PL, 7, PsI, Coping and Adaptation

4. (3) Signs of *circulatory* constriction include blanching (delayed capillary refill) and cyanosis, swelling of the toes, pain that is out of proportion for the type of fracture, and temperature changes. Tingling and numbness (**Answer 1**), loss of movement (**Answer 2**), and constant pain (**Answer 4**) are symptoms associated with constriction or pressure on a peripheral nerve.

> **Test-taking tip**—Requires knowledge of difference between motor, sensory, and circulatory signs/symptoms.

AS, 6, PhI, Reduction of Risk Potential

5. (3) Paralytic ileus is characterized by diminished, absent, or uncoordinated bowel sounds due to inappropriate or absent autonomic nervous system (vagal) stimulation of the intestinal tract. Paralytic ileus may occur due to anesthetic interruption of autonomic outflow or hypokalemia. Edema of the intestinal mucosa (**Answer 1**) is usually found with inflammation or ulcerative colitis. Acute dilation of the colon (**Answer 2**) and high, tinkling bowel sounds (**Answer 4**) are associated with large-bowel obstruction.

> **Test-taking tip**—Look for words in the answer that define "paralysis."

AN, 8, PhI, Physiological Adaptation

6. (2) The three-point gait is appropriate when weight bearing is not allowed on the affected limb. The swing-to and swing-through crutch gaits may also be used when only one leg can be used for weight bearing. **Answers 1** and **3** are utilized when weight bearing is allowed on both feet. **Answer 4**, the tripod gait, is utilized when the patient has little or no sensation or movement (paralysis) in the lower limbs.

> **Test-taking tip**—Need to know which limbs are used with each gait. Key words: "no weight bearing."

PL, 3, PhI, Basic Care and Comfort

7. (3) Patients are NPO and encouraged not to smoke or take medications the morning of an upper GI series. Patients are NPO for 6–8 hours, *not* 24 hours (**Answer 1**). Enemas and cathartics (**Answer 2**) are *not* administered before an upper GI series; however, they are given *after* the series, to aid in the elimination of the barium. The test involves an x-ray, using a barium swallow as contrast medium. Gastroscopy (**Answer 4**) is the direct visualization of the stomach.

> **Test-taking tip**—Note the time element: *before*; this eliminates #2. Eliminate #1 because being NPO for 24 hours is excessive. #4 is the description for a different test, not for *UGI* series.

IMP, 4, PhI, Reduction of Risk Potential

8. (2) Deep partial-thickness burns involve both the epidermis and some of the dermis. They have a pink-red appearance and are characterized by moisture or blisters. Deep partial-thickness burns are very painful, because nerve endings remain and may be exposed to the air. A *superficial* partial-thickness burn involves only the epidermis (**Answer 1**). An example is sunburn: the skin is usually red and dry. In *full*-thickness burns, subcutaneous tissue, muscle, and even bone are also involved (**Answers 3** and **4**). Typically, a full-thickness burn is white, gray, or charred in color and is dry and leathery in appearance. Nerve endings have been destroyed, so the area is painless.

> **Test-taking tip**—The key word is "deep." Three of the choices are not deep.

AN, 1, PhI, Physiological Adaptation

Key to codes following rationales: *Nursing process:* **AS**, Assessment; **AN**, Analysis; **PL**, Plan; **IMP**, Implementation; **EV**, Evaluation. *Category of human function:* **1**, Protective; **2**, Sensory-perceptual; **3**, Comfort, Rest, Activity, and Mobility; **4**, Nutrition; **5**, Growth and Development; **6**, Fluid-Gas Transport; **7**, Psychosocial-Cultural; **8**, Elimination. **Client need: SECE**, Safe, Effective Care Environment; **PhI**, Physiological Integrity; **PsI**, Psychosocial Integrity; **HPM**, Health Promotion/Maintenance. See appendices for full explanation.

9. **(2)** Some authorities believe that the psychosomatic issue contributing to ulcers is an unresolved dependence-independence conflict. This conflict frequently prevents the patient from accepting a dependent role, even on a temporary basis. However, the unresolved dependency wish that many of these people have frequently results in irritable, angry behavior when treatments are not exactly on time. Other psychosomatic research has linked anxiety and neurotic behavior (**Answer 1**) with the occurrence of *angina pectoris;* repressed anger and hostility (**Answer 3**) with the development of *rheumatoid arthritis;* and compulsive time orientation (**Answer 4**) (type A personality) with onset of *myocardial infarction.*

   Test-taking tip—Ask which emotional response would most likely stimulate a parasympathetic (stress) response.
   AN, 7, PsI, Coping and Adaptation

10. **(3)** Increased carbohydrates are needed for healing and tissue repair. Anorexia, *not increased appetite* (**Answer 1**), is a problem. Increased, *not decreased* protein catabolism is present (**Answer 2**). Digestive enzyme secretion is decreased, *not increased* (**Answer 4**).

    Test-taking tip—Need to know the effects of immobility on metabolism. Selecting **Answer 2** would be too obvious!
    AN, 4, PhI, Basic Care and Comfort

11. **(1)** Glaucoma is an *imbalance* between the rate of secretion of intraocular fluids and the rate of their absorption. Glaucoma may be acute/closed-angle (obstruction of the angle between the cornea and iris) or chronic/open-angle (obstruction occurs proximal or distal to the angle). It is characterized by increased intraocular pressures. Narrowing of the arterioles and retinal ischemia (**Answer 2**) are the result of prolonged hypertension. Clouding of the cornea (**Answer 3**) is not seen in glaucoma. Buckling of the retina (**Answer 4**) is associated with retinal detachment.

    Test-taking tip—Only one choice describes a problem of imbalance, the major problem in glaucoma that leads to increased intraocular pressure related to the imbalance.
    AN, 2, PhI, Physiological Adaptation

12. **(1)** Patients experiencing dumping syndrome should be advised to ingest liquids between meals rather than with meals (**Answer 2**) or at any time they desire (**Answer 3**). Taking fluids between meals allows for adequate hydration, reduces the amount of bulk ingested with meals, and aids in preventing rapid gastric emptying. Six small meals rather than three large meals, as well as resting after eating, are also measures used to prevent the occurrence of symptoms, which usually disappear over time. There is no need to restrict the quantity of fluids (**Answer 4**), just the timing.

    Test-taking tip—Key point is a *time* factor *(when).* Decreasing volume at meal time, not in general, is the key. Fluid spreads the process.
    PL, 4, PhI, Basic Care and Comfort

13. **(2)** Daily weights are taken following nephrectomy. Daily increases of 2 lb or more are indicative of fluid retention and should be reported to the physician. Intake and output records may also reflect this imbalance. Increased specific gravity of urine (**Answer 1**) indicates that the patient is *underhydrated* rather than overhydrated. A urinary output of 50 mL/hr (**Answer 3**) is the *desired* minimum following renal surgery. Periorbital edema (**Answer 4**) is a *later* sign of excess fluid retention.

    Test-taking tip—Key word: "early" indicator. Daily weight is the best indicator.
    AS, 8, PhI, Reduction of Risk Potential

14. **(1)** The Miller-Abbott tube is a double-lumen tube, with one lumen leading to the inflatable balloon and the other lumen used for aspiration of intestinal contents. **Answer 2** is an example of a *Levin* tube, used for gastric suction. **Answer 3**

is an example of a *Harris* tube, and **Answer 4,** a *Cantor* tube, both used for intestinal decompression, like the Miller-Abbott.

   Test-taking tip—Need to know which tubes are single vs. double lumen.
   IMP, 8, PhI, Reduction of Risk Potential

15. **(2)** The narrow QRS complexes are normal, within 0.12 second, but there are no regular P waves for each QRS. The baseline appears "wavy" and the rhythm is "regularly irregular, " which describes atrial fibrillation. The second and fifth QRS complexes are wide and bizarre but alike, indicating a unifocal origin. **Answer 1** is incorrect because there is not one P wave for every QRS, and the multifocal PVCs would look different in configuration. Even though the rate is 100, **Answer 3** is incorrect because the impulse is not originating from the SA node, which is necessary for a sinus rhythm. **Answer 4** is incorrect because atrial tachycardia is more rapid and regular, and though the P waves are difficult to see, they are present. Also, the PVCs are unifocal, not multifocal, in origin.

    Test-taking tip—Look for the normal components of an ECG—PQRS. Only one choice has no P waves like the strip.
    AN, 6, PhI, Physiological Adaptation

16. **(2)** If treatment with thyroid hormone is effective, there should be an *overall increase* in metabolic rate and a decrease in fluid retention; that is, increased blood pressure, pulse rate, pulse pressure, temperature, and rate and depth of respirations. As a result of improved renal blood flow, glomerular filtration and urine output should also increase, thus reducing the weight gain due to fluid retention. **Answers 1, 3,** and **4** are incorrect because each contains at least one outcome that is not consistent with improved status.

    Test-taking tip—Know the physiological effect of the thyroid on the body. ↑Thyroid function = ↑BP, P, T, R, pulse pressure = ↓fluid retention.
    EV, 3, PhI, Pharmacological and Parenteral Therapies

17. **(2)** Aldosterone secretion by the adrenal cortex is stimulated by decreases in cardiac output. Aldosterone acts to conserve sodium in the kidney tubules, passively increasing water reabsorption and improving fluid volume balance. Normally, if the patient had only a water loss, he or she would also be hypernatremic because of this mechanism. However, in burns the patient's hypovolemia (hemoconcentration) is due to both fluid and electrolyte loss in edema fluids, as well as through the denuded areas of skin. **Answer 1** is not the best answer because, although ADH is being released, its action has not at this time prevented hemoconcentration. **Answer 3** is incorrect because very little sodium is released due to cellular disruption. Sodium is the main cation of the extracellular fluid. **Answer 4** is incorrect because increased serum-potassium levels stimulate the release of aldosterone.

    Test-taking tip—Think fluid shift and hemoconcentration early in burns.
    AN, 6, PhI, Physiological Adaptation

18. **(4)** Because the patient's ability to react to stress is decreased, maintaining a quiet environment becomes a nursing priority. Dehydration is a common problem in Addison's disease, so close observation of the patient's hydration level is crucial. To promote optimal hydration and sodium intake, fluid intake is *increased,* particularly fluids containing electrolytes, such as broths, carbonated beverages, and juices. **Answer 1** is incorrect because it limits sodium. **Answer 2** is incorrect because it limits fluids. Daily weights and intake and output records are essential for monitoring fluid balance. Drug therapy in Addison's disease is directed toward oral replacement of adrenocorticosteroids such as cortisone, prednisone, and fludrohydrocortisone (Florinef). Insulin (**Answer 3**) is *not* required.

Test-taking tip—Addison's is the *reverse* of Cushing's syndrome. Note the pattern in the options: three relate to physical aspects of care; one deals with stress. In this case, choose the one that is different.

IMP, 3, PhI, Basic Care and Comfort

19. (3) The vagus nerve stimulates an increase in both hydrochloric acid secretion and gastric motility. Vagotomy not only decreases hydrochloric acid secretion but also alters the motility of the stomach and intestines; this may result in a sensation of fullness after meals, eructation, and abdominal distention. **Answer 1** is incomplete. **Answers 2 and 4** are the reverse of effects of vagal action.

Test-taking tip—Look for a choice that would be similar to the problem that led to the gastrectomy. Note that both #1 and #3 are correct, but #3 incorporates #1.

AN, 4, PhI, Reduction of Risk Potential

20. (3) Potassium is transported back into the cells along with glucose; therefore the administration of insulin and glucose will facilitate the movement of potassium back into the cell. Sodium polystyrene sulfonate (Kayexalate) (**Answer 2**) is a resin that attacks and binds potassium. It may be given either orally or as an enema; however, its use would *not* be indicated in this case *unless* more conservative means were unsuccessful. Morphine sulfate (**Answer 1**) and synthetic aldosterone (**Answer 4**) are *not* indicated for the management of hyperkalemia.

Test-taking tip—The "choice" would always be to move K⁺ back into the cell, not get rid of it through diarrhea.

PL, 6, PhI, Pharmacological and Parenteral Therapies

21. (2) Alcohol is extremely drying and contributes to skin breakdown. An emollient lotion should be used. Bed cradles (**Answer 1**) keep the pressure of bed clothing off pressure points. High-protein diet (**Answer 3**) aids in the healing process. Assessment of skin (**Answer 4**) is vital, to recognize any red areas.

Test-taking tip—Think of the effect of each choice on the skin, using a true-or-false approach regarding prevention of decubitus. Note that the question asks for *least* appropriate.

PL, 1, PhI, Basic Care and Comfort

22. (1) The hypovolemia and shock that accompany burns greatly increase the body's stress response. Increased serum levels of norepinephrine, epinephrine, and aldosterone facilitate venous return and thus assist in maintaining cardiac output and blood pressure. The pituitary is also stimulated in the stress response to increase circulating levels of ADH (decreases water output) and cortisol. Increased levels of the latter hormone are implicated in the development of Curling's ulcer (stress ulcer), which may develop in patients of all ages and with both minor and major burns. Generally, H₂ antagonists and antacids are used to reduce its occurrence. **Answer 2** is incorrect because *negative* nitrogen balance occurs due to protein mobilization for healing. Patients with burns are given high-protein, high-calorie meals and supplemental vitamins to promote wound healing. **Answer 3** is incorrect because hemolysis of red blood cells and decreased hematocrit are primarily *due to the injury* itself *rather than* to epinephrine agglutination. In thermal burns, up to 40% of the red blood cell mass may be hemolyzed. Hypothermia is a problem in the postburn period but is the *result of the loss of skin areas;* hence **Answer 4** is incorrect. The patient treated by the open or exposed method of burn therapy is particularly susceptible to chilling. Increased thermostat settings and radiant heat lamps may be employed to aid in maintaining normal body temperature.

Test-taking tip—Burns are a major *stress;* ulcers are caused by stress (Curling's ulcer is also known as stress ulcer).

EV, 1, PhI, Physiological Adaptation

23. (1) Ventricular tachycardia occurs most commonly in patients with acute MI and coronary artery disease. Of immediate significance to the patient, if untreated, are the hemodynamic dysfunction, a *drop* in blood pressure rather than an increase (**Answer 2**), and the possibility of progressing to ventricular fibrillation. **Answer 3** is incorrect because if pain does result it will be *angina, not MI* pain. **Answer 4** is incorrect because ventricular tachycardia is potentially *life threatening* and requires intervention.

Test-taking tip—"V-tach" is life threatening. Look for another life-threatening choice (ventricular fibrillation).

AN, 6, PhI, Reduction of Risk Potential

24. (3) Bivalving the cast involves full-length splitting of the cast on each side. The underlying padding is also cut, because blood-soaked padding shrinks and can also cause circulatory constriction. After the cast is cut, it is spread sufficiently to relieve constriction. This procedure does not disturb reduction of the bone. The cast is then reapplied (**Answer 1**) *after* the *swelling* has gone down. **Answer 2** is the technique used when the cast is *removed.* The patient's limb should always be *elevated* (**Answer 4**) after bivalving, because the underlying condition (edema, i.e., swelling) is best relieved by elevation of the limb, ice packs, and isometric exercises.

Test-taking tip—Look for the best method for relieving pressure. Look at two similar options (#2 and #3) and how they differ ("split and spread down the *middle*" vs. "on *each side*"). Note that the word "bivalve" in the question is similar to "split/spread cast in each side" ("bi" = 2; each side = 2 sides).

IMP, 3, PhI, Reduction of Risk Potential

25. (2) The tube will be inserted with greater ease if the patient is sitting up with head slightly flexed. The tube should be lubricated and will be passed into the stomach with greater accuracy if the patient is given water to drink through a straw; at the same time that the patient is swallowing, the tube is advanced. **Answer 1** is not correct because the tube should be irrigated with saline, *not* water, to prevent electrolyte imbalances. **Answer 3** is not correct because pressure must *not* be used during irrigation. If resistance is met, the physician should be notified immediately. Ice chips (**Answer 4**) should be used *sparingly, not* as often as desired, to prevent electrolyte imbalances from excessive hypotonic water ingestion.

Test-taking tip—One choice involves tube insertion; the others involve tube management (although not correct).

IMP, 4, PhI, Reduction of Risk Potential

26. (3) Eyedrops should be instilled into the conjunctival sac to prevent medication from hitting the sensitive cornea. The patient should then be instructed to close the eye, but not squeeze shut, so that the medication can be distributed evenly over the eye. **Answers 1 and 4** are incorrect because instillation on these structures would increase corneal irritation. **Answer 2** is incorrect because drops instilled into the inner canthus are likely to run down the outer aspects of the nose or be absorbed systemically through the tear duct.

Test-taking tip—The correct choice is more indirect placement of drops; the other choices are all *direct* locations.

IMP, 2, PhI, Pharmacological and Parenteral Therapies

27. (3) The main treatment for patients with myasthenia gravis is anticholinesterase drugs. These drugs increase the response of muscles to nerve impulses and improve muscle strength by inhibiting the rapid removal of acetylcholine from the myoneural junction. **Answer 1** is partially correct, in that adrenergic drugs such as ephedrine sulfate are administered to improve muscle tone but these drugs *do not inhibit cholinesterase* at the myoneural junction. Likewise, anticholinergic drugs (**Answer 2**) such as atropine *are* also used in the treatment of myasthenia, primarily to *reduce* the

incidence of *side effects* of the anticholinesterase drugs and to reverse their effect if "cholinergic crisis" occurs. Cholinergic drugs (**Answer 4**) are *not* indicated in the treatment of myasthenia gravis.

> **Test-taking tip**—Need to know effects of broad drug classes. Clue: two drugs look similar (#2 and #3); #2 is used if there are side effects from #3—the drugs of choice.

PL, 3, PhI, Pharmacological and Parenteral Therapies

28. (3) Patients with burns limited to an extremity are generally treated by a closed method; that is, wounds are covered with a layer of sterile, fine mesh gauze impregnated with an antibacterial agent such as mafenide 1%. Wounds are cleansed one or more times per day, and dressing are reapplied using strict sterile technique. Patients treated by the closed or semi-open method do *not* have to be *isolated* (**Answer 1**). Patients treated by the open method (wounds completely exposed to the air) require strict isolation to prevent infection. The open method is usually used for minor burns, areas difficult to dress (burns of trunk, perineum), or new skin grafts. **Answer 2** is incorrect because *sterile* technique must be used. Heat lamp (**Answer 4**) is incorrect because the wound is covered in the *closed* method.

> **Test-taking tip**—Two choices are "closed" to the air, and only one uses aseptic technique.

IMP, 1, PhI, Reduction of Risk Potential

29. (4) Although 70–80% of patients having subtotal gastrectomies may experience some symptoms of dumping syndrome, it is a significant problem for only a small percentage (5–10%). The term *dumping* is used because the symptoms are believed to be due to the rapid emptying of the gastric contents into the small intestine. This produces gastric distention, and some authorities believe that large amounts of extracellular fluid then enter the intestines to dilute the hypertonic stomach contents. The subsequent lowering of the blood volume produces shocklike symptoms, such as weakness, diaphoresis, faintness, and palpitations. **Answers 1, 2,** and **3** are incorrect percentages.

> **Test-taking tip**—Select the smaller percentage; you would remember if *most* patients develop a "significant" problem.

AN, 4, PhI, Physiological Adaptation

30. (2) Patients with hyperthyroidism have an increased basal metabolic rate (BMR) and increased T_3 and T_4. Increased serum cholesterol (**Answer 1**), increased TSH (**Answer 3**), and increased menstrual volume (**Answer 4**) are findings consistent with *hypothyroidism*. Menstruation in hyperthyroidism characteristically is *decreased* in volume. Cycle lengths may be shortened or prolonged, but eventually amenorrhea develops.

> **Test-taking tip**—Look for an answer with a change in metabolism.

AN, 3, PhI, Physiological Adaptation

31. (2) Pilocarpine constricts the pupil by causing contraction of the ciliary muscles, thus widening the outflow channels and increasing aqueous flow. **Answer 1** is incorrect because pilocarpine is a parasympathomimetic; that is, it mimics the action of acetylcholine at cholinergic nerve endings, thus *decreasing* pupil size. **Answer 3** is incorrect, in that *diuretics* such as acetazolamide (Diamox), a carbonic anhydrase inhibitor, are used to decrease aqueous production, not pilocarpine. **Answer 4** does not describe the actions of any medication used in glaucoma therapy.

> **Test-taking tip**—Look for a choice that would let the pressure "out."

EV, 2, PhI, Pharmacological and Parenteral Therapies

32. (1) Hyponatremia, or decreased serum sodium, may develop in patients with burns because sodium tends to move with water into edema fluids and into denuded areas of skin.

Answers 2 and **4** are incorrect because both these mechanisms tend to increase sodium reabsorption by the kidney tubules. Inadequate fluid replacement (**Answer 3**) would tend to mask hyponatremia because of hemoconcentration.

> **Test-taking tip**—Look for the only answer that relates to destruction of skin (longest answer *might* be a hint). Also, *hypo*natremia is similar to the word "loss" in the correct option.

AN, 6, PhI, Physiological Adaptation

33. (3) Patients with high abdominal incisions are prone to atelectasis following surgery because they tend to breathe shallowly to prevent incisional pain. However, the nurse must also institute measures to prevent thrombophlebitis (**Answer 1**), wound infection, and dehiscence. Abdominal distention due to air swallowing (**Answer 2**) is *unlikely* because the patient has a nasogastric tube in place. Urinary retention after surgery (**Answer 4**) is generally due to the *effects of anesthesia* on the autonomic nervous system *rather than* to the *residual effects* of anticholinergic medications.

> **Test-taking tip**—Think postoperative pain. Which answer would *pain cause*?

EV, 6, PhI, Reduction of Risk Potential

34. (2) The nasogastric tube is removed after bowel sounds have been reestablished (generally around the third day) and after the patient has passed flatus or stool. **Answers 1** and **3** are incorrect because they do not include the return of bowel sounds. Before removal, the tube is frequently clamped for 2–4 hours—*not 2 days* (**Answer 4**)—to test the patient's tolerance. Gastric residue is measured after this period. If it is more than 100 mL, the nasogastric tube is left in place. Likewise, if the patient experiences any pain, nausea, vomiting, or distention during this period, the tube is left in. If no symptoms occur and there is a minimal amount of gastric residue, the tube is removed.

> **Test-taking tip**—The "time" depends on the patient's bowel sounds. Follow the logic: GI surgery, NG tube → "bowel sounds" (#2). Correct choice is the *only* one without a specific time.

EV, 8, PhI, Basic Care and Comfort

35. (2) Age is important baseline information because IV infusion rates to maintain appropriate quantity and specific gravity of urinary output differ; for example, 10–20 mL/hr for infants versus 50–70 mL/hr for adults. Weight is significant if the Evans or Brooke formula is used for fluid replacement therapy. Both of these formulas use both the size of the burn and the weight of the patient to calculate the amount of fluid to be replaced. Vital signs and skin turgor are both important measures of the degree or extent of hypovolemia. As dehydration develops, skin turgor becomes poor, mucous membranes dry, and the eyeballs feel soft. Likewise, the pulse may become thready and the blood pressure may decrease. Size (weight), as discussed, *not sex* would determine therapy (**Answer 1**). Level of mentation (**Answer 3**) is *less* helpful in this particular situation because of the fear, pain, and acute anxiety experienced by some patients. Quantity and specific gravity of urine output (**Answer 4**) are important in assessing the adequacy of fluid *replacement rather than* as part of the initial *assessment*.

> **Test-taking tip**—Look for an answer with "body weight."

AS, 6, PhI, Pharmacological and Parenteral Therapies

36. (3) Dilantin (phenytoin, diphenylhydantoin) is consistently found to be effective against most types of seizures except absence seizures. Its precise action is unknown, but it appears to stabilize cell membranes by altering intracellular sodium concentrations. Plasma levels of the drug are checked frequently to avoid toxicity and to determine effective dosage. Side effects include gastritis and nervousness, and at toxic levels the drug may cause ataxia. Phenobarbital

(**Answer 1**) is also used in *conjunction* with diphenylhydantoin. Diazepam (**Answer 2**) may be used as *adjunct* therapy in seizure disorders. Trimethadione (**Answer 4**) is used in the control of absence seizures.

> **Test-taking tip**—"Drug of choice" means first line of drugs used to decrease seizures (Dilantin *decreases* seizures).

IMP, 2, PhI, Pharmacological and Parenteral Therapies

37. (**2**) After arterial punctures, the *first* nursing priority is to observe for bleeding or hematoma formation, particularly in the first 4 hours after the procedure. Vital signs (**Answer 1**) are monitored. The specific gravity and urinary output (**Answer 3**) are monitored, but this is *not as significant as* observing the puncture site. The peripheral pulse distal to the puncture site (**Answer 4**) is also monitored. Because of the size of the vessel, bleeding can quickly cause volume depletion and shock.

> **Test-taking tip**—This is a priority question—look for the choice with the most immediate risk to the patient (bleeding).

AN, 6, PhI, Reduction of Risk Potential

38. (**2**) With the exception of the Evans formula, whole blood is administered to patients with burns *only when the hematocrit* begins to manifest *red blood cell loss.* Several fluid formulas have been developed to serve as a guideline for fluid replacement in the patient with burns. The *Evans* formula is the oldest and is based on both the size of the wound and the patient's weight. Colloids (blood, dextran, plasma) and crystalloids (electrolyte solutions) *are* administered during the *first 48 hours.* The *Brooke* formula is similar, except that blood is not given until the hematocrit level has fallen and the need is demonstrated. The *Parkland* formula is based on the premise that volume expansion is dependent on the rate of infusion rather than the type of replacement. During the first 24 hours, fluid volume *is* replaced with electrolyte solutions (Ringer's lactate) only (**Answer 1**). Colloids are used *only* if urine output is not maintained (**Answer 3**). During the first or *second 24 hours,* dextrose and water (**Answer 4**) *are* used to maintain fluid volume.

> **Test-taking tip**—Keep in mind the *time* period: within *first* 24 hours. Question also asks for *least* likely choice. With burns, think volume (water) loss is what needs to be replaced, not blood.

IMP, 6, PhI, Pharmacological and Parenteral Therapies

39. (**3**) Removal of gastric secretions incurs the *loss* of sodium, potassium, and hydrochloric acid ions. The loss of these ions may lead not only to metabolic alkalosis ($\downarrow H^+$) but also to *hypo*kalemia. **Answers 1** and **2** are incorrect because hypernatremia and hyperkalemia indicate an *excess* in sodium and potassium ions. Hypoproteinemia (**Answer 4**) occurs with liver dysfunctions and is *not* a side effect of nasogastric suctioning.

> **Test-taking tip**—The key word is *prolonged.* Acid will be lost; therefore, think alkalosis.

AN, 4, PhI, Physiological Adaptation

40. (**2**) Because the flank incision in nephrectomy is directly below the diaphragm, deep breathing is painful. Additionally, there is a greater incisional pull each time the person moves than there is with abdominal surgery. Incisional pain following nephrectomy generally requires analgesic administration every 3–4 hours for 24–48 hours after surgery. Therefore turning, coughing, and deep-breathing exercises should be planned to maximize the analgesic effects. The patient may be on *either side,* as long as drainage tubes are not kinked and gravity flow is uninhibited (**Answer 1**). A *low* Fowler's or *semi*-Fowler's position is generally more comfortable for the patient and of sufficient height to encourage gravity flow from drainage tubes (**Answer 3**). Fluid administration is directed toward maintaining *blood* volume and *urinary* output (**Answer 4**).

> **Test-taking tip**—Think patient comfort (analgesics) to reduce patient complications. Note that the words "deep breathing and coughing" in the *stem also* are in the *correct* option (#2).

PL, 6, PhI, Reduction of Risk Potential

41. (**1**) Hemorrhage may follow nephrectomy because of the difficulty in securing ligatures in the short renal-artery stump. It may occur on the day of surgery or 8–12 days postoperatively, when normal tissue sloughing occurs with healing. Dressing and urine are observed for bright-red bleeding, vital signs are monitored, and the patient is continually observed for any other indications of shock. Hyperkalemia (**Answer 2**), tetany (**Answer 3**), and polyuria (**Answer 4**) are *not* common complications after nephrectomy.

> **Test-taking tip**—After any surgery, bleeding is a potential problem.

AS, 6, PhI, Reduction of Risk Potential

42. (**4**) It is important to recognize that the loss of anatomical integrity initiates a grieving process. Allowing the patient to express feelings of depression, apathy, or disinterest indicates that such feelings are acceptable and not uncommon. **Answer 1** is always appropriate and should be consistently carried out; however, in the situation depicted it would *follow* the verbalization of feelings. **Answers 2** and **3** are also alternatives the nurse may wish to employ *after* assessing the patient's major concerns.

> **Test-taking tip**—First priority—what is concerning the patient? First, *feelings.*

IMP, 7, PsI, Coping and Adaptation

43. (**1**) Chilling the tube *before* insertion assists in relieving some of the nasal discomfort. Water-soluble lubricants along with viscous lidocaine (Xylocaine) may also be used. It is usually only lightly lubricated before insertion. The patient may be administered a sedative (**Answer 2**) on physician's orders to reduce *apprehension during* insertion. Warming the tube (**Answer 3**) has *no* advantages. The patient is *usually positioned* (**Answer 4**) in *high* Fowler's position during insertion to aid in swallowing the tube.

> **Test-taking tip**—Note two contradictory options: "chill" vs. "warm" the tube. Think patient comfort: cold reduces pain.

IMP, 8, PhI, Basic Care and Comfort

44. (**3**) The symptoms of dumping syndrome are most likely to occur following the ingestion of large amounts of sugars or carbohydrates. Therefore a diet that is high in protein and fats and low in carbohydrates is recommended, to reduce symptomatology and to provide the patient with essential energy requirements. **Answers 1** and **4** are incorrect because they do not supply sufficient protein for energy and tissue repair. High protein intake is essential after surgery and most prolonged illnesses for rebuilding tissue. **Answers 2** and **4** are incorrect because they list *high* carbohydrates.

> **Test-taking tip**—Look for foods that slow the movement of food out of the stomach (e.g., $\downarrow$CHO, $\uparrow$fat).

PL, 4, PhI, Basic Care and Comfort

45. (**2**) Because the dysfunction in myasthenia gravis occurs at the myoneural junction, it is considered a lower neuron lesion. Upper motor neuron lesions (**Answer 1**) involve cranial neurons and their axons in the spinal cord. Combined lesions (**Answer 3**) generally occur with spinal injury when axons of cranial neurons are destroyed, resulting in hyperreflexia and increased muscle tone below the level of the lesion, and destruction of motor neurons at the level of the injury, which in turn leads to hyporeflexia, decreased muscle tone, and muscle atrophy in those muscles normally innervated by these neurons. Myasthenia gravis is *not* an inherited disorder (**Answer 4**). Recent evidence suggests an autoimmune basis.

Test-taking tip—Think of the symptoms—which answer best explains myasthenia gravis? Eliminate #3 and #4. Is it upper or lower motor?

AN, 3, PhI, Physiological Adaptation

46. **(2)** The patient should be cautioned to limit the number of ice cubes he or she sucks on because the nasogastric suction will remove not only the increased water ingested from the melted cubes but also essential electrolytes. **Answers 1, 3, and 4** *are* appropriate mouth care measures for a patient who has a nasogastric tube.

Test-taking tip—One answer is different from the others (teeth, tongue, mouth, gums, lips)—it involves swallowing melted *ice*. Note the key term *with caution*.

IMP, 1, PhI, Basic Care and Comfort

47. **(2)** Hyperkalemia (excesses in serum potassium) occurs in burns due to three separate mechanism: (1) cellular injury resulting in the movement of potassium from the intracellular space into the extracellular space; (2) decreased glomerular filtration and urine output preventing excretion of increased serum potassium; and (3) inadequate tissue metabolism resulting in increased hydrogen ion formation (metabolic acidosis). In the kidney tubules, hydrogen and potassium ions are exchanged for sodium ions. In metabolic acidosis, more hydrogen ions are excreted than potassium ions. Exudate formation *itself does not* significantly affect serum-potassium levels (**Answer 1**). During physical and emotional stress, aldosterone levels are *increased*, thereby *lowering* serum potassium (**Answer 3**). Hyperbilirubinemia *itself does not* affect potassium concentration (**Answer 4**), though red blood cell destruction probably increases the amount of circulating potassium, because potassium is the major intracellular cation.

Test-taking tip—Look for an answer that describes destruction of tissue or cells ("disruption of cell membrane").

EV, 6, PhI, Physiological Adaptation

48. **(4)** Recognizing the patient's concern is essential both in maintaining rapport and in keeping the lines of communication open. Having done this, the nurse can then assure the patient that one kidney is sufficient to handle renal functions. This statement can then be followed by other discharge instructions, such as the need for adequate fluid intake, avoiding infections, and untoward signs that the patient needs to observe for. **Answers 1, 2, and 3** do not recognize the patient's concern or facilitate open communication.

Test-taking tip—The best answer acknowledges the patient's concern. Eliminate "call the doctor" (#3) because a nurse *can* discuss the patient's concerns. Eliminate #1 and #2 because they are trite clichés that close off elaboration.

IMP, 7, PsI, Coping and Adaptation

49. **(1)** A freshly applied cast generates heat as moisture evaporates and the cast hardens. To facilitate drying, keep it exposed to the air. Do not use plastic covers or Chux on pillows to elevate the limb, because these tend to slow drying. **Answer 2** is incorrect; signs of increased pressure are numbness and tingling, pain, and loss of movement. **Answer 3** is an inappropriate response to the question because it fails to recognize the patient's cognitive needs. **Answer 4** does not take into account that discomfort and apprehension can be reduced if the patient understands what is to be expected.

Test-taking tip—The question asks *expected outcome* with a new cast. Eliminate #3 because #1 gives the same information without offering a trite cliché.

IMP, 3, PhI, Basic Care and Comfort

50. **(3)** Edrophonium (Tensilon) is a short-acting anticholinesterase compound. A positive Tensilon test result (a prompt and dramatic increase in muscle strength) is consistent with the diagnosis of myasthenia gravis. **Answer 1** is

incorrect because an exacerbation of symptoms would indicate another cause for the muscle dysfunction. **Answer 2** is partially correct: ptosis is relieved, but so is sagging of the other facial muscles. **Answer 4** is incorrect because the increase in muscle strength is accompanied by *decreased* fatigability as long as the drug continues to circulate.

Test-taking tip—Look for improvement as a result. Eliminate "slight" (#4) and partial relief (#2) in favor of "prompt and dramatic."

EV, 3, PhI, Pharmacological and Parenteral Therapies

51. **(2)** The normal range of intraocular pressures is 12–22 mm Hg. **Answer 1** is *below* the range of normal pressures and may occur in hypovolemia (soft eyeballs) or dehydration. **Answer 3** is incorrect because ocular pressures are measured in *millimeters* of mercury. **Answer 4** is incorrect because pressures above 22 mm Hg are considered *elevated*.

Test-taking tip—Watch for the correct unit of measure (mm, not cm). Eliminate too low (#1), too high (#4).

EV, 2, HPM, Prevention and Early Detection of Disease

52. **(3)** It is not uncommon for a patient to feel that she will no longer be able to fulfill her role and needs as a woman following a hysterectomy. Verbalization of feelings allows the nurse to assess the patient's coping mechanisms and encourages the patient to deal with her emotional response. **Answer 3** is an open-ended question that allows the patient room to respond. **Answers 1 and 2** avoid the problem initially. **Answer 2** may be appropriate if, after talking to the patient, the nurse assesses that her responses represent a more significant or deep-seated problem. **Answer 4** would be appropriate *after* the patient has aired her feelings.

Test-taking tip—Use therapeutic communication—first, explore patient's comment. Eliminate MD and meds as initial responses. First, focus on feelings!

IMP, 7, PsI, Coping and Adaptation

53. **(2)** Desperation and panic may strike while the injury is occurring but *rarely* occur *during* the recovery period. During the acute stage of burn recovery, anxiety is common due to the stress and pain of injury and dressing changes. Anxiety decreases the individual's ability to perceive situations realistically, which may result in an altered mental state (**Answer 1**). During the intermediate phase of burn recovery, patients may react to continued pain, changes in body image, and financial stress with various psychological responses, ranging from withdrawal and depression (**Answer 3**) to acting out anger by refusing to cooperate with the medical regimen and by dependency (**Answer 4**).

Test-taking tip—Note "least likely" in the stem, meaning "which one is incorrect." Also note time period: *during* recovery.

AS, 7, PsI, Coping and Adaptation

54. **(2)** Though nausea may occur following the administration of narcotics, if it is accompanied by the absence of bowel sounds and upper abdominal distention, gastric or small-intestine dilation should be suspected and the nurse's findings reported to the physician. Changing the patient's position (**Answer 1**) and insertion of a rectal tube (**Answer 3**) are *not* helpful if peristalsis is not present (bowel sounds). Administering morphine (**Answer 4**) is *not* indicated until the source of the patient's discomfort is diagnosed.

Test-taking tip—Note the *time* of the event following surgery. What functions should return within 48 hours? Only one option deals with *assessment* (auscultate); the other three are implementation responses (change, insert, administer).

IMP, 8, PhI, Reduction of Risk Potential

55. **(1)** In the use of crutches, all weight bearing should be on the hands. Constant pressure in the axilla from weight bearing can lead to damage of the brachial plexus nerves and produce crutch paralysis. **Answers 2, 3, and 4** *are appropriate*

instructions to give to the patient preparing for crutch walking.

Test-taking tip—The best answer is the wrong thing to teach.

IMP, 3, PhI, Basic Care and Comfort

56. **(2)** Epileptic seizures or convulsions are the result of excessive, simultaneous, disordered neuronal discharge in the brain. This dysrhythmic electrical discharge may be focal (jacksonian seizure) or widely dispersed (grand mal seizures). **Answers 3** and **4** are incorrect because theories for the initiation of these convulsions vary from *decreased* (**Answer 3**) intracellular K^+ to *decreased* (**Answer 4**) cerebrospinal fluid to alteration in neuronal defense due to trauma, toxins, or inflammation. Depending on existing potential in the individual, **Answer 1** *may* be a precipitating factor.

Test-taking tip—Look for the key word: "neuronal."

AN, 2, PhI, Physiological Adaptation

57. **(2)** After the tube has been inserted into the stomach, its movement into the duodenum is first facilitated by having the patient lie on the *right* side for 2 hours, then on the back with head *elevated* for 2 hours, and finally on the left side for 2 hours. After the tube has passed the pylorus (this is usually checked by x-ray), *ambulating* the patient will help move the tube to the point of obstruction. *After* positioning and ambulation, the physician or the nurse may advance the tube 1–4 inches at specified time intervals (**Answer 1**) to provide slack for peristaltic action. Remaining quiet or flat in bed (**Answers 3** and **4**) will *not* facilitate the advancement of the tube either through the pylorus or through the small intestine.

Test-taking tip—Focus on the two positioning options: right vs. flat supine. Understand the concept of peristalsis and think of the sequence of positioning (right → supine in semi-Fowler's → left).

IMP, 8, PhI, Basic Care and Comfort

58. **(4)** The hypovolemia that occurs in the initial stage of burns is the result of fluid lost from denuded areas of skin and edema in and around the burned surface area. Edema formation is due to a shift of plasma fluids to the interstitial space. **Answers 1, 2,** and **3** are incorrect because when tissues are burned, a change in the permeability of both tissue and capillary membranes occurs. This change and increased vasodilation result in a shift of excessively large amounts of extracellular fluid (electrolytes and proteins) into the burned area. Most of this fluid loss occurs deep in the wound, where fluid moves into the deeper tissue. Burns of a highly vascular area (muscle, face) are believed to cause more severe fluid volume shifts than comparable burns to other areas of the body.

Test-taking tip—Where was fluid before the burn? Where would it go after the burn? Note the time period: *initial* stage.

AN, 6, PhI, Physiological Adaptation

59. **(2)** Vigorous activities such as brushing the teeth and brushing the hair are generally discouraged during periods of acute distress. These activities tend to increase aqueous production and therefore pressures because they activate sympathetic nervous system stimulation of the vasculature. Quiet activities such as watching TV (**Answer 1**), moderate activities such as reading, self-feeding (**Answer 3**), and passive range-of-motion exercises (**Answer 4**) *are* encouraged.

Test-taking tip—Look for the activity most likely to increase pressure in the eyes or head. Look for what is *not* OK because the stem says "to avoid." Three activities are quiet, passive; one is active (brushing).

IMP, 2, PhI, Basic Care and Comfort

60. **(2)** Diphenylhydantoin (phenytoin, Dilantin) must be injected IV slowly and in small increments to prevent vasodepression and circulatory collapse. Respiratory depression (**Answer 1**) is generally associated with *morphine sulfate*. *Adrenergic* (alpha) drugs such as norepinephrine bitartrate (Levophed) may cause vein and tissue necrosis (**Answer 3**) and have only *rarely* caused sudden malignant increases in blood pressure (**Answer 4**).

Test-taking tip—Know the *expected effects* of IV Dilantin. Think circulatory.

IMP, 2, PhI, Pharmacological and Parenteral Therapies

61. **(3)** Generally the patient with chronic, or open-angle glaucoma has few complaints of intense symptomatology. The usual onset of this condition is slow, silent, and painless. However, some patients experience *prodromal* symptoms, such as aching and discomfort around the eye, disturbed accommodation to darkness, and blurring of peripheral vision (**Answer 1**). Any complaint of pain or increasing discomfort with radiation to the forehead and temporal area is a grave sign of a sudden increase in pressure. Difficulty with close vision (**Answer 2**) is *not* characteristic of glaucoma. Halos around lights (**Answer 4**) occur *less commonly.*

Test-taking tip—Key word is *sudden*—complaint of eye pain often indicates an acute (sudden) change in intraocular pressure.

EV, 2, PhI, Physiological Adaptation

62. **(1)** Patients are ambulated as soon as possible to prevent the complications of bed rest; generally ambulation can begin as soon as 24 hours after surgery. In some instances, such as when the patient is severely debilitated or has complications due to ulcer perforation, bed rest may be prolonged, as in **Answers 2** and **3**. If this is the case, the nurse will need to observe closely for signs of complications (atelectasis, thrombophlebitis, etc.) and institute measures to prevent them. The patient is *rarely* if ever gotten up immediately after awakening, as in **Answer 4**.

Test-taking tip—Look for the best general *timing* to prevent complications and ensure patient safety. Key term: "usually," meaning typically (not rarely, or under special circumstances).

PL, 3, PhI, Basic Care and Comfort

63. **(1)** In cholinergic crisis, all anticholinesterase drugs are withdrawn and atropine (an anticholinergic drug) is given in 2 mg doses IV every hour until signs of atropine toxicity develop (dry mouth, blurred vision, tachycardia, rash or flushing of the skin, and elevated temperature). **Answers 2, 3,** and **4** are incorrect because they do *not* act to decrease cholinergic responses. Ephedrine (**Answer 2**) is used in myasthenia gravis to *increase* muscle tone; potassium chloride (**Answer 3**) is used to *increase* serum K^+ because it is believed that adequate serum-potassium levels potentiate the effects of cholinergic drugs; and neostigmine bromide (**Answer 4**) *is* an anticholinesterase that acts to improve cholinergic transmission of impulses at the myoneural junction.

Test-taking tip—Look for the antidote (an anticholinergic drug) to counteract untoward effects.

IMP, 3, PhI, Pharmacological and Parenteral Therapies

64. **(3)** Critical burns are classified as *deep* partial-thickness *over 30%* of the body or *full* thickness *over 10%* of the body. Extensive burns involving the face, hands, and feet or those associated with respiratory injuries are also considered critical. The most frequently used method of calculating the extent of a burn is the "rule of nines." Although this method is fairly simple to apply, it is somewhat inaccurate. This is particularly true when it is applied to children because allowances are not made for the proportional differences in head size and extremity size between children and adults. Hence superficial partial-thickness burns (**Answer 1**) are not serious unless large areas are involved or the patient is very young or old. Deep partial-thickness burns (**Answer 2**) are

classified as a major burn if over *25%* of the body is involved. The fourth-degree burn classification is *not* routinely used (**Answer 4**).

> **Test-taking tip**—First, eliminate what is least (superficial) and not used (#4).Then, think proportion—greater depth (*full thickness*) *and* less area.

EV, 6, PhI, Physiological Adaptation

65. (3) In chronic, or open-angle glaucoma, the obstruction to aqueous outflow is due to degenerative changes in either the trabeculum, Schlemm's canal, or the aqueous veins. Closed-angle glaucoma is characterized by obstruction of aqueous outflow due to narrowing of the angle between the anterior chamber and the root of the iris. The other answers are incorrect because chronic, or open-angle, glaucoma occurs *more frequently* than *closed-angle* (**Answer 1**), is characterized by slow, insidious, painless onset *rather than* the acute symptoms of closed-angle glaucoma (**Answer 2**), and *is* certainly familial, if not hereditary (**Answer 4**). Due to this latter characteristic, family members of patients with open-angle glaucoma should be encouraged to have their intraocular pressure assessed annually, particularly past age 40.

> **Test-taking tip**—Look for similarity between the condition ("open-angle") and clues in the choice that says "does not close," meaning it is *open*. The question asks how *open* angle is different.

AN, 2, PhI, Physiological Adaptation

66. (2) Although each of the listed measures *can* be used to assess the adequacy of the fluid replacement, hourly urine outputs and vital signs provide significant information on fluid balance in the acute burn period. Decreased urine output, increased pulse rate, and restlessness are early signs of inadequate fluid replacement. Increase in blood pressure, pulse, respirations, and urine output are early signs of circulatory overload. Changes in daily weights provide accurate data over the *long run* and are extremely important in monitoring fluid volumes in patients on diuretic therapy, such as patients with congestive heart failure or cirrhosis. **Answers 1, 3,** and **4** are *not* the *best* indicators.

> **Test-taking tip**—Key words: *best* and *early*. Look for indication of adequate volume. Note the two options that include "urinary output," and choose the one that also has *vital* signs that are *vital* to assess ↓fluid volume and overload.

EV, 6, PhI, Physiological Adaptation

67. (3) The most frequent cause of noncompliance to the medical treatment of chronic, or open-angle glaucoma is the miotic effects of pilocarpine. Pupillary constriction impedes normal accommodation, making night driving difficult and hazardous, reducing the patient's ability to read for extended periods, and making participation in games with fast-moving objects impossible. **Answer 1** is incorrect because *daytime* driving is *not* restricted. **Answer 2** is incorrect because this process is *painless*. The fact that the process is painless and insidious may in fact increase patients' noncompliance because they do not usually experience any adverse reactions if they do not instill their eyedrops. Nausea and vomiting are *rare* toxic effects of pilocarpine and are usually very mild; hence **Answer 4** is incorrect.

> **Test-taking tip**—Try KIS—Keep it simple: glaucoma is a problem with vision; hence, "decreased . . . vision" in #3 looks good. In addition, the stem mentions "medical treatment"; pilocarpine is a *specific* drug mentioned in #3. Recognize expected effects of miotics.

EV, 2, PhI, Pharmacological and Parenteral Therapies

68. (4) Profuse perspiration, diaphoresis, is one of a group of symptoms that happen 5–30 minutes after a high-carbohydrate meal or when liquid is taken with the meal. This is caused by entrance of food into the jejunum before it

has had a chance to begin the digestive process. Other symptoms include a feeling of fullness, *not hunger* (**Answer 1**); diarrhea, *not* constipation (**Answer 2**); and weakness, *not* increased strength (**Answer 3**).

> **Test-taking tip**—Stem asks what would the nurse *see* (objective). Three choices are subjective. Choose the one that is different.

EV, 4, PhI, Physiological Adaptation

69. (2) It is not safe to insert any foreign object under a cast, because the skin may break and become infected. Scratching also disturbs the padded surface under the cast, causing it to become wrinkled, which may lead to skin irritation and breakdown. Itching under the cast can be relieved by directing air (from a blower) under the cast. Oral medication is *not* generally effective in relieving this type of skin irritation (**Answer 1**). Rolling the cast (**Answer 3**) while the patient scratched would only *increase* the risk of skin damage. Taking the pencil from the patient (**Answer 4**) would *deny* his or her ability both to understand the rationale and to take responsibility for actions.

> **Test-taking tip**—Patient safety is a priority (reduce risk of damage to skin).

IMP, 3, PhI, Reduction of Risk Potential

70. (2) The primary dysfunction in myasthenia gravis occurs at the myoneural junction (the synapse between the end of a myelinated nerve fiber and a skeletal muscle fiber). Normally, acetylcholine is secreted by the nerve ending, which counts on the muscle fiber membrane by increasing its permeability to sodium. If sufficient sodium enters the muscle fiber membrane, an action potential is promulgated and causes the muscle fiber to contract. To enable the muscle fiber to repolarize, the acetylcholine in the synaptic junction is destroyed by cholinesterase. In myasthenia gravis, these normal impulses are blocked at the myoneural junction. **Answer 1** is incorrect because degeneration of the basal ganglia results in increased muscle tone, as occurs with *Parkinson's disease*. **Answer 3** is incorrect because increased stimulation of muscle fibers by anterior motor neurons would also increase muscle contractions. **Answer 4** is *partially* correct, in that there does seem to be a *familial* tendency toward the development of myasthenia; however, if myasthenia is *generalized*, it usually affects *not only* facial and mastication muscles but *also* ocular movement (diplopia and ptosis), as well as muscles of the neck, trunk (respirations), and limbs.

> **Test-taking tip**—Look for clues—*myo* (muscle); *neural* (nerve). Major problem is muscle weakness.

IMP, 3, PhI, Physiological Adaptation

71. (1) The diuretic stage of burns occurs 48–72 hours after injury. The fluid shift is the opposite of that in the initial stage. Fluids, electrolytes, and proteins may move very rapidly from the interstitial space back into the vascular compartment. Unless renal damage has occurred and there is *no indication* (**Answer 2**), diuresis ensues, due to the increased blood volume and renal blood flow. Serum electrolytes and hematocrit are decreased due to hemodilution. If urine output is insufficient at this time, symptoms of circulatory overload and cardiac failure will occur. There are *no data to support* **Answer 3**. The sodium value is within *normal* limits (**Answer 4**).

> **Test-taking tip**—Clue: time frame—after the initial phase (54 hours). Think *expected* changes over time in fluid balance (major shifts). Recognize normal serum Na⁺ value and eliminate #4. With *increased output*, you can eliminate #2 and #3.

AN, 8, PhI, Physiological Adaptation

72. (1) The most common side effects of pyridostigmine (Mestinon) and neostigmine bromide (Prostigmin) include anorexia, nausea, diarrhea, and abdominal cramps. These

symptoms are due to increased gastrointestinal secretions, smooth-muscle contractions (peristalsis), and irritation of the gastric mucosa. **Answer 2** is incorrect because increased cholinergic discharge increases bladder tone and contraction, thus *facilitating* voiding. **Answers 3** and **4** are incorrect because the symptoms listed are consistent with increased adrenergic, *not* cholinergic, discharge or stimulation.

> **Test-taking tip**—Need to know expected *common outcomes*. Think *GI* system: nausea is a *common* side effect with many drugs. Other options are *more severe*.

AS, 4, PhI, Pharmacological and Parenteral Therapies

73. **(4)** In response to direct questioning by the patient, the nurse needs to provide brief, accurate information. Some patients who have had gastrectomies are able to tolerate three meals a day before discharge from the hospital. However, for the majority of patients, it takes 6–12 months before their surgically reduced stomach has stretched enough to accommodate a larger meal. **Answer 1** is incorrect because it does not answer the question. **Answer 2** is correct as far as it goes, but still does not answer the patient's question. If the nurse does not know the answer to a question, he or she should admit it but try to get the information. **Answer 3** is incorrect because it gives *inaccurate* information.

> **Test-taking tip**—The correct choice *answers* what the patient asked; #2 and #4 are similar, but #4 gives more specific information (6–12 months as opposed to "a little longer").

IMP, 4, PsI, Coping and Adaptation

74. **(1)** The most common cause of hypothyroidism is excess thyroid tissue destruction due to radioactive iodine therapy for hyperthyroidism. Spontaneous hypothyroidism is believed to be due to an autoimmune response. Several studies have revealed a high incidence of antibodies for thyroid antigen in patients with spontaneous atrophy (**Answer 2**). Other, *less common* causes include surgical removal (**Answer 3**), Hashimoto's thyroiditis, overuse of antithyroid drugs (**Answer 4**), and pituitary tumors or insufficiency that decrease the circulating levels of thyroid-stimulating hormone.

> **Test-taking tip**—Use a process of elimination and keep *two common* causes in mind.

AN, 3, PhI, Physiological Adaptation

75. **(3)** In order to take full advantage of the effects of anticholinesterase drugs, they should generally be scheduled 20–30 minutes before eating. **Answers 1** and **2** are not totally incorrect, in that these drugs generally act over a 3-hour period; however, *peak action* occurs *quickly*, and patients with dysphagia *need time* to eat, chew, and swallow during meals. Rushing at meals causes unnecessary fatigue. **Answer 4** may not allow *enough* time for the drug to take effect.

> **Test-taking tip**—Clue: time frame. First, eliminate the extremes (#1, #4); look for a midpoint. Most drugs take effect within 30 min. What is the desired outcome? Improve swallowing of food.

IMP, 3, PhI, Pharmacological and Parenteral Therapies

76. **(2)** Body image changes are the most frequent basis for psychological responses during the recuperative phase. This is particularly true if the patient is young or has sustained facial or neck burns. Also, self-esteem is often lowered. The patient needs to be encouraged to talk about the perceived changes between what he or she was, and what he or she is now. Sessions with a psychiatric nurse specialist may be helpful. Occasionally individual or group therapy is indicated. Pain and immobility (**Answer 1**) create problems in the *acute* phase of burns. Financial concerns (**Answer 3**) may affect responses during the recuperative phase, but they are *not* a significant concern for all patients. Anger (**Answer 4**) may be a response during *each phase* as the patient reacts to various real and imagined losses.

> **Test-taking tip**—Clue: time frame ("recuperative stage"), not acute stage. The reality of disfigurement fits the time period.

EV, 7, PsI, Coping and Adaptation

77. **(2)** Signs of "cholinergic crisis" include pupils constricted to less than 2 mm, severe diarrhea, nausea, vomiting, hypersalivation, lacrimation, pallor, and hypotension. Bradycardia may occur but is uncommon. In severe cases, confusion progressing to coma may occur due to blockage of cerebral synapses. **Answers 1** and **3** are symptoms related to increased *adrenergic* discharge. **Answer 4** is only partially correct.

> **Test-taking tip**—The "eyes" have it! First decide that *constricted* pupils occur (this means that #1 and #3 are eliminated). The expected effects of too much medication in this condition would eliminate #4 (not *dry* mucous membranes, but *hyper*salivation).

AS, 2, PhI, Pharmacological and Parenteral Therapies

78. **(3)** A deficiency of thyroid hormone causes widespread metabolic changes. Alterations in fluid and electrolyte balance due to increased capillary permeability lead to fluid retention that results in edema, particularly of the eyelids, hands, and feet. **Answer 1** is incorrect because the lowered metabolic rate decreases cellular oxygen consumption; as a result, the heart rate, pulse pressure, and blood pressure are *reduced*. **Answer 2** is incorrect because there is eyelid edema, *not* facial edema. The basal metabolic rate is reduced, causing symptoms of anorexia, constipation, and intolerance to cold due to a lowered body temperature. **Answer 4** is incorrect because it includes diarrhea. Reduced cerebral blood flow affects both perception and coordination and results in symptoms of lethargy, generalized weakness, and *slowing* of both intellectual and motor functions.

> **Test-taking tip**—Note *hypo* (↓), not hyper (↑). Associate metabolic changes with the thyroid. Increased (↑) sluggishness (#3) really means *slow down* (↓).

AS, 3, PhI, Physiological Adaptation

79. **(1)** The patient with hyperthyroidism has an increased metabolic rate due to excess serum thyroxine leading to symptoms of systolic hypertension, heat intolerance, widened pulse pressure, and emotional excitability. **Answer 2** is incorrect because the diastolic blood pressure *reduces* due to decreased peripheral resistance. Weight *loss* (not gain, as in **Answer 3**) occurs because of increased catabolism despite an increase in appetite. Anorexia in **Answer 4** is incorrect because the patient has *increased* appetite.

> **Test-taking tip**—Note *hyper*—metabolism speeds up. Three options have both a correct and an incorrect element. Look for the option in which both parts are correct (#1).

AS, 3, PhI, Physiological Adaptation

80. **(4)** Myasthenia gravis is a rare disease of unknown cause but is suspected to have autoimmune characteristics. **Answer 1** is not correct because thymectomy has *often* resulted in remission or improvement (in approximately 70% of patients), *not* rarely. **Answer 2** is not correct because myasthenia gravis runs a *chronic* and progressive, *not* acute and rapid course. One of the major symptoms is muscle weakness, *not* increased strength (**Answer 3**).

> **Test-taking tip**—Use process of elimination, with a true-or-false approach as you look at key words in the options: *rarely, acute, increased* muscle strength.

AN, 3, PhI, Physiological Adaptation

81. **(1)** A nasogastric tube will be inserted early on the surgical day to monitor GI contents. **Answer 2** is not correct because the patient will *not* be allowed anything by mouth; all medications will be administered by *injection* in the immediate preoperative period. **Answer 3** is not correct because, although it is important for the *physician* (not a *nursing*

intervention) to explain possible complications when obtaining permission to perform the surgery, the timing is inappropriate for any lengthy descriptions of possible complications. **Answer 4** is not a good choice because the patient should be *encouraged,* not discouraged, to take an appropriate amount of pain medications so he or she will be able to cough, turn, and deep breathe to avoid respiratory complications.

> **Test-taking tip**—Choose the best answer to *present* complication during or after surgery. Clue: because it is *gastric* surgery; look at the option that has "naso*gastric* tube."

IMP, 1, PhI, Reduction of Risk Potential

82. **(1)** The primary pathology in Cushing's syndrome is increased serum cortisol, which acts to accelerate the rate of gluconeogenesis in the body, thus mobilizing stored fats and proteins. Serum glucose is increased, stimulating insulin secretion by the pancreas and resulting in abnormalities in fat metabolism and deposition. Weight gain is common; the torso enlarges and fat pads develop on the back of the neck and in the cheeks, giving the patient the characteristic "buffalo hump" and "moon facies." Increased epinephrine secretion (**Answer 2**) is associated with *pheochromocytoma.* Increased aldosterone **Answer 3** is associated with *primary aldosteronism.* Decreased ACTH secretion (**Answer 4**) is associated with dysfunctions of the *pituitary* gland.

> **Test-taking tip**—Cushing's and cortisol both start with *C.*

AN, 3, PhI, Physiological Adaptation

83. **(2)** Lassitude and muscle weakness are early clinical signs of Cushing's syndrome. Catabolism from gluconeogenesis occasionally results in a marked decrease in skeletal mass, and the patient's extremities may appear wasted. **Answer 1** is incorrect because gluconeogenesis from excess cortisol secretion results in *hyperglycemia.* **Answer 3** is *partially correct:* hypersecretion of aldosterone in Cushing's disease is *rare;* however, large quantities of cortisol tend to increase sodium and water retention and potassium excretion. Edema and hypokalemia occur only in *severe* cases. Discoloration and hyperpigmentation (**Answer 4**) occur with *adrenal insufficiency.*

> **Test-taking tip**—Visualize the patient with Cushing's—skinny legs (wasting) and buffalo hump (fat mobilization).

EV, 3, PhI, Physiological Adaptation

84. **(1)** Signs and symptoms of Addison's disease include hypotension, hypoglycemia, muscular weakness, fatigue, weight loss, hyperkalemia, and depression. These symptoms are primarily due to disturbances in sodium, water, and potassium imbalances that cause severe dehydration. **Answer 2** includes symptoms of *Cushing's syndrome.* **Answer 3** is incorrect because hyperglycemia and weight gain are consistent also with *Cushing's Syndrome.* **Answer 4** also includes symptoms of *Cushing's* syndrome.

> **Test-taking tip**—Look for signs of a *deficiency* (*hypo*, weight *loss*, ↓ energy). If one part of an option is incorrect, the entire option is incorrect (e.g., weight *gain* in #3 makes the entire option incorrect, although *hypo*tension is correct).

AS, 3, PhI, Physiological Adaptation

85. **(1)** Iron deficiency anemia is characterized by a decrease in red blood cell color due to a decrease in iron (hypochromic) and an increase in immature red blood cells (microcytic). **Answer 2** describes the red blood cells in *pernicious anemia.* **Answers 3 and 4** describe *no* particular conditions.

> **Test-taking tip**—Look for similar meanings in stem and answer—*deficiency* in the stem, and *hypo* and *micro* in the correct option (#1).

AN, 6, PhI, Physiological Adaptation

86. **(1)** In assessing any patient's emotional responses, the nurse should first assess the patient's ego strength, body image, and coping abilities for life situations in general. The manner in which the patient views himself or herself will greatly affect attitudes toward disease and emotional response. If the patient normally denies or represses threatening information or situations, desirable outcomes may be difficult to achieve. Research indicates that social supports are extremely important in maintaining health. The relationship between the patient and the patient's mother (**Answer 2**) should be assessed. However, if the patient has a strong self-image, the issues between mother and adult child should be resolvable either alone or with objective outside help. **Answer 3** is *incomplete.* Economic status and work history (**Answer 4**), depending on their value to the patient, *may not* be important determinants of emotional response.

> **Test-taking tip**—Select the broadest, most inclusive answer that covers them all. When in doubt about the best psychosocial option, choose the "self-image, self-concept" type of answer.

AN, 7, PsI, Coping and Adaptation

87. **(1)** The primary fluid and electrolyte imbalances in Addison's disease are *hypo*natremia, *hypo*volemia, and *hyper*kalemia. These imbalances are caused by *decreased* aldosterone secretion. **Answers 2 and 3** are incorrect because they occur with *excessive* secretion of this hormone. Calcium levels are *not* affected by this condition (**Answer 4**).

> **Test-taking tip**—Need to know relationship with sodium (↓) and potassium (↑). Key word is *decreased* aldosterone secretion.

EV, 6, PhI, Physiological Adaptation

88. **(2)** Mafenide 1% (Sulfamylon) is a white antibacterial ointment applied once or twice daily. Besides causing pain on application, this medication is a carbonic anhydrase inhibitor that interferes with the kidney's ability to excrete hydrogen ions and thus may cause metabolic acidosis, *not* metabolic alkosis (**Answer 3**). Patients who are treated with mafenide 1% need to have their acid-base balance monitored by blood gas determinations. Clinical signs of metabolic acidosis are increased rate and depth of respirations. *Silver nitrate* causes black discoloration of linens, and its hypotonicity causes electrolyte imbalances (**Answers 1 and 4**). Patients treated with silver nitrate need supplemental sodium, potassium, and chloride.

> **Test-taking tip**—Recognize expected desired and untoward *metabolic* effects. This eliminates #1; #4 is a side effect of a different drug.

EV, 1, PhI, Pharmacological and Parenteral Therapies

89. **(3)** The best early intervention would be to increase fluid intake, because constipation is common when activity is decreased or usual routines have been interrupted. **Answer 1** is incorrect because this may not be necessary and also *requires a doctor's order.* **Answer 2** is incorrect because this is a great deal of exertion when the patient is not expressing an urge to defecate. Although activity usually helps bowel evacuation, it would be *impossible* to exercise extremities that have unhealed fractures (**Answer 4**).

> **Test-taking tip**—Priority *nursing* action is to prevent and correct constipation: ↑ fluids →↑ *fecal* movement.

IMP, 8, PhI, Basic Care and Comfort

90. **(1)** Thyroid storm may be precipitated by a number of stresses, such as infection, real or threatened loss of a loved one, or thyroid surgery undertaken before the patient was prepared adequately with antithyroid drugs. A change heralding thyroid storm is a fever: the patient's temperature may rise as high as 106°F (41°C). **Answers 2, 3,** and **4** *are* symptoms of hyperthyroidism and become *exaggerated* during thyroid storm. Without treatment, the patient progresses from delirium to coma; death ensues as the result of heart failure.

> **Test-taking tip**—Key word is *cardinal*—most important; what you will note *first.*

AS, 3, PhI, Physiological Adaptation

91. **(2)** Bloody drainage from the nasogastric tube more than 12 hours after surgery should be considered unusual and reported to the surgeon. Prolonged bleeding may be indicative of a slow bleeder, a blood dyscrasia, or problems with incisional closure. Any of these may increase blood loss and lead to shock. **Answers 1, 3,** and **4** are incorrect because they are *normal* findings in the *early* postgastrectomy period.

> **Test-taking tip**—The key element is a *time* factor, *not* color (i.e., not greenish-yellow, red). Choose an answer indicating the greatest risk to the patient (*prolonged* bleeding).

EV, 6, PhI, Reduction of Risk Potential

92. **(2)** Calculating the correct rate requires computation of the hourly volume (290 mL) and the minute volume (5 mL), and then multiplying the rate, in mL/min, by the drop factor (15 gtt/mL). (The hourly and minute volumes have been rounded to the nearest whole number.) **Answers 1** and **3** are *not fast enough* to deliver this large a volume in the prescribed period. **Answer 4** is *too rapid.* A quick method of computing the drip rate is to use the first two numbers in the 24-hour fluid volume, i.e., 7000 mL in 24 hours = 70 gtt/min. This shortcut may be useful when initially starting an infusion, before mathematically calculating the rate. Use only with 15 gtt/mL factor.

> **Test-taking tip**—Use basic IV calculation. Eliminate the extremes (#1 and #3 are too slow; #4 is too fast); select the midpoint here.

IMP, 6, PhI, Pharmacological and Parenteral Therapies

93. **(1)** Osteoblastic activity (bone growth) requires the stress and strain of weight bearing to be proportional to osteoclastic activity (bone breakdown). When the patient is immobilized for an extended period of time, bone breakdown takes place. Although dietary intake is important, it is not recommended that there be an increase in calcium intake (**Answer 2**) due to the potential for kidney stones as a result of immobilization. Osteoporosis is related to a *deficit* of calcium, not an excess (**Answer 3**). Bone growth is dependent on weight bearing, *not lack* of it (**Answer 4**).

> **Test-taking tip**—Focus on two options with "lack of weight bearing." Recognize expected outcome of immobilization—look for *loss* of bone density.

AN, 3, PhI, Physiological Adaptation

94. **(4)** Sinus arrhythmias is the most frequent arrhythmia and occurs as a *normal* phenomenon, often related to the respiratory cycle. **Answer 1** is incorrect because lidocaine is used to treat *life-threatening ventricular* arrhythmias. **Answer 2** is incorrect because exercise, which increases the heart rate, will abolish the arrhythmia, so rest or limited activity is *not indicated.* **Answer 3** is incorrect because the arrhythmia originates in the *sinoatrial* node, *not* in the atrioventricular node, and digoxin is the treatment for *atrial arrhythmias.*

> **Test-taking tip**—Is this ECG pattern OK or not OK? Is it "Oh! Oh!" or is it "Eh!"?

EV, 6, PhI, Reduction of Risk Potential

95. **(2)** Hematocrit is reduced due to hemodilution and volume overload resulting from the interstitial-to-plasma fluid shift. Erythropoietin factor (**Answer 1**) is produced by the kidneys and would *only* be reduced *if* there were kidney failure. Metabolic acidosis (**Answer 3**) does increase red blood cell fragility, but it is *not applicable* in this situation. Hypoalbuminemia (**Answer 4**) causes loss of oncotic pressures in the vascular compartment. The primary effect of this phenomenon is movement of fluid from the vascular compartment to the interstitial space, the outcome of which is hemo*concentration.*

> **Test-taking tip**—Read answers to find clues—low hematocrit and hemodilution.

AN, 6, PhI, Physiological Adaptation

96. **(3)** Pernicious anemia may occur following subtotal gastrectomy (when large portions of the stomach are removed) due to the loss of tissue that produces the intrinsic factor. Loss of this factor necessitates the parenteral administration of *vitamin B_{12},* the *extrinsic* factor. **Answer 1** is incorrect because the extrinsic factor is found in *food.* **Answers 2** and **4** are incorrect because it is the *loss of intrinsic* factor that results in the malabsorption of vitamin B_{12}.

> **Test-taking tip**—Note the pattern in the responses: two extrinsic factors, one intrinsic; choose the one that is different. Need to know reason for expected problem.

EV, 4, PhI, Physiological Adaptation

97. **(1)** The gastric distress that occurs as a side effect of these medications can be reduced by administering the drugs along with milk, soda crackers, or antacids. The nursing actions in **Answer 2** are consistent with *elimination* problems (urinary retention); those in **Answer 3** are consistent with *central nervous system* excitation (flushing, irritability); and the action in **Answer 4** is consistent with *cardiac arrhythmias* (palpitations, PVCs).

> **Test-taking tip**—Relate the system affected (GI) to the intervention (food).

IMP, 4, PhI, Pharmacological and Parenteral Therapies

98. **(2)** Generalized tonic-clonic (grand mal) seizures are characterized by auras preceding the convulsive spasms of all muscle groups, loss of consciousness, and loss of sphincter control. Brief, abrupt loss of consciousness, with a characteristic "blank stare," is indicative of *absence (petit mal) seizures* (**Answer 1**). *Focal or partial seizures* usually involve only a portion of the brain and reflect the area of the brain activated by abnormal discharge (such as tonic and clonic contractions of the large muscles in an arm or leg) (**Answer 3**). Localized twitching of facial muscles, especially of the angle of the mouth, or within a finger or toe, is characteristic of a *jacksonian seizure* (**Answer 4**).

> **Test-taking tip**—Look at "minutes" vs. "seconds"; "generalized" in the stem goes with the *longer* time period. Look for key words in stem and answer—"*generalized*" and "*all motor muscle groups.*"

AS, 2, PhI, Physiological Adaptation

99. **(3)** The speed (velocity) of nerve impulses decreases with aging, making responses slower. The amount of change varies with individuals, so a *specific* change according to age is *not predictable* (**Answers 1** and **2**). Sensory conduction decreases faster over time compared with motor conduction; some areas are less sensitive (ankle malleolus), but the change is not generalized throughout the body (**Answer 4**).

> **Test-taking tip**—The key word in the stem is "normal," and the correct choice must apply to all older adults. Choose the most inclusive Answer: #3 includes #1 and #2.

AS, 2, HPM, Growth and Development

100. **(2)** Pain management requires the nurse and physician to collaborate to achieve optimal relief for the patient. The use of analgesics for pain requires a physician's order. The nurse assesses the patient's response to drug therapy and alerts the MD to needed changes. The nurse may also recommend nondrug interventions to promote patient comfort (progressive relaxation, massage). **Answers 1** and **3** are manageable by *independent* nursing actions—careful assessment, ROM, proper positioning. **Answer 4** is *not a nursing diagnosis,* but a medical problem to be corrected by surgery.

> **Test-taking tip**—The key words in the stem are *best* outcome and *collaboratively.* Although independent nursing actions could be planned for each option, look for the one that requires physician's orders to implement care.

AN, 3, SECE, Management of Care

101. **(3)** There is an increase in body fat and a decrease in lean muscle mass, which increases the duration of drug effects. There is a decrease in the percentage of body water (**Answer 1**) in the elderly; however, it is the changes in the kidney that affect drug excretion, resulting in drug toxicity. *Enzymes* in the liver, *not* hormones (**Answer 2**) are diminished, which

affects the metabolism of drugs. The CNS effects (**Answer 4**) are usually *increased* in the elderly because of problems with drug accumulation, duration of effects, and toxicity.

> **Test-taking tip**—Eliminate the options that are not true first (#2, #4). Know normal processes of drug metabolism regardless of age.

AN, 5, PhI, Pharmacological and Parenteral Therapies

102. (3) All of the diagnoses are problems in the AIDS patient. Providing optimum pain management and keeping the patient comfortable must be a priority, particularly over skin integrity (**Answer 1**). Pain control will also have an impact on patient anxiety (**Answer 2**) and breathing (**Answer 4**).

> **Test-taking tip**—When all the answers are correct, use Maslow's hierarchy to establish priorities. With three good choices, choose the one that could cover two other options (#3 covers #2 and #4).

AN, 3, PhI, Basic Care and Comfort

103. (2) Heat cramps occur when fluids are lost through excessive sweating and water is replaced without sodium replacement. A balanced solution or sources of water and sodium should be ingested. Sodium chloride tablets may be taken, but they may cause stomach irritation. If there was a prior history (**Answer 1**) and another admission, there is still a need for patient teaching. **Answers 3 and 4** are not incorrect; fluids *are* important for evaporative cooling, and potassium and magnesium *may be* lost, *but* the role of *sodium* is *most important* to prevent future problems.

> **Test-taking tip**—The stem asks for the *most* important. When all of the options are correct, use a process of elimination to select the one that will make the greatest difference—prevent harm (#2)—or incorporates other options.

IMP, 6, PhI, Basic Care and Comfort

104. (1) Tachycardia and urine output less than 30 mL per hour are classic indicators of low circulating volume—hypovolemic shock. Both the cardiac and renal systems are compensating for the low perfusion state. **Answer 2** is partially correct; pitting edema, however, is seen with fluid retention and volume *excess*. **Answer 3** indicates dehydration, also a state of fluid deficit, but the signs would *not be classic* of shock. **Answer 4** describes a state of fluid volume excess.

> **Test-taking tip**—Turn each option into a true-or-false question: e.g., would a patient in shock have an increased pulse? True? Or false?

AN, 6, PhI, Physiological Adaptation

105. (2) In a patient who is immune-suppressed, the oral mucous membranes are often a source of infection; therefore, a complaint of a sore throat is an important early indication of a potential problem. With immunosuppression the body is often *unable* to respond to an infection with the characteristic indicators, such as a fever (**Answer 1**). The drugs used to suppress the immune system *mask* the signs of infection (**Answer 3**). **Answer 4** is *not* a sign of infection.

> **Test-taking tip**—The key word is *early*. Know the concept of immunosuppression and what this may affect (e.g., *mask* some infections, reduce ability to *fight* infection with fever, allow opportunistic infections to *take hold* [mucous membranes]).

AN, 1, PhI, Physiological Adaptation

106. (1) Peritonitis is the most serious complication of CAPD. How to maintain aseptic or sterile technique to prevent bacteria from entering the peritoneal cavity is the most important information to teach the patient. **Answer 2, 3, and 4** are also important to teach the CAPD patient *after* the nurse determines that the patient will be able to safely perform sterile technique.

> **Test-taking tip**—This is a "rank order of priority" question. When all of the options are correct, which one prevents the patient from the greatest potential risk?

IMP, 8, SECE, Safety and Infection Control

107. (1) A witnessed or unwitnessed cardiac arrest starts with establishing the state of consciousness of the patient. It is important to determine if the patient is awake before proceeding with emergency CPR. **Answers 2 and 4** are the *next* steps in initiating CPR. **Answer 3**, although not part of the ABCs of CPR, would be done *after* establishing a pulse.

> **Test-taking tip**—This is a "rank order of priority" question. Remember "shake and shout," *then* your ABCs.

AS, 6, PhI, Physiological Adaptation

108. (4) The patient's signs are consistent with an increase in venous pressure. Pericardial effusion or cardiac tamponade impairs the ventricles from adequately filling during diastole. Venous pressure increases and stroke volume decreases. **Answers 1 and 2** would result in signs and symptoms consistent with left-sided heart failure, and difficulty breathing would likely be present. Hypertrophy (**Answer 3**) is *not* reduced, but rather *managed* through drug therapy.

> **Test-taking tip**—Look for patterns in the options. Three of the choices involve the ventricles—how could you choose just one?

PL, 6, PhI, Physiological Adaptation

109. (3) The priority with status epilepticus is the adequacy of the patient's airway and breathing. Measuring the patient's blood gases would be important in determining the need for more aggressive management. **Answers 1, 2, and 4** are not priority concerns.

> **Test-taking tip**—This is a priority question—if airway is affected, assessing the status will be the best answer. Also note a pattern in the responses: three options have "time," one does not. Choose the one that is different (#3).

AS, 2, PhI, Physiological Adaptation

110. (2) As cerebral hypoxia develops, the patient becomes restless and drowsy well before any of the characteristic signs and symptoms of increasing intracranial pressure are present. **Answers 1, 3, and 4** are all consistent with increasing intracranial pressure but occur much *later,* after there has been significant cerebral herniation and distortion of the brain.

> **Test-taking tip**—The key word in the stem is *early.* A "change" in level of consciousness (could be restlessness or a lack of responsiveness) is almost always the best answer with neurological problems. A key word in the best option is *change.*

AN, 2, PhI, Physiological Adaptation

111. (4) Frequently patients complain of severe itching from the opioids used with epidural analgesia. Antihistamines and comfort measures are effective for many patients, as well as reduction in the dosage or administering Narcan to control itching without reversing the analgesic effects. Respiratory depression (**Answer 1**) is not a common problem with careful titration of standard dosages. Only when the patient becomes sedated does the respiratory function become a concern. **Answers 2 and 3** are *not* expected side effects (however, postural hypotension and constipation are potential problems).

> **Test-taking tip**—The clue in the stem is "most common." Look for something annoying but not serious. Otherwise epidural analgesia would not be used as often as it is.

EV, 3, PhI, Pharmacological and Parenteral Therapies

112. (1) Maintaining perfusion is the priority in the early postoperative period. Pain (**Answer 2**) would also be important; however, it is *not* life threatening. **Answers 3 and 4** are also important nursing diagnoses, but they are *not actual* problems, although there is risk *potential.*

> **Test-taking tip**—This is a priority question. Consider the *greatest* risk to the patient, meaning the possibility of a life-threatening problem (cardiac).

AN, 6, PhI, Physiological Adaptation

113. (1) There is a risk to the patient with COPD if the O_2 flow rate is too high. The patient with COPD has a hypoxic respi-

ratory drive. If the liter flow is above 2 L, there is a risk for respiratory depression. **Answers 2, 3,** and **4** are important nursing actions to determine the *effectiveness* of oxygen therapy.

Test-taking tip—Look for patterns in the options. Three options assess the *effectiveness* of the treatment. One validates the *appropriateness* of the order. Choose the one that is different.

AS, 6, PhI, Reduction of Risk Potential

114. **(1)** Tuberculosis is an airborne infectious disease. Preventing further spread of the disease would be a priority for care. Covering the mouth when coughing, proper disposal of tissues, and hand washing must be reinforced. **Answers 2, 3,** and **4** are important actions *after* preventing disease transmission.

Test-taking tip—This is a priority question. Think *prevention before* treatment.

PL, 6, SECE, Safety and Infection Control

115. **(3)** A pneumothorax exerts a "pushing" pressure on the heart and unaffected lung. Function is compromised. Semi-Fowler's is optimal positioning for chest expansion. **Answers 1, 2,** and **4** would *inhibit* chest expansion partially.

Test-taking tip—Visualize each position and how ventilation would be affected. The best position is one that maximizes ventilation and minimizes lung restriction.

IMP, 6, PhI, Reduction of Risk Potential

116. **(2)** Intestinal obstructions are medical emergencies because of the risk for severe fluid and electrolyte imbalance and the development of hypovolemia. The obstruction prevents normal fluid and electrolyte reabsorption in the small intestine. Although there may be gastric distention and vomiting, which might result in aspiration (**Answer 1**), it is *not* a priority or a *direct* result of the obstruction. Nutrition would be altered (**Answer 3**), but there would be a *deficit* of electrolytes (hypokalemia). Nausea (**Answer 4**) may be present, but it is neither a priority *nor* stated as a *nursing diagnosis*.

Test-taking tip—This is a priority question (fluid volume deficit vs. aspiration). Look at the *direct* result of the obstruction.

AN, 8, PhI, Physiological Adaptation

117. **(4)** The post-MI patient with left-sided heart failure, which is also cardiogenic shock, would be experiencing metabolic acidosis. The pH would decrease, consistent with acidosis. **Answers 1, 2,** and **3** would all *increase* as a result of the myocardial damage.

Test-taking tip—Note the key word: *decrease*. Know the clinical relevance of laboratory tests. Think what effect myocardial damage would have on each test.

EV, 6, PhI, Physiological Adaptation

118. **(1)** The patient is most likely in shock. Bicarbonate is needed with metabolic acidosis, which will develop. The compensatory tachycardia will result in poor oxygenation. Although the question does not indicate difficulty breathing, the patient is not being perfused well (pulselessness) and may go into cardiac arrest if emergency treatment is not begun. CPR (**Answers 2** and **4**) would not be done because there *is* a heart rhythm, although perfusion is ineffective. Atropine (**Answer 3**) would not be given because it *increases* heart rate.

Test-taking tip—Use a process of elimination—CPR is not indicated. Therefore, eliminate #2 and #4. Do you give atropine or sodium bicarbonate for shock?

PL, 6, PhI, Reduction of Risk Potential

119. **(2)** Oxygen therapy is important to the prevention and treatment of life-threatening arrhythmias, which occur often as a result of myocardial ischemia. The ineffective contraction of the heart may result in reduced cardiac output and poor perfusion, leading to hypotension. Acid-base abnormalities and enzymes (**Answer 1**) do *not* improve with O_2. Hyperox-

emia (**Answer 3**) would *not require* additional oxygen. Hypertension (**Answer 4**) is *not* expected with an MI; and conduction defects are due to damage to the conduction system and do *not* respond to O_2.

Test-taking tip—Phrase each option as a true-false question and determine if oxygen would improve the patient problem.

AS, 6, PhI, Physiological Adaptation

120. **(4)** Surgery is usually a stressful situation that increases anxiety. Administration of an anxiolytic such as midazolam (Versed), lorazepam (Ativan), or diazepam (Valium) during the preoperative period may be necessary to lower the blood pressure and prevent any complications. Antihypertensive agents (**Answer 1**) are usually *held* before surgery to reduce the risk of hypotension from an adverse interaction with anesthesia. Checking vital signs (**Answer 2**), although not wrong, would not resolve the patient's preoperative anxiety and stress. An elevated BP possibly related to preoperative stress would *not* be a reason to cancel surgery (**Answer 3**). That may only further increase the patient's stress.

Test-taking tip—Do something for the patient's stress first. Only one option deals with the preoperative stress.

IMP, 3, PhI, Reduction of Risk Potential

121. **(2)** During cardioversion the patient is awake but sedated. The anticipation of the procedure may be anxiety producing. Auscultation (**Answer 1**) would *not* be necessary, because the patient will be monitored. There should *not* be any *pain* (**Answer 3**) or *infection* (**Answer 4**).

Test-taking tip—Look at the time frame. Choose an option that addresses the patient need *before* the procedure.

IMP, 6, PhI, Pharmacological and Parenteral Therapies

122. **(3)** Total normal output for a 24-hour period is 2500 mL, with 1500 mL from urine and 1000 mL from skin, lungs, and feces. **Answer 1** is the *minimum* amount of urine output that is acceptable for a 24-hour period. **Answer 2** is acceptable, but *not normal*, and **Answer 4** would be *excessive*; it occurs with diuresis or diabetes insipidus (2–3 L in 24 hours).

Test-taking tip—The key word is *normal*. Recall that the minimum amount of urine desired for 1 hour is 30 mL, and 3 L is excessive. When numbers (i.e., amounts) are involved, avoid the extremes (too low and too high).

EV, 8, PhI, Physiological Adaptation

123. **(3)** The blood gases are consistent with compensated respiratory alkalosis. The patient is *hyperventilating*, breathing rapidly and blowing off carbon dioxide. A slower rate, not deeper, will increase the CO_2 level. **Answer 1** will prevent hypoventilation. **Answer 2** will prevent complications from immobility (e.g., pneumonia), which would produce an elevated CO_2, not O_2, level. Fluids (**Answer 4**) will *not* improve a blood gas alteration that is the result of a respiratory response.

Test-taking tip—Look at the two options that deal with breathing (deep breaths, breathe slowly). Consider how each option will increase CO_2 level. Know normal blood gas ranges.

IMP, 6, PhI, Reduction of Risk Potential

124. **(3)** The first action is to measure the glucose level, start an IV, and prepare to give glucose or insulin. A dangerously low blood sugar level is life threatening and must be corrected immediately. **Answers 1, 2,** and **4** are not incorrect nursing actions; however, they are *not the first* priority.

Test-taking tip—The key word is *first*. Only one option takes a direct action to determine the cause of unconsciousness.

IMP, 4, PhI, Reduction of Risk Potential

125. **(2)** Toxoplasmosis is an opportunistic infection and a parasite of birds and mammals. The oocysts remain infectious in moist soil for about 1 year. Eating raw or undercooked meat, *not vegetables* (**Answer 1**), is a mode of transmission. The

parasite is transmitted through ingestion, *not air* (**Answer 3**). Ingestion of oocysts from cat feces is the most common mode of oral infection in the United States. Cats do *not* have to be avoided (**Answer 4**), *but handling of litter* should be avoided, and hand washing would be essential for a patient who is immunocompromised.

Test-taking tip—When preventing infection, two options are usually desirable choices—wearing gloves and hand washing.

IMP, 1, SECE, Safety and Infection Control

126. (2) Pneumoccocal pneumonia vaccine is given to anyone at high risk for pneumococcal pneumonia or its complications. One immunization is recommended for lifetime protection, although revaccination every 6 years should be considered for high-risk patients. A booster for tetanus and diphtheria (**Answer 1**) is only needed every *10* years to maintain lifelong immunity. **Answer 3**, influenza, is given *annually* for high-risk individuals. Measles and mumps (**Answer 4**) is indicated for *anyone* born after 1956 with an uncertain immune status.

Test-taking tip—Use the process of elimination and what you know about normal pediatric immunization patterns to figure out adult variations.

IMP, 1, HPM, Prevention and Early Detection of Disease

127. (3) Polycythemia vera is a chronic myeloproliferative disorder characterized mainly by erythrocytosis (increased RBC mass). Hemoglobin and hematocrit will be elevated. **Answers 1, 2,** and **4** are also laboratory findings, but they are considered *minor* criteria in this condition.

Test-taking tip—Know the major physiological abnormality and important diagnostic indicator.

AS, 6, PhI, Physiological Adaptation

128. (1) The development of atrial fibrillation, although not life threatening, will have the greatest impact on hemodynamics; and the patient may experience chest pain, dyspnea, and heart failure following an MI. The patient may automatically revert back to a sinus rhythm; however, the effect of the rhythm change must be assessed. **Answers 2, 3** and **4** do not indicate the need for treatment or immediate response on the part of the nurse.

Test-taking tip—Consider which change presents the greatest risk to the patient (e.g., fibrillation). Know the acceptable parameters of cardiac functioning (i.e., what is OK vs. not OK).

AN, 6, PhI, Physiological Adaptation

129. (1) Use of eye patches may be continued postoperatively, depending on surgeon preference. This is done to achieve >90% success rate of the surgery. A moderate amount of pain *is* expected (**Answer 2**). Positioning (**Answer 3**) *depends* on the location and severity of the detachment; prone or face down positioning may be required. Vision is usually blurred because accommodation has been paralyzed. A return to normal vision (**Answer 4**) *cannot* be predicted preoperatively.

Test-taking tip—Time sequence (preoperative) points to the best choice. Only one option says "may" be done; the other choices are *too definitive* ("is expected," "will be used").

IMP, 2, PsI, Coping and Adaptation

130. (2) The nurse *leading*, without holding, the patient is the correct approach. The nurse is the "sight" for the patient, and being ahead of the individual who is blind is more secure and safe for the patient. **Answers 1, 3,** and **4** all have the nurse holding the patient, rather than the patient holding onto the nurse.

Test-taking tip—Look for patterns in the options. Only one has the patient being *led* by the nurse.

IMP, 3, PhI, Basic Care and Comfort

131. (3) Most falls in the elderly, including those with Parkinson's disease, occur in the bathroom. There is a loss of muscle strength in legs with normal aging. Combined with muscle rigidity and postural instability in Parkinson's, the risk for falls is great. **Answers 1** and **2**, *as stated*, are not the most important ways to reduce falls. *Nonskid* soles and proper fit (not necessarily snug) are safety concerns. **Answer 4** improves posture, not necessarily reducing the risk for falling.

Test-taking tip—*Visualize* each option and how *stability* would be improved.

IMP, 3, PhI, Basic Care and Comfort

132. (1) Pain from passive movement or stretching of the fingers is characteristic of the development of compartment syndrome. The cast is acting as a "space-limiting" sleeve around the muscle, nerves, and blood vessels, resulting in increased tissue pressure. Skin color, temperature, capillary refill, and quality of peripheral pulses are not reliable clinical indicators of compartment syndrome. The fracture is too recent for disuse (**Answer 2**). Increasing pain is *not normal* (**Answer 3**). Nerve compression (**Answer 4**) would cause paresthesia or paralysis.

Test-taking tip—Use process of elimination and knowledge of usual signs and symptoms of circulatory, sensory, and motor impairment.

AN, 2, PhI, Physiological Adaptation

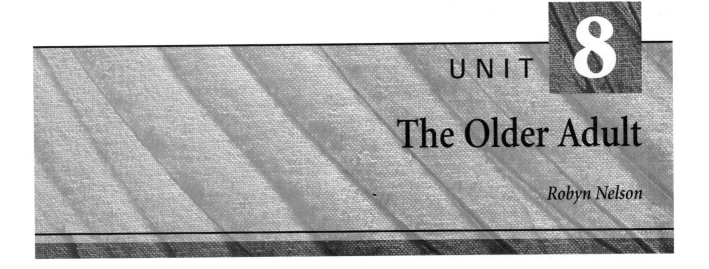

UNIT 8

The Older Adult

Robyn Nelson

Introduction

This unit is unique in that the primary objective is to present **practical**, concise information of **clinical** relevance for the beginning practitioner that is not covered elsewhere. The focus is on 12 significant problems and concerns associated with the older adult (e.g., *falls, use of restraints, thermoregulation, sleep disturbance, skin breakdown, polypharmacy,* specific types of *hearing changes,* age-related *macular degeneration, incontinence, sexual neglect, caregiver burden,* warning signs of *poor nutrition*).

The unit begins with health assessment of the older adult, system by system, highlighting the most common changes associated with the aging process; it ends with several functional rating scales to assist in management of care in the home or community.

Covered elsewhere in this book are other age-relevant problems and test questions. Refer to **Unit 6** for mental health conditions common in the older adult (e.g., dementia, Alzheimer's, depression). **Unit 7** covers common age-relevant problems related to immobility, bladder and bowel dysfunction, hip fracture, use of assistive devices, cardiovascular conditions (stroke, hypertension), cataracts, and glaucoma. Also covered in **Unit 7** are health problems that have more serious consequences in the older adult, such as pneumonia and osteoporosis. Nutritional needs of the elderly are included in **Unit 9**.

I. Health assessment of the older adult (also see Unit 7)

A. *Skin*
1. Decrease in elasticity → wrinkles and lines, dryness.
2. Loss of fullness → sagging.
3. Generalized loss of adipose and muscle tissue → wasting appearance.
4. Decrease of adipose tissue on extremities, redistributed to hips and abdomen in middle age.
5. Bony prominences become visible.
6. Excessive pigmentation → age spots.
7. Dry skin and deterioration of nerve fibers and sensory endings → pruritus.
8. Decreased blood flow → pallor and blotchiness.
9. Overgrowth of epidermal tissue → lesions (some benign, some premalignant, some malignant).

B. *Nails:*
1. Dry, brittle.
2. Increased susceptibility to fungal infections.
3. Decreased growth rate.
4. Toenails thick, difficult to cut.

C. *Hair:*
1. Loss of pigment → graying, white.
2. Decreased density of hair follicles → thinning of hair.
3. Decreased blood flow to skin and decreased estrogen production → baldness.
   a. Hair distribution: thin on scalp, axilla, pubic area, upper and lower extremities.
   b. Decreased facial hair in *men.*
4. Decreased estrogen production → increased facial (chin, upper lip) hair in *women.*

D. *Eyes:*
1. Loss of soluble protein with loss of lens transparency → development of *cataracts.*
2. Decrease in pupil size limits amount of light entering the eye → elderly need more light to see.
3. Decreased pupil reactivity → decrease in rate of light changes to which a person can readily adapt.
4. Decreased accommodation to darkness and dim light → diminished night vision.
5. Loss of orbital fat → sunken appearance.
6. Blink reflex—slowed.
7. Eyelids—loose.
8. Visual acuity—diminished.
9. Peripheral vision—diminished.
10. Visual fields—diminished.

11. Lens accommodation—decreased; requires corrective lenses.
12. *Presbyopia*—lens may lose ability to become convex enough to accommodate to nearby objects; starts at age 40 (*farsightedness*).
13. Color of iris—fades.
14. Conjunctiva—thins, looks yellow.
15. Increased intraocular pressure → *glaucoma*.

E. *Ears:*
1. Changes in cochlea → decrease in average pitch of sound.
2. Hearing loss—greater in left ear than right; greater in higher frequencies than in lower.
3. Tympanic membrane—atrophied, thickened → hearing loss.
4. Presbycusis—progressive loss of hearing in old age.

F. *Mouth:*
1. Dental caries.
2. Poor-fitting dentures.
3. Cancer of the mouth—increased risk.
4. Decrease in taste buds → inability to taste sweet/salty foods.
5. Olfactory bulb atrophies → decreased ability to smell.

G. *Cardiovascular:*
1. Lack of elasticity of vessels → increased resistance to blood flow; decreased diameter of arteries → increased blood pressure.
2. Atherosclerotic plaques → thrombosis.
3. Valves become sclerotic, less pliable → reduced filling and emptying.
4. Diastolic murmurs heard at base of heart.
5. Loss of elasticity, decreased contractility → decreased cardiac output.
6. Changes in the coronary arteries → pooling of blood in systemic veins and shortness of breath → reduced pumping action of the heart.
7. Disturbance of the autonomic nervous system → dysrhythmias.
8. Extremities—arteriosclerotic changes → weaker pedal pulses, colder extremities, mottled color.

H. *Respiratory:*
1. Efficiency reduced with age.
2. Greater residual air in lungs after expiration.
3. Decreased vital capacity.
4. Weaker expiratory muscles → decreased capacity to cough.
5. Decreased ciliary activity → stasis of secretions → susceptibility to infections.
6. Oxygen debt in the muscles → dyspnea on exertion.
7. Reduced chest wall compliance.

I. *Breasts:*
1. Atrophy.
2. Cancer risk—increased with age.

J. *Gastrointestinal:*
1. Lack of intrinsic factor → pernicious anemia.

2. Gastric motility—decreased.
3. Esophageal peristalsis—decreased.
4. Hiatal hernia—increased incidence.
5. Digestive enzymes—gradual decrease of ptyalin (which converts *starch*), pepsin and trypsin (which digest *protein*), lipase (*fat*-splitting enzyme).
6. Absorption—decreased.
7. Improper diet → constipation.

K. *Endocrine:*
1. Basal metabolism rate lowered → decreased temperature.
2. Cold intolerance.
3. Women: decreased ovarian function → increased gonadotropins.
4. Decreased renal sensitivity to ADH → unable to concentrate urine as effectively as younger persons.
5. Decreased clearance of blood glucose after meals → elevated postprandial blood glucose.
6. Risk of *diabetes mellitus* increases with age.

L. *Urinary:*
1. Renal function—impaired due to poor perfusion.
2. Filtration—impaired due to reduction in number of functioning nephrons.
3. Urgency and frequency: *men*—often due to prostatic hyperplasia; *women*—due to perineal muscle weakness.
4. Nocturia—*both* men and women.
5. Urinary tract infection—increased incidence.
6. Incontinence—especially with dementia.

M. *Musculoskeletal:*
1. Muscle mass—decreased.
2. Bony prominences—increased.
3. Demineralization of bone.
4. Narrowing of intervertebral space → shortening of trunk.
5. Posture—normal; some kyphosis.
6. Range of motion—limited.
7. Osteoarthritis—related to extensive physical activities and joint use.
8. Gait—altered.
9. Osteoporosis related to menopause, immobilization, elevated levels of cortisone.
10. Calcium, phosphorus, and vitamin D decreased.

N. *Neurological:*
1. Voluntary, automatic reflexes—slowed.
2. Sleep pattern—changes.
3. Mental acuity—changes.
4. Sensory interpretation and movement—changes.
5. Pain perception—diminished.
6. Dexterity and agility—lessened.
7. Reaction time—slowed.
8. Memory—past more vivid than recent memory.
9. Depression.
10. Alzheimer's disease.

O. *Sexuality:*
1. *Women:*
   a. Estrogen production—decreased with menopause.
   b. Breasts atrophy.
   c. Vaginal secretions—reduced lubricants.
   d. Sexuality—drive continues; sexual activity declines.
2. *Men:*
   a. Testosterone production—decreased.
   b. Testes—decrease in size; decreased sperm count.
   c. Libido and sexual satisfaction—no changes.

◆ **II. General nursing diagnoses in the older adult**
   A. *Risk for loneliness* related to isolation and loss of many friends and family members due to separation and death.
   B. *Self-care deficit* related to inability to complete activities of daily living.
   C. *Impaired verbal communication* related to hearing loss.
   D. *Fluid volume* deficit related to low fluid intake.
   E. *Impaired skin integrity* related to prolonged back-lying position and inability to turn self.
   F. *Body image disturbance* related to physical changes associated with the aging process.
   G. *Sleep pattern disturbance* related to concern about outcomes of pending diagnostic tests.

III. Problems associated with the older adult*
   A. *Falls:*
   ◆ 1. **Assessment.** *Risk factors:*
      a. Gait changes—prone to trip and stumble; do not pick feet up as high.
      b. Postural instability—tendency to lose balance; older adults take steps to correct balance and increase possibility of falling.
      c. Impaired muscular control—inability to recover from trip or unexpected step; weaker muscle cushioning and slowed righting reflexes.
      d. Deterioration of vision and hearing—impaired obstacle avoidance.
      e. Loss of short-term memory—prone to trip over forgotten objects.
      f. Environmental:
         (1) Home: unstable furniture and appliances; stairs with poor rails; throw rugs and frayed carpets; poor lighting; low beds and toilets; pets; objects on floor; medications.
         (2) Institutions: recent admission or trans-

fer; furniture; slick, hard floors; unsupervised activities; meal times; absence of hand rails; inadequate lighting.
   ◆ 2. **Nursing goal/implementation:** reduce risk of falling in the older adult with fall-prevention measures.
      a. Treat underlying condition (e.g., muscle weakness, imbalance, pain).
      b. Reduce risk factors (e.g., visual problems, orthostasis).
      c. Reduce environmental hazards.
      d. Increase leg range-of-motion (ROM) exercises.
      e. Develop an individualized exercise plan.
      f. Support adequate nutrition.
   B. *Use of restraints:*
   1. *Definition*—any device, material, or equipment attached to the patient that cannot be easily removed by the patient; restricts free movement; includes leg restraints, arm restraints, hand mitts, soft ties or vests, wheelchair safety bars, "geri-chairs."
   ◆ 2. **Assessment** of problems resulting from use of restraints:
      a. Increased agitation, confusion.
      b. Falls.
      c. Pressure sores.
      d. Bone density loss (demineralization).
      e. Immobility hazard.
      f. Death from strangulation.
   ◆ 3. **Nursing goal/implementation:** provide restraint-free care with alternatives to restraints:
      a. *Physical:* recliners; medications for pain relief; seating adaptations (physical therapy/occupational therapy); chairs with deep seats.
      b. *Psychosocial:* active listening; increased or decreased sensory stimulation; increased visiting; reality orientation.
      c. *Activity:* structured daily routines; wandering/pacing permitted; physical exercise; nighttime activities.
      d. *Environmental:* door buzzers; limb bracelet alarms; signs.
      e. *Structural:* exit alarms; increased lighting; enclosed courtyards.
      f. *Supervision:* family, nursing; volunteer; security.
      g. Sedation.
   C. *Thermoregulation*—normal oral temperature for >75 years: 96.9–98.3°F; rectal, 98–99°F. Decreased or absence of increased temperature in infection or dehydration.
   ◆ 1. **Assessment** of causes:
      a. Factors affecting the *hypothalmus:* decreased—muscle activity, metabolic rate, food and fluid intake, subcutaneous fat; changes in peripheral blood flow; diseases; medications.

*Source: Dr. Cheryl Osborne, EdD, RN, Professor of Nursing, Director of Gerontology, California State University–Sacramento.

b. *External factors:* environmental temperature; humidity; airflow; type and amount of clothing.

◆ 2. **Nursing goal/implementation:** prevent hypothermia and hyperthermia.

a. Ensure adequate fluid and food intake.

b. Maintain constancy in environmental temperature: *avoid* drafts, overheating, prolonged exposure to cold.

c. Monitor ventilation: provide airflow (air conditioners, fans; safe sources of heat).

d. Use layered clothing (remove when warm; add when cold).

D. *Sleep disturbances.*

◆ 1. **Nursing goal/implementation:** promote restful sleep and prevent sleep deprivation with sleep care strategies:

a. Maintain normal sleep pattern: arrange medications and therapies to minimize sleep interruptions.

b. Encourage daytime activity; discourage daytime naps.

c. Support bedtime routines/rituals: bedtime reading, listening to music, quiet television.

d. Promote comfort: mattress, pillows, wrinkle-free linen, loose bed covering.

e. Promote relaxation: warm milk or soup if not contraindicated, back rub.

f. *Avoid*/minimize stimulation before bedtime: *no* caffeine after dinner, reduce fluid intake before sleep, refrain from smoking.

g. *Avoid*/minimize drugs that negatively influence sleep, such as ranitidine, diltiazem, atenolol, nifedipine.

h. Create a restful environment: turn off lights, reduce or eliminate noise, minimize disruptions for therapy or monitoring.

E. *Skin breakdown.*

◆ 1. **Assessment:**

a. *Age-related changes:* slower rate of epidermal proliferation; thinner dermis; *decreased*—dermal blood supply, melanocytes (gray hair), moisture, sweat and sebaceous glands.

b. Predisposing *risk factors:* exposure to ultraviolet rays (sunlight, excessive tanning); adverse medication effects; personal hygiene habits (too frequent bathing); limited activity, heredity.

c. *Functional consequences:* dry skin; skin wrinkles; delayed wound healing; *increased*—susceptibility to burns, injury, infection, altered thermoregulation, skin cancer, cracking nails.

◆ 2. **Nursing goal/implementation:** treatment for pressure sores.

a. *Stage I*—reddened broken skin: *cover* and *protect* (use sprays, gels, transparent films, transparent occlusive wafers).

b. *Stage II*—blister or partial-thickness skin loss: *cover, protect, hydrate, insulate,* and *absorb* exudate (use transparent films, occlusive wafer dressings, calcium alginate for absorbing exudate; polyurethane foam, moistened gauze dressing).

c. *Stage III*—full-thickness skin loss: *cover, protect, hydrate, insulate, absorb, cleanse, prevent infection,* and *promote granulation* (use occlusive wafer dressings, absorption dressing, calcium alginate, and moistened gauze dressings).

d. *Stage IV*—full-thickness skin loss involving muscle, tendon, and bone: same as stage III except before *promote granulation dead eschar (tissue) is removed* (use absorption dressing, calcium alginate, and moistened gauze dressings).

F. *Polypharmacy*—concurrent use of several drugs increasing the potential for adverse reactions, drug interactions, and self-medication errors (Table 8–1).

1. Reasons for polypharmacy:

a. Lack of communication among multiple health care providers.

b. Lack of information about over-the-

TABLE 8–1 Medications That Should *Not* be Used by Older Adults

Medication Category	Contraindicated Medications
Antidepressants	Elavil
	Triavil
Cardiovascular	Aldomet
	Catapres
	Cyclospasmol
	Pavabid
	Serpasil
	Trental
Pain and arthritis medications	Bufferin
	Darvocet
	Darvon
	Feldene
	Talwin
Gastrointestinal	Colace
	Dialose-Plus
	Donnatal
	Doxidan
	Mylanta
	Surfak
	Tigan
Tranquilizers and hypnotics	Ativan
	Dalmane
	Halcion
	Librium
	Nembutal
	Restoril
	Valium
	Xanax
Neurological	Artane
	Cogentin

counter drug use.

c. Lack of information about patient non-compliance.

d. Use of complementary (alternative, folk medicine) therapies and fear of telling health care provider.

e. Assumption that once medication is started, it should be continued indefinitely and not changed.

f. Assumption that if there are no early side effects, there will not be any later.

g. Changes in daily habits (smoking, activity, diet/fluid intake).

h. Changes in mental-emotional status that may affect consumption patterns.

i. Changes in health status.

j. Financial limitations (drug substitution).

◆ 2. **Nursing goal/implementation:** assist the older adult to use medications safely and try nonpharmacological interventions for common health problems.

a. *Constipation:* exercise, relaxation, biofeedback; increase fluid and fiber intake.

b. *Stress incontinence:* pelvic muscle exercises, biofeedback.

c. *Anxiety, depression:* counseling, exercise, meditation, relaxation techniques; touch, music, and pet therapy.

d. *Arthritis:* acupuncture, heat therapy, therapeutic exercise, postural or alignment aids; touch, music, and pet therapy.

e. *Chronic neuromuscular problems:* massage, body work, touch and music therapy.

f. *Sleep problems:* see **D.** Sleep disturbances.

G. *Hearing changes*—external auditory canal atrophies, resulting in thinner walls and increased cerumen buildup; degenerative changes in ossicular joints leading to slower/stiffer movements; loss of hair cells and cochlear neurons in inner ear.

1. Types:

a. *Presbycusis*—bilateral loss of high-pitched tones; slightly less severe in women than in men.

b. *Impaired pitch discrimination*—after 55 yr, makes localizing and understanding sounds difficult; impaired ability to understand consonants.

c. *Decline in speech discrimination*—after 60 yr, speech intelligibility declines; slowing of memory and slowing of mental processes with advancing age may also affect speech, hearing, and understanding.

d. *Diminished vestibular function*—deficits in equilibrium and greater fall risk.

◆ 2. **Nursing goal/implementation:** improve communication for hearing-impaired person.

a. *Compensate with other senses*—face listener; make eye contact if culturally acceptable; get person's attention before

talking; use touch if culturally appropriate; help with hearing aid; *avoid* walking around room while talking; write down key words if person can read.

b. *Alter stimulus and behavior*—speak in normal volume of voice or slightly lower, *avoid* shouting; use short sentences; separate important words with pauses; allow more time for communication; have person repeat to show understanding; repeat; teach person to be more assertive about impairment.

c. *Modify environment*—eliminate or reduce background noise (turn off running water, close doors, lower TV or radio); select areas with sound-absorbing abilities for conversations (carpets, drapes); amplify telephone; allow for adequate light on speaker's face.

H. *Visual impairment.*

1. *Age-related macular degeneration* (AMD)—leading cause of irreversible and legal blindness for those over 65 yr; blurred far and near vision; loss of central vision; difficulty going up and down steps and stairs; parts of words and letters disappear when reading; straight lines appear to be wavy. Acuity: 20/200 or less.

a. **Risk factors:** increased age, women, Caucasian, smoking, UV light exposure, diabetes, diet (low in leafy green vegetables and antioxidants).

b. Prevention: UV light filters, aspirin, vitamins A and B, beta carotene, zinc.

c. Prognosis: no treatment or cure; laser may prevent spread of AMD in some patients.

◆ d. **Nursing goal:** assist patient to maintain independent functioning.

2. See **Unit 7** for other causes of visual problems in the older adult, such as stroke, p. 561; glaucoma, p. 553; cataracts, p. 554; and diabetes, p. 525.

I. *Loss of urinary control*—neurological mechanism controlling bladder emptying does not work effectively and results in incontinence; a symptom, *not* a diagnosis.

◆ 1. **Assessment.** *Risk factors:*

a. Immobility.

b. Cognitive and functional impairments—Parkinson's disease, Alzheimer's disease, multiple sclerosis, alcoholism, stroke, vitamin B deficiency, inability to walk and transfer to toilet.

c. Medications.

d. Institutionalization.

e. Pathological conditions—*men:* hyperplasia leading to infection, incomplete emptying, urgency, and frequency; *women:* weakening of pelvic floor postmenopause,

leading to residual urine and infection; atrophy of vaginal and trigonal tissue, leading to frequency, urgency, and incontinence.
  f. Childbirth.
  2. Incontinence—possible symptom of urinary tract infection, impaction, chronic constipation, dementia, inability to walk and transfer by self to toilet, dehydration.
◆ 3. **Nursing goal/implementation:** minimize incontinence episodes and reduce urinary tract infections.
  a. Regular toileting schedule—every 2 hr, with some exceptions at night; or personalize regimen based on assessment.
  b. Modify environment—location of toilet, good lighting, prompt response to calls for assistance, use of Velcro closures on clothing, raised toilet seats with safety bars.
  c. Monitor fluid intake; adequate hydration—1–2 L during day; *avoid* alcohol and caffeine and restrict fluids at bedtime.
  d. *Avoid* medications contributing to incontinence.
  e. *Avoid* use of indwelling catheters if possible.
  f. Use usual undergarments; be positive about continence; use absorbent pads to improve perineal hygiene if other measures fail.
  g. Treat constipation.
J. *Sexual neglect*—many myths exist about sexuality and aging.
  1. *Facts* about sexuality in the older adult:
    a. Sexual desire can and does exist in advanced age.
    b. If in good health, a satisfying sex life can extend into the eighties and beyond; if sexually active in youth and middle age, vigor and interest will be retained into old age.
    c. Sexual attractiveness has little to do with age and the appearance of partner.
    d. Less than 1% of sudden coronary deaths occur during sexual intercourse; greater anxiety and tension exists if sex is restricted.
    e. Vaginal lubrication is decreased because of menopause, but sexual pleasure still exists.
    f. Sex may actually be better in later years; partners have an appreciation of intimate sharing and caring.
    g. Sexual activity is a good form of exercise and helps maintain flexibility and stamina.
    h. Older adults have a strong interest in sexual activity and physical and mental well-

being; older adults should be encouraged to continue sexual interests without guilt.
    i. Male erections can continue into the eighties and beyond.
◆ 2. **Nursing goal:** assist the patient to reduce barriers to a satisfying sexual experience.
    a. *Barriers* to a satisfying sexual experience:
      (1) Loss of sexual responsiveness—*causes:* monotony of a "same old" sexual relationship; mental or physical fatigue; overindulgence in food or drink; preoccupation with career or economic pursuits; physical or mental infirmities of either partner; performance anxiety.
      (2) *Changes with aging*—hormonal; decreased muscle tone and elasticity; prostate hyperplasia; sclerosing arteries and veins; increased time needed for arousal and rearousal; medications (e.g., antihypertensives); surgery (e.g., prostatectomy); response to menopause; availability of a partner.
K. *Caregiver burden*—80–90% of the care given to dependent adults is given by family and friends, especially middle-age women.
  1. *Negative* consequences of caregiving:
    a. Infringement on privacy.
    b. Decreased social contact.
    c. Loss of income and assets.
    d. Increased family conflict and distress.
    e. Little or no time for personal or recreational activities.
    f. Increased use of alcohol and psychotropic drugs.
    g. Changes in living arrangements (sharing households).
    h. Likelihood of decreasing or giving up job responsibilities.
    i. Increased risk of clinical depression.
    j. Feelings of anger, guilt, anxiety, grief, depression, helplessness, chronic fatigue, emotional exhaustion.
    k. Poor health and increased stress-related illness and injuries.
  2. *Positive* consequences of caregiving:
    a. Family becomes closer.
    b. Making a difference in the quality of care.
    c. Companionship for dependent adult and caregiver.
    d. Better understanding of the dependent adult's needs.
    e. Feeling useful and worthwhile.
    f. Improved relationship between caregiver and dependent adult.
  3. Impact of hospitalization of older adult on caregiver:
    a. Frustration with delays in older adult being admitted.

b. Perception of poor care; complaints about rudeness; upset that call lights and questions are not answered in a timely manner.

c. Lack of involvement in decision making.

d. Lack of preparation for discharge; too much information given too quickly; problems coordinating services (e.g., home visits, needed equipment).

e. Fatigue/stress from going back and forth to hospital.

◆ 4. **Nursing goal/implementation:** assist the caregiver in achieving control and a sense of satisfaction.

   a. Strategies to minimize caregiver burden:

     (1) Develop and maintain a routine.

     (2) Concentrate on the present.

     (3) Talk about the reasons for being a caregiver.

     (4) Use respite care as needed.

L. *Poor nutrition.*

◆ 1. **Assessment** of warning signs:

   a. Disease, illness, or chronic condition that changes eating habits/pattern; also emotional problems: confusion, depression, or sadness.

   b. Eating too little or too much, skipping meals, drinking more than 1–2 alcoholic beverages daily.

c. Missing, loose, or rotten teeth or ill-fitting dentures.

d. Spending less than 25–30 dollars per week on food.

e. Living alone.

f. Taking multiple medications with increased chance for side effects (change in taste, constipation, weakness, drowsiness, diarrhea, nausea).

g. Unplanned weight loss or gain.

h. Problems with self-care (walking, shopping, buying and preparing food).

i. Age >80 (frail elderly).

◆ 2. **Nursing goal:** promote optimal nutritional health for the older adult. (See **Unit 9** for additional information on nutrition in the older adult.)

M. See **Unit 6** for discussion of *depression, elder abuse,* and causes of *impaired cognition,* such as dementia, Alzheimer's and delirium.

IV. Use the *functional rating scale for the older adult* to rate social resources, economic resources, mental health, physical health, and activities of daily living (Table 8–2).

V. Use the *functional screening examination* to help determine dependent/independent status for planning home care (Table 8–3).

Adult

TABLE 8–2 **Functional Rating Scale for the Older Adult**

SOCIAL RESOURCES RATING SCALE

Rate the current social resources of the person being evaluated along the six-point scale presented below. Circle the *one* number that best describes the person's present circumstances.

1. **Excellent social resources.** Social relationships are very satisfying and extensive; at least one person would take care of him or her indefinitely.
2. **Good social resources.** Social relationships are fairly satisfying and adequate, and at least one person would take care of him or her indefinitely; *or* social relationships are very satisfying and extensive, and only short-term help is available.
3. **Mildly socially impaired.** Social relationships are unsatisfactory, of poor quality, few, but at least one person would take care of him or her indefinitely; *or* social relationships are fairly satisfactory, adequate, and only short-term help is available.
4. **Moderately socially impaired.** Social relationships are unsatisfactory, of poor quality; few, and only short-term care is available; *or* social relationships are at least adequate or satisfactory; but help would only be available now and then.
5. **Severely socially impaired.** Social relationships are of poor quality, few; and help would only be available now and then; *or* social relationships are at least satisfactory or adequate; but help is not even available now and then.
6. **Totally socially impaired.** Social relationships are unsatisfactory, of poor quality, few, and help is not even available now and then.

ECONOMIC RESOURCES RATING SCALE

Rate the current economic resources of the person being evaluated along the six-point scale presented below. Circle the *one* number that best describes the person's present circumstances.

1. **Economic resources are excellent.** Income is ample and person has reserves.
2. **Economic resources are satisfactory.** Income is ample but person has no reserves; *or* income is adequate and person has reserves.
3. **Economic resources are mildly impaired.** Income is adequate but person has no reserves; *or* income is somewhat inadequate but person has reserves.
4. **Economic resources are moderately impaired.** Income is somewhat inadequate and person has no reserves.
5. **Economic resources are severely impaired.** Income is totally inadequate and person may or may not have reserves.
6. **Economic resources are completely impaired.** Person is destitute, completely without income or reserves.

MENTAL HEALTH RATING SCALE

Rate the current mental functioning of the person being evaluated along the six-point scale presented below. Circle the *one* number that best describes the person's present functioning.

1. **Outstanding mental health.** Intellectually alert and clearly enjoying life. Manages routine and major problems with ease and is free from any psychiatric symptoms.
2. **Good mental health.** Handles both routine and major problems satisfactorily and is intellectually intact and free of psychiatric symptoms.
3. **Mildly mentally impaired.** Has mild psychiatric symptoms and/or mild intellectual impairment. Continues to handle routine, though not major, problems satisfactorily.
4. **Moderately mentally impaired.** Has definite psychiatric symptoms and/or moderate intellectual impairment. Able to make routine commonsense decisions, but unable to handle major problems.
5. **Severely mentally impaired.** Has severe psychiatric symptoms and/or severe intellectual impairment that interferes with routine judgments and decision making in everyday life.
6. **Completely mentally impaired.** Grossly psychotic or completely impaired intellectually. Requires either intermittent or constant supervision because of clearly abnormal or potentially harmful behavior.

PHYSICAL HEALTH RATING SCALE

Rate the current physical functioning of the person being evaluated along the six-point scale presented below. Circle the *one* number that best describes the person's present functioning.

1. **In excellent physical health.** Engages in vigorous physical activity, either regularly or at least from time to time.
2. **In good physical health.** No significant illnesses or disabilities. Only routine medical care such as annual checkups required.
3. **Mildly physically impaired.** Has only minor illnesses and/or disabilities that might benefit from medical treatment or corrective measures.
4. **Moderately physically impaired.** Has one or more diseases or disabilities that are either painful or require substantial medical treatment.
5. **Severely physically impaired.** Has one or more illnesses or disabilities that are either severely painful or life threatening or require extensive medical treatment.
6. **Totally physically impaired.** Confined to bed and requires full-time medical assistance or nursing care to maintain vital bodily functions.

PERFORMANCE RATING SCALE FOR ACTIVITIES OF DAILY LIVING (ADL)

Rate the current performance of the person being evaluated on the six-point scale presented below. Circle the *one* number that best describes the person's present performance.

1. **Excellent ADL capacity.** Can perform all ADL without assistance and with ease.
2. **Good ADL capacity.** Can perform all ADL without assistance.
3. **Mildly impaired ADL capacity.** Can perform all but one to three ADL. Some help is required with one to three, but not necessarily every day. Can get through any single day without help. Is able to prepare own meals.
4. **Moderately impaired ADL capacity.** Regularly requires assistance with at least four ADL but is able to get through any single day without help; *or* regularly requires help with meal preparation.
5. **Severely impaired ADL capacity.** Requires help each day but not necessarily throughout the day or night with many ADL.
6. **Completely impaired ADL capacity.** Requires help throughout the day and/or night to carry out ADL.

Summary of Ratings		Projected Outcome
Social resources	_____	>15—Requires help
Economic resources	_____	12–15—Intermediate
Mental health	_____	supports
Physical health	_____	<11—Independent
Activities of daily living	_____	living
Cumulative impairment score (sum of the five ratings)	_____	

Source: Adapted from University of California Davis Medical Center, Alzheimer's Center, Sacramento, Calif.

TABLE 8–3   Functional Screening Examination

Test Request	Function Tested	Able Normal	Limited but Able	Unable
Put both hands together, behind your head	Shoulder external rotation, flexion, abduction; elbow flexion; wrist extension; gross strength (managing clothing, hair combing, washing back)	☐	☐	☐
Put both hands together, behind your back	Shoulder internal rotation, adduction; elbow flexion; gross strength (managing clothing, washing lower back)	☐	☐	☐
Sitting, touch great toe with opposite hand	Back, hip, knee flexion, gross strength, balance (lower extremity dressing and hygiene)	☐	☐	☐
Squeeze my two fingers, each hand	Grasp; approximately 20 lb grasp needed for functional activities (e.g., holding a pan)	☐	☐	☐
Hold paper between thumb and lateral side of index finger (while examiner tries to pull it out)	Pinch; approximately. 3 lb grip needed for functional activities (e.g., turning a key)	☐	☐	☐
Show me your medicines	Cognition; knowledge; visual acuity, hand function; compliance; polypharmacy; effective management of health problems; access to health care; support system; finances; polyproviders	☐	☐	☐
Get up from the chair without using your hands, walk 10 ft down hall, turn around, stand with your eyes closed (examiner nudges to determine balance), sit down without using hands	Hip strength; gait, symmetry in posture velocity, step height; balance, ability to withstand sudden changes in position; fall risk; cardiovascular and pulmonary status; transfer ability; motion; fear of falls; judgment and cognition; environmental awareness; need for assistance/equipment; flexibility; endurance; ability to walk and function at home	☐	☐	☐
Take off your shoes and socks	Balance; fine motor skills; dexterity; hearing and receptive language; visual acuity; judgment; registration and attention span; low back flexibility and mobility; weight shifting; safety and adequacy of footware; social support if nails are cut by someone else; pain and comfort on movement	☐	☐	☐
Observe a meal being prepared/eaten	Nutritional intake; intactness of reflexes; use of utensils; hand/oral motor function; sequencing skills, visual acuity; use of utensils and equipment; ability to get needed help; ability to handle food and liquid; ability to compensate for limitations	☐	☐	☐

Summary and conclusions:

_____

_____

_____

_____

_____

_____

_____

_____

_____

_____

Adult

Source: Dr. Cheryl Osborne, EdD, RN, Professor of Nursing, Director of Gerontology, California State University, Sacramento.
NOTE: *Totally independent*—total score of 9 in Able or Limited columns; *dependent* >1 in Unable column.

▪ Review of Nutrition

Sally L. Lagerquist, Bobbi Morrison, Robyn Nelson, and Janice Stecchi

NUTRITION DURING PREGNANCY AND LACTATION

Table 9–1 gives a summary of nutrient needs (maternal and fetal) during pregnancy.

I. **Milk group**—important for calcium, protein of high biological value, and other vitamins and minerals.
   A. *Pregnancy*—three to four servings (four to five for adolescents).
   B. *Lactation*—four to five servings.
   C. *Count as one serving*—1 cup milk; ½ cup undiluted evaporated milk; ¼ cup dry milk; 1¼ cups cottage cheese; 2 cups low-fat cottage cheese; 1½ oz cheddar or Swiss cheese; or 1½ cups ice cream.

II. **Meat, poultry, fish, dry beans, nuts, and eggs group**—important for protein, iron, and many B vitamins.
   A. *Pregnancy*—three servings.
   B. *Lactation*—three servings.
   C. *Count as one serving*—½ cup cooked dry beans, 1 egg, or 1½ tbsp peanut butter is equivalent to 1 oz meat; use peanut butter or nuts rarely to *avoid* excessive fat intake; limit eggs to reduce cholesterol intake; trim fat from meat, and remove skin from poultry.

III. **Vegetable and fruit group**—vitamins and minerals (especially vitamins A and C) and roughage.
   A. *Vegetables:*
      1. *Pregnancy*—three to four servings.
      2. *Lactation*—three to five servings.
      3. *Count as one serving*—1 cup raw leafy greens, ½ cup of others.
   B. *Fruits:*
      1. *Pregnancy*—two to four servings.
      2. *Lactation*—two to four servings.
      3. *Count as one serving*—½ medium grapefruit; 1 medium apple, banana, or orange; ¾ cup fruit juice.
   C. *Good sources (vitamin C)*—citrus, cantaloupe, mango, papaya, strawberries, broccoli, and green and red bell peppers.
   D. *Fair sources (vitamin C)*—tomatoes, honeydew melon, asparagus tips, raw cabbage, collards, kale, mustard greens, potatoes (white and sweet), spinach, and turnip greens.
   E. *Good sources (vitamin A)*—dark-green or deep-yellow vegetables and a few fruits (apricots, broccoli, pumpkin, sweet potato, spinach, cantaloupe, carrots, and winter squash).
   F. *Good sources of folic acid*—dark-green *foliage*-type vegetables.

IV. **Bread and cereal group**—good for thiamine, iron, niacin, and other vitamins and minerals.
   A. *Pregnancy*—6 to 11 servings.
   B. *Lactation*—6 to 11 servings.
   C. *Count as one serving*—1 slice bread, 1 oz ready-to-eat cereal, ½–¾ cup cooked cereal, cornmeal, grits, macaroni, noodles, rice, or spaghetti.

V. **Note:** use dark-green leafy and deep-yellow vegetables often; eat dry beans and peas often; count ½ cup cooked dry beans or peas as a serving of vegetables or 1 oz from meat group.

TABLE 9–1 Nutrient Needs During Pregnancy

Nutrient	Maternal Need	Fetal Need	Food Source
Protein	Maternal tissue growth: uterus, breasts, blood volume, storage	Rapid fetal growth	Milk and milk products; animal meats—muscle, organs; grains, legumes; eggs
Calories	Increased BMR	Primary energy source for growth of fetus	Carbohydrates: 4 kcal/g Proteins: 4 kcal/g Fats: 9 kcal/g
Minerals Calcium (and phosphorus)	Increase in maternal Ca^{2+} metabolism	Skeleton and tooth formation	Milk and milk products, especially natural cheese*
Iron	Increase in RBC mass Prevent anemia Decrease infection risk	Liver storage (especially in third trimester)	Organ meats—liver, animal meat; egg yolk; whole or enriched grains; green leafy vegetables; nuts
Vitamins A	Tissue growth	Cell development—tissue and bone growth and tooth bud formation	Butter, cream, fortified margarine; green and yellow vegetables
B	Coenzyme in many metabolic processes	Coenzyme in many metabolic processes	Animal meats, organ meats; milk and cheese; beans, peas, nuts; enriched grains
Folic acid	Meet increased metabolic demands in pregnancy Production of blood products	Meet increased metabolic demands, including production of cell nucleus material Prevent neural tube defects	Liver; deep-green, leafy vegetables
C	Tissue formation and integrity Increase iron absorption	Tissue formation and integrity	Citrus fruit, berries, melons; peppers; green, leafy vegetables; broccoli; potatoes
D	Absorption of Ca^{2+}, phosphorus	Mineralization of bone tissue and tooth buds	Fortified milk and margarine
E	Tissue growth; cell wall integrity; RBC integrity	Tissue growth; cell integrity; RBC integrity	Widely distributed: meat, milk, eggs, grains, leafy vegetables, vegetable oils

*Natural cheese contains less lactose; therefore it is a good source for those with lactose intolerance. Tofu (soybean cake) also is high in calcium, and contains *no* lactose.

NUTRITIONAL NEEDS OF THE NEWBORN

I. Calories—108 kcal/kg/day.

II. Protein—2.2 g/kg/day (1 g protein = 1 oz milk).

III. Fluids—3.5 oz/kg/day.

IV. Vitamin D—400 IU daily for bottle-fed babies after week 2.

V. Fluoride—0.25 mg daily up to 3 years old when local water supply has less than 0.3 ppm content.

RECOMMENDED DIETARY ALLOWANCES: PEDIATRIC, ADULT, PREGNANCY, LACTATION

Table 9–2.

ETHNIC FOOD PATTERNS

Tables 9–3 and 9–4.

COMMON VITAMINS AND RELATED DEFICIENCIES

Table 9–5.

Nutrition

TABLE 9–2 Recommended Dietary Allowances[a]

Age (Years)	Weight (kg)	Weight (lb)	Height (cm)	Height (inches)	Protein (g)	Vitamin A (µg RE)[c]	Vitamin D (µg)[d]	Vitamin E (mg α-TE)[e]	Vitamin K (µg)	Vitamin C (mg)	Thiamin (mg)	Riboflavin (mg)	Niacin (mg NE)[f]	Vitamin B$_6$ (mg)	Folate (µg)	Vitamin B$_{12}$ (µg)	Calcium (mg)	Phosphorus (mg)	Magnesium (mg)	Iron (mg)	Zinc (mg)	Iodine (µg)	Selenium (µg)	Average Energy Allowance (kcal)
Infants																								
0.0–0.5	6	13	60	24	13	375	7.5	3	5	30	0.3	0.4	5	0.3	25	0.3	400	300	40	6	5	40	10	650
0.5–1.0	9	20	7	28	14	375	10	4	10	35	0.4	0.5	6	0.6	35	0.5	600	500	60	10	5	50	15	850
Children																								
1–3	13	29	90	35	16	400	10	6	15	40	0.7	0.8	9	1.0	50	0.7	800	800	80	10	10	70	20	1300
4–6	20	44	112	44	24	500	10	7	20	45	0.9	1.1	12	1.1	75	1.0	800	800	120	10	10	90	20	1800
7–10	28	62	132	52	28	700	10	7	30	45	1.0	1.2	13	1.4	100	1.4	800	800	170	10	10	120	30	2000
Men																								
11–14	45	99	157	62	45	1000	10	10	45	50	1.3	1.5	17	1.7	150	2.0	1200	1200	270	12	15	150	40	2500
15–18	66	145	176	69	59	1000	10	10	65	60	1.5	1.8	20	2.0	200	2.0	1200	1200	400	12	15	150	50	3300
19–24	72	160	177	70	58	1000	10	10	70	60	1.5	1.7	19	2.0	200	2.0	1200	1200	350	10	15	150	70	2900
25–50	79	174	176	70	63	1000	5	10	80	60	1.5	1.7	19	2.0	200	2.0	800	800	350	10	15	150	70	2900
51+	77	170	173	68	63	1000	5	10	80	60	1.2	1.4	15	2.0	200	2.0	800	800	350	10	15	150	70	2300
Women																								
11–14	46	101	157	62	46	800	10	8	45	50	1.1	1.3	15	1.4	150	2.0	1200	1200	280	15	12	150	45	2200
15–18	55	120	163	64	44	800	10	8	55	60	1.1	1.3	15	1.5	180	2.0	1200	1200	300	15	12	150	50	2200
19–24	58	128	164	65	46	800	10	8	60	60	1.1	1.3	15	1.6	180	2.0	1200	1200	280	15	12	150	55	2200
25–50	63	138	163	64	50	800	5	8	65	60	1.1	1.3	15	1.6	180	2.0	800	800	280	15	12	150	55	2200
51+	65	143	160	63	50	800	5	8	65	60	1.0	1.2	13	1.6	180	2.0	800	800	280	10	12	150	55	1900
Pregnant					60	800	10	10	65	70	1.5	1.6	17	2.2	400	2.2	1200	1200	320	30	15	175	65	+300
Lactating																								
1st 6 months					65	1300	10	12	65	95	1.6	1.8	20	2.1	280	2.6	1200	1200	355	15	19	200	75	+500
2nd 6 months					62	1200	10	11	65	90	1.6	1.7	20	2.1	260	2.6	1200	1200	340	15	16	200	75	+500

Source: From Recommended Dietary Allowances, © 1989, Food and Nutrition Board, National Research Council, Washington, DC.

[a]The allowances, expressed as average daily intakes over time, are intended to provide for individual variations among most normal persons as they live in the United States under usual environmental stresses. Diets should be based on a variety of common foods in order to provide other nutrients for which human requirements have been less well defined.

[b]Weights and heights of Reference Adults are actual medians for the U.S. population of the designated age, as reported by National Health and Nutrition Examination Survey II. The use of these figures does not imply that the height-to-weight ratios are ideal.

[c]Retinol equivalents. 1 retinol equivalent = 1 µg retinol or 6 µg β-carotene.

[d]As cholecalciferol. 10 µg cholecalciferol. 400 IU of vitamin D.

[e]α-Tocopherol equivalents. 1 mg d-α tocopherol = 1 α-TE.

[f]1 NE (niacin equivalent) is equal to 1 mg of niacin or 60 mg of dietary tryptophan.

Nutrition

TABLE 9–3 **Ethnic Food Patterns**

Ethnic Group	Cultural Food Patterns	Dietary Excesses or Omissions
Mexican (native)	Basic sources of protein—dried beans, flan, cheese, many meats, fish, eggs Chili peppers and many deep-green and yellow vegetables Fruits include: zapote, guava, papaya, mango, citrus Tortillas (corn, flour); sweet bread; fideo; tacos, burritos, enchiladas	*Limited* meats, milk, and milk products Some are using flour tortillas more than the more nutritious corn tortillas *Excessive* use of lard (manteca), sugar Tendency to boil vegetables for long periods of time
Filipino (Spanish-Chinese influence)	Most meats, eggs, nuts, legumes Many different kinds of vegetables Large amounts of rice and cereals	May *limit* meat, milk, and milk products (the latter may be due to lactose intolerance) Tend to prewash rice Tend to fry many foods
Chinese (mostly Cantonese)	Cheese, soybean curd (tofu), many meats, chicken and pigeon eggs, nuts, legumes Many different vegetables, leaves, bamboo sprouts Rice and rice-flour products; wheat, corn, millet seed; green tea Mixtures of fish, pork, and chicken with vegetables—bamboo shoots, broccoli, cabbage, onions, mushrooms, pea pods	Tendency among some immigrants to use *excess* grease in cooking May be *low* in protein, milk, and milk products (the latter may be due to lactose intolerance) Often wash rice before cooking Large amounts of soy and oyster sauces, both of which are *high in salt*
Puerto Rican	Milk with coffee Pork, poultry, eggs, dried fish; beans (habichuelas) Viandas (starchy vegetables; starchy ripe fruits) Avocados, okra, eggplant, sweet yams Rice, cornmeal	Use *large* amounts of lard for cooking *Limited* use of milk and milk products *Limited* amounts of pork and poultry
African American	Milk with coffee Pork, poultry, eggs *Fruit:* strawberries, watermelon *Vegetables:* turnip, collard, mustard greens; kale, okra, sweet potatoes Cereals (including grits, hominy, cornbread, hot breads) Molasses (dark molasses is especially good source of calcium, iron, vitamins B_1 and B_2, and niacin)	*Limited* use of milk group (lactose intolerance) Extensive use of frying, "smothering," simmering for cooking *Large* amounts of fat: salt pork, bacon drippings, lard, gravies May have *limited* use of citrus and enriched breads
Middle Eastern (Greek, Syrian, Armenian)	Yogurt Predominantly lamb, nuts, dried peas, beans, lentils Deep-green leaves and vegetables; dried fruits Dark breads and cracked wheat	Tend to use *excessive* sweeteners, lamb fat, olive oil Tend to fry meats and vegetables *Insufficient* milk and milk products (almost no butter—use olive oil, which has no nutritive value except for calories) *Deficiency* in fresh fruits
Middle European (Polish)	Many milk products Pork, chicken Root vegetables (potatoes), cabbage, fruits Wheat products Sausages, smoked and cured meats, noodles, dumplings, bread, cream with coffee	Tend to use *excessive* sweets and to overcook vegetables *Limited* amounts of fruits (citrus), raw vegetables, and meats
Native American (American Indian—much variation)	If "Americanized," use milk and milk products Variety of meats: game, fowl, fish; nuts, seeds, legumes Variety of vegetables, some wild Variety of fruits, some wild, rose hips; roots Variety of breads, including tortillas, cornmeal, rice	*Nutrition-related problems:* obesity, diabetes, dental problems, iron deficiency anemia; alcoholism *Limited* quantities of high-protein foods depending on availability (flocks of game, fowl) and economic situation *Excessive* use of sugar
Italian	Staples are pasta with sauces; bread; eggs; cheese; tomatoes; and vegetables such as artichokes, eggplant, greens, and zucchini Only small amount of meat is used	*Limited* use of whole grains *Insufficient* servings from milk group Tendency to overcook vegetables Enjoy sweets

TABLE 9–4   Hot-Cold Theory of Disease Treatment*

Hot Diseases or Conditions	Cold Diseases or Conditions	Hot Foods	Cold Foods	Hot Medicines and Herbs	Cold Medicines and Herbs
Constipation	Cancer	Beverages, aromatic	Barley water	Anise	Bicarbonate of soda
Diarrhea	Common cold	Cereal grains	Cod	Aspirin	Linden
Infections	Earache	Cheese	Dairy products	Castor oil	Milk of magnesia
Kidney diseases	Headache	Chili peppers	Fruits, tropical	Cinnamon	Orange flower water
Liver complaints	Joint pain	Chocolate	Honey	Cod liver oil	Sage
Skin eruptions	Malaria	Coffee	Meats (goat, fish, chicken)	Garlic	
Throat (sore)	Menstrual period	Eggs	Milk, bottled	Ginger root	
Ulcers	Paralysis	Fruits, temperate zone	Raisins	Iron preparations	
Warts	Pneumonia	Goat milk	Vegetables, fresh	Mint	
	Rheumatism	Hard liquor		Penicillin	
	Stomach cramps	Meats (beef, water fowl, mutton)		Tobacco	
	Teething	Oils		Vitamins	
	Tuberculosis	Onions			
		Peas			

Source: Adapted from Wilson, HS, and Kneisl, CR: Psychiatric Nursing, ed. 2. Addison-Wesley, Menlo Park, Calif., 1983, p. 774.
*A Latin American, particularly Puerto Rican, approach to treating diseases. A "hot" disease is treated with "cold" treatments (foods, medicines) and vice versa.

TABLE 9–5   Physiological Functions and Deficiency Syndromes of Common Vitamins

Vitamin	Chief Functions	Results of Deficiency	Characteristics	Good Sources

Vitamin A
Retinol (animal source)
Carotene
Beta-carotene
	Essential for maintaining the integrity of epithelial membranes
	Helps maintain resistance to infections
	Necessary for the formation of rhodopsin and prevention of night blindness
	Necessary for proper bone growth
	Facilitates RNA formation from DNA
	Thought to be cancer preventive because of antioxidant properties associated with control of free radical damage to DNA and cell membranes
		Mild:
		Retarded growth
		Increased susceptibility to infection
		Abnormal function of gastrointestinal, genitourinary, and respiratory tracts due to altered epithelial membranes
		Skin dries, shrivels, thickens; sometimes pustule formation
		Night blindness
		Severe:
		Xerophthalmia, a characteristic eye disease, and other local infections
			Fat soluble
			Not destroyed by ordinary cooking temperatures
			Is destroyed by high temperatures when oxygen is present
			Marked capacity for storage in the liver
			NOTE: Excessive intake of carotene, from which vitamin A is formed, may produce yellow discoloration of the skin *(carotenemia)*; excessive vitamin A intake causes symptoms similar to those of deficiency conditions
				Liver
				Animal fats:
				  Butter
				  Cheese
				  Cream
				  Egg yolk
				  Whole milk
				Fish liver oil
				Liver
				Vegetables:
				  Green leafy, especially escarole, kale, parsley
				  Yellow, especially carrots
				Artificial:
				Concentrates in several forms
				Irradiated fish oils

Vitamin D
Calciferol
Ergocalciferol
Cholecalciferol
Calcitriol
Antirachitic factor
	Hormone-like regulation of calcium and phosphorus metabolism by promotion of:
	  Gastrointestinal absorption
	  Bone and tooth mineralization
	  Renal reabsorption
	  Skeletal reserves
	  Antirachitic
		Mild:
		Interferes with utilization of calcium and phosphorus in bone and tooth formation
		Irritability
		Weakness
		Severe:
		Rickets in young children
		Osteomalacia in adults
			Soluble in fats and organic solvents
			Relatively stable under refrigeration
			Stored in liver
			Often associated with vitamin A
				Formed in the skin by exposure to sunlight
				Fortified milk and dairy products
				Egg yolk
				Fish liver oils
				Fish having fat distributed through the flesh, salmon, tuna, herring, sardines
				Liver
				Oysters
				Artificially prepared forms

Continued

Nutrition

TABLE 9–5   Physiological Functions and Deficiency Syndromes of Common Vitamins—cont'd

Vitamin	Chief Functions	Results of Deficiency	Characteristics	Good Sources
Vitamin E Alpha-tocopherol Beta-tocopherol Gamma-tocopherol	Important antioxidant that: Prevents red blood cell hemolysis Protects vitamin A and unsaturated fatty acids from oxidation Promotes cell membrane integrity Improves immune response May protect against cancer	Red blood cell resistance to rupture is decreased, but deficiency seldom occurs except in *premature* infants and people with *chronic fat malabsorption*	Soluble in fat Stable to heat in absence of oxygen and ultraviolet light Unstable under freezing and processing	Vegetable oils Margarine Whole grain or fortified cereals Wheat germ Green leafy vegetables
Vitamin K Menadione Phylloquinone Menaquinone	Promotes synthesis of clotting factors	Prolonged clotting time, resulting in bleeding NOTE: Seldom occurs in the absence of anticoagulant drugs; in addition to food sources, intestinal bacteria manufacture approximately half the body's requirement Fat malabsorption can cause deficiency Synthetic form (menadione) does not depend on fat absorption	Soluble in fat Stable to heat	Green leafy vegetables Meats Dairy products Intestinal bacteria
Vitamin C Ascorbic acid	Essential to formation of intracellular cement substances in a variety of tissues including skin, dentin, cartilage, and bone matrix Important in healing of wounds and bone fractures Prevents scurvy Facilitates absorption of iron Protects folate Antioxidant Promotes capillary permeability	*Mild:* Lowered resistance to infections Joint tenderness Susceptibility to dental caries, pyorrhea, and bleeding gums Delayed wound healing Bruising *Severe:* Hemorrhage Anemia Scurvy NOTE: Many drugs affect availability	Soluble in water Easily destroyed by oxidation; heat hastens the process Lost in cooking, particularly if water in which food was cooked is discarded; loss is greater if cooked in iron or copper utensils Quick-frozen foods lose little of their vitamin C Stored in the body to a limited extent	Abundant in most fresh fruits and vegetables, especially citrus fruit and juices, tomato and orange *Artificial:* Ascorbic acid Cevitamic acid
Thiamine Vitamin B$_1$	Important role in carbohydrate metabolism Essential for maintenance of normal appetite Essential for normal functioning of nervous tissue Coenzyme for cellular energy production	*Mild:* Loss of appetite Impaired metabolism of starches and sugars Emaciation Irritability *Severe:* Various nervous disorders Loss of coordinating power of muscles Beriberi Paralysis in humans	Soluble in water Not readily destroyed by ordinary cooking temperatures Destroyed by exposure to heat, alkali, or sulfites Not stored in body NOTE: Deficiency is often associated with alcoholism	Widely distributed in plant and animal tissues but seldom occurs in high concentration, except in brewer's yeast Enriched or whole grain cereals Pork Peas, beans Nuts *Artificial:* Concentrates from yeast Rice polishings Wheat germ

TABLE 9–5 Physiological Functions and Deficiency Syndromes of Common Vitamins—cont'd

Vitamin	Chief Functions	Results of Deficiency	Characteristics	Good Sources
Riboflavin Vitamin B$_2$	Important as coenzyme in cellular oxidation Essential to normal growth Participates in light adaptation Vital to protein metabolism Associated with niacin and vitamin B$_6$ functions	Impaired growth Lassitude and weakness Cheilosis Glossitis Dermatitis Anemia Photophobia Cataracts	Water soluble Alcohol soluble Not destroyed by heat in cooking unless with alkali Unstable in light, especially in presence of alkali	Milk and milk products Enriched foods Whole grain breads and cereals Liver Meats Eggs
Niacin Nicotinic acid Nicotinamide Antipellagra vitamin	As the component of two important enzymes, it is important in glycolysis, tissue respiration, fat synthesis, and cellular energy production Nicotine acid, but not nicotinamide, causes vasodilation and flushing Prevents pellagra	Pellagra Gastrointestinal disturbances Mental disturbances NOTE: Associated with alcoholism	Soluble in hot water and alcohol Not destroyed by heat, light, air, or alkali Not destroyed in ordinary cooking	Milk Eggs Meats Legumes Enriched foods Whole grain cereals Nuts NOTE: Also formed in the body from dietary tryptophan (amino acid)
Vitamin B$_6$ Pyridoxine Pyridoxal Pyridoxamine	Used in hemoglobin synthesis Essential for metabolism of tryptophan to niacin Needed for utilization of certain other amino acids	Anemias Depressed immunity Dermatitis around eyes and mouth Neuritis Anorexia, nausea, and vomiting	Soluble in water and alcohol Rapidly inactivated in presence of heat, sunlight, or air	Meats Cereal grains Some fruits Nuts
Folate Folacin Folic acid	Essential for normal functioning of hematopoietic system Important coenzyme for RNA and DNA synthesis Important in fetal development Functions interrelated with those of vitamin B$_{12}$	Anemia NOTE: Neural tube defects (e.g., *spina bifida*) are associated with maternal deficiency; alcohol and contraceptives interfere with absorption	Slightly soluble in water Easily destroyed by heat in presence of acid Decreases when food is stored at room temperature NOTE: A large dose may prevent appearance of anemia in a case of pernicious anemia but still permit neurological symptoms to develop	Liver Green leafy vegetables Peas, beans Some fruits
Vitamin B$_{12}$ Cyanocobalamin Hydroxycobalamin	Necessary for myelin synthesis Essential for normal development of red blood cells Associated with folate metabolism	Pernicious anemia Neurological disorders	Soluble in water or alcohol Unstable in hot alkaline or acid solutions	Found only in animal products (e.g., meats, eggs, dairy products) Most of vitamin B$_{12}$ required by humans is synthesized by intestinal bacteria; can also be recycled

Source: Thomas, CL (ed): Taber's Cyclopedic Medical Dictionary, ed. 18, FA Davis, Philadelphia, 1997, pp. 2236–2239.

Nutrition

NUTRITIONAL NEEDS OF THE OLDER ADULT

I. *Calories*—1500–2000 kcal/day to maintain ideal weight; 12% of calories from protein sources; 50–60% of calories from carbohydrates; 20–30% of calories from fats.

II. *High fiber*—prevent or alleviate constipation and dependence on laxatives.

III. *Sodium*—3–4 g/day according to cardiac and renal status.

IV. *Fats*—limit to help retard the development of cancer, atherosclerosis, obesity, and other diseases.

V. *Fluids*—6–8 glasses/day.

VI. *Common deficiencies:* calories; calcium; folic acid; iron; thiamine; vitamins A, B_{12}, C, and D; niacin; zinc.

VII. Factors contributing to food preferences:
  A. Physical ability to prepare, shop for, and eat food.
  B. Income.
  C. Availability of food if dependent on others.
  D. Food intolerances.

VIII. Table 9–6 provides interventions for common eating problems in the older adult.

TABLE 9–6   Eating Problems of the Older Adult and Ways to Improve Nutrition

Problem	Cause	Dietary Interventions

Within the mouth	Impaired taste buds
	Dental caries
	Chewing difficulty due to:
	  Poorly fitting dentures
	  No dentures
	  No saliva
	Paralysis
	Metallic taste from medications
		Referral for correction of dental problems
		Mouthwash/oral care before meals
		Food prepared to meet patient's needs (chopped, pureed, soft)

In the upper GI tract	Swallowing difficulty Paralysis due to stroke Food causing GI distress	Thickened and jellied liquids Soft, chopped foods Small, frequent meals Presentation important (how food looks on serving plate) *Avoid* expressions such as "baby food" (negative connotation)
In the lower GI tract	Constipation Diarrhea Bloating	Add fruits/liquids to restore bowel function (see bowel training) *Avoid* foods that cause diarrhea Plan meals at appropriate times for ease of digestion *Avoid* salt
Psychosocial	Loneliness Meals no longer social event Depression Anorexia	Encourage attendance at meal program if available Arrange group meals/activities when possible Emphasize best nutrition when appetite is at peak (breakfast) Allow time to complete meal Interact with others whenever possible
In the environment	Inability to shop for, prepare, or cook food Impaired vision Lack of resources Difficulty in feeding self Acute or chronic illnesses present (e.g., arthritis, stroke)	Refer to Meals-on-Wheels Encourage family involvement; describe how food is arranged on plate Refer to social services Assess need for assistive devices Assess ability to grasp utensils and guide food to mouth Open packages and milk cartons; butter the bread; cut meat and vegetables

Source: Thomas, CL (ed): Taber's Cyclopedic Medical Dictionary, ed. 18, FA Davis, Philadelphia, 1997.

Nutrition

RELIGIOUS CONSIDERATIONS IN MEAL PLANNING

I. Orthodox Jews:
   A. Kosher meat and poultry.
   B. *No* shellfish, eels, or pork products.
   C. Milk and dairy products *cannot* be consumed with meat or poultry; requires separate utensils.
   D. *No* eggs with a blood spot may be eaten. Eggs may be used with either meat or dairy meals

II. Conservative and Reform Jews: dietary practices may vary from religious laws.

III. Muslims: *no* pork or alcohol.

IV. Hindus: vegetarians (cows are sacred).

V. Seventh-day Adventists:
   A. Vegetarianism is common (lacto-ovo).
   B. *No* shellfish or pork products.
   C. *Avoid* stimulants (coffee, tea, other caffeine sources).
   D. No alcohol.

VI. Mormons: *no* coffee, tea, or alcohol.

SPECIAL DIETS

I. **Low-carbohydrate diet**—ketogenic: low carbohydrate, high fat; *dumping syndrome:* low carbohydrate, high fat, high protein.

II. **Gluten-free diet**—elimination of all foods made from oats, barley, wheat, and rye; used for *celiac* disease.

III. **High-protein diet**—lean meat, cheese, and green vegetables.
   A. *Nephrotic* syndrome (may also be on low-sodium diet).

B. *Acute leukemia* (combined with high-calorie and soft-food diets).
C. *Neoplastic* disease.

IV. **Low-protein diet:**
   A. Usually accompanied by high-carbohydrate diet and normal fats and calories.
   B. *Renal* failure, uremia, anuria, acute glomerulonephritis.

V. **Low-sodium diet:**
   A. *Heart* failure.
   B. *Nephrotic* syndrome.
   C. *Acute glomerulonephritis* (varies with degree of oliguria).

COMMON THERAPEUTIC DIETS

I. **Clear-liquid diet**
   A. *Purpose:* relieve thirst and help maintain fluid balance.
   B. *Use:* postsurgically and following acute vomiting or diarrhea.
   C. *Foods allowed:* carbonated beverages; coffee (caffeinated and decaffeinated); tea; fruit-flavored drinks; strained fruit juices; clear, flavored gelatins; broth, consommé; sugar; popsicles; commercially prepared clear liquids; and hard candy.
   D. *Foods avoided:* milk and milk products, fruit juices with pulp, and fruit.

II. **Full-liquid diet**
   A. *Purpose:* provide an adequately nutritious diet for patients who cannot chew or who are too ill to do so.
   B. *Use:* acute infection with fever, gastrointestinal upsets, after surgery as a progression from *clear liquids.*
   C. *Foods allowed:* clear liquids, milk drinks, cooked cereals, custards, ice cream, sherbets, eggnog, all

strained fruit juices, vegetable juices, creamed vegetable soups, puddings, mashed potatoes, instant breakfast drinks, yogurt, mild cheese sauce or pureed meat, and seasonings.
D. *Foods avoided:* nuts, seeds, coconut, fruit, jam, and marmalade.

III. Soft diet

A. *Purpose:* provide adequate nutrition for those who have trouble chewing.
B. *Use:* patients with no teeth or ill-fitting dentures; transition from full-liquid to general diet; and for those who cannot tolerate highly seasoned, fried, or raw foods following acute infections or gastrointestinal disturbances, such as gastric ulcer or cholelithiasis.
C. *Foods allowed:* very tender minced, ground, baked, broiled, roasted, stewed, or creamed beef, lamb, veal, liver, poultry, or fish; crisp bacon or sweetbreads; cooked vegetables; pasta; all fruit juices; soft raw fruits; soft breads and cereals; all desserts that are soft; and cheeses.
D. *Foods avoided:* coarse whole-grain cereals and breads; nuts; raisins; coconut; fruits with small seeds; fried foods; high-fat gravies or sauces; spicy salad dressings; pickled meat, fish, or poultry; strong cheeses; brown or wild rice; raw vegetables, as well as lima beans and corn; spices such as horseradish, mustard, and catsup; and popcorn.

IV. Sodium-restricted diet

A. *Purpose:* reduce sodium content in the tissues and promote excretion of water.
B. *Use:* heart failure, hypertension, renal disease, cirrhosis, toxemia of pregnancy, and cortisone therapy.
C. *Modifications:* mildly restrictive 2 g sodium diet to extremely restricted 200 mg sodium diet.
D. *Foods avoided:* table salt; all commercial soups, including bouillon; gravy, catsup, mustard, meat sauces, and soy sauce; buttermilk, ice cream, and sherbet; sodas; beet greens, carrots, celery, chard, sauerkraut, and spinach; *all canned* vegetables; frozen peas; all baked products containing salt, baking powder, or baking soda; potato chips and popcorn; fresh or canned shellfish; all cheeses; smoked or commercially prepared meats; salted butter or margarine; bacon; olives; and commercially prepared salad dressings.

V. Renal diet

A. *Purpose:* control protein, potassium, sodium, and fluid levels in body.
B. *Use:* acute and chronic renal failure, hemodialysis.
C. *Foods allowed:* high-biological proteins such as meat, fowl, fish, cheese, and dairy products—range between 20 and 60 mg/day. Potassium is usually limited to 1500 mg/day. Vegetables such as cabbage, cucumber, and peas are lowest in potassium. Sodium is restricted to 500 mg/day. Fluid intake is restricted to the daily urine volume plus 500 mL, which represents insensible water loss. Fluid intake measures water in fruit, vegetables, milk, and meat.
D. *Foods avoided:* cereals, bread, macaroni, noodles, spaghetti, avocados, kidney beans, potato chips, raw fruit, yams, soybeans, nuts, gingerbread, apricots, bananas, figs, grapefruit, oranges, percolated coffee, Coca-Cola, Orange Crush, sport drinks, and breakfast drinks such as Tang or Awake.

VI. High-protein, high-carbohydrate diet

A. *Purpose:* corrects large protein losses and raises the level of blood albumin. May be modified to include low-fat, low-sodium, and low-cholesterol diets.
B. *Use:* burns, hepatitis, cirrhosis, pregnancy, hyperthyroidism, mononucleosis, protein deficiency due to poor eating habits, geriatric patients with poor food intake, nephritis, nephrosis, and liver and gallbladder disorders.
C. *Foods allowed:* general diet with added protein. In adults, high-protein diets usually contain 135–150 g protein.
D. *Foods avoided:* restrictions depend on modifications added to the diet. These modifications are determined by the patient's condition.

VII. Purine-restricted diet

A. *Purpose:* designed to reduce intake of uric acid–producing foods.
B. *Use:* high uric acid retention, uric acid renal stones, and gout.
C. *Foods allowed:* general diet plus 2–3 quarts of liquid daily.
D. *Foods avoided:* cheese containing spices or nuts, fried eggs, meat, liver, seafood, lentils, dried peas and beans, broth, bouillon, gravies, oatmeal and whole wheats, pasta, noodles, and alcoholic beverages. *Limited* quantities of meat, fish, and seafood allowed.

VIII. Bland diet

A. *Purpose:* provision of a diet low in fiber, roughage, mechanical irritants, and chemical stimulants.
B. *Use:* gastritis, hyperchlorhydria, functional GI disorders, gastric atony, diarrhea, spastic constipation, biliary indigestion, and hiatus hernia.
C. *Foods allowed:* varied to meet individual needs and food tolerances.
D. *Foods avoided:* fried foods, including eggs, meat, fish, and seafood; cheese with added nuts or spices; commercially prepared luncheon meats; cured meats such as ham; gravies and sauces; raw vegetables; potato skins; fruit juices with pulp; figs; raisins; fresh fruits; whole wheats; rye bread; bran cereals; rich pastries; pies; chocolate; jams with seeds; nuts; seasoned dressings; caf-

feinated coffee; strong tea; cocoa; alcoholic and carbonated beverages; and pepper.

IX. Low-fat, cholesterol-restricted diet

A. *Purpose:* reduce hyperlipidemia, provide dietary treatment for malabsorption syndromes and patients having acute intolerance for fats.

B. *Use:* hyperlipidemia, atherosclerosis, pancreatitis, cystic fibrosis, sprue, gastrectomy, massive resection of the small intestine, and cholecystitis.

C. *Foods allowed:* nonfat milk; low-carbohydrate, low-fat vegetables; most fruits; breads; pastas; cornmeal; lean meats; unsaturated fats such as corn oil; desserts made without whole milk; and unsweetened carbonated beverages.

D. *Foods avoided:* **remember to avoid the five C's of cholesterol—cookies, cream, cake, coconut, chocolate;** whole milk and whole-milk or *cream* products, avocados, olives, commercially prepared *baked* goods such as donuts and muffins, poultry skin, highly marbled meats, shellfish, fish canned in oil, nuts, *coconut,* commercially prepared meats, butter, ordinary margarines, olive oil, lard, pudding made with whole milk, *ice cream,* candies with *chocolate, cream,* sauces, gravies, and commercially fried foods.

X. Diabetic diet

A. *Purpose:* maintain blood glucose as near normal as possible; prevent or delay onset of diabetic complications.

B. *Use:* diabetes mellitus.

C. *Foods allowed:* choose foods with low *glycemic index;* composed of 45–55% carbohydrates, 30–35% fats, and 10–25% protein. Foods are divided into groups from which exchanges can be made. Coffee, tea, broth, bouillon, spices, and flavorings can be used as desired. Exchange groups include: *milk, vegetables, fruit, starch/bread* (includes starchy vegetables), *meat* (divided into lean, medium fat, and high fat), and *fat* exchanges. The number of exchanges allowed from each group is dependent on the total number of calories allowed. Nonnutritive sweeteners (aspartame) if desired. Nutritive sweeteners (sorbitol) in moderation with controlled, normal-weight diabetics.

D. *Foods avoided:* concentrated sweets or regular soft drinks.

XI. Acid and alkaline ash diet

A. *Purpose:* furnish a well-balanced diet in which the total acid ash is greater than the total alkaline ash each day.

B. *Use:* retard the formation of renal calculi. The type of diet chosen depends on laboratory analysis of the stones.

C. *Acid and alkaline ash food groups:*
   1. *Acid ash:* meat, whole grains, eggs, cheese, cranberries, prunes, plums.

   2. *Alkaline ash:* milk, vegetables, fruit (except cranberries, prunes, and plums).
   3. *Neutral:* sugars, fats, beverages (coffee and tea).

D. *Foods allowed:* all the patient wants of the following.
   1. Breads: any, preferably whole grain; crackers; rolls.
   2. Cereals: any, preferably whole grain.
   3. Desserts: angel food or sunshine cake; cookies made without baking powder or soda; cornstarch pudding, cranberry desserts, custards, gelatin desserts, ice cream, sherbet, plum or prune desserts; rice or tapioca pudding.
   4. Fats: any, such as butter, margarine, salad dressings, Crisco, Spry, lard, salad oils, olive oil, etc.
   5. Fruits: cranberries, plums, prunes.
   6. Meat, eggs, cheese: any meat, fish, or fowl, two servings daily; at least one egg daily.
   7. Potato substitutes: corn, hominy, lentils, macaroni, noodles, rice, spaghetti, vermicelli.
   8. Soup: broth as desired; other soups from foods allowed.
   9. Sweets: cranberry or plum jelly; sugar; plain sugar candy.
   10. Miscellaneous: cream sauce, gravy, peanut butter, peanuts, popcorn, salt, spices, vinegar, walnuts.

E. *Restricted foods:* no more than the amount allowed each day.
   1. Milk: 1 pint daily (may be used in other ways than as beverage).
   2. Cream: ⅓ cup or less daily.
   3. Fruits: one serving of fruit daily (in addition to the prunes, plums, and cranberries); certain fruits listed under *Foods avoided,* following, are *not allowed at any time.*
   4. Vegetables, including potatoes: two servings daily; certain vegetables listed under *Foods avoided,* following, are *not allowed at any time.*

F. *Foods avoided:*
   1. Carbonated beverages, such as ginger ale, cola, root beer.
   2. Cakes or cookies made with baking powder or soda.
   3. Fruits: dried apricots, bananas, dates, figs, raisins, rhubarb.
   4. Vegetables: dried beans, beet greens, dandelion greens, carrots, chard, lima beans.
   5. Sweets; chocolate or candies other than those listed under *Foods allowed,* preceding; syrups.
   6. Miscellaneous: other nuts, olives, pickles.

XII. High-fiber diet

A. *Purpose:* soften stool; exercise digestive tract muscles; speed passage of food through digestive tract to prevent exposure to cancer-causing agents in food; lower blood lipids; prevent sharp rise in blood glucose after eating.

B. *Use:* diabetes, hyperlipidemia, constipation, diverticulosis, anticarcinogenic (colon).

C. *Foods allowed:* recommended intake about 6 g crude fiber daily: all bran cereals; watermelon, prunes, dried peaches, apple with skin; parsnips, peas, brussels sprouts; sunflower seeds.

XIII. Low-residue (low-fiber) diet
A. *Purpose:* reduce stool bulk and slow transit time.

B. *Use:* bowel inflammation during acute diverticulitis or ulcerative colitis, preparation for bowel surgery, esophageal and intestinal stenosis.

C. *Foods allowed:* eggs; ground or well-cooked tender meat, fish, poultry; milk; mild cheeses; strained fruit juice (except prune); cooked or canned apples, apricots, peaches, pears; ripe bananas; strained vegetable juice; canned, cooked, or strained asparagus, beets, green beans, pumpkin, acorn squash, spinach; white bread; refined cereals (Cream of Wheat).

FOOD LIST FOR READY REFERENCE IN MENU PLANNING

I. High-cholesterol foods—over 50 mg/100 g portion: beef, butter, cheese, egg yolks, shellfish, kidney, liver, pork, veal.

II. High-sodium foods—over 500 mg/100 g portion: bacon—cured, Canadian; beef—corned, cooked, canned, dried, creamed; biscuits, baking powder; bouillon cubes; bran, added sugar and malt; bran flakes with thiamine; raisins; breads—wheat, French, rye, white, whole wheat; butter, cheese—cheddar, Parmesan, Swiss, pasteurized American; cocoa; cookies, gingersnaps; cornflakes; cornbread; crackers—graham, saltines; margarine; milk—dry, skim; mustard; oat products; olives—green, ripe; peanut butter; pickles, dill; popcorn with oil and salt; salad dressing—blue cheese, Roquefort, French, Thousand Island; sausages—bologna, frankfurters; soy sauce; tomato catsup; tuna in oil.

III. High-potassium foods—more than 400 mg/100 g portion: almonds; bacon, Canadian; baking powder, low-sodium; beans—white, lima; beef, hamburger; fruits, fruit juices; bran with sugar and malt; cake—fruitcake, gingerbread; cashew nuts; chicken, light meat; cocoa; coffee, instant; cookies, gingersnaps; dates; garlic; milk—skim, powdered; peanuts, roasted; peanut butter; peas; pecans; potatoes, boiled in skin; scallops; tea, instant; tomato puree; turkey, light meat; veal; walnuts, black; yeast, brewer's.

IV. Foods high in B vitamins
A. *Thiamine:* pork, dried beans, dried peas, liver, lamb, veal, nuts, peas.

B. *Riboflavin:* liver, poultry, milk, yogurt, whole-grain cereals, beef, oysters, tongue, fish, cottage cheese, veal.

C. *Niacin:* liver, fish, poultry, peanut butter, whole grains and enriched breads, lamb, veal, beef, pork.

V. Foods high in vitamin C: oranges, strawberries, dark-green leafy vegetables, potatoes, grapefruit, tomato, cabbage, broccoli, melon, liver.

VI. Foods high in iron, calcium, and residue
A. *Iron:* breads—brown, corn, ginger; fish, tuna; poultry; organ meats; whole-grain cereals; shellfish; egg yolk; fruits—apples, berries; dried fruits—dates, prunes, apricots, peaches, raisins; vegetables—dark-green leafy, potatoes, tomatoes, rhubarb, squash; molasses; dried beans and peas; peanut butter; brown sugar; noodles; rice.

B. *Calcium:* milk—dry, skim, whole, evaporated, buttermilk; cheese—American, Swiss, hard; vegetables—kale, turnip greens, mustard greens, collards; tofu.

C. *Residue:* whole-grain cereals—oatmeal, bran, shredded wheat; breads—whole wheat, cracked wheat, rye, bran muffins; vegetables—lettuce, spinach, Swiss chard, raw carrots, raw celery, corn, cauliflower, eggplant, sauerkraut, cabbage; fruits—bananas, figs, apricots, oranges.

VII. Foods to be used in low-protein and low-carbohydrate diets
A. *Low protein* (these proteins are allowed in various amounts in controlled-protein diets for *renal decompensation*): milk—buttermilk, reconstituted evaporated, low-sodium, skim, and powdered; meat—chicken, lamb, turkey, beef (lean), veal; fish—sole, flounder, haddock, perch; cheese—cheddar, American, Swiss, cottage; eggs; fruits—apples, grapes, pears, pineapple; vegeta-

bles—cabbage, cucumbers, lettuce, tomatoes; cereals—cornflakes, puffed rice, puffed wheat, farina, rolled oats.

B. *Low carbohydrate:* all meats; cheese—hard, soft, cottage; eggs; shellfish—oysters, shrimp; fats—bacon, butter, French dressing, salad oil, mayonnaise, margarine; vegetables—asparagus, green beans, beet greens, broccoli, brussels sprouts, cabbage, celery, cauliflower, cucumber, lettuce, green pepper, spinach, squash, tomatoes; fruits—avocados, strawberries, cantaloupe, lemons, rhubarb.

VIII. **Food guide pyramid**—guide to daily food selection (Figure 9–1)

    A. *Fats, oils:* use sparingly.

    B. *Milk group:* two to three servings.

    C. *Meat group:* two to three servings.

    D. *Fruit group:* two to four servings.

    E. *Vegetable group:* three to five servings.

    F. *Bread/cereal group:* 6 to 11 servings.

FIGURE 9-1 Food guide pyramid—guide to daily food choices. (US Department of Agriculture.)

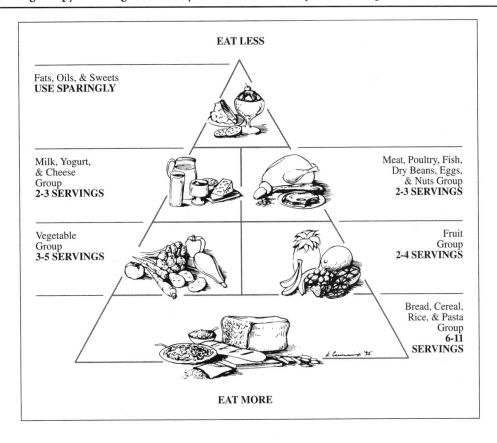

Nutrition

Questions

Select the one best answer for each question.

1. A patient who is diabetic states that she is a "peanut butter freak." Which exchange would be equivalent to 2 tbsp peanut butter?
   1. 8 oz whole milk.
   2. 2 tbsp butter.
   3. ¼ cup cottage cheese.
   4. 2 tbsp cream cheese.
2. A patient is placed on an 1800-calorie diabetic diet; a typical lunch would include two meat exchanges, two bread exchanges, one vegetable exchange, one fruit exchange, one fat exchange, and one milk exchange. Given these allowances, which would be inappropriate for this patient to consume at a birthday luncheon?
   1. A piece of plain sponge cake.
   2. An 8 oz glass of Coca-Cola.
   3. A taco (tortilla, meat, cheddar cheese, lettuce).
   4. Avocado and orange salad.
3. A patient has been placed on a high-protein diet. Which food would the nurse suggest this patient select?
   1. Rice (1 cup).
   2. Eggnog (8 oz).
   3. Cheddar cheese (1 oz).
   4. Broccoli (1 cup).
4. Which food would the nurse recommend be *avoided* by a patient experiencing dumping syndrome?
   1. Liver and bacon.
   2. Orange and avocado salad.
   3. Creamed chicken.
   4. Glazed donuts and coffee.
5. Dietary restriction of protein in chronic renal failure is used to prevent the accumulation of nitrogenous wastes and resulting azotemia. Which food containing amino acids would be allowed in a diet for a patient with chronic renal failure?
   1. Roast beef.
   2. Milk and eggs.
   3. Chicken and turkey.
   4. Shellfish.
6. Which food may be more likely to cause discomfort in a patient with cholecystitis?
   1. Whole milk.
   2. Cottage cheese.
   3. Whole-grain breads.
   4. Eggs.
7. Which food should the nurse advise a patient with a colostomy to *avoid*?
   1. Carbonated drinks.
   2. Fresh-cooked green beans.
   3. Liver and bacon.
   4. Cooked cereals.
8. A patient is a 30-year-old gravida 3 para 2 who is 4 weeks pregnant. She has been a vegetarian for 8 years. She eats no eggs or dairy products (vegan vegetarian). When assessing the adequacy of this patient's diet, to which food group would the nurse pay particular attention?
   1. Grains.
   2. Protein foods.
   3. Vitamin C–rich foods.
   4. Fruits and vegetables.
9. A patient is a 17-year-old primigravida. At 30 weeks of gestation she is diagnosed with iron deficiency anemia. The patient takes her iron and vitamin supplements sporadically due to unacceptable GI side effects but eats many foods high in iron. In planning diet teaching, which nutrient will the nurse emphasize to promote heme production?
   1. Niacin.
   2. Vitamin A.
   3. Vitamin D.
   4. Folic acid.

Answers/Rationale

1. **(3)** A diabetic diet is most often based on an exchange system. Foodstuffs in this system are divided into six types. Foods from within each list can be substituted for another in the same list because they have approximately the same food value. Peanut butter is in the *meat* exchange list, as is cottage cheese, and therefore these can be substituted for one another. Whole milk (**Answer 1**) is on the milk exchange list. Butter and cream cheese (**Answers 2** and **4**) are considered to be fats.
   Test-taking tip—Think "substitute" for a high-protein source.
   IMP, 4, PhI, Basic Care and Comfort
2. **(2)** Given the patient's food allowances, all these foods (**Answers 1, 3,** and **4**) would be allowed *except* for the Coca-Cola. All concentrated sweets and regular soft drinks are contraindicated on a diabetic diet.
   Test-taking tip—Try matching each exchange with the options—one will have *no* match. The question calls for what is *not* OK to eat.
   PL, 4, PhI, Basic Care and Comfort
3. **(2)** Eggs and milk are two sources of protein with the highest biological values (high-quality proteins). Eggnog (8 oz) contains 15 g protein. Rice (**Answer 1**) contains only 4 g, cheddar cheese (**Answer 3**) contains only 7 g, and broccoli (**Answer 4**) contains only 5 g. Meat, fish, and legumes contain more protein than does eggnog, but their percent of protein utilization is lower, making them almost equal in value to eggnog.
   Test-taking tip—With two possible choices, choose the one with more sources of protein (egg *and* milk).
   IMP, 4, PhI, Basic Care and Comfort
4. **(4)** Concentrated sugars and carbohydrates should be avoided by these patients. Likewise, fluid ingestion with meals or snacks should also be avoided to prevent rapid emptying of the stomach. **Answers 1, 2,** and **3** are examples of high-protein, high-fat, low-carbohydrate foods, which *are* appropriate.
   Test-taking tip—Know two things to *avoid* with meals—carbohydrates and fluids.
   PL, 4, PhI, Reduction of Risk Potential

Key to codes following rationales *Nursing process:* **AS,** Assessment; **AN,** Analysis; **PL,** Plan; **IMP,** Implementation; **EV,** Evaluation. *Category of human function:* **1,** Protective; **2,** Sensory perceptual; **3,** Comfort, Rest, Activity, and Mobility; **4,** Nutrition; **5,** Growth and Development; **6,** Fluid-Gas Transport; **7,** Psychosocial-Cultural; **8,** Elimination. **Client need: SECE,** Safe, Effective Care Environment; **PhI,** Physiological Integrity; **PsI,** Psychosocial Integrity; **HPM,** Health Promotion/Maintenance. See appendices for full explanation.

5. **(2)** The diet for patients with chronic renal failure is restricted in total amount of protein and amino acid content. Eggs and milk are generally included in the diet because they contain *all the essential* amino acids. Meats from animals (**Answer 1**), fowl (**Answer 3**), and fish (**Answer 4**) are restricted due to their sulfur-containing, *nonessential* amino acids.

> **Test-taking tip**—Know that an egg is considered a *perfect* protein, so it is often a correct choice.

PL, 4, PhI, Basic Care and Comfort

6. **(1)** Whole milk has a *high fat* content, so a patient with cholecystitis is generally advised to switch to low-fat or skim milk. Cottage cheese (**Answer 2**), whole-grain breads (**Answer 3**), and eggs (**Answer 4**) *are* allowed in a low-fat diet, although eggs may be limited to four per week.

> **Test-taking tip**—Look for the food that is *not* OK to have. Use a true-false approach option by option to find the item that is high fat and *not* OK to have.

IMP, 4, PhI, Reduction of Risk Potential

7. **(1)** Carbonated drinks, cabbage, sauerkraut, and nuts tend to increase *flatulence,* and most patients feel uncomfortable passing flatus into the colostomy bag, because it causes the bag to inflate. Onions, cheese, and fish may cause *odorous* drainage. Generally the initial diet following a colostomy is a low-fiber diet for several weeks. As the diet is increased, the individual patient can determine more accurately which foods cause constipation, diarrhea, flatus, or dyspepsia. **Answers 2, 3,** and **4** are *not troublesome* to most such patients.

> **Test-taking tip**—With diet and bowel disorders, look for *causes* of *gas.*

PL, 4, PhI, Reduction of Risk Potential

8. **(2)** Pregnant vegetarians who omit dairy foods may be unable to meet the requirement for an additional 30 g protein per day over their nonpregnant needs. **Answer 1** is incorrect because individuals who have been vegetarians for some time usually have evolved diets *adequate* in *grain* intake. **Answers 3** and **4** are incorrect because individuals who are vegan vegetarians usually ingest a wide variety of fruits and vegetables to meet pregnancy requirements for vitamin C, fiber, and other nutrients.

> **Test-taking tip**—Think about the food group for milk, dairy, and meat—protein. Recall protein requirements during pregnancy and lactation.

AS, 4, PhI, Basic Care and Comfort

9. **(4)** Folic acid (folacin) is essential for increased heme production for hemoglobin and prevention of megaloblastic anemia. **Answer 1** is incorrect because niacin has *no* direct or indirect role in erythropoiesis or heme production. **Answer 2** is incorrect because vitamin A is essential for *fetal bone growth* and *tooth* development. **Answer 3** is incorrect because vitamin D is essential for *mineralization* of bone tissue and *calcium and phosphorus absorption.*

> **Test-taking tip**—Know the nutritional benefit of common vitamins and minerals.

PL, 4, PhI, Basic Care and Comfort

UNIT 10

Review of Pharmacology

Geraldine Colombraro, Sally L. Lagerquist, Bobbi Morrison,
Robyn Nelson, and Janice Stecchi

GUIDELINES FOR ADMINISTERING MEDICATIONS TO INFANTS AND CHILDREN

I. Developmental considerations

- **A.** Be honest. Do *not* bribe or threaten child to obtain cooperation.
- **B.** When administering medication, do so in the least traumatic manner possible.
- **C.** Describe any sensations child may expect to experience, e.g., "pinch" of needle during IM.
- **D.** Explain how child can "help" nurse, e.g., "Lie as still as you can."
- **E.** Tell child that it is OK to cry; provide privacy.
- **F.** Offer support, praise, and encouragement during and after giving medication.
- **G.** Allow child opportunity for age-appropriate therapeutic play to work through feelings and experiences, to clarify any misconceptions, and to teach child more effective coping strategies.

II. Safety considerations

- **A.** Be absolutely sure dose you are giving is both safe (check recommended mg/kg) and accurate (have another nurse check your calculations). Remember: dose should generally be smaller than adult dose.
- **B.** Check identification band or ask parent or another nurse for child's first and last name.
- **C.** Restrain child to avoid injury while giving medication; a second person is often required to help hold child.

III. Oral medications

- **A.** Use syringe without needle to draw up medication.
- **B.** *Position:* upright or semireclining.
- **C.** Place tip of syringe along the side of infant's tongue, and give medication slowly, in small amounts, allowing infant to swallow. Medicine cups can be used for older infants and children. *Never* pinch infant or child's nostrils to force him or her to open mouth.
- **D.** When giving tablets or capsules (that are *not* enteric coated), crush and mix into smallest possible amount of food or liquid to ensure that child takes entire dose. Do *not* mix with essential food or liquid (e.g., milk); select an "optional" food, such as applesauce.

IV. Ophthalmic installations

- **A.** *Position:* supine or sitting with head extended.
- **B.** For eye drops: hold dropper 1–2 cm above middle of conjunctival sac.
- **C.** For eye ointment: squeeze 2 cm of ointment from tube onto conjunctival sac.
- **D.** After giving drops or ointment, encourage child to keep eyes closed briefly, to maximize contact with eyes. Child should be asked to look in all directions (with eyes closed) to enhance even distribution of medication.
- **E.** Whenever possible, administer eye ointments at nap time or bedtime, due to possible blurred vision.

V. Otic installations

- **A.** *Position:* head to side so that affected ear is uppermost.
- **B.** For child **under** 3 yr of age: pull pinna gently **down** and back.
- **C.** For child 3 yr of age and **over:** pull pinna gently **up** and back.

Pharmacology

D. After administering ear drops, encourage child to remain with head to side with affected ear uppermost, to maximize contact with entire external canal to reach eardrum. Gentle massage of area in front of ear will facilitate entry of ear drops into canal.

E. If ear drops are kept in refrigerator, allow to warm to room temperature before instilling.

VI. Dermatological installations

A. Remember: young child's skin is more permeable; therefore there is increased risk for medication absorption and resultant systemic effects; monitor for systemic effects.

B. Apply thin layer of cream or ointment, and confine it to portions of skin where it is essential.

VII. Rectal medication

A. Prepare child emotionally and physically; rectal route is invasive and embarrassing, particularly for children.

B. *Position:* side-lying with upper leg flexed.

C. Lubricate rounded end of suppository and insert past anal sphincter with gloved fingertip (wear gloves when inserting rectal medication).

D. Remove fingertip but hold child's buttocks gently together until child no longer strains or indicates urge to expel medication.

VIII. Intramuscular medication

A. Because the infant or child is much smaller physically than an adult, the nurse should select a shorter needle, generally ⅝ inch (infant) to 1 inch (child).

B. Preferred injection sites are on the thigh: vastus lateralis—lateral aspect; rectus femoris—anterior aspect. The deltoid muscle, though small, provides easy access and can be used in children with adequate muscle mass.

C. **Avoid** posterior gluteal muscle in children under age 4.

D. Because of vast differences in size, muscle mass, and subcutaneous tissue, it is especially important to note bony prominences as landmarks for intramuscular injections.

E. Have a second adult present to help restrain the child.

F. Once the nurse has told the child he or she is to receive an injection, the procedure should be carried out as quickly and skillfully as possible.

Pharmacology

COMMON PSYCHOTROPIC DRUGS

I. Antipsychotics (also called *neuroleptics, major tranquilizers*)

A. **Phenothiazines** (prochlorperazine [Compazine], promazine HCl [Sparine], chlorpromazine HCl [Thorazine], thioridazine [Mellaril], trifluoperazine HCl [Stelazine], perphenazine [Trilafon], triflupromazine HCl [Vesprin], fluphenazine enanthate [Prolixin]).

B. **Butyrophenones** (haloperidol [Haldol, Serenace], droperidol fentanyl citrate [Innovar]).

C. **Thiothixenes** (chlorprothixene [Taractan], thiothixene [Navane]) —chemically related to phenothiazines, with similar therapeutic effects.

D. **Dibenzoxazepines**—atypical antipsychotics (clozapine [Clozaril], loxapine succinate [Loxitane])
1. *Use*—those who do not respond to other neuroleptic antipsychotic drugs; offers relief from schizophrenic symptoms: hallucinations, delusions, flat affect, apathy.
2. *Assessment*—*side effects:*
   a. Most serious is *agranulocytosis* (potentially fatal; reversible if diagnosed within 1–2 wk of onset).
   (1) *Symptoms* of agranulocytosis: infection, high fever, chills, sore throat, malaise, ulceration of mucous membranes.
   (2) Lab value: Discontinue drug with WBC <2000 μL or granulocyte <1000 μL.
   b. Other side effects: seizures, tachycardia, orthostatic hypotension.
   c. *Caution:* must have weekly blood tests for WBC; do *not* resume clozapine once it is discontinued, due to side effects.

E. **Benzisoxazole derivative**—risperidone (Risperdal)
1. *Use*—incremental increases for first 3 days to manage psychotic symptoms. *Benefit:* less incidence of extrapyramidal symptoms.
2. *Assessment*—*side effects:* same as for phenothiazines.

F. **General use**—acute and chronic psychoses; most useful in cases of disorganization of thought or behavior; to decrease panic, fear, hostility, restlessness, aggression, and withdrawal.

G. **General assessment**—*side effects:*
1. *Hypersensitivity* effects:
   a. *Blood dyscrasia*—agranulocytosis, leukopenia, granulocytopenia.
   b. *Skin reactions*—solar sensitivity, allergic dermatitis, flushing, blue-gray skin.
   c. *Obstructive jaundice.*

2. *Extrapyramidal symptoms (EPS)* affecting voluntary movement and skeletal muscles
   a. *Parkinsonism* (also called pseudoparkinsonism)—tremors, cogwheel rigidity, shuffling gait, pill-rolling, masklike facies, salivation, and difficulty starting muscular movement (dyskinesia).
   b. *Dystonia*—limb and neck spasms (torticollis), extensive rigidity of back muscles (opisthotonos), oculogyric crisis, speech and swallowing difficulties, and protrusion of tongue.
   c. *Akathisia*—motor restlessness, pacing, foot tapping, inner tremulousness, and agitation.
   d. ***Tardive dyskinesia (TD)***—excessive blinking; vermiform tongue movement; stereotyped, abnormal, involuntary sucking, chewing, licking, and pursing movements of tongue and mouth; grimacing, blinking, frowning, rocking.
   (1) *Cause*—long-term use of high doses of antipsychotic drugs.
   (2) *Predisposing factors*—age, women, organic brain syndrome (OBS); history of electroconvulsive therapy (ECT) or use of tricyclics or anti-Parkinson drugs.
3. *Potentiates* central nervous system depressants.
4. *Orthostatic hypotension* (less with butyrophenones).
5. *Anticholinergic effects* (atropine-like)—dry mouth, stuffy nose, blurred vision, urinary retention, and constipation.
6. Pigment retinopathy—ocular changes (lens and corneal opacity).
7. ***Neuroleptic malignant syndrome (NMS)***
   a. *Description:* a rare complication of antipsychotic drugs, with a rapid progression (1–3 days) and a 20% mortality rate. It is a serious medical emergency for which early recognition of symptoms is critical. *Onset:* at start, after change, or dose increase, when used with combination of medications.
   b. ***Assessment:***
   (1) ↑Vital signs: extreme temperature of 107°F (leading to seizures, diaphoresis, confusion, stupor, and coma), fluctuating BP, tachycardia.
   (2) Lab values: *increased* creatine phosphokinase (CPK), *increased* potassium, leukocytosis (↑WBC).
   (3) Renal failure.
   (4) Muscular: parkinsonian rigidity (lead pipe skeletal muscle rigidity) that leads to dyspnea and dysphagia, tremors, dyskinesia.

Pharmacology

(5) *At risk:* patients with organic brain disorders and severe dehydration.
◆ c. *Medical treatment*
  (1) Discontinue all drugs *stat.*
  (2) Institute supportive care.
  (3) Administer Parlodel or Dantrium, dopamine function–enhancing substances (e.g., levodopa, carbidopa, bromocriptine, amantadine).
H. **Antipsychotic agents—comparison of side effects** (Table 10–1)
◆ I. **General nursing care plan/implementation:**
  1. Goal: *anticipate, observe for, and check for side effects.*
    a. Protect the person's skin from *sunburn* when outside.
    b. For *hypotension:* take BP and have person lie down for 30 min, especially after an injection.
    c. Watch for signs of *blood dyscrasia:* sore throat, fever, malaise.
    d. Observe for symptoms of *hypothermic* or *hyperthermic* reaction due to effect on heat-regulating mechanism.
    e. Observe for, withhold drug for, and report early symptoms of *jaundice* and bile tract obstruction, high fever, upper abdominal pain, nausea, diarrhea, rash; monitor *liver function.*
    f. Relieve excessive *mouth dryness:* mouth rinse, increase fluid intake, gum or hard candy.
    g. Relieve gastric irritation, *constipation:* take with and *increase fluids* and *roughage* in diet.
    h. Observe for and report changes in carbohydrate metabolism (glycosuria, weight gain, polyphagia): change diet.

  2. Goal: *health teaching.*
    a. Dangers of drug potentiation with alcohol or sleeping pills.
    b. Advise about driving or occupations where blurred vision may be a problem.
    c. Caution against abrupt cessation at high doses.
    d. Warn regarding dark urine (sign of jaundice, urinary retention).
    e. Have client with respiratory disorder breathe deeply and cough (drug is a cough depressant).
    f. Need for continuous use of drug and follow-up care.
    g. Prompt reporting of hypersensitivity symptoms: fever, laryngeal edema; abdominal distention (constipation, urinary retention); jaundice; blood dyscrasia.
◆ J. **General evaluation/outcome criteria:**
  1. Behavior is less agitated.
  2. Knows side effects to observe for, lessen, and/or prevent.
  3. Continues to use drug.

II. Antidepressants
A. **Tricyclic antidepressants (TCAs)**—(imipramine HCl [Tofranil], desipramine HCl [Norpramine, Pertofrane], nortriptyline HCl [Pamelor, Aventyl], trimipramine [Surmontil], clomipramine [Anafranil], amitriptyline HCl [Elavil, Endep], amitriptyline HCl/perphenazine [Triavil], protriptyline HCl [Vivactil], doxepin HCl [Sinequan, Adapin], bupropion (Wellbutrin), trazodone (Desyrel), amoxapine (Asendin)—effective in 2–4 wk.
  1. *Use*—elevate mood in depression, increase physical activity and mental alertness; may

TABLE 10–1 Antipsychotic Agents—Comparison of Side Effects

Classification	Name Generic	Trade	Extrapyramidal Symptoms (EPS)	Sedation	Anticholinergic	Orthostatic Hypotension
Phenothiazine	Chlorpromazine	Thorazine	3	4	3	4
	Fluphenazine	Prolixin	5	2	2	2
	Perphenazine	Trilafon	4	2	2	2
	Prochlorperazine	Compazine	4	3	2	2
	Promazine	Sparine	3	3	4	3
	Thioridazine	Mellaril	2	4	4	4
	Triflupromazine	Vesprin	3	4	4	3
Butyrophenone	Haloperidol	Haldol	5	1	1	1
Thioxanthene	Thiothixene	Navane	4	2	2	2
Dibenzoxazepine	Clozapine	Clozaril	1	5	5	4
	Loxapine	Loxitane	4	3	2	3
Benzisoxazole	Risperidone	Risperdal	1	1	1	3

1 = very low; 2 = low; 3 = moderate; 4 = high; 5 = very high.

bring relief of symptoms of depression so that client can attend individual or group therapy; bipolar disorder, depressed; dysthymic disorder; sleep disturbance; agitation.

◆ 2. **Assessment**—*side effects:*
   a. *Behavioral*—activation of latent schizophrenia (hallucinations); hypomania; suicide attempts; mental *confusion.* Withhold drug if observed.
   b. *Central nervous system* (CNS)—*tremors, seizures,* ataxia, jitteriness, irritability.
   c. *Autonomic nervous system* (ANS)—*dry mouth,* nasal congestion, aggravation of glaucoma (blurred vision), constipation, urinary retention, edema, paralysis, *ECG* changes (flattened T waves; **arrhythmia** severe in overdose).

◆ 3. **Nursing care plan/implementation:**
   a. Goal: *assess risk of suicide during initial improvement:* careful, close observation.
   b. Goal: *prevent risk of tachycardia and cardiac arrhythmias and orthostatic hypotension:* use caution with client with cardiovascular disease, hyperthyroidism, having ECT or surgery (gradually discontinue 2–3 days *before* surgery). Monitor BP, pulse twice a day; ECGs, 2–3/wk until dose adjusted.
      (1) *Avoid* long hot showers or baths.
   c. Goal: *observe for signs of urinary retention, constipation:* monitor I&O and *weight gain* (encourage exercise).
      (1) Fiber diet.
      (2) Reduced calories.
   d. Goal: *cautious drug use with glaucoma or history of seizures.* Observe seizure precautions due to lowered seizure threshold.
   e. Goal: *health teaching:*
      (1) Advise against driving car or participating in activities requiring mental alertness, due to *sedative* effects.
      (2) Encourage increased fluid intake and frequent mouth rinsing to combat dry mouth; use candy, ice; take with food.
      (3) *Avoid* smoking, which decreases drug effects.
      (4) *Avoid* use of alcohol and other drugs, due to adverse interactions, especially OTC (e.g., antihistamines).
      (5) Advise of *delay* in desired effect (2–4 wk).
      (6) Instruct gradual discontinuance to *avoid* withdrawal symptoms.

◆ 4. **Evaluation/outcome criteria:** diminished symptoms of agitated depression and anxiety.

B. **Monoamine oxidase inhibitors** (MAOIs) (phenelzine sulfate [Nardil], isocarboxazid [Marplan], tranylcypromine sulfate [Parnate], iproniazid [Marsilid], pargiline HCl [Eutonyl], nialamide [Niamid]).

◆ 1. **Assessment**—*side effects:*
   a. *Behavioral*—may activate latent schizophrenia, mania, excitement.
   b. *CNS*—tremors; **hypertensive crisis** (*avoid:* cheese, colas, caffeine, red wine, beer, yeast, chocolate, chicken liver, and other substances high in *tyramine or pressor amine,* e.g., amphetamines and cold and hay fever medication); *intracerebral hemorrhage; hyperpyrexia.*
   c. *ANS*—*dry mouth,* aggravation of glaucoma, bowel and bladder control problems; edema, paralysis, ECG changes (arrhythmia severe in overdose).
   d. *Allergic* hepatocellular jaundice.

◆ 2. **Nursing care plan/implementation:**
   a. Goal: *reduce risk of hypertensive crisis:* diet restrictions of foods high in *tyramine* content.
   b. Goal: *observe for urinary retention:* measure I&O.
   c. Goal: *health teaching.*
      (1) Therapeutic response takes 2–3 wk.
      (2) *Food and alcohol restrictions:* avocado, bananas, raisins, licorice, chocolate, aged cheese, yogurt, sour cream, papaya, figs, over-ripe fruit, sausages, liver, herring, soy sauce, meat tenderizers, red wine, beer, caffeine, cola, yeast, chocolate.
      (3) Change position gradually to prevent postural hypotension.
      (4) Report any stiff neck, palpitations, chest pain, headaches because of possible hypertensive crises (can be fatal).
      (5) Take *no nonprescribed* drugs.

◆ 3. **Evaluation/outcome criteria:**
   a. Improvement in sleep, appetite, activity, interest in self and surroundings.
   b. Lessening of anxiety and complaints.

C. **Selective serotonin reuptake inhibitors** (SSRIs) (fluoxetine [Prozac], paroxetine [Paxil], sertraline [Zoloft], fluvoxamine [Luvox]). SSRIs are generally the first line choice because of fewer side effects, do not require blood monitoring, and are safe in overdose.

◆ 1. **Assessment**—*side effects: CNS stimulation*— insomnia, agitation, headache (especially with Prozac); weight loss; sexual dysfunction (men: impotence; women: loss of orgasm). Other side effects are similar to TCAs (dry mouth, sedation, nausea).

◆ 2. **Nursing care plan/implementation:**
   a. Goal: *reduce insomnia, agitation:* take early in day; *avoid* alcohol, caffeine; teach relaxation before sleeptime.
   b. Goal: *reduce headaches:* give analgesics.
   c. Goal: *prevent weight loss:* weigh every day or every other day, same time and scale; do *not* use with patients who are anorexic.

◆ 3. Evaluation/outcome criteria:
  a. Improvement in mood and hygiene, thought and communication patterns.
  b. Has not harmed self.
  c. No significant anticholinergic and cardiovascular side effects.

● III. **Antianxiety (also called** *anxiolytics, minor tranquilizers*) **(Table 10–2)**
  A. Chlordiazepoxide (Librium)
    1. *Use*—acute alcohol withdrawal, tension, and irrational fears; anxiety disorders, preoperative sedation; has muscle relaxant and anticonvulsant properties.
    ◆ 2. Assessment—*side effects:* hypotension, drowsiness, motor uncoordination, confusion, skin eruptions, edema, menstrual irregularities, constipation, extrapyramidal symptoms, blurred vision, lethargy; increased or decreased libido.

◆ 3. **Nursing care plan/implementation:**
  a. Goal: *administer cautiously, because drug may:*
    (1) Be habituating (causing withdrawal convulsions; therefore gradual withdrawal necessary).
    (2) Potentiate CNS depressants.
    (3) Have adverse effect on pregnancy.
    (4) Be dangerous for those with suicidal tendencies or severe psychoses, narrow angle glaucoma, elderly or debilitated.
  b. Goal: *reduce GI effects:* crush tablet or take with meals or milk; give *antacids* 1 hr before.
  c. Goal: *monitor effects on liver function:*

> Periodic liver function tests and blood counts, especially with upper respiratory infection, hepatic or renal dysfunction.

TABLE 10–2   Antianxiety Agents: Comparison

Drug	Use	Side Effects/Cautions
Acetylinic Alcohol *Placidyl* (ethchlorvynol, a sedative-hypnotic)		*See* Propanediol Carbamates; also: Confusion Ataxia Hypotension Exaggerated depression (muscle weakness and deep sleep)
Benzodiazepines *Ativan* (Lorazepam) *Librium* (chlordiazepoxide) *Serax* (oxazepam) *Valium* (diazepam) *Tranxene* (clorazepate) *Restoril* (temazepam) *Xanax* (alprazolam) *Klonopin* (clonazepam) *Halcion* (triazolam)	Short-term, for specific stress	Drowsiness Lethal overdose with alcohol High risk for dependency with long-term use; taper gradually over 2–6 wk Symptoms with abrupt withdrawal: irritability, dizziness Do *not* use in pregnancy
Beta-Adrenergic Blocker *Inderal* (propranolol hydrochloride)	Stage fright Relief of physical signs of anxiety (tachycardia)	Hypotension Bradycardia No risk of dependence or abuse
Buspirone Hydrochloride *BuSpar*	Long-term use	Less sedation; no risk of dependence *Delayed* effect (3 wk); no CNS depression
Diphenylmethane Antihistamine *Atarax* (hydroxyzine hydrochloride) *Vistaril* (hydroxyzine pamoate)	Safe for long-term use	No risk of physical dependency or abuse; minimal toxicity May cause drowsiness
Propanediol Carbamates *Equanil* (meprobamate, a sedative-hypnotic)	Rarely used	Drowsiness High risk for tolerance, addiction, and overdose *Withdrawal symptoms:* insomnia, anxiety, hallucination, seizures CNS depressant
Tricyclic Antidepressants (TCAs) *Anafranil* (clomipramine) *Tofranil* (imipramine)	Prevention of panic attacks Severe obsessive-compulsive disorder	Dry mouth Blurred vision Constipation Weight gain Abrupt withdrawal may cause **seizures, cardiac arrhythmias**

Source: Adapted from Lagerquist S: Nurse Notes: Psychiatric-Mental Health, Philadelphia, Lippincott, 1997, p. 69.

d. Goal: *health teaching.*
   (1) Advise against suddenly stopping drug (withdrawal symptoms begin in 5–7 days).
   (2) Talk with physician if plans to be or is pregnant or lactating.
   (3) Urge to drink fluids.
   (4) *Avoid:* alcohol, OTC drugs, and heavy smoking and caffeine.

◆ 4. **Evaluation/outcome criteria:** decreased alcohol withdrawal symptoms or preoperative anxiety; no seizures or confusion.

B. Diazepam (Valium)
1. *Use*—muscle relaxant; *not* used for psychotic behavior.

◆ 2. **Assessment**—*side effects:* same as for chlordiazepoxide, plus double or blurred vision, difficult speech, headache, hypotension, incontinence, tremor, urinary retention, liver damage.

◆ 3. **Nursing care plan/implementation:**
   a. Goal: *anticipate, observe for, and check for side effects,* especially depression, suicidal risk, and constipation.
   b. Goal: *reduce risk of hypotension, respiratory depression, phlebitis, venous thrombosis.* Give IM: in large muscles, slowly, and rotate sites, have client lie down; IV: over 1 min period.
   c. Goal: *observe for psychological and physical dependence: avoid* abrupt discontinuation.
   d. Goal: *health teaching:* sedative effects, potentiation of other CNS-depressant drugs and alcohol, and problem of habituation.

◆ 4. **Evaluation/outcome criteria:** relief of tension, anxiety, skeletal muscle spasm.

IV. Antimanic
A. **Lithium** (Eskalith, Lithane, Lithobid)—effect occurs 1–3 wk after first dose.
1. *Use*—acute manic attack and prevention of recurrence of cyclic manic-depressive episodes of bipolar disorders.

◆ 2. **Assessment**—*side effects:* levels from 1.6–2.0 mEq/L may cause blurred vision, tinnitus, tremors, nausea and vomiting, severe diarrhea, polyuria, polydipsia; ataxia. levels >2 mEq/L may cause motor weakness, headache, edema, and lethargy; *signs of severe toxicity:* arrhythmias, MI, cardiovascular collapse, oliguria/anuria; *neurological* (twitching, marked drowsiness, slurred speech, dysarthria, athetotic movements, convulsions, delirium, stupor, coma) with levels >2.5 mEq/L.
   a. *Precautions*—cautious use with clients on *diuretics;* with abnormal *electrolytes* (sweating, dehydrated, and postoperative clients); with *thyroid* problems, on *low-salt diets;* with *heart failure;* with *impaired*

renal function; with *pregnancy and lactation;* risk of suicide.

b. *Dosage*—**therapeutic** level 0.8–1.6 mEq/L; dose for maintenance 300–1200 mg/day; *toxic* level >2.0 mEq/L; blood sample drawn in acute phase 10–14 hr after last dose, taken tid.

◆ 3. **Nursing care plan/implementation:**
   a. Goal: *anticipate, observe for, and check for signs and symptoms of toxicity.*
      (1) Reduce GI symptoms: take *with meals.*
      (2) Check for edema: daily weight, I&O.
      (3) Monitor blood levels (1.6–2.0 mEq/L) for signs of *toxicity:* nausea, vomiting, diarrhea, anorexia, ataxia, weakness, drowsiness, fine tremor or muscle twitching, slurred speech.
      (4) Monitor results from repeat thyroid and kidney function tests.
      (5) Withhold drug and notify MD when 1.5 mEq/L is reached.
      (6) Monitor vital signs 2–3 times/day (pulse irregularities, hypotension, arrhythmias).
   b. Goal: *report immediately fever, diarrhea, prolonged vomiting.*
   c. Goal: *monitor effect* (therapeutic and toxic) through blood samples taken:
      (1) 10–14 hr after last dose.
      (2) Every 2–3 days until 1.6 mEq/L is reached.
      (3) Once a week while in hospital.
      (4) Every 2–3 mo to maintain blood levels <2 mEq/L.
   d. Goal: *health teaching.*
      (1) Advise client 1–3 wk lag time for effect.
      (2) Urge to drink adequate *liquids* (2–3 L/day), ice; strict oral hygiene.
      (3) Report: *polyuria* and polydipsia.
      (4) *Diet:* avoid caffeine, crash diets, diet pills, self-prescribed low-salt diet, alcohol, antacids, high-sodium foods (which increase lithium excretion and reduce drug effect); take *with meals.* Use sugarless candy.
      (5) Caution against driving, operating machinery that requires mental alertness until drug is effective.
      (6) Warn *not* to change or omit dose.

◆ 4. **Evaluation/outcome criteria:**
   a. Changed facial affect.
   b. Improved posture, ability to concentrate, sleep patterns; mood is stabilized.
   c. Assumption of self-care.
   d. No signs of lithium toxicity.

V. Antiparkinsonian agents
  A. Trihexphenidyl HCl (Artane).
  B. Benztropine mesylate (Cogentin).
    1. *Use*—counteract drug-induced extrapyramidal reactions.
  ◆ 2. **Assessment:**
      a. Trihexyphenidyl HCl
        (1) *Side effects*—anticholinergic: *dry mouth, blurred vision,* dizziness, nausea, *constipation,* drowsiness, *urinary hesitancy* or *retention;* pupil dilation; headache; weakness; *tachycardia.*
        (2) *Precautions*—cautious use with: cardiac, liver, or kidney disease or obstructive gastrointestinal-genitourinary disease, BPH, or myasthenia gravis. Do *not* give if glaucoma present.
      b. Benztropine mesylate—*side effects:* same as for trihexyphenidyl HCl *plus:*
        (1) Effect on *body temperature* (hyperpyrexia) may result in life-threatening state (heatstroke).
        (2) *Gastrointestinal (GI) distress.*
        (3) Inability to concentrate, memory difficulties, and mild confusion (often mistaken for senility); *drowsiness.*
        (4) May lead to toxic *psychotic* reactions.
        (5) *Subjective sensations*—light or heavy feelings in legs, numbness and tingling of extremities, *light-headedness* or tightness of head, and giddiness.

  ◆ 3. **Nursing care plan/implementation:**
      a. Goal: *relieve GI distress* by giving *after* or *with* meals or at bedtime.
      b. Goal: *monitor adverse effects:*
        (1) Hypotension, tachycardia: check pulse, blood pressure; increased temperature; decreased sweating.
        (2) Constipation and fecal impaction: add roughage to *diet.*
        (3) Dry mouth: increase *fluid* intake; encourage frequent mouth rinsing; offer sugarless candy or gum, ice.
        (4) Blurred vision, dizziness: assist with ambulation; use side rail.
        (5) Urinary retention: maintain I&O.
      c. *Health teaching:*
        (1) *Avoid* driving, and limit activities requiring alertness.
        (2) Delayed drug effect (2–3 days).
        (3) Potential abuse due to hallucinogenic effects.
        (4) *Avoid* alcohol and other CNS depressants; *avoid* hot weather.
        (5) Take with food.
        (6) Do *not* stop drug abruptly.
  ◆ 4. **Evaluation/outcome criteria:**
      a. Less rigidity, drooling, and oculogyric crisis.
      b. Improved gait, balance, posture.
      c. Has not experienced symptoms of hyperthermia.

ABSORPTION RATES

Table 10–3.

TABLE 10–3 Rates of Absorption by Different Routes

Route of Administration	Time Until Drug Takes Effect*
Topical	Hours to days
Oral	30–90 min
Rectal	5–30 min (unpredictable)
Subcutaneous injection	15–30 min
Intramuscular injection	10–20 min
Sublingual tablet	3–5 min
Sublingual injection	3 min
Inhalation	3 min
Endotracheal	3 min
Intravenous	30–60 sec
Intracardiac	15 sec

*In a healthy person with normal perfusion.

REGIONAL ANALGESIA-ANESTHESIA IN LABOR AND DELIVERY

Table 10–4.

MIND-ALTERING SUBSTANCES

Major substances used by the public to alter mental states are compared in Table 10–5.

COMMON DRUGS

Table 10–6.

TABLE 10–4   Regional Analgesia-Anesthesia for Labor and Birth

Types	Characteristics	Nursing Implications
Common Agents in 0.5–1.0% Solution Lidocaine (Xylocaine) Bupivacaine (Marcaine) HCl Tetracaine (Pontocaine) HCl Mepivacaine HCl (Carbocaine) Chloroprocaine HCl (Nesacaine)	Used with epinephrine (or other vasoconstrictor drug) to delay absorption, prolong anesthetic effect, and decrease chance of hypotension	*Note any history of allergy;* note response: allergic reaction, hypotension, and lack of wearing off of anesthetic effect; observe for hypertensive crisis if agent combined with epinephrine and oxytocin is also being given
Peripheral Nerve Block Pudendal (5–10 mL each side) anesthetizes lower two-thirds of vagina and perineum	Perineal anesthesia of short duration (30 min); local anesthesia; simple and safe; does not depress neonate; may inhibit bearing-down reflex	To get cooperation, give explanation during procedure
Paracervical (uterosacral) block (5–10 mL given into each side) anesthetizes cervix and upper two-thirds of vagina; *note:* used more for gynecological surgery than for labor	May be given between 3 and 8 cm by physician when woman is having at least three contractions in 10 min; lasts 45–90 min; can be repeated; can be followed by local, epidural, or other; may cause temporary fetal bradycardia	Explain: especially length and type of needle; take maternal vital signs and FHR; have her void; help position; monitor FHR continuously; monitor contractions; and watch for return of pain
Local infiltration	Useful for perineal repairs	No special nursing care
Epidural lumbar block	Useful during first and second stages; can be given "one shot" or continuously; T-10 to S-5 for vaginal birth; T-8 to S-1 for abdominal birth; complete anesthesia for labor and birth	*Hypotension* (with resultant fetal bradycardia): (a) turn from supine to lateral, or *elevate* legs, (b) administer humidified oxygen by mask at 8–10 L/min, (c) increase rate of IV fluids (use infusate *without* oxytocin); will need coaching to push and low forceps may be required
Subarachnoid spinal Continuous	Useful during first or second stage of labor, or for abdominal surgery	Instruct when to bear down
Low spinal ("saddle," "one shot") block	Same as continuous	Same as continuous
Intrathecal (spinal): morphine, fentanyl, Sufentanil	0.5 mg produces marked analgesia for 12–24 hr; onset in 20–30 min Fentanyl and Sufentanil produce short-acting analgesia (1½–3½ hr)	*Side effects:* respiratory depression, pruritus, nausea, vomiting, sleepiness, urinary retention; keep *naloxone* 0.4 mg at bedside and respiratory support equipment readily available

Pharmacology

TABLE 10–5 Major Substances Used for Mind Alteration

Official Name	Slang Name	Usual Single Adult Dose/Duration	Legitimate Medical Uses (Present and Projected)	Short-Term Effects	Long-Term Effects
Alcohol—whisky, gin, beer, wine	Booze, hooch, suds, moonshine, firewater, nightcap	1½ oz gin or whiskey, 12 oz beer/2–4 hr	Rare: sometimes used as a sedative (for tension)	CNS depressant; relaxation (sedation); euphoria; drowsiness; impaired judgment, reaction time, coordination, and emotional control; frequent aggressive behavior and driving accidents; loss of inhibitions; slurred speech	Diversion of energy and money from more creative and productive pursuits; habituation; possible obesity with chronic excessive use; irreversible damage to brain and liver; addiction with severe withdrawal illness (DTs) with heavy use; many deaths
Caffeine—coffee, tea, Coca-Cola, No-Doz, APC	Java, mud, brew	1–2 cups, 1 bottle, 5 mg/2–4 hr	Mild stimulant; treatment of some forms of coma	CNS stimulant; increased alertness; reduction of fatigue	Sometimes insomnia, restlessness, or gastric irritation; habituation
Nicotine (and coal tar)—cigarettes, cigars, pipe tobacco, snuff	Fags, nails, weeds, butts, chaw, cancer sticks	1–2 cigarettes/1–2 hr	None (used as an insecticide)	CNS stimulant; relaxation or distraction	Lung (and other) cancer, heart and blood vessel disease, cough, etc.; higher infant mortality rate; many deaths; habituation; diversion of energy and money; air pollution; fire
SEDATIVES Alcohol—see above	Downers				
Barbiturates—amobarbital (Amytal, Tuinal), pentobarbital (Nembutal), secobarbital (Seconal), phenobarbital	Barbs, blue angel, blue devils, yellow jackets, yellow birds, dolls, red devils, red birds, phennies, goofers, jelly beans, tooies	50–100 mg	Treatment of insomnia and tension; Induction of anesthesia; As an anticonvulsant	CNS depressants; sleep induction; relaxation (sedation); sometimes euphoria; drowsiness; impaired judgment, reaction time, coordination, and emotional control; relief of anxiety/tension; muscle relaxation	Irritability, weight loss, addiction with severe withdrawal illness (like DTs); diversion of energy and money; habituation, addiction
Glutethimide (Doriden)	Gorilla pills, CBs, D	500 mg			
Chloral hydrate (Noctec)	Peter, Mickey	500 mg			
Meprobamate (Miltown, Equanil)	Dolls, dollies	400 mg/4 hr[a]			
STIMULANTS Caffeine—see above Nicotine—see above	Uppers				
Amphetamines Amphetamine (Benzedrine) Methamphetamine (Methedrine, Pesoxyn) Dextroamphetamine (Dexedrine)	Pep pills, wake-ups, Bennies, splash, peaches Water crystal, speed, meth, Dexies, uppers	2.5–15.0 mg	Treatment of obesity, narcolepsy, fatigue, depression, hyperkinesia	CNS stimulants; increased alertness; reduction of fatigue; loss of appetite; insomnia; often euphoria, agitation	Restlessness, weight loss, toxic psychosis (mainly paranoid); diversion of energy and money; habituation; extreme irritability, toxic psychosis

Continued

Drug	Slang names	Dose	Medical use	Action/effects	Adverse effects/overdose
Phenmetrazine HCl (Preludin)	Diet pills	25 mg			*Symptoms of overdose:* hallucinations, convulsions; cardiac, respiratory failure; coma; pulmonary edema
Cocaine	Coke, snow, blow, happy gold dust, toot, lady, flake, crack, cecil, girl, C	Variable/4 hr[a]	Anesthesia of the eye and throat		
TRANQUILIZERS					
Chlordiazepoxide (Librium)	Green and whites, roaches	5–25 mg	Treatment of anxiety, tension, alcoholism, neurosis, psychosis, psychosomatic disorders, and vomiting	Selective CNS depressants; relaxation, relief of anxiety/tension; suppression of hallucinations or delusions, improved functioning	Sometimes drowsiness, dryness of mouth, blurring of vision, skin rash, tremor; occasionally jaundice, agranulocytosis, or death
Phenothiazines					
Chlorpromazine HCl (Thorazine)		10–50 mg			
Perchlorperazine (Compazine)		5–10 m			
Trifluoperazine HCl (Stelazine)		2–5 mg			
Reserpine (rauwolfia)		0.10–0.25 mg/4–6 h[a]	Treatment of depression, tension, loss of appetite, high blood pressure, nausea and vomiting from chemotherapy		
Marijuana or cannabis	Pot, grass, Texas tea, weed, stuff, joint, reefers, Mary Jane, MJ, hay, locoweed	Variable—1 cigarette or pipe, or 1 drink or cake (India)/4 hr[a]		Relaxation, euphoria, increased appetite, some alteration of time perception, possible impairment of judgment and coordination; mixed CNS depressant-stimulant; lowered inhibitions	Usually none; possible diversion of energy and money; habituation; occasional acute panic reactions (with paranoia, delusions, hallucinations)
Hashish[b]	Hash, rope, Sweet Lucy				
ANTIDEPRESSANTS					
Ritalin	Speed, uppers, eye opener	5–10 mg; 25 mg, 10 mg	Treatment of moderate to severe depression	Relief of depression (elevation of mood), stimulation	Basically the same as tranquilizers above
Dibenzazepine (imipramine [Tofranil], amitriptyline HCl [Elavil])		10 mg, 15 mg/4–6 h[a]	Treatment of severe depression		
MAO inhibitors (phenelzine sulfate [Nardil], tranylcypromine sulfate [Parnate])					
NARCOTICS (OPIATES, ANALGESICS)					
Opium	Op, black, poppy, tar, Big O	10–12 "pipes" (Asia)/4 hr[a]	Treatment of severe pain, diarrhea, and cough	CNS depressants; sedation, euphoria, relief of pain, impaired intellectual functioning and coordination	Constipation, loss of appetite and weight, temporary impotency or sterility; habituation, addiction with unpleasant and painful withdrawal illness
Heroin	Horse, H, smack, shit, junk, brown, pcag, TNT, M, white stuff, Miss Emma	Variable—bag or paper with 5–10% heroin			
Morphine (Astramorph)		10–15 mg			
Codeine	Terp, robo, romo, syrup	15–30 mg	Topical anesthetic		
Aspirin/oxycodone HCl (Percodan)	Perks, Perkies	1 tablet			
Meperidine HCl (Demerol)	Doctors	50–100 mg			

[a]Time given pertains to all drugs listed.
[b]Hashish or charas is a more concentrated form of the active ingredient THC (tetrahydrocannabinol) and is consumed in smaller doses, analogous to vodka-beer ratios.

Pharmacology

Pharmacology

TABLE 10–5 Major Substances Used for Mind Alteration—cont'd

Official Name	Slang Name	Usual Single Adult Dose/Duration	Legitimate Medical Uses (Present and Projected)	Short-Term Effects	Long-Term Effects
NARCOTICS (OPIATES, ANALGESICS)—cont'd					
Methadone (Dolophine)	Dollies, done	2.5–40.0 mg			
Cough syrups (Cheracol, Hycodan, Romilar, etc.)		2–4 oz (for euphoria)/4–6 hr^a			
Dilaudid	DLs, 4s, lords, little D				
HALLUCINOGENS					
LSD (Lysergic acid diethylamide)	Acid, sugar cube, trip, big D	150 µg/10–12 hr	Experimental study of mind and brain function; enhancement of creativity and problem solving; treatment of alcoholism, mental illness, and reduction of intractable pain in the dying person; chemical warfare	Production of visual imagery, increased sensory awareness, anxiety, nausea, impaired coordination; sometimes consciousness expansion	Usually none; sometimes precipitates or intensifies an already existing psychosis (hallucinations); more commonly can produce a panic reaction (extreme hyperactivity)
Psilocybin	Magic mushrooms, God's flesh, rooms	25 mg			
STP	Serenity, tranquility, peace				
DMT	Businessman's Trip	6 mg			
Mescaline (peyote)	Cactus, mesc, mescal, half moon, big chief, bad seed	350 mg/12–14 hr			
PCP (Phencyclidine)	Angel dust, hog, rocket fuel				
MDMA	Ecstasy, XTC, Adam				
MISCELLANEOUS					
Glue, gasoline, and solvents		Variable	None except for antihistamines used for allergy and amyl nitrite for fainting	When used for mind alteration generally produces a "high" (euphoria) with impaired coordination and judgment	Variable—some of the substances can seriously damage the liver or kidney, and some produce hallucinations
Amyl nitrite		1–2 ampules			
Antihistamines		25–50 mg			
Nutmeg		Variable/2 hr			
Nonprescription "sedatives" (Compoze)					
Catnip					
Nitrous oxide					

TABLE 10–6   Common Drugs

Drug and Dosage	Use	Action	◆ Assessment: Side Effects
Adrenergics			
Alpha and beta agonists Epinephrine (Adrenalin)—SC or IM 0.1–1 mg in 1:1000 solution; IV—intracardiac 1:10,000 solution; ophthalmic 1:1000–1:50,000 solution	Asystole, bronchospasm, anaphylaxis, glaucoma	Stimulates pacemaker cells; inhibits histamine and mediates bronchial relaxation; ↓ intraocular pressure	Ventricular arrhythmias, fear, anxiety, anginal pain, decreased renal blood flow, burning of eyes, headache
NURSING IMPLICATIONS: Use TB syringe for greater accuracy; massaging injection site hastens action; repeated injections may cause tissue necrosis; *avoid* injection in buttocks because bacteria in area may lead to gas gangrene; may make mucous plugs in lungs more difficult to dislodge			
Norepinephrine (Levophed)—IV 8–12 µg/min titrated to desired response	Acute hypotension, cardiogenic shock	Increases rate and strength of heartbeat; increases vasoconstriction	Palpitations, pallor, headache, hypertension, anxiety, insomnia, dilated pupils, nausea, vomiting, glycosuria, tissue sloughing
NURSING IMPLICATIONS: Observe vital signs, mentation, skin temperature, and color (earlobes, lips, nailbeds); tissue necrosis occurs with infiltration; antidote is phentolamine 5–10 mg in 10–15 mL normal saline			
Beta agonists Dobutamine (Dobutrex)—IV 1.5–10 µg/kg/min	Acute heart failure	Stimulates cardiac contractile force (positive inotropy); fewer changes in heart rate than dopamine or isoproterenol	Tachycardia, arrhythmias
NURSING IMPLICATIONS: Mix with 5% dextrose; do *not* dilute until ready to use; protect from light; administer with infusion pump; check vital signs constantly; extravasation can produce tissue necrosis; see Norepinephrine			
Dopamine (Inotropin)—IV 1–5 µg/kg/min titrated to desired response; gradually increase to 1–4 µg/kg/min increments at 10–30 min intervals; must maintain at 20 µg/kg/min or less	Acute heart failure	↑ Cardiac contractility; ↑ renal blood flow	Ectopic beats, nausea, vomiting, tachycardia, anginal pain, dyspnea, hypotension
NURSING IMPLICATIONS: Monitor vital signs, urine output, and signs of peripheral ischemia; will cause tissue sloughing if infiltration occurs			
Isoproterenol (Isuprel)—10–15 mg sublingually; IV 0.5–5.0 µg/min in solution	Cardiogenic shock, heart block, bronchospasm—asthma, emphysema	↑ Cardiac contractility; facilitates AV conduction and pacemaker automaticity	Tachyarrhythmias, hypotension, headache, flushing of skin, nausea, tremor, dizziness
NURSING IMPLICATIONS: Monitor vital signs, ECG; oral inhalation solutions must *not* be injected			
Analgesics (see Table 10–10 for Equianalgesic Dosing) Acetaminophen (Tylenol, Datril, Panadol)—PO 325–650 mg q4h	Simple fever or pain	Analgesic and antipyretic actions; no anti-inflammatory or anticoagulant effects	No remarkable side effects when taken for a short period
NURSING IMPLICATIONS: Consult with physician if no relief after 4 d of therapy			
Aspirin (acetylsalicylic acid)—PO or rectal 0.3–0.6 g	Minor aches and pains; fever from colds and influenza; rheumatoid arthritis; anticoagulant therapy	Selectively depresses subcortical levels of CNS	Erosive gastritis with bleeding, coryza, urticaria, nausea, vomiting, tinnitus, impaired hearing, and respiratory alkalosis
NURSING IMPLICATIONS: Administer *with food or after meals;* observe for nasal, oral, or subcutaneous bleeding; push fluids; check *Hct, Hgb, prothrombin times* frequently; *avoid* use in children with flu			

Continued

TABLE 10–6   Common Drugs—cont'd

Drug and Dosage	Use	Action	◆ Assessment: Side Effects
Analgesics—cont'd (see Table 10–10 for Equianalgesic Dosing)			
Butorphanol (Stadol) IM: 1–2 mg IV: 0.5–2 mg	**Obstetric use:** Control pain, especially during labor. *Avoid* in opioid-addicted patients.	30–40 times more potent than meperidine; onset: 2–15 min; duration: 0.5–2 hr	No excessive sedation. Neonatal respiratory depression less than with meperidine. Sinusoidal FHR pattern after administration.
NURSING IMPLICATIONS: Care must be taken that drug is *not* given with meperidine, as it may potentiate effects of meperidine; *avoid* in opioid-addicted patients			
Codeine—PO, IM, or SC 15–60 mg (gr ¼ to 1)	Control pain; may be used during the puerperium	Nonsynthetic narcotic analgesic	Of little use during labor; allergic response; constipation; GI upset
NURSING IMPLICATIONS: Note response to the medication; less respiratory depression; preferred for head injury patient			
Ecotrin (enteric-coated aspirin)	See Aspirin	See Aspirin	See Aspirin
NURSING IMPLICATIONS: See Aspirin; do *not* take with milk or dairy			
Etodolac (Lodine)—PO 400–1200 mg/day, 300–400 q6–8h	Management of osteoarthritis; mild to moderate pain	Inhibits prostaglandin synthesis; suppression of inflammation and pain (NSAID)	Dyspepsia, asthma, drowsiness, dizziness, rash, tinnitus, anaphylaxis
NURSING IMPLICATIONS: Give 30 min *before or* 2 hr *after* meals for rapid effect; may be taken with food to decrease GI irritation			
Fentanyl transdermal (Duragesic)—25–100 μg/hr	Chronic pain; not recommended for postoperative pain **Obstetric use:** Short-acting pain control during labor	Binds to opiate receptors in the CNS to alter response and perception of pain	Drowsiness, confusion, weakness, constipation, dry mouth, nausea, vomiting, anorexia, sweating
NURSING IMPLICATIONS: Apply to upper torso, flat, nonirritated surface; when applying, hold firmly with palm of hand 10–20 sec			
Hydrocodone/Acetaminophen (Vicodin)—PO 5–10 mg q4–6h	Moderate to severe pain	Bind to opiate receptors in CNS; alter perception of and response to painful stimuli	Confusion, sedation, hypotension, constipation
NURSING IMPLICATIONS: Assess: type, location, and intensity of pain before and 1 hr (peak) after giving; prolonged use may lead to physical and psychological dependence; give with *food or milk* to reduce GI irritation			
Hydromorphone (Dilaudid)— PO 2–4 mg q3–6h; IM 1–2 mg q3–6h up to 2–4 mg q4–6h; IV 0.5–1.0 mg q3h	Moderate to severe pain; antitussive	Bind to opiate receptors in the CNS; alter perception and response to pain	Sedation, confusion, hypotension, constipation
NURSING IMPLICATIONS: Give PO with *food or milk;* give IV 2 mg over 3–5 min; *fluids, bulk,* and laxatives to minimize constipation			
Ibuprofen (Motrin)—300–800 mg oral 3–4/day not to exceed 3200 mg/day	Nonsteroid anti-inflammatory, antirheumatic used in chronic arthritis pain	Inhibition of prostaglandin synthesis or release	GI upset, leukopenia; sodium/water retention
NURSING IMPLICATIONS: Give on *empty stomach* for best result; may mix with food if GI upset severe; teach caution when using other medications			
Indomethacin (Indocin)—PO 25 mg 3–4/day; increase to max 200 mg daily in divided doses	Rheumatoid arthritis; bursitis; gouty arthritis	Antipyretic/anti-inflammatory action; inhibits prostaglandin biosynthesis	GI distress, bleeding; rash; headache; blood dyscrasias; corneal changes
NURSING IMPLICATIONS: Monitor GI side effects; administer *after* meals for best effect or *with* food, milk, or antacids if GI symptoms severe			

Pha

TABLE 10–6   Common Drugs—cont'd

Drug and Dosage	Use	Action	◆ Assessment: Side Effects
Analgesics—cont'd			
Ketorolac (Toradol)—PO, IV 10 mg q4–6h; IM 30–60 mg initially, then 15–30 mg q6h; ophthalmic 1 gtt qid for 1 wk	Short-term management of pain; ocular itching due to allergies (NSAID)	Inhibits prostaglandin synthesis producing peripherally mediated analgesia; antipyretic/anti-inflammatory	Drowsiness, dizziness, dyspnea, prolonged bleeding time, dyspepsia

NURSING IMPLICATIONS: May be given routinely or prn; *advise* dentist or MD before any procedure

Meperidine HCl (Demerol)—PO or IM 50–100 mg q3–4h	Pain due to trauma or surgery; allay apprehension before surgery	Acts on CNS to produce analgesia, sedation, euphoria, and respiratory depression	Palpitations, bradycardia, hypotension, nausea, vomiting, syncope, sweating, tremors, convulsions

NURSING IMPLICATIONS: Check *respiratory rate* and depth before giving drug; give IM, because subcutaneous administration is painful and can cause local irritation

	Obstetric use: maternal relaxation may either slow labor or speed up labor	Depresses CNS, maternal and fetal; allays apprehension; PO peak action—1–2 hr; IM peak action first hour	Maternal side effects same as above; also can depress fetus

NURSING IMPLICATIONS: Monitor maternal vital signs, contractions, progress of labor, and response to drug; fetal heart rate; if delivery occurs during peak action, prepare to give narcotic antagonist to mother or neonate or both

Morphine SO₄—PO 10–30 mg (Roxanol, MS Contin); SC 8–15 mg; IV 4–10 mg; rectal 10–20 mg	Control pain and relieve fear, apprehension, restlessness, as in pulmonary edema	Depresses CNS reception of pain and ability to interpret stimuli; depresses respiratory center in medulla	Nausea, vomiting, flushing, confusion, urticaria, depressed rate and depth of respirations, decreased blood pressure

NURSING IMPLICATIONS: Check rate and depth of *respirations* before administering drug; observe for gas pains and *abdominal distention*; smaller doses for aged; monitor vital signs; observe for postural hypotension

	Obstetric use: preeclampsia, eclampsia; uterine dysfunction; pain relief	Increases cerebral blood flow; provides antihypertensive action; CNS depressant	Respiratory and circulatory depression in mother and neonate; may depress contractions

NURSING IMPLICATIONS: Observe for level of sedation, respirations, arousability, and deep-tendon reflex; give narcotic antagonist as necessary; check I&O (*urinary retention* possible)

Nalbuphine (Nubain) IV: 1 mg at 6–10 min intervals	**Obstetric use:** pain relief during labor. *Avoid* in opioid-addicted patients.	Onset: 2–15 min; duration: 1–4 hr	Increased sedation and limited ceiling effect; ceiling effect for neonatal respiratory depression

NURSING IMPLICATIONS: Less nausea and vomiting and sedation if given with PCA. Prophylactic nalbuphine seems unable to prevent pruritis

Naproxen (Naprosyn)—PO 250–500 mg bid	Mild to moderate pain; dysmenorrhea; rheumatoid arthritis; osteoarthritis (NSAID)	Inhibits prostaglandin synthesis; suppression of inflammation	Headache, drowsiness, dizziness, nausea, dyspepsia, constipation, bleeding

NURSING IMPLICATIONS: Take with a full glass of *water; avoid* exposure to sun

Oxycodone HCl (Percodan, Tylox)—PO 3–20 mg; SC 5 mg	**Postpartum use:** control pain; may be used during puerperium; 5–6 times more potent than codeine .	Less potent and addicting than morphine; for moderate pain—episiotomy and "afterpains"; peak action 1 hr	See Morphine SO₄

NURSING IMPLICATIONS: Administer per order and observe for effect

Continued

TABLE 10–6 Common Drugs—cont'd

Drug and Dosage	Use	Action	◆ Assessment: Side Effects
Analgesics—cont'd			
Pentazocine (Talwin)—PO 50–100 mg; IM 30–60 mg q3–4h	Relief of moderate to severe pain	Narcotic antagonist, opioid antagonist properties, equivalent to codeine	Respiratory depression, nausea, vomiting, dizziness, lightheadedness, seizures
NURSING IMPLICATIONS: Monitor *respirations,* BP; *caution* with patients with MI, head injuries, COPD			
Antacids (see Antiulcer)			
Antiadrenal			
Aminoglutethimide (Cytadren)—250 mg q6h	Cushing's	Inhibits enzymatic conversion of cholesterol to pregnenolone, thus reducing synthesis of adrenal glucocorticoids/mineralocorticoids	Cortical hypofunction, hypotension, hypothyroidism
NURSING IMPLICATIONS: Monitor: vital signs, lab values, disease signs and symptoms; observe frequently during periods of stress			
Antianemics	Iron deficiency anemia; prophylactically during infancy, childhood, pregnancy	Corrects nutritional iron deficiency anemia	Nausea, vomiting, anorexia, constipation, diarrhea; yellow-brown discoloration of eyes, teeth
Ferrous sulfate (Feosol, Fer-in-Sol)—adults, PO 300 mg–1.2 g qd; children under 6 yr, PO 75–225 mg qd; 6–12 yr, PO 120–600 mg qd			
NURSING IMPLICATIONS: To minimize GI distress, give *with* meals; do *not* give with antacids or tea; liquid form should be taken through straw to prevent *staining* of teeth; causes dark-green/black stool			
Antianginals	Hypertension: angina; arrhythmias	Blocks (cardiac) beta-adrenergic receptors	Fatigue, weakness, bradycardia, heart failure, pulmonary edema
Atenolol (Tenormin)—PO 50–150 mg daily; IV 5 mg initially, wait 10 min, then another 5 mg			
NURSING IMPLICATIONS: Give 1 mg/min IV; check vital signs; assess for signs of fluid *overload*			
Isosorbide dinitrate (Isordil, Isorbid)—sublingual 2.5–10.0 mg q5–10min for 3 doses; PO 5–10 mg initially, 10–40 mg q6h	Acute angina: long-term prophylaxis for angina; heart failure	Produces vasodilation, decreases preload	Headache, dizziness, hypotension, tachycardia
NURSING IMPLICATIONS: *Avoid* eating, drinking, or smoking until sublingual tablets are dissolved; change positions *slowly;* aspirin or acetaminophen for headache			
Nitroglycerin—sublingual 0.25–0.6 mg prn; transdermal (patch) 2.5–15.0 mg/day; topical 2–3 inches q8h; IV 10–20 µg/min	Angina pectoris; adjunctive treatment in MI, heart failure, hypertension (IV form)	Directly relaxes smooth muscle, dilating blood vessels; lowers peripheral vascular resistance; increases blood flow	Faintness, throbbing headache, vomiting, flushing, hypotension, visual disturbances
NURSING IMPLICATIONS: Instruct patient to sit or lie down when taking drug, to reduce *hypotensive* effect; onset 1–3 min; may take 1–3 doses at 5 min intervals to relieve pain; up to *10/day* may be allowed; if headache occurs, tell patient to expel tab as soon as pain relief occurs; keep drug at bedside or on person; watch *expiration* dates—tabs lose potency with exposure to air and humidity; *alcohol* ingestion soon after taking may produce shocklike syndrome from drop in BP; *smoking* causes vasoconstricting effect; causes burning under tongue; may crush between teeth to ↑ absorption			
Antiarrhythmics (also see Calcium Channel Blockers)			
Bretylium (Bretylol)—IV 0.5–10 mg/kg q6h; IM 5–10 mg/kg (max 250 mg in one site)	Ventricular fibrillation; ventricular tachycardia	Inhibits norepinephrine release from sympathetic nerve endings; increased fibrillation threshold	Worsening of arrhythmia; tachycardia and increased BP initially; nausea, vomiting; hypotension later
NURSING IMPLICATIONS: Monitor BP and cardiac status closely; *rotate* IM injection sites; no more than 5 mL/site			

TABLE 10–6 Common Drugs—cont'd

Drug and Dosage	Use	Action	◆ Assessment: Side Effects
Antiarrhythmics—cont'd			
Diphenylhydantoin (Dilantin)—PO 100–200 mg 3–4 times daily; IV loading dose 10–15 mg/kg (not to exceed 50 mg/min), 50–100 mg over 5–10 min	Digitalis toxicity; ventricular ectopy	Depresses pacemaker activity in SA node and Purkinje tissue without slowing conduction velocity	Severe pain if administered in small vein; ataxia, vertigo, nystagmus, seizures, confusion, skin eruptions, hypotension if administered too fast

NURSING IMPLICATIONS: With IV use monitor vital signs; observe for CNS side effects; have O_2 on hand; seizure precautions (padded side rails, nonmetal airway; suction, mouth gag); also see Anticonvulsants

Lidocaine HCl—IV 50–100 mg; bolus; 1–4 mg/kg/min, IV drip	Ventricular tachycardia; PVCs	Depresses myocardial response to abnormally generated impulses	Drowsiness, dizziness, nervousness, confusion, paresthesias

NURSING IMPLICATIONS: Monitor vital signs; observe for signs of CNS toxicity; monitor ECG for *prolonged PR* interval

Procainamide HCl (Pronestyl)—PO, IM 500–1000 mg 4–6 times qd; IV 1 g	Atrial and ventricular arrhythmias; PVCs; overdose of digitalis; general anesthesia	Depresses myocardium; lengthens conduction time between atria and ventricles	Polyarthralgia, fever, chills, urticaria, nausea, vomiting, psychoses, rapid decrease in BP

NURSING IMPLICATIONS: Check pulse rate *before* giving; monitor heart action during IV administration

Propranolol HCl (Inderal)—0.5–3.0 mg IV push (up to 3 mg); 20–60 mg orally 3–4 times daily	Ventricular ectopy; angina unresponsive to nitrites, paroxysmal atrial tachycardia; hypertension	Beta-adrenergic blocker, ↓ cardiac contractility, ↓ heart rate, ↓ myocardial oxygen requirements	Bradycardia, hypotension, vertigo, paresthesia of hands

NURSING IMPLICATIONS: Instruct patient to take pulse *before* each dose; do *not* give to patients with history of asthma or chronic obstructive pulmonary disease; no smoking, because hypertension may occur

Quinidine SO_4—PO 0.2–0.6 g q2h loading dose; maintenance: 400–1000 mg tid–qid; IV 5–10 mg/kg over 30–60 min	Atrial fibrillation; PAT; ventricular tachycardia; PVCs	Lengthens conduction time in atria and ventricles; blocks vagal stimulation of heart	Nausea, vomiting, diarrhea, vertigo, tremor, headache, abdominal cramps, AV block, cardiac arrest

NURSING IMPLICATIONS: *Count pulse before* giving; report changes in rate, quality, or rhythm; give drug *with food*; monitor BP daily

Antiasthmatics			
Cromolyn sodium—inhale, 1 cap 4 times qd	Perennial bronchial asthma (not acute asthma or status asthmaticus)	Inhibits release of bronchoconstrictors—histamine and SRS-A; suppresses allergic response	Cough, hoarseness, wheezing, dry mouth, bitter aftertaste, urticaria, urinary frequency

NURSING IMPLICATIONS: Instruct on use of inhaler—exhale; tilt head back; inhale rapidly, deeply, steadily; remove inhaler; exhale—repeat until dose is taken; gargle or drink water after treatment

Anticholelithics			
Ursodeoxycholic (Actigal)	Gallstones	Dissolves gallstones	Diarrhea, *avoid* concurrent use with bile acid sequestrants

NURSING IMPLICATIONS: *Monitor* for pain, GI distress

Anticholinergics (antimuscarinics)			
Atropine, SO_4—0.3–1.2 mg PO, SC, IM, or IV; ophthalmic 0.5–1.0% up to 6 times qd	Peptic ulcer; spasms of GI tract, Stokes-Adams syndrome; control excessive secretions during surgery	Blocks parasympathomimetic effects of acetylcholine on effector organs	Dry mouth, tachycardia, blurred vision, drowsiness, skin flushing, urinary retention; *contraindications:* glaucoma and paralytic ileus

NURSING IMPLICATIONS: Observe for postural *hypotension* in ambulating patients; administer cautiously in aged; and monitor vital signs for pulse and respiratory rate changes

Continued

Pharmacology

TABLE 10–6   Common Drugs—cont'd

Drug and Dosage	Use	Action	◆ Assessment: Side Effects
Anticholinergics (antimuscarinics)—cont'd			
Dicyclomine (Bentyl) 10–20 mg 3–4 × day	Diverticulosis	Antispasmodic	Blurred vision, constipation, dry eyes, dry mouth
NURSING IMPLICATIONS: Report symptoms listed under side effects, abdominal pain			
Glycopyrrolate (Robinul)—PO 1-2 mg bid/tid; IM, IV 4.4 mcg/kg (preop); 100-200 mcg qid (ulcer)	Inhibit salivation and respiratory secretions; peptic ulcer disease	Inhibits action of acetylcholine (antimuscarinic action)	Tachycardia, dry mouth, urinary hesitancy
NURSING IMPLICATIONS: Give 30-60 min. *before* meals; do *not* give within 1 h of antacids; IM or IV may be given undiluted.			
Hyoscyamine (Levsinex) 0.125–0.5 mg 3-4 × day; or 0.375 mg twice a day in released tablets	Diverticulosis	Manages spasms of irritable bowel syndrome	Constipation, dry mouth, blurred vision
NURSING IMPLICATIONS: *Monitor* for: pain, bleeding, constipation, drug reaction			
Propantheline bromide (Pro-Banthine)—PO 15 mg qid; IM or IV 30 mg	Decreases hypertonicity and hypersecretion of GI tract; ulcerative colitis; peptic ulcer	Blocks neural transmission at ganglia of autonomic nervous system and at parasympathetic effector organs	Nausea, gastric fullness, constipation, mydriasis
NURSING IMPLICATIONS: Give *before* meals; observe urinary output to *avoid retention,* particularly in elderly; mouth care to relieve dryness; *contraindicated* with glaucoma			
Tincture of belladonna— 0.3–0.6 mL tid	Hypermotility of stomach; bowel, biliary, and renal colic; prostatitis	Blocks parasympathomimetic effects of acetylcholine	Dry mouth, thirst, dilated pupils, skin flushing, elevated temperature, delirium
NURSING IMPLICATIONS: Administer 30–60 min *before* meals; observe for side effects; *physostigmine salicylate* is antidote			
Anticoagulants			
Enoxaparin (Lovenox)— 30–40mg bid SC, 7–10 days; or 1 mg/kg q12h	Deep vein thrombosis; prophylaxis before knee and abdominal surgery	Potentiates inhibitory effect of antithrombin	Bleeding, anemia, thrombocytopenia
NURSING IMPLICATIONS: Observe injection sites for: hematomas, ecchymosis, or inflammation; *ice cube massage* at site prior to injection may lessen bruising			
Heparin—initial dose: IV 5,000–20,000–40,000 U followed by infusion over 24 hr	Acute thromboembolic emergencies	Prevents thrombin formation	Hematuria, bleeding gums, ecchymosis
NURSING IMPLICATIONS: Observe clotting times—should be 20–30 min; antagonist is *protamine sulfate*			
Warfarin sodium (Coumadin)—initial dose: PO 10–15 mg; maintenance dose: PO 2–10 mg qd	Venous thrombosis; atrial fibrillation with embolization; pulmonary emboli; myocardial infarction	Depresses liver synthesis of prothrombin and factors VII, IX, and X	Minor or major hemorrhage, alopecia, fever, nausea, diarrhea, dermatitis
NURSING IMPLICATIONS: Drug effects last 3–4 days; antagonist is vitamin K; *avoid* foods high in vitamin K; *no* aspirin			
Anticoagulant Antidotes			
Protamine sulfate 1%—IV 10 mg/mL slowly; 1 mg/100 U heparin	Overdose of heparin	Positive electrostatic charge inactivates negatively charged heparin molecules	Excessive coagulation; hypotension, bradycardia, dyspnea
NURSING IMPLICATIONS: Slow IV; no more than 50 mg in 10 min period; monitor VS continuously; check APTT for effectiveness			

TABLE 10–6   Common Drugs—cont'd

Drug and Dosage	Use	Action	◆ Assessment: Side Effects
Anticoagulant Antidotes—cont'd			
Vitamin K₁ (Aquamephyton, Konakion)—PO, IM, SC 2.5–25.0 mg; 0.5–1.0 mg in newborns	Warfarin (Coumadin) hypoprothrombinemia; hemorrhagic disease in newborns	Counteracts the inhibitory effects of oral anticoagulants on hepatic synthesis of vitamin K–dependent clotting factors	Flushing, hypotension, allergic reactions; reappearance of clotting problems (high doses)

> NURSING IMPLICATIONS: Give IV only if absolutely necessary; dilute with preservative-free 0.9% NaCl, D₅W, or D₅NaCl; protect solution *from light;* repeat injection may cause redness and pain; check PT for drug effect

Anticonvulsants			
Carbamazepine (Tegretol) 200 mg twice/day (range: 600–1200/day in divided doses)	Multiple sclerosis	Decreases synaptic transmission in CNS by affecting sodium channels in neurons	Contraindicated in hypersensitivity, bone marrow depression; drowsiness, ataxia, agranulocytosis, aplastic anemia

> NURSING IMPLICATIONS: *Monitor:* CBC, liver function, ECG. Therapeutic levels should be 6–12 mcg/mL; take medication as directed around the clock; use sunscreen due to photosensitivity

Clonazepam (Klonopin)—PO 1.5 mg in 3 doses initially, 0.5–1.0 mg every third day	Absence seizures (petit mal seizures, myoclonic seizures)	Produces anticonvulsant and sedative effects in the CNS, mechanism unknown	Drowsiness, ataxia, behavioral changes

> NURSING IMPLICATIONS: Give *with* food; evaluate *liver enzymes, CBC,* and *platelets; avoid* abrupt withdrawal—may cause status epilepticus

Diazepam (Valium)—PO 2–10 mg bid–qid; IM or IV 5–10 mg	All types of seizures	Induces calming effect on limbic system, thalamus, and hypothalamus	Drowsiness, ataxia, paradoxical increase in CNS excitability

> NURSING IMPLICATIONS: IV may cause phlebitis; give IV injection slowly, because respiratory arrest can occur; inject IM deeply into tissue

Ethosuximide (Zarontin)—PO 500 mg/day, increase by 250 mg/day until effective	Absence seizures	Depresses motor cortex and reduces CNS sensitivity to convulsive nerve stimuli	GI distress: nausea, vomiting, cramps, diarrhea, anorexia; blood dyscrasias

> NURSING IMPLICATIONS: Administer *with* meals; regular *CBC;* precautions to avoid injury from drowsiness

Magnesium salts 4–5 g by IV infusion	Cirrhosis	Osmotically active in GI tract	Use caution in renal failure; *contraindicated* in: hypermagnesemia, anuria, heart block

> NURSING IMPLICATIONS: *Monitor:* vital signs, seizure precautions, I&O; *respiratory rate must be 16* before administration

Magnesium sulfate—PO 1–5 g/IM or IV 1–4 g loading dose, followed by continuous infusion (2–3 g/hr.)	Control seizures in pregnancy, epilepsy; relief of acute constipation; reduces edema, inflammation, and itching of skin; may inhibit preterm contractions	Depresses CNS and smooth, cardiac, and skeletal muscle; promotes osmotic retention of fluid	Flushing, sweating, extreme thirst, complete heart block, dehydration, depressed or absent reflexes, ↓ respirations

> NURSING IMPLICATIONS: If given IV, monitor vital signs continuously; I&O; use with caution in patients with *impaired renal* function; observe mother and newborn for signs of toxicity if given near birth; antidote: calcium gluconate

Phenytoin or diphenylhydantoin (Dilantin) SO₄—PO 30–100 mg 3–4 times qd; IM 100–200 mg 3–4 times qd; IV 150–250 mg	Psychomotor epilepsy, convulsive seizures; ventricular arrhythmias	Depresses motor cortex by preventing spread of abnormal electrical impulses	Nervousness, ataxia, gastric distress, nystagmus, slurred speech, hallucinations, gingival hyperplasia

> NURSING IMPLICATIONS: Give *with* meals *or* pc; frequent and diligent mouth care; advise patient that urine may turn *pink to red-brown;* teach patient signs of adverse reactions; mix IV with normal saline (precipitates with D₅W)

Continued

TABLE 10–6   **Common Drugs—cont'd**

Drug and Dosage	Use	Action	◆ Assessment: Side Effects
Anticonvulsants—cont'd			
Primidone (Mysoline)—PO 100–250 mg, increase over 10 days not to exceed 2 g/day.	Tonic-clonic, focal, or local seizures	Inhibits abnormal brain electrical activity; dose-dependent CNS depression	Excessive sedation or ataxia, vertigo
NURSING IMPLICATIONS: Careful neurological, cardiovascular, and respiratory assessment; have resuscitation equipment available			
Valproic acid (Depakene)—PO 15 mg/kg/day, increase up to 60 mg/kg/day	Absence, tonic-clonic, myoclonic, focal, or local seizures	Inhibits spread of abnormal discharges through brain	Nausea, vomiting, diarrhea (disappear over time); drowsiness or sedation if taken in combination with other anticonvulsants
NURSING IMPLICATIONS: Assess responses; monitor blood levels; precautions against excessive sedation; *discourage alcohol* use			
Antidiarrheals			
Diphenoxylate HCl with atropine sulfate (Lomotil)—PO 5–10 mg tid–qid	Diarrhea	Increases intestinal tone and decreases propulsive peristalsis	Rash, drowsiness, dizziness, depression, abdominal distention, headache, blurred vision, nausea
NURSING IMPLICATIONS: May *potentiate* action of barbiturates, opiates, and other depressants; closely observe patients receiving these drugs, and administer narcotic antagonists such as levallorphan tartrate (Lorfan), naloxone HCl (Narcan), and nalorphine HCl (Naline) as ordered; administer cautiously to patients with hepatic dysfunction—may precipitate *hepatic coma*			
Kaolin with pectin (Kaopectate)—adults, PO 60–120 mL after each bowel movement (BM); children over 12, PO 60 mL; 6–12 yr, PO 30–60 mL; 3–6 yr, P0 15–30 mL after each BM	Diarrhea	Reported to absorb irritants and soothe	Granuloma of the stomach
NURSING IMPLICATIONS: Do *not* administer for more than 2 days, in presence of fever, or to children younger than 3 yr			
Paregoric or camphorated opium tincture—5–10 mL q2h, not more than qid	Diarrhea	Acts directly on intestinal smooth muscle to increase tone and decrease propulsive peristalsis	Occasional nausea; prolonged use may produce dependence
NURSING IMPLICATIONS: Contains approximately 1.6 mg morphine or 16 mg opium and is subject to federal narcotic regulations; administer with partial glass of water to facilitate passage into stomach; observe number and consistency of stools—discontinue drug as soon as diarrhea is controlled; keep in tight *light-resistant* bottles			
Antiemetics			
Chlorpromazine (Thorazine)—preop IM 12.5–25.0 g 1–2 hr before; IV 25–50 mg; PO 10–25 mg q4–6h; IM 25–50 mg q3–4h; suppository 50–100 mg q6–8h	Nausea, vomiting, hiccups, preoperative sedation, psychoses	Alters the effects of dopamine in the CNS; anticholinergic, alpha-adrenergic blocking	Sedation, extrapyramidal reactions, dry eyes, blurred vision, hypotension, constipation, dry mouth, photosensitivity
NURSING IMPLICATIONS: Keep *flat* 30 min after IM; change positions slowly; frequent mouth care; may turn urine *pink* to *red-brown*			
Prochlorperazine dimaleate (Compazine)—5–30 mg qid PO, IM, rectal	Nausea, vomiting, and retching	See Trimethobenzamide HCl	Drowsiness, orthostatic hypotension, palpitations, blurred vision, diplopia, headache
NURSING IMPLICATIONS: Use *cautiously* in children, pregnant women, and patients with liver disease			

TABLE 10–6   Common Drugs—cont'd

Drug and Dosage	Use	Action	◆ Assessment: Side Effects
Antiemetics—cont'd			
Trimethobenzamide HCl (Tigan)—250 mg qid, PO, IM, rectal	Nausea; vomiting	Suppresses chemoreceptors in the trigger zone located in the medulla oblongata	Drowsiness, vertigo; diarrhea, headache, hypotension; jaundice; blurred vision; rigid muscles

NURSING IMPLICATIONS: Give deep IM to prevent escape of solution; can cause edema, pain, and burning

Antifungal			
Amphotericin B (Fungizone)—IV 5 mg/250 mL dextrose over 4–6 hr (to 1 mg/kg body weight)	Severe fungal infections; histoplasmosis	Fungistatic or fungicidal; binds to sterols in fungal cell membrane, altering cell permeability	Febrile reactions; chills, nausea, vomiting; muscle/joint pain; renal damage; hypotension, tachycardia, arrhythmias; hypokalemia

NURSING IMPLICATIONS: Monitor for side effects; thrombophlebitis at IV site; BUN >40; creatinine >3; stop drug because of *nephrotoxicity*

Ketoconazole (Nizoral)—oral 200–400 mg daily	Histoplasmosis, systemic fungal infections	Antifungal	Headache, fatigue, dizziness; nausea, vomiting; decreased libido, impotence; gynecomastia, especially in men

NURSING IMPLICATIONS: Administer *with* food; *avoid* concomitant use of antacids, H_2 blockers; advise to report side effects

Nystatin (Nilstat, Mycostatin)—PO, rectal, vaginal: 100,000–1,000,000 U 3–4 times qd	Skin, mucous membrane infections *(Candida albicans)*; oral thrush, vaginitis; intestinal candidiasis	Fungistatic and fungicidal; binds to sterols in fungal cell membrane	Nausea, vomiting, GI distress, diarrhea

NURSING IMPLICATIONS: *Oral* use—clear mouth of food; keep medication in mouth several minutes before swallowing; *vaginal*—usually requires 2 wk therapy; continue use during menses; consult physician before using anti-infective douches; determine predisposing factors to infection (diabetes, pregnancy, antibiotics, tight-fitting nylon pantyhose)

Antigout			
Allopurinol (Lopurin, Zyloprim)—PO 100 mg initially, 300 mg daily with meals or pc	Primary hyperuricemia, secondary hyperuricemia with cancer therapy	Lowers plasma and urinary uric acid levels; no analgesic, anti-inflammatory, or uricosuric actions	Rash, itching; nausea, vomiting; anemia; drowsiness

NURSING IMPLICATIONS: Report side effects, particularly *rash*, because drug must be stopped; *avoid* driving or other complex tasks until drug effects known; give at least *3000 mL* fluid daily; minimum urine output of *2000 mL/day*; keep urine neutral or *alkaline* with sodium bicarbonate or potassium citrate; use *cautiously* with: liver disease, impaired renal function, history of peptic ulcers, lower GI disease, or bone marrow depression

Colchicine—PO 1.0–1.2 mg acute phase; 0.5–2.0 mg nightly with milk or food; IV 1–2 mg initially	Gouty arthritis, acute gout	Inhibits leukocyte migration and phagocytosis in gouty joints; nonanalgesic, nonuricosuric	Nausea, vomiting, diarrhea, abdominal pain, peripheral neuritis, bone marrow depression (sore throat, bleeding gums, sore mouth), tissue and nerve necrosis with IV use

NURSING IMPLICATIONS: Do *not* dilute IV form with normal saline or 5% dextrose—use sterile water to prevent precipitation; infuse over 3–5 min IV; potentiate drug action with *alkaline ash foods* (milk, most fruits and vegetables)

Probenecid (Benemid)—PO 0.25–0.50 g twice daily pc	Chronic gouty arthritis, no value in acute; adjuvant therapy with penicillin to increase plasma levels	Inhibits renal tubular resorption of uric acid; no analgesic or anti-inflammatory activity; competitively inhibits renal tubular secretion of penicillin and many weak organic acids	Headache, nausea, vomiting, anorexia, sore gums, urinary frequency, flushing

NURSING IMPLICATIONS: Give *with* food, milk, or prescribed antacid; 3000 mL/day fluids; *avoid* alcohol, which increases serum urates; do *not* take with aspirin—inhibits action of drug; renal function and hematology should be evaluated frequently; during acute gout, give with colchicine

Continued

Pharmacology

TABLE 10–6 Common Drugs—cont'd

Drug and Dosage	Use	Action	◆ Assessment: Side Effects
Antihistamines Astemizole (Hismanal)—PO 10 mg/day	Relief of allergic symptoms (rhinitis, urticaria); less sedating	Blocks the effects of histamine	Drowsiness, headache, fatigue, stimulation, dry mouth, rash, increased appetite (none of these are frequent)
NURSING IMPLICATIONS: Take *1 hr before* or *2 hr after* eating; good oral hygiene; may need to reduce calories			
Chlorpheniramine maleate (Chlor-Trimeton)—PO 2–4 mg tid–qid; SC, IM, or IV 10–20 mg	Asthma; hay fever; serum reactions; anaphylaxis	Inhibits action of histamine	Nausea, gastritis, diarrhea, headache, dryness of mouth and nose, nervousness, irritability
NURSING IMPLICATIONS: IV may drop BP; give slowly; caution patient about drowsiness			
Diphenhydramine HCl (Benadryl)—PO 25–50 mg tid–qid; IM or IV 10–20 mg	Allergic and pyrogenic reactions; motion sickness; radiation sickness; hay fever; Parkinson's disease	Inhibits action of histamine on receptor cells; decreases action of acetylcholine	Sedation, dizziness, inability to concentrate, headache, anorexia, dermatitis, nausea, diplopia, insomnia
NURSING IMPLICATIONS: *Avoid* use in newborn or preterm infants and patients with glaucoma; supervise ambulation; caution against driving or operating mechanical devices; excitation or hallucinations may occur in children			
Nedocromil (Tilade) inhalation, 2 sprays	Asthma	Prevents the release of histamine from sensitized mast cells	Hypersensitivity, acute asthma attacks; does not relieve (may accelerate) bronchospasm
NURSING IMPLICATIONS: Monitor pulmonary function; use only as prescribed; if symptoms increase, notify health care professional; teach proper use of metered-dose inhaler			
Terfenadine (Seldane)—PO 60 mg 2 times daily	Relief of allergic symptoms, nasal and dermatoses	Blocks the effects of histamine	Drowsiness, sedation, headache, nausea, abdominal pain, dry mouth
NURSING IMPLICATIONS: Risk of *arrhythmias* if taking certain antibiotics; false-negative skin test reactions; take *with* food or milk			
Antihyperglycemics *Alpha-glucosidase inhibitor* Acarbose (Precose) 25 mg 3 × day; may be increased q4–8wk (range: 50–100 mg 3 × day)	Diabetes	Alpha-glucosidase inhibitors/oral hypoglycemic	Overdose signs: flatulence, diarrhea, abdominal discomfort
NURSING IMPLICATIONS: Observe for side effects of hypoglycemia; take same time each day; do *not* double dose; therapy is long term			
Biguanide Metformin (Glucophage) 500 mg 2 × day; may increase by 500 mg to 2000 mg/day	Diabetes	Decreases hepatic production of glucose; decreases intestinal absorption of glucose	Lactic acidosis; nausea, vomiting, diarrhea, abdominal bloating
NURSING IMPLICATIONS: Monitor glucose levels; take medication as directed; dietary compliance; metallic taste resolves spontaneously			
Sulfonylureas Acetohexamide (Dymelor)— PO 200–1500 mg qd; 1–2/day; duration 12–24 hr	Oral hypoglycemic; antidiabetic	Lowers blood glucose by stimulating insulin release from beta cells; effective only if pancreas has ability to produce insulin	Hypoglycemia (profuse sweating, hunger, headache, nausea, confusion, ataxia, coma), skin rashes, bone marrow depression, liver toxicity
NURSING IMPLICATIONS: Drug therapy must be combined with diet therapy, weight control, and planned, graded exercise; alcohol intolerance may occur (disulfiram reaction—flushing, pounding headache, sweating, nausea, vomiting); should *not* be taken at bedtime unless specifically ordered (nocturnal hypoglycemia more likely); take at *same time* each day; *contraindicated* in liver disease, renal disease, pregnancy			

TABLE 10–6   Common Drugs—cont'd

Drug and Dosage	Use	Action	◆ Assessment: Side Effects
Antihyperglycemics—cont'd			
Chlorpropamide (Diabinese)—PO 100–500 mg maintenance; not to exceed 750 mg/day; duration 30–60 hr	See Acetohexamide	See Acetohexamide	See Acetohexamide
NURSING IMPLICATIONS: See Acetohexamide			
Glimepiride (Amaryl), glipizide (Glucotrol); 1–2 mg once daily; increase slowly up to 8 mg in one dose; 15 mg/day in divided dose	Diabetes mellitus, adult onset	Stimulate release of insulin from pancreas	Photosensitivity, hypoglycemia; ingestion of alcohol may induce reaction
NURSING IMPLICATIONS: Observe for signs of hypoglycemia; long-term therapy; *avoid* aspirin, alcohol; follow prescribed diet/exercise program			
Glyburide (Micronase)—PO 2.5–5 mg initially; 1.25–20 mg/day	See Acetohexamide	See Acetohexamide	See Acetohexamide
NURSING IMPLICATIONS: See Acetohexamide			
Tolazamide (Tolinase)—PO 100–500 mg; 1/day; duration 10–14 hr	See Acetohexamide	See Acetohexamide	See Acetohexamide
NURSING IMPLICATIONS: See Acetohexamide			
Tolbutamide (Orinase)—PO 500–3000 mg; 2–3/day; duration 6–12 hr	See Acetohexamide	See Acetohexamide	See Acetohexamide
NURSING IMPLICATIONS: See Acetohexamide			
Insulin—rapid acting Crystalline zinc (Regular) (Humulin R) (clear)—onset 0.5–1.0 hr; peak 2–4 hr; duration 6–8 hr	Poorly controlled diabetes; trauma; surgery, coma	Enhances transmembrane passage of glucose into cells; promotes carbohydrate, fat, and protein metabolism	Hypoglycemia (profuse sweating, nausea, hunger, headache, confusion, ataxia, coma), allergic reaction at injection site
NURSING IMPLICATIONS: Monitor blood and urine for glucose and acetone levels; insulin currently being used can be kept at *room temperature for 1 mo;* refrigerate stock insulin only; rotate injection sites; cold insulin leads to lipodystrophy, reduced absorption, and local reaction; only form of insulin that is given IV			
Prompt insulin zinc suspension (Semilente) purified pork (cloudy)—onset 1–2 hr; peak 4–10 hr; duration 12–16 hr	Patients allergic to Regular; used in combination with longer-lasting insulin	See Crystalline zinc (Regular)	See Crystalline zinc (Regular)
NURSING IMPLICATIONS: See Crystalline zinc (Regular); compatible with all Lente preparations			
Insulin—intermediate acting NPH insulin (isophane insulin suspension) purified pork (Humulin N$^+$) (cloudy)—onset 1–2 hr; peak 5–12 hr; duration 18–24 hr	Patients who can be controlled by one dose per day	See Crystalline zinc (Regular)	See Crystalline zinc (Regular)
NURSING IMPLICATIONS: Gently rotate vial between palms, invert several times to mix; do *not* shake; see Crystalline zinc (Regular)			

Pharmacology

Continued

TABLE 10–6 Common Drugs—cont'd

Drug and Dosage	Use	Action	◆ Assessment: Side Effects
Antihyperglycemics—cont'd			
Insulin zinc suspension (Lente insulin) (cloudy)—onset 1–3 hr; peak 6–12 hr; duration 18–24 hr	Patients allergic to NPH	See Crystalline zinc (Regular)	See Crystalline zinc (Regular)
NURSING IMPLICATIONS: See Crystalline zinc (Regular)			
Insulin—slow acting Extended insulin zinc suspension (Ultralente, Humulin U) purified beef (cloudy)—onset 4–8 hr; peak 12–24 hr; duration 36 hr	Often mixed with Semilente for 24 hr curve	See Crystalline zinc (Regular)	See Crystalline zinc (Regular)
NURSING IMPLICATIONS: See Crystalline zinc (Regular)			
Antihypertensives			
Captopril (Capoten)—PO 50 mg tid	Hypertension, heart failure	Prevents production of angiotensin II; vasodilation	Hypotension, loss of taste perception, proteinuria, rashes
NURSING IMPLICATIONS: Monitor VS and weight; take 1 hr *before* and 2 hr *after* meals; change positions slowly; *avoid* salt and salt substitutes			
Clonidine (Catapres)—PO 200–600 mcg/day; transdermal 100–300 mcg applied every 7 days	Mild to moderate hypertension; also used for epidural pain management	Stimulates alpha-adrenergic receptors in CNS	Drowsiness; dry mouth; postural hypotension
NURSING IMPLICATIONS: Instruct patient to take same time each day; *avoid* sudden position changes; *report:* mental depression, swelling of feet, paleness or cold feeling in fingertips or toes, vivid dreams or nightmares			
Guanadrel (Hylorel)—PO 5 mg bid (range: 20–75 mg/d)	Moderate to severe hypertension	Prevents release of norepinephrine in response to sympathetic stimulation	Confusion; fainting; fatigue; diarrhea; orthostatic hypotension; dizziness
NURSING IMPLICATIONS: Give with *diuretics* to minimize tolerance and fluid retention; *weigh* twice weekly; less side effects after 8 wk of therapy			
Guanfacine hydrochloride (Tenex)—PO 1 mg daily to maximum dose of 3 mg/day	Hypertension, in combination with thiazide-like diuretics	Centrally acting alpha-adrenergic receptor agonist	Drowsiness; weakness; dizziness; dry mouth; constipation; impotence
NURSING IMPLICATIONS: Warn patient *not* to drive or perform activities requiring alertness; take at *bedtime* to minimize sedation; monitor BP and pulse			
Guanethidine SO$_4$ (Ismelin)—PO 10–50 mg qd in divided doses	Severe to moderately severe hypertension	Blocks norepinephrine at postganglionic synapses	Orthostatic hypotension, diarrhea, inhibition of ejaculation
NURSING IMPLICATIONS: *Postural hypotension* is marked in the morning and *accentuated* by hot weather, alcohol, and exercise; teach to rise slowly, with assistance			
Hydralazine HCl (Apresoline)—PO 10–50 mg qid	Moderate hypertension	Dilates peripheral blood vessels, increases renal blood flow	Palpitations, tachycardia, angina pectoris, tremors, depression
NURSING IMPLICATIONS: Encourage moderation in exercise and identification of stressful stimuli			
	Obstetric use: preeclampsia, eclampsia	Relaxes peripheral blood vessels (opens vascular bed—physiological dehydration)	Headache, heart palpitation, gastric irritation, coronary insufficiency, edema, chills, fever, severe depression
NURSING IMPLICATIONS: Side rails up; must *not* stand without assistance; may be given with diuretics; observe carefully; IM route only; monitor BP; IV for severe hypertension and preeclampsia; in pregnancy, must *not* decrease arterial pressure too much or too rapidly, otherwise will jeopardize uteroplacental perfusion			

TABLE 10–6   Common Drugs—cont'd

Drug and Dosage	Use	Action	◆ Assessment: Side Effects
Antihypertensives—cont'd			
Methyldopa (Aldomet)—PO 500 mg–2 g in divided doses	Severe to moderately severe hypertension	Inhibits formation of dopamine, a precursor of norepinephrine	Initial drowsiness, depression with feelings of unreality, edema, jaundice, dry mouth
NURSING IMPLICATIONS: *Contraindicated* in acute and chronic liver disease; encourage not to drive car if drowsy			
Minoxidil (Loniten)—PO 5 mg/day (range: 10–40 mg/day)	Severe hypertension; end-stage organ failure	Relaxes vascular smooth muscle	ECG changes; tachycardia; Na$^+$, water retention; hypertrichosis
NURSING IMPLICATIONS: Depilatory cream may minimize increased hair growth; report resting pulse *increase more than 20 beats/min;* caution patient to change positions slowly			
Phentolamine hydrochloride (Regitine)—PO 50 mg 4–6 doses daily; IV, IM, or local 5–10 mg, diluted in minimum 10 mL normal saline	Prevents dermal necrosis; hypertensive crisis; pheochromocytoma	Blocks alpha-adrenergic receptors	Weakness, dizziness, orthostatic hypotension, nausea, vomiting, abdominal pain
NURSING IMPLICATIONS: When giving parenterally, patient should be *supine;* monitor for overdosage (precipitous drop in BP); do *not* give with epinephrine			
Prazosin (Minipress)—PO 6–15 mg/d bid or tid	Mild to moderate hypertension	Dilates arteries and veins by blocking postsynaptic alpha$_1$-adrenergic receptors	Dizziness, headache, weakness, palpitations; orthostatic hypotension with first dose
NURSING IMPLICATIONS: Monitor: I&O, VS, and *weight* at beginning of therapy; teach patient/family to check BP at least weekly; need to comply with other interventions (wt. reduction, diet, smoking cessation, exercise)			
Reserpine (Serpasil)—PO 0.25 mg qd	Mild to moderate hypertension	Depletes catecholamines and decreases peripheral vasoconstriction, heart rate, and BP	Depression, nasal stuffiness, increased gastric secretions, rash, pruritus
NURSING IMPLICATIONS: Watch for signs of *mental depression;* closely monitor pulse rates of patients also receiving digitalis; *avoid* alcohol			
	Obstetric use: Pre-eclampsia-eclampsia	CNS-depressant tranquilizer; sedation is major effect; decreases neural transmission to nerves; decreases tone in blood vessels	Low level of toxicity; weight gain; diarrhea; allergic reactions—dry mouth, itching, skin eruptions
NURSING IMPLICATIONS: Side rails up; must not stand up without assistance; observe carefully; monitor *BP*			
Timolol (Timoptic)—PO 20–40 mg/day; ophthalmic 1 gtt 1–2 times/day	Hypertension, migraine, glaucoma	Blocks stimulation of myocardial (beta$_1$) and pulmonary/vascular (beta$_2$) receptors	Fatigue, weakness, depression, insomnia, peripheral vasoconstriction, diarrhea, nausea, vomiting
NURSING IMPLICATIONS: Check VS and evidence of heart failure; do *not* take if pulse <50; *avoid* OTC cold remedies, coffee, tea, and cola			
Metaraminol (Aramine)— 2–10 mg IM or 15–100 mg in 500 mL sodium	Adrenalectomy	Elevated systolic and diastolic BP by vasoconstriction	Hypertension, cardiac arrhythmias; may cause hypertensive crisis, if on MAO inhibitors or antidepressants
NURSING IMPLICATIONS: *Monitor* VS frequently (q3–5min); observe for side effects; have *phentolamine available as antidote*			
Anti-infectives			
Cefazolin (Ancef, Kefzol)—IM or IV 250 mg–1.5 g q6–12h	*Staphylococcus aureus; Escherichia coli; Klebsiella;* group A and B *Streptococcus; Pneumococcus*	Bactericidal	Allergic reaction; urticaria, rash; abnormal bleeding
NURSING IMPLICATIONS: See Penicillin; may cause *false-positive* lab tests (Coombs, urine glucose); oral probenecid may be taken concurrently to prolong effects of drug			

Continued

Pharmacology

TABLE 10–6 Common Drugs—cont'd

Drug and Dosage	Use	Action	◆ Assessment: Side Effects
Anti-infectives—cont'd			
Cephalexin (Keflex)—PO 1–4 g daily in 2–4 equally divided doses	Infections caused by gram-positive cocci; infections: respiratory, biliary, urinary, bone, septicemia, abdominal; surgical prophylaxis	Bactericidal effects on susceptible organisms; inhibition of bacterial cell wall synthesis	Nausea, vomiting; urticaria; toxic paranoid reactions; dizziness; increased alkaline phosphatase; nephrotoxicity; bone marrow suppression

NURSING IMPLICATIONS: Peak blood levels delayed when given with food; *report* nausea, flushing, tachycardia, headache; monitor for *nephrotoxicity* and for bleeding

Drug and Dosage	Use	Action	Assessment: Side Effects
Cephalothin (Keflin, Seffin)—IM, IV 2–12 g/day in 4–6 equally divided doses	Same as cephalexin except not recommended for biliary tract infections	Same as Cephalexin	See Cephalexin

NURSING IMPLICATIONS: Same as Cephalexin; pain at site of IM; given in large muscle; rotate sites

Drug and Dosage	Use	Action	Assessment: Side Effects
Ciprofloxacin (Cipro)—PO 250–750 mg q12h; IV 200–400 mg q12h; ophthalmic 1–2 gtt q15–30min, then 4–6 times daily	Lower respiratory tract infections; skin, bone, and joint infections; UTI	Inhibits bacterial DNA synthesis	Restlessness, nausea, diarrhea, vomiting, abdominal pain

NURSING IMPLICATIONS: Give PO on an *empty stomach* unless GI irritation occurs, then take with food; *do not* take with milk or yogurt; IV over 60 min

Drug and Dosage	Use	Action	Assessment: Side Effects
Clarithromycin (Biaxin)—7.5 mg/kg q12h; usual 500 mg q12h	Peptic ulcer	Inhibits protein synthesis of bacterial ribosome	Hypersensitivity to other antibiotics; use with caution in *liver/renal* impairment

NURSING IMPLICATIONS: Take medication around the clock; report signs of superinfection, diarrhea; do *not* take during pregnancy

Drug and Dosage	Use	Action	Assessment: Side Effects
Cloxacillin (Tegopen)—PO 250–500 mg q6h	Penicillinase-producing staphylococci infections: respiratory, sinus, and skin	Binds to bacterial cell wall, leading to cell death	Nausea, vomiting, diarrhea, rashes, allergic reactions, seizures (high doses)

NURSING IMPLICATIONS: *Give around the clock* on an *empty* stomach; observe for signs of *superinfection* (black, furry tongue, vaginal itching, loose stools)

Drug and Dosage	Use	Action	Assessment: Side Effects
Co-trimoxazole (Bactrim, Septra)—PO 160 mg twice daily or 20 mg/kg/day for *P. carinii* pneumonia	Acute otitis media; urinary tract infection; shigellosis; *P. carinii* pneumonia; prostatitis	Bacteriostatic; anti-infective; antagonizes folic acid production; combination of sulfamethoxazole and trimethoprim	Hypersensitivity; see Sulfisoxazole

NURSING IMPLICATIONS: IV administration can cause phlebitis and *tissue damage* with extravasation

Drug and Dosage	Use	Action	Assessment: Side Effects
Doxycycline (Vibramycin)—PO 100 mg q12h on day 1; then 100 mg/day × 7 days; IV—200 mg in 1–2 inf. on day 1; then 100–200 mg/day	Chlamydia, other STDs Lyme disease	Inhibits bacterial protein of the 30S bacterial ribosome	Urticaria, diarrhea; nausea, vomiting; photosensitivity

NURSING IMPLICATIONS: Take prescribed medications as ordered; use sunscreen or protective clothing due to photosensitivity; report signs of superinfection, if original symptoms not improved

Drug and Dosage	Use	Action	Assessment: Side Effects
Erythromycin—adults, PO 250 mg q6h; children, PO 30–50 mg/kg qd	Pneumonia; pelvic inflammatory disease; intestinal amebiasis; ocular infections; used if allergic to penicillin	Inhibits protein synthesis of microorganism; more effective against gram-positive organisms	Abdominal cramping, distention, diarrhea

NURSING IMPLICATIONS: Be sure culture and sensitivity done *before* treatment; give on *empty* stomach 1 hr before or 3 hr after meals; do *not* crush or chew tabs; do *not* give with fruit juice

TABLE 10–6   Common Drugs—cont'd

Drug and Dosage	Use	Action	◆ Assessment: Side Effects
Anti-infectives—cont'd			
Gentamicin (Garamycin)— IM, IV 3–5 mg/kg/day in 3–4 divided doses; topical; skin, eye	Serious gram-negative infections; possible *S. aureus,* uncomplicated urinary infections	Bactericidal effects on susceptible gram-positive and gram-negative organisms and mycobacteria	Serious toxic effects: kidneys, ear; causes muscle weakness/paralysis
NURSING IMPLICATIONS: Monitor *plasma* levels (peak is 4–10 µg/mL); patients with burns, cystic fibrosis may need higher doses			
Metronidazole (Flagyl) 7.5 mg/kg q6h (not to exceed 4 g/day)	Diverticulosis	Disrupts DNA and protein synthesis in susceptible organisms	Cimetidine may decrease metabolism; seizures, dizziness, abdominal pain
NURSING IMPLICATIONS: Administer with *food or milk* to decrease GI symptoms; *avoid* alcohol; has unpleasant metallic taste; *avoid* OTC medication while on this drug			
Penicillin—penicillin G, penicillin G potassium, penicillin G procaine, ampicillin 400,000–1.2 mil U q8h × 10 days, or single dose of 2.4 mil U	*Streptococcus; Staphylococcus; Pneumococcus; Gonococcus; Treponema pallidum*	Primarily bactericidal	Dermatitis and delayed or immediate anaphylaxis
NURSING IMPLICATIONS: Outpatients should be observed for *20 min after injection;* hospitalized patients should be observed at frequent intervals for 20 min after injection			
Pentamidine (Pentam)—IV 4 mg/kg once daily; inhale 300 mg via nebulizer	Prevention or treatment of *P. carinii* pneumonia	Appears to disrupt DNA or RNA synthesis to protozoa	Anxiety, headache, bronchospasm, cough, hypotension, arrhythmias, nephrotoxicity, hypoglycemia, leukopenia, thrombocytopenia, anemia, chills
NURSING IMPLICATIONS: Assess for infection and respiratory status; unpleasant metallic taste may occur (not significant)			
Sulfisoxazole (Gantrisin), sulfamethizole (Thiosulfil), and sulfisomidine (Elkosin)— PO 2.4 g loading dose, then 1–2 g qid × 7–10 days	Acute, chronic, and recurrent urinary tract infections	Bacteriostatic and bactericidal	Nausea, vomiting, oliguria, anuria, anemia, leukopenia, dizziness, jaundice, skin rashes, and photosensitivity
NURSING IMPLICATIONS: Maintenance of blood levels is important; encourage *fluids* to prevent crystal formation in kidney tubules—push up to 3000 mL/day; *avoid* in later stage of pregnancy and first month of life for newborn (may cause kernicterus)			
Tetracyclines—doxycycline hyclate (Vibramycin), oxytetracycline (Terramycin), tetracycline HCl (Sumycin)—PO 250–500 mg q6h; IM 250 mg/day; or IV 250–500 mg q8–12h	Broad-spectrum antibiotic	Primarily bacteriostatic	GI upsets such as diarrhea, nausea, vomiting; sore throat; black, hairy tongue; glossitis; inflammatory lesions in anogenital region
NURSING IMPLICATIONS: *Phototoxic* reactions have been reported; patients should be advised to stay out of direct sunlight; medication should *not* be given with milk or snacks, because food interferes with absorption of tetracyclines; do *not* give to pregnant women and children under 8 yr			
Trimethoprim (TMP)/ sulfamethoxazole (SMZ) (Bactrim)—PO 160 mg TMP or 800 mg SMZ q12h for 14–21 days; IV 8–10 mg/kg TMP/40–50 mg/kg SMZ q6–12h	Bronchitis, *Shigella* enteritis, otitis media, *P. carinii* pneumonia, UTI, traveler's diarrhea	Combination inhibits the metabolism of folic acid in bacteria; bactericidal	Nausea, vomiting, rashes, phlebitis at IV site, aplastic anemia, hepatic necrosis
NURSING IMPLICATIONS: Check IV site frequently; do *not* give IM; give PO on *empty stomach;* take *around the clock; avoid* exposure to sun			

Pharmacology

Continued

TABLE 10–6 **Common Drugs—cont'd**

Drug and Dosage	Use	Action	◆ Assessment: Side Effects
Anti-inflammatory			
Gastrointestinal Mesalamine (Asacol, Pentusa, Rowasa)—800 mg 3 × day for 6 wk	Ulcerative colitis	Local-acting anti-inflammatory in GI tract	*Contraindicated* if patient has allergy to sulfonamides or salicylates; acceleration of symptoms; abdominal pain
NURSING IMPLICATIONS: *Monitor* for: abdominal pain, diarrhea, blood in stools, superinfection; if no improvement notify health care professional; may need diagnostic studies			
Olsalazine (Dipentum)—see mesalamine—PO 1 g/day in 2 divided doses	See Mesalamine	See Mesalamine	See Mesalamine
NURSING IMPLICATIONS: See Mesalamine			
Sulfasalazine (Azulifidine)—see mesalamine—PO 3–4 g/day in divided doses	See Mesalamine	See Mesalamine	See Mesalamine
NURSING IMPLICATIONS: See Mesalamine			
Glucocorticoids—inhalants Beclomethasone (Beclovent, Vanceril)—42–50 μg/spray; 2 metered sprays 3–4 × day	Emphysema	Glucocorticoid (inhalation)	Headache, hypersensitivity to fluorocarbon propellant; used with *caution* in diabetes or glaucoma
NURSING IMPLICATIONS: Do *not* exceed 1 mg/day			
Flunisolide (AeroBid) 42–50 μg/spray; 2 metered sprays 2–4/day	Emphysema	Potent locally acting anti-inflammatory and immune modifier	Headache, dysphonia, fungal infections; adrenal suppression with long-term use
NURSING IMPLICATIONS: *Monitor* respiratory status and lung sounds; *assess* patients changing from systemic to inhaled glucocorticoids for signs of *adrenal insufficiency* (anorexia, nausea, weakness, hypotension, hypoglycemia)			
Triaminolone (Azmacort)—See Beclomethasone	Asthma	See Beclomethasone	See Beclomethasone
NURSING IMPLICATIONS: See Beclomethasone			
Glucocorticoids—systemic Cortisone acetate—PO or IM 20–100 mg qd in single or divided doses	ACTH insufficiency; rheumatoid arthritis; allergies; ulcerative colitis; nephrosis	Anti-inflammatory effect of unknown action	Moon facies, hirsutism, thinning of skin, striae, hypertension, menstrual irregularities, delayed healing, psychoses
NURSING IMPLICATIONS: Give oral form pc, with snack at bedtime; give deep IM (*never* deltoid); monitor vital signs; observe for behavior changes; skin care and activity to tolerance; *diet*—salt restricted, high protein, KCl supplement; protect from injury			
Desoxycorticosterone acetate (hydrocortisone)—IM/IV 100–500 mg q2–6h; PO 3–5 mg bid qid	Addison's disease; burns; surgical shock; adrenal surgery	Promotes reabsorption of sodium; restores plasma volume, BP, and electrolyte balance	Edema, hypertension, pulmonary congestion, hypokalemia
NURSING IMPLICATIONS: Salt restriction according to BP readings; *monitor* vital signs; weigh daily			
Dexamethasone (Decadron)—PO 0.5–5.0 mg qd; IM or IV 4–20 mg qd	Addison's disease; allergic reactions; leukemia; Hodgkin's disease; iritis; dermatitis; rheumatoid arthritis	Anti-inflammatory effect	See Cortisone acetate
NURSING IMPLICATIONS: *Contraindicated* in tuberculosis; see Cortisone acetate for nursing care			

TABLE 10–6   Common Drugs—cont'd

Drug and Dosage	Use	Action	◆ Assessment: Side Effects
Glucocorticoids—systemic—cont'd			
Methylprednisolone sodium (Solu-Medrol)—IV, IM, 10–40 mg, slowly	Glucocorticoid, corticosteroid	See Dexamethasone	See Dexamethasone
NURSING IMPLICATIONS: See Dexamethasone			
Prednisolone (Deltsone)—5–60 mg/day single or divided dose	Multiple sclerosis	Suppress inflammation and normal immune response	Depression, euphoria; peptic ulceration; thromboembolism
NURSING IMPLICATIONS: *Monitor* for *Homans' sign*, abdominal pain, vomiting, tarry stools, mental status or mood changes			
Prednisone—PO 2.5–15.0 mg qd	Rheumatoid arthritis; cancer therapy	Anti-inflammatory effect of unknown action	Insomnia and gastric distress
NURSING IMPLICATIONS: See Cortisone acetate			
Antilipemics			
Cholestyramine (Questran)—PO 4 g 1–4 times/day	Hypercholesterolemia; pruritus from increased bile	Binds bile acids in GI tract, increased clearance of cholesterol	Nausea, constipation, abdominal discomfort
NURSING IMPLICATIONS: Take *before* meals; do *not* take with other medications; give others 1 hr before or 4–6 hr after			
Gemfibrozil (Lopid)—PO 1200 mg/day	Hypercholesterolemia	May inhibit peripheral lipolysis and reduce triglyceride synthesis in liver	GI upset (abdominal pain, epigastric pain, diarrhea, nausea, vomiting), rash, headache, dizziness, blurred vision
NURSING IMPLICATIONS: Use *caution* when driving or doing tasks requiring alertness; take *before* meals			
Lovastatin (Mevacor)—PO 20–80 mg daily with evening meal	Primary hypercholesterolemia	Inhibits enzyme that catalyzes synthesis of cholesterol; decreases synthesis of LDL	Headache, constipation, diarrhea, altered taste, blurred vision, muscle cramps
NURSING IMPLICATIONS: Give *with* food; *restrict* fat, cholesterol, carbohydrates, and alcohol in diet			
Niacin (vitamin B_3, nicotinic acid)—PO 1.5–6.0 g	Hypercholesterolemia	Decreases liver's production of LDLs and synthesis of triglycerides	GI upset, flushing, pruritus, hyperuricemia, hyperglycemia
NURSING IMPLICATIONS: Take the drug *with* meals; prevent flushing by taking an *aspirin 30 min before*; monitor closely during first year of therapy			
Simvastatin (Zocor)—10–20 mg qd	See Lovastatin	See Lovastatin	See Lovastatin
NURSING IMPLICATIONS: Give once in the *evening* with or without food			
Antineoplastics			
6 mercaptopurine (Purinethol)—PO 2.5 mg/kg/day; may increase to 5 mg/kg after 4 wk; maintenance 1.5–2.5 mg/kg/day	Leukemia (ulcerative)	Antineoplastic	Bone marrow depression, severe hepatotoxicity
NURSING IMPLICATIONS: *Monitor:* bleeding, infection, *liver* function tests, skin care, nausea and vomiting			
Methotrexate (Rheumatrex) 15–30 mg/day for 5 days; repeat after 1 wk for 3–5 courses	Leukemia Breast, lung cancer	Interferes with folic acid metabolism, resulting in inhibition of DNA synthesis and cell reproduction	Pulmonary fibrosis, hepatotoxicity, stomatitis, signs and symptoms of chemotherapy side effects
NURSING IMPLICATIONS: Monitor *liver* function; *assess* respiratory status; see nursing care of patients receiving chemotherapy			

Pharmacology

Continued

TABLE 10–6   Common Drugs—cont'd

Drug and Dosage	Use	Action	◆ Assessment: Side Effects
Antineoplastics—cont'd			
Mitotane (Lysodren) 9–10 g/day in 3–4 divided doses initially; decrease for maintenance	Adrenocortical carcinoma	Affects pituitary disorders	GI complaints; lethargy, somnolence
NURSING IMPLICATIONS: *Monitor:* signs of disease progression, GI abnormalities, abdominal pain			
Antiparkinson Agents			
Benztropine (Cogentin)—1–2 mg/day (range: 0.5–6 mg/day)	Parkinson's disease	Blocks cholinergic activity in CNS	Blurred vision, dry eyes; constipation; *caution* with antihistamines, phenothiazines
NURSING IMPLICATIONS: Take as directed for best results; monitor for drowsiness, dizziness, orthostatic hypotension; good mouth care; use *caution* with OTC drugs, overheating (drug causes a decrease in perspiration)			
Carbidopa/levodopa (Sinemet)—10/100, 25/100, 25/250 carbidopa/levodopa ratio	Parkinson's disease	Levodopa is converted to dopamine in CNS, where it serves as a neurotransmitter	Use with MAO inhibitors; may result in hypertensive crisis; some drugs can reverse effects, e.g., phenothiazines, reserpine
NURSING IMPLICATIONS: Assess parkinsonian symptoms; monitor *hepatic, renal* function; teach about orthostatic hypotension, gastric irritation, drowsiness			
Biperiden (Akineton)—2 mg 3–4×/day; *not to exceed* 16 mg/day	Parkinson's disease	Restores natural balance of neurotransmitters in CNS	Same as Benztropine (Cogentin)
NURSING IMPLICATIONS: See Benztropine			
Trihexyphenidyl (Artane)—1–2 mg daily; usual maintenance dose: 5–15 mg/day in divided dose	Parkinson's disease	Inhibits action of acetylcholine	Dizziness, nervousness, blurred vision, mydriasis
NURSING IMPLICATIONS: Monitor symptoms; *avoid* orthostatic hypotension; mouth care			
Antiplatelet			
Clopidogrel (Plavix)—PO 75 mg qd	Reduce risk of atherosclerotic event (MI, stroke)	Inhibits platelet aggregation	Bleeding; neutropenia; reactions similar to aspirin
NURSING IMPLICATIONS: Give once daily without regard to food; *avoid* aspirin, NSAIDs; observe for symptoms of: stroke, peripheral vascular disease, MI			
Dipyridamole (Persantine)—PO 70–100 mg 4 times/day; IV 570 µg/kg	Prevent thromboembolism; surgical graft patency; *diagnostic* agent in myocardial perfusion studies	Decreases platelet aggregation; coronary vasodilator	Headache, dizziness, hypotension, nausea; MI, arrhythmias with IV
NURSING IMPLICATIONS: Take at *evenly* spaced intervals; *avoid* use of alcohol; if no GI irritation, take 1 hr before or 2 hr after meals			
Ticlopidine (Ticlid)—PO 250 mg bid	Stroke prevention; prevent early restenosis of coronary stents	Inhibits platelet aggregation; prolongs bleeding time	Diarrhea, rashes, bleeding, intracerebral bleeding
NURSING IMPLICATIONS: Give *with* food or immediately *after* eating			
Antituberculous*			
First-line drugs			
Isoniazid—5–10 mg/kg up to 300 mg PO or IM	Tuberculosis	Suppresses or interferes with biosynthesis; bacteriostatic	Peripheral neuritis, hepatitis, hypersensitivity
NURSING IMPLICATIONS: Give pyridoxine (B$_6$) 10 mg as prophylaxis for neuritis; 50–100 mg as treatment			

*Note: To minimize resistant strains, combination therapy is used long term.

TABLE 10–6   Common Drugs—cont'd

Drug and Dosage	Use	Action	◆ Assessment: Side Effects
First-line drugs—cont'd Ethambutol—15–25 mg/kg PO	See Isoniazid	See Isoniazid	Optic neuritis (reversible with discontinuation of drug; very rare at 15 mg/kg); skin rash

NURSING IMPLICATIONS: Use with caution with renal disease or when eye testing is not feasible; used *in combination with* other drug

Rifamate combination (isoniazid with rifampin) Rifater combination (isoniazid and pyrazinamide with rifampin)—see Rifampin	See Rifampin	See Rifampin	See Rifampin

NURSING IMPLICATIONS: See Rifampin

Rifampin—10–20 mg/kg PO 600 mg IV	Tuberculosis, meningitis, *H. influenzae*	Impairs RNA synthesis; bactericidal	Hepatitis, febrile reaction, purpura (rare)

NURSING IMPLICATIONS: *Orange* urine color; *negates* effect of birth control pills

Streptomycin—15–20 mg/kg up to 1 g IM	Tuberculosis, endocarditis, tularemia	Inhibits protein synthesis; bactericidal	*Eighth cranial* nerve damage, *nephrotoxicity*

NURSING IMPLICATIONS: Use with caution in *older* patients or those with *renal* disease

Pyrazinamide—15–30 mg/kg up to 3 g PO	Tuberculosis	Bactericidal	Hyperuricemia, hepatotoxicity

NURSING IMPLICATIONS: Loss of glycemic control in those with diabetes

Antiulcer			
Aluminum hydroxide gel (Amphojel)—PO 5–10 mL q2–4h or 1 hr pc	Gastric acidity; peptic ulcer; phosphatic urinary calculi; ↓ phosphorus level in chronic renal failure	Buffers HCl in gastric juices without interfering with electrolyte balance	Constipation and fecal impaction

NURSING IMPLICATIONS: *Shake well* before administering; encourage *fluids* to prevent impaction and milk–alkali syndrome

Calcium carbonate (Titralac)—PO 1–2 g taken with H_2O after meals and at bedtime	Peptic ulcer and chronic gastritis	Reduces hyperacidity	Constipation or laxative effect

NURSING IMPLICATIONS: See Aluminum hydroxide gel

Cimetidine (Tagamet)—PO 300–600 mg q6h (qid); IM, IV 300 mg q6h	Duodenal ulcers, GERD, gastric hypersecretion; peptic acid gastritis, heart burn; esophagitis	Inhibits action of histamine at H_2-receptor site, inhibits gastric acid secretion; neutralizes and absorbs excess acid	Confusion, dizziness; nausea; rash; diarrhea, constipation; hypermagnesemia

NURSING IMPLICATIONS: Give *with* meals or immediately *after; avoid* smoking; *avoid* prolonged administration to patients with renal insufficiency

Cisapride (Propulsid)—5–10 mg 3–4×/day	Peptic ulcer	Enhances the release of acetylcholine at the myenteric plexus	Anticholinergics will decrease effects; effects of alcohol accelerated

NURSING IMPLICATIONS: Take as directed; do *not* miss dose even if feeling well; *avoid* mixing with OTC drugs; *avoid* alcohol (may cause drowsiness)

Continued

Pharmacology

TABLE 10–6 **Common Drugs—cont'd**

Drug and Dosage	Use	Action	◆ Assessment: Side Effects
Antiulcer—cont'd			
Famotidine (Pepcid)—40 mg/day at bedtime or 20 mg twice a day	Peptic ulcer	Inhibits gastric acid secretion by inhibiting histamine at H_2-receptor site	Use with caution: elderly, renal failure; confusion, arrhythmias, agranulocytosis, aplastic anemia
NURSING IMPLICATIONS: Assess for: epigastric pain, blood in stool or emesis; monitor lab values to avoid side effects; take medication for full course of treatment; *avoid* self medication with OTC drugs; *avoid* smoking			
Lansoprazole (Prevacid)—15 mg/day; with *H. pylori*: 30 mg twice a day with amoxicillin	Peptic ulcer	Binds to an enzyme in presence of gastric acid; prevents final transport of hydrogen ions into gastric lumen	Hypersensitivity; use with caution in elderly; dose change needed with hepatic impairment
NURSING IMPLICATIONS: *Avoid* alcohol; *report* signs of: GI bleeding, cramping, abdominal pain, vomiting			
Magnesium and aluminum hydroxides (Maalox suspension)—PO 5–30 mL q1–3h pc and hs	Gastric hyperacidity; peptic ulcer; heartburn; reflux esophagitis	Neutralizes and binds gastric acids, heals ulcers	Constipation from aluminum hydroxide; diarrhea from magnesium hydroxide
NURSING IMPLICATIONS: Encourage fluid intake; *contraindicated* for debilitated patients or those with renal insufficiency			
Misoprostol (Cytotec) 200 mcg 4 × day	Peptic ulcer	Prostaglandin analogue	Hypersensitivity to prostaglandins; diarrhea; *avoid* during pregnancy
NURSING IMPLICATIONS: Monitor effectiveness of the drug; report increase in abdominal pain, bleeding			
Nizatidine (Axid) see cimetidine	See Cimetidine	See Cimetidine	See Cimetidine
NURSING IMPLICATIONS: See Cimetidine			
Omeprazole (Prilosec) 20 mg once daily	Peptic ulcer GERD	Gastric acid–pump inhibitor	Abdominal pain; *contraindicated*: hypersensitivity
NURSING IMPLICATIONS: May cause drowsiness, dizziness. *Avoid*: alcohol, aspirin, NSAIDs, foods that cause GI irritation			
Ranitidine (Zantac)—PO 150 mg bid; IM 50 mg q6–8h; IV 50 mg q6–8h	Duodenal ulcer, gastric ulcer, GERD, gastric hyper secretion	Inhibits action of histamine at H_2-receptor site, inhibits gastric acid secretion	Headache, malaise, nausea, constipation, diarrhea
NURSING IMPLICATIONS: Food does *not* affect absorption; give 1 hr *apart* from antacids; *smoking* interferes with action			
Sucralfate (Carafate)—PO 1 g qid	Prevention and treatment of duodenal ulcer	Reacts with gastric acid to form a thick paste that adheres to the ulcer surface	Constipation
NURSING IMPLICATIONS: Give 1 hr *before* and *at bedtime;* do *not* crush or chew tablets; take *antacids* 30 min before or 1 hr after sucralfate; increase *fluids and dietary* bulk			
Antiviral			
Acyclovir (Zovirax)—PO 200 mg, 3–5 times/day; IV 5 mg/kg q8h over 1 hr; topical 6 times daily for 1 wk	Herpes simplex (1, 2)	Converts to an active cytotoxic metabolite that inhibits viral DNA replication	Headache, nausea, vomiting, diarrhea, increased serum BUN and creatinine
NURSING IMPLICATIONS: Measure I&O q8h; ensure adequate *hydration;* assess for common side effects; apply topical with *finger cot* or rubber glove; refer for counseling			

TABLE 10–6   Common Drugs—cont'd

Drug and Dosage	Use	Action	◆ Assessment: Side Effects
Antiviral—cont'd			
Indinavir (Crixivan)—PO 800 mg q8h	HIV; possible prevention in combination therapy	Inhibits action of HIV protease and cleavage of viral polyproteins	Ketoacidosis; kidney stones; hyperglycemia; altered taste; acid regurgitation
NURSING IMPLICATIONS: Give with *water or other liquids* (skim milk, coffee, tea, juice) *1 hr before* or *2 hr after* meal; *avoid* high-fat, high-protein meal within 2 hr; with concurrent therapy, may need to take drugs 1 hr apart; capsules are sensitive to moisture—keep desiccant in bottle			
Nevirapine (Viramune)—PO 200 mg qd for 2 wk, then bid	HIV; delays disease progression	Binds to the enzyme reverse transcriptase; disrupts DNA synthesis	Rash; *Stevens-Johnson syndrome* (severe erythema multiforme)
NURSING IMPLICATIONS: Give with or without food; drug does not cure AIDS—decreases opportunistic infections			
Zidovudine (AZT, Retrovir)—PO 200 mg q4h	AIDS and related disorders	Inhibits HIV replication	Blood disorders, especially anemia and granulocytopenia; headache; nausea; insomnia; myalgia
NURSING IMPLICATIONS: Monitor for signs of opportunistic infection and adverse drug effects; drug must be taken *around the clock;* regular blood tests (q2wk)			
Blood Viscosity–Reducing Agent			
Pentoxifylline (Trental)—PO 400 mg tid	Peripheral vascular disease (intermittent claudication)	Increases flexibility of RBCs; inhibits platelet aggregation	Nausea, vomiting, GI upset; drowsiness; dizziness; headache
NURSING IMPLICATIONS: Give *with* meals to minimize GI irritation; take tablets whole; report persistent GI or CNS side effects			
Bronchodilators			
Albuterol (Ventolin)—PO 2–6 mg 3–4 times/day; inhale q4–6h or 2 puffs 15 min before exercise	Bronchodilator	Results in accumulation of cyclic adenosine monophosphate (cAMP) at beta-adrenergic receptors	Nervousness, restlessness, tremor, hypertension, nausea
NURSING IMPLICATIONS: Give *with* meals; allow 1 min *between* inhalations; rinse mouth with water *after* inhalation			
Aminophylline—PO 250 mg bid–qid; rectal 250–500 mg; IV 250–500 mg over 10–20 min	Rapid relief of bronchospasm; asthma; pulmonary edema	Relaxes smooth muscles and increases cardiac contractility; interferes with reabsorption of Na^+ and Cl^- in proximal tubules	Nausea, vomiting, cardiac arrhythmias, intestinal bleeding, insomnia, restlessness, and rectal irritation from suppository
NURSING IMPLICATIONS: Give oral *with* or *after meals;* monitor *vital signs* for changes in BP and pulse; weigh daily; IM injections are painful			
Ephedrine SO_4—PO, SC, or IM 25 mg tid–qid	Asthma: allergies; bradycardia; nasal decongestant	Relaxes hypertonic muscles in bronchioles and GI tract	Wakefulness, nervousness, dizziness, palpitations, hypertension
NURSING IMPLICATIONS: Monitor vital signs; *avoid* giving dose near bedtime; *check urine* output in older adults			
Ipratropium (Atrovent) 1–4 inhalations	Emphysema	Inhibits cholinergic receptors in bronchial smooth muscle	Nasal dryness, epistaxis; fluorocarbon toxicity when used with other inhalants
NURSING IMPLICATIONS: Instruct proper use of inhaler; do *not* use more than 12 metered doses in 12 hr; if severe bronchospasm occurs, consult physician/nurse practitioner			
Isoproterenol HCl (Isuprel)—inhalation of 1:100 or 1:200 solution	Mild to moderately severe asthma attack; bronchitis; pulmonary emphysema	Relaxes hypertonic bronchioles	Nervousness, tachycardia, hypertension, insomnia
NURSING IMPLICATIONS: Monitor vital signs *before and after* treatment; teach patient how to use nebulizer			

Pharmacology

Continued

TABLE 10–6   Common Drugs—cont'd

Drug and Dosage	Use	Action	◆ Assessment: Side Effects
Bronchodilators			
Metaproterenol (Alupent) 20 mg 3–4 times/day; inhalation 2–3 metered-dose inhalations	Asthma	Bronchodilation	Nervousness, restlessness, tremor, paradoxical bronchospasm
NURSING IMPLICATIONS: Assess lung sounds; observe for wheezing (paradoxical bronchospasm); observe patients' respiratory signs and symptoms; refer to health care professional if symptoms persist or shortness of breath continues			
Salmeterol (Serevent)—50 μg twice a day (two inhalations)	Asthma	Produces accumulation of cAMP at beta-adrenergic receptors	Headache, palpitations, abdominal pain; *avoid* when using beta-adrenergic agents (decreases effectiveness)
NURSING IMPLICATIONS: Assess lung sounds; *monitor* pulmonary function; do *not* use for acute symptoms			
Theophylline—PO 400 mg/day in divided doses; max adult dose: 900 mg divided dose	Treatment/prevention of emphysema, asthma (bronchoconstriction); chronic bronchitis	Bronchodilation	Restlessness; increased respiration, heart rate; palpitations, arrhythmias; nausea, vomiting; increased urine output → dehydration
NURSING IMPLICATIONS: Monitor theophylline levels: 10–20 μg/mL; monitor signs of toxicity; take with 8 oz water or *with* meals to decrease GI symptoms			
Terbutaline (Brethine)—PO 2.5–5.0 mg q6h (*not* to exceed 20 mg/24 hr); SC 0.25 mg, repeat 15–30 min (*not* to exceed 0.5 mg/hr); inhalation—2 puffs (0.2 mg each) q4–6h	Bronchospasm **Obstetric use:** may be used for premature labor; currently not FDA approved for use as tocolytic agent, but widely used	See Isoproterenol	See Isoproterenol If used in pregnancy: maternal and fetal tachycardia
NURSING IMPLICATIONS: See Isoproterenol			
Zafirlukast (Accolate)—20 mg twice daily	Asthma	Antagonizes the effects of leukotrienes	Headache, fever, infection, pain
NURSING IMPLICATIONS: *Monitor* lung sounds, respiratory function			
Zileuton (Zyflo)—600 mg qid	Asthma	Enzyme inhibitor	Headache, dizziness; chest pain; increases blood level of theophylline, propranolol, warfarin
NURSING IMPLICATIONS: Assess lung sounds; do *not* discontinue or reduce dosage without consulting health care professional; not used to treat acute attack			
Calcium Channel Blockers			
Amlodipine (Norvasc)—PO 5–10 mg qd	Hypertension, angina pectoris, vasospastic angina (Prinzmetal's), muscle cells	Inhibits the transport of calcium into myocardial and vascular smooth muscle	Arrhythmias, peripheral edema, heart failure, photosensitivity, gingival hyperplasia
NURSING IMPLICATIONS: Instruct patient to: monitor pulse, report rate <50 beats/min, take with or without food			
Diltiazem (Cardizem)—PO 30–120 mg 3–4 times/day; IV 5–15 mg/hr	Angina, hypertension, atrial arrhythmias	Inhibits excitation-contraction; decreased SA, AV node conduction	Headache, fatigue, arrhythmias, edema, hypotension, constipation, rash
NURSING IMPLICATIONS: May take *with* meals; take pulse; do *not* give drug if pulse <50 beats/min; change positions slowly; may take nitroglycerin sublingually concurrently			

TABLE 10–6   Common Drugs—cont'd

Drug and Dosage	Use	Action	◆ Assessment: Side Effects
Calcium Channel Blockers—cont'd			
Metoprolol (Lopressor)—100 mg/day up to 450 mg/day	Hypertension	Blocks stimulation of myocardial adrenergic receptors (beta$_1$)	*Contraindicated* in: CHF, pulmonary edema; *caution* with renal impairment
NURSING IMPLICATIONS: Monitor vitals, especially BP; prevent *orthostatic hypotension; avoid* self-medication with OTC; may cause drowsiness; medication may increase *sensitivity to cold*			
Nicardipine (Cardene)—PO 20–40 mg tid	Angina, hypertension	Calcium channel blocker, inhibits excitation-contraction	Dizziness, light-headedness, headache, peripheral edema, flushing
NURSING IMPLICATIONS: Give on an *empty* stomach; chest pain may occur 30 min after dose (temporary, from *reflex tachycardia*)			
Nifedipine (Procardia)—PO 10–30 mg tid (*not* to exceed 180 mg/day); sublingual 10 mg repeated in 15 min	Angina, hypertension **Obstetric use:** may be used for premature labor. Currently not FDA approved for use as tocolytic agent	Calcium channel blocker, vasodilation	Dizziness, light-headedness, giddiness, headache, nervousness, nasal congestion, sore throat, dyspnea, cough, wheezing, nausea, flushing, warmth
NURSING IMPLICATIONS: May take *with* meals; make position changes slowly; angina may occur 30 min after dose (temporary)			
Verapamil (Calan, Isopten)—PO 240–480 mg, 3–4 times/day; IV 75–150 µg/kg over 2 min	Angina; supraventricular arrhythmias; essential hypertension	Inhibits calcium movement into smooth-muscle cells; lowers pressure by reducing cardiac contractility	Constipation, AV block, hepatotoxicity
NURSING IMPLICATIONS: Monitor VS and ECG for *bradycardia* and *arrhythmias;* observe for *jaundice, abdominal pain;* encourage *fluids* and *bulk-forming* foods			
Cardiac Glycosides			
Digitoxin—digitalizing dose: PO 200 µg twice/day; IM or IV 200–400 µg; maintenance dose: PO 50–300 µg qd	Heart failure: atrial fibrillation and flutter; supraventricular tachycardia	Increases force of cardiac contractility, slows heart rate, decreases right atrial pressures, promotes diuresis	Arrhythmias; nausea, vomiting; anorexia, malaise; color vision, yellow or blue
NURSING IMPLICATIONS: Hold medication if pulse rate less than *50* or over *120;* encourage foods high in *potassium* (e.g., bananas, orange juice); observe for signs of electrolyte depletion, apathy, disorientation, and anorexia			
Digoxin (Lanoxin)—digitalizing dose: PO 10–15 µg/kg; IV 0.6–1 mg/kg; maintenance dose: PO 0.125–0.375 mg qd	See Digitoxin	See Digitoxin	See Digitoxin
NURSING IMPLICATIONS: See Digitoxin			
Chemotherapy (see Tables 7–41 and Antineoplastics 10–8)			
Cholinergic			
Bethanechol chloride (Urecholine)—PO 5–30 mg; SC 2.5–5.0 mg	Postoperative abdominal atony and distention; bladder atony with retention; postsurgical or postpartum urinary retention; myasthenia gravis	Increases GI and bladder tone; decreases sphincter tone	Belching, abdominal cramps, diarrhea, nausea, vomiting, incontinence, profuse sweating, salivation, respiratory depression
NURSING IMPLICATIONS: Check *respirations;* have urinal or bedpan close at hand and answer calls quickly; atropine SO$_4$ is the *antidote* for cholinergic drugs			

Continued

Pharmacology

TABLE 10–6 **Common Drugs—cont'd**

Drug and Dosage	Use	Action	◆ Assessment: Side Effects
Cholinergic—cont'd			
Edrophonium (Tensilon)—IV 2 mg; IM 10 mg	Diagnosis of myasthenia gravis; reversal of neuromuscular blockers	Inhibits breakdown of acetylcholine; anticholinesterase, cholinergic	Excess secretions, bronchospasm, bradycardia, abdominal cramps, vomiting, diarrhea, excess salivation, sweating
NURSING IMPLICATIONS: Effects last up to 30 min; give IV *undiluted* with *TB* syringe			
Neostigmine (Prostigmin)— PO 15–30 mg q3–4h; SC, IM 0.25–1 mg	Myasthenia gravis, postoperative bladder distention, urinary retention, reversal of neuromuscular blockers	Inhibits breakdown of acetylcholine; cholinergic	Excess secretions, bronchospasm, bradycardia, abdominal cramps, nausea, vomiting, diarrhea, excess salivation, sweating
NURSING IMPLICATIONS: Take oral form *with* food or milk; with chewing difficulty, take 30 min before eating			
Pilocarpine HCl—1–2 gtts 1–2% solution up to 6 times/day	Chronic open-angle and acute closed angle glaucoma	Contraction of the sphincter muscle of iris, resulting in miosis	Brow ache, headache, ocular pain, blurring and dimness of vision, allergic conjunctivitis, nausea, vomiting, profuse sweating; bronchoconstriction in patients with bronchial asthma
NURSING IMPLICATIONS: Initially the medication may be irritating; teach proper sterile technique for instilling drops—wipe excess solution to prevent systemic symptoms; discard cloudy solutions			
Physostigmine salicylate (Eserine)—0.1 mL of 0.25–10% solution: not more than qid; IM, IV 0.5–3 mg	Glaucoma, reverse effects of tricyclic antidepressants, overdose, toxic effects of atropine and diazepam	Increases concentration of acetylcholine	Sweating, marked miosis, lacrimation, nausea, diarrhea
NURSING IMPLICATIONS: If brown eyed, may require stronger solution or more frequent dose			
Pyridostigmine (Mestinon)— PO 60 mg/day × 3 days; IM, IV 2 mg q2–3h Maintenance: 60–150 mg/day	Myasthenia gravis, reversal of neuromuscular blockers	Inhibits breakdown of acetylcholine and prolongs its effects	See Neostigmine
NURSING IMPLICATIONS: See Neostigmine			
Central Nervous System Stimulants			
Amphetamine SO$_4$—PO 5–60 mg qd in divided doses	Mild depressive states; narcolepsy; postencephalitic parkinsonism; obesity control; minimal brain dysfunction in children (attention deficit disorder)	Raises BP, decreases sense of fatigue, elevates mood	Restlessness, dizziness, tremors, insomnia; increased libido; suicidal and homicidal tendencies; palpitations; anginal pain
NURSING IMPLICATIONS: Give *before* 4 P.M. to avoid sleep disturbance; dependence on drug may develop; *contraindicated* with MAO inhibitors, hyperthyroidism, and psychotic states			
Methylphenidate hydrochloride (Ritalin)—PO 0.3 mg/kg/day or adults 20–60 mg in divided doses	Childhood hyperactivity; narcolepsy; attention deficit disorder in children	Mild CNS and respiratory stimulation	Anorexia, dizziness, drowsiness, insomnia, nervousness, BP and pulse changes
NURSING IMPLICATIONS: To avoid insomnia take last dose 4–5 hr before bedtime; monitor vital signs; check weight 2–3 times weekly and report weight losses			

TABLE 10–6   Common Drugs—cont'd

Drug and Dosage	Use	Action	◆ Assessment: Side Effects
Decongestants			
Phenylephrine (Neo-Synephrine, Sinex)—SC, IM 2–5 mg q10–15min not to exceed 5 mg; IV 40–60 μg/min; nasal 2–3 gtts or 1–2 sprays q3–4h; ophthalmic 3 gtt/day	Shock, hypotension, decongestant, adjunct to spinal anesthesia, mydriatic	Constricts blood vessels by stimulating alpha-adrenergic receptors	Dizziness, restlessness, dyspnea, tachycardia, arrhythmias; ophthalmological: burning, photophobia, tearing

NURSING IMPLICATIONS: Check for correct concentration; protect eyes from *light sensitivity;* blow nose before using; *rebound congestion* will occur with prolonged use

Pseudoephedrine (Sudafed)—PO 60 mg q4–6h	Nasal congestion, allergies, chronic ear infections	Produces vasoconstriction in respiratory tract and possibly bronchodilation	Nervousness, anxiety, palpitations, anorexia

NURSING IMPLICATIONS: Give at least 2 hr before bedtime to minimize *insomnia*

Diuretics			
Acetazolamide (Diamox)—PO 250–1000 mg/day; IV 500 mg	Glaucoma; heart failure; convulsive disorders	Weak diuretic; produces acidosis; self-limiting effect; increases bicarbonate excretion	Electrolyte depletion symptomatology—lassitude, apathy, decreased urinary output, mental confusion

NURSING IMPLICATIONS: Weigh daily; I&O; assess edema; give *early* in day to allow sleep at night; observe for side effects; replace electrolytes as ordered

Ethacrynic acid (Edecrin)—PO 50–200 mg qd in divided doses	Pulmonary edema; ascites; edema of heart failure	Inhibits the reabsorption of Na⁺ in the ascending loop of Henle	Nausea, vomiting, diarrhea, hypokalemia, hypotension, gout, dehydration, deafness, metabolic acidosis

NURSING IMPLICATIONS: Assess for dehydration—skin turgor, neck veins; hypotension; *KCl* supplement

Furosemide (Lasix)—PO 40–80 mg qd in divided doses	Edema and associated heart failure; cirrhosis; renal disease; nephrotic syndrome: hypertension	Inhibits Na⁺ and Cl⁻ reabsorption in the loop of Henle	Dermatitis, pruritis, paresthesia, blurring of vision, postural hypotension, nausea, vomiting, diarrhea, dehydration, electrolyte depletion, hearing loss (usually reversible)

NURSING IMPLICATIONS: Assess for weakness, lethargy, leg cramps, anorexia; peak action in 1–2 hr; duration 6–8 hr; do *not* give at bedtime; supplemental *KCl* indicated; may induce *digitalis toxicity*

Hydrochlorothiazide (HydroDIURIL and Esidrix 25–100 mg tid)—PO Diuril 0.5–1.0 qd	Edema; heart failure; Na⁺ retention in steroid therapy; hypertension	Inhibits NaCl and water reabsorption in the distal ascending loop and the distal convoluted tubule of the kidneys	Hypokalemia, nausea, vomiting, diarrhea, dizziness, paresthesias; may exacerbate diabetes

NURSING IMPLICATIONS: Watch for muscle weakness; give well-diluted potassium chloride supplement; *monitor* urine for changes in sugar and acetone

Mannitol (Osmitrol)—50–100 gm/24 hr as 15–20% solution	Cerebral edema, oliguria, acute renal failure, drug intoxication	Hypertonic solution that kidney tubules cannot reabsorb, thereby causing obligatory water loss	Diarrhea; water intoxication, thirst, headache

NURSING IMPLICATIONS: Usually Foley catheter required; monitor *cardiac and respiratory* status; a rate of infusion to elicit 30–50 mL urine/hr

Spironolactone (Aldactone)—PO 25 mg bid–qid	Cirrhosis of liver; when other diuretics are ineffective	Inhibits effects of aldosterone in distal tubules of kidney	Headache, lethargy, diarrhea, ataxia, skin rash, gynecomastia

NURSING IMPLICATIONS: Potassium-sparing drug; do *not* give supplemental KCl; monitor for signs of electrolyte imbalance

Continued

Pharmacology

TABLE 10–6   Common Drugs—cont'd

Drug and Dosage	Use	Action	◆ Assessment: Side Effects
Emetic			
Ipecac syrup—PO 15–30 mL for emesis, followed by 1–2 glasses H$_2$O (adults and children >1 yr); 5–10 mL followed by ½–1 glass H$_2$O (children <1 yr)	Emergency emetic for poison ingestion	NH$_4$ ions cause gastric irritation	Violent emesis, tachycardia, decreased BP, dyspnea
NURSING IMPLICATIONS: *Contraindicated* in liver and renal disease; if given for emesis, follow dose with as much *water* as patient will drink			
Enzyme			
Pancrelipase (Viokase)—adults, PO 325 mg–1 g qd, during meals; children, PO 300–600 mg tid	Chronic pancreatitis; cystic fibrosis; gastrectomy; pancreatectomy; sprue	Assists in digestion of starch, protein, and fats; decreases nitrogen and fat content of stool	Anorexia, nausea, vomiting, diarrhea, buccal/anal soreness (infants), sneezing, skin rashes, diabetes
NURSING IMPLICATIONS: May be taken with antacid or cimetidine; do *not* crush or chew tabs; *monitor* I&O, weight; be alert for signs of diabetes; children may use sprinkles			
Expectorants			
Guaifenesin (Robitussin)—100–400 mg q4h	Respiratory congestion	Increases expectoration by causing irritation of gastric mucosa; reduces adhesiveness/surface tension of respiratory tract fluid	Low incidence of GI upset; drowsiness
NURSING IMPLICATIONS: Encourage to stop smoking; increase fluid intake; respiratory hygiene			
Terpin hydrate—PO 5–10 mL, q3–4h	Bronchitis; emphysema	Liquefies bronchial secretions	Nausea, vomiting, gastric irritation
NURSING IMPLICATIONS: Give undiluted; *push* fluids			
Fibrinolytic Agents			
Alteplase, recombinant (Activase, tPA)—IV bolus 100 mg over 90 min: 15 mg bolus given over 1–2 min; then 50 mg over 30 min; then 35 mg over 60 min	Acute MI; under investigation for pulmonary emboli, deep-vein thrombosis, and peripheral artery thrombosis	Promotes conversion of plasminogen to plasmin, which is fibrinolytic	Internal or local bleeding; urticaria; dysrhythmias related to reperfusion; hypotension; nausea, vomiting
NURSING IMPLICATIONS: Assess for signs of reperfusion (relief of chest pain, no ST segment elevation); observe for *bleeding; avoid* IM injection; do *not* mix other medications in line			
Streptokinase—IV 1.5 million U diluted to 45 mL infused over 60 min	Lysis of pulmonary or systemic emboli or thrombi; acute MI	Reacts with plasminogen, dissolves fibrin clots	Prolonged coagulation; allergic reactions; mild fever
NURSING IMPLICATIONS: Monitor for signs of excessive *bleeding,* particularly at injection sites; *avoid* nonessential handling of patient			
Urokinase—IV 4400 IU/kg over 10 min; 1.0–1.8 mL of 5000 IU/mL into catheter	Massive pulmonary emboli, coronary artery thrombi, occluded IV catheter	Directly activates plasminogen	Bleeding, anaphylaxis, rash
NURSING IMPLICATIONS: Vital signs; check *q15min* for bleeding during first hr; q15–30min for 8 hr; have *epinephrine* ready			
Fibrinolytic Antidote			
Aminocaproic acid (Amicar)—PO, IV 5 g loading dose; 1 g/hr to 30 g in 24 hr	Management of streptokinase or urokinase overdose	Inhibits plasminogen activator and antagonizes plasmin	Hypotension, bradycardia, cardiac arrhythmias
NURSING IMPLICATIONS: Give slowly IV to prevent side effects; not recommended for DIC			

TABLE 10–6   Common Drugs—cont'd

Drug and Dosage	Use	Action	◆ Assessment: Side Effects
Hormones			
Chlorotrianisene (TACE), estrogen—PO 12–50 mg	Prostatic cancer; menopause	Nonsteroidal synthetic estrogen	Rare after one course of treatment; thromboembolism; impotence and gynecomastia in men

NURSING IMPLICATIONS: Supply patient with package insert; *contraindicated* in blood coagulation disorders

Diethylstilbestrol (DES)—PO or IM 0.2–5.0 mg qd; vaginal suppository 0.1–0.5 mg at bedtime	Prostate carcinoma; menopausal symptoms; osteoporosis; pain; mammary carcinoma; atrophic vaginitis	Synthetic nonsteroidal compound with estrogenic effects on pituitary, ovaries, myometrium, endometrium, and other tissues	Anorexia, nausea, vomiting, headache, diarrhea, dizziness, fainting—many side effects with long-term use

NURSING IMPLICATIONS: *Never* give if woman is pregnant—predisposes to vaginal cancer in female offspring at puberty

Estradiol—PO 1–2 mg for replacement therapy; up to 10 mg for cancer qd–tid; cyclic (on 3 wk, off 1 wk)	Menopausal symptoms; osteoporosis; hypogenitalism; sexual infantilism; breast and prostatic carcinoma	Inhibits release of pituitary gonadotropins; promotes growth of female genital tissues	Anorexia, nausea, vomiting, diarrhea, fluid retention, mental depression, headache, thromboembolism; feminization in men

NURSING IMPLICATIONS: Baseline VS; weigh daily; encourage frequent physical checkups to check serum lipids; teach breast self-examination

Medroxyprogesterone (Provera)—PO 2.5–10.0 mg; IM 400–1000 mg weekly	Amenorrhea; functional uterine bleeding; threatened abortion; dysmenorrhea; adjunctive and palliative with renal cancer and endometriosis; PMS	Similar to progesterone, but can be taken orally; thickens uterine decidua	Drowsiness, cyclic menstrual withdrawal bleeding, GI upset, headache, edema, breast congestion

NURSING IMPLICATIONS: Teach patient regarding self–administration; breast self-examination for possible breast changes

Menotropins (Pergonal)—IM 1 amp (FSH + LH)/day for 9–12 days (followed by 5000–10,000 U HCG, if ovulation does not occur, repeat with 2 amp)	**Infertility use:** treatment of secondary anovulation; stimulation of spermatogenesis	Human gonadatropic responses; induces ovulation; sperm stimulation	Abortions occur in 25%; failure rate 55–80% of patients; possible multiple births; ovarian enlargement; gynecomastia in men

NURSING IMPLICATIONS: Assist in collection of urine to assess estrogen levels; counsel regarding couple's need to have daily intercourse from day of HCG injection until ovulation

Progesterone—SC or IM 5–10 mg qd; sublingual 5–10 mg	Amenorrhea; dysmenorrhea; endometriosis; habitual abortion	Converts endometrium into secreting structure; prevents ovulation; stimulates growth of mammary tissue	Nausea, vomiting, dizziness, edema, headache, protein metabolism

NURSING IMPLICATIONS: Give deep IM and rotate sites; weigh daily to ascertain fluid retention

Testosterone—PO 5–10 mg qd; IM 25–50 mg 2–3 times/wk; 200–400 mg IM q2–4wk for breast cancer	Hypogonadism; eunuchism; impotence; advanced cancer of breast	Growth of sex organs and appearance of secondary male sex characteristics; counteracts excessive amounts of estrogen	Nausea, dyspepsia, masculinization, hypercalcemia, menstrual irregularities, renal calculi; Na^+, K^+, and H_2O retention

NURSING IMPLICATIONS: Observe for edema; weigh daily; I&O; *push fluids* for bedridden patients, to prevent renal calculi

Vasopressin (Pitressin)—IM/SC 5–10 μ bid/qid; IM/SC 2.5–5 μ q2–3d for chronic therapy	Diabetes insipidus	Antidiuretic	Nausea, flatus, tremor, pounding in head, water intoxication

NURSING IMPLICATIONS: *Monitor* fluid balance, vital signs

Pharmacology

Continued

TABLE 10–6 Common Drugs—cont'd

Drug and Dosage	Use	Action	◆ Assessment: Side Effects
Immune Modifiers			
Glatiramer acetate (Copaxone)—20 mg/day	Multiple sclerosis	Management of relapsing-remitting MS	Allergic reactions, anxiety, chest pain, weight gain, cough
NURSING IMPLICATIONS: Monitor for side effects; new drug to attempt to control signs and symptoms of progressing multiple sclerosis			
Interferon β-1b (Betaseron)—30 μg once a week	Multiple sclerosis	Reduce incidence of relapse	Seizures, GI symptoms, flulike symptoms, neutropenia, injection site reactions
NURSING IMPLICATIONS: Monitor progress of multiple sclerosis; determine if drug is effective in reducing incidence of relapse; provide information about multiple side effects			
Immunosuppressant Agents			
Azathioprine (Imuran)—3–5 mg/kg/day initially; maintenance: 1–3 mg/kg/day	Prevent renal transplant rejection Ulcerative colitis Rheumatoid arthritis	Antagonizes purine metabolism/inhibition of DNA/RNA synthesis	Hypersensitivity; additive myelosuppression with antineoplastics; hepatotoxicity, leukopenia
NURSING IMPLICATIONS: Assess for infection; monitor I&O and *daily weight*			
Cyclosporine (Sandimmune)—PO 5–10 mg/kg several hours before surgery; daily for 2 weeks; reduce dosage by 2.5 mg/kg/week to 5–10 mg/kg/day. IV 5–6 mg/kg several hours before surgery daily; switch to PO form as soon as possible	Prevent organ rejection Ulcerative colitis Rheumatoid arthritis	Inhibits interleukin-2, which is necessary for initiation of T-cell activity	Hypersensitivity; *caution* with alcohol, renal impairment
NURSING IMPLICATIONS: *Monitor:* I&O, daily weight, blood pressure; take as directed (time of day and with food); observe *nephrotoxicity, gingival hyperplasia; avoid* self administration of OTC drugs			
Muromonab-CD3 (Orthoclone OKT3)—IV 5 mg/day, 10–14 days	Renal, liver, or cardiac transplant rejection	Immunosuppression of T-cell function	Tremor; dyspnea, shortness of breath; wheezing; chest pain; diarrhea; nausea, vomiting; chills, fever
NURSING IMPLICATIONS: Draw solution into filter; give IV push over <1 min; do *not* give as IV infusion; do *not* mix with other medications			
Mycophenolate (CellCept)—PO 1 g bid	Prevent renal transplant rejection	Inhibits purine synthesis; suppresses T and B lymphocytes	Diarrhea; vomiting; leukopenia; sepsis
NURSING IMPLICATIONS: Give initial dose *within* 72 hr of transplant; give on *empty* stomach 1 hr before or 2 hr after meals; do *not* open, crush, or chew capsules; do *not* give with *magnesium* or *aluminum* antacids			
Tracrolimus—PO 0.075–0.15 mg/kg q12h; IV 0.05–0.1 mg/kg/day	Prevent rejection in liver transplant	Inhibits T-lymphocyte activation	Headache, insomnia, tremor, ascites, hypertension, peripheral edema, abdominal pain, rash, hyperglycemia, anemia
NURSING IMPLICATIONS: Give 6 *hr after* transplant; oral therapy is preferred because of anaphylaxis with IV; therapy is lifelong			
Mineralocorticoid Agent			
Fludrocortisone (Florinef)—PO 0.1–0.2 mg qd	Addison's	Causes sodium reabsorption, hydrogen and potassium excretion, and water retention	Heart failure; adrenal suppression, hypertension
NURSING IMPLICATIONS: Do *not* miss dose; therapy is lifelong; high potassium; *report:* weight gain, muscle weakness, cramps, nausea, anorexia, dizziness			

Pharmacology

TABLE 10–6   Common Drugs—cont'd

Drug and Dosage	Use	Action	◆ Assessment: Side Effects
Mucolytic Agent			
Acetylcysteine (Mucomyst)—1–5 mL of 20% solution or 1–10 mL of 10% solution per nebulizer tid	Emphysema; pneumonia; tracheostomy care; atelectasis; cystic fibrosis	Lowers viscosity of respiratory secretions by opening disulfide linkages in mucus	Stomatitis, nausea, rhinorrhea, bronchospasm

NURSING IMPLICATIONS: Observe *respiratory rate;* maintain open airway with suctioning as necessary; observe asthmatics carefully for *increased bronchospasm;* discontinue treatment immediately if this occurs; odor disagreeable initially

Drug and Dosage	Use	Action	Assessment: Side Effects
Muscle Relaxants			
Baclofen (Lioresal)—5 mg tid up to 10–20 mg 4 times/day maintenance dose	Relief of spasticity of multiple sclerosis, spinal cord injury	Centrally acting skeletal-muscle relaxant; depresses polysynaptic afferent reflex activity at spinal cord level	Pruritis, tinnitus; nausea, vomiting; diarrhea or constipation; drowsiness

NURSING IMPLICATIONS: Administer *with* food if GI symptoms; monitor for safety when ambulating; do *not* discontinue abruptly

Drug and Dosage	Use	Action	Assessment: Side Effects
Dantrolene sodium (Dantrium)—25 mg/day to 25 mg bid–tid to 100 mg qid max	See Baclofen	See Baclofen	See Baclofen

NURSING IMPLICATIONS: See Baclofen

Drug and Dosage	Use	Action	Assessment: Side Effects
Narcotic Antagonist			
Naloxone HCl (Narcan)—IV 0.1–0.2 mg repeated q2–3 min prn up to 0.4–2 mg for narcotic-induced respiratory depression	Reverses respiratory depression due to narcotics	Reverses respiratory depression of morphine SO_4, meperidine HCl, and methadone HCl; does not itself cause respiratory depression, sedation, or analgesia	No common side effects; tachycardia, hypertension, nausea and vomiting with high doses

NURSING IMPLICATIONS: Note time, type of narcotic, dosage received; not useful with CNS depression from other drugs; respiratory depression *may return;* monitor closely

Drug and Dosage	Use	Action	Assessment: Side Effects
Sedatives and Hypnotics			
Chlordiazepoxide HCl (Librium)—PO 5–10 mg; IM or IV 50–100 mg	Psychoneuroses; preoperative apprehension; chronic alcoholism; anxiety	CNS depressant resulting in mild sedation; appetite stimulant; anticonvulsant	Ataxia, fatigue, blurred vision, diplopia, lethargy, nightmares, confusion

NURSING IMPLICATIONS: Ensure anxiety relief by allowing patient to verbalize feelings; advise patient to *avoid* driving and alcoholic beverages

Drug and Dosage	Use	Action	Assessment: Side Effects
Chloral hydrate—PO 250 mg tid; hypnotic: PO 0.5–1.0 g; rectal supplement 0.3–0.9 g	Sedation for elderly; delirium tremens; pruritus; mania; barbiturate and alcohol withdrawal	Depresses sensorimotor areas of cerebral cortex	Nausea, vomiting, gastritis; pinpoint pupils; delirium; rash; decreased BP, pulse, respirations, temperature; hepatic damage

NURSING IMPLICATIONS: *Caution:* should not be taken in combination with alcohol; dependency is possible

Drug and Dosage	Use	Action	Assessment: Side Effects
Diazepam (Valium)—PO 2–10 mg tid–qid; IM or IV 2–10 mg q3–4h	Anxiety disorders; alcohol withdrawal; adjunctive therapy in seizure disorders; status epilepticus; tetanus, preoperative or preprocedural sedation (also see Midazolam)	Induces calming effect on limbic system, thalamus, and hypothalamus	CNS depression—sedation or ataxia (dose related); dry mouth; blurred vision; mydriasis; constipation; urinary retention

NURSING IMPLICATIONS: Do *not* mix with other drugs; IM injection painful; observe for *phlebitis;* monitor response; measures to ensure patient safety (e.g., falls); high potential for abuse; *contraindicated* in acute closed-angle glaucoma and porphyria

Continued

Pharmacology

TABLE 10–6 **Common Drugs—cont'd**

Drug and Dosage	Use	Action	◆ Assessment: Side Effects
Sedatives and Hypnotics—cont'd			
Flurazepam (Dalmane)—PO >15 yr, 30 mg hs; elderly or debilitated, 15 mg hs	Hypnotic	Fastest acting; see Diazepam	See Diazepam
NURSING IMPLICATIONS: See Diazepam			
Hydroxyzine pamoate (Vistaril)—PO 25–100 mg qid	See Chlordiazepoxide (Librium); antiemetic in postoperative conditions; adjunctive therapy	CNS relaxant with sedative effect on limbic system and thalamus	Drowsiness, headache, itching, dry mouth, tremor
NURSING IMPLICATIONS: Give deep IM only; *potentiates* action of warfarin (Coumadin), narcotics, and barbiturates			
Lorazepam (Ativan)—PO 1–2 mg bid–tid (up to 10 mg); 2–4 mg hs; IM 4 mg max; IV 2 mg max	Anxiety disorders; insomnia; alternative to diazepam for status epilepticus; preanesthesia	See Diazepam	See Diazepam
NURSING IMPLICATIONS: See Diazepam			
Meprobamate (Equanil, Miltown)—PO 400 mg tid–qid	Anxiety; stress; absence seizures	See Hydroxyzine pamoate (Vistaril)	Voracious appetite, dryness of mouth, ataxia
NURSING IMPLICATIONS: Older patients prone to drowsiness and hypotension; observe for *jaundice*			
Midazolam (Versed)—IM 0.05–0.08 mg/kg; IV 0.1–0.15 mg/kg	Preanesthesia; prediagnostic procedures; induction of general anesthesia	Penetrates blood-brain barrier to produce sedation and amnesia	Respiratory depression, apnea, disorientation, behavioral excitement
NURSING IMPLICATIONS: Monitor ventilatory status and oxygenation; prevent injuries from CNS depression; nonirritating to vein			
Phenobarbital—sedative, PO 20–30 mg tid; hypnotic, PO 50–100 mg; IV or IM 100–300 mg; butabarbital (Butisol), pentobarbital (Nembutal), secobarbital (Seconal)	Preoperative sedation; emergency control of convulsions; absence seizures	Depresses CNS, promoting drowsiness	Cough, hiccups, restlessness, pain, hangover; CNS and circulatory depression
NURSING IMPLICATIONS: Observe for hypotension during IV administration; put up side rails on bed of older patients; observe for increased tolerance			
Promethazine (Phenergan)—IV, IM, PO 25–50 mg	Preoperative sedation; postoperative sedation	Antihistaminic; sedative, antiemetic, anti–motion sickness	Drowsiness; coma; hypotension, hypertension; leukopenia; photosensitivity; irregular respirations; blurred vision; urinary retention; dry mouth, nose, throat
NURSING IMPLICATIONS: Administer PO *with* food, milk; IM deep into large muscles, rotate sites; verify compatibility with other drugs; safety concerns due to sedative effect			
Serum			
Immune globulin—IM 0.02 mL/kg	Hepatitis	Provides passive immunity	Do *not* use if patient is hypersensitive
NURSING IMPLICATIONS: Should be administered within *2 wk* of exposure			
Thyroid Hormone Inhibitors			
Lugol's solution—PO 2–6 drops tid 10 days before thyroidectomy	To reduce size, vascularity of thyroid before thyroid surgery; emergency treatment of thyroid storm; or control of hyperthyroid symptoms after radioiodine (^{131}I) therapy	Inhibits thyroid hormone secretion, synthesis	GI distress; stained teeth; increased respiratory secretions; rashes, acne
NURSING IMPLICATIONS: *Dilute in juice,* give through *straw;* bloody diarrhea/vomiting indicates acute poisoning			

Pharmacology

TABLE 10–6   Common Drugs—cont'd

Drug and Dosage	Use	Action	◆ Assessment: Side Effects
Thyroid Hormone Inhibitors—cont'd			
Propylthiouracil—PO 300–400 mg/day, divided initial dose; 100–150 mg/day maintenance dose; methimazole (Tapazole) 15–60 mg/day initial dose; 5–15 mg/day maintenance dose	Hyperthyroidism; return patient to euthyroid state; also used preoperatively	Inhibits functional thyroid hormone synthesis by blocking reactions; responsible for iodide conversion to iodine; inhibition of T_4 conversion to T_3	Blood dyscrasias, hepatotoxicity, hypothyroidism
NURSING IMPLICATIONS: Teach importance of compliance with medication protocol; *avoid* iodine-rich foods (seafood, iodized salt); caution when using other drugs			
Saturated potassium iodide (SSKI)—300 mg tid–qid	See Lugol's solution	See Lugol's solution	See Lugol's solution
NURSING IMPLICATIONS: See Lugol's solution			
Thyroid Hormone Replacement			
Levothyroxine (Levothroid, Synthroid)—PO 0.05–0.10 mg/day; IV 200–500 μg	Hypothyroidism	Replacement therapy to alleviate symptoms	Symptoms of hyperthyroidism
	Myxedema coma	Emergency replacement therapy	
NURSING IMPLICATIONS: Teach signs and symptoms of hyperthyroidism, hypothyroidism; monitor bowel activity; teach diet to combat constipation; keep medication in tight light-proof container; *avoid foods* that inhibit thyroid secretion (turnips, cabbage, carrots, peaches, peas, strawberries, spinach, radishes)			
Liothyronine (Cytomel)—PO 25 μg/day to maintenance dose 25–75 μg	Mild hypothyroidism in adults	Replacement therapy	See Levothyroxine
NURSING IMPLICATIONS: See Levothyroxine			
Uterine Contractants			
Ergonovine maleate (Ergotrate)—PO, IM, IV 0.2 mg (gr 1/320)	Postabortal or postpartum hemorrhage; promotes involution after delivery of placenta	Stimulates uterine contractions for 3 hr or more	Nausea, vomiting; occasional transient hypertension, especially if given IV; cramping
NURSING IMPLICATIONS: Store in *cool* place; monitor maternal BP and pulse; *do not use in labor*			
Methylergonovine maleate (Methergine)—PO 0.2 mg; IM, IV, 0.2 mg (gr 1/320)	Postpartum hemorrhage, after delivery of placenta	Stimulates stronger and longer contractions than ergonovine maleate (Ergotrate)	Nausea, vomiting, transient hypertension, dizziness, tachycardia; cramping
NURSING IMPLICATIONS: Do *not* give if mother is hypertensive; do *not* use if solution is discolored; *do not use in labor*			
Oxytocin (Pitocin, Syntocinon)—IM 0.3–1.0 mL; IV 1 mL (10 U) in 1000 mL solution	Stimulates rhythmic contractions of uterus	Induces labor; augments contractions; prevents or controls postpartum atony; antidiuretic effect	Tetanic contractions, uterine rupture, cardiac arrhythmias, FHR deceleration
NURSING IMPLICATIONS: *Contraindicated* if cervix is unripe, in CPD, abruptio placentae, and cardiovascular disease; *monitor:* FHR, contractions, maternal BP, pulse, I&O; watch for signs of water intoxication with prolonged IV use; drug of choice in presence of hypertension; *never* use undiluted; DC if tetanic contractions occur; *antidote:* propranolol			
Volume Expander			
Albumin—IV 5%, 25% 500 mL as needed	Cirrhosis	Provides colloidal oncotic pressure, which mobilizes fluid from extracellular back into intravascular space	Hypersensitivity, CHF, hepatic failure
NURSING IMPLICATIONS: Monitor progress of disease; monitor for signs of shock; if fever, tachycardia, or hypotension occur, *stop* treatment and call physician			

Pharmacology

FOOD AND FLUID CONSIDERATIONS WITH DRUGS

Table 10–7.

ANTINEOPLASTIC DRUG CLASSIFICATIONS

Table 10–8.

TABLE 10–7 Food and Fluid Considerations with Drugs

Key:
1. Take with food or milk
2. Take on empty stomach (1h ac or 2h pc)
3. Don't drink milk or eat dairy products
4. Take with full glass of water
5. Take ½ h before meals
6. Take with or without food

A
Albuterol 1
Allopurinol 1
Aminophylline 1
Amlodipine 6
Amiodarone 1
Amoxicillin 6
Ampicillin 2
Aspirin 1
Augmentin 6
Azo Gantrisin 4,6

B
Baclofen 1
Bactrim 4,6
Belladonna 5
Benemid 1,4
Bisacodyl 3

C
Captopril 2
Cefaclor 6
Cefuroxime axetil 6

Cephalexin 6
Cholestyramine 5
Chlorothiazide 1
Cimetidine 1
Ciprofloxacin 4,6
Clonazepam 1
Clopidogrel 6
Cloxacillin 2
Co-trimoxazole 4,6
Cyclosporine 1

D
Demeclocycline 2,3
Diltiazem 1
Diuril 1
Donnatal 5
Dopar 1
Doxycycline hyclate 3,6
Dulcolax 3

E
Ecotrin 3
Enalapril 6
Ethosuximide 1
Etodolac 2
Eythromycin stearate 2

F
Famotidine 6
Feldene 1
Ferrous sulfate 3
Flecainide 6
Fluoxetine 6

G
Gantrisin 4,6
Gemfibrozil 5
Glycopyrrolate 5

H
Hismanyl 2
Hydrocodone/acetaminophen 1
Hydromorphone 1

I
Ibuprofen 1,2
Ilosone 6
Indinavir 2,4
Indomethacin 1
Isoniazid 2

K
Keflex 6
Ketoconazole 1
Ketoprofen 1
K-Lor 1

L
Levodopa 1
Libium 1
Lisinopril 6
Lovastatin 1

M
Macrodantin 1
Marax 1
Metronidazole 1
Mexiletine 1
Mycophenolate 2

N
Nafcillin 2
Naproxen 4
Neostigmine 5
Niacin 1
Nicardipine 5
Nitrofurantoin 1

P
Parlodel 1
Penicillamine 2
Penicillin G 2
Penicillin V 2
Persantine 2
Phenylbutazone 1
Phenytoin 1
Prednisone 1
Pro-Banthine 5
Probenecid 4

Q
Quinidine 1

R
Ranitidine 6
Rifampin 2
Robinul 5

S
Simvastatin 6
Sinemet 1
Slow-K 1
Sucralfate 2
Sulfisoxazole 4,6

T
Tedral 1
Tetracycline 2,3
Theophylline 1,4
Ticlopidine 1
Trimethoprim 2

V
Vasotec 6

Z
Zestril 6

TABLE 10–8 Antineoplastic Drug Classifications

I. **Alkylating agents**
   A. Alkyl sulfonates
      1. Busulfan *(Myleran)*
   B. Ethylenimines
      1. Thiotepa
   C. Nitrosoureas
      1. Carmustine (BCNU, *BiCNU*)
      2. Lomustine (CCNU, *CeeNu*)
      3. Semustine (methyl-CCNU)
      4. Streptozocin *(Zanosar,* streptozotocin)
   D. Nitrogen mustards
      1. Mechlorethamine hydrochloride *(Mustargen,* HN_2, nitrogen mustard)
      2. Cyclophosphamide *(Cytoxan)*
      3. Chlorambucil *(Leukeran)*
      4. Melphalan *(Alkeran, L-PAM,* L-phenylalanine mustard)
      5. Ifosfamide *(Ifex)*
   E. Triazenes
      1. Dacarbazine *(DTIC-Dome)*
II. **Antibiotics**
   A. Anthracyclines
      1. Doxorubicin hydrochloride *(Adriamycin)*
      2. Daunorubicin (daunomycin, *Cerubidine)*
      3. Idarubicin *(Idamycin)*
   B. Bleomycins
      1. Bleomycin sulfate *(Blenoxane)*
   C. Dactinomycin (actinomycin D, *Cosmegen)*
   D. Mitomycin (mitomycin C, *Mutamycin)*
   E. Plicamycin *(Mithracin)*
III. **Antimetabolites**
   A. Folate antagonist
      1. Methotrexate *(Folex, Mexate)*
   B. Purine analogues
      1. Thioguanine (6-TG, 6-thioguanine)
      2. Mercaptopurine (6-MP, *Purinethol)*
      3. Fludarabine *(Fludara)*
      4. Pentostatin (deoxycoformycin, *Nipent)*
      5. Cladribine (2-chloro-deoxyadenosine, *Leustatin)*
   C. Pyrimidine analogues
      1. Cytarabine (cytosine arabinoside, *Cytosar-U,* ara-C)
      2. Fluorouracil (5-FU, 5-fluorouracil)

IV. **Cellular growth factors**
   A. Filgrastim *(Neupogen)*
   B. Sargramostim *(Leukine, Prokine)*
V. **Enzymes**
   A. L-Asparaginase *(Elspar)*
VI. **Hormonal agents**
   A. Androgens/antiandrogens
      1. Flutamide *(Eulexin)*
   B. Estrogens/antiestrogens
      1. Tamoxifen citrate *(Nolvadex)*
      2. Estramustine phosphate sodium *(Emcyt)*
   C. Glucocorticoids
   D. Luteinizing hormone–releasing hormone (LH-RH) antagonists
      1. Buserelin *(Suprefact)*
      2. Leuprolide *(Lupron)*
   E. Octreotide acetate *(Sandostatin)*
VII. **Immunomodulating agents**
   A. Levamisole *(Ergamisol)*
   B. Interferons
      1. Interferon alfa-2a *(Roferon-A)*
      2. Interferon alfa-2b *(Intron A)*
   C. Interleukins: aldesleukin (interleukin-2, IL-2, *Proleukin)*
VIII. **Miscellaneous agents**
   A. Carboplatin *(Paraplatin)*
   B. Cisplatin *(cis-*platinum II, *Platinol)*
   C. Hexamethylmelamine (HMM)
   D. Hydroxyurea *(Hydrea)*
   E. Mitotane (o,p'-DDD, *Lysodren)*
   F. Mitoxantrone *(Novantrone)*
   G. Procarbazine (N-methylhydrazine, *Matulane, Natulan)*
IX. **Monoclonal antibodies**
X. **Plant-derived products**
   A. Vinca alkaloids
      1. Vincristine *(Oncovin)*
      2. Vinblastine *(Velban)*
   B. Epipodophyllotoxins
      1. Etoposide *(Vepesid)*
      2. Teniposide *(Vumon)*
   C. Taxanes: paclitaxel *(Taxol)*

Pharmacology

PROPERTIES OF SELECTED ANALGESIC AGENTS

Table 10–9.

EQUIANALGESIC DOSING FOR OPIOID ANALGESICS

Table 10–10.

TABLE 10–9   Properties of Selected Analgesic Agents

Specific Group	Analgesic	Antipyretic	Anti-inflammatory
Nonopioid			
Acetaminophen	*	*	0
Ibuprofen	*	*	*
Naproxen	*	*	*
Fenoprofen	*	*	*
Flurbiprofen	*	*	*
Ketoprofen	*	*	*
Nonsteroidal			
Aspirin	*	*	*
Indomethacin	*	*	*
Sulindac	*	0	*
Meclofenamate	*	0	*
Tolmetin	*	*	*
Diflunisal	*	0	*
Piroxicam	*	*	*
Diclofenac	*	*	*
Etodolac	*	0	*
Nabumetone	*	*	*

* = possesses the property assigned; 0 = lacks the property assigned.

TABLE 10–10 Equianalgesic Dosing for Opioid Analgesics

Drug	Approximate Equianalgesic Dose		Recommended Starting Dose (adults >50 kg body weight)		Recommended Starting Dose (children and adults <50 kg body weight)[a]	
	Oral	Parenteral	Oral	Parenteral	Oral	Parenteral
Opioid Agonist[b]						
Morphine[b]	30 mg q3–4h (around-the-clock dosing) 60 mg q3–4h (single dose or inter-mittent dosing)	10 mg q3–4h	30 mg q3–4h	10 mg q3–4h	0.3 mg/kg q3–4h	0.1 mg/kg q3–4h
Codeine[c]	180–200 mg q3–4h	130 mg q3–4h	60 mg q3–4h	60 mg q2h (intramuscular/subcutaneous)	1mg/kg q3–4h[d]	Not recommended
Hydrocodone (in Lorcet, Lortab, Vicodin, others)	30 mg q3–4h	Not available	10 mg q3–4h	Not available	0.2 mg/kg q3–4h[d]	Not available
Hydromorphone[b] (Dilaudid)	7.5 mg q3–4h	1.5 mg q3–4h	6 mg q3–4h	1.5 mg q3–4h	0.06 mg/kg q3–4h	0.015 mg/kg q3–4h
Levorphanol (Levo-Dromoran)	4 mg q6–8h	2 mg q6–8h	4 mg q6–8h	2 mg q6–8h	0.04 mg/kg q6–8h	0.02 mg/kg q6–8h
Meperidine (Demerol)	300 mg q2–3h	100 mg q3h	Not recommended	100 mg q3h	Not recommended	0.75 mg/kg q2–3h
Methadone (Dolophine, others)	20 mg q6–8h	10 mg q6–8h	20 mg q6–8h	10 mg q6–8h	0.2 mg/kg q6–8h	0.1 mg/kg q6–8h
Oxycodone (Roxicodone, also in Percocet, Percodan, Tylox, others)	30 mg q3–4h	Not available	10 mg q3–4h	Not available	0.2 mg/kg q3–4h[d]	Not available
Oxymorphone[b] (Numorphan)	Not available	1 mg q3–4h	Not available	1 mg q3–4h	Not recommended	Not recommended
Opioid Agonist-Antagonist and Partial Agonist						
Buprenorphine (Buprenex)	Not available	0.3–0.4 mg q6–8 h	Not available	0.4 mg q6–8h	Not available	0.004 mg/kg q6–8h
Butorphanol (Stadol)	Not available	2 mg q3–4h	Not available	2 mg q3–4h	Not available	Not recommended
Dezocine (Dalgan)	Not available	10 mg q3–4h	Not available	10 mg q3–4h	Not available	Not recommended
Nalbuphine (Nubain)	Not available	10 mg q3–4h	Not available	10 mg q3–4h	Not available	0.1 mg/kg q3–4h
Pentazocine (Talwin, others)	150 mg q3–4h	60 mg q3–4h	50 mg q4–6h	Not recommended	Not recommended	Not recommended

Adapted from Acute Pain Management Guideline Panel: *Acute Pain Management in Adults: Operative Procedures. Quick Reference Guide for Clinicians.* Agency for Health Care Policy and Research, Public Health and Human Services, Rockville, MD, 1992. AHCPR Publication No. 92-0019.

Note: Published tables vary in the suggested doses that are equianalgesic to morphine. Clinical response is the criterion that must be applied for each patient; titration to clinical response is necessary. Because there is not complete cross-tolerance among these drugs, it is usually necessary to use a lower than equianalgesic dose when changing drugs and to retitrate to response.

Caution: Recommended doses do not apply to patients with renal or hepatic insufficiency or other conditions affecting drug metabolism and kinetics.

[a]Caution: Doses listed for patients with body weight less than 50 kg cannot be used as initial starting doses in babies less than 6 mo of age.

[b]For morphine, hydromorphone, and oxymorphone, rectal administration is an alternate route for patients unable to take oral medications, but equianalgesic doses may differ from oral and parenteral doses because of pharmacokinetic differences.

[c]**Caution:** Codeine doses above 65 mg often are not appropriate because of diminishing incremental analgesia with increasing doses but continually increasing constipation and other side effects. Oral doses refer to combination with aspirin or acetaminophen.

[d]**Caution:** Doses of aspirin and acetaminophen in combination opioid/NSAID preparations must also be adjusted to the patient's body weight.

Pharmacology

Questions

Select the one best answer for each question.

1. A patient has meperidine, 75 mg every 3–4 hours prn, ordered for postoperative pain. Before administering this narcotic, the nurse should:
   1. Position in a semi-Fowler's position to minimize respiratory effects.
   2. Assess the type, location, and intensity of discomfort.
   3. Evaluate whether the pain is real.
   4. Try other measures to relieve discomfort, such as position change.

2. Neostigmine bromide (Prostigmin), 0.5 mg subcutaneously stat, is ordered by a patient's physician to relieve urinary retention. The nurse knows that this drug is classified as:
   1. A cholinergic.
   2. An anticholinesterase.
   3. An anticholinergic.
   4. A beta blocker.

3. The nurse explains to a patient that although salicylates are given to relieve pain in rheumatoid arthritis, they also function as an:
   1. Analgesic.
   2. Anti-inflammatory.
   3. Anticholinergic.
   4. Antiadrenergic.

4. Drug therapy goals for a patient include strengthening cardiac contraction and increasing glomerular filtration rate. Which medication would the nurse prepare to accomplish both goals?
   1. Epinephrine.
   2. Digoxin.
   3. Furosemide (Lasix).
   4. Hydralazine.

5. Which outcome is the best indicator that digoxin has been effective?
   1. Increased systolic and diastolic pressures.
   2. Unlabored respirations and increased urinary output.
   3. Decreased pulse rate and increased urinary output.
   4. Increased blood pressure and decreased pulse rate.

6. Patient teaching includes the early side effects of theophylline administration, which are:
   1. Tachycardia and palpitations.
   2. Anorexia, nausea, and vomiting.
   3. Restlessness and tremors.
   4. Headache and insomnia.

7. Based on the peak action of furosemide (Lasix) PO, the nurse will evaluate the drug's effects in:
   1. 30–60 minutes.
   2. 1–2 hours.
   3. 3–4 hours.
   4. 6–8 hours.

8. The nurse administers sodium polystyrene sulfonate (Kayexalate) knowing that the drug reduces hyperkalemia by:
   1. Exchanging sodium ions for potassium ions in the GI tract, thereby increasing potassium excretion in the feces.
   2. Inhibiting potassium absorption sites in the GI tract.
   3. Promoting diarrhea, thereby decreasing potassium absorption from the gut.
   4. Altering the effects of aldosterone in the kidney tubules.

9. The nurse knows that the best time to give oral iron preparations is:
   1. With meals, to decrease gastric upset.
   2. 1 hour before eating, to enhance absorption.
   3. 1 hour after eating, to slow absorption.
   4. At bedtime.

10. A patient is instructed to report the following side effect of neomycin administration:
    1. Deafness.
    2. Nausea.
    3. Diarrhea.
    4. Anaphylaxis.

11. Before administering morphine sulfate, the nurse should check:
    1. Apical and radial pulse.
    2. Respiratory rate.
    3. Urinary output.
    4. Skin color and turgor.

12. The nurse administers spironolactone (Aldactone) knowing that it is classified as:
    1. An aldosterone antagonist.
    2. A carbonic anhydrase inhibitor.
    3. A thiazide.
    4. An osmotic diuretic.

13. Which supplement would the nurse not ordinarily administer to the patient receiving spironolactone?
    1. Vitamin B_6.
    2. Potassium chloride.
    3. Ascorbic acid.
    4. Calcium carbonate.

14. The primary objective in giving prednisone along with aspirin for acute rheumatoid arthritis is:
    1. To inhibit the autoimmune factors associated with rheumatoid arthritis.
    2. To prevent further joint destruction.
    3. To decrease inflammation and suppress symptomatology.
    4. To increase glucose levels for tissue repair.

15. The nurse would recognize prednisone toxicity if which of the following occurred?
    1. Tinnitus.
    2. Exfoliative dermatitis.
    3. Glucosuria.
    4. Nausea and vomiting.

16. Propantheline bromide (Pro-Banthine) is given to patients with cholelithiasis and cholecystitis because it:
    1. Reduces gastric secretions and intestinal hypermobility.
    2. Decreases bile secretion by the liver and gallbladder.
    3. Slows the emptying of the stomach, thereby reducing chyme in the duodenum.
    4. Inhibits contraction of the gallbladder and the bile duct.

17. The nurse would most likely give papaverine HCl for relief of gallbladder pain rather than morphine SO_4 because:
    1. Morphine depresses gallbladder contractions, thereby decreasing bile secretions.
    2. Opiates tend to mask symptoms in patients with acute abdomen.
    3. Morphine tends to increase contractions of the sphincter of Oddi, thereby increasing intraductal pressures.
    4. Morphine relaxes smooth muscles, thereby increasing bile production.

18. The nurse can anticipate side effects of hydrochlorothiazide because it is classified as:
    1. An aldosterone inhibitor.
    2. A carbonic anhydrase inhibitor.
    3. A potassium-sparing drug.
    4. A potassium-wasting drug.

19. The nurse knows that hydrochlorothiazide exerts its primary effect on:
    1. The proximal and distal tubules of the kidney.
    2. The distal convoluted tubule of the kidney only.
    3. The distal ascending loop of Henle and the distal tubule of the kidney.
    4. The descending loop of Henle and the proximal tubule of the kidney.

20. Assessment for the side effects of hydrochlorothiazide includes signs of:
    1. Hypernatremia.
    2. Hyperkalemia.
    3. Hypochloremia.
    4. Hypouricemia.
21. A 2-year-old child (diagnosis: meningitis) is to be sedated with phenobarbital, 18 mg PO q6h. The label reads "20 mg per 5 mL." How much phenobarbital should the nurse administer to this child?
    1. 4 mL.
    2. 4.3 mL.
    3. 4.5 mL.
    4. 4.8 mL.
22. A patient's CSF culture is positive for *Haemophilus influenzae* meningitis. To protect other members of the patient's family who have been exposed to meningitis, the nurse should explain that they may be given:
    1. Amoxicillin/clavulanate potassium (Augmentin).
    2. Sulfisoxazole.
    3. Rifampin.
    4. Immune serum globulin.
23. The nurse is to administer pancreatin to a child with cystic fibrosis. To evaluate the effect of this medication, the nurse should know that the primary purpose of this medication is to increase the absorption of:
    1. Glucose.
    2. Vitamin C.
    3. Sodium chloride.
    4. Fats.
24. The nurse about to administer medication to a 5-year-old patient notes that the child has no ID bracelet. The best way for the nurse to identify this patient would be to ask:
    1. The child, "Is your name _____?"
    2. The adult visiting, "The child's name is _____?"
    3. The other children in the room what the child's name is.
    4. Another staff nurse to identify this child.
25. Elixir of digoxin (Lanoxin) is available with 0.05 mg of the drug in 1 mL of solution. How much of this elixir should the nurse administer if the physician's order reads "0.125 mg PO bid"?
    1. 2 mL.
    2. 2.25 mL.
    3. 2.5 mL.
    4. 2.75 mL.
26. In teaching a parent how to administer Cortisporin eye drops to an infant, the nurse would be most correct in advising the parent to place the drops:
    1. Directly onto the infant's sclera.
    2. In the inner canthus of the infant's eye.
    3. In the outer canthus of the infant's eye.
    4. In the middle of the lower conjunctival sac of the infant's eye.
27. The doctor orders ferrous sulfate (Fer-in-Sol), 0.6 mL PO tid. For maximum absorption, the nurse should plan to administer this medication:
    1. Between meals.
    2. Before meals.
    3. During meals.
    4. After meals.
28. Two weeks after starting an oral iron supplement, the patient's mother tells the nurse that the child's stools are black. The nurse should advise the mother:
    1. "This is a normal side effect and means the medication is working."
    2. "I will notify the doctor, who will probably decrease the dosage slightly."
    3. "I will need a specimen to check the stool for possible bleeding."
    4. "You sound quite concerned. Would you like to talk about this further?"
29. A pregnant woman's history reveals 12 weeks of gestation, severe pruritus, dysuria, and thick creamy vaginal discharge for the past 3 days. Which assessment factor is considered predisposing to the development of monilial vaginitis?
    1. Pregnancy.
    2. Late adolescence.
    3. High-carbohydrate diet.
    4. Sickle cell anemia.
30. Health teaching for a patient with vaginal infection with *Candida albicans* should be planned and implemented to ensure her consistent and appropriate use of the prescribed medication. Which medication is effective in the treatment of monilial (yeast) vaginitis?
    1. Metronidazole (Flagyl) oral tablets.
    2. Nystatin (Mycostatin) vaginal suppositories.
    3. Local applications of podophyllin.
    4. Antibiotic (bacitracin) ointment.
31. Reviewing the results of a patient's routine prenatal lab work, the nurse notes that her VDRL is positive. To protect the fetus from congenital syphilis, the patient must receive treatment before weeks 18–20. History suggests possible allergy to penicillin. Which drug would be ordered to treat venereal disease in the penicillin-allergic patient?
    1. Streptomycin.
    2. Sulfisoxazole (Gantrisin).
    3. Chloramphenicol (Chloromycetin).
    4. Erythromycin.
32. Health teaching regarding uncomfortable signs and symptoms of side effects of oral antibiotic therapy includes:
    1. Tinnitus (ringing in the ears).
    2. Nausea, vomiting, and abdominal pain.
    3. Nausea and glossitis.
    4. Nausea, diarrhea, and vaginal yeast infections.
33. Which medication is ordered most commonly to attempt to inhibit premature labor?
    1. Diazepam (Valium).
    2. Betamethasone.
    3. Ritodrine (Yutopar).
    4. Bromocryptine mesylate (Parlodel).
34. In evaluating a patient's response to beta-mimetic therapy used to inhibit premature labor, to which sign of side effects must the nurse be alert?
    1. Maternal hypertension.
    2. Fetal bradycardia.
    3. Maternal and fetal tachycardia.
    4. Uterine hypertonia.
35. When a parturient is given a paracervical block, the nurse can expect:
    1. Low forceps birth.
    2. Depression of contractions, maternal hypotension, fetal bradycardia, postnatal uterine atony.
    3. Depression of contractions and fetal bradycardia.
    4. Loss of bearing-down reflex, low forceps birth.
36. When a parturient is given epidural (or caudal) anesthesia, the nurse could expect:
    1. Maternal hypotension, low forceps birth, need to remain flat in bed for several hours after birth.
    2. Loss of bearing-down reflex, depression of contractions, maternal hypotension, fetal bradycardia, low forceps birth.
    3. Loss of bearing-down reflex, depression of contractions, maternal hypotension, fetal bradycardia, low forceps birth, postnatal bladder atony, postnatal uterine atony.
    4. Depression of contractions, maternal hypotension.

37. When a parturient is given saddle block (low spinal) anesthesia, the nurse can expect:
    1. Loss of bearing-down reflex, maternal hypotension, low forceps birth, need to remain flat in bed for several hours after birth.
    2. Fetal bradycardia, low forceps birth, postnatal uterine atony, need to remain flat in bed for several hours after birth.
    3. Loss of bearing-down reflex, low forceps birth, postnatal bladder atony, postnatal uterine atony.
    4. Loss of bearing-down reflex, maternal hypotension, low forceps birth, need to remain flat in bed for several hours after birth, fetal bradycardia, postnatal uterine atony, postnatal bladder atony.

38. A patient is receiving tetracycline preoperatively in preparation for bowel surgery. Which *common* side effect should the nurse instruct the patient to expect with tetracycline?
    1. Urticaria.
    2. Urinary retention.
    3. Jaundice.
    4. Deafness.

39. The following activities have been planned for a patient who is mute and autistic. In which activity will it be important for the nursing staff to take precautionary measures for a common side effect of Thorazine (chlorpromazine), which has been prescribed for this patient?
    1. Shopping in an enclosed mall after lunch.
    2. Attending the symphony on Wednesday evening.
    3. A day at the beach, if the weather permits.
    4. A morning at the art museum.

40. Some patients who are on phenothiazines are also given benztropine mesylate (Cogentin). The nurse administers this medication in order to:
    1. Prevent skin reactions.
    2. Increase the effectiveness of the phenothiazines.
    3. Decrease motor restlessness.
    4. Reduce extrapyramidal side effects.

41. A patient has been on IM fluphenazine (Prolixin) for 3 years. This patient has recently complained of frequent sore throats and malaise. What potentially serious side effect might these symptoms indicate to the nurse?
    1. Agranulocytosis.
    2. Akathisia.
    3. Dystonia.
    4. Dyskinesia.

42. When nialamide (Niamid) or isocarboxazid (Marplan) is administered, what must the nurse know about the effects of these drugs?
    1. They lower the threshold for seizures.
    2. They potentiate the effects of many other drugs and common foods.
    3. They decrease muscular contractions.
    4. They commonly cause obstructive jaundice.

43. Lithium salts are frequently used to treat manic disorders. What side effect is the nurse *least* likely to observe?
    1. Slurred speech.
    2. Twitching and athetotic movements.
    3. Motor weakness.
    4. Tardive dyskinesia.

44. A 9-month-old patient has been diagnosed with Hirschsprung's disease. At this time, the child is admitted to the hospital for a temporary colostomy; preoperatively, the doctor orders kanamycin. The nurse caring for this child should know that kanamycin is being given to:
    1. Increase peristalsis.
    2. Decrease amount of GI secretions.
    3. Promote passage of stool and flatus.
    4. Decrease number of intestinal flora.

45. A 22-month-old patient is admitted to the pediatric unit for observation following accidental ingestion of 17 children's acetaminophen (Tylenol) caplets. In the first 2–3 days following this child's admission, it is essential that the nurse plan to observe the child closely for signs of:
    1. Hepatic failure.
    2. Renal failure.
    3. Hyperthermia.
    4. Hemorrhage.

46. In an acetaminophen (Tylenol) overdose situation, the nurse should have on hand the antidote to acetaminophen, which is:
    1. Acetylcysteine (Mucomyst).
    2. Potassium chloride.
    3. Aspirin.
    4. Heparin.

47. The doctor orders aminophylline, 100 mg via IV, for a child who is having an acute asthmatic attack. The nurse should know that the main reason the doctor ordered aminophylline is because it is a(n):
    1. Bronchodilator.
    2. Anticholinergic.
    3. Expectorant.
    4. Mucolytic agent.

48. The nurse is to administer 100 mg of aminophylline IV. The ampule contains 500 mg (gr 7½) of aminophylline in 10 mL of solution. How much solution should the nurse withdraw from the ampule?
    1. 2 mL.
    2. 4 mL.
    3. 6 mL.
    4. 8 mL.

49. While aminophylline is infusing, the nurse should plan to closely monitor the patient's:
    1. Level of consciousness.
    2. Blood pressure.
    3. Cardiac rhythm.
    4. Temperature.

50. The nurse should know that, to prevent future asthmatic attacks, a patient will most likely receive:
    1. Theophylline.
    2. Cromolyn sodium.
    3. Prednisone.
    4. Diphenhydramine.

51. A 15-year-old patient is admitted to the hospital with a diagnosis of infectious hepatitis (type A). To protect other members of this patient's family who have been exposed to infectious hepatitis, the nurse should explain that they may be given:
    1. Amoxicillin/clavulanate potassium (Augmentin).
    2. Sulfisoxazole.
    3. Rifampin.
    4. Immune globulin.

52. A 17-month-old child has retropharyngeal abscess and is to receive ampicillin four times a day. The child weighs 15 kg (33 lb). The nurses' reference indicates that the correct dosage is 75 mg/kg/day. Which dose should the nurse give to this patient at 10 A.M.?
    1. 11 mg.
    2. 28 mg.
    3. 280 mg.
    4. 1125 mg.

53. A 4-year-old patient is scheduled for repair of a left undescended testicle. To administer a pentobarbital sodium (Nembutal) suppository preoperatively to this patient, in which position should the nurse place him?
    1. Prone with legs abducted.
    2. Sitting on a potty seat.

3. Supine with foot of bed elevated.

4. Side-lying with upper leg flexed.

54. A 4-year-old boy appears very anxious and frightened before receiving a rectal suppository as a preoperative medication. Which statement by the nurse would be most appropriate in helping the child take this medication?

    1. "Be a big kid! Everyone's waiting for you."
    2. "You look so scared. Want to know a secret? This won't hurt a bit!"
    3. "Lie still now and I'll let you have one of your presents before you even have your operation."
    4. "Take a nice, big, deep breath and then let me hear you count to five."

55. A 4-year-old patient is scheduled for surgery. In preparing this child's preop injections, which size needle should the nurse select to administer this child's IM injection?

    1. 25 G, ⅝ inch.
    2. 22 G, 1 inch.
    3. 20 G, 1½ inch.
    4. 18 G, 1½ inch.

56. Meperidine hydrochloride (Demerol) would be preferred over morphine sulfate for a patient with a chest tube because Demerol:

    1. Causes less nausea and vomiting.
    2. Reduces anxiety and respiratory rate more effectively.
    3. Causes less smooth muscle spasms.
    4. Causes less respiratory depression.

57. A patient with diabetes has been giving herself NPH and regular insulin daily in two separate injections. The nurse would be accurate in telling the patient that:

    1. One injection, mixing the insulins, is safe, and injection sites will be used less.
    2. Her method is the best way to ensure accurate administration.
    3. It does not really make any difference if she uses one or two syringes.
    4. More mistakes are made when mixing insulins.

58. Before administering a blood transfusion, the tubing should be flushed with:

    1. 5% dextrose in water.
    2. Dextran.
    3. 5% dextrose, 0.5 normal saline.
    4. Lactated Ringer's.

59. Which patient information, documented during an assessment, would be a contraindication to the patient receiving verapamil (Calan)?

    1. Epigastric pain and treatment for a peptic ulcer.
    2. Hypertension and angina on exertion.
    3. History of asthma and allergic bronchitis.
    4. Hypotension associated with bradycardia.

60. A patient is receiving heparin IV for acute thrombophlebitis. The activated partial thromboplastin time (APTT) is >110 sec. The best nursing action would be to:

    1. Stop the heparin infusion.
    2. Give protamine sulfate.
    3. Call the MD to report the APTT.
    4. Do nothing; this is the desired level.

61. A transfusion reaction is suspected. The transfusion is stopped and the MD notified. The next appropriate nursing action would be to:

    1. Change all IV tubing to prevent additional infusion of blood cells.
    2. Keep the IV line open with saline until further orders.
    3. Arrange for the laboratory to pick up the remaining unit of blood.
    4. Collect a urine specimen from the patient.

62. A patient with a history of arthritis and peptic ulcer disease is receiving misoprostol (Cytotec). Patient teaching about the drug would include:

1. Take the medication three times a day before meals and at bedtime.

2. Importance of using this drug when NSAIDs are also being taken by the patient.

3. Purpose of drug is to reduce *H. pylori* bacteria in the stomach.

4. Take a laxative to prevent side effect of constipation.

63. Magnesium hydroxide (Milk of Magnesia) is the routine laxative order to prevent or correct constipation. For which patient would the nurse question the order?

    1. An elderly woman with potential for fecal impaction.
    2. A patient with chronic renal failure who is admitted for shunt revision.
    3. A male patient who is recovering from total knee replacement.
    4. An older male patient who is being treated for pneumonia.

64. A patient is admitted to the emergency department (ED) in acute distress from asthma. Theophylline and 5% dextrose are being infused IV. The patient is experiencing hypotension and an irregular pulse. The first nursing action would be to:

    1. Stop the medication and call the ED physician.
    2. Check the BP and pulse frequently while the drug infuses.
    3. Increase IV rate to reverse possible hypovolemia.
    4. Slow infusion rate and notify the ED physician.

Answers/Rationale

1. **(2)** Before administering any narcotic, the nurse should assess the type, location, and intensity of pain, as well as factors that seem to precipitate or relieve it. Meperidine, like morphine, has hypotensive and respiratory depressant effects. Positioning in anticipation of respiratory changes is not indicated (**Answer 1**). Pain and discomfort are subjective symptoms that are always real to the patient (**Answer 3**). Based on the information gained in **Answer 2**, it is then possible to decide whether the patient needs supportive measures (such as back rub or position change as in **Answer 4**), the bedpan, and/or the administration of a narcotic.

    Test-taking tip—Choose the first step in the nursing process—*assess.*

    AS, 3, PhI, Pharmacological and Parenteral Therapies

2. **(2)** Neostigmine bromide (Prostigmin) is an anticholinesterase. It enhances bladder tone and contraction, enabling complete emptying of the bladder. It is also used in the treatment of myasthenia gravis. Bethanechol chloride (Urecholine) is an example of a cholinergic drug (**Answer 1**), also used to treat postoperative urinary retention. Atropine is an example of an antcholinergic drug (**Answer 3**), which would act to inhibit initiation of urination. Beta blockers (**Answer 4**) such as propranolol do *not* affect the bladder.

    Test-taking tip—Know *expected* effects of common drug classifications.

    PL, 8, PhI, Pharmacological and Parenteral Therapies

Key to codes following rationales *Nursing process:* **AS,** Assessment; **AN,** Analysis; **PL,** Plan; **IMP,** Implementation; **EV,** Evaluation. *Category of human function:* **1,** Protective; **2,** Sensory perceptual; **3,** Comfort, Rest, Activity, and Mobility; **4,** Nutrition; **5,** Growth and Development; **6,** Fluid-Gas Transport; **7,** Psychosocial-Cultural; **8,** Elimination. **Client need: SECE,** Safe, Effective Care Environment; **PhI,** Physiological Integrity; **PsI,** Psychosocial Integrity; **HPM,** Health Promotion/Maintenance. See appendices for full explanation.

3. **(2)** Salicylates, particularly acetylsalicylic acid (aspirin), are given in divided doses after each meal and at bedtime for their analgesic (reduced pain), anti-inflammatory (reduced swelling), and antipyretic (reduced fever) effects. **Answer 1** is incorrect because relief of pain was already described in the question. **Answers 3 and 4** are incorrect because salicylates neither inhibit nor stimulate the autonomic nervous system synapses.

> **Test-taking tip**—Consider why the drug relieves pain—decreased inflammation.

IMP, 3, PhI, Pharmacological and Parenteral Therapies

4. **(2)** Digoxin increases the force and velocity of cardiac contraction and *slows* the heart rate by delaying conduction through the atrioventricular node. The hemodynamic effects of its action include *increased cardiac output,* decreased right atrial and venous pressures, decreased left ventricular filling pressure, and increased excretion of sodium and water. Epinephrine **(Answer 1)** increases the force of cardiac contractions but also increases heart rate, which in this case would increase cardiac embarrassment. Furosemide (Lasix) **(Answer 3)** is a rapidly acting diuretic that enhances excretion of sodium and water. However, although its use is indicated to reduce fluid volume during the acute phase of pulmonary edema, it has *no known direct effects* on the cardiac musculature. Hydralazine **(Answer 4)** is a peripheral vasodilator used in hypertensive therapy. It is *not* indicated in this situation.

> **Test-taking tip**—Know the expected therapeutic effects. Would increased or *decreased* heart *rate* improve cardiac output and renal blood flow?

PL, 6, PhI, Pharmacological and Parenteral Therapies

5. **(3)** The best indicator that digoxin has been effective in strengthening cardiac contraction and increasing glomerular filtration is a decrease in heart rate (vagal effect) and increased urinary output. As a result of these drug effects, cardiac output is improved, raising blood pressure and decreasing pulmonary congestion. **Answers 1, 2, and 4** are only partially correct.

> **Test-taking tip**—Look for *one* expected effect (increased urinary output) to help eliminate two other options.

EV, 6, PhI, Pharmacological and Parenteral Therapies

6. **(2)** Theophylline relaxes bronchial smooth muscles, which helps relieve the wheezing and coughing associated with bronchospasm. Side effects are rare, but the earliest signs of overdose are usually anorexia, nausea, and vomiting. Tachycardia **(Answer 1)**, restlessness and tremors **(Answer 3)**, headache and insomnia **(Answer 4)**, are side effects associated with bronchodilators.

> **Test-taking tip**—Know expected outcomes of drug therapy—desired and untoward effects.

IMP, 6, PhI, Pharmacological and Parenteral Therapies

7. **(2)** Furosemide is a rapidly acting diuretic with a peak action in 1–2 hours and a duration of 6–8 hours. The peak time is too rapid for **Answer 1** and too long for **Answers 3 and 4.**

> **Test-taking tip**—Notice the time overlap—the option that includes both is better.

EV, 8, PhI, Pharmacological and Parenteral Therapies

8. **(1)** Sodium polystyrene sulfonate (Kayexalate) is a cation-exchange resin. As it passes along the intestine or is retained in the colon after enema administration, sodium ions are partially released and replaced by potassium ions, allowing for fecal excretion of potassium ions. This drug is extremely unpalatable and may be administered in syrup, chilled, or mixed in the diet, and if necessary, administered directly into the stomach per nasogastric tube. Side effects of administration include anorexia, nausea, vomiting, constipation, hypokalemia, hypocalcemia, and sodium retention. **Answers 2, 3, and 4** are *not* actions of sodium polystyrene sulfonate.

> **Test-taking tip**—Know the common therapies for increased K^+—*ion exchange;* also glucose and insulin, sorbitol. Focus on the options that include *increasing* K^+ *excretion* rather than decreasing K^+ absorption **(Answers 2 and 3).**

IMP, 8, PhI, Pharmacological and Parenteral Therapies

9. **(1)** *Ideally,* oral iron preparations should be taken on an empty stomach **(2)**. However, they tend to irritate the gastric mucosa, so they should be administered *with* or *immediately after* meals to ensure patient compliance. Thus **Answers 2, 3, and 4** are *not* the *best* answers. Patients may complain of constipation or loose stools. Stools will change color (dark green to black). Ferrous sulfate is apt to deposit on teeth and gums, so frequent oral hygiene is necessary, and therapy will need to continue even after hemoglobin levels return to normal, to ensure adequate iron stores in the body.

> **Test-taking tip**—Key word is *best* time. **Answer 1** is better than **Answer 3.** Iron is harsh on the stomach.

PL, 4, PhI, Pharmacological and Parenteral Therapies

10. **(1)** Toxic doses of neomycin may result in eighth cranial nerve damage much like that produced by streptomycin. Kidney damage may also occur, extending from milk albuminuria to elevation in blood urea nitrogen. Nausea **(Answer 2)** is common with ingestion of antibiotics, though not specific to neomycin. Erythromycin most commonly causes nausea, vomiting, and diarrhea **(Answer 3)**. Anaphylactic reactions **(Answer 4)** are associated most commonly with penicillin administration.

> **Test-taking tip**—Use a process of elimination—find a *specific, serious* side effect that can occur. *Drug would not be given* in the first place with known allergic potential (because of anaphylaxis); GI upset is common to most antibiotics, and not specific to neomycin.

EV, 2, PhI, Pharmacological and Parenteral Therapies

11. **(2)** Morphine strongly depresses the medullary respiratory centers. Therefore, before administering the narcotic, the nurse should assess the patient's respiratory rate and depth to prevent severe respiratory depression. **Answers 1, 3, and 4** are not affected by morphine.

> **Test-taking tip**—Know which systems (in this case, respiratory) respond to commonly used drugs—particularly pain medications.

AS, 6, PhI, Pharmacological and Parenteral Therapies

12. **(1)** Spironolactone (Aldactone) is an aldosterone inhibitor, inhibiting the effects of hyperaldosteronemia, which is common in cirrhosis. This drug safely increases sodium and water excretion but does not cause concomitant losses of potassium as do other diuretics. For this reason, potassium supplements are not generally given to the patient. An example of a carbonic anhydrase inhibitor **(Answer 2)** is acetazolamide (Diamox); an example of a thiazide **(Answer 3)** is chlorothiazide (Diuril) or hydrochlorothiazide (HydroDIURIL); and an example of an osmotic diuretic **(Answer 4)** is mannitol.

> **Test-taking tip**—Look for clues from the stem, such as similarity in words—aldac*tone* and aldoster*one.*

IMP, 6, PhI, Pharmacological and Parenteral Therapies

13. **(2)** Potassium chloride is not given since the patient is on spironolactone (Aldactone), which does *not* cause concomitant *losses* of potassium as do other diuretics. For this reason, potassium supplements are *not* generally given to the patient. Spironolactone would *not* contraindicate the administration of vitamin B_6 **(Answer 1)**, ascorbic acid **(Answer 3)**, or calcium gluconate **(Answer 4)**.

> **Test-taking tip**—Know the expected outcome of *potassium*-sparing diuretics. Know drug classifications.

PL, 4, PhI, Pharmacological and Parenteral Therapies

14. **(3)** The primary objective in giving corticosteroids is to lessen the symptoms of the disease process. Most patients initially respond well to these drugs; however, as the disease progresses, higher and higher doses are required to relieve symptoms. **Answers 1 and 2** are incorrect because corticosteroids have no curative effects, only palliative. Many of the side effects of corticosteroid administration are due to the effects of these drugs on glucose metabolism **(Answer 4)**, such as Cushing-like syndrome.

Test-taking tip—Look for an option that will improve an "itis"—inflammation.

AN, 3, PhI, Pharmacological and Parenteral Therapies

15. **(3)** Side effects of prednisone therapy mimic the manifestations of Cushing's syndrome (moon facies, abnormal fat deposits, purple striae, hyperglycemia with glucosuria, hypertension, obesity, and emotional disturbances). Side effects of *other drugs* used in the management of rheumatoid arthritis include tinnitus (**Answer 1**), from aspirin; nausea, vomiting (**Answer 4**), headaches, and vertigo with indomethacin (Indocin) administration; and dermatitis ranging from erythema to exfoliative dermatitis (**Answer 2**) with gold salts therapy.

Test-taking tip—Know the untoward effects of excessive *steroids* on the body.

EV, 8, PhI, Pharmacological and Parenteral Therapies

16. **(4)** Although the primary use of propantheline bromide in many clinical situations involving the gastrointestinal tract is to reduce gastric secretions and intestinal hypermotility, it is used in gallbladder disease because of its antispasmodic effects an the gallbladder and bile duct. **Answer 1** is therefore correct, but *not the best* choice. **Answers 2** and **3** are incorrect because propantheline bromide does *not* reduce bile secretions; its calming effect on gastric motility does *not* reduce the amount of chyme entering the duodenum.

Test-taking tip—Look for an option that alleviates and explains a possible cause of gallbladder *pain.*

IMP, 4, PhI, Pharmacological and Parenteral Therapies

17. **(3)** Morphine sulfate causes spasms of the sphincter of Oddi, thereby increasing intraductal pressures and abdominal pain. Papaverine and meperidine, both synthetic opiates, as well as nitroglycerin, may be administered to relieve pain associated with gallbladder disease. **Answer 1** is incorrect because the effect of morphine is to increase spasms in the gallbladder. **Answer 2,** though correct, is not the *best* answer Opiates are withheld when a patient has an acute abdomen and the diagnosis is unknown or tentative. In this case, the patient has an established history of gallbladder disease and specific symptomatology. **Answer 4** is incorrect, in that although morphine does relax vascular smooth muscle, this effect does not increase bile synthesis in the liver.

Test-taking tip—Look for options that are opposites— *increase* or decrease contractions. Which would likely cause pain?

EV, 3, PhI, Pharmacological and Parenteral Therapies

18. **(4)** Hydrochlorothiazide is a thiazide diuretic that promotes the excretion of water, sodium, and chloride by inhibiting the reabsorption of sodium ions in the distal ascending limb of the loop of Henle and in the distal convoluted tubule of the nephron. Natriuresis promotes the secondary loss of potassium, so this drug is classified as potassium wasting. Spironolactone is an example of an aldosterone inhibitor and is a potassium-sparing diuretic (**Answers 1, 3**). Acetazolemide (Diamox) is the most frequently employed carbonic anhydrase inhibitor (**Answer 2**).

Test-taking tip—Know the common side effects of frequently used diuretics. *Potassium* is *usually* lost (wasted). Focus on two contradictory options. You know potassium is involved; decide whether it is spared or wasted.

EV, 8, PhI, Pharmacological and Parenteral Therapies

19. **(3)** Hydrochlorothiazide is a thiazide diuretic that promotes the excretion of water, sodium, and chloride by inhibiting the reabsorption of sodium ions in the distal ascending limb of the loop of Henle and in the distal convoluted tubule of the nephron. Natriuresis promotes the secondary loss of potassium, so this drug is classified as potassium wasting. **Answer 1** describes the effect of the carbonic anhydrase inhibitors, e.g., acetazolemide (Diamox). **Answer 2** would be the effect of the potassium-sparing diuretics such as spironolactone

(Aldactone). **Answer 4** is the site for the osmotic diuretics, e.g., mannitol, urea.

Test-taking tip—Picture a functional nephron unit from a physiology book—know the action point for the most common diuretics.

AN, 8, PhI, Pharmacological and Parenteral Therapies

20. **(3)** Thiazide diuretics promote the excretion of sodium, chloride, bicarbonate, and potassium. However, chloride excretion tends to be proportionately greater than bicarbonate excretion, so therapy may result in hypochloremic alkalosis. Hyponatremia, *not* hypernatremia (**Answer 1**), occurs. Hypokalemia, *not* hyperkalemia (**Answer 2**), may develop, especially with brisk diuresis. Supplemental KCl therapy and/or increased dietary intake of potassium is indicated with thiazide therapy. **Answer 4** is incorrect because it says hypouricemia and hyperuricemia result, which may precipitate frank gout.

Test-taking tip—When potassium loss (*hypo*kalemia) is not a choice, think what else goes with K⁺ to *balance* the shift (Cl⁻).

AS, 8, PhI, Pharmacological and Parenteral Therapies

21. **(3)** The formula for finding the correct answer is Dose desired/Dose on hand = x/Amount on hand.

$18/20 = x/5$

$20x = 18(5)$

$x = 18(5)/20$

$x = 4.5$ mL

Test-taking tip—The age of the patient is a distractor. Know the formula; the dose on hand is 5 mL.

IMP, 2, PhI, Pharmacological and Parenteral Therapies

22. **(3)** Rifampin is the drug of choice for the prophylactic treatment of *Haemophilus influenzae* meningitis. The usual dose is 20 mg/kg/day in a single dose for 4 days. Amoxicillin/clavulanate potassium (Augmentin) (**Answer 1**) sulfisoxazole (**Answer 2**) and immune serum globulin (**Answer 4**) are not the drugs of choice to prevent *H. influenzae* meningitis.

Test-taking tip—Use the process of elimination—the stem says *prevent;* two options are treatment for infections, and one option has minimal effect in many situations (immune globulin). Select a broad-spectrum antibiotic for prophylaxis.

IMP, 1, PhI, Pharmacological and Parenteral Therapies

23. **(4)** Pancreatin (Viokase) is an exocrine pancreatic supplement used as a digestive aid in cystic fibrosis; its primary use is to promote the absorption of fats. Pancreatin has no effect on the absorption of glucose (**Answer 1**), vitamin C (**Answer 2**), or sodium chloride (**Answer 3**).

Test-taking tip—Know the digestive problem (fat) with cystic fibrosis.

AN, 4, PhI, Pharmacological and Parenteral Therapies

24. **(4)** The only acceptable way to identify a 5-year-old patient is to have a parent or another staff member identify the patient. **Answer 1** is incorrect because most 5-year-old children, under the age of reason, cannot legally be held accountable for self-identification. **Answer 2** is incorrect unless the nurse is sure this adult is this patient's parent. Also, it would be better to ask, "What is the child's name?" **Answer 3** is also incorrect; children cannot legally be held accountable for identifying other children.

Test-taking tip—Look for the person with the *legal* responsibility—parent or, if not present, staff.

IMP, 1, SECE, Management of Care

25. **(3)** The correct answer is found using the following formula: Dose desired/Dose on hand = x/Amount on hand.

$0.125/0.05 = x/1$

$0.05x = 0.125(1)$

$x = 0.125(1)/0.05$

$x = 2.5$ mL

Test-taking tip—Know the formula; it works every time. Use extra care with decimal points.

IMP, 6, PhI, Pharmacological and Parenteral Therapies

26. (4) The recommended procedure for administering eyedrops to any patient calls for the drops to be placed in the middle of the lower conjunctival sac. Placing drops directly onto the sclera (**Answer 1**) is irritating and less effective. Placing drops in the inner canthus of the eye (**Answer 2**) may lead to systemic effects from absorption via tear ducts. Placing drops in the outer canthus of the eye (**Answer 3**) results in loss of medication and may also cause infection.

    Test-taking tip—The age or size of the patient is a distractor: *correct* technique for eyedrops does not change.
    IMP, 2, PhI, Pharmacological and Parenteral Therapies

27. (1) Maximum absorption of Fer-in-Sol occurs between meals, when hydrochloric acid is freely available in the stomach. When given before meals (**Answer 2**), it may cause GI upset, which will interfere with eating. When given during meals (**Answer 3**) or after meals (**Answer 4**), there is slowed absorption of the drug; however, GI upset is minimized.

    Test-taking tip—The stem says *maximum:* when is HCl readily available? The question does not ask about avoiding GI upset.
    PL, 4, PhI, Pharmacological and Parenteral Therapies

28. (1) When oral iron preparations are given correctly, the stools normally turn dark green or black. Parents of children receiving this medication should be advised that this side effect indicates the medication is being absorbed and is working well. **Answers 2, 3,** and **4** would only increase the parents' anxiety and lead them to believe that the stool color was abnormal.

    Test-taking tip—Know the expected outcome of drug therapies, particularly changes in urine or feces color. Iron and black stools = a good thing!
    EV, 8, PhI, Pharmacological and Parenteral Therapies

29. (1) Normal pregnancy *alters vaginal pH* and favors the growth of yeast organisms *(Candida).* **Answer 2** is wrong because *age is not a factor* in the development of yeast vaginitis. **Answer 3** is wrong because ingestion of large amounts of *carbohydrates* does *not* alter vaginal pH. **Answer 4** is wrong because sickle cell anemia is *not* a predisposing factor in yeast vaginitis.

    Test-taking tip—Use a process of elimination. Use what you *do* know about risk factors of monilia in pregnant women (*not* age or sickle cell anemia). What alters the pH of the vagina?
    AS, 5, HPM, Prevention and Early Detection

30. (2) Nystatin is the drug of choice for treatment of vaginal infections caused by *Candida albicans.* **Answer 1** is wrong because metronidazole is used in treatment of *trichomonal vaginitis.* **Answer 3** is wrong because podophyllin is used in treating *venereal warts.* **Answer 4** is wrong because bacitracin ointment is used in treating *skin* infections.

    Test-taking tip—Method of administration is a clue (i.e., "vaginal" in the stem and "vaginal" in the option)
    IMP, 1, PhI, Pharmacological and Parenteral Therapies

31. (4) Erythromycin or tetracycline is commonly used in treating penicillin-allergic patients with venereal disease. **Answer 1** is wrong because streptomycin is used in treating *tuberculosis.* **Answer 2** is wrong because sulfisoxazole is most commonly used to treat *urinary tract* infections. Further, its use is *contraindicated* in pregnancy. **Answer 3** is wrong because chloramphenicol is used in treating *Salmonella* infections and is also *contraindicated* during pregnancy.

    Test-taking tip—Match drugs listed with primary conditions for which each are used. Eliminate two of the drugs that are contraindicated during pregnancy. Recognize erythromycin as the choice when penicillin is indicated but *allergy* exists.
    PL, 1, PhI, Pharmacological and Parenteral Therapies

32. (4) Prolonged, heavy doses of oral antibiotics are irritating to the GI tract and result in nausea and diarrhea; yeast infections are common sequelae of antibiotic therapy. **Answer 1** is

wrong; tinnitus is a symptom of streptomycin toxicity. **Answer 2** is wrong because abdominal pain is more commonly associated with sulfisoxazole therapy. **Answer 3** is wrong because glossitis and stomatitis are associated with chloramphenicol therapy.

    Test-taking tip—Recognize *commonly* occurring side effects of antibiotics. Prepare patient to manage.
    IMP, 1, PhI, Pharmacological and Parenteral Therapies

33. (3) Ritodrine is the drug of choice when attempting to inhibit labor. **Answer 1** is wrong because diazepam is used most commonly as an *anticonvulsant.* **Answer 2** is wrong because betamethasone is used to stimulate production of *fetal pulmonary surfactant.* **Answer 4** is wrong because bromocriptine mesylate is used to *inhibit lactation in nonbreastfeeding* mothers.

    Test-taking tip—Know the *main use* for each of the four drugs listed in order to eliminate the three that are wrong.
    PL, 5, PhI, Pharmacological and Parenteral Therapies

34. (3) Persistent maternal tachycardia (over 140 beats/min) is a sign of impending pulmonary edema in patients receiving beta-mimetic drugs; fetal tachycardia is a common result of ritodrine therapy. **Answer 1** is wrong because ritodrine commonly results in maternal *hypotension.* **Answer 2** is wrong because the common fetal reaction to beta-mimetics is *tachycardia.* **Answer 4** is wrong because ritodrine is given to *reduce* uterine hyperirritability and threatened premature labor.

    Test-taking tip—Look for clues. *Mimetic* looks like *mimic*—which option mimics beta effects? Choose the option that includes mother *and* fetus. Know effects of drug classes generally.
    EV, 5, PhI, Pharmacological and Parenteral Therapies

35. (3) Depression of contractions and fetal bradycardia are expected effects of paracervical block. **Answer 1** is incorrect because the bearing-down reflex is not affected by this anesthesia and therefore low forceps birth is usually *not needed.* **Answer 2** is incorrect because *maternal* blood pressure and *postnatal* uterine contractility are *not* affected by paracervical block. **Answer 4** is incorrect because the bearing-down reflex is not affected, and therefore forceps birth is usually not needed.

    Test-taking tip—Recognize *expected* effects. Eliminate choices 1 and 4 that would increase risk to the infant (forceps). Review why fetal bradycardia occurs.
    AN, 5, PhI, Pharmacological and Parenteral Therapies

36. (3) The medication never mixes with cerebrospinal fluid, and therefore there is *no need* for the woman to lie flat for several hours after receiving this form of anesthesia (**Answer 1**). **Answers 2** and **4** are incorrect because the lists are incomplete.

    Test-taking tip—Choose the most complete list in this question, where **Answer 3** incorporates 2 and 4.
    AN, 5, PhI, Pharmacological and Parenteral Therapies

37. (4) All of the listed effects are to be expected following spinal anesthesia: loss of bearing-down reflex, depression of contractions, maternal hypotension, fetal bradycardia, low forceps birth, postnatal bladder atony, need to remain flat in bed for several hours after birth, and postnatal uterine atony. **Answers 1, 2,** and **3** are incorrect because the lists are incomplete.

    Test-taking tip—Choose the option that includes all the others.
    AN, 1, PhI, Pharmacological and Parenteral Therapies

38. (1) Hypersensitivity reactions (urticaria and hives) are common drug reactions. Photosensitization (exaggerated sunburn) in certain hypersensitive persons may also occur with exposure to direct or artificial sunlight during tetracycline use. Urinary retention (**Answer 2**) is a side effect of anticholinergic and antihistamine drugs. Jaundice (**Answer 3**) from drug toxicity is more common with isoniazid (INH),

acetaminophen, phenothiazines (chlorpromazine [Thorazine]), sulfonamides, and antidiabetic drugs (e.g., tolbutamide [Orinase]). Hepatotoxicity may occur with tetracycline, but it is less common. **Answer 4,** deafness (ototoxicity), is a major side effect of the aminoglycoside antibiotics (e.g., gentamicin, neomycin, streptomycin, tobramycin) and diuretics, such as furosemide and ethacrynic acid.

> **Test-taking tip**—This is an *expected* common side effect. Only one would be clinically acceptable, although annoying (rash).

IMP, 1, PhI, Pharmacological and Parenteral Therapies

39. (3) The patient needs to be protected against photosensitivity and dermatitis when exposed to the sun; a sunscreen preparation should be applied to exposed parts of the skin, and the patient should wear long sleeves and cover-up clothing. **Answers 1, 2,** and **4** refer to *indoor* activities, where there is no danger of sunburn.

> **Test-taking tip**—Which answer is not like the others? Look at patterns: three indoor activities and one outdoor. Select the one that is different.

PL, 1, PhI, Reduction of Risk Potential

40. (4) This is the best choice because it *encompasses* **Answer 3. Answers 1** and **2** are definitely incorrect.

> **Test-taking tip**—When two options are correct, choose the one that covers them both.

PL, 7, PhI, Pharmacological and Parenteral Therapies

41. (1) Blood dyscrasias often are overlooked when first symptoms of possible adverse drug effects appear in the form of a minor cold. **Answers 2, 3,** and **4** refer to extrapyramidal tract symptoms that are *not* life threatening.

> **Test-taking tip**—Which answer is not like the others? One option is potentially life threatening (hematological system); three are not life threatening and relate to the musculoskeletal system.

AN, 6, PhI, Pharmacological and Parenteral Therapies

42. (2) Hypertensive crisis can be precipitated by combining this drug with common cold medications and foods high in tyramine or pressor amines (e.g., yogurt, Chianti wine, cheese, Coca-Cola, coffee). All other options are incorrect.

> **Test-taking tip**—Application of knowledge about side effects of these two drugs and the drug classification (monoamine oxidase inhibitor) will lead you to the only correct answer.

EV, 6, PhI, Pharmacological and Parenteral Therapies

43. (4) This effect is seen in patients taking a *major tranquilizer*. All of the other options are *likely* side effects of lithium salts.

> **Test-taking tip**—Note the word "least" likely. Recall that **Answer 4** is a symptom of a *different* drug category than lithium (Phenothiazine).

EV, 7, PhI, Pharmacological and Parenteral Therapies

44. (4) Kanamycin is an antibiotic that, although poorly absorbed in the GI tract, is often used as part of bowel prep before abdominal surgery. It acts as a bacteriocidal agent, thus significantly decreasing the number of intestinal flora and reducing risk of peritonitis in the postop period. Kanamycin does not increase peristalsis (**Answer 1**), promote passage of stool or flatus (**Answer 3**), or decrease amount of GI secretions (**Answer 2**).

> **Test-taking tip**—The age and diagnosis do not matter. Why would *any* patient need an antibiotic preoperatively? "Mycins" such as Kana*mycin*, erythro*mycin*, strepto*mycin* are antibiotics that decrease bacterial growth.

AN, 1, PhI, Pharmacological and Parenteral Therapies

45. (1) The major toxic effect of an overdose of acetaminophen (Tylenol) is liver failure; liver function should be closely monitored during the first 2–3 days following the ingestion of acetaminophen. Renal failure (**Answer 2**) may occur as a *late* complication of acetaminophen toxicity, as may bleeding and hemorrhage (**Answer 4**). Hyperthermia (**Answer 3**) is not a major symptom of this type of ingestion; it is more common in salicylate ingestion.

> **Test-taking tip**—Know the functions of the liver, including detoxification of substances such as medications.

PL, 1, PhI, Pharmacological and Parenteral Therapies

46. (1) Acetylcysteine (Mucomyst) is the antidote for acetaminophen poisoning: it serves to protect the liver. It is usually given orally in a carbonated beverage (e.g., cola), but it can also be given via nasogastric tube. A loading dose is followed by q4h doses until a total of 18 doses have been given. KCl (**Answer 2**), aspirin (**Answer 3**), and heparin (**Answer 4**) are not antidotes for acetaminophen and do not serve to protect the child's liver.

> **Test-taking tip**—Use a process of elimination. The potential adverse effects of three of the options would likely preclude use as an antidote.

IMP, 1, PhI, Pharmacological and Parenteral Therapies

47. (1) Aminophylline, a bronchodilator that acts as a smooth-muscle relaxant, is used to prevent and relieve symptoms of bronchial asthma. Anticholinergics (**Answer 2**) are used to treat muscle spasms along the GI tract. Aminophylline is neither an expectorant (**Answer 3**), which would assist in the removal of mucus from the respiratory tract, nor a mucolytic agent (**Answer 4**), which would help thin out viscid secretions.

> **Test-taking tip**—Know the drug classifications of frequently used medications. Remember that in asthma, bronchioles *constrict*; therefore, a broncho*dilator* is used.

AN, 6, PhI, Pharmacological and Parenteral Therapies

48. (1) The formula for finding the correct answer is Dose desired/Dose on hand = *x*/Amount on hand.
$100/500 = x/10$
$500x = 100(10)$
$x = 100(10)/500$
$x = 2$ mL

> **Test-taking tip**—Know the formula and the answer is easy; the dose on hand is 10 mL.

IMP, 6, PhI, Pharmacological and Parenteral Therapies

49. (3) A transient side effect of IV aminophylline is an increase in heart rate; toxic effects include a prolonged increase in heart rate and abnormalities in cardiac rhythm. While receiving IV aminophylline, the patient should be on a cardiac monitor, and both rate and rhythm should be closely monitored and documented by the nurse. Aminophylline may also cause a transient change in the blood pressure (**Answer 2**), but this is not as much a concern as the patient's cardiac rhythm. Aminophylline should not affect level of consciousness (**Answer 1**) or temperature (**Answer 4**); thus there is no particular need for the nurse to monitor these specifically at this time.

> **Test-taking tip**—With two potentially correct answers, select the more encompassing choice—change in heart function will ultimately affect BP. The words "closely monitor" in the stem usually call for a *priority* answer (cardiac is usually a priority).

PL, 6, PhI, Pharmacological and Parenteral Therapies

50. (2) Cromolyn sodium, an uncategorized drug used as an adjunct in the treatment of asthma, is used only after the acute attack is relieved; its primary intent is prophylaxis, i.e., to prevent future attacks. Cromolyn is used in an inhaler. It is absorbed into the systemic circulation after its inhalation into the lungs. It acts on the mast cells and also inhibits the release of histamine. Theophylline (**Answer 1**), prednisone (**Answer 3**), and diphenhydramine (**Answer 4**) do *not prevent future* asthmatic attacks and have no prophylactic value.

> **Test-taking tip**—Look for a pattern: three of the options are used for *acute* episodes; choose the one that meets the condition of the stem (future prevention).

AN, 6, PhI, Pharmacological and Parenteral Therapies

51. **(4)** Immune serum globulin (ISG) offers the family members some protection against type A infectious hepatitis. It contains antibodies against the organism and will aid the family members in resisting this infectious disease. Amoxicillin/clavulanate potassium (Augmentin) (**Answer 1**) and sulfisoxazole (**Answer 2**) are antibiotics used for a variety of infections, but they would not prevent hepatitis. Rifampin (**Answer 3**) is used prophylactically for *Haemophilus influenzae* meningitis and to treat TB but would not prevent hepatitis.

    Test-taking tip—Know when immune globulin may be effective (infectious hepatitis) and when it is not (*H. influenzae* meningitis). Remember that protection for hepatitis exposure is achieved through passive immunity (i.e., immune serum globulin).
    IMP, 1, HPM, Prevention and Early Detection

52. **(3)** The nurse should give 280 mg at 10 A.M. Using the formula of 75 mg/kg/day, 75 mg (15 kg = 1125 mg per day, to be divided into 4 doses. 1125 mg divided by 4 doses = 280 mg per dose.

    Test-taking tip—Use basic math. Do not forget to divide the daily dose of 1125 mg by the total number of doses per day to get the amount to be given for a single dose at 10:00 A.M.
    IMP, 1, PhI, Pharmacological and Parenteral Therapies

53. **(4)** The recommended position to administer rectal medications to children is side-lying with the upper leg flexed. This position allows the nurse to safely and effectively administer the medication while promoting comfort for the child. If the child were to lie prone (**Answer 1**), the nurse could not administer the medication as safely or effectively, even if the legs were abducted; further, this position would most likely cause the child some discomfort. If the child were sitting on a potty seat (**Answer 2**), the nurse could not reach the rectum to insert the suppository, and it is likely the suppository would be immediately expelled. If the child were to lie supine (**Answer 3**), the nurse could not administer the medication comfortably for the child.

    Test-taking tip—Do not use "real world" experience to answer this question (i.e., how you may have seen a mother do it!) Visualize the positions; then choose one based on patient comfort and nursing effectiveness.
    IMP, 1, PhI, Pharmacological and Parenteral Therapies

54. **(4)** Preschool children commonly experience fears and fantasies regarding invasive procedures. The nurse should attempt to momentarily distract the child with a simple task that can be easily accomplished while the child remains in the side-lying position. The suppository can be slipped into place while the child is counting, and then the nurse can praise the child for cooperating, while holding the buttocks together to prevent expulsion of the suppository. The nurse should *not pressure* the child into acting like a "big kid" (**Answer 1**) in such a frightening situation (use of the word "kid" is also *not appropriate*). The nurse should *not lie,* breaking a trust by saying something "won't hurt a bit" (**Answer 2**). The nurse should *never "bribe"* a child with gifts to ensure cooperation (**Answer 3**).

    Test-taking tip—Maximize patient control over the situation and use age-appropriate distraction techniques.
    IMP, 5, PsI, Coping and Adaptation

55. **(2)** In selecting the correct needle to administer an IM injection to a young child, the nurse should always look at the child and use judgment in evaluating muscle mass and amount of subcutaneous fat. A medium-gauge needle (22 G) that is 1 inch long would be most appropriate for a young child. A ⅝ inch needle (**Answer 1**) would be too small, and a 1½ inch (18–20 G) needle would be too long and unnecessarily large (**Answers 3, 4**). A 23 or 25 G needle would be too

thin to use on most children (**Answer 1**) and would be better suited for use with a newborn or an infant.

    Test-taking tip—Visualize the "average" size of a 4-year-old. *Medium* size is safe.
    IMP, 1, PhI, Pharmacological and Parenteral Therapies

56. **(4)** Both drugs have depressant effects; however, morphine sulfate affects rate and depth of respirations and cough reflex, which would be undesirable following chest tube insertion. *Both* drugs cause nausea and vomiting (**Answer 1**). Morphine sulfate is used to reduce anxiety and respiratory rate (**Answer 2**), particularly in pulmonary edema. Demerol does cause fewer smooth muscle spasms (**Answer 3**); however, that is *not the concern* in this situation, but it would be with GI surgery such as cholecystectomy.

    Test-taking tip—Choose "respiratory" over GI symptoms, anxiety, or muscle spasm. Know *expected* effects of opioid analgesics, and what the greatest concern is for this patient situation (respiratory effectiveness).
    PL, 3, PhI, Pharmacological and Parenteral Therapies

57. **(1)** Regular and intermediate-acting insulins are normally mixed to avoid the need to use injection sites twice as often. Rotation of sites is important, and the same site should not be used more often than every 2 to 4 weeks to avoid the development of lipodystrophies. **Answer 2** may ensure accuracy; however, it is *not standard* practice or necessary. Although not unsafe, use of two syringes does increase the potential for lipodystrophy; therefore, it does make a difference (**Answer 3**). There is *no evidence* that more errors are made when insulin types are mixed (**Answer 4**).

    Test-taking tip—Know the "clear to cloudy" rule with mixing insulins; therefore, one syringe is all you need.
    IMP, 4, PhI, Pharmacological and Parenteral Therapies

58. **(4)** Blood and a solution containing glucose (dextrose) will result in precipitation when mixed outside the body. Saline is often the solution of choice. However, lactated Ringer's, an electrolyte-balanced solution without dextrose, is acceptable. **Answers 1, 2,** and **3** contain glucose (dextrose).

    Test-taking tip—Look for patterns in the options. Three of the choices contain dextrose. Choose the one that does not.
    IMP, 6, PhI, Pharmacological and Parenteral Therapies

59. **(4)** Verapamil, a calcium channel blocker, is indicated for the management of hypertension and arrhythmia with rapid ventricular rates. Blood pressure and pulse should be taken before administration, and the medication would most likely be held or changed with persistent hypotension and bradycardia. **Answers 1, 2,** and **3** would *not* be contraindications; the medication may be given to patients with these existing conditions.

    Test-taking tip—To narrow the choices, focus on two contradictory options: *hyper*tension vs. *hypo*tension. Know expected therapeutic and side effects of drug classifications.
    AN, 6, PhI, Pharmacological and Parenteral Therapies

60. **(3)** The APTT is greater than 3 times the normal level. Therapeutic levels are 1.5 to 2.5 times the normal (control) level. With a potential medical emergency, the nurse must notify the MD; care decisions are collaborative. **Answers 1** and **2** are not independent nursing actions. **Answer 4** is incorrect and could be life threatening for the patient.

    Test-taking tip—Focus on two contradictory options: "do nothing" vs. "call the MD." Know normal laboratory values and expected therapeutic levels and realize this is an "Oh! Oh!" situation.
    AN, 6, PhI, Reduction of Risk Potential

61. **(2)** The priority is to keep the IV site open. Medications may need to be given to reverse the patient's untoward reaction to the transfusion. **Answers 1, 3,** and **4** will eventually be done, but *not before* the patency of the IV is determined and maintained.

Test-taking tip—Take care of the patient's safety first, then changing the equipment and laboratory tests.

IMP, 6, PhI, Pharmacological and Parenteral Therapies

62. **(2)** Cytotec prevents gastric mucosal injury related to chronic NSAID therapy in high-risk patients (elderly, debilitated, or history of ulcers). The medication is taken *with* meals, *not before* (**Answer 1**). The drug has *no effect* on *H. pylori* (**Answer 3**). The drug decreases gastric acid secretion and increases production of protective mucus. A side effect of the drug is diarrhea, *not* constipation (**Answer 4**).

Test-taking tip—Look for clues in the stem (a possible link between arthritis and ulcer disease).

IMP, 4, PhI, Pharmacological and Parenteral Therapies

63. **(2)** Metabolism and excretion of the drug are done primarily by the kidneys. In chronic renal failure, the kidneys would be unable to regulate electrolyte balance and the patient would be at higher risk for the development of an electrolyte imbalance. Another classification of laxative should be used in the renal patient. This laxative is *not* contraindicated for others (**Answers 1, 3,** and **4**).

Test-taking tip—Use the process of elimination. Would an electrolyte-based laxative (magnesium) adversely affect one of these patients more?

IMP, 8, PhI, Pharmacological and Parenteral Therapies

64. **(4)** Hypotension and arrhythmias are expected side effects of too-rapid administration of theophylline or aminophylline. An infusion pump should be used for administration to ensure an accurate and safe dosage. **Answer 1** is not appropriate because the drug is needed to improve breathing. **Answer 2** is incorrect because it does not respond to the side effects. **Answer 3** would *increase* the *adverse* drug effects.

Test-taking tip—Before contacting the MD, look for a nursing action that ensures patient safety. The choice is between "stop" or "slow" before calling the MD. Choose "slow," because "stop" may stop the benefit of this drug (to improve breathing).

IMP, 6, PhI, Pharmacological and Parenteral Therapies

Common Diagnostic Procedures, Intravenous and Oxygen Therapy, Isolation Precautions, and Hands-on Nursing Care

Bobbi Morrison, Robyn Nelson, and Janice Stecchi

COMMON DIAGNOSTIC PROCEDURES

I. **Noninvasive diagnostic procedures** are those procedures that provide an indirect assessment of organ size, shape, and/or function; these procedures are considered safe, are easily reproducible, require less complex equipment for recording, and generally do not require the written consent of patient or guardian.

◆ **A. General nursing responsibilities:**

1. Reduce patient's anxieties and provide emotional support by:
   a. Explaining purpose and procedure of test.
   b. Answering questions regarding safety of the procedure, as indicated.
   c. Remaining with patient during procedure when possible.
2. Use procedures in the collection of specimens that avoid contamination and facilitate diagnosis—clean-catch urine and sputum specimens after deep breathing and coughing, for example.

B. Graphic studies of heart and brain:

1. *Electrocardiogram (ECG)*—graphic record of electrical activity generated by the heart during depolarization and repolarization; *used to* diagnose abnormal cardiac rhythms and coronary heart disease.
2. *Echocardiography* (ultrasound cardiography) —graphic record of motions produced by cardiac structures as high-frequency sound vibrations are echoed through chest wall into the heart; transesophageal echocardiography produces a clearer image, particularly in obese, barrel-chested, or patients with chronic obstructive pulmonary disease (COPD); *used to* demonstrate valvular or other structural deformities, detect pericardial effusion, diagnose tumors and cardiomegaly, or evaluate prosthetic valve function.
3. *Phonocardiogram*—graphic record of heart sounds; *used to* keep a permanent record of patient's heart sounds before and after cardiac surgery.
4. *Electroencephalogram (EEG)*—graphic record of the electrical potentials generated by the physiological activity of the brain; *used to* detect surface lesions or tumors of the brain and presence of epilepsy.
5. *Echoencephalogram*—beam of pulsed ultrasound is passed through the head, and returning echoes are graphically recorded; *used to* detect shifts in cerebral midline structures caused by: subdural hematomas, intracerebral hemorrhage, or tumors.

C. Roentgenological studies (x-ray)

1. *Chest—used to* determine size, contour, and position of the heart; size, location, and nature of pulmonary lesions; disorders of thoracic bones or soft tissue; diaphragmatic contour and excursion; pleural thickening or effusions; and gross changes in the caliber or distribution of pulmonary vasculature.

2. *Kidney, ureter, and bladder (KUB)*—used to determine size, shape, and position of kidneys, ureters, and bladder.

3. *Mammography*—examination of the breast with or without the injection of radiopaque substance into the ducts of the mammary gland; *used to* determine the presence of tumors or cysts. *Patient preparation:* no deodorant, perfume, powders, or ointment in underarm area on day of x-ray. May be uncomfortable due to pressure on the breast.

4. *Skull*—outline configuration and density of brain tissues and vascular markings; *used to* determine the size and location of: intracranial calcifications, tumors, abscesses, or vascular lesions.

D. **Roentgenological studies (fluoroscopy)**—require the ingestion or injection of a radiopaque substance to visualize the target organ.

◆ 1. *Additional nursing responsibilities* may include:

▶ a. Administration of *enemas or cathartics* before the procedure and a laxative after.

b. Keeping the patient *NPO* 6–12 hr before examination; check with MD regarding oral medications.

c. Ascertaining patient's *history of allergies* or allergic reactions (e.g., iodine, seafood).

d. Observing for *allergic* reactions to contrast medium following procedure.

e. Providing fluid and food following procedure, to counteract dehydration.

f. Observing stool for color and consistency until barium passes.

2. Common fluoroscopic examinations:

a. *Upper GI*—ingestion of barium sulfate or meglumine diatrizoate (Gastrografin, a white, chalky, radiopaque substance), followed by fluoroscopic and x-ray examination; *used to* determine:

(1) Patency and caliber of *esophagus;* may also detect esophageal varices.

(2) Mobility and thickness of *gastric* walls, presence of ulcer craters, filling defects due to tumors, pressures from outside the stomach, and patency of pyloric valve.

(3) Rate of passage in small bowel and presence of structural abnormalities.

b. *Lower GI*—rectal instillation of barium sulfate followed by fluoroscopic and x-ray examination; *used to* determine contour and mobility of colon and presence of any space-occupying tumors; perform before

◆ upper GI. *Patient preparation:* explain purpose; *no food after evening meal* the evening before test; *stool softeners, laxatives, enemas, and suppositories* to cleanse the bowel before the test; *NPO after midnight* before test; oral medications *not*

permitted day of test. *After completion of exam:* food, *increased liquid* intake, and rest; *laxatives for at least 2 days* or until stools are normal in color and consistency.

c. *Cholecystogram* (done if gallbladder not seen with ultrasound)—ingestion of organic iodine contrast medium Telepaque (iopanoic acid), or Oragrafin (preparation of calcium or sodium salt of ipodate) followed in 12 hr by x-ray visualization; gallbladder disease is indicated with *poor* or no visualization of the bladder; accurate only if GI and liver function is intact; perform before barium enema or upper

◆ GI. *Patient preparation:* explain purpose; administer large amount of *water* with contrast capsules; *low-fat meal* evening *before* x-ray; *oral laxative or stool softener after meal; no food* allowed after contrast capsules; water, tea, or coffee, with no cream or sugar, usually allowed. *After completion of exam:* fluids, food, and rest; observe for any signs of allergy to contrast medium.

d. *Cholangiogram*—intravenous injection of a radiopaque contrast substance, followed by fluoroscopic and x-ray examination of the bile ducts; failure of the contrast medium to pass certain points in the bile duct pinpoints *obstruction.*

e. *Intravenous urography (IVU) or pyelography (IVP)*—injection of a radiopaque contrast medium, followed by fluoroscopic and x-ray films of kidneys and urinary tract; *used to* identify lesions in kidneys and ureters and provide a rough estimate of kidney function.

f. *Cystogram*—installation of radiopaque medium through a catheter into the bladder; *used to* visualize bladder wall and evaluate ureterovesical valves for reflux.

g. *Phlebography* (lower limb venography)—determines patency of the tibial-popliteal, superficial femoral, common femoral, and saphenous veins. A contrast medium is injected into the superficial and/or deep veins of the involved extremity, followed by x-rays, while the leg is placed in a variety of positions; *used to* detect deep-vein thrombosis and to select a vein for use in arterial bypass grafting; localized clotting may result.

E. **Computed tomography (CT)**—an x-ray beam sweeps around the body, allowing measurement of various tissue densities; provides clear radiographic definition of structures that are not visible by other techniques, permitting earlier diagnosis and treatment and more effective and efficient follow-up. Initial scan may be followed

Treatments

by "contrast enhancement" using an injection of an intravenous contrast agent (iodine), followed
◆ by a repeat scan. *Patient preparation:* instructions for eating before test vary. Clear liquids up to 2 hr before are usually permitted.

F. **Magnetic resonance imaging (MRI)**—noninvasive, nonionic technique produces cross-sectional images by exposure to magnetic energy sources. Provides superior contrast of soft tissue, including healthy, benign, and malignant tissue, along with veins and arteries; uses no contrast medium; takes 30–90 min to complete; patient must *stay still* for periods of 5–20 min at a time—equipment often very noisy. *Patient*
◆ *preparation:* patient can take food and medications except for low abdominal and pelvic studies (food/fluids withheld 4–6 hr to decrease peristalsis). *Restrictions:* patients who have metal implants, permanent pacemakers, or implanted medication pumps such as insulin, or who are pregnant or on life support systems. Patients who are obese may not be able to have full-body MRI because they may not fit in the scanner tunnel. Patients who are claustrophobic may need distraction (e.g., music) or may be referred to a facility that has an MRI chamber that is more open.

G. **Multiple-gated acquisition scan (MUGA)**—also known as blood pool imaging. Red blood cells are tagged with a radioactive isotope. A computer-operated camera takes sequential pictures of actual heart wall motion; *complement* to cardiac catheterization; *used to* determine valvular effectiveness, follow progress of heart disease, diagnose cardiac aneurysms, detect coronary artery disease, determine effects of cardiovascular drug therapy. No special preparation. Painless, except for injections. Wear *gloves* if contact with patient urine occurs within 24 hr after scan.

H. **Ultrasound (sonogram)**—scanning by ultrasound is used to diagnose disorders of the thyroid, kidney, liver, uterus, gallbladder, and fetus and the intracranial structures in the neonate. It is not useful when visualization through air or bone is required (lung studies). In some agencies the sonogram has taken the place of the oral cholecystogram in diagnosing gallbladder dis-
◆ ease, bile duct distention, and calculi. *Patient preparation* is minimal, i.e., NPO for at least 8 hr for gallbladder studies. No x-rays. Thirty-two ounces of water PO 30 min before studies of lower abdomen or uterus.

I. **Pulmonary function studies:**
1. Ventilatory studies—utilization of a spirometer to determine how well the lung is ventilating.
   a. *Vital capacity (VC)*—largest amount of air that can be expelled after maximal inspiration.

(1) *Normally* 4000–5000 mL.
(2) *Decreased* in restrictive lung disease.
(3) May be normal, slightly increased, or decreased in chronic obstructive lung disease.
   b. *Forced expiratory volume (FEV$_T$)*—percentage of vital capacity that can be forcibly expired in 1, 2, or 3 sec.
(1) *Normally 81–83% in 1 sec, 90–94% in 2 sec, and 95–97% in 3 sec.*
(2) *Decreased* values indicate expiratory airway obstruction.
   c. *Maximum breathing capacity (MBC)*—maximum amount of air that can be breathed in and out in 1 min with maximal rate and depth of respiration.
(1) Best overall measurement of ventilatory ability.
(2) *Reduced* in restrictive and chronic obstructive lung disease.
2. Diffusion studies—measure the rate of exchange of gases across alveolar membrane. Carbon monoxide single-breath, rebreathing, and steady-state techniques—used because of special affinity of hemoglobin for carbon monoxide; *decreased* when fluid is present in alveoli or when alveolar membranes are thick or fibrosed.

J. **Sputum studies:**
1. Gross sputum evaluations—collection of sputum samples to ascertain quantity, consistency, color, and odor.
2. *Sputum smear*—sputum is smeared thinly on a slide so that it can be studied microscopically; *used to* determine cytological changes (malignant cell) or presence of pathogenic bacteria, e.g., tubercle bacilli.
3. *Sputum culture*—sputum samples are implanted or inoculated into special media; *used to* diagnose pulmonary infections.
4. *Gastric lavage or analysis*—insertion of a nasogastric tube into the stomach to siphon out swallowed pulmonary secretions; *used to* detect organisms causing pulmonary infections; especially useful for detecting tubercle bacilli in children.

K. **Examination of gastric contents:**
1. *Gastric analysis*—aspiration of the contents of the fasting stomach for analysis of free and total acid.
   a. Gastric acidity is generally *increased* in presence of duodenal ulcer.
   b. Gastric acidity is usually *decreased* in pernicious anemia, cancer of the stomach.
2. Stool specimens—*examined for:* amount, consistency, color, character, and melena; *used to* determine presence of: urobilinogen, fat, nitrogen, parasites, and other substances.

L. **Thermography**—a picture of the surface temperature of the skin using infrared photography (non-ionizing radiation) detects the circulation pattern of areas in the breasts. Tumors produce more heat than normal breast tissue. Useful with large tumors, but may not detect small or deep lesions. Requires expensive equipment and is difficult to interpret accurately.

M. Doppler ultrasonography—*used to* measure blood flow in the major veins and arteries. The transducer of the test instrument is placed on the skin, sending out bursts of ultra-high-frequency sound. The ratio of ankle to brachial systolic pressure (API $\geq$ 1) provides information about vascular insufficiency. Sound varies with respiration and the Valsalva maneuver. No discomfort to the patient.

N. Caloric stimulation test—*used to* evaluate the vestibular portion of the eighth cranial nerve, identify the impairment or loss of thermally induced nystagmus. Reflex eye movements (nystagmus) result in response to cold or warm irrigations of the external auditory canal if the nerve is intact. A *diminished or absent* response occurs with Meniere's or acoustic neuroma. Nausea, vomiting, or dizziness can be precipitated by the test.

O. 24-hour urine collection—a true and accurate evaluation of kidney function, primarily glomerular filtration. Substances excreted by the kidney are excreted at different rates, amounts, and times of day or night. Timed urine collection is done for *protein, creatinine, electrolytes, urinary steroids,* etc. A large container is used with or without preservative. Label with patient name, type of test, and exact time test starts and ends. Not usually necessary to measure urine. Have patient void, discard urine; test starts at this time. Have patient void as close to the end of the 24 hr period as possible. If refrigeration is required, urine may be stored in iced container.

P. Glucose testing—to detect disorder of glucose metabolism, such as diabetes.

1. *Fasting (FBS):* blood sample is drawn after a 12 hr fast (usually overnight). Water is allowed. If diabetes is present, value will be 126 mg/dL.

2. *2 hr postprandial (PPBS):* blood is taken after a meal. For best results, patient should be on a high-carbohydrate diet for 2–4 days before testing. Patient fasts overnight, eats a high-carbohydrate breakfast; blood sample is drawn 2 hr after eating. Patient should rest during 2 hr interval. Smoking and coffee may increase glucose level.

3. *Glucose tolerance test (GTT):* done when sugar in urine, or FBS or 2 hr PPBS is not conclusive. A timed test, usually 2 hr. High-carbohydrate diet is eaten 3 days before test. Blood is drawn after overnight fast. Patient drinks a very sweet glucose liquid. All of the solution must be taken. Blood and urine sam-

ple usually taken at 30 min, 1 hr, 2 hr, and sometimes 3 hr after drinking solution. Blood glucose peaks in 30–60 min, and returns to normal, usually within 3 hr.

II. Invasive diagnostic procedures—procedures that directly record the size, shape, or function of an organ and that are often complex or expensive or require utilization of highly trained personnel; these procedures may result in morbidity and occasionally death of the patient and therefore require the written consent of the patient or guardian.

◆ **A. General nursing responsibilities:**

1. *Before procedure:* institute measures to provide for patient's safety and emotional comfort.

   a. Have patient sign permit for procedure.

   b. Ascertain and report any patient history of allergy or allergic reactions.

   c. Explain procedure briefly, and accurately advise patient of any possible sensations, such as flushing or a warm feeling, as when a contrast medium is injected.

   d. Keep patient NPO 6–12 hr before procedure if anesthesia is to be used.

   e. Allow patient to verbalize concerns, and note attitude toward procedure.

   f. Administer preprocedure sedative, as ordered.

   g. If procedure done at bedside:

      (1) Remain with patient, offering frequent reassurance.

      (2) Assist with optional positioning of patient.

      (3) Observe for indications of complications—shock, pain, or dyspnea.

2. *After procedure:* institute measures to avoid complications and promote physical and emotional comfort.

   a. Observe and record vital signs.

   b. Check injection cut-down or biopsy sites for bleeding, infection, tenderness, or thrombosis.

      (1) Report untoward reactions to physician.

      (2) Apply warm compresses to ease discomfort, as ordered.

   c. If topical anesthetic is used during procedure (e.g., gastroscopy, bronchoscopy), do *not* give food or fluid until gag reflex returns.

   d. Encourage relaxation by allowing patient to discuss experience and verbalize feelings.

B. Procedures to evaluate the cardiovascular system:

1. *Angiocardiography*—intravenous injection of a radiopaque solution or contrast medium for the purpose of studying its circulation through the patient's heart, lungs, and great

vessels; *used to* check the competency of heart valves, diagnose congenital septal defects, detect occlusions of coronary arteries, confirm suspected diagnoses, and study heart function and structure before cardiac surgery.

2. *Cardiac catheterization*—insertion of a radiopaque catheter into a vein to study the heart and great vessels.

   a. *Right-heart catheterization*—catheter is inserted through a cut-down in the antecubital vein into the superior vena cava, through the right atrium and ventricle, and into the pulmonary artery.

   b. *Left-heart catheterization*—catheter may be passed retrograde to the left ventricle through the brachial or femoral artery; it can be passed into the left atrium after right-heart catheterization by means of a special needle that punctures the septa; or it may be passed directly into the left ventricle by means of a posterior or anterior chest puncture.

   c. Cardiac catheterizations are *used to*:
      (1) Confirm diagnosis of heart disease and determine the extent of disease.
      (2) Determine existence and extent of congenital abnormalities.
      (3) Measure pressures in the heart chambers and great vessels.
      (4) Obtain estimate of cardiac output.
      (5) Obtain blood samples to measure oxygen content and determine presence of cardiac shunts.

   ◆ d. *Specific nursing interventions*:
      (1) *Preprocedure patient teaching*:
         (a) Fatigue due to lying still for 3 hr or more is a common complaint.
         (b) Some fluttery sensations may be felt—occur as catheter is passed backward into the left ventricle.
         (c) Flushed, warm feeling may occur when contrast medium is injected.
      (2) *Postprocedure observations*:
         (a) Monitor ECG pattern for arrhythmias.
         (b) Check extremities for color and temperature, peripheral pulses (femoral and dorsalis pedis) for quality.

3. *Angiography (arteriography)*—injection of a contrast medium into the arteries to study the vascular tree; *used to* determine obstructions or narrowing of peripheral arteries.

4. *Pericardiocentesis (pericardial aspiration)*—puncture of the pericardial sac is performed to remove fluid accumulating with pericardial effusion. The goal is to prevent cardiac tamponade (compression of the heart). *Nursing responsibilities*: monitor ECG and CVP

during the procedure, have resuscitative equipment ready. Head of bed elevated to ▱ *45–60 degrees*. Maintain peripheral IV with saline or glucose. Following the procedure, monitor BP, CVP, and heart sounds for recurrence of tamponade (pulsus paradoxus).

C. Procedures to evaluate the respiratory system:

1. *Pulmonary circulation studies*—*used to* determine regional distribution of pulmonary blood flow.

   a. *Lung scan*—injection of radioactive isotope into the body, followed by lung scintiscan, which produces a graphic record of gamma rays emitted by the isotope in lung tissues; *used to* determine lung perfusion when space-occupying lesions or pulmonary emboli and infarction are suspected.

   b. *Pulmonary angiography*—x-ray visualization of the pulmonary vasculature after the injection of a radiopaque contrast medium; *used to* evaluate pulmonary disorders, e.g., pulmonary embolism, lung tumors, aneurysms, and changes in the pulmonary vasculature due to such conditions as emphysema or congenital defects.

2. *Bronchoscopy*—introduction of a special lighted instrument (bronchoscope) into the trachea and bronchi; *used to* inspect tracheobronchial tree for pathological changes, remove tissue for cytological and bacteriological studies, remove foreign bodies or mucous plugs causing airway obstruction, assess functional residual capacity of diseased lung, and apply chemotherapeutic agents.

   ◆ a. *Prebronchoscopy nursing actions*:
      (1) Oral hygiene.
      (2) Postural drainage is indicated.

   b. *Postbronchoscopy nursing actions*:
      (1) Instruct patient *not* to swallow oral secretions but to let saliva run from side of mouth.
      (2) Save expectorated sputum for laboratory analysis, and observe for frank bleeding.
      (3) NPO until gag reflex returns.
      (4) Observe for subcutaneous emphysema and dyspnea.
      (5) Apply ice collar to reduce throat discomfort.

3. *Thoracentesis*—needle puncture through the chest wall and into the pleura; *used to* remove fluid and occasionally air from the pleural ◆ space. *Nursing responsibilities before* thoracentesis:

   ▱ a. *Position*: high Fowler's position or sitting up on edge of bed, with feet supported on chair to facilitate accumulation of fluid in the base of the chest.

✒ b. If patient is unable to sit up—turn onto *unaffected* side.

c. Evaluate continually for signs of shock, pain, cyanosis, increased respiratory rate, and pallor.

▯ **D. Procedures to evaluate the renal system:**

1. *Renal angiogram*—small catheter is inserted into the femoral artery and passed into the aorta or renal artery, radiopaque fluid is instilled, and serial films are taken.

   a. *Used to* diagnose renal hypertension and pheochromocytoma and differentiate renal cysts from renal tumors.

   ◆ b. *Postangiogram nursing actions:* check pedal pulse for signs of decreased circulation.

2. *Cystoscopy*—visualization of bladder, urethra, and prostatic urethra by insertion of a tubular, lighted, telescopic lens (cystoscope) through the urinary meatus.

   a. *Used to* directly inspect the bladder; collect urine from the renal pelvis; obtain biopsy specimens from bladder and urethra; remove calculi; and treat lesions in the bladder, urethra, and prostate.

   ◆ b. *Nursing actions following* procedure:

   (1) Observe for urinary retention.

   (2) Warm sitz baths to relieve discomfort.

3. *Renal biopsy*—needle aspiration of tissue from the kidney for the purpose of microscopic examination.

▯ **E. Procedures to evaluate the digestive system:**

1. *Celiac angiography, hepatoportography, and umbilical venography*—injection of a contrast medium into the portal vein or related vessel; *used to* determine patency of vessels supplying target organ or detect lesions in the organs that distort the vasculature.

2. *Esophagoscopy and gastroscopy*—visualization of the esophagus, the stomach, and sometimes the duodenum by means of a lighted tube inserted through the mouth.

3. *Proctoscopy*—visualization of rectum and colon by means of a lighted tube inserted through the anus.

4. *Peritoneoscopy*—direct visualization of the liver and peritoneum by means of a peritoneoscope inserted through an abdominal stab wound.

5. *Liver biopsy*—needle aspiration of tissue for the purpose of microscopic examination; *used to* determine tissue changes, facilitate diagnosis, and provide information regarding a disease course. *Nursing action:* place patient ✒ on *right side* and position pillow for pressure, to prevent bleeding.

6. *Paracentesis*—needle aspiration of fluid from the peritoneal cavity; *used to* relieve excess fluid accumulation or for diagnostic studies.

   ◆ a. *Specific nursing actions before paracentesis:*

   (1) Have patient void—to prevent possible injury to bladder during procedure.

   ✒ (2) *Position*—sitting up on side of bed, with feet supported by chair.

   (3) Check vital signs and peripheral circulation frequently throughout procedure.

   (4) Observe for signs of hypovolemic shock—may occur due to fluid shift from vascular compartment following removal of protein-rich ascitic fluid.

   ◆ b. *Specific nursing actions following paracentesis:*

   (1) Apply pressure to injection site and cover with sterile dressing.

   (2) Measure and record amount and color of ascitic fluid; send specimens to lab for diagnostic studies.

7. *Small-bowel biopsy*—a specimen is obtained by passing a tube through the oral cavity and is microscopically examined for changes in
◆ cellular morphology. *Nursing responsibilities: no* food or fluids 8 hr before procedure. Obtain written consent. Remove dentures if present. Monitor vital signs before, during, and after procedure for indications of hemorrhage. Procedure takes approximately 1 hour.

▯ **F. Procedures to evaluate the reproductive system in women:**

1. *Culdoscopy*—surgical procedure in which a culdoscope is inserted into the posterior vaginal cul-de-sac; *used to* visualize: uterus, fallopian tubes, broad ligaments, and peritoneal contents.

2. *Hysterosalpingography*—x-ray examination of uterus and fallopian tubes following insertion of a radiopaque substance into the uterine cavity; *used to* determine patency of fallopian tubes and detect pathology in uterine cavity.

3. *Breast biopsy*—needle aspiration or incisional removal of breast tissue for microscopic examination; *used to* differentiate among benign tumors, cysts, and malignant tumors in the breast.

4. *Cervical biopsy and cauterization*—removal of cervical tissue for microscopic examination and cautery; *used to* control bleeding or obtain additional tissue samples.

5. *Uterotubal insufflation (Rubin's test)*—injection of carbon dioxide into the cervical canal; *used to* determine fallopian tube patency.

▯ **G. Procedures to evaluate the neuroendocrine system:**

1. *Radioactive iodine uptake test (iodine 131 uptake)*—ingestion of a tracer dose of ^{131}I, followed in 24 hr by a scan of the thyroid for amount of radioactivity emitted.

a. *High* uptake indicates hyperthyroidism.
b. *Low* uptake indicates hypothyroidism.

2. *Eight-hour intravenous ACTH test*—administration of 25 units of ACTH in 500 mL of saline over an 8 hr period.

   a. *Used to* determine function of adrenal cortex.
   b. 24 hr urine specimens are collected, before and after administration, for measurement of 17-ketosteroids and 17-hydroxycorticosteroids.
   c. In *Addison's* disease, urinary output of steroids does *not increase* following administration of ACTH; *normally* steroid excretion *increases threefold to fivefold* following ACTH stimulation.
   d. In *Cushing's* syndrome, hyperactivity of the adrenal cortex *increases* the urine output of steroids in the second urine specimen *tenfold*.

3. *Cerebral angiography*—fluoroscopic visualization of the brain vasculature after injection of a contrast medium into the carotid or vertebral arteries; *used to* localize lesions (tumors, abscesses, intracranial hemorrhages, and occlusions) that are large enough to distort cerebrovascular blood flow.

4. *Myelogram*—through a lumbar-puncture needle, a contrast medium is injected into the subarachnoid space of the spinal column to visualize the spinal cord; *used to* detect herniated or ruptured intervertebral disks, tumors, or cysts that compress or distort spinal cord.

◼◆ *Nursing responsibilities: elevate head of bed* with water-soluble contrast; *flat* with oil contrast; check for bladder distention with metrizamide (water soluble); vital signs every 4 hr for 24 hr.

5. *Brain scan*—intravenous injection of a radioactive substance, followed by a scan for emission of radioactivity.

   a. *Increased* radioactivity at site of abnormality.
   b. *Used to* detect brain tumors, abscesses, hematomas, and arteriovenous malformations.

6. *Lumbar puncture*—puncture of the lumbar subarachnoid space of the spinal cord with a needle to withdraw samples of cerebrospinal fluid (CSF); *used to* evaluate CSF for infections and determine presence of hemorrhage. *Not* done if increased intracranial pressure (ICP) suspected.

❚ **H. Procedures to evaluate the skeletal system.** *Arthroscopy*—examination of a joint through a fiberoptic endoscope called an arthroscope. Usually done in the OR (same-day surgery) under aseptic conditions using a local anesthetic, although a general anesthetic may be used. A tourniquet is used to reduce blood flow to the area while the scope is introduced through a cannula. Saline is used as the viewing medium. Biopsy or removal of loose bodies from the joint may be done. A compression dressing (e.g., Ace bandage) is applied. Restrictions vary according to surgeon preference and nature of procedure. Weight bearing may be immediate or restricted for 24 hr. Teach patient to observe for signs of infection.

DIAGNOSTIC TESTS TO EVALUATE FETAL WELL-BEING

Table 11–1.

NEWBORN SCREENING PROCEDURES

Table 11–2.

TABLE 11–1 ☐ **Diagnostic Tests to Evaluate Fetal Well-being**

Test	Implications of Results	Risks
Nonstress Test (NST) Requires electronic fetal monitoring Correlates fetal movements with FHR and intact fetal CNS; 90% of gross fetal movements associated with accelerations of the FHR	*Reactive test*—indicates intact CNS. *Nonreactive test*—does not meet criteria for reactivity. May indicate fetal jeopardy.	Noninvasive procedure No known contraindications
Contraction Stress Test (CST) Correlates fetal heart rate response to induced uterine contractions; indicator of *uteroplacental insufficiency*	Increased doses of oxytocin are administered to stimulate uterine contractions. Interpretation: *Negative results* indicate absence of abnormal deceleration with all contractions. Reassurance that the fetus is likely to survive if labor occurs in 1 wk. *Positive results* indicate abnormal FHR decelerations with contractions. May indicate *uteroplacental insufficiency* and that the fetus is at increased risk for perinatal morbidity and death.	Invasive procedure Risk for uterine hyperstimulation and jeopardy to the fetus
Ultrasound Passage of high-frequency sound waves through uterus to obtain data regarding fetal growth, placental position, and uterine cavity; can be done abdominally or vaginally	May be *used for:* pregnancy confirmation, fetal viability, estimation of fetal age, placental location, detection of fetal abnormalities, identification of multiple gestation, and confirmation of fetal death.	Noninvasive procedure Inconclusive evidence of harmful effects on humans
Biophysical Profile (BPP) Assessment of five fetal biophysical variables: tone, breathing movements, gross body movement, amniotic fluid volume, and FHR reactivity (NST); first four variables assessed by ultrasound; score of 2 assigned to each normal finding, and 0 to each abnormal; maximum score 10	Used to assess the fetus at risk for intrauterine compromise. *Normal* fetal biophysical activities indicate that the CNS is functional and the fetus is not hypoxemic. *Abnormal* findings with oligohydramnios indicate fetal jeopardy (acidosis and impending death) and necessity for immediate delivery. *Normal:* 8–10 (if amniotic fluid volume (AFV) adequate). Equivocal: 6. Abnormal: <4.	Noninvasive procedures No known contraindications
Amniocentesis Invasive procedure for amniotic fluid analysis; needle placed through abdominal wall to obtain designated amount of fluid for examination; ultrasound *always precedes* this procedure; possible after 14 weeks of gestation	Amniotic fluid (fetal cells) might be analyzed for chromosomal studies to detect: aberrations, inborn errors of metabolism; determine fetal lung maturity, fetal age, presence of isoimmune disease, alpha-fetoprotein (AFP) levels for determination of neural tube defects, and presence of meconium.	Complications: <1%, but risks might include: onset of contractions, infections; placental, cord, fetal, or bladder puncture Fetomaternal hemorrhage with possible Rh isoimmunization Rh negative mothers should receive RhoGAM following the procedure
Percutaneous Umbilical Blood Sampling (PUBS; also called *cordocentesis*) Technique used to obtain pure fetal blood from the umbilical cord while the fetus is in utero; ultrasound done first to locate umbilical cord, then a needle is inserted through the maternal abdomen and into the fetal umbilical vein; done in *second and third trimesters*; a paralytic agent, such as Pavulon, may be given to prevent fetal movement during the procedure	*Indications* for fetal blood sampling: ■ Rapid fetal karyotyping. ■ Diagnosis of fetal infection. ■ Platelet disorders. ■ Fetal blood grouping. ■ Diagnosis and treatment of isoimmunization. ■ Assessment of fetal well-being (pH, P_{O_2}). ■ Fetal metabolic disorders. ■ Fetal blood transfusion. ■ Administration of fetal medications.	Overall fetal loss risk <2%; complication rate after PUBS: <0.5% *Complications* include: failure to obtain sample, bleeding, premature rupture of membranes, chorioamnionitis, fetal bradycardia, Rh isoimmunization (Rh negative women given RhoGAM).
Chorionic Villus Sampling (CVS) Involves obtaining a small sample of chorionic villi from edge of developing placenta between 10 and 12 weeks of gestation; can be accomplished either transcervically or transabdominally; use sterile procedure; chorionic tissue aspirated into a syringe	Because chorionic villi originate in zygote, it reflects the genetic makeup of the fetus. *Indications for CVS:* ■ Advanced maternal age (>35 yr). ■ Biochemical and molecular assays for infections. ■ Assays for metabolic disorders.	Vaginal bleeding, spontaneous abortion (SAB), rupture of membranes, limb anomalies (increased risk if done <10 weeks of gestation); intrauterine infection, Rh isoimmunization (Rh negative women given RhoGAM)

Treatments

TABLE 11–2 ▌ **Newborn Screening Procedures**

Test	Implications of Results	Nursing Priorities
Cord blood type, group, and Coombs' test	Sample of cord blood is collected at delivery to determine newborn's *blood type* and *group* (Rh positive or negative). Coombs' test is done, especially for those whose mothers have type O or Rh-negative blood, or for neonates who are considerably jaundiced. Direct Coombs' test will determine *if antibodies* are present in the neonate's blood.	1. Review prenatal record to determine risk for ABO and Rh incompatibility. 2. Assess for jaundice. Age of the neonate in hours or days at the onset of jaundice is essential to diagnose underlying clinical causes. 3. Provide support and information to the family regarding screening procedures.
Phenylketonuria (PKU)	PKU is an autosomal recessive disease of protein synthesis in which the blood level of the amino acid phenylalanine becomes very high; the disorder results in *mental retardation*. If test is positive, retardation can be prevented through dietary control. Test is done with blood sample from neonate's heel 24–36 hr after having milk. Usually repeat screening recommended, especially if discharged early.	1. Review family history for incidence of inborn errors of metabolism. 2. Observe neonate for: lethargy, apnea, poor feeding, poor muscle tone, jaundice, enlarged tongue, diarrhea, and unusual (musty) body odor. 3. Provide support and information regarding screening procedures. Stress importance of follow-up testing.
Hypothyroidism	Mass neonatal screening for hypothyroidism is a cost-effective measure for preventing mental retardation caused by thyroid dysfunction. Sample of neonate's blood is taken for analysis (may be done with PKU analysis).	1. Review family history for thyroid dysfunction. 2. Provide support and information regarding screening procedures.
Galactosemia	Galactosemia is an autosomal recessive disease in which the inborn error of metabolism involves the body's inability to convert galactose to glucose. Surplus of galactose causes *liver* and *brain damage*. May be done with blood sample for PKU.	1. Review family history for inborn errors of metabolism. 2. Provide support and information regarding screening procedures.
Sickle cell disease	Sickle cell is an autosomal recessive disorder occurring in certain ethnic groups, most commonly African-American. Other ethnic origins may include: Mediterranean, Caribbean, Arabian, East Indian, and South and Central American. Disease is marked by crescent-shaped RBCs caused by defective hemoglobin. Severe, life-threatening attacks (crises) begin in childhood (fever and abdominal pain). Blood sample is taken after birth.	1. Review family history for autosomal blood disorders, especially if member of high-risk ethnic group. 2. Provide support and information to parents regarding genetic screening. 3. Provide support and information to the family.

INTRAVENOUS THERAPY

I. Infusion systems

A. Plastic bag:
1. Contains no vacuum—needs no air to replace fluid as it flows from container.
2. Medication can be added with syringe through a resealable latex port.
   a. During infusion, administration set should be completely clamped before medications are added.
   b. Prevents undiluted, and perhaps toxic, dose from entering administration set.

B. Closed system:
1. Requires partial vacuum—however, only filtered air enters container.
2. Medication may be added during infusion through air vent in administration set.

C. Administration sets:
1. *Standard sets*—deliver 10–15 drops/mL.
2. *Pediatric or minidrop sets*—deliver 60 drops/mL.
3. *Controlled-volume sets*—permit accurate infusion of measured volumes of fluids.
   a. Particularly valuable when piggybacked into primary infusion.
   b. Solutions containing drugs can then be administered intermittently.
4. *Y-type administration sets*—allow for simultaneous or alternate infusion of two fluids.
   a. May contain filter and pressure unit for blood transfusions.
   b. *Air embolism* significant hazard with this type of administration set.
5. *Positive-pressure sets*—designed for rapid infusion of replacement fluids.
   a. In emergency, built-in pressure chamber increases rate of blood administration.
   b. Pump chamber *must* be filled at all times to avoid air embolism.
   c. Application of positive pressure to infusion fluids is responsibility of *physician*.
6. *Infusion pumps*—used to deliver small volumes of fluid or doses of high-potency drugs.
   a. Used primarily in neonatal, pediatric, and adult intensive care units.
   b. Have increased the safety of parenteral therapy and reduced nursing time.

II. Fluid administration

A. Factors influencing rate:
1. Patient's size.
2. Patient's physical condition.
3. Age of patient.
4. Type of fluid.
5. Patient's tolerance to fluid.
6. Patient's position.

B. Flow rates for parenteral infusions can be computed using the following formula:

$$\frac{\text{gtt/mL of given set}}{60 \text{ min/hr}} \times \text{total volume/hr} = \text{gtt/min}$$

E.g., if 1000 mL is to be infused in an 8 hr (125 mL/hr) period and the administration set delivers 15 gtt/mL, the rate is 31.2 gtt/min:

$$\frac{15}{60} \times 125 = \frac{1}{4} \times 125 = 31.2 \text{ gtt/min}$$

C. Generally the type of fluid administration set determines its rate of flow.
1. *Fluid* administration sets—approximately 15 gtt/min.
2. *Blood* administration sets—approximately 10 gtt/min.
3. *Pediatric* administration sets—approximately 60 gtt/min.
4. Always check information on the administration set box to determine the number of gtt/mL before calculating; varies with manufacturer.

D. Factors influencing flow rates:
1. *Gravity*—a change in the height of the infusion bottle will increase or decrease the rate of flow; for example, raising the bottle higher will increase the rate of flow, and vice versa.
2. *Blood clot* in needle—stopping the infusion for any reason or an increase in venous pressure may result in partial or total obstruction of needle by clot due to:
   a. *Delay* in changing infusion bottle.
   b. Blood pressure cuff on, or restraints *on* or *above* infusion needle.
   c. Patient *lying on arm* in which infusion is being made.
3. Change in *needle position*—against or away from vein wall.
4. *Venous spasm*—due to cold blood or irritating solution.
5. *Plugged vent*—causes infusion to stop.

III. Fluid and electrolyte therapy

A. Types of therapy:
1. *Maintenance therapy*—provides water, electrolytes, glucose, vitamins, and in some instances protein to meet daily requirements.
2. *Restoration of deficits*—in addition to maintenance therapy, fluid and electrolytes are added to replace *previous* losses.
3. *Replacement therapy*—infusions to replace *current* losses in fluid and electrolytes.

B. Types of intravenous fluids (Table 11–3):
1. *Isotonic solutions*—fluids that approximate the osmolarity (280–300 mOsm/L) of normal blood plasma.

TABLE 11–3 Commonly Used Intravenous Fluids

IV Solution	Na (mEq/L)	K (mEq/L)	Ca (mEq/L)	Cl (mEq/L)	Lactate (mEq/L)	Calories/L
0.9% NaCl (NS)	154	0	0	154	0	0
5% Dextrose (D_5W)	0	0	0	0	0	170
5% Dextrose + 0.9% NaCl (D_5NS)	154	0	0	154	0	170
5% Dextrose + 0.45% NaCl ($D_5\frac{1}{2}NS$)	77	0	0	77	0	170
Lactated Ringer's solution	130	4	3	109	28	9
3% NaCl	462	0	0	462	0	0
5% NaCl	770	0	0	770	0	0
0.45% NaCl	69.3	0	0	69.3	0	0
10% Dextrose ($D_{10}W$)	0	0	0	0	0	340

a. Sodium chloride (0.9%)—normal saline.
  (1) *Indications:*
    (a) Extracellular fluid replacement when Cl^- loss is equal to or greater than Na^+ loss.
    (b) Treatment of metabolic alkalosis.
    (c) Na^+ depletion.
    (d) Initiating and terminating blood transfusions.
  (2) Possible *side effects:*
    (a) Hypernatremia.
    (b) Acidosis.
    (c) Hypokalemia.
    (d) Circulatory overload.
b. Five percent dextrose in water (D_5W).
  (1) *Provides calories* for energy, *sparing body protein* and *preventing* ketosis resulting from fat breakdown.
    (a) 3.75 calories are provided per gram of glucose.
    (b) USP standards require use of monohydrated glucose, so only 91% is actually glucose.
    (c) D_5W yields 170.6 calories; D_5W means 5 g glucose/100 mL water.

> $50 \times 3.75 = 187.5$ calories/L
> $0.91 \times 187.5 = 170.6$ calories/L

  (2) *Indications:*
    (a) Dehydration.
    (b) Hypernatremia.
    (c) Drug administration.
  (3) Possible *side effects:*
    (a) Hypokalemia.
    (b) Osmotic diuresis—dehydration.
    (c) Transient hyperinsulinism.
    (d) Water intoxication.
c. Five percent dextrose in normal saline.
  (1) *Prevents* ketone formation and *loss of* potassium and intracellular water.
  (2) *Indications:*
    (a) Hypovolemic shock—temporary measure.
    (b) Burns.
    (c) Acute adrenocortical insufficiency.
  (3) Same *side effects* as normal saline.

d. Isotonic multiple-electrolyte fluids—*used for* replacement therapy; ionic composition approximates blood plasma.
  (1) Types—Plasmanate, Polysol, and lactated Ringer's.
  (2) *Indicated in:* vomiting, diarrhea, excessive diuresis, and burns.
  (3) Possible *side effect*—circulatory overload.
  (4) Lactated Ringer's is *contraindicated* in severe metabolic acidosis and/or alkalosis and liver disease.
  (5) Same *side effects* as normal saline.
2. *Hypertonic solutions*—fluids with an osmolarity much higher than 310 mOsm (+50 mOsm); increase osmotic pressure of blood plasma, thereby drawing fluid from the cells.
  a. Ten percent dextrose in normal saline.
    (1) Administered in large vein to dilute and prevent venous trauma.
    (2) *Used for* nutrition and to replenish Na^+ and Cl^-.
    (3) Possible *side effects:*
      (a) Hypernatremia (excess Na^+).
      (b) Acidosis (excess Cl^-).
      (c) Circulatory overload.
  b. Sodium chloride solutions, 3% and 5%.
    (1) Slow administration essential to prevent overload (100 mL/hr).
    (2) *Indicated in* water intoxication and severe sodium depletion.
3. *Hypotonic solutions*—fluids whose osmolarity is significantly less than that of blood plasma (−50 mOsm); these fluids lower plasma osmotic pressures, causing fluid to enter cells.
  a. 0.45% sodium chloride—used for replacement when requirement for Na^+ use is questionable.
  b. 2.5% dextrose in 0.45% saline, also 5% D in 0.2% NaCl—common rehydrating solution.
    (1) *Indications:*
      (a) Fluid replacement when some Na^+ replacement is also necessary.
      (b) Encourage diuresis in patients who are dehydrated.

Treatments

(c) Evaluate kidney status before instituting electrolyte infusions.
(2) Possible *side effects:*
    (a) Hypernatremia.
    (b) Circulatory overload.
    (c) Use with *caution* in edematous patients with cardiac, renal, or hepatic disease.
    (d) After adequate renal function is established, appropriate electrolytes should be given to *avoid hypokalemia.*

4. *Alkalizing agents*—fluids used in the treatment of *metabolic acidosis:*
  a. Ringer's:
    (1) Administration—rate usually not more than 300 mL/hr.
    (2) *Side effects*—observe carefully for signs of *alkalosis.*
  b. Sodium bicarbonate:
    (1) *Indications:*
      (a) Replace excessive loss of bicarbonate ion.
      (b) Emergency treatment of life-threatening acidosis.
    (2) Administration:
      (a) Depends on patient's weight, condition, and carbon dioxide level.
      (b) Usual dose is 500 mL of a 1.5% solution (89 mEq).
    (3) *Side effects:*
      (a) Alkalosis.
      (b) Hypocalcemic tetany.
      (c) Rapid infusion may induce cellular acidity and death.

5. *Acidifying solutions*—fluids used in treatment of *metabolic alkalosis.*
  a. Types:
    (1) Normal saline (see **B.** 1. Isotonic solutions, p. 756).
    (2) Ammonium chloride.
  b. Administration—dosage depends on patient's condition and serum lab values.
  c. *Side effects:*

(1) Hepatic encephalopathy in presence of decreased liver function because ammonia is metabolized by liver.
(2) Toxic effects of irregular respirations, twitching, and bradycardia.
(3) *Contraindicated* with renal failure.
6. *Blood and blood products* (Table 11–4).
  a. *Indications:*
    (1) Maintenance of blood volume.
    (2) Supply red blood cells to maintain oxygen-carrying capacity.
    (3) Supply clotting factors to maintain coagulation properties.
    (4) Exchange transfusion.

IV. Intravenous cancer chemotherapy
  A. Usual sites: forearm, dorsum of hand, wrist, antecubital fossa.
  B. Procedure:
    1. Normal saline infusion usually started first, to verify vein patency, position of needle. Chemotherapy "piggybacked" into IV line that is running.
    2. Rate: usually 1 mL/min. Running slowly decreases nausea, vomiting, and the degree of vein damage.
    3. Check vein patency every 3–5 min.
    4. If more than one drug is to be infused, normal saline should be infused between drugs.
    5. *Never* infuse against resistance.
    6. *Stop* treatment if patient reports pain at needle site. Extravasation (infiltration of toxic drugs into tissue surrounding vessel) may be present.
▶   7. If extravasation present, begin protocol appropriate to drug administered (e.g., flushing of line with saline, applying ice or heat, local injection of site with antidote drugs, topical application of steroid creams).
    8. Once treatment is completed, remove needle, apply Band-Aid, exert pressure to prevent hematoma formation.

V. Complications of IV therapy: Table 11–5.

Treatments

TABLE 11–4   Transfusion with Blood or Blood Products

Blood or Blood Product	Indications	◆ Assessment: Side Effects	◆ Nursing Care Plan/ Implementation
Whole blood	1. Acute hemorrhage 2. Hypovolemic shock	1. Hemolytic reaction 2. Fluid overload 3. Febrile reaction 4. Pyrogenic reaction 5. Allergic reaction	1. See **Unit 7**, Table 7–22 (pp. 508–509), for complete discussion of nursing responsibilities 2. Protocol for checking blood before transfusion is begun varies with each institution; however, at least *two* RNs must verify that the unit of blood has been crossmatched for a specific patient
Red blood cells, packed	1. Acute anemia with hypoxia 2. Aplastic anemia 3. Bone marrow failure due to malignancy 4. Patients who need red blood cells but not volume	See Whole blood	See Whole blood
Red blood cells, frozen	1. See Red blood cells, packed 2. Patients sensitized by previous transfusions	1. Less likely to cause antigen reaction 2. Decreased possibility of transmitting hepatitis	See Whole blood
White blood cells (leukocytes)	Currently being used in severe leukopenia with infection (research still being done)	1. Elevated temperature 2. Graft-versus-host disease	1. Careful monitoring of temperature 2. *Must* be given as soon as collected
Platelet concentrate	1. Severe deficiency 2. Patients who have thrombocytopenia and are bleeding, with platelet counts *below* 10,000/μL.	1. Fever, chills 2. Hives 3. Development of antibodies that will destroy platelets in future transfusions *Contraindications:* 1. Idiopathic thrombocytopenic purpura 2. Disseminated intravascular coagulation (DIC)	Monitor temperature
Single-donor fresh plasma	1. Clotting deficiency or concentrates not available or deficiency not fully diagnosed 2. Shock	1. Side effects rare 2. Heart failure 3. Possible hepatitis	Use sterile, pyrogen-free filters
Plasma removed from whole blood (up to 5 days after expiration date, which is 21 days)	1. Shock due to loss of plasma 2. Burns 3. Peritoneal injury 4. Hemorrhage 5. While awaiting blood crossmatch results	See Single-donor fresh plasma	See Single-donor fresh plasma
Freeze-dried plasma	See Plasma removed from whole blood	See Single-donor fresh plasma	Must be reconstituted with sterile water before use
Single-donor fresh-frozen plasma	1. See Single-donor fresh plasma 2. Inherited or acquired disorders of coagulation 3. Preoperatively for hemophilia	See Single-donor fresh plasma	1. Notify blood bank to thaw about 30 min before administration 2. Give *immediately*
Cryoprecipitate concentrate (factor VIII—antihemophilic factor)	For hemophilia: 1. Prevention 2. Preoperatively 3. During bleeding episodes	Rare	0.55 mL of cryoprecipitate concentrate has same effect on serum level as 1600 mL of fresh-frozen plasma
Factors II, VII, IX, and X compiled	Specific deficiencies	Hepatitis	Commercially prepared

Continued

Treatments

TABLE 11–4   Transfusion with Blood or Blood Products—cont'd

Blood or Blood Product	Indications	◆ Assessment: Side Effects	Nursing Care Plan/ ◆ Implementation
Fibrinogen (factor I)	Fibrinogen deficiency	Increased risk of hepatitis because the hepatitis virus combines with fibrinogen during fractionation	1. Reconstitute with sterile water 2. Do *not* warm fibrinogen or use hot water to reconstitute 3. Do *not* shake 4. Must be given with a filter
Albumin or salt-poor albumin	1. Shock due to hemorrhage, trauma, infection, surgery, or burns 2. Treatment of cerebral edema 3. Low serum-protein levels	None; these are heat-treated products	Commercially prepared
Dextran	Hypovolemic shock	1. Rare allergic reaction 2. Patients with heart or kidney disease susceptible to heart failure or pulmonary edema	Commercially prepared

TABLE 11–5   Complications of IV Therapy

| Complication | Assessment | | ◆ Nursing Care Plan/Implementation |
	Subjective Data	Objective Data	
Infiltration—fluid infusing into surrounding tissue rather than into vessel	Pain around needle insertion	1. Infusion rate slow 2. Swelling, hardness, coolness, blanching of tissue at site of needle 3. Blood does not return into tubing when bag/bottle lowered 4. Puffiness under surface of arm	1. Stop IV 2. Apply warm towel to area 3. Restart at another site 4. Record
Thrombophlebitis—inflammatory changes in vessel; *thromboemboli*—the development of venous clots within the inflamed vessel	Pain along the vein	Redness, swelling around affected area (red line)	1. Stop IV 2. Notify physician 3. Cold compresses or warm towel, as ordered 4. Restart in another site 5. *Rest affected limb; do not rub* 6. See nursing care of thrombophlebitis, **Unit 7**, pp. 463–464
Pyrogenic reaction—contaminated equipment/solution	1. Headache 2. Backache 3. Nausea 4. Anxiety	1. ↑ temperature 2. Chills 3. Face flushed 4. Vomiting 5. ↓ BP 6. Cyanosis	1. Discontinue IV 2. Vital signs 3. Send equipment for culture/analysis 4. Antibiotic ointment, as ordered, at injection site 5. *Prevention:* change tubing q24–48h; meticulous sterile technique; check for precipitation, expiration dates, damage to containers, tubings, etc.; refrigerate hyperalimentation fluids; discard hyperalimentation fluids that have been at room temperature for 8–12 hr and use new bag regardless of amount left in first bag (change, to prevent infection—excellent medium for bacterial growth)
Fluid overload—excessive amount of fluid infused; infants/elderly at risk	1. Headache 2. Shortness of breath 3. Syncope 4. Dyspnea	1. ↑ pulse, venous pressure 2. Venous distention 3. Flushed skin 4. Coughing 5. ↑ respirations 6. Cyanosis, pulmonary edema 7. Shock	1. Stop IV 2. Semi-Fowler's *position* 3. Notify physician 4. Be prepared for diuretic therapy 5. *Preventive measures:* monitor flow rate and patient's response to IV therapy (see **Unit 7**, Fluid volume excess, p. 470, for subjective and objective data)
Air emboli—air in circulatory system	Loss of consciousness	1. Hypotension, cyanosis 2. Tachycardia 3. ↑ venous pressure 4. Tachypnea	1. Turn on *left* side, with head *down* 2. Administer oxygen therapy 3. **Medical emergency—call physician**
Nerve damage—improper position of limb during infusion or *tying* limb down too tight during infusion → damage to nerve	Numbness: fingers, hands	Unusual position for limb	1. Untie 2. Passive ROM exercises 3. Monitor closely for return of function 4. Record limb status
Pulmonary embolism—blood clot enters pulmonary circulation and obstructs pulmonary artery	Dyspnea	1. Orthopnea 2. Signs of circulatory and cardiac collapse	1. Slow IV to keep vein open (rate: 5–6 drops/min) 2. Notify physician 3. **Medical emergency** 4. Be prepared for lifesaving measures and anticoagulation therapy

OXYGEN THERAPY

I. **Purpose**—to relieve hypoxia and provide adequate tissue oxygenation.

II. **Clinical indications:**
   A. Any patient who is likely to have significant *shunt* from:
      1. Fluid in the alveoli.
         a. Pulmonary edema.
         b. Pneumonia.
         c. Near-drowning.
         d. Chest trauma.
      2. Collapsed alveoli (atelectasis).
         a. Airway obstruction.
            (1) Any unconscious patient.
            (2) Choking.
         b. Failure to take deep breaths.
            (1) Pain (rib fracture).
            (2) Paralysis of the respiratory muscles (spine injury).
            (3) Depression of the respiratory center (head injury, drug overdose).
         c. Collapse of an entire lung (pneumothorax).
      3. Other gases in the alveoli.
         a. Smoke inhalation.
         b. Toxic inhalations.
         c. Carbon monoxide poisoning.
      4. Respiratory arrest.
   B. Cardiac arrest.
   C. Shock.
   D. Shortness of breath.
   E. Signs of respiratory insufficiency.
   F. Breathing fewer than 10 times per minute.
   G. Chest pain.
   H. Stroke.
   I. Anemia.
   J. Fetal decelerations during labor.

III. **Precautions:**
   A. Patients with COPD should receive oxygen at *low* flow rates (usually 1–3 L/min), to prevent inhibition of hypoxic respiratory drive.
   B. *Excessive* amounts of oxygen for prolonged periods of time will cause *retrolental fibroplasia* and blindness in premature infants.
   C. Oxygen delivered *without* humidification will result in drying and irritation of respiratory mucosa, decreased ciliary action, and thickening of respiratory secretions.
   D. Oxygen supports combustion, and *fire* is a potential hazard during its administration.
      1. Ground electrical equipment.
      2. Prohibit smoking.
      3. Institute measures to decrease static electricity.
   E. *High* flow rates of oxygen delivered by ventilator or cuffed tracheostomy and endotracheal tubes can produce signs of oxygen toxicity in 24–48 hr:

      1. Cough, sore throat, decreased vital capacity, and substernal discomfort.
      2. Pulmonary manifestations due to:
         a. Atelectasis.
         b. Exudation of protein fluids into alveoli.
         c. Damage to pulmonary capillaries.
         d. Interstitial hemorrhage.

IV. **Oxygen administration:**
   A. Oxygen is dispensed from cylinder or piped-in system.
   B. Methods of delivering oxygen:
      1. Nasal prongs/cannula.
         a. Comfortable and simple, and allows patient to move about in bed.
         b. Delivers 25–40% oxygen at flow rates of 4–6 L/min.
         c. Difficult to keep in position unless patient is alert and cooperative.
      2. Jet mixing Venturi mask.
         a. Allows for accurate delivery of prescribed concentration of oxygen.
         b. Delivers 24–50% oxygen at flow rates of 4–8 L/min.
         c. Useful in long-term treatment of COPD.
      3. Simple O_2 face mask.
         a. Poorly tolerated—used for short periods of time; feeling of "suffocation."
         b. Delivers 50–60% oxygen at flow rates of 8–12 L/min.
         c. Significant rebreathing of carbon dioxide at low oxygen flow rates.
         d. Hot—may produce pressure sores around nose and mouth.
      4. Continuous positive airway pressure (CPAP) mask.
         a. Increases pulmonary volume; opens alveoli; may improve V/Q mismatch.
         b. Used with sleep apnea with or without O_2 source.
      5. Nonrebreather reservoir mask.
         a. Reservoir bag has one-way valve preventing the patient from exhaling back into the bag.
         b. Oxygen flow rate prevents collapse of bag during inhalation.
         c. Delivers 90–95% oxygen at flow rates of 10–12 L/min.
         d. Ideal for severe hypoxia, but patient may complain of feelings of suffocation.
      6. T-tube.
         a. Provides humidification and enriched oxygen mixtures to tracheostomy or endotracheal tube.
         b. Delivers up to 100% oxygen at flow rates at least two times minute ventilation.

V. **Intubation and mechanical ventilation:**
   A. *Indications:*
      1. Apnea.

2. Inadequate upper airway or inability to clear secretions.
3. Worsening respiratory acidosis ($PaCO_2 > 50$ mm Hg) and hypoventilation.
4. $PaO_2 < 55$ mm Hg.
5. Absent gag reflex.
6. Heavy sedation or paralysis.
7. Imminent respiratory failure (respiratory rate <8–10 breaths/min or >30–40 breaths/min).
8. Chest wall trauma.
9. Profound shock.
10. Controlled hyperventilation (e.g., increased ICP).

B. *Types of positive pressure ventilators:*
1. Pressure cycled—gas flows into the patient until a predetermined airway pressure is reached. Tidal volume is not constant.
2. Time cycled—gas flows for a certain percentage of time during ventilatory cycle.
3. Volume cycled—most common ventilators used; tidal volume is determined, and a fixed volume is delivered with each breath.

C. *Ventilator modes:*
1. Controlled—machine delivers a breath at a fixed rate regardless of patient's effort or demands.
2. Assist-controlled—machine senses a patient's efforts to breathe and delivers a fixed tidal volume with each effort.
3. Intermittent mandatory ventilation (IMV)—breaths are delivered by the machine, but the patient may also breathe spontaneously without machine assistance.
4. Pressure support—patient breathes spontaneously and determines ventilator rate. Tidal volume determined by inflation pressure and patient's lung-thorax compliance.

D. *Minute ventilation*—determined by the respiratory rate and the tidal volume. A respiratory rate of 10-15 breaths per minute is considered appropriate. Close monitoring is required to achieve desired (not necessarily normal) $PaCO_2$.

E. *Positive end-expiratory pressure* (PEEP)—maintenance of positive airway pressure at the end of expiration. Applied in the form of continuous positive airway pressure (CPAP) for the patient breathing spontaneously or continuous positive pressure ventilation (CPPV) for the patient receiving mechanical breaths. Applied in 3–5 cm H_2O increments. Levels >10–15 cm H_2O are associated with *cardiovascular dysfunction* and *hemodynamic* compromise.

Treatments

POSITIONING THE PATIENT

Table 11–6. Figure 11–1, **Common Patient Positions.**

COMMONLY USED TUBES

Table 11–7.

COLOSTOMY CARE ▸

Tables 11–8 and 11–9.

TABLE 11–6   Positioning the Patient for Specific Surgical Conditions ◢

Surgical Condition	Key Points	Rationale
Amputation: lower extremity	*No* pillows under stump after first 24 hr; turn patient *prone* several times a day	Prevents flexion deformity of the limb
Appendicitis: ruptured	Keep in *Fowler's* position—*not* flat in bed	Keeps infection from spreading upward in the peritoneal cavity
Burns (extensive)	Usually *flat* for first 24 hr	Potential problem is hypovolemia, which will be more symptomatic in a sitting position
Cast, extremity	Keep extremity *elevated*	Prevents edema
Craniotomy	Head *elevated* with supratentorial incision; *flat* with cerebellar or brainstem incision	Reduces cerebral edema, which contributes to increased intracranial pressure
Flail chest	Position on *affected* side	Reduces the instability of the chest wall that is causing the paradoxical respiratory movements
Gastric resection	Lie down *after* meals	May be useful in preventing dumping syndrome
Hiatal hernia (*before* repaired)	Head of bed *elevated* on shock blocks	Prevents esophageal irritation from gastric regurgitation
Hip prosthesis	1. Keep affected leg in *abduction* (splint or pillow between legs) 2. *Avoid* adduction and flexion of the hip 3. Use trochanter roll along outside of femur anterior joint capsule incision to keep affected leg turned slightly *inward;* no trochanter roll with posterior joint capsule incision as leg is turned slightly *outward*	If affected hip is flexed and allowed to adduct and internally rotate, the head of the femur may be displaced from the socket
Laminectomy; fusion	*Avoid* twisting motion when getting out of bed, ambulating	Prevents any shearing force on the spine
Liver biopsy	Place on *right* side, and position pillow for pressure	Prevents bleeding
Lobectomy	Do *not* put in Trendelenburg position. Position of comfort—sides, back	Pushes abdominal contents against diaphragm; may cause respiratory embarrassment
Mastectomy	1. Do *not* abduct arm first few days 2. Elevate hand and arm *higher* than shoulder if lymph glands removed	Puts tension on suture line Prevents lymphedema
Pneumonectomy	Turn *only* toward operative side for short periods; *no* extreme lateral positioning	1. Gives unaffected lung room for full expansion 2. Prevents mediastinal shift 3. In case of bleeding there will be no drainage into the unaffected bronchi
Radium implantation in cervix	Bed rest—usually may *elevate* head to 30 degrees	*Must* keep radium insert positioned correctly
Respiratory distress	*Orthopnea* position usually desirable	Allows for maximum expansion of lungs
Retinal detachment	1. Affected area toward bed—*complete bed rest* 2. No *sudden* movements of head 3. *Face down* if gas bubble in place	1. Gravity may help retina fall in place; prevents further tearing 2. Any sudden increase in intraocular pressure may further dislodge retina
Traction Straight traction	Check specific orders about how much head may be elevated	Body is used as the countertraction—this must not be less than the pull of the traction
Balanced suspension	May give patient more freedom to move about than in straight traction	In balanced suspension additional weights supply countertraction
Unconscious patient	Turn on side with head slightly *lowered*—"coma" position	1. Important to let secretions drain out by gravity 2. *Must* prevent aspiration
Vascular Ileofemoral bypass; arterial insufficiency	1. Do *not* elevate legs 2. *Avoid* hip flexion—walk or stand, but do *not* sit	1. Arterial flow is helped by gravity 2. Flexion of the hip compresses the vessels of the extremity
Vein strippings; vein ligations	1. Keep legs *elevated* 2. Do *not* stand or sit for long periods	1. Prevents venous stasis 2. Prevents venous pooling

Source: Jane Vincent Corbett, RN, MS, EdD, Professor, School of Nursing, University of San Francisco. Used with permission.

Treatments

FIGURE 11–1 ◪ **Common patient positions.** *(A)* **Dorsal recumbent** (back-lying), legs up—used in gynecological and obstetrical procedures such as forcep delivery or vaginal exam; legs down—for comfort and following spinal anesthesia. *(B)* **Prone**—may be used in unconscious patients to promote drainage from mouth and prevent flexion contractures. *(C)* **Fowler's**—semi-sitting; 45–60 degrees; knees may or may not be bent. Facilitates breathing and drainage. *(D)* **Sims'**—position of choice for enemas and rectal examination, prevents aspiration in unconscious patients, comfortable sleeping position for pregnant woman.

POSITIONS

A. DORSAL RECUMBENT POSITION

B. PRONE POSITION

KNEES MAY BE BENT

C. FOWLER'S POSITION

D. SIMS' POSITION

FIGURE 11–1—cont'd *(E)* **Knee-chest** or **genupectoral**—used for gynecological and obstetrical conditions such as impacted fetal head or transverse presentation. *(F)* **Trendelenburg**—used in abdominal surgery. **Modified Trendelenburg** (torso flat and feet elevated) preferred in shock. *(G)* **Lithotomy or dorsosacral**—used in genital tract operations and vaginal hysterectomy. *(H)* **Right lateral recumbent**—side-lying, relieves pressure on sacrum and heels.

POSITIONS

E. KNEE-CHEST OR GENUPECTORAL POSITION

F. TRENDELENBURG POSITION

G. LITHOTOMY OR DORSOSACRAL POSITION

H. RIGHT LATERAL RECUMBENT POSITION

Treatments

TABLE 11–7 **Review of the Use of Common Tubes**

Tube or Apparatus	Purpose	Examples of Use	Key Points
Chest tubes	1. *Anterior tube* drains mostly air from pleural space 2. *Posterior tube* drains mostly fluid from pleural space 3. Removal of fluid and air from pleural space is necessary to reestablish negative intrapleural pressure	1. *Thoracotomy* 2. *Open heart surgery* 3. *Spontaneous pneumothorax* 4. *Traumatic pneumothorax*	1. See Key Points for each of the three entries under Drainage system, below 2. *Sterile* technique is used when changing dressings around the tube insertions ◪ 3. Fowler's *position* to facilitate air and fluid removal ⬤ 4. Cough, deep breathe q1h; splint chest; medicate for pain 5. Manage pain carefully in order *not* to depress respirations 6. Prepare for removal when there is little or no drainage, air leak disappears, or fluctuations stop in water seal; have suture set, air-occlusive dressing, and sturdy elastic tape ready; medicate for pain before removal; monitor breathing after removal (breath sounds, rate, chest pain)
Drainage system (see Figure 11–2, p. 771) #1: drainage compartment	Collects drainage		1. Mark level in bottle each shift to keep accurate record—*not* routinely emptied; replaced when full 2. *Never* raise container above the level of the chest; otherwise backflow will occur
#2: water-seal chamber	Water seal prevents flow of atmospheric air into pleural space; essential to prevent recollapse of the lung		1. Air bubbles from postoperative residual air *will* continue for 24–48 hr 2. *Persistent* large amounts of air bubbles in this compartment indicate an *air leak* between the alveoli and the pleural space 3. Clamp tube(s) *only* to verify a leak; replace a broken, cracked, or full drainage unit; or verify readiness of patient for tube removal; not necessary to clamp when ambulating if water seal intact 4. If tube becomes disconnected, place tubing end in sterile water or saline; if dislodged from chest, seal insertion site *immediately* on expiration if possible; use *sterile air-occlusive* dressing 5. If air leak is present, clamping the tube for very long (more than 10 sec) may cause a tension pneumothorax 6. Fluctuation of the fluid level in this bottle is *expected* (when the suction is turned off) because respiration changes the pleural pressure: if there is *no fluctuation* of the fluid in the tube of this bottle (when the suction is turned off), either the lung is fully expanded or the tube is blocked by kinking or by a clot 7. Although not routinely used, milking (gently squeezing) the tubes, if ordered, will prevent blockage from clots or debris; otherwise gravity drainage is sufficient to maintain patency 8. Drainage of more than 100 mL in 1 hr should be *reported* to physician
#3: suction control—connected to wall suction	Level of the column of water (i.e., 15–20 cm) is used to control the amount of suction applied to the chest tube—if the water evaporates to only *10 cm* depth, this will be the *maximum* suction generated by the wall suction		1. Air *should continuously bubble* through this compartment when the suction is on; the bubbles are from the atmosphere—not the patient; when the wall suction is turned higher, the bubbling will increase, but the increased pulling of air is from the atmosphere and *not* from the pleural space 2. Because the level of H_2O determines the maximum negative pressure that can be obtained, make sure the water does *not* evaporate—keep filling the bottle to keep the ordered level; if there is *no* bubbling of air through this container, the wall suction is *too low*

Treatments

TABLE 11–7   Review of the Use of Common Tubes—cont'd

Tube or Apparatus	Purpose	Examples of Use	Key Points
Heimlich flutter valve	1. Has a one-way valve so fluids and air can drain out of the pleural space but cannot flow back 2. Eliminates the need for a water seal—no danger when tube is unclamped below the valve	Same as for other chest tubes	1. Can be connected to suction if ordered 2. Sometimes can just drain into portable bag so patient is more mobile
Tracheostomy tube	1. Maintains patent airway and promotes better O_2–CO_2 exchange 2. Makes removal of secretions by suctioning easier 3. Cuff on trach is necessary if need airtight fit for assisted ventilation	1. *Acute respiratory distress* due to poor ventilation 2. *Severe burns of head and neck* 3. *Laryngectomy* (trach is permanent)	1. Use oxygen *before* and *after* each suctioning 2. Humidify oxygen 3. *Sterile* technique in suctioning; clean technique at home 4. Cleanse inner cannula as needed—only leave out 5–10 min 5. Hemostat handy if outer cannula is expelled—have obturator taped to bed and another trach set handy 6. Cuff must be deflated periodically to prevent necrosis of mucosa, unless low-pressure cuff used
Penrose drain	Soft collapsible latex rubber drain inserted to drain serosanguineous fluid from a surgical site; usually brought out to the skin via a stab wound	*Bowel resection*	1. Expect drainage to progress from serosanguineous to more serous 2. *Sterile* technique when changing dressing—do often 3. Physician will advance tube a little each day
Nasogastric (NG) tubes Levin tube and small-bore feeding tubes	1. Inserted into stomach to decompress by removing gastric contents and air—prevents any buildup of gastric secretions, which are continuous 2. Used when stomach must be washed out (lavage) 3. Used for feedings when patient is unable to swallow (gavage)	1. Any abdominal or other *surgery after which peristalsis is absent* for a few days 2. *Overdoses* 3. *Gastrointestinal hemorrhage* 4. *Cancer of the esophagus* 5. *Early postoperative care for patient who had a laryngectomy or radical neck dissection*	1. Connect to *low* intermittent suction 2. Irrigate prn with normal saline or puffs of air 3. Clean, but *not* sterile, procedure 4. Mouth care needed 5. Report *"coffee ground"* material (digested blood) 6. For overdose, stomach is pumped out as *rapidly* as possible 7. For hemorrhage, tepid normal saline may be used to lavage 8. Critical to make sure tube still in stomach *before* beginning feeding; listen for air passing into stomach, and if possible aspirate gastric contents; small-bore tubes require placement check by x-ray 9. Follow feeding with some water to rinse out the tube 10. Clamp tube when ambulating 11. With larger-bore tubes, determine residuals and withhold feeding if large residuals obtained
Salem sump	Double-lumen tube with vent to *protect gastric mucosa* from trauma of suctioning	Same as Levin tube	1. Irrigate vent (blue tubing) with air only 2. See Levin tube
Gastrostomy tube	1. Inserted into stomach via abdominal wall 2. May be used for decompression 3. Used *long term for feedings*	Conditions affecting *esophagus* in which it is impossible to insert a nasogastric tube	1. Principles of tube feedings same as with Levin nasogastric tube, *except* no danger that tube is in trachea 2. If permanent, tube may be replaceable

Treatments

Continued

TABLE 11–7   Review of the Use of Common Tubes—cont'd

Tube or Apparatus	Purpose	Examples of Use	Key Points
Miller-Abbott tube Cantor tube	Longer than Levin tube—has mercury or air in bags so tube can be used to *decompress the lower intestinal tract*	1. *Small-bowel obstructions* 2. *Intussusception* 3. *Volvulus*	1. Care similar to that for Levin NG tube—irrigated 2. Connected to suction, *not* sterile technique 3. Orders will be written on how to advance the tube, gently pushing tube a few inches each hour; patient position may affect advancement of tube 4. X-rays determine the desired location of tube
T-tube	To *drain bile* from the common bile duct *until* edema has subsided	*Cholecystectomy* when a common duct exploration (CDE) or choledochostomy was also done	1. Bile drainage is influenced by *position* of the drainage bag 2. Clamp tube as ordered to see if bile will flow into duodenum normally
Hemovac	A type of closed-wound drainage connected to suction—used to *drain a large amount* of serosanguineous drainage from under an incision	1. *Mastectomy* 2. *Total hip procedures* 3. *Total knee procedures*	1. May compress unit, and have portable vacuum or connect to wall suction 2. Small drainage tubes may get clogged—physician may irrigate these at times
Jackson-Pratt	1. A method of closed-wound suction drainage—indicated when tissue displacement and tissue trauma may occur with rigid drain tubes (e.g., Hemovac) 2. See Hemovac	1. *Neurosurgery* 2. *Neck surgery* 3. *Mastectomy* 4. *Total knee and hip replacement* 5. *Abdominal surgery* 6. *Urological procedures*	1. Empty reservoir when full, to prevent loss of wound drainage and back-contamination 2. See Hemovac.
Three-way Foley	To provide avenues for *constant irrigation and constant drainage* of the urinary bladder	1. Transurethral resection (TUR) 2. *Bladder* infections	1. Watch for blocking by clots—causes bladder spasms 2. Irrigant solution often has *antibiotic* added to normal saline or sterile water 3. *Sterile* water rather than normal saline may be used for lysis of clots
Suprapubic catheter	To *drain bladder* via an opening through the abdominal wall above the pubic bone	*Suprapubic* prostatectomy	May have orders to irrigate prn or continuously
Ureteral catheter	To *drain urine* from the pelvis of one kidney, or for *splinting* ureter	1. *Cystoscopy* for diagnostic workups 2. *Ureteral surgery* 3. *Pyelotomy*	1. *Never* clamp the tube—pelvis of kidney only holds 4–8 mL 2. Use *only* 5 mL sterile normal saline if ordered to irrigate

Note: This review focuses on care of tubes, not on total patient care.
Source: Jane Vincent Corbett, RN, MS, EdD, Professor, School of Nursing, University of San Francisco. Used with permission.

Treatments

TABLE 11–8 ▶ Emptying Colostomy Appliance

Check for drainage in appliance at least twice during each shift. If drainage present (diarrhea-type stool):

Do	Do Not
1. Unclamp the bottom of bag	1. Remove appliance each time it needs emptying
2. Drain into bedpan	2. Use any materials that could irritate bowel
3. Use a squeeze-type bottle filled with warm water to rinse inside of appliance	3. Ignore patient's needs
4. Clean off clamp if soiled	
5. Put a few drops of deodorant in appliance if not odorproof	
6. Fasten bottom of appliance securely (fold bag over clamp 2–3 times before closing)	
7. Check for leakage under appliance every 2–4 hr	
8. Communicate with patient while attending to appliance	

TABLE 11–9 ▶ Changing Colostomy Appliance

Gather equipment: gloves, skin prep packet, colostomy appliance measured to fit stoma properly (if new surgical stoma, it will continue to shrink with the healing process; use stoma measuring guide), skin barrier, warm water and soap, face cloth/towel, plastic bag for disposal of old equipment. Remember that bowel is very fragile; also, working near bowel increases peristalsis, and feces and flatulence may be expelled.

Do	Do Not
1. Remove old appliance carefully, pulling from area with least drainage to area with most drainage	1. Tear appliance quickly from skin
2. Wash skin area with soap and water	2. Wash stoma with soap; put anything dry onto stoma
3. Observe skin area for potential breakdown	3. Irritate skin or stoma
4. Use packet of skin prep on the skin around the stoma; allow skin prep solution to dry on skin before applying colostomy appliance	4. Put skin prep solution onto stoma; it will cause irritation
5. Apply skin barrier you have measured and cut to size	5. Make opening too large (increases risk of leakage)
6. Put appliance on so that the bottom of the appliance is easily accessible for emptying (e.g., if patient is out of bed most of the time, put the bottom facing the feet; if patient is in bed most of the time, have bottom face the side); picture-frame the adhesive portion of the appliance with 1-inch tape	6. Have appliance attached so patient cannot be involved in own care
7. Put a few drops of deodorant in appliance if not odorproof	7. Use any materials that would irritate bowel
8. Use clamp to fasten bottom of appliance	8. Avoid conversation/eye contact
9. Talk to patient (or communicate in best way possible for patient) during and after procedure	9. Contaminate other incisions
10. Use good hand-washing technique	

FIGURE 11–2 Chest drainage system.

To suction

From patient

Drainage collection

Suction control

Water seal

BASIC PROSTHETIC CARE ▶

Tables 11–10 and 11–11.

TABLE 11–10   ▶ Care of Dentures

Wear gloves
If patient cannot remove own dentures, grasp upper plate at the front teeth and move up and down gently to release suction
Lift the lower plate up one side at a time
Use extreme care not to damage dentures while cleaning
Use tepid, *not* hot, water to clean
Avoid soaking for long periods of time
Inspect for sharp edges
Do oral cavity assessment
Replace moistened dentures in patient's mouth
Use appropriately labeled container for storage when dentures are to remain out of patient's mouth

TABLE 11–11   ▶ Caring for an Artificial Eye

With gloved hand pull lower eyelid down over the infraorbital bone and exert pressure below the eyelid
Pressure will make the eye pop out
Handle eye prosthesis carefully
Using *aseptic* technique, cleanse socket with saline-moistened gauze, stroking from inner to outer canthus
Wash the prosthesis in warm normal saline
To reinsert, gently pull the patient's lower lid down, raise the upper lid if necessary, slip the saline-moistened eye prosthesis gently into the socket, and release the lids

GUIDELINES FOR ISOLATION PRECAUTIONS ⊙

Table 11–12.

TABLE 11–12 ⟐ Guidelines for Isolation Precautions

The Hospital Infection Control Advisory Committee and the Centers for Disease Control and Prevention (1996) have concluded that some fluids, secretions, and excretions not covered under Universal Precautions (UP) represent a potential source of nosocomial and community-acquired infections. The term *Universal Precautions* has been replaced in the hospital setting by a two-tiered system of isolation: **Standard Precautions** for control of nosocomial infections; and **Transmission-based Precautions** for patients known or suspected to be infected with highly transmissible pathogens. *Standard Precautions* incorporate the major components of blood and body fluid precautions from Universal Precautions. *Transmission-based Precautions* may be combined for diseases that have multiple routes of transmission and are used in addition to *Standard Precautions*.

Standard Precautions

Use **Standard Precautions**, or the equivalent, for the care of all patients.

1. *Hand washing.*
   a. Wash hands after touching: blood, body fluids, secretions, excretions, and contaminated items, whether or not gloves are worn. Wash hands immediately after gloves are removed, between patient contacts, and when otherwise indicated to avoid transfer of microorganisms to other patients or environments. It may be necessary to wash hands between tasks and procedures on the same patient to prevent cross-contamination of different body sites.
   b. Use a plain (non-antimicrobial) soap for routine hand washing.
   c. Use an antimicrobial agent or a waterless antiseptic agent for specific circumstances (e.g., control of outbreaks or hyperendemic infections), as defined by the infection control program. (See *Contact Precautions* for additional recommendations on using antimicrobial and antiseptic agents.)
2. *Gloves.* Wear gloves (clean, nonsterile gloves are adequate) when touching: blood, body fluids, secretions, excretions, and contaminated items. Put on clean gloves just before touching mucous membranes and nonintact skin. Change gloves between tasks and procedures on the same patient after contact with material that may contain a high concentration of microorganisms. Remove gloves promptly after use, before touching noncontaminated items and environmental surfaces, and before going to another patient; wash hands immediately to avoid transfer of microorganisms to other patients or environments.
3. *Mask, eye protection, face shield.* Wear a mask and eye protection or a face shield to protect mucous membranes of the eyes, nose, and mouth during procedures and patient care activities that are likely to generate splashes or sprays of blood, body fluids, secretions, and excretions.
4. *Gown.* Wear a gown (a clean, nonsterile gown is adequate) to protect skin and to prevent soiling of clothing during procedures and patient care activities that are likely to generate splashes or sprays of blood, body fluids, secretions, or excretions. Select a gown that is appropriate for the activity and amount of fluid likely to be encountered. Remove a soiled gown as promptly as possible, and wash hands to avoid transfer of microorganisms to other patients or environments.
5. *Patient care equipment.* Handle used patient care equipment soiled with blood, body fluids, secretions, and excretions in a manner that prevents skin and mucous membrane exposures, contamination of clothing, and transfer of microorganisms to other patients and environments. Ensure that reusable equipment is not used for the care of another patient until it has been cleaned and reprocessed appropriately. Ensure that single-use items are discarded properly.
6. *Environmental control.* Ensure that the hospital has adequate procedures for the routine care, cleaning, and disinfection of environmental surfaces, beds, bed rails, bedside equipment, and other frequently touched surfaces, and ensure that these procedures are being followed.
7. *Linen.* Handle, transport, and process used linen soiled with blood, body fluids, secretions, and excretions in a manner that prevents skin and mucous membrane exposures and contamination of clothing, and that avoids transfer of microorganisms to other patients and environments.
8. *Occupational health and blood-borne pathogens.*
   a. Take care to prevent injuries when using needles, scalpels, and other sharp instruments or devices; when handling sharp instruments after procedures; when cleaning used instruments; and when disposing of used needles. *Never* recap used needles, or otherwise manipulate them using both hands, or use any other technique that involves directing the point of a needle toward any part of the body; rather, use either a one-handed "scoop" technique or a mechanical device designed for holding the needle sheath. Do *not* remove used needles from disposable syringes by hand, and do *not* bend, break, or otherwise manipulate used needles by hand. Place used disposable syringes and needles, scalpel blades, and other sharp items in appropriate puncture-resistant containers that are located as close as practical to the area in which the items were used, and place reusable syringes and needles in a puncture-resistant container for transport to the reprocessing area.
   b. Use mouthpieces, resuscitation bags, or other ventilation devices as an alternative to mouth-to-mouth resuscitation methods in areas where the need for resuscitation is predictable.
9. *Patient placement.* Place a patient who contaminates the environment or who does not (or cannot be expected to) assist in maintaining appropriate hygiene or environmental control in a private room. If a private room is not available, consult with infection control professionals regarding patient placement or other alternatives.

Transmission-Based Precautions
Airborne Precautions

In addition to **Standard Precautions**, use Airborne Precautions, or the equivalent, for patients known or suspected to be infected with microorganisms transmitted by airborne droplet nuclei (small-particle residue [5 microns or smaller in size] of evaporated droplets containing microorganisms that remain suspended in the air and that can be dispersed widely by air currents within a room or over a long distance).

1. *Patient placement.* Place the patient in a private room that has (1) monitored negative air pressure in relation to the surrounding area, (2) 6 to 12 air changes per hour, and (3) appropriate discharge of air outdoors or monitored high-efficiency filtration of room air before the air is circulated to other areas in the hospital. Keep the room door closed and the patient in the room. When a private room is not available, place the patient in a room with a patient who has active infection with the same microorganism, unless otherwise recommended, but with no other infection. When a private room is not available and cohorting is not desirable, consultation with infection control professionals is advised before patient placement.
2. *Respiratory protection.* Wear respiratory protection when entering the room of a patient with known or suspected infectious pulmonary tuberculosis. Susceptible persons should not enter the room of patients known or suspected to have *measles* (rubeola) or *varicella* (chickenpox) if other immune caregivers are available. If susceptible persons must enter the room of a

Continued

TABLE 11–12   Guidelines for Isolation Precautions—cont'd

patient known or suspected to have measles (rubeola) or varicella, they should wear respiratory protection. Persons immune to measles (rubeola) or varicella need not wear respiratory protection.

3. *Patient transport.* Limit the movement and transport of the patient from the room to essential purposes only. If transport or movement is necessary, minimize patient dispersal of droplet nuclei by placing a surgical mask on the patient, if possible.

4. *Additional precautions for preventing transmission of tuberculosis.* Consult CDC "Guidelines for Preventing the Transmission of Tuberculosis in Health-Care Facilities" (*MMWR* 43:1–132, 1994; *Fed Reg* 59:54242–54303, 1994) for additional prevention strategies.

Droplet Precautions

In addition to **Standard Precautions,** use **Droplet Precautions,** or the equivalent, for a patient known or suspected to be infected with microorganisms transmitted by droplets (large-particle droplets [larger than 5 microns in size] that can be generated by the patient during coughing, sneezing, talking, or the performance of procedures).

1. *Patient placement.* Place the patient in a private room. When a private room is not available, place the patient in a room with a patient who has active infection with the same microorganism but with no other infection (cohorting). When a private room is not available and cohorting is not achievable, maintain spatial separation of at least 3 ft between the infected patient and other patients and visitors. Special air handling and ventilation are not necessary, and the door may remain open.

2. *Mask.* In addition to standard precautions, wear a mask when working within 3 ft of the patient. (Logistically, some hospitals may want to implement the wearing of a mask to enter the room.)

3. *Patient transport.* Limit the movement and transport of the patient from the room to essential purposes only. If transport or movement is necessary, minimize patient dispersal of droplets by masking the patient, if possible.

Contact Precautions

In addition to **Standard Precautions,** use **Contact Precautions,** or the equivalent, for specified patients known or suspected to be infected or colonized with epidemiologically important microorganisms that can be transmitted by direct contact with the patient (hand or skin-to-skin contact that occurs when performing patient care activities that require touching the patient's dry skin) or indirect contact (touching) with

environmental surfaces or patient care items in the patient's environment.

1. *Patient placement.* Place the patient in a private room. When a private room is not available, place the patient in a room with a patient who has active infection with the same microorganism but with no other infection (cohorting). When a private room is not available and cohorting is not achievable, consider the epidemiology of the microorganism and the patient population when determining patient placement. Consultation with infection control professionals is advised before patient placement.

2. *Gloves and hand washing.* In addition to wearing gloves as outlined under **Standard Precautions,** wear gloves (clean, nonsterile gloves are adequate) when entering the room. During the course of providing care for a patient, change gloves after having contact with infective material that may contain high concentrations of microorganisms (fecal material and wound drainage). Remove gloves before leaving the patient's environment and wash hands immediately with an antimicrobial agent or a waterless antiseptic agent. After glove removal and hand washing, ensure that hands do *not* touch potentially contaminated environmental surfaces or items in the patient's room to avoid transfer of microorganisms to other patients or environments.

3. *Gown.* In addition to wearing a gown as outlined under **Standard Precautions,** wear a gown (a clean, nonsterile gown is adequate) when entering the room if you anticipate that your clothing will have substantial contact with the patient, environmental surfaces, or items in the patient's room; or if the patient is incontinent or has diarrhea, an ileostomy, a colostomy, or wound drainage not contained by a dressing. Remove the gown before leaving the patient's environment. After gown removal, ensure that clothing does *not* contact potentially contaminated environmental surfaces to avoid transfer of microorganisms to other patients or environments.

4. *Patient transport.* Limit the movement and transport of the patient from the room to essential purposes only. If the patient is transported out of the room, ensure that precautions are maintained to minimize the risk of transmission of microorganisms to other patients and contamination of environmental surfaces or equipment.

5. *Patient care equipment.* When possible, dedicate the use of noncritical patient care equipment to a single patient (or cohort of patients infected or colonized with the pathogen requiring precautions) to avoid sharing between patients. If use of common equipment or items is unavoidable, adequately clean and disinfect them before use for another patient.

Source: Centers for Disease Control and Prevention and Hospital Infection Control Practices Advisory Committee, 1996; adapted from Garner, JS, Guidelines for isolation precautions in hospitals. *Infect Control Hosp Epidemiol* 17:53–80, 1996.

BLADDER TRAINING

Table 11–13.

TABLE 11–13 Bladder Training

1. Determine patient's desire/capacity to participate in such a program.
2. Encourage patient to void at certain times throughout the day (e.g., q2h then q3h, when getting up in morning, after meals, before bedtime).
3. Do *not* decrease fluid intake (would put patient at risk for infection).
4. Encourage patient to resist voiding when bladder is not full (use a technique such as counting while voiding and trying to increase that number to a desired level).
5. Encourage patient to ask for assistance when needed, to avoid falls when attempting to get to toilet alone while unsteady on feet.
6. Respond to requests for assistance.
7. *Decrease caffeine* and *alcohol* in diet.
8. Monitor for skin breakdown in patients who are incontinent.
9. Have patient practice Kegel exercises to improve tone and function of pelvic floor.
10. Refer to physical therapist who specializes in this area, if necessary.

BOWEL TRAINING

Table 11–14.

TABLE 11–14 Bowel Training

1. Verify that the patient is not impacted.
2. Determine patient's desire/capacity to participate in the program.
3. Determine normal bowel habits.
4. Increase fiber and fluids in the diet.
5. Establish a routine: same time each day.
6. Give stool softener, cathartic, or suppository as ordered.
7. Offer patient a hot drink before set time for defecation.
8. Provide time and privacy.
9. Encourage position that will facilitate defecation (sitting position is best, leaning forward without straining).
10. Document interventions that are successful.

Treatments

Questions

Select the one best answer for each question.

1. A patient's laboratory values indicate hemoconcentration secondary to fluid loss. Which of the following intravenous solutions should the nurse anticipate will be ordered as the most appropriate during initial fluid replacement therapy?
   1. 10% dextrose and saline.
   2. 5% dextrose and water with 60 mEq KCl.
   3. 5% dextrose and water only.
   4. Distilled water.

2. Before surgery, a patient was instructed in the use of an incentive spirometer. The *primary* purpose of this activity is:
   1. To encourage coughing.
   2. To arouse and stimulate the patient.
   3. To encourage deep breathing.
   4. To measure tidal volume and expiratory reserve volume.

3. The nurse explains to a patient's family that humidification is given with oxygen administration because:
   1. Oxygen is highly permeable in water, thereby increasing gaseous diffusion.
   2. Oxygen is very drying to the mucous membranes.
   3. The partial pressures of oxygen are increased by water dilution, allowing more oxygen to reach the alveoli.
   4. Water acts as a carrier substance facilitating movement of oxygen across the respiratory membrane.

4. To correctly administer 1000 mL of 5% dextrose/water in 10 hours using a standard 15-drop administration set, the nurse would adjust the infusion rate to:
   1. 32 drops per minute.
   2. 25 drops per minute.
   3. 20 drops per minute.
   4. 15 drops per minute.

5. The nurse would conclude that a patient's fasting serum-glucose levels are normal if the results are:
   1. 30–60 mg/dL of blood.
   2. 80–126 mg/dL of blood.
   3. 126–140 md/dL of blood.
   4. 140–200 mg/dL of blood.

6. A laboratory test to measure serum- and urine-glucose levels before and after ingestion of a glucose load has been ordered. The nurse knows that the test to be done is called:
   1. Fasting blood sugar.
   2. Glucose tolerance test.
   3. Postprandial blood glucose.
   4. Tolbutamide response test.

7. After a glucose tolerance test, the nurse would look for the blood-glucose levels to return to normal in about how many hours?
   1. One.
   2. Two.
   3. Three.
   4. Four.

8. Following a gastroscopy, the nurse will plan to offer the patient food or fluid:
   1. As soon as he or she returns to the room.
   2. One hour later, or after he or she is fully alert.
   3. Three to 4 hours later, or when the gag reflex returns.
   4. Six to 8 hours later to prevent the electrolyte imbalance that may occur with this procedure.

9. The nurse knows that a 24-hour urine-for-creatinine clearance measures which of the following kidney functions?
   1. Filtration fraction.
   2. Glomerular filtration rate.
   3. Renal blood flow.
   4. Quantity and specific gravity of urinary output.

10. A patient asks why an intravenous pyelogram (IVP) is being done. The nurse tells the patient the purpose is to:
    1. Determine the size, shape, and placement of the kidneys.
    2. Test renal tubular function and the patency of the urinary tract.
    3. Measure renal blood flow.
    4. Outline the kidney vasculature.

11. The nursing care of a patient before an IVP includes:
    1. Telling the patient that the contrast medium may produce a warm, flushed feeling in the face and a salty taste in the mouth.
    2. Administering radiopaque capsules 6 hours before the test.
    3. Ascertaining whether or not the patient has any allergies to mercury.
    4. Pushing fluids until 2 hours before the test, to prevent dehydration.

12. The nurse's preparation of the patient undergoing IV cholangiogram includes:
    1. Administering radiopaque tablets the evening before the examination.
    2. A fatty meal the evening before the examination.
    3. Forcing fluids for 6–8 hours before the examination.
    4. Informing the patient that he or she may experience a feeling of warmth, flushing of face, and/or a salty taste when the contrast medium is injected.

13. The nurse knows that the most important effect of intermittent positive-pressure breathing (IPPB) is:
    1. Mobilization of bronchial secretions.
    2. Increased alveolar ventilation.
    3. Prevention of atelectasis.
    4. Decreased airway resistance.

Answers/Rationale

1. **(3)** Initial fluid therapy is directed toward increasing fluid volume and urine output. **Answer 1**, being a hypertonic solution that would act to increase intracellular dehydration, is therefore *contraindicated*. Once adequate urinary output has been established, potassium salts are added (**Answer 2**) to relieve hypokalemia. The amount of added potassium chloride depends on the extent of hypokalemia. **Answer 4**, distilled water, is a hypotonic solution; that is, it does not contain any additional electrolytes. Hypotonic solutions, such as 0.45% sodium chloride, are frequently given to relieve hypertonic syndromes. However, distilled water is *never* given in fluid replacement therapy.

   Test-taking tip—The key word is *initial*. Use H_2O to replace fluid loss. Focus on two similar options that have 5% D/W (**2, 3**). Eliminate the option with *KCl* (**1**) because it is added *later*.

   AN, 8, PhI, Pharmacological and Parenteral Therapies

2. **(3)** The purpose of the incentive spirometer is to encourage deep breathing. The patient is able to directly visualize progress by the number and height of balls he or she is able to raise. *Aftereffects* of this activity may indeed be coughing up sputum (**Answer 1**) and arousal (**Answer 2**) as the patient

---

Key to codes following rationales *Nursing process:* **AS**, Assessment; **AN**, Analysis; **PL**, Plan; **IMP**, Implementation; **EV**, Evaluation. *Category of human function:* **1**, Protective; **2**, Sensory-perceptual; **3**, Comfort, Rest, Activity, and Mobility; **4**, Nutrition; **5**, Growth and Development; **6**, Fluid-Gas Transport; **7**, Psychosocial-Cultural; **8**, Elimination. **Client need:** **SECE**, Safe, Effective Care Environment; **PhI**, Physiological Integrity; **PsI**, Psychosocial Integrity; **HPM**, Health Promotion/Maintenance. See appendices for full explanation.

competes with himself or herself. Incentive spirometry can be used as a rough measure of tidal volume and expiratory reserve volume (**Answer 4**) because the patient breathes in deeply and exhales completely into the incentive spirometer.

> **Test-taking tip**—Key word is *primary* (or first) purpose. Patients are *first* taught to deep breathe.

PL, 6, PhI, Reduction of Risk Potential

3. (2) Humidification of oxygen is extremely important in reducing its drying effects on the mucous membranes of the bronchial tree. Humidification of oxygen is generally provided by a water nebulizer. **Answers 1, 3,** and **4** are incorrect because oxygen is *not highly permeable* in water; thus, water tends to *inhibit* rather than facilitate oxygen diffusion across the respiratory membrane. Humidification expands the volume of the inhaled gas, but by doing so it *decreases* the partial pressure of the gas in the alveoli. Normal alveolar partial pressures of oxygen are approximately 100 mm Hg, whereas the partial pressures of oxygen in the atmosphere are approximately 135 mm Hg.

> **Test-taking tip**—The question is asking why O_2 is given with humidification. Look for a simple answer. *Humid*ification provides *moisture* because O_2 is *drying*.

PL, 6, PhI, Reduction of Risk Potential

4. (2) Maintenance of infusion rates as ordered is extremely important. In this example, the nurse can use the following equation:

$$\frac{\text{gtts/mL of given set}}{60 \text{ min/hr}} \times \text{total volume/hr} = \text{gtts/min}$$

Thus,

$$\frac{15}{60} \times 100 = \frac{1}{4} \times 100 = 25 \text{ gtts/min}$$

> **Test-taking tip**—Divide 1000 mL by 10 to determine how many mL per hour; then use this formula to calculate drops per minute.

IMP, 6, PhI, Pharmacological and Parenteral Therapies

5. (2) Normal fasting serum-glucose levels are 80–126 mg/dL of blood. Levels below 60 (**Answer 1**) indicate hypoglycemia; levels above 126 mg/dL (**Answers 3, 4**) indicate hyperglycemia.

> **Test-taking tip**—Key term is *normal*. First eliminate the extreme numbers (too low and too high). "Normal" tends to be a low-midpoint value.

IMP, 4, PhI, Reduction of Risk Potential

6. (2) Procedurally, the patient to receive the glucose tolerance test consumes a high-carbohydrate diet for 3 days *before* the test. All drugs that may influence the test are discontinued during this period (oral contraceptives, aspirin, steroids). On the day of the test, fasting blood (**Answer 1**) and urine specimens are collected *before* the test, to provide control glucose levels. *After* ingestion of a glucose load, specimens of blood and urine are collected at hourly intervals for 3 hours. In diabetes mellitus, glucose levels are elevated. The postprandial blood glucose (**Answer 3**) is determined by giving the patient an oral glucose load only. Blood-glucose levels are then evaluated in 2 hours. Usually glucose levels will return to normal during this period of time. The tolbutamide response test (**Answer 4**) may also be used to confirm diabetes. After the patient fasts overnight, a baseline fasting blood sample is drawn. Intravenous tolbutamide is then given, and blood samples are drawn in 20–30 minutes. After this test the patient should be given orange juice and instructed to eat breakfast.

> **Test-taking tip**—Key phrase is *before and after;* FBS (**1**) is done only *before.* Postprandial means *after* a meal. Glucose tolerance (**2**) has *both* a "before" and an "after" component.

AN, 4, PhI, Reduction of Risk Potential

7. (3) Within 3 hours the patient's serum-glucose levels should not only have returned to normal, but some hypoglycemia should be expected. **Answers 1, 2,** and **4** are incorrect.

> **Test-taking tip**—Eliminate the extremes (**1, 4**). Recall that the procedure calls for *3 days* of high carbohydrate; you will make a good guess by selecting *3 hours.*

EV, 4, PhI, Reduction of Risk Potential

8. (3) Following gastroscopy, food and fluids are withheld until the gag reflex returns (generally 2–3 hours) in order to prevent aspiration. The gag reflex is inactivated by either an anesthetic spray or an oral preparation gargled by the patient before insertion of the gastroscopy tube. Inhibition of the gag reflex facilitates insertion. **Answers 1** and **2** are incorrect because the period of time is *too brief.* **Answer 4** is incorrect not only because it is generally unnecessary to wait 6–8 hours for the gag reflex to return, but because this procedure does *not precipitate* an electrolyte imbalance.

> **Test-taking tip**—Note that *time frame* is key here. Eliminate the extremes (**1, 2** are too soon; **4** is too long, as well as an incorrect reason).

PL, 4, PhI, Reduction of Risk Potential

9. (2) Decreased amounts of creatinine in the urine are a reflection of the glomerular filtration rate, indicating the *ability* of the kidney to clear the renal blood of this substance. The filtration fraction is simply the *amount* of glomerular filtrate entering the tubules (**Answer 1**). Renal blood flow is estimated by measuring *renal excretion of para-aminohippuric acid (PAH)* (**Answer 3**). Though the amount and specific gravity of urine may be determined, it is *not the primary* function of this laboratory test (**Answer 4**).

> **Test-taking tip**—Key words in the stem: measure *kidney functions,* meaning measure kidney's *ability* to "do its job," i.e., to clear (filter). Choose **2** over **1** (both options have "filtration") because **1** is the *amount* entering.

AS, 8, PhI, Reduction of Risk Potential

10. (2) Intravenous pyelogram tests both the function and patency of the kidneys. After the intravenous injection of a radiopaque contrast medium, the size, location, and patency of the kidneys can be observed by roentgenogram, as well as the patency of the urethra and bladder as the kidneys function to excrete the contrast medium. **Answer 1** is an example of a *KUB,* or flat plate of the abdomen, which can reveal gross structural changes in the kidneys and urethra. Renal blood flow (**Answer 3**) is determined by the injection of *para-aminohippuric acid (PAH)* and measurement of its excretion in the urine. **Answer 4** is an example of *renal angiogram.*

> **Test-taking tip**—Match other common renal system tests (KUB, PAH, renal angiogram) with the descriptions, to identify one that does not fit. Choose the option that describes a test that gives more than anatomical information (eliminate **1, 4**). **Answer 2** provides more data (tubular function and patency of urinary tract) than **Answer 3** (blood flow).

IMP, 8, SECE, Management of Care

11. (1) Patient teaching includes telling the patient that a warm, flushed sensation and salty taste may occur from the contrast medium. The contrast medium is given by IV injection during the procedure, *not in capsule* form (**Answer 2**). **Answer 3** is incorrect because allergies to *iodine, not to mercury,* are the concern. Fluids are not pushed before this procedure; they are *withheld* for up to 8 hours before testing, to produce a slight dehydration that aids in concentrating the contrast medium in the kidneys and urinary system (**Answer 4**).

> **Test-taking tip**—Eliminate **Answer 2** because the test is done intravenously (intravenous pyelogram), not with capsules. Eliminate **Answer 3** because the potential allergy is to *iodine.* Eliminate **Answer 4** because the opposite is needed for the test.

IMP, 8, PhI, Reduction of Risk Potential

12. **(4)** The patient is informed of possible reaction to injection of the contrast medium, which is administered by an IV injection at the time of the test, *not by tablets* the evening before (**Answer 1**). **Answer 2** is incorrect because if patients are given anything by mouth they are given a *low-fat* meal the evening before IV cholangiogram or oral cholecystogram. The patient is usually quite ill at this time and may not be able to tolerate oral intake. In order to have a clear visualization of the gallbladder, the bowel is cleansed, and food and fluids are *withheld, not* forced (**Answer 3**), for 6–8 hours.

   Test-taking tip—Note the name of the procedure: *IV* cholangiogram, meaning that the contrast medium will be injected. Eliminate the three other options that refer to oral intake.

   PL, 4, PhI, Reduction of Risk Potential

13. **(2)** The most important effect of intermittent positive-pressure breathing (IPPB) is increased alveolar ventilation. It *also* helps mobilize secretions (**Answer 1**), decrease the occurrence of atelectasis (**Answer 3**), and decrease airway resistance (**Answer 4**) through *mechanical* bronchodilation.

   Test-taking tip—When all options are correct, choose the one (alveolar ventilation) that encompasses the three other effects.

   EV, 6, PhI, Physiological Adaptation

Answers/Rationale

UNIT 12

Practice Test

Geraldine Colombraro, Sally L. Lagerquist, Bobbi Morrison,
Robyn Nelson, and Janice Stecchi

INTRODUCTION

The **Practice Test** is a *follow-up assessment* tool designed to assess areas of improvement from your initial self-assessment using the **Pre Test.** Take the **Practice Test** immediately after reading the specific *content* areas related to your indi-

vidual problem areas as identified by the **Pre Test.** Determine that you are now able to meet the goal of 80% correct answers in this integrated exam.

After taking this **Practice Test,** use the units in this book again to fill in any "gaps" this test reveals in your preparation. Then take the **Final Test** to assess your readiness for NCLEX-RN.

QUESTIONS

Select the one best answer for each question.

1. For an adolescent boy, the main life-stage task is:
   1. Developing a sense of trust in others and in his environment.
   2. Finalizing his goals and plans for the future.
   3. Striving to attain independence and identity.
   4. Resolving inner conflicts and turmoil.
2. A child lying on the stretcher during admission suddenly complains of nausea and begins to vomit. The nurse should immediately:
   1. Turn the child's head to the side.
   2. Suction the child's oropharynx.
   3. Raise the head of the stretcher.
   4. Insert an NG tube.
3. A woman is in active labor; her membranes ruptured spontaneously 2 hours ago. While auscultating for the point of maximum intensity (PMI) of fetal heart tones before applying an external fetal monitor, the nurse counts 100 beats per minute. Which action should the nurse take *immediately?*

   1. Examine the woman for signs of a prolapsed cord.
   2. Turn the woman on her left side to increase placental perfusion.
   3. Take the woman's radial pulse while still auscultating the FHR.
   4. Start oxygen by mask to reduce fetal distress.
4. The nurse explains that a flexible sigmoidoscopy involves:
   1. Instillation of a radiopaque contrast medium into the lower gastrointestinal tract.
   2. Insertion of a fiber-optic scope that allows for direct visual examination of the anal canal, rectum, and sigmoid colon.
   3. Insertion of a fiber-optic scope that allows for direct visualization of the sigmoid colon, transverse colon, and ileocecal valve.
   4. Surgical removal of polyps and biopsy of suspicious gastrointestinal mucosa.
5. A viable 7-pound, 12-ounce boy is born. Apgar scores are 7 and 9. In assessing the baby, the nurse notes he appears slightly cyanotic. What should the nurse perform *first?*
   1. Wrap him in another blanket, to reduce heat loss.

2. Stimulate him to cry, to increase oxygenation.

3. Aspirate his mouth and nose with bulb syringe.

4. Elevate his head to promote gravity drainage of secretions.

6. A 32-year-old mother of three adolescents has increased her consumption of alcoholic beverages to 24 oz of 80-proof drinks per day. She gets angry with the children very quickly, cries spontaneously several times every day, and complains of headaches constantly. In planning her care, what would be considered the *least* appropriate nursing intervention?

1. Stimulating her to work at a concrete task.

2. Encouraging her to cry.

3. Providing her with someone to talk to.

4. Isolating her from stimuli.

7. The nurse explains to a patient that bronchitis is characterized by:

1. Hypertrophy of the bronchial mucous glands and the production of mucoid sputum sometimes difficult to expectorate.

2. Bronchoconstriction and edema of the wall of the bronchioles.

3. Exudate in the alveoli.

4. Increasing lung stiffness.

8. Which assessment finding indicates a need for further assessment of a pregnant woman's general health status at 18 weeks of gestation?

1. Rheumatic fever at age 12.

2. Rubella titer negative.

3. Family history of multifetal births.

4. Treatment for chlamydial infection before pregnancy validation.

9. If a child's nasogastric tube is functioning properly after an emergency appendectomy, the nurse should expect to make which observation?

1. There is no drainage on the surgical dressing.

2. The child's abdomen is soft.

3. The child is able to swallow saliva.

4. There are bowel sounds in all four quadrants.

10. At 38 weeks of gestation, a woman's cervix is dilated 4 cm and effaced 60%. She does not speak English and has no prenatal record. Which nursing diagnosis is least likely to prove a problem during this woman's labor and birth?

1. *Pain* related to uterine contractions and fear.

2. *Impaired verbal communication* related to language barrier.

3. *Anxiety/fear* related to poor communication and labor.

4. *Altered nutrition, less than body requirements*.

11. The nurse plans care for an adolescent based on the knowledge that this patient least needs:

1. External control on his or her behavior by adults.

2. Limit setting based on fear and reprimands.

3. Adult role models for identification.

4. Stable relationships and interactions.

12. A patient has been admitted to the hospital with acute rheumatoid arthritis. The hands are painful and edematous, and there is severe pain in the left hip. The temperature is 101°F orally; pulse, 96; respirations, 22. ASA grx̄ qid has been ordered. The nurse can expect this patient's temperature and pulse to be elevated because of:

1. Increased fluid losses.

2. Inflammation of the hand and hip joints.

3. Stress response.

4. Side effect of salicylate therapy.

13. Which factor should the nurse identify as the most probable cause of a child's lice?

1. The child washes the hair only once a week.

2. The child shares the comb and brush with a friend.

3. The child wears a hat to school every day.

4. The child's hair is long, thick, and curly.

14. A 45-year-old man is assessed as having an obsessive-compulsive disorder. Which behavior would the nurse *least* expect him to exhibit?

1. Working 50- to 60-hour weeks.

2. Smoking two packs of cigarettes a day.

3. Showing flexibility in decision making.

4. Exhibiting a low level of concentration.

15. The nurse knows that a colostomy begins functioning:

1. Immediately.

2. 2–3 days postoperatively.

3. 1 wk postoperatively.

4. 2 wk postoperatively.

16. A woman is seen in clinic complaining of amenorrhea, fatigue, urinary frequency, and morning nausea. She states that her LMP was 7 weeks ago and that her menses have been normal except for one episode following a spontaneous abortion at 8 weeks of gestation. She states she has a 5-year-old boy and 3-year-old twin girls at home. Which would accurately describe this woman if she is pregnant now?

1. Gravida 4 para 2.

2. Gravida 5 para 3.

3. Gravida 4 para 3.

4. Gravida 3 para 2.

17. The *least* appropriate nursing intervention for a client experiencing alcohol withdrawal delirium would be:

1. Reinforcing time, place, and person.

2. Providing consistent and concrete answers to questions.

3. Administering ordered vitamins and glucose.

4. Applying and maintaining physical restraints.

18. The nurse is discussing nutrition in pregnancy with a group of women in the prenatal clinic. Which comment indicates a lack of understanding that requires the nurse's intervention?

1. "I'll be drinking six to eight glasses (1500–2000 mL) of water, milk, and juices every day."

2. "Since I am overweight, I am maintaining a weight gain of two-thirds of a pound a week during the last 6 months of pregnancy."

3. "Since our nutrient needs can't be met through dietary sources, I am taking plenty of vitamin and mineral supplements."

4. "Since I am a vegetarian, I am working with a registered dietitian to plan meals with complementary protein combinations."

19. Following above-the-knee amputation, a patient verbalizes feelings of decreased self-worth and of being less of a person. Acceptance of the surgery is largely dependent on:
1. What the doctor says.
2. How the patient's family is reacting.
3. How the nursing staff reacts and responds to the patient's behavior.
4. The patient's ability to grieve.

20. After being in a community mental health day treatment center for 3 weeks, an adolescent client has become apathetic and withdrawn. The client generally sits alone and stares into space. The most appropriate nursing intervention would include:
1. Selecting a group activity for the client to participate in.
2. Stimulating self-growth by providing challenging activities for the client.
3. Allowing the client to spend at least 3 hours a day in the room, for inner reflection.
4. Encouraging staff members to sit with the client during group activities until there is voluntary socialization.

21. The nurse recognizes that the pattern of pulmonary dysfunction reflected by increased total lung capacity (TLC), functional residual capacity (FRC), and residual volume (RV) is characteristic of:
1. Restrictive lung disease.
2. Obstructive lung disease.
3. Vascular lung disease.
4. A combination of restrictive and obstructive lung disease.

22. A 15-year-old girl is seen in clinic with complaints of severe vulvovaginal itching, burning on urination, and thin, watery vaginal discharge for the past 4 days. During the history and physical examination, she appears very embarrassed and upset. Looking at the floor, she admits to being sexually active. She says, "Do you think I'm pregnant, or have something awful? How can I tell my mother?" Which nursing diagnosis is *least likely* to apply in this situation?
1. *Anxiety/fear* related to the perceived possibility of diagnosis of pregnancy or sexually transmitted disease.
2. *Ineffective individual coping* related to situational crisis.
3. *Self-esteem disturbance* related to inability to reconcile expectations of peers and family; situational crisis.
4. *Powerlessness* related to lifestyle of helplessness.

23. A patient, age 25, has been scheduled for surgery to remove the lesions at the footplate of the stapes, associated with *otosclerosis*. A patient who is scheduled for a *stapedectomy* should be told to expect:
1. Tinnitus for several weeks after surgery.

2. Rhinitis as the edema from surgery resolves.
3. The hearing loss to continue for a while.
4. Showering and swimming not to be permitted.

24. A 16-year-old hospitalized in a psychiatric unit for 10 days disappears from the hospital after an argument with a staff member. The client is found walking about a mile from the hospital grounds. In planning care for this client after this incident, the nurse would consider which factor most significant? The client's need to:
1. Be reprimanded for deviant behavior.
2. Be medicated to calm down.
3. Be listened to in order to identify feelings.
4. Understand the consequences of his or her actions.

25. The physician orders prednisone, 10 mg every morning, for a patient with rheumatoid arthritis. Which precaution should the nurse advise the patient of during predischarge teaching?
1. Take oral preparations of prednisone before meals.
2. Never stop or change the amount of the medication without medical advice.
3. Have periodic complete blood counts while on the medication.
4. Wear sunglasses if exposed to bright light for an extended period of time.

26. External fetal monitor tracings show consistent fetal decelerations of uniform shape, which begin with the contraction and return to baseline as the contraction subsides. What is the correct interpretation of these data?
1. Acute fetal distress.
2. Uteroplacental insufficiency.
3. Umbilical cord compression.
4. Physiological fetal bradycardia.

27. A woman with active tuberculosis (TB) wants to become pregnant. The nurse knows that further teaching is necessary when the woman states:
1. "Pulmonary TB may jeopardize my pregnancy."
2. "Spontaneous abortion may occur in one out of five women who are infected."
3. "I can get pregnant after I have been free of TB for 6 months."
4. "I know that I may not be able to have close contact with my baby until contagion is no longer a problem."

28. The nurse can increase the ventilatory efficiency of a patient with COPD by positioning the patient as follows:
1. High Fowler's.
2. Prone.
3. Sitting up and leaning slightly forward.
4. Trendelenburg.

29. During the adolescent period, the *least* important task to complete is:
1. Developing an individualized personality.
2. Attaining adequate defense mechanisms.
3. Establishing an ego identity.
4. Refining and stabilizing the superego.

30. The nurse would position a patient with *ruptured appendix* in:
    1. Semi-Fowler's.
    2. Trendelenburg.
    3. Left Sims'.
    4. Dorsal recumbent.

31. A woman wants to breastfeed her baby. Which hormone, normally secreted during the postpartum period, influences both the milk ejection reflex and uterine involution?
    1. Estrogen.
    2. Progesterone.
    3. Relaxin.
    4. Oxytocin.

32. A 7-year-old is admitted to the burn unit in serious condition with deep partial-thickness burns over the head, face, neck, and anterior chest. On the first night in the hospital, the nurse enters the room and finds the child crying softly and moaning in pain. Recognizing the extent of the injuries, the nurse should:
    1. Do nothing at this time.
    2. Offer two acetaminophen (Tylenol) pills as ordered and a glass of warm milk.
    3. Give an IM injection of 40 mg of meperidine HCl (Demerol) as ordered.
    4. Inject 25 mg of meperidine HCl (Demerol) as ordered via central IV line.

33. Suddenly, during a labor contraction, a woman's water breaks. Which assessment finding indicates a deviation from normal labor patterns?
    1. Dark-colored amniotic fluid.
    2. The woman complains of nausea and vomits.
    3. Fetal bradycardia with contractions.
    4. The woman becomes diaphoretic and irritable.

34. The most important nursing intervention in planning care for a client with increasing symptoms of depression and alcoholism would include:
    1. Referring to an alcohol rehabilitation program.
    2. Identifying how the client has coped with anxiety in the past.
    3. Arranging for inpatient hospitalization.
    4. Requesting a prescription for an antidepressant.

35. What should the nurse recognize as an *inappropriate* method of treating *hyperthyroidism*?
    1. Subtotal thyroidectomy.
    2. Administration of propylthiouracil.
    3. Radioiodine therapy.
    4. Administration of thyroglobulin.

36. A pregnant woman returns for a routine visit at 12 weeks of gestation. Which nursing assessment could the nurse use to verify the EDB and estimate uterine/fetal growth?
    1. Leopold's maneuvers.
    2. Weight-gain pattern.
    3. Vital signs and fetal heart tones.
    4. Height of the fundus.

37. A teenager has a history of setting fires. These arson attempts may exhibit which behavior?
    1. Acting out.
    2. Depression.
    3. Paranoia.
    4. Mania.

38. Which statement by the nurse correctly describes a wheeze?
    1. A high-pitched musical sound produced by airflow in narrowed bronchioles.
    2. Rarely considered pathological.
    3. A medium-pitched sonorous sound produced by airflow in obstructed bronchi.
    4. A high-pitched crowing sound produced by edema in the trachea.

39. A 32-year-old client is diagnosed as having a mood disorder. What drug is usually administered in treating such disorders?
    1. Lithium (lithium carbonate).
    2. Librium (chlordiazepoxide HCl).
    3. Prolixin (fluphenazine hydrochloride).
    4. Mellaril (thioridazine).

40. The primary purpose of the nurse performing passive range-of-motion exercises to an acute rheumatoid arthritis patient's affected limbs is to:
    1. Prevent contractures and limited range of motion.
    2. Continually evaluate the patient's functional abilities.
    3. Assess the patient's pain tolerance.
    4. Evaluate the effectiveness of drug therapy.

41. A pregnant woman's last menstrual period began on April 3. Which is an accurate estimate of her EDB?
    1. January 3.
    2. January 10.
    3. January 27.
    4. December 10.

42. After 24 hours of hospitalization for a suicide attempt, the client begins to verbalize more and has interacted with other clients on the inpatient psychiatric unit. The nurse should realize that this increase in energy level may indicate that the client:
    1. Needs less individual attention.
    2. Needs more individual attention.
    3. Needs a decrease in antidepressant medications.
    4. Is presently motivated to get well.

43. The appropriate nursing action with a patient experiencing expressive aphasia following a CVA would be:
    1. Help the patient and family accept this permanent disability.
    2. Associate words with physical objects.
    3. Wait indefinitely for the patient to verbalize.
    4. Tell the family that the patient cannot communicate.

44. Which action by the nurse would be most helpful in preparing a 5-year-old for cardiac catheterization?
    1. Describe the procedure in very simple terms.

2. Take the child to the lab to observe such a procedure.

3. Answer only those questions the child asks.

4. Use puppets to dramatize the procedure for the child.

45. The number of first-time pregnancies in women between ages 35 and 40 years has increased by 40%. The nurse conducting a parent education class for these women, in the last trimester of pregnancy, should include discussion of:

1. Energy and stamina to meet demands of parenting.

2. Feeling troubled by pregnancy and being less adjusted during the last trimester of pregnancy.

3. The longer labor experienced by older mothers.

4. The greater number of labor/birth complications experienced by older mothers.

46. The nurse explains to a patient that the colostomy appliance for a double barrel colostomy should be changed:

1. Every day.

2. When drainage leaks through the seal.

3. Once a week.

4. At a time selected by the visiting nurse.

47. A woman in labor expresses concern about her baby's status. If the nurse identifies the presence of early decelerations, which intervention should be instituted?

1. Elevate the woman's hips, and start oxygen by mask.

2. Lower the head of the bed, and place the woman in supine position.

3. Mark the tracing in red, and check for dislodged electrode.

4. Reassure the woman that this represents a normal tracing.

48. A patient is scheduled for a temporary colostomy due to severe diverticulitis. Preoperative preparation of this patient includes administration of neomycin SO_4. The nurse expects that this antibiotic will:

1. Combat postoperative wound infection.

2. Decrease bacterial count of the colon.

3. Reduce the size of the suspected tumor before surgery.

4. Stimulate peristalsis and facilitate action of cleansing enemas.

49. A 35-year-old person takes an overdose of sleeping pills and alcohol, and is brought to the emergency department in an ambulance called by a neighbor, who discovered the person unconscious on the living room sofa. On admission, the client is unconscious. Vital signs are TPR 98–60–10 and BP 90/50. Reflexes are dull. The emergency department nurse's initial response should include:

1. Administering a central nervous system stimulant.

2. Paging the resident on call.

3. Maintaining a patent airway.

4. Assessing the patient's neurological signs.

50. After nebulizer treatment with isoproterenol (Isuprel), the following pulmonary function data were obtained:

	TLC	FRC	RV	VC	FEV_1
Before treatment	7000	5000	4200	2800	2000
After treatment	7000	4000	3000	3800	2500

The nurse would conclude that the change in lung volumes indicates:

1. Improvement.

2. Deterioration.

3. No change.

4. Data inadequate to decide.

51. A vaginal examination disclosed several painful red papules on the inner surfaces of the labia minora and in the vagina. Lesions were extremely painful on gentle touch with an applicator. Discharge had a very foul odor. Inflammatory regional lymph nodes were easily palpated. With which infectious organism are these assessment findings associated?

1. *Trichomonas vaginalis.*

2. *Candida albicans.*

3. Herpesvirus type 2.

4. *Neisseria gonorrhoeae.*

52. A 15-year-old in a day treatment center begins to mutilate the forearms with lighted cigarettes and scratch the wrists with thumbtacks and staples found on the unit. What is the *least* appropriate nursing goal?

1. Supervising closely.

2. Avoiding confrontations regarding this behavior.

3. Removing all items that could be used for destructive purposes.

4. Assisting the teenager to increase self-esteem.

53. A woman asks the nurse what makes a pregnancy test "turn positive." The nurse's best response is based on the knowledge that the biological marker for pregnancy tests is:

1. Human placental lactogen.

2. Human chorionic gonadotropin.

3. Luteinizing hormone.

4. Alpha-fetoprotein.

54. A woman who does not speak English is in active labor, with moderate to strong contractions every 2–3 minutes, lasting 45 seconds. She appears very frightened. By which modality can the nurse convey caring and allay anxiety?

1. Asking her husband to translate all interactions.

2. Touching, smiling, and speaking in a calm, assured voice.

3. Speaking slowly, loudly, and clearly, to facilitate her understanding.

4. Offering to notify the doctor on call.

55. After an adolescent has been in a mental health day treatment center for a year and a half, the professional staff are considering discharging this client. The client asks the nurse whether other people must be told about the time spent in a mental health center. The

most appropriate response the nurse could make would be:
1. "Yes, especially to all future school officials."
2. "Yes, especially to all prospective employers."
3. "No, this is an individual decision."
4. "No, there is no specific requirement."

56. A peripheral iridectomy is the surgical procedure of choice following an acute episode of closed-angle glaucoma. Which nursing measure is *inappropriate* for a patient who has had an *iridectomy*?
    1. Instill eyedrops to mobilize the affected pupil by alternate dilation and constriction.
    2. Ambulate the patient as soon as possible after the surgery.
    3. Reinforce the surgical dressing as needed to prevent infection.
    4. If ordered, instruct the patient to massage the affected eye.

57. A woman who is pregnant complains of constipation. What should the nurse recommend to relieve her symptoms of constipation?
    1. Regular bedtime use of mild laxatives such as mineral oil.
    2. Limit fluid intake to 1000 mL daily.
    3. Increase dietary intake of fresh fruit and salads.
    4. Begin Kegel exercises to increase tone.

58. In monitoring the postop course of an adolescent who has had surgery for a ruptured appendix, the nurse would be most correct in expecting that this patient will:
    1. Have severe pain for 24 hours.
    2. Be discharged within 48 hours.
    3. Make a slow, steady recovery.
    4. Make a fairly rapid and complete recovery.

59. An adolescent may exhibit depression differently from an adult. An adolescent who is depressed is most likely to exhibit which behavior?
    1. Withdrawal.
    2. Apathy.
    3. Violence.
    4. Regression.

60. The nurse needs to know that the woman likely to be at highest risk for pelvic inflammatory disease (PID) is one who:
    1. Uses an intrauterine device (IUD) for contraception.
    2. Acquired gonorrhea from a fomite.
    3. Has had multiple sex partners.
    4. Drinks one alcoholic beverage per day (e.g., glass of wine).

61. Nursing actions that will facilitate a COPD patient's medical therapy include:
    1. Limiting fluid intake to prevent volume overload and right-sided heart failure.
    2. Oral and endotracheal suctioning as necessary.
    3. Instructing the patient in deep breathing and coughing techniques and pursed-lip exhalations.

4. Maintenance of bed rest and activity restrictions to reduce acidosis.

62. When a newborn is nearly 24 hours old, a nursing assessment notes that the infant's skin is dry and flaking and that there are several areas of an apparent macular rash. The nurse charts this as:
    1. Erythema toxicum.
    2. Milia.
    3. Icterus neonatorum.
    4. Multiple hemangiomas.

63. What is a reliable index of the exercise tolerance of a patient who has rheumatoid arthritis?
    1. Pulse and respiratory rate.
    2. Occurrence and duration of pain in the affected joint.
    3. Mobility of joints.
    4. Decreased redness and swelling of joints.

64. In planning nursing care for a hospitalized client who is suicidal, what is the *least* appropriate nursing action?
    1. Searching personal effects for toxic agents.
    2. Removing straps from clothing.
    3. Placing the client in small groups for observation.
    4. Removing sharp objects from the environment.

65. In positioning a child with burns of the head, face, neck, and anterior chest during recovery, the nurse should:
    1. Avoid head flexion.
    2. Keep the child as still as possible.
    3. Avoid sitting the child up in a chair.
    4. Place two firm pillows under the child's head.

66. A woman in labor, with an interest in using Lamaze for labor and birth, appears tired, tense, and uncomfortable. She complains that her back aches, the monitor "bothers" her, and she wants people to leave her alone and let her rest. Which nursing intervention, implemented by the nurse, demonstrates *proper* nursing judgment?
    1. Offer to get an order for some pain medication.
    2. Reposition the woman and apply sacral pressure.
    3. Turn monitor off audible reading.
    4. Darken room and leave her alone for 5 minutes.

67. A patient's arterial blood gases reveal: pH 7.38, PO_2 65, PCO_2 55, HCO_3 32. The nurse's interpretation of this patient's blood gases is that he or she has:
    1. Uncompensated respiratory acidosis.
    2. Compensated respiratory acidosis.
    3. Uncompensated metabolic alkalosis.
    4. Compensated metabolic alkalosis.

68. An adolescent's parents have decided that they would rather have their child placed outside of the home when discharged from the mental health day treatment center. The most appropriate intervention the nurse could make would include:
    1. Asking the parents to reassess their feelings about this decision.
    2. Suggesting that the parents discuss this decision with the entire family.

3. Referring the parents to a social worker to assist in finding an alternative placement.

4. Assisting the parents in finding an appropriate discharge placement.

69. Which laboratory test result or parameter(s) would be increased on assessment of a patient with acute rheumatoid arthritis?

1. Hemoglobin and hematocrit.
2. Sedimentation rate and C-reactive protein.
3. Wasserman test result.
4. Platelet count.

70. Anticipatory guidance may be indicated to help expectant parents achieve the normal developmental tasks of the beginning family. What is *least likely* to cause anxiety and stress at 18 weeks of gestation?

1. Economic demands of having a child.
2. Change in intrafamily relationships.
3. Increasing awareness of the need to be responsible for another individual (the baby).
4. Feelings of having to "compete" for attention.

71. The teaching plan for a patient with COPD should emphasize:

1. Smoking and alcohol restrictions.
2. Nutrition, fluid balance, and ways to stop smoking.
3. Vocational rehabilitation programs available in the community.
4. Activity restrictions and pulmonary physiology.

72. To establish a relationship with a 14-year-old boy who is hospitalized in a private, coed, inpatient mental hospital unit, what would be inappropriate for the nurse to consider?

1. Boys in early adolescence feel threatened by women authority figures.
2. Enforced inactivity will deprive the adolescent of a major avenue for relieving frustration.
3. Impulse control is a major problem for men.
4. Fear and ambivalence will usually dissipate with the passage of time.

73. When a woman uses Norplant implants for contraception, it is essential for the nurse to discuss the fact that she:

1. Is likely to have breakthrough bleeding.
2. Is not protected against most sexually transmitted diseases.
3. Will be more at risk for endometrial cancer.
4. Is likely to experience some weight loss.

74. A woman who is pregnant states, "I don't feel like myself lately." Further assessment identifies feelings of discomfort due to mood swings, tingling, tender breasts, and fluctuating sexual desire. Which nursing diagnosis is *most* appropriate?

1. *Body image disturbance* related to second trimester physiological and psychological adaptations.
2. *Altered nutrition, less than body requirements,* related to increased need for vitamin B_6 during pregnancy.

3. *Ineffective individual coping* related to perceived need to alter lifestyle, role change.
4. *Personal identity disturbance* related to introspection and self-focusing.

75. An adolescent client in a mental health day treatment center for depression exhibits frequent outbursts of maladaptive behavior. This client started hitting other clients and even struck a nurse. In assessing this client's behavior, the nurse should consider which fact to be most relevant?

1. Hitting others makes the client feel satisfied because the client is then in control of the situation.
2. Hitting others provides an escape from feelings of hopelessness.
3. Hitting others is a mechanism for alleviating anxiety.
4. Hitting others allows this client to instill fear in others.

76. Chronic obstructive pulmonary disease can progress to respiratory failure. A patient with emphysema becomes increasingly drowsy, tachypneic, and tachycardic. The nurse should first:

1. Prepare IV aminophylline.
2. Position the patient in high Fowler's.
3. Give 2 liters of O_2 per nasal cannula.
4. Administer 60% O_2 via mask.

77. A woman who is pregnant complains her nausea is very "bothersome" in the morning, when she must prepare breakfast for her family. Which action should the nurse recommend?

1. Avoid eating before retiring.
2. Drink a glass of fruit juice immediately on rising.
3. Eat one or two soda crackers before rising.
4. Make and eat her breakfast first.

78. A child is to have daily debridement and whirlpool therapy for burns. In cleansing the burns, the nurse would be most correct in selecting sterile:

1. 4×4 gauze pads.
2. Cotton balls.
3. Washcloths.
4. Telfa pads.

79. A patient with a history of alcohol abuse is hospitalized after an overdose of sleeping pills. The nurse should be aware that in the first 72 hours following admission to the hospital the patient is most likely to exhibit:

1. Withdrawal delirium.
2. Suspiciousness.
3. Mood swings.
4. The use of coping mechanisms such as reaction formation.

80. A patient has a smoking history of 25 years and a recent episode of 5 days of increased breathlessness. On physical examination, the patient is found to have a barrel chest, medium-pitched crackles, and wheezes in the right upper lobe and both lower lung lobes. The nurse observes that this patient demonstrates the "in-

creased work of breathing" during this acute period by:

1. Increasing the rate and depth of respirations.
2. Increasing diaphragmatic excursion.
3. Using pursed-lip exhalations.
4. Using accessory muscles for ventilation.

81. A woman who is pregnant complains of severe "charley horses" during the night. Which action should the nurse recommend to provide symptomatic relief?
    1. Drink a glass of milk at bedtime.
    2. Extend affected leg and dorsiflex the foot.
    3. Increase dietary intake of vitamin C.
    4. Mild exercise every evening, such as walking.

82. Two days before above-the-knee amputation, an adult patient expresses a desire to learn more about the surgery and outcome. Preoperative teaching is directed toward:
    1. Discussing the possibility of another vocation.
    2. Learning crutch walking.
    3. Instruction in postoperative exercises.
    4. Encouraging the patient to verbalize fears and concerns.

83. A 14-year-old boy with a history of setting fires has developed a homosexual relationship with a 16-year-old boy. In planning care, the nurse should *primarily*:
    1. Avoid confronting him about attention-getting behavior.
    2. Validate his rationale for establishing the relationship.
    3. Explore his thoughts, feelings, and attitudes.
    4. Enforce limits on interactions between the two patients.

84. A male adolescent (age 15) complains of having nothing to do while he is recovering from an appendectomy. The nurse should:
    1. Ask him to place routine lab slips in the charts.
    2. Refer him to the tutor and arrange for him to get his school books and homework.
    3. Bring in several board games, and encourage him and his 14-year-old roommate to start playing with one of them.
    4. Introduce him to the two 15-year-old girls in the room next door.

85. Health teaching for a woman infected with herpes simplex 2 should include:
    1. "Abstain from intercourse until lesions heal."
    2. "Penicillin is the drug of choice for treatment."
    3. "Therapy is curative."
    4. "The organism is associated with later development of hydatidiform mole."

86. Which statement by the nurse correctly describes a double-barrel colostomy?
    1. It is the least common type of colostomy, and it discharges liquid or unformed stool.
    2. A single loop of the transverse colon is exteriorized and supported by a glass rod. There are two openings, a proximal loop and a distal loop.
    3. It has two stomas. A proximal loop discharges feces, and a distal loop discharges mucus.
    4. It is most often permanent and is done to treat disorders of the sigmoid colon.

87. When administering lithium to a client with a mood disorder, what is the *least* relevant consideration?
    1. If the client's urinary output decreases significantly, diuretics should be ordered.
    2. The client must be given a complete physical examination before administering the drug.
    3. If the client experiences nausea, vomiting, and muscle weakness, the dosage may require regulating.
    4. If the client exhibits symptoms of mania during the first 10 days of receiving the drug, haloperidol (Haldol) may also be administered.

88. A woman in labor suddenly screams and shouts in Spanish. Her husband translates that she has a "terrible pain in her calf," a charley horse. What should the nurse do *immediately*?
    1. Inform the doctor that the woman has signs of abruptio placentae.
    2. Administer oxygen by mask to expedite conversion of muscle lactic acid.
    3. Straighten the woman's knee and dorsiflex her foot.
    4. Turn the woman on her left side to increase placental perfusion.

89. A 7-year-old child is fitted for a pressure stockinette to cover her head, face, and neck to minimize scarring as her burns are healing. To help the child cope with her injuries, treatment, and recuperation, the nurse should ask her parents to bring:
    1. Her favorite toys and stuffed animals.
    2. Some of her friends for a short visit.
    3. Her favorite foods, including pizza and ice cream.
    4. Colorful scarves and hats.

90. A 14-year-old boy is likely to experience several biological and psychosocial changes at this time. Which behavior would the nurse expect to see?
    1. An increase in imaginative thinking.
    2. An increased ability to learn by rote.
    3. An increase in academic achievement.
    4. An increased ability to cope with frustration.

91. The nursing goal for a non–English-speaking woman who has just given birth is demonstration of confidence and competence in caring for her newborn. Which modality will be most effective in facilitating and evaluating her achievement of this goal?
    1. Giving her a booklet in her language, describing basic techniques of baby care.
    2. Discussing the pattern and procedure of basic newborn care with her.
    3. Demonstrating basic baby care procedures and having her perform them with her husband.
    4. Referring her to the public health department nurses in her community.

92. The nurse identifies methods to reduce flatus and odor for a patient with a double-barrel colostomy. What would be the *least* effective method to achieve this?

1. Avoid eating broccoli and cabbage.
2. Use *Banish* deodorant drops in bottom of appliance.
3. Put pinhole in appliance to let flatus escape.
4. Empty feces and gas from appliance as necessary.

93. A woman in labor says, "I can't stand it any longer. I have to push." On vaginal examination, her cervix has dilated to 8 cm and the head is at station 0. For which reason should the nurse encourage this woman to pant, or breathe naturally, with her contractions?

1. Pushing now could cause the cord to prolapse.
2. She should increase her oxygen level before completion of the first stage.
3. Pushing before complete dilation may cause cervical edema and may prolong labor.
4. Panting will speed cervical dilation.

94. Pulmonary function data were collected on a patient. The results were:

	TLC	FRC	RV	VC	FEV$_1$
Predicted	6000	3000	2000	4000	3000
Observed	7000	5000	4200	2800	2000

The nurse's analysis of these data reveals:

1. Hyperinflation.
2. Hyperventilation.
3. Hyperpnea.
4. Hypercapnia.

95. The nurse should teach the parents of a child with lice that to prevent other members of the family from getting lice:

1. The child should sleep alone and in her or his own bed.
2. All family members should get a very short haircut.
3. The child should wear a hair net for a few days.
4. All family members should comb their hair with a fine-toothed comb after regular shampooing.

96. An 18-year-old with acting-out behaviors has been living in a group home for the past 2 months. The patient has asked permission to visit a friend in the psychiatric hospital. The nurse should:

1. Allow the patient to visit.
2. Assess the patient's motives.
3. Ask parents' permission.
4. Consult with the hospital staff.

97. Which nursing intervention should be implemented to reduce a pregnant woman's stress in the first trimester regarding her feelings about mood swings, tingling, tender breasts, and fluctuating sexual desire?

1. Validate normalcy of emotional lability.
2. Recommend high-protein, high-vitamin diet.
3. Refer her to a psychologist for counseling.
4. Reinforce positive feelings about the pregnancy.

98. A complication of chronic obstructive pulmonary disease is the possible rupture of an emphysematous bleb. The nurse suspects that the patient has a right tension pneumothorax. What signs would the nurse expect to see?

1. Flushed appearance from elevated blood pressure.
2. Tracheal deviation to the unaffected side.
3. Hyporesonance on the affected side.
4. Medial shift of the heart.

99. A 15-year-old's behavior is becoming increasingly combative. The teenager hits other clients and the nursing staff at least once or twice each day. What is an inappropriate nursing goal? Help the teenager:

1. Develop impulse control.
2. Manage feelings appropriately.
3. Learn socially acceptable behavior.
4. Internalize feelings.

100. To reduce symptoms of early morning stiffness in a patient who has rheumatoid arthritis, the nurse can encourage the patient to:

1. Take a hot tub bath or shower in the morning.
2. Put joints through passive ROM before trying to move them actively.
3. Sleep with a hot pad.
4. Take two aspirins before arising, and wait 15 minutes before attempting locomotion.

ANSWERS/RATIONALE

1. **(3)** The adolescent is striving to attain a sense of independence and identity. Trust (**Answer 1**) is usually developed during infancy and matures as the individual develops. Goals and plans (**Answer 2**) are made during the adolescent period, but they are rarely finalized realistically until late adulthood. During this period, inner conflicts (**Answer 4**) are rarely resolved and are usually heightened.

    Test-taking tip—Know age-appropriate psychosocial tasks.

    EV, 5, HPM, Growth and Development

2. **(1)** To prevent aspiration, the first and immediate action the nurse should take is to turn the child's head to the side. All of the other actions (**Answers 2, 3, 4**) may also prevent aspiration but will take considerably longer and are not effective immediately.

    Test-taking tip—Patent airway is the primary concern in this question; note the use of the word *immediately*, meaning an instant action.

    IMP, 1, PhI, Reduction of Risk Potential

3. **(3)** Taking the mother's pulse while listening to the FHR will differentiate between the maternal and fetal heart rates and rule out fetal bradycardia. **Answer 1** is wrong because although the cord may prolapse at any time before the oncoming head occludes the cervix, the most common time of occurrence is *when* the membranes *rupture*. **Answer 2** is wrong because fetal bradycardia has *not yet been determined*; the nurse needs to differentiate maternal from fetal heart rate. **Answer 4** is wrong because if the fetal heart rate is normal, there is no need for supplemental oxygen therapy.

    Test-taking tip—Think priority, which is to assess and determine if there is a problem with *fetal* pulse rate. Differentiate between maternal and fetal pulse rates. Recall normal fetal rate vs. bradycardia.

    IMP, 6, PhI, Reduction of Risk Potential

4. **(2)** Sigmoidoscopy involves the insertion of a flexible instrument into the anus that allows direct visualization of the anal canal, rectum, and sigmoid colon. The patient is usually prepared for this procedure with enemas. **Answer 1** is an example of a lower GI study. **Answer 3** describes a colonoscopy, and **Answer 4** describes two of the procedures that can be accomplished with a colonoscope.

    Test-taking tip—Read the choices closely looking for clues. Visualize (oscopy) and think of the anatomy.

    IMP, 8, PhI, Reduction of Risk Potential

5. **(3)** Gentle aspiration of mucus helps maintain a patent airway, required for effective gas exchange. **Answer 1** is wrong because the *first priority is a patent airway*. **Answer 2** is wrong because the baby may aspirate mucus, which would *occlude* the airway. **Answer 4** is wrong because gravity drainage is accomplished in *head-dependent* position.

    Test-taking tip—Apply the ABCs: *airway* first. Review the plan of care for an infant immediately after delivery. Prioritize procedures, and choose the answer you would do *first*, to maintain a patent airway.

    IMP, 6, PhI, Reduction of Risk Potential

6. **(4)** Isolation may lead to withdrawal and depression. She needs positive reinforcement and reassurance to increase her self-esteem. Isolation may also lead to an increase in her

drinking and depression. Based on the symptoms she is exhibiting, involving her in simple, concrete tasks (**Answer 1**) may help her feel useful. Crying (**Answer 2**) helps her alleviate anxiety through the physical expression of her feelings. Encouraging the verbalization of her feelings (**Answer 3**) will demonstrate that someone cares for her enough to listen, and may decrease her anxiety level.

    Test-taking tip—Note key phrase: "least appropriate."

    PL, 7, PsI, Psychosocial Adaptation

7. **(1)** The basic pathophysiological changes associated with chronic bronchitis are hypertrophy of the mucous glands lining the bronchi and the production of increased amounts of mucus (sometimes thick and difficult to expectorate) that tend to narrow the airway and trap air distal to the mucus. Bronchoconstriction and edema of the bronchial walls (**Answer 2**) are characteristic of *asthma*. Exudate in the alveoli (**Answer 3**) and increasing lung stiffness (**Answer 4**) are consistent with *pneumonia*.

    Test-taking tip—Look for inflammation ("-itis") in the bronchials.

    IMP, 6, PhI, Physiological Adaptation

8. **(1)** Definitive (30%) increase in blood volume occurs at this point in pregnancy; rising cardiac load imposes stress on the heart valves (e.g., mitral stenosis) affected during the episode of rheumatic fever. **Answer 2** is wrong because *first-trimester* rubella infection presents the greatest hazard to the fetus, and immunization should be planned for the immediate postpartum period. **Answer 3** is wrong because diagnosis of multifetal pregnancy would be based *not* on discussions of *general* health status but on *physical evidence* (fundal height, ultrasound). **Answer 4** is wrong because once treatment is *ended,* infection is *gone.*

    Test-taking tip—The key is timing: *second* trimester, not *first* (2). Recall cardiac risks of rheumatic fever and how pregnancy places a woman at increased risk. Note that the stem asks for *general* health status; therefore, eliminate specific physical assessment called for in **Answer 3**. Eliminate **Answer 4** because a *prior* treated infection is *not* a second-trimester concern.

    AS, 1, PhI, Reduction of Risk Potential

9. **(2)** The main purpose of a nasogastric tube is to drain fluid and gas from the stomach; if it is functioning properly, the child's abdomen should be soft, and the tube should drain stomach contents, including bile. The nasogastric tube will not affect the drainage on the dressing (**Answer 1**) or the bowel sounds (**Answer 4**). The child may complain of a sore throat from this tube, but it should not affect the ability to swallow saliva (**Answer 3**).

    Test-taking tip—What should the nasogastric tube do? What would be the *expected* outcome?

    EV, 8, PhI, Reduction of Risk Potential

10. **(4)** Although hydration may be affected by the physiological stress of labor, the duration is insufficient to significantly affect nutritional status. **Answer 1** is wrong because discomfort generally *does* accompany labor. **Answer 2** is wrong because the inability to communicate clearly *affects* nurse-patient relationships and may induce or augment anxiety. **Answer 3** is wrong because labor *is* commonly accompanied by anxiety.

    Test-taking tip—This question asks for the nursing diagnosis that is *least* likely to be a problem. First, eliminate the three options that *are* likely to be a problem at 38 weeks of gestation with a cervix that is 4 cm dilated and 60% effaced.

    AN, 5, SECE, Management of Care

11. **(2)** Limits *do* need to be set, but they should be based on *mutual respect* rather than fear. Adult (or external) controls on behavior (**Answer 1**) are essential and must be consistent. Role models serve to stimulate the identification process (**Answer 3**) both consciously and unconsciously. Stable relationships (**Answer 4**) *are* essential if the adolescent is to mature and develop a sense of trust.

Key to codes following rationales *Nursing process:* **AS,** Assessment; **AN,** Analysis; **PL,** Plan; **IMP,** Implementation; **EV,** Evaluation. *Category of human function:* **1,** Protective; **2,** Sensory perceptual; **3,** Comfort, Rest, Activity, and Mobility; **4,** Nutrition; **5,** Growth and Development; **6,** Fluid-Gas Transport; **7,** Psychosocial-Cultural; **8,** Elimination. **Client need: SECE,** Safe, Effective Care Environment; **PhI,** Physiological Integrity; **PsI,** Psychosocial Integrity; **HPM,** Health Promotion/Maintenance. See appendices for full explanation.

PL, 5, HPM Growth and Development

12. (2) Fever and increased pulse rates occur in rheumatoid arthritis due to the systemic inflammatory process of this dysfunction. If the fever is high or prolonged, increased fluid losses could occur due to insensible water loss (**Answer 1**); however, the effects on body temperature would be secondary to the primary inflammatory response. Though the stress response (**Answer 3**) does increase pulse rate, normally it does not significantly affect body temperature. **Answer 4** is incorrect because salicylates have an antipyretic effect.

Test-taking tip—Look for a choice consistent with an "itis" (inflammation).
EV, 3, PhI, Physiological Adaptation

13. (2) Lice are spread by direct or indirect contact: sharing combs and brushes, sharing hats, sleeping together, etc. It is generally unrelated to frequency of hair washing (**Answer 1**), wearing a hat (**Answer 3**), or having long hair (**Answer 4**).

Test-taking tip—Because lice are contagious, the best answer focuses on *prevention* of *spread* to *others*. Only one option involves *others*.
AS, 1, HPM, Prevention and Early Detection of Disease

14. (3) Most obsessive-compulsive individuals are highly *inflexible* and resist change because change stimulates anxiety and they are unable to cope with stress. **Answers 1, 2,** and **4** are all *likely* behaviors.

Test-taking tip—Note key phrase: "*least* expect."
AS, 7, PsI, Coping and Adaptation

15. (2) The stomas will begin to secrete mucus within 48 hours, and the proximal loop should begin to drain fecal material within 72 hours. Ileostomies (**Answer 1**) begin to drain immediately. **Answers 3** and **4** are incorrect because peristalsis generally returns within 48–72 hours postoperatively.

Test-taking tip—Know when bowel sounds (peristalsis) return following general anesthesia.
EV, 8, PhI, Physiological Adaptation

16. (1) History of three pregnancies plus current pregnancy (gravida 4). Parity refers to the number of pregnancies carried to viability, *not* the number of babies. Two pregnancies were carried past viability (para 2). This formula does not allow for indicating the number of abortions or living children. **Answers 2, 3,** and **4** are wrong based on the definitions of gravida and parity.

Test-taking tip—Be able to determine a woman's obstetric history by defining gravida and para. Use the acronym GTPAL (gravida, term, preterm, abortions, living children).
AN, 5, HPM, Growth and Development

17. (4) The psychological effect of being restrained can be severe. Therefore, any form of restraint should be applied as a last resort. Isolating the client from other clients during the initial adjustment period would serve to decrease stimuli and possibly prevent the need for restraints. **Answers 1, 2,** and **3** are all more appropriate interventions.

Test-taking tip—Note key phrase: "*least* appropriate."
IMP, 7, PsI, Psychosocial Adaptation

18. (3) The nurse should find out what "plenty of vitamins and mineral supplements" means. Hypervitaminosis has an *adverse* effect on the woman's immune system response and fetal development. **Answer 1** is not the answer because 1500–2000 mL of fluids per day *is* recommended. **Answer 2** is not the answer because the recommended weight gain, with a good diet, *is* two-thirds of a pound per week for the last 6 months of pregnancy. **Answer 4** is not the answer because a registered dietitian *is* recommended to assist vegetarian women with complementary protein combinations.

Test-taking tip—When a question asks for the answer that requires further teaching because of a lack of understanding on the patient's part, look for the incorrect answer. Review basic nutrient and fluid needs in pregnancy and lactation.
EV, 4, HPM, Prevention and Early Detection

19. (4) The loss of a limb is significant. The patient facing the amputation must deal with self-perception, incorporate the changes in body image, and be allowed to grieve. The nurse must be sensitive to the patient's stage of grieving and provide information as asked for, at a level consistent with the patient's ability to comprehend. Although the attending physician (**Answer 1**), family (**Answer 2**), and nursing staff (**Answer 3**) may affect the patient's perception of a situation, the work of grieving is primarily personal, with movement both forward and backward as the patient progresses through the stages.

Test-taking tip—Focus on the patient's needs first.
AN, 7, PsI, Coping and Adaptation

20. (4) The adolescent *initially* needs the staff's help in one-to-one socialization. The client *next* must be stimulated by the staff to participate in minimally demanding group activities (**Answer 1**). Allowing a minimum of 3 hours of isolated behavior (**Answer 3**) will probably increase the withdrawal. Perhaps the nurse could establish a behavior-modification program involving a trade-off of 15 minutes alone for every 45 minutes spent socializing and interacting with others. If activities are too challenging (**Answer 2**), the client may become frustrated and feel incompetent, which would lead to a decrease in self-esteem.

Test-taking tip—Note key phrase: "*most* appropriate."
PL, 7, PsI, Psychosocial Adaptation

21. (2) Increased lung volumes (TLC, FRC, RV) and decreased airflow—vital capacity (VC) and forced expiratory volume in 1 second (FEV_1)—are functional problems consistent with obstructive lung disease. In restrictive lung disease (**Answer 1**), volumes generally are decreased. Vascular lung disease (**Answer 3**) has no effect on ventilatory capacity but directly affects diffusion of gases; that is, pulmonary infarction decreases blood flow to the lungs, so some alveoli that are ventilated are no longer perfused. Restrictive lung disease is incorrect (**Answer 4**).

Test-taking tip—Visualize a lung with *increased* capacities: hyperinflated, trapped air (COPD).
AN, 6, PhI, Physiological Adaptation

22. (4) Adolescents rarely demonstrate a lifestyle characterized by helplessness; rather, they are striving to gain control over their own lives. **Answer 1** is wrong because the teenager *has* verbalized anxiety and fear over possible diagnoses. **Answer 2** is wrong because the threat of adolescent pregnancy evidently presents a situational crisis for her. **Answer 3** is wrong because either diagnosis *will* provide her with evidence that she failed to meet family expectations, and precipitates situational crisis.

Test-taking tip—Pay attention to key phrase: "least likely."
AN, 7, PsI, Coping and Adaptation

23. (3) Stapedectomy is the surgical procedure for the treatment of otosclerosis. Its success cannot be determined in the immediate postoperative period. The patient must be told that hearing is affected for a while after surgery because of edema. Tinnitus (**Answer 1**) is a postoperative complication that must be reported, but is *not* expected. The resolution of postoperative edema (**Answer 2**) does *not* result in rhinitis. Once the ear has healed, normal activities *are* permitted, including showering and swimming (**Answer 4**). With an upper respiratory infection, deep-sea diving and flying are usually restricted.

Test-taking tip—Use a process of elimination. Ringing in the ears is *never* normal, which leaves short-term hearing impairment, given the surgery.
IMP, 2, PhI, Reduction of Risk Potential

24. **(3)** The adolescent client is probably very frightened and angry. The client needs to feel that his side will be considered in order to cope effectively with these feelings and with this behavior. **Answers 1, 2,** and **4** are all staff oriented and provide little psychological support for the client as an individual striving for independence.

   Test-taking tip—Choose the "*most* significant" need.

   AN, 7, PsI, Psychosocial Adaptation

25. **(2)** In preparing the patient for discharge on prednisone therapy, the nurse should caution him or her to (a) take oral preparations after meals; (b) remember that routine checks of vital signs, weight, and lab studies are critical; (c) never stop or change the amount of medication without medical advice; and (d) store the medication in a light-resistant container. **Answer 1** is incorrect because prednisone, as well as other medications given in rheumatoid arthritis therapy, is irritating to the GI tract and should be taken after meals. **Answer 3** is incorrect because although fluid, electrolyte, and serum-glucose levels need frequent evaluation during prednisone therapy, CBCs need regular checking if the patient is on phenylbutazone (Butazolidin), oxyphenbutazone (Tandearil), or ibuprofen (Motrin) therapy. **Answer 4** is a precaution given to patients on hydroxychloroquine SO_4 (Plaquenil) or chloroquine (Aralen) therapy.

   Test-taking tip—Think patient safety. The greatest risk is discontinuing or altering dose.

   IMP, 4, PhI, Pharmacological and Parenteral Therapies

26. **(4)** Early decelerations represent the normal fetal response to head compressions during contractions. **Answer 1** is wrong because head compression does not cause fetal distress. **Answers 2** and **3** are wrong because there are no signs of late or variable decelerations.

   Test-taking tip—First, decide if this is *OK* or not *OK*. Note the word "physiological," which implies an anticipated outcome. You can eliminate options with "insufficiency" and "distress," which mean there is a problem.

   AN, 6, HPM, Growth and Development

27. **(3)** Intervention is needed when the woman thinks that she needs to wait only 6 months after being free of TB before she can get pregnant. She needs to wait 1.5–2 years after she is declared to be free of TB before she should attempt pregnancy. **Answer 1** is not the answer because pregnancy *may* be jeopardized by TB. **Answer 2** is not the answer because spontaneous abortion *does* occur in one of five women who are infected. **Answer 4** is not the answer because she will *not* have close contact with her baby until contagion is no longer a problem.

   Test-taking tip—The focus of the best answer is not *what* may occur, but *when*. The *time* period is the problem here.

   EV, 1, SECE, Safety and Infection Control

28. **(3)** The position that allows for the greatest amount of lung expansion is sitting up and leaning slightly forward. This position can be facilitated by allowing the patient to rest his or her arms on a bedside table. The position that also facilitates lung expansion, but not to the same degree, is high Fowler's (**Answer 1**). Both the prone position (**Answer 2**) and the Trendelenburg position (**Answer 4**) tend to decrease full lung expansion due to increased pressure of abdominal contents on the diaphragm.

   Test-taking tip—When two options are plausible, choose the most comprehensive (two actions instead of just one).

   IMP, 6, PhI, Basic Care and Comfort

29. **(4)** The superego may never be completely refined or stabilized. Some individuals may achieve an optimal level of functioning some time in late adulthood; however, rarely will the superego become stabilized during adolescence. As stated in **Answer 1,** the individual *does* strive to develop an independent and unique personality during adolescence. To maintain a steady state of functioning, the adolescent must learn to use defense mechanisms (**Answer 2**) in an appropriate manner. Developing a positive ego identity (**Answer 3**) is one of the major goals of adolescence.

   Test-taking tip—Key words: "least important," means eliminate the three options that *are* age related.

   PL, 5, HPM, Growth and Development

30. **(1)** The patient is placed in a semi-Fowler's position to promote the flow of drainage to the pelvic region, where a localized abscess can be drained or be resolved by the body's normal defenses. The elevated position also keeps the infection from spreading upward in the peritoneal cavity. **Answers 2, 3,** and **4** are incorrect because none of them elevates the trunk of the body.

   Test-taking tip—Look for a pattern. Only one choice has the patient sitting up.

   IMP, 3, PhI, Physiological Adaptation

31. **(4)** Contraction of the milk ducts and the let-down reflex occur under the stimulation of *oxytocin* released by the posterior pituitary gland. **Answers 1, 2,** and **3** are wrong because these hormones have no effect on the let-down reflex or uterine involution.

   Test-taking tip—Know the hormones responsible for initiation and continuation of lactation. You can also select the correct answer by recalling the hormone involved in *uterine involution* (also included in the question).

   AN, 5, HPM, Growth and Development

32. **(4)** The nurse should know that deep partial-thickness (second-degree) burns cause severe pain. The nurse should also know that during the first 48–72 hours after a serious burn, there is a very poor peripheral circulation due to hypovolemia; therefore, medications should be given via the IV route. PO (**Answer 2**) and IM (**Answer 3**) medications are generally contraindicated during this time. To do nothing (**Answer 1**) would be inappropriate, given the nature and extent of the injuries.

   Test-taking tip—Think impaired peripheral circulation; think IV, not IM; eliminate PO due to burns on face and neck.

   IMP, 3, PhI, Pharmacological and Parenteral Therapies

33. **(1)** Normal amniotic fluid is essentially colorless; any color may signify fetal or maternal problems. For example, green amniotic fluid indicates meconium released due to fetal hypoxia; bloody amniotic fluid may indicate abruptio placentae. **Answer 2** is wrong because nausea with or without emesis *is common* in labor, due to physiological stress. **Answer 3** is wrong because fetal bradycardia *commonly* manifests at contraction acme, due to head compression. **Answer 4** is wrong because diaphoresis and irritability *are* signs of transitional phase of labor.

   Test-taking tip—Choose the answer here that is *not* normal. Know normal and expected findings (**2, 3, 4**), and then identify the one that is not normal.

   AS, 5, PhI, Reduction of Risk Potential

34. **(2)** Past coping mechanisms are important in assessing the client's ability to return to a steady state of functioning. Strengths and weaknesses in the client's ability to rationally assess and cope with feelings need to be explored. Referrals may need to be made (**Answer 1**), but an initial assessment of the client needs to be completed first. Inpatient hospitalization may be needed (**Answer 3**); however, the assessment of ability to cope with the situation may assist in identifying whether hospitalization is needed. Obtaining a prescription for an antidepressant at this time (**Answer 4**) may prove to be detrimental. Even if the client does not decide to overdose, medication without psychological support is generally ineffective.

   Test-taking tip—Choose an assessment intervention as a most important priority (e.g., "identifying").

   IMP, 7, PsI, Psychosocial Adaptation

35. (4) Thyroglobulin (Proloid) is a purified extract of pig thyroid and is used in the treatment of *hypothyroidism*. **Answers 1, 2,** and **3** *are* current methods for treating Graves' disease, or hyperthyroidism.

> **Test-taking tip**—Key word is "inappropriate," which means select the *wrong* treatment. Another key term is *hyper*thyroidism, not hypothyroidism.

IMP, 3, SECE, Management of Care

36. (4) At 12 weeks of gestation, fundus should be palpable at the pubic symphysis. **Answer 1** is wrong because of inability to palpate due to current uterine size and position. **Answer 2** is wrong because weight-gain patterns provide no information regarding uterine or fetal growth. **Answer 3** is wrong because maternal vital signs are not diagnostic of gestational age or uterine growth, and fetal heart tones may be heard with a Doppler as early as 9–10 weeks.

> **Test-taking tip**—Key terms: timing (12 wk gestation) and uterine and fetal *growth*. Eliminate **Answer 1** because it is too early to do; eliminate **Answers 2** and **3** because they do not give information about gestation and *fetal growth*.

AS, 5, HPM, Prevention and Early Detection

37. (1) Acting out is the expression through behavior (rather than through words) of emotions that occur when the client relives or reproduces the feelings, wishes, or conflicts that are operating unconsciously. The client may be feeling frustrated, angry, ambivalent, etc., for numerous reasons, such as conflict between self and parents, a reaction to parents' marital conflicts, sibling rivalry, or frustration due to poor self-esteem. By definition, **Answers 2, 3,** and **4** are incorrect.

> **Test-taking tip**—Review definition of *acting out*.

AS, 7, PsI, Coping and Adaptation

38. (1) A wheeze is a high-pitched, musical chest sound produced by airflow in narrowed bronchioles. It is primarily an expiratory sound and is always, *not* rarely (**Answer 2**), considered pathological. *Rhonchi* are medium-pitched sonorous sounds (**Answer 3**) produced by airflow obstruction in larger airways. *Stridor* is a high-pitched crowing sound (**Answer 4**) on inspiration and is due to an upper-airway obstruction, such as edema, adhesions, or tracheal hypertrophy.

> **Test-taking tip**—Think "wheeze" is a "squeeze"—only one choice includes narrowing.

IMP, 6, PhI, Physiological Adaptation

39. (1) Lithium is used to treat affective disorders. Thioridazine (Mellaril) (**Answer 4**) is a major tranquilizer used to treat schizophrenia. Thioridazine has been used to treat the manic phase of bipolar affective disorders, but it is not the primary drug. Chlordiazepoxide HCl (Librium) (**Answer 2**) is a minor tranquilizer used to relieve the mild or moderate anxiety usually associated with affective and somatoform disorders. Fluphenazine HCl (Prolixin) (**Answer 3**) is a long-acting psychotropic used primarily to treat schizophrenia. It can be administered biweekly in an injection for a long-term effect.

> **Test-taking tip**—Review types of common medications for each psychiatric disorder.

IMP, 7, PhI, Pharmacological Therapy

40. (1) The *primary* purpose of passive range-of-motion exercises is to prevent contractures and decreased range of motion. *Secondarily,* passive range-of-motion exercises assist the nurse in evaluating functional abilities (**Answer 2**), pain tolerance (**Answer 3**), and the effectiveness of drug therapy (**Answer 4**).

> **Test-taking tip**—The stem asks for a *purpose* (goal). Three of the options are nursing actions.

IMP, 3, PhI, Basic Care and Comfort

41. (2) By calculation of EDB using Nägele's rule of counting back 3 months and adding 7 days to the date of LMP: 4th month − 3 months = 1st month (January); third day plus 7 days = tenth day; January 10 is her EDB. **Answer 1** is wrong

because of failure to add 7 days to LMP. **Answer 3** is wrong because 7 days were subtracted from date of LMP. **Answer 4** is wrong because of counting back 4 months instead of 3.

> **Test-taking tip**—Mathematical accuracy is the key to the right answer, using Nägele's rule. Use the formula for calculating the EDB.

AN, 5, HPM, Growth and Development

42. (2) An increase in the client's energy level may provide enough motivation to make another suicide attempt. Generally, depressed clients do not kill themselves because their energy level is very low. Therefore, the one-to-one relationship needs to be maintained and stressed at this time. **Answers 1, 3,** and **4** are dangerous assumptions at this time.

> **Test-taking tip**—Focus on two contradictory options (less attention vs. more attention); select "more attention."

EV, 7, PsI, Psychosocial Adaptation

43. (2) The patient needs an opportunity to receive word images. Point to the object and clearly enunciate its name, e.g., "spoon." Also, the patient with expressive aphasia needs the chance to practice repeating words. Begin with simple words, such as *yes* and *no*, and then progress to complete phrases. Recovery from aphasia depends on the area of the brain involved and the extent of damage. There may be spontaneous recovery or improvement with speech therapy 2 years after the stroke. To consider the impairment permanent (**Answer 1**) would be premature. **Answer 3** is incorrect because waiting may increase the patient's frustration. Try to anticipate the patient's needs to reduce feelings of helplessness. The nurse plays an important part in showing the family members how to communicate and in not discouraging communication (**Answer 4**).

> **Test-taking tip**—Only one option shows "action" to improve patient communication.

IMP, 2, PsI, Coping and Adaptation

44. (4) A preschooler would probably respond best to the use of puppets to dramatize the procedure. Any description of the procedure alone (**Answer 1**), no matter how simple, would probably not be enough to enable most preschoolers to understand what will happen to them. Taking a patient to the operating room or the catheterization lab (**Answer 2**) would probably be unnecessarily frightening for any patient, especially a child. The child may not ask any questions himself or herself (**Answer 3**), and if the child does not, the nurse would be unable to do any teaching.

> **Test-taking tip**—Growth and development stage at preschool calls for therapeutic play (i.e., dramatic). Cognitive input is *not age appropriate.*

IMP, 5, PsI, Coping and Adaptation

45. (1) The nurse needs to address the amount of energy and stamina needed to meet the demands of parenting. Older women have commented that the lack of energy and stamina came as a surprise. **Answer 2** is incorrect because older women tend to be *less troubled* by pregnancy and remain better adjusted during the last trimester. Older mothers, as a group, do *not* have longer labor (**Answer 3**), nor, with good prenatal care, do they show a greater number of labor/birth complications (**Answer 4**).

> **Test-taking tip**—Focus on the *general expected* concerns for this age group and this trimester. You can eliminate options that focus on "troubled" feelings, "*longer* labor," "*greater* number of . . . complications."

PL, 5, HPM, Growth and Development

46. (2) Appliance should be changed every 2–3 days or as soon as there is leakage. Drainage can excoriate the skin; therefore, a new appliance needs to be applied as soon as leakage appears. **Answer 1** is wrong because every day is too often; there will be damage to the skin from pulling the appliance off so often. **Answer 3** is wrong because 1 week is too long for the skin to go without being examined and cleansed.

Answer 4 is incorrect; the visiting nurse does not determine when the appliance should be changed.

> **Test-taking tip**—Look for a choice that reflects individual differences and patient control.

PL, 8, PhI, Reduction of Risk Potential

47. **(4)** Early decelerations represent the normal fetal response to contractions. **Answer 1** is wrong because this action would be taken to relieve possible cord compression. **Answer 2** is wrong because use of the Trendelenburg position is *not* necessary. **Answer 3** is an inaccurate interpretation of the assessment data.

> **Test-taking tip**—First decide if this is *OK* or not OK. Because it is OK, choose psychosocial rather than repositioning (**1, 2**) or looking for a problem (**3**, dislodged electrode). Review the differences and nursing interventions between early, late, and variable decelerations of the FHR. Know expected outcomes and risks of each, and choose appropriate interventions.

IMP, 5, HPM, Growth and Development

48. **(2)** Neomycin sulfate is used preoperatively because it is poorly absorbed in the intestinal tract and acts to decrease the bacteria count in the colon. As the result of this action, postoperative infection is reduced (**Answer 1**). Neomycin does not reduce tumor size (**Answer 3**) or directly affect peristalsis (**Answer 4**).

> **Test-taking tip**—Timing is important (preop) and purpose of drug classification—antibiotic

EV, 8, PhI, Pharmacological and Parenteral Therapies

49. **(3)** The first priority with any client who is unconscious is to maintain a patent airway. The nurse would need a physician's order to administer any medication or stimulant (**Answer 1**), which may not be appropriate in this situation. The emergency department nurse would see that the attending resident was paged (**Answer 2**), but this task could be delegated while the nurse administered primary care. Monitoring neurological signs (**Answer 4**) is also essential but can be done *after* ensuring that the client can breathe.

> **Test-taking tip**—Remember the ABCs: *airway* first.

IMP, 6, PhI, Physiological Adaptation

50. **(1)** Treatment with bronchodilators such as isoproterenol will decrease bronchoconstriction, *improving* the movement of air in and out of the lungs. **Answers 2, 3,** and **4** are incorrect because these pulmonary function studies indicate that the patient has been able to increase inspiratory capacity by 1000 mL (VC 2800–3800) and expiratory capacity (RV decreased, FRC decreased, and FEV_1 increased).

> **Test-taking tip**—Know vital capacity (VC)—the amount of air in a breath.

EV, 6, PhI, Physiological Adaptation

51. **(3)** Painful, red, papular lesions associated with foul-smelling vaginal discharge are characteristic of herpesvirus type 2 infection. **Answer 1** is wrong because *discrete* lesions do *not* accompany trichomonal infections; discharge usually is *thin, frothy, and gray or yellow-green* and usually has a foul odor (like rotting fish). **Answer 2** is wrong because monilial vaginal infections produce a *characteristic white, cheesy* discharge. **Answer 4** is wrong because gonorrhea in women is often totally *asymptomatic* or may produce a *purulent vaginal* discharge.

> **Test-taking tip**—Only by knowing signs and symptom (especially color of discharge) for each infectious lesion will you be able to identify the organism involved. Review causes and treatments for herpesvirus type 2. Know the potential risks during pregnancy and delivery for the fetus/newborn.

AS, 1, PhI, Physiological Adaptation

52. **(2)** Confrontation *could* help the 15-year-old client identify the inappropriateness of mutilation and other destructive behaviors as attention-getting devices. **Answers 1, 3,** and **4** *are* all *appropriate* interventions.

> **Test-taking tip**—Note the key phrase: *"least* appropriate."

PL, 7, PsI, Psychosocial Adaptation

53. **(2)** Human chorionic gonadotropin (HCG) is the biological marker used in pregnancy tests. This hormone is produced by the fertilized ovum and the chorionic villi and maintains the corpus luteum's production of estrogen and progesterone for the first 8–10 weeks of pregnancy. The hormone reaches maximum level at 50–70 days. **Answer 1** is incorrect because human placental lactogen is produced by the *placenta*. Luteinizing hormone (**Answer 3**) is the primary anterior pituitary hormone during the *second "half"* of the *menstrual cycle*. Alpha-fetoprotein (**Answer 4**) is a biological marker for assessing for open neural tube *defects* in the *fetus*.

> **Test-taking tip**—Because the HCG is produced by the *fertilized* ovum, it is the marker for a positive *pregnancy*.

AN, 5, HPM, Growth and Development

54. **(2)** Touch, facial expression, and tone of voice may be used effectively to reduce anxiety, apprehensions, and fear in situations where verbal communication is inhibited by language barriers. **Answer 1** is wrong because the continual use of an intermediary (her husband) may impede establishing the rapport necessary for a successful labor experience. **Answer 3** is wrong because incomprehensible words become no more understandable if spoken slowly or distinctly; loud voices are disconcerting during labor. **Answer 4** is inappropriate because the *nurse,* not the MD, is there to provide ongoing care and allay anxiety.

> **Test-taking tip**—Because she is *not verbal* (in English), use *nonverbal* communication.

PL, 7, PsI, Coping and Adaptation

55. **(3)** Although there *are* several specific forms that elicit disclosure of this information, there is no law that mandates disclosure (**Answer 4**). The client has to make this decision independently. The nurse should provide therapeutic support for whatever decision. **Answers 1** and **2** are untrue statements.

> **Test-taking tip**—Note the key phrase "*most* appropriate"; it provides therapeutic support for patient's decision.

IMP, 7, PsI, Coping and Adaptation

56. **(3)** An iridectomy is performed in the upper segment of the iris and is covered by the upper eyelid, as normally. The excision in the iris is occluded, which decreases discomfort. Infection is less likely because bacteria are carried in the tears, by gravity, to the lower cul-de-sac. The need for a dressing is usually indicated, to decrease infection or eye movement. Because infection is *not* likely and mobilization of the eye (**Answer 1**) *is* desirable to prevent posterior synechiae (adhesion of iris to cornea or lens), no dressing is needed. **Answers 2** and **4** *are* appropriate actions. Massage of the eye, if ordered, encourages continuous flow of fluids through the surgical opening.

> **Test-taking tip**—The key word is *inappropriate*. Although dressings prevent infection, *reinforcing* the dressing would be necessary for bleeding, which is *not* indicated.

IMP, 2, PhI, Basic Care and Comfort

57. **(3)** Increased dietary bulk and adequate fluids relieve symptoms of constipation naturally, by stimulating peristalsis. **Answer 1** is wrong because regular use of laxatives *reduces normal bowel functions;* mineral oil contributes to loss of fat-soluble vitamins A, D, and E. **Answer 2** is wrong because *adequate* fluid intake is needed to avoid dry, packed stools associated with constipation. **Answer 4** is wrong because Kegel exercises increase sphincter control and do *not* encourage defecation.

> **Test-taking tip**—Think diet, not laxatives or Kegel exercises.

PL, 8, PhI, Basic Care and Comfort

58. **(4)** Adolescents who have had an appendectomy are expected to make a complete, rapid recovery; they should have *minimal* to moderate pain during the first 24 hours

(**Answer 1**). Discharge time frame varies, not necessarily within 48 hours, or after a *slow* recovery (**Answers 2, 3**).

> **Test-taking tip**—Consider age-appropriate expected outcome.

EV, 8, SECE, Management of Care

59. (**3**) Hostility and aggression are considered the underlying factors in the psychogenesis and psychodynamics of depression. The adolescent is in a stage of development in which he or she experiences extensive anger due to frustration. The adolescent has a greater energy level because of the increased libidinal energy available in his or her system. To expend this energy, many adolescents act out their feelings of depression in violent ways rather than become withdrawn, apathetic, or regressive (**Answers 1, 2, 4**).

> **Test-taking tip**—Choose the option that is different: violence is different from withdrawal, apathy, and regression.

AS, 7, PsI, Coping and Adaptation

60. (**3**) PID is more common in women who have multiple sex partners. **Answer 1** is incorrect because there is an increased incidence of *infection* (*not* PID) in women during the first month after insertion of an IUD. Gonorrhea (**Answer 2**) can cause PID *whether* it is acquired through skin-to-skin contact *or* from a fomite (a fomite is a nonliving material on which disease-producing organisms can be conveyed, e.g., bed linens or washcloths). **Answer 4** is incorrect because a pattern of *heavy* alcohol consumption is associated with certain nutritional deficiencies (e.g., vitamin B complex) that decrease a person's immune responsiveness to vaccines and depress the cell-mediated and humoral lymphocytic activity.

> **Test-taking tip**—Think inflamed pelvis from multiple sex partners.

AN, 1, HPM, Prevention and Early Detection

61. (**3**) Deep breathing, coughing, and pursed-lip exhalations are all techniques that the nurse can teach the patient to improve ventilation. *Adequate* fluid intake (**Answer 1**) is essential for keeping sputum liquefied; however, very hot and very cold drinks should be avoided because they may cause bronchospasm. Patients with COPD also need to be taught to avoid exposure to infections, early signs of infection, and the need to seek medical intervention promptly should symptoms occur. **Answers 2** and **4** are not indicated in this patient's therapy.

> **Test-taking tip**—Look for an option that makes the patient an active participant in the care.

IMP, 6, PhI, Physiological Adaptation

62. (**1**) Erythema toxicum is the normal, nonpathological macular newborn rash. **Answer 2** is wrong because milia are small *white* nodules due to clogged sebaceous glands. **Answer 3** is wrong because *icterus neonatorum* is the term for normal physiological *jaundice* of the newborn, which occurs *48–72 hours after birth*. **Answer 4** is wrong because hemangiomas are small elevated clusters of capillaries ("stork bites").

> **Test-taking tip**—The clue to the correct answer is time (24 hours old) and type of rash (macular), not yellow (**3**) or white (**2**).

IMP, 5, HPM, Growth and Development

63. (**2**) Patients should not be encouraged to do exercises to the point of unusual pain, and pain should not last longer than one-half hour after exercise. If pain lasts longer than this, the exercises are too strenuous. **Answer 1** is incorrect because pulse and respiratory rates are affected not only by physical stress but also by emotional and psychological stress. **Answers 3** and **4** indicate that therapy has been effective.

> **Test-taking tip**—Read the choices. Look for an indication that the exercise was appropriate or excessive.

EV, 3, PhI, Basic Care and Comfort

64. (**3**) The client should be placed under one-to-one, not group, observation to ensure effective protection against suicidal behaviors. **Answers 1, 2,** and **4** are all appropriate actions.

> **Test-taking tip**—Note the key phrase: "*least* appropriate."

IMP, 7, PsI, Psychosocial Adaptation

65. (**1**) In positioning the child during recovery, the nurse should avoid those positions in which contractures and flexion deformities may occur. With burns on the neck, the nurse should keep the neck extended and help the child avoid flexing the neck (**Answer 4**). Keeping the child still (**Answer 2**) will predispose him or her to complications of immobility. There is no reason why the child cannot sit in a chair (with help as needed) during recovery (**Answer 3**).

> **Test-taking tip**—Burned tissue should always be positioned in either neutral or extended position for healing, *never* flexed.

IMP, 3, PhI, Basic Care and Comfort

66. (**2**) The woman is demonstrating signs of beginning transition. Sacral pressure and back rubs assist in reducing her discomfort at this time. **Answer 1** is wrong because assessment indicates irritability, *not* pain. Further, she has expressed a desire to use Lamaze for labor and birth. **Answer 3** is wrong because it is important to maintain continual assessment of fetal status during the transitional stage. **Answer 4** is wrong because the woman should be attended continually during transition.

> **Test-taking tip**—First, you need to recognize the symptoms of transition; therefore, positioning is the best answer. Eliminate the three other options because pain medication is not used as a first intervention when she wants to use "natural childbirth" (i.e., Lamaze). **Answers 3** and **4** are contraindicated during transition.

IMP, 3, PhI, Basic Care and Comfort

67. (**2**) To read blood gases, first note the pH. In this case, pH is 7.38, which is within the normal range (7.35–7.45) but is on the acidotic side. Next, look at the PCO_2 and HCO_3 to see which one is causing the shift to acidosis. In this case the PCO_2 is 55 (acidosis) and the HCO_3 is 32 (alkalosis). Therefore, the patient has compensated respiratory acidosis because the kidneys have been able to conserve enough bicarbonate to keep pH within normal range. In this case a pH below 7.35 would indicate uncompensated respiratory acidosis (**Answer 1**). If the patient had uncompensated metabolic alkalosis (**Answer 3**), pH would be above 7.45. If the patient had compensated metabolic alkalosis (**Answer 4**), pH would be between 7.41 and 7.45.

> **Test-taking tip**—Look at each component to determine normal, increased, or decreased. If pH is normal, it has to be *compensated*. Below 7.4 = acidosis; above 7.4 = alkalosis.

AN, 6, PhI, Physiological Adaptation

68. (**2**) Although the adolescent's parents may perceive this as a parental decision, it is important for the entire family to be included in the decision-making process because the entire family system will be affected by this change. Asking the parents to reassess their feelings (**Answer 1**) may help them evaluate the situation, but it avoids facing the issue as a family decision. A referral may be appropriate (**Answers 3, 4**); however, all parties involved in the decision must be listened to before making a referral or searching for an alternative placement.

> **Test-taking tip**—Key phrase: "*most* appropriate." It is most appropriate to involve the *family* system in decision making related to an adolescent.

IMP, 7, PsI, Coping and Adaptation

69. (**2**) In rheumatoid arthritis both the erythrocyte sedimentation rate and C-reactive protein levels are increased. Anemia is common, so hemoglobin and hematocrit are usually decreased, not increased (**Answer 1**). The Wasserman test result (**Answer 3**) is normally negative. The platelet count (**Answer 4**) is not affected.

> **Test-taking tip**—Only one option measures inflammation. Know appropriate lab tests.

AN, 1, PhI, Physiological Adaptation

Practice Test

70. **(4)** During pregnancy, attention is focused on the expectant parents; feelings of competition for attention with the baby arise during the *postpartum* period. **Answer 1** is wrong because pressures of present and anticipated expenses associated with childbearing *do* impose stress on the family. **Answer 2** is wrong because both expectant parents *must adjust* to changing relationships between themselves and their extended families. **Answer 3** is wrong because both parents may *experience* stress on recognizing the need to be totally responsible for the health and development of a baby and the concomitant need to change their lifestyle to meet those obligations.

   Test-taking tip—The key is *timing*: 18 weeks of gestation. Review the normal developmental tasks of pregnancy by trimester, especially the adjustments of the family. The question asks for the *least likely* cause, so choose an *incorrect answer* because these feelings would occur in the postpartum period, *not* at 18 weeks.

   AN, 7, PsI, Coping and Adaptation

71. **(2)** Although it is not possible to make a patient stop smoking, the patient should be presented with information about methods used by other people who were successful in stopping. Although most people are aware of the deleterious effects of smoking, patients need to be reminded of the relationship between smoking and their present condition. Fluid intake and nutrition should be discussed and adapted to individual needs. Patients should be able to identify drugs, giving the name, correct dosage, timing, and potential side effects. Alcohol in moderation is not restricted (**Answer 1**). Vocational rehabilitation should be present as an option but not emphasized (**Answer 3**). Activities should be encouraged to tolerance (**Answer 4**).

   Test-taking tip—Look for the option that is broadest and encompasses the most areas for teaching.

   IMP, 6, PhI, Physiological Adaptation

72. **(4)** The passage of time will *not* help him cope effectively with his feelings of fear and ambivalence. These feelings are a normal part of the maturation process, and *only* with effective limit setting and psychological support will the adolescent's ability to cope be strengthened. In early adolescence boys generally *are* intolerant of women authority figures (**Answer 1**). They perceive these women as a threat to their emerging masculine identity. Adolescents *need* physical activity to alleviate tension (**Answer 2**). Men in general have problems dealing with impulse control (**Answer 3**) and need consistent limits set on their behaviors.

   Test-taking tip—Note the word "inappropriate" and think of the four options in this question as true or false. It is *false* that with passage of time, fear and ambivalence will dissipate.

   AN, 7, PsI, Coping and Adaptation

73. **(2)** Norplant implants do not provide protection against sexually transmitted diseases. Couples should also receive information about the need to use condoms for prevention of transmission of STDs. **Answer 1** is incorrect because some women *may* experience breakthrough bleeding, but many will *not*. If they do, it usually is only temporary. **Answer 3** is incorrect because there is *no* correlation between use of long-acting Progestin implants and endometrial cancer. **Answer 4** is incorrect because women may experience weight *gain*, usually *not* weight loss.

   Test-taking tip—Choose the answer that is the most critical to know about so that she can use *protection*. Eliminate **Answers 3** and **4** because they are theoretically incorrect.

   IMP, 1, PhI, Pharmacological and Parenteral Therapies

74. **(1)** This woman's behavior typifies patterns expressed during the second trimester. **Answer 2** is wrong because her symptoms are related both to fluctuating hormone levels and to

psychological reevaluation of self and marriage. **Answers 3** and **4** are wrong because of the *physiological* component of her symptoms.

   Test-taking tip—Look for the expected body image changes related to *second-trimester* pregnancy, covering *both* physiological and psychological components.

   AN, 7, HPM, Growth and Development

75. **(2)** Hitting others provides the adolescent with an outlet for feelings of hopelessness and despair. Although this behavior may not make a person feel happy or satisfied, it does provide a defense against feeling unhappy. **Answers 1, 3,** and **4** are not primary motivations of this behavior.

   Test-taking tip—Note the phrase "most relevant" and turn this question into a "true or false." Note a relationship between *depression* in the stem and *hopelessness* in **Answer 2**.

   AN, 7, PsI, Coping and Adaptation

76. **(2)** Position the conscious patient sitting upright in a supported, forward-leaning position (high Fowler's, orthopneic) to improve ventilation and oxygenation. A calm and reassuring approach will decrease hyperactivity of the patient and oxygen need. Acute respiratory failure is a medical emergency. Aminophylline (**Answer 1**) is indicated to combat bronchospasm, but it is *not an independent nursing* action. Low-flow oxygen (2 L) is also administered to the patient in respiratory failure; however, nasal cannulas (**Answer 3**) do not provide predictable O_2 concentrations. A Venturi mask would be more appropriate. **Answer 4** is incorrect because the higher concentration of O_2 (60%) may lead to respiratory depression unless the patient is maintained on controlled mechanical ventilation.

   Test-taking tip—Focus on the patient first, then the equipment.

   AN, 6, PhI, Physiological Adaptation

77. **(3)** Dry soda crackers absorb gastric juices and increase blood sugar, thereby reducing nausea. **Answer 1** is wrong because eating before retiring has no effect on morning nausea. **Answer 2** is wrong because drinking fruit juice on an empty stomach may increase nausea. **Answer 4** is wrong because demands of physical activity may increase nausea.

   Test-taking tip—Narrow your focus to the two options for *what*, not when, to eat/drink. One item is a dry food (crackers), the other is liquid (but acidic). Eliminate the acidic liquid because it can be a gastric irritant.

   IMP, 4, PhI, Basic Care and Comfort

78. **(1)** The best topical cleansing material to use in debriding burns are sterile 4×4 gauze pads. Cotton balls (**Answer 2**) may pull and stick to burned tissue. Washcloths (**Answer 3**) are too harsh and may damage new healing tissue. Telfa pads (**Answer 4**) are too smooth and will not cleanse the area as well as gauze pads.

   Test-taking tip—Think of the most effective texture and eliminate cotton, terrycloth, Telfa.

   IMP, 7, PhI, Reduction of Risk Potential

79. **(1)** Individuals who have used alcohol habitually over an extended time period usually exhibit symptoms of withdrawal delirium when the alcohol intake is severely decreased or curtailed. **Answers 2, 3,** and **4** are less likely reactions.

   Test-taking tip—Note the phrase "most likely to exhibit" and review signs and symptoms of alcohol withdrawal.

   AS, 7, PsI, Psychosocial Adaptation

80. **(4)** Indications of respiratory distress and the increased work of breathing in this patient are characterized by the use of the accessory muscles of respiration, the sternocleidomastoid and trapezius muscles. Using these muscles enables the patient to *increase the size* of the thorax, thus allowing air to move in. Patients with chronic bronchitis and air trapping generally are not able to increase the depth of breathing (**Answer 1**) by increasing diaphragmatic excursion (**Answer 2**). Some patients may be using pursed-lip exhalations

(**Answer 3**), but these help maintain open airways for the expulsion of gases.

Test-taking tip—Visualize the patient. If the patient was "working" to take in a breath, what would you see?

AS, 6, PhI, Physiological Adaptation

81. (**2**) "Charley horse" pain (cramp in gastrocnemius muscle) is due to sudden spasm and acute flexion of leg muscles; it is relieved by dorsiflexing the foot, which reduces the muscle spasm. **Answer 1** is wrong because such action will not eliminate the possibility of muscle spasm during pregnancy. **Answer 3** is wrong because the actions of vitamin C do not affect muscle spasms. **Answer 4** is wrong because exercise does not prevent muscle spasm.

Test-taking tip—Key concept is *timing*. Choose the option that can produce on-the-spot *symptomatic relief* (key words in the item).

IMP, 3, HPM, Prevention and Early Detection

82. (**3**) Although the patient expresses a willingness to learn, apprehension will limit the ability to assimilate much. The patient must be taught specific arm and leg exercises, including frequent repositioning onto the abdomen to prevent contracture. Before discharge, alternative vocational pursuits (**Answer 1**) may be discussed, as indicated. In the *postoperative* period the focus changes to crutch walking (**Answer 2**). Encouraging the patient to verbalize fears and concerns (**Answer 4**) is not a specific teaching strategy but rather an intervention designed to give support, as well as identify potential problems.

Test-taking tip—The stem says "learn;" therefore something to *teach* before surgery is the best choice.

PL, 1, PhI, Basic Care and Comfort

83. (**3**) His thoughts, feelings, and attitudes toward sexual relationships need to be explored to assess his level of maturity in deciding his sexual preference. *Confrontation*, rather than avoidance of confrontation (**Answer 1**), could help him identify his use of homosexual behavior as an attention-seeking device. Validation of his rationale for seeking homosexual relationships (**Answer 2**) may be identified more appropriately through exploring his thoughts, feelings, and attitudes regarding his sexual orientation. Enforcing limits on his relationships (**Answer 4**) will only make him angry and is in any case an invasion of his right to privacy and freedom of choice. As long as neither client is forcing himself on the other, their relationship should not be interfered with. However, if it is determined that for some appropriate reason this relationship is detrimental to either individual's optimal level of functioning, limits should be set.

Test-taking tip—Focus on the phrase "*primary* concern," which calls for exploring thoughts, feelings, and attitudes.

PL, 7, HPM, Growth and Development

84. (**3**) A male adolescent will most likely prefer the companionship of another boy close to his age. Although he may be interested in girls (**Answer 4**), being introduced to them would not necessarily prove helpful for him. Adolescents cannot be relied on to place materials into hospital charts (**Answer 1**). Because his recovery is expected to be rapid and complete, he will miss little school, and there is no need to get him involved with in-hospital tutoring (**Answer 2**); he can easily catch up with his schoolwork when he gets home.

Test-taking tip—Remember age-relevant growth and development stage: socialization with peers is the most important social influence for the adolescent.

IMP, 5, PsI, Coping and Adaptation

85. (**1**) Abstinence will eliminate any unnecessary pain during intercourse and will reduce the possibility of transmitting infection to one's sexual partner. **Answer 2** is wrong because the current drug of choice is *acyclovir* (Zovirax). **Answer 3** is

wrong because currently available therapy is *only palliative*; the virus remains in the body after symptoms subside. **Answer 4** is wrong because hydatidiform mole has a *genetic* basis.

Test-taking tip—Look for the option that reduces chances of transmission of herpes simplex 2.

IMP, 1, HPM, Prevention and Early Detection

86. (**3**) A double-barrel colostomy has two stomas that may or may not be separated by skin. The proximal loop discharges feces, and the distal loop discharges mucus. The closure of this temporary colostomy usually occurs in approximately 6 months. **Answer 1** is an example of an ascending colostomy, **Answer 2** describes a transverse loop colostomy, and **Answer 4** describes a descending colostomy.

Test-taking tip—Visualize two gun barrels. Which option describes two round openings?

PL, 8, PhI, Physiological Adaptation

87. (**1**) Lithium is excreted through the kidneys. Consequently, the kidneys must function adequately to avoid lithium toxicity. Diuretics should *not* be given concurrently with lithium because they may potentiate sodium and fluid depletion, which may lead to lithium toxicity. Haloperidol (Haldol) (**Answer 4**) is a major tranquilizer that is sometimes administered simultaneously with lithium during the first week to 10 days to control manic symptoms. Nausea, vomiting, and muscle weakness (**Answer 3**) are all possible side effects of lithium. They indicate a need for close observation and regulation of the drug if they disrupt the person's level of functioning. Every client should be screened before the administration of any medication (**Answer 2**). However, because lithium is a drug that is taken over a long period of time, blood levels must be consistently regulated and physical examinations routinely scheduled (every 3 months initially, then every 6 months once the client appears to be regulated).

Test-taking tip—Note the phrase "least relevant" and turn this into a "true or false" question. Know that lithium is a salt depleter; therefore, diuretics should *not* be given.

EV, 7, PhI, Pharmacological Therapy

88. (**3**) Sudden spasm and extreme flexion of the calf muscles are relieved by forcibly extending the muscle by hyperextension of the knee and dorsiflexion of the foot. **Answer 1** is wrong because her complaint is due to muscle spasm. **Answer 2** is wrong because relief is accomplished by stretching the muscle; the pain is not due to lowered levels of oxygen in the muscle. **Answer 4** is wrong because increasing placental perfusion will be ineffective in relieving the muscle spasm.

Test-taking tip—Because the complaint is the leg, the best answer is an intervention that deals with the leg, for immediate symptom relief.

IMP, 3, PhI, Reduction of Risk Potential

89. (**4**) To help the child cope with body image changes associated with her burns, the nurse should work with her parents to help her with her physical appearance. Colorful scarves and hats will cover her hairless scalp and pressure stockinette, making her look more like other school-age children. It may also boost her morale. Stuffed animals (**Answer 1**) may harbor bacteria and be a possible source of infection. Her friends (**Answer 2**) will probably not be allowed to visit in the hospital, especially in the burn unit, which is a frightening place for most children. They can call her or send cards and pictures instead; they can visit her when she returns home. Favorite foods (**Answer 3**) will not specifically help the child cope with her injuries and treatment; therefore, this is not a good choice.

Test-taking tip—Think body image concerns that are *age* typical for school-age children, who are influenced by their peers and usually want to "fit in."

IMP, 5, PsI, Coping and Adaptation

90. **(1)** Adolescents are preoccupied with their changing bodies, their relationships, and their fantasies. Although they have difficulty with rote learning (**Answer 2**), they have an increased potential for imaginative thinking. During this period they are less able to concentrate on their academic work (**Answer 3**), which leads to increased feelings of frustration that are usually *not* accompanied by an increased ability to cope (**Answer 4**).

> **Test-taking tip**—Know age-appropriate behavior.

EV, 7, HPM, Growth and Development

91. **(3)** Assisting the mother to develop basic skills in infant care under comfortable professional supervision is the most effective way of increasing a woman's confidence and competence in caring for her infant. **Answer 1** is wrong because although the booklet is a helpful adjunct to teaching, skills are most effectively gained by actual experience. *Note:* Always sensitively assess her ability to read. **Answer 2** is wrong because clear, meaningful communication is inhibited by the language barrier, and actual experience in providing care will be of most assistance to her. **Answer 4** is wrong because basic infant care techniques should be mastered before the mother leaves the hospital with her newborn.

> **Test-taking tip**—Note the use of the word "demonstration" in the stem and in the correct option (**3**). The best answer is a nonverbal, hands-on activity.

IMP, 7, PsI, Coping and Adaptation

92. **(3)** Putting a pinhole in the appliance is the least effective method because it allows flatus to escape immediately and the patient has no control. **Answer 1** is incorrect because foods that cause increased flatus, such as cabbage and broccoli, *should* be avoided. **Answer 2** is incorrect because any deodorant that is safe for mucous membranes *can* be used, or the patient can purchase appliances that have an odor barrier. **Answer 4** is incorrect because emptying the appliance *does* protect the seal in that extra weight from a full pouch will pull at a seal; once the seal is broken, odor can escape.

> **Test-taking tip**—The stem says "least" effective; one option does not *reduce* the gas problem, it just releases the gas.

PL, 8, PhI, Basic Care and Comfort

93. **(3)** Pushing on an incompletely dilated cervix may contribute to development of cervical edema and/or or lacerations. **Answer 1** is wrong because an engaged head occludes the cervix. Neither panting nor normal breathing increases oxygen level (**Answer 2**). **Answer 4** is wrong because breathing patterns do *not* affect cervical dilation.

> **Test-taking tip**—Key information in the stem: head at station 0 (eliminates **1**) and 8 cm dilation (incomplete dilation; same as "before complete dilation" in the correct option **3**). Focus on "normal"; focus on the *time* element (first trimester).

AN, 5, PhI, Reduction of Risk Potential

94. **(1)** The observed total lung capacity (TLC), functional residual capacity (FRC), and residual volume (RV) are all increased over expected values. These values indicate that the patient is hyperinflated, a common phenomenon with air obstruction and air trapping. Hyperventilation is characterized by an increase in P_{O_2} and pH (**Answer 2**). Hyperpnea is simply an increase in respiratory rate (**Answer 3**). Hypercapnia is identified when P_{CO_2} is elevated (**Answer 4**).

> **Test-taking tip**—Look at the *total* capacity (TLC). Visualize a balloon—hyperinflated.

AN, 6, PhI, Physiological Adaptation

95. **(1)** Lice are spread by direct or indirect contact; the child should sleep alone to prevent other family members from also getting lice. In addition, the family should be taught to wash the linens in hot soapy water to kill any lice that are on them. Having the family all get short haircuts (**Answer 2**) or

use a fine-toothed comb (**Answer 4**), or having the child wear a hair net (**Answer 3**), would not necessarily prevent the other family members from getting lice.

> **Test-taking tip**—The focus is on what the *child* needs to do to prevent the spread, not the unaffected *family* members.

IMP, 1, HPM, Prevention and Early Detection of Disease

96. **(2)** The 18-year-old may have valid reasons for wanting to visit a friend, but allowing the patient to visit without assessing motives (**Answer 1**) may prove detrimental to the patient, to the friend, and to the staff. The parents (**Answer 3**) essentially relinquished their decision-making authority by allowing their child to live in the group home. The hospital staff would have to be consulted before the visit, regardless of the patient's motive. However, **Answer 4** is too vague, in that it does not specify what issues would be covered in the consultation.

> **Test-taking tip**—Key word: "assess," the first step of the nursing process.

IMP, 7, PsI, Psychosocial Adaptation

97. **(1)** Understanding the reasons for disconcerting symptoms and receiving assurance of their normalcy assist in coping. **Answer 2** is wrong because although diet may improve the general sense of well-being, diet will *not affect feelings* generated by the developmental tasks of pregnancy. **Answer 3** is wrong because the woman is demonstrating *normal* behavioral changes associated with the first trimester of pregnancy. **Answer 4** is wrong because it does not address the problem.

> **Test-taking tip**—Because these *are normal* physiological and psychological changes that are expected during the first trimester of pregnancy, choose the answer that says these are normal.

IMP, 7, HPM, Growth and Development

98. **(2)** Indications of mediastinal shift and tension pneumothorax include cyanosis, severe dyspnea, and deviation of the trachea and larynx from the normal midline position toward the side of the chest *opposite* the pneumothorax (the unaffected side). Because no blood is available for cardiac output, the blood pressure is absent, not elevated (**Answer 1**). **Answer 3** is incorrect because the lung has collapsed on the affected side, resulting in tympany on percussion, reduced or absent breath sounds, and *hyperresonance*. With a right tension pneumothorax, the heart will shift *laterally* from the normal midclavicular line. If the *left* lung were involved, the heart would shift medially (**Answer 4**).

> **Test-taking tip**—Define the key problem: *pneumo* (air) *thorax* (chest cavity)—pushing on left lung. What would deviate?

AS, 6, PhI, Physiological Adaptation

99. **(4)** It is important for the client who is angry to express feelings overtly. Internalizing them would cause increased feelings of frustration and anxiety and would therefore be counterproductive. **Answers 1, 2,** and **3** *are* all appropriate goals.

> **Test-taking tip**—The question asks for an *inappropriate* nursing goal.

PL, 7, PsI, Psychosocial Adaptation

100. **(1)** A hot tub bath or shower in the morning helps many patients limber up and reduces the symptoms of early morning stiffness. Cold and ice packs are used to a lesser degree, though some patients state that cold decreases localized pain, particularly during acute attacks. Passive ROM exercises (**Answer 2**) may be helpful, but this is not the response of choice because they cannot be done by the patient. Sleeping with a hot pad (**Answer 3**) may cause localized injury. Some patients, however, have found electric blankets helpful in reducing early morning stiffness. Taking salicylates on an empty stomach (**Answer 4**) may increase gastric irritation and distress.

> **Test-taking tip**—Look for nonpharmacological actions that address the *immediate* need.

IMP, 3, PhI, Basic Care and Comfort

UNIT 13

Final Test

Geraldine Colombraro, Sally L. Lagerquist, Bobbi Morrison,
Robyn Nelson, and Janice Stecchi

WHAT IS THE FINAL TEST?

The **Final Test** is a multiple-choice exam designed to assess your baseline nursing knowledge and evaluate your ability to apply that knowledge to various clinical situations and to items presented in a simulated NCLEX-RN exam. Self-analysis of your scores will help you prioritize what to study by identifying your individual problem areas.

Written to reflect the content framework and the purpose of the NCLEX-RN Test Plan (to measure a candidate's ability to practice safely and effectively as a Registered Nurse in an entry-level position), the **Final Test** can be used as preparation and review for the licensure examination. It can also be used for review by *nurses returning to active practice* and by international nurses who are *graduates of nursing schools outside of the United States* and are preparing for qualifying examinations.

Each question on the **Final Test** was field tested in a pilot test given to NCLEX-RN candidates representing a wide geographic distribution, as well as various types of nursing programs.

Selection of Content and Distribution of the Questions

The **Final Test** is composed of 200 content-integrated, multiple-choice questions, each with four options. *One* of the answers is most complete and therefore the best choice. The other three answers (distractors) are not always wrong but are usually not as complete or as important as the best answer.

Using a nursing process framework, the questions on the **Final Test** reflect nursing situations that involve different clinical areas and diagnoses. As on the NCLEX-RN, the number of questions for each content area varies. The percentage distribution of items in this test related to client needs follows the NCLEX-RN blueprint (see **Table 1–1** in **Unit 1,** Orientation, for percentages).

Based on the blueprint for the *Test Plan for The National Council Licensure Examination* (NCLEX-RN) published by the National Council of State Boards of Nursing, Inc., the **Final Test** assesses your knowledge, skills, and abilities in the five phases of the *nursing process:* Assessment (AS), Analysis (AN), Plan (PL), Implementation (IMP), and Evaluation (EV), and four broad areas of *client needs:* Safe, Effective Care Environment (SECE), Physiological Integrity (PhI), Psychosocial Integrity (PsI), and Health Promotion and Maintenance (HPM); and 10 *subcategories* of client needs, including eight detailed areas of *human functions* (Protective, Sensory-Perceptual, Comfort, Rest, Activity and Mobility, Nutrition, Growth and Development, Fluid-Gas Transport, Psychosocial-Cultural, Elimination). Each question in the **Final Test** has been classified according to the above categories.

Timing

Allow about 1 minute per question. Time yourself and plan to complete the 200-question test in no more than 3.5 hours. Simulate test-taking conditions by having uninterrupted time of 3.5 hours, or divide the exam into two sessions of 100 questions for 1 hour and 45 minutes for each session.

Test Results

When you check your answers, keep track not only of how many are incorrect, but also how many are incorrect in *each category* of nursing process, client needs, and human functions.

Suggestions for Further Study

You can use your test results, in combination with the following appendices, to assess your NCLEX-RN strengths and weaknesses.

I.	When you have problems with *types* of questions	Refer to Appendix:
	A. Nursing process	
	1. Definitions/Descriptions	F
	2. Index to nursing process *questions*	G

II.	When you have problems with *content*/subject areas	Refer to Appendix:
	A. Client needs (4 broad categories and 10 subcategories)	
	1. Definitions/Descriptions	B
	2. Index to *content*	C
	3. Index to *practice questions that cover these content areas*	D, E
	B. Human functions (8 specific concepts and detailed areas)	
	1. Definitions/Descriptions	H
	2. Index to *content*	I
	3. Index to *practice questions that cover these content areas*	J

You now have an individualized evaluation with which to develop your plan for *what* you need to study and *where* to find the material for further study. Our good wishes for your success!

QUESTIONS

Select the one best answer for each question.

1. Which statement by the nurse would correctly characterize essential hypertension?
    1. Forty percent of the American adult population is affected by hypertension.
    2. Essential hypertension is more severe in men than women.
    3. American blacks develop hypertension at an earlier age than whites but have a lower mortality rate.
    4. Given newer screening devices, most persons with hypertension are now being detected.

2. In assessing a woman's reasons for suspecting she may be 3 months pregnant, the most relevant question for the nurse to ask would be:
    1. "Are you currently taking oral contraceptives?"
    2. "When was your last menstrual period?"
    3. "How much weight have you gained?"
    4. "Have you been pregnant before?"

3. When caring for a child who has experienced severe burn(s) of the oral cavity and possibly of the esophagus, pharynx, and larynx, the primary nursing intervention should be:
    1. Observe for symptoms of shock.
    2. Check airway for signs of obstruction.
    3. Maintain adequate hydration by offering small amounts of clear liquid.
    4. Initiate intravenous therapy immediately.

4. A patient with a history of substance abuse is admitted to the hospital after being brought there by police; the patient had been found on school property running around in the nude with several other students. The patient appeared to be hallucinating. The nurse who admits this patient to the unit should be primarily concerned with:
    1. Providing a general orientation to the unit.
    2. Maintaining a quiet environment.
    3. Taking precautions against seizures.
    4. Taking vital signs every 4 hours.

5. A patient with a history of severe abdominal cramping and vomiting a moderate amount of blood arrives at the emergency department. The nurse's *primary* concern should be:
    1. Observing for signs and symptoms of shock.
    2. Immediately paging the physician on call.
    3. Filling out the appropriate assessment tool.
    4. Immediately administering CPR.

6. The nurse considers information regarding smoking cigarettes and marijuana essential for pregnant women because it is well established that these activities may lead to:
    1. Retarded infants.
    2. Low-birth-weight infants.
    3. Deformed infants.
    4. Malnourished infants.

7. The nurse finds a post-MI patient slumped on the side rails of the bed. The patient does not respond when the nurse shakes the patient's shoulders and loudly calls the patient's name. The nurse's next action is to:
    1. Call for help and note the time.
    2. Clear the airway.
    3. Give two sharp thumps to the precordium.
    4. Administer two quick breaths.

8. Postoperative orders include "IV of D5 ¼ NS at 75 mL per hour." At 7:00 P.M., a new 1000 mL bag of fluid is hung. If the IV infuses at the prescribed rate, how much fluid should be left in the bag at 7:00 A.M.?
    1. 100 mL.
    2. 900 mL.
    3. Nothing should be left; bag should be empty.
    4. Not enough information is given to determine this.

9. As a cardiac patient gets up to use the commode, he turns ashen and diaphoretic. Vital signs are as follows: BP 128/60, pulse 42, respirations 24. ECG shows patterns of complete heart block. The nurse knows that the patient's signs and symptoms are related to:
    1. Inability of heart to increase its rate during exertion.
    2. Insufficient blood flow to the coronary arteries.
    3. Increased stroke volume.
    4. Inability of the circulatory reflexes to increase venous return.

10. A woman is in labor; she and the father learn that the fetus is in the transverse position. The father tells the nurse that they had counted on his being with her throughout their baby's birth. The nurse's most therapeutic response would be to:
    1. Refer him to the attending physician for permission to attend the birth.
    2. Ask if he has attended childbirth education classes.
    3. Check with the attending physician and relay the response to the couple.
    4. Tell the father to dress and meet the nurse in the cesarean room.

11. Parents of an infant on an apnea monitor ask the nurse what the monitor will do. The nurse's most appropriate response would be:
    1. "It will stimulate your baby's breathing."
    2. "It will monitor your baby's vital signs."
    3. "It will sound an alarm if your baby's breathing stops."
    4. "It will maintain your baby's respirations."

12. Preoperative teaching includes deep breathing and coughing. What is the *least* desired outcome of the teaching plan? The patient:
    1. States the rationale for repeating these exercises every 1–2 hours postoperatively.
    2. Demonstrates coughing technique.
    3. Inhales through both nose and mouth and raises abdomen with each respiration.
    4. States she recognizes the need to repeat exercises until she is feeling light-headed.

Questions

13. A patient's blood gases are as follows: Po_2 85, Pco_2 37, pH 7.35, HCO_3 19. The nurse's analysis of this patient's blood gases indicate:
    1. Compensated metabolic acidosis.
    2. Hyperventilation.
    3. Uncompensated metabolic acidosis.
    4. Alveolar hypoventilation.

14. In doing a child's admission assessment, the nurse should be alert to note which signs/symptoms of chronic lead poisoning?
    1. Irritability and seizures.
    2. Dehydration and diarrhea.
    3. Bradycardia and hypotension.
    4. Petechiae and hematuria.

15. A woman is hospitalized with mild preeclampsia. In planning the woman's care during this hospitalization, which nursing order is *least* likely to be implemented?
    1. Vital signs and FHR and rhythm q4h while awake.
    2. Daily weight.
    3. Deep-tendon reflexes once per shift.
    4. Absolute bed rest.

16. The nurse prepares a patient for tracheostomy based on the knowledge that the purpose of a tracheostomy is to:
    1. Decrease patient anxiety by increasing the size of the airway.
    2. Provide more controlled ventilation and ease removal of secretions the patient is unable to handle.
    3. Provide increased cerebral oxygenation, thereby preventing further respiratory depression.
    4. Facilitate nursing care, because tracheal tubes have fewer side effects than nasotracheal tubes.

17. A teenager with a history of substance abuse is hospitalized for hallucinatory behavior. The mother is very upset. She is in the waiting room crying uncontrollably. The most appropriate nursing action would be to:
    1. Provide privacy for her.
    2. Ask the physician to order diazepam (Valium) for her.
    3. Contact her husband.
    4. Offer to sit with her.

18. The pressure dressing placed after modified mastectomy encircles the patient's chest and fits very snugly. The nurse should anticipate difficulty in which postoperative nursing function?
    1. Maintaining good body alignment.
    2. Initiating arm exercises.
    3. Promoting deep breathing and coughing.
    4. Taking vital signs.

19. The nurse must be on the alert constantly for anaphylaxis, an immediate hypersensitivity reaction, characterized by local reactions such as:
    1. Angioedema.
    2. Cardiovascular collapse.
    3. Nausea, vomiting, diarrhea.
    4. Asthma-like symptoms.

20. If the first day of a pregnant woman's last menstrual period (LMP) was July 10, what is her baby's expected date of birth (EDB)?
    1. April 17.
    2. May 30.
    3. March 14.
    4. June 1.

21. At 7:00 A.M., the night nurse hangs a new 500 mL bag of D5 ½ NS and adjusts the flow rate to 35 mL/hr per MD order. If the IV infuses at the proper rate, how much fluid should be left in the bag when the day nurse makes rounds at 11:30 A.M., halfway through the shift?
    1. 160 mL.
    2. 250 mL.
    3. 340 mL.
    4. Unable to determine.

22. An adolescent patient with a history of substance abuse asks the nurse, "Have you ever used drugs?" The most appropriate nursing response would be:
    1. "Yes, once I tried grass."
    2. "Why do you want to know?"
    3. "How will my answer help you?"
    4. "No, I don't think so."

23. A woman is in labor; her membranes are ruptured by the attending physician. The nurse should expect the amniotic fluid to:
    1. Be slightly bloody.
    2. Have a slightly pungent odor.
    3. Have a thick consistency.
    4. Turn litmus paper blue.

24. The nurse should know that the majority of amputations are attributed to:
    1. Chemical burns.
    2. Diabetic ulcers.
    3. Arteriosclerosis obliterans.
    4. Bone tumors.

25. A 15-year-old is admitted to the hospital with a compound fracture of the left tibia and patella following a minibike accident. The fractures are repaired surgically, and a long leg cast is applied. During the first night in the hospital, the patient complains of severe pain in the left leg. At this time, it would be most appropriate for the nurse to:
    1. Obtain more information about the characteristics of the pain.
    2. Give the patient a dose of "Demerol 50 mg IM prn q4–6h" as ordered.
    3. Reassure the patient that the pain will diminish in a few days.
    4. Distract the patient by turning on the television.

26. When caring for a child who has received a diazepam (Valium) "IV push" × 2 during a procedure, which vital sign should the nurse evaluate *first*?
    1. Temperature.
    2. Pulse.

3. Respirations.

4. Blood pressure.

27. Several weeks after the funeral of one of her twin infants, a mother tells the community health nurse that she is experiencing difficulty producing enough breast milk to satisfy the other infant. The most appropriate response for the nurse to make would be:

    1. "You probably have a virus and should see a doctor right away."

    2. "Your baby is probably reacting to the loss of a sibling and not sucking long enough to stimulate an adequate supply."

    3. "Milk production may decrease with an increase in stress."

    4. "The lactation ducts may be occluded."

28. When parents ask how their baby might have gotten pyloric stenosis, the nurse should tell them that:

    1. Their baby was born with this condition.

    2. Their baby acquired it due to a formula allergy.

    3. Their baby developed this condition during the first few weeks of life.

    4. There is no way to determine this preoperatively.

29. Morphine sulfate, 0.6 mg, has been ordered to relieve the chest pain of a patient who has had an anterior MI. The nurse would give this narcotic to:

    1. Increase the threshold for pain tolerance and decrease arterial resistance.

    2. Increase arterial resistance and reduce apprehension and anxiety, as well as pain.

    3. Relieve apprehension, anxiety, and pain and stimulate medullary respiratory centers.

    4. Reduce venous capacitance and reduce pain threshold.

30. A pregnant woman with severe preeclampsia is at 38 weeks of gestation; she is in active labor, with contractions every 10 minutes, and her membranes ruptured 45 minutes ago. Her husband is with her. The nurse's primary intervention would be to:

    1. Teach the couple about the stages of labor.

    2. Prepare the woman for birth.

    3. Assess the couple's degree of preparation.

    4. Answer any questions the couple may have.

31. In preparing preop injections for a 3-year-old, which size needle would the nurse be most correct in selecting to administer the IM injection?

    1. 25 G, ⅝ inch.

    2. 21 G, 1 inch.

    3. 18 G, 1 inch.

    4. 18 G, 1½ inch.

32. The physician orders the insertion of a permanent pacemaker for a patient with complete heart block. In preparing a preoperative teaching plan for this patient, the nurse would initially:

    1. Assess the patient's interest in learning about the procedure and current understanding.

    2. Invite the patient's family to join the preoperative teaching session.

    3. Ascertain from the physician the amount of information she or he has given the patient.

    4. Have the operative permit signed, then institute the teaching plan.

33. Following administration of preoperative medication, it is important for the nurse to:

    1. Position the patient in high Fowler's position to improve ventilation.

    2. Let the patient know that the patient will be asleep when the nurse leaves the unit.

    3. Tell the patient that a nurse will be there when the patient returns.

    4. Get the patient up to the bathroom when he or she complains of bladder fullness.

34. In the first few hours after cardiac catheterization, which nursing measure would be most essential?

    1. Checking pedal pulse in the extremity used for the cut-down.

    2. Encouraging the patient to cough and deep breathe hourly.

    3. Keeping the patient sedated to maintain the pressure dressing.

    4. Monitoring the patient's urine output.

35. The nurse has established the unresponsiveness of a patient. After the airway is opened, the next nursing action would be to:

    1. Look, listen, and feel for breathing.

    2. Pinch the patient's nostrils and give two full breaths.

    3. Check the patient's carotid pulse for 5–10 seconds.

    4. Finger sweep the patient's mouth for any foreign object.

36. While the nurse is changing a CVP dressing, the patient becomes tachypneic and complains of chest pain. The nurse suspects the symptoms are related to an air embolism. The first nursing priority would be to position the patient:

    1. In Trendelenburg.

    2. On the left side, head down.

    3. On the right side, head up.

    4. Supine, in high Fowler's.

37. A pregnant woman is in active labor and has not received any anesthesia. She is in the transitional phase of the first stage of labor. During this time the nurse would expect her to be:

    1. Irritable.

    2. Excited.

    3. Euphoric.

    4. Serious.

38. An adolescent patient's girlfriend comes to visit him in the hospital. The nurse suspects that they may become intimate. What is the most appropriate nursing intervention?

    1. Do not allow his girlfriend to visit.

    2. Inform the couple that "necking" is prohibited.

    3. Provide privacy from staff and other clients.

    4. Allow visitation with supervision.

39. A patient is to be discharged on a 2 g sodium diet. The nurse would know that the patient understands the dietary limitations if he or she selected:
    1. Filet of sole, tossed salad with lemon juice, coffee.
    2. Chow mein, fried rice, tea.
    3. Canned tomato soup, unsalted crackers, skim milk.
    4. Two hot dogs with mustard, macaroni salad, ginger ale.

40. A patient complains of increasing shortness of breath with exercise. On physical examination, the patient is found to be moderately overweight and has BP 152/105, pulse 81, respirations 16, and fine basilar crackles in both lung fields, and the point of maximal impulse (PMI) is shifted to the left and down by 1.5 cm. The best explanation the nurse could offer this patient is that this shortness of breath is most likely related to:
    1. Inadequate functioning of the left ventricle.
    2. Insufficient blood return to the right side of the heart.
    3. Asynergistic pumping of the left ventricle.
    4. Obesity and sedentary lifestyle.

41. The best approach for the nurse to take in administering a preop injection to a preschooler would be to:
    1. Ask the mother to explain the injection to the child.
    2. Simply give the injection as quickly as possible without telling the child anything, because it may scare the child.
    3. Give a short and simple explanation immediately before giving the injection.
    4. Tell the child the injection must be given and then the mother can read a story.

42. The nurse explains that the *primary* objective of a preoperative skin prep is:
    1. To clean the skin of excess oils and hair.
    2. To prevent postoperative infection by sterilizing the skin.
    3. To prevent postoperative infection by reducing the number of microorganisms on the skin.
    4. To provide a clear field for the incision.

43. Because a patient who hallucinates is not in touch with reality, the most appropriate nursing intervention would be to:
    1. Maintain a safe environment.
    2. Establish a trusting relationship.
    3. Orient the patient to time, place, and person.
    4. Isolate the patient from other patients.

44. Which hobby will most likely be restricted for an adult following recovery from pacemaker insertion?
    1. Swimming.
    2. Fashioning lamps from driftwood and metal.
    3. Operating ham radio.
    4. Playing golf.

45. During the first 24–48 hours after admission, the most appropriate diet for a patient who has GI bleeding is likely to be:
    1. NPO.
    2. Clear liquids.
    3. A soft, bland diet.
    4. Skim or regular milk.

46. If a woman is pregnant for the second time, but her first pregnancy did not reach viability, what would be her parity using the four-digit scoring system?
    1. 1-0-0-1.
    2. 0-0-1-0.
    3. 0-1-0-0.
    4. 0-1-0-1.

47. After determining that a patient is pulseless, the nurse would begin adult one-person CPR at a minimum compression rate of:
    1. 60 compressions per minute.
    2. 80 compressions per minute.
    3. 90 compressions per minute.
    4. 100 compressions per minute.

48. A patient has had an appendectomy, following a ruptured appendix. During postop care, the nurses' notes in this patient's chart should include documentation of:
    1. Teaching to prevent dumping syndrome and to promote early ambulation.
    2. Frequent mouth care and dressing changes, including drainage.
    3. Bowel sounds, intake and output, and the need for a low-residue diet.
    4. Dressing changes, intake and output, and bowel sounds.

49. Three hours after admission to the CCU for anterior myocardial infarction (MI), a patient develops increasing ventricular ectopy, followed by a short burst of ventricular tachycardia. The first nursing action is to:
    1. Notify the attending physician.
    2. Increase the flow of O_2 from 4 to 8 liters.
    3. Administer a bolus of lidocaine, per order.
    4. Repeat the morphine sulfate, per order.

50. Sudden infant death syndrome (SIDS) occurs most frequently with which risk factor?
    1. Hispanic.
    2. Low birth weight.
    3. Midrange socioeconomic status.
    4. Breastfeeding.

51. After a patient returns from surgery following craniotomy, the nurse knows that the optimum positioning of a neurosurgery patient, unless otherwise indicated, would be:
    1. Flat on back.
    2. Head elevated 30 degrees.
    3. Head elevated 45 degrees.
    4. Head elevated 90 degrees.

52. Immediately before a woman is to give birth, her husband expresses anxiety about staying with her. The *most* appropriate response the nurse could make would be:
    1. "Many people feel frightened at this time."
    2. "You'll do fine, don't worry."

3. "Think of your wife. How will she feel if you don't stay?"

4. "Once things get going, you'll forget about being afraid."

53. Which type of anesthesia should the nurse anticipate will be used for an amputation?
    1. IV regional.
    2. Spinal.
    3. General intravenous and inhalation anesthesia.
    4. Muscle relaxant.

54. To facilitate the proper drying of a long leg cast, the nurse should include which measure in the plan of care?
    1. Leave the cast exposed to the air.
    2. Encourage the patient to remain in one position.
    3. Place the patient on a bedboard.
    4. Use only tips of the fingers to handle the cast.

55. Which nursing care procedure is *least* important during the period before insertion of the pacemaker?
    1. Providing sedation to relieve anxiety and promote relaxation as needed.
    2. Instituting arm and leg range-of-motion exercises to prevent postinsertion complications.
    3. Establishing an intravenous line and having emergency equipment and medications available.
    4. Weighing the patient and instituting intake and output records.

56. On turning a patient who has had a right modified mastectomy to her left side, the nurse notes a moderately large amount of serosanguineous drainage on the bedsheets. The nurse should:
    1. Remove the dressing to ascertain the origin of the bleeding.
    2. Milk the Hemovac tubing, using a downward motion.
    3. Note vital signs, reinforce the dressing, and notify the surgeon immediately.
    4. Recognize that this is a frequent occurrence with this type of surgery.

57. Immediately following birth, an infant's condition is assessed. The respirations do not establish readily, there is slight cyanosis, and there is some muscle flaccidity. The most appropriate nursing action would be to:
    1. Initiate CPR immediately.
    2. Clear airway and administer oxygen.
    3. Reassure the parents.
    4. Check the mother's chart for her last medication (drug, time, and amount).

58. Which nursing action is essential to prevent hypoxemia during tracheal suctioning?
    1. Removing oral and nasal secretions.
    2. Encouraging the patient to deep breathe and cough to facilitate removal of upper-airway secretions.
    3. Administering 100% oxygen to reduce the effects of airway obstruction during suctioning.

4. Auscultating the lungs to determine the baseline data to assess the effectiveness of suctioning.

59. An expectant couple is informed that a cesarean will be performed immediately. The couple inquire whether the mother must be put to sleep. The most appropriate nursing response would be to:
    1. Refer the couple to the anesthesiologist.
    2. Ask the attending physician to explain the procedure to the couple.
    3. Tell the couple that she probably will receive general anesthesia.
    4. Inform the couple that most women who have a cesarean birth receive spinal anesthesia.

60. A client is hospitalized for substance abuse and hallucinatory behavior. During the admission procedure, in assessing this client's mother, the nurse would expect her initial reaction to be:
    1. Anger.
    2. Denial.
    3. Acceptance.
    4. Shock.

61. What should the nurse see in the vomitus that is characteristic of infants with pyloric stenosis?
    1. Stomach contents only.
    2. Stomach contents plus bile.
    3. Stomach contents streaked with blood.
    4. Stomach contents with flecks of feces.

62. At 36 weeks, a pregnant woman's preeclamptic condition changes: she has hyperreflexia, generalized edema, and ataxia. If she begins to have a convulsion, the nurse's *primary* action should be:
    1. Maintain patent airway.
    2. Observe for bowel or bladder evacuation.
    3. Administer cardiopulmonary resuscitation.
    4. Maintain a safe environment.

63. An assessment finding in a patient with an MI that would be an early indicator of the extent of tissue necrosis in the heart is:
    1. The duration of sinus tachycardia.
    2. CPK and ALT (SGOT) enzyme measures.
    3. The duration of chest pain.
    4. The occurrence of primary ventricular fibrillation.

64. Which system should the nurse monitor carefully for possible toxic effects of EDTA?
    1. Neurological.
    2. Renal.
    3. Cardiovascular.
    4. Hematological.

65. The nurse knows that a modified radical mastectomy involves removal of:
    1. The breast only.
    2. The breast and axillary nodes.
    3. The breast, pectoralis major muscle, and axillary lymph nodes.
    4. The breast, underlying chest muscle, axillary lymph nodes, and internal mammary lymph nodes.

66. An adolescent patient's friend brings a marijuana cigarette. The nurse finds the cigarette under the patient's pillow. The most appropriate nursing action would be to:
    1. Ignore the situation.
    2. Inform the police.
    3. Discuss the incident with the patient's parents.
    4. Confront the patient.

67. On the first postoperative day following an above-the-knee amputation, a patient's surgeon ordered rehabilitation exercises to begin. Which is most important for the nurse to initiate *first*?
    1. External rotation of the stump.
    2. Hyperextension of the thigh and stump.
    3. Lifting the buttock and stump off the bed while the patient is lying flat on the back.
    4. Arm exercises to prepare for crutch walking.

68. A toddler is admitted to the hospital with severe eczema lesions on the face, scalp, neck, and arms. The best nursing intervention to prevent the toddler from scratching the affected areas would be to apply:
    1. Clove-hitch restraints to the hands.
    2. Elbow restraints to the arms.
    3. Mittens to the hands.
    4. A posey jacket to the torso.

69. During the first stage of labor, maternal and fetal vital signs must be closely monitored. The best time to observe maternal vital signs is:
    1. Immediately before a contraction.
    2. Between contractions.
    3. Immediately after a contraction.
    4. Any time the mother feels totally comfortable.

70. A child admitted to rule out intussusception is scheduled for a barium enema. The nurse should teach the child's parents that the major purpose of this procedure is to:
    1. Confirm the diagnosis.
    2. Reduce the telescoping.
    3. Ease the passage of stool.
    4. Provide symptomatic relief.

71. If a woman is 3 months pregnant, what symptom or symptoms would the nurse's assessment most likely discover?
    1. Quickening.
    2. Lightening.
    3. Breast tingling and tenderness.
    4. Nausea and vomiting.

72. A patient is to have a breast biopsy and possible mastectomy. Before going to see this patient the morning of surgery, the nurse assigned to assist her in the final preparations for surgery should first:
    1. Prepare the preoperative medication.
    2. Check to be sure the operative permit has been signed.
    3. Check to see if the preoperative laboratory reports have been placed in the chart.
    4. Check the diet orders to be sure the patient has been placed on the NPO list.

73. The attending physician and anesthesiologist decide to administer spinal anesthesia for a cesarean birth. The nurse knows the amount of anesthesia used will be as minimal as possible because spinal anesthesia:
    1. Produces severe fetal depression.
    2. Causes maternal hypotension.
    3. Rapidly crosses the placenta.
    4. Depresses maternal respirations.

74. A client's mother asks the nurse what caused her son to take drugs. The most therapeutic response would be:
    1. "He probably wanted to be like his peers."
    2. "Inappropriate limits were probably set on his behavior."
    3. "It involves many factors."
    4. "He felt isolated and unloved."

75. At 2:30 A.M., the nurse hangs a 1000 mL bottle of IV fluid. If the IV infuses at 110 mL per hour as ordered, how much fluid should infuse by 6:00 A.M.?
    1. 385 mL.
    2. 500 mL.
    3. 615 mL.
    4. 740 mL.

76. When teaching the parents about an apnea monitor, the nurse should stress:
    1. "Always respond to the monitor alarm immediately."
    2. "Initiate CPR whenever the alarm sounds."
    3. "A responsible adult must remain in the room with the infant at all times."
    4. "Call the emergency department during any episodes of apnea."

77. On admission to the recovery room, a patient is very restless. The respirations are deep and somewhat irregular; the patient startles easily and moans at the nurse's touch. The best nursing action is:
    1. Continue to stimulate the patient by saying that the operation is over.
    2. Raise the side rails and remain quietly in attendance.
    3. Administer meperidine (Demerol) HCl, 100 mg IM.
    4. Check the nailbeds for cyanosis.

78. On the third day of hospitalization following an anterior MI, a patient becomes increasingly restless. Pulse rate has increased to 126 beats per minute. The first nursing action is to:
    1. Do a partial physical assessment, which includes vital signs, pulmonary auscultation, and cognitive functions.
    2. Ask if the patient is upset, because depression is common on the third day of hospitalization.
    3. Readminister oxygen per nasal catheter (prongs or tongs) at 6 liters, because restlessness is an early sign of cerebral hypoxia.
    4. Decrease the rate of intravenous infusion to prevent fluid volume overload.

79. While observing a patient throughout a blood transfusion, the nurse should be alert to which possible sign of a hemolytic reaction?
    1. Urticaria.
    2. Polyuria.
    3. Flank pain.
    4. Hypothermia.
80. A patient is awaiting the insertion of a pacemaker. The blood pressure is 128/60. Which medication should the nurse have available during this patient's preoperative period?
    1. Lidocaine (Xylocaine).
    2. Atropine sulfate.
    3. Digoxin.
    4. Propranolol hydrochloride (Inderal).
81. In considering the equipment for Bryant's traction, the nurse should expect to see:
    1. A Kirschner wire in the fractured femur.
    2. A Steinmann pin in the fractured femur.
    3. Adhesive material taped to the skin of both legs.
    4. Adhesive material taped to the skin of the fractured leg only.
82. In providing health teaching for an expectant couple, what should the nurse tell them is a *probable* sign of pregnancy?
    1. Fetal heart sounds.
    2. Positive pregnancy test.
    3. Fetal movements felt by examiner.
    4. Outline of fetus on sonogram.
83. The physician suspects that a patient has a peptic ulcer. The nurse should expect the physician to order which diet after the first 48–72 hours?
    1. Small feedings of bland food.
    2. Frequent feedings of clear liquids.
    3. A regular diet given frequently in small amounts.
    4. NPO.
84. A patient tells the nurse that there are big white ants crawling all over the wall. The most appropriate nursing response would be:
    1. "Where are they? I'll kill them for you."
    2. "You must be seeing things."
    3. Silence.
    4. "I don't see any ants; but you seem afraid."
85. In assisting a patient to prepare for immediate surgery, what would the nurse do?
    1. Remove the patient's wedding band.
    2. Begin exploring the patient's fears and anxieties about surgery.
    3. Assist in removing dentures and nail polish.
    4. Remind the patient to void following preoperative medication.
86. A patient is to be discharged on the antihypertensive drug reserpine. The nurse's instructions to avoid intermittent hypotension would include:
    1. "Rise slowly from sitting or lying."
    2. "Ingest alcohol to prevent hypotension."
    3. "Avoid cold weather, which precipitates attacks."
    4. "Exercise to decrease sudden vasodilation."

87. The nurse administers preop medication, atropine (0.15 mg) IM. Fifteen minutes later, the patient is breathing rapidly and has a flushed, red face. The nurse should:
    1. Administer the atropine antidote stat.
    2. Give the patient a cool sponge bath.
    3. Tell the patient these are normal side effects of atropine.
    4. Page and advise the surgeon of the patient's condition before transporting the patient to the operating room.
88. The nurse has discussed important aspects of breast-feeding with a new mother. To evaluate the effects of the teaching, the nurse asks her to put it in her own words. Which response indicates a need for further teaching?
    1. "Rest and relaxation are essential."
    2. "An adequate diet is important."
    3. "Large breasts produce more milk."
    4. "Birth control is necessary throughout breastfeeding if I don't want to become pregnant."
89. A patient who has had a modified mastectomy begins to demonstrate some early signs of shock, such as increased pulse, cool, clammy skin, and restlessness. The nurse could enhance venous return by:
    1. Administering oxygen via mask to reduce restlessness.
    2. Keeping trunk flat and raising foot of bed.
    3. Placing her in Trendelenburg position.
    4. Wrapping her entire body in warmed blankets.
90. In discussing what clothes a toddler with eczema should wear, both in the hospital and at home, the nurse would be most correct in teaching the mother that this child should wear only:
    1. Cotton.
    2. Linen.
    3. Natural wool.
    4. Polyester blend.
91. The physician orders a soapsuds enema for a woman in preterm labor whose membranes have ruptured. The most appropriate nursing action would be to:
    1. Administer the enema as soon as possible.
    2. Recheck the order for the type of enema.
    3. Refuse to administer the enema because this is a preterm labor and membranes have ruptured.
    4. Ask the physician to check the fetal position before giving the enema.
92. While doing chest compressions during CPR on an adult, the nurse hears a "cracking" sound. The appropriate response would be to:
    1. Stop chest compressions immediately and ventilate only.
    2. Compress no more than 1.5 inch.
    3. Check for proper hand placement and continue.
    4. Have someone else who is not as strong do compressions.

93. A pregnant woman verbalizes concern about the possibility of having to remain hospitalized for the next 8 weeks because of her preeclampsia. The *most* therapeutic response the nurse could make would be:
  1. "It may not be that bad if you keep busy."
  2. "Tell me how you are feeling."
  3. "I'll sit with you a while."
  4. "Maybe you should tell your doctor how you are feeling."

94. A patient should be able to describe signs of pacemaker malfunction. Which behavior would indicate that this goal has been met?
  1. Counts pulse correctly and identifies need to monitor rate daily.
  2. Counts pulse correctly and identifies the significance of drainage or discoloration around the battery insertion site.
  3. Counts pulse correctly, states the estimated life of the battery, and understands need for prophylactic replacement.
  4. Counts pulse correctly and identifies need to report rate changes and symptoms such as dizziness, palpitations, and hiccoughs.

95. A pregnant woman is in early labor; she has a history of drinking alcohol and of smoking cigarettes and marijuana, although she stopped when she learned she was pregnant. Her husband expresses some concern over his wife's previous smoking habits. The nurse should inform him that:
  1. Although she no longer smokes, she was exposed to cigarette and marijuana smoke, which could affect her pregnancy.
  2. She is assured of a healthy infant because she stopped smoking as soon as she knew she was pregnant.
  3. The early labor is probably due to her smoking marijuana.
  4. Alcohol is considered much safer than marijuana.

96. A patient with a left leg fracture is to be taught the three-point gait before discharge. This patient should be given which instruction by the nurse?
  1. "Advance your right crutch, swing the left foot forward, advance the left crutch, and then bring the right foot forward."
  2. "Move your right crutch and left foot forward together, and then swing the right foot and left crutch in one movement."
  3. "While partially bearing weight on your left leg, advance both crutches and then bring your right leg forward."
  4. "Using one movement, advance your left foot and both crutches and then bring your right leg forward."

97. Immediately postoperative, after general anesthesia, a patient has an airway in place and is in a supine position. To prevent airway obstruction, the nurse should:
  1. Leave the airway tube in and turn the patient's head to the side.
  2. Maintain the patient's present position.
  3. Remove the airway tube and turn the patient's head to the side.
  4. Remove the airway tube and maintain the patient's prone position.

98. A patient with a history of substance abuse asks the nurse not to tell anyone about the patient smoking a marijuana joint in the hospital room, and the patient promises to never do it again. The nurse should realize that this patient is *mostly*:
  1. Being sincere and wanting to change.
  2. Seeking attention.
  3. Being manipulative.
  4. Trying to avoid punishment.

99. The nurse can expect increased restlessness in a patient with tachycardia following an anterior myocardial infarction because:
  1. Decreased ventricular filling time results in decreased venous return and cerebral edema.
  2. Palpitations result in anxiety.
  3. Decreased ventricular filling time always results in decreased cardiac output and tissue perfusion.
  4. A significant decrease in stroke volume may occur, causing a decrease in cardiac output.

100. To evaluate a mother's understanding of the discussion about Down syndrome, the nurse would ask her to explain the syndrome in her own words. Which response indicates a need for further health teaching?
  1. "Down syndrome is an abnormality that can result from an extra chromosome."
  2. "Only children born to older women have Down syndrome."
  3. "A test can be done to diagnose Down syndrome while the fetus is still in utero."
  4. "Down syndrome includes a form of mental retardation."

101. A patient is to have an above-the-knee (AK) amputation for severe vascular insufficiency and gangrene of the foot. The best explanation by the nurse for why the patient is to have this amputation would be:
  1. The degree of vascular insufficiency is extensive.
  2. AK amputees are better suited for a prosthesis.
  3. The higher the amputation, the less energy required for rehabilitation of balance and walking.
  4. Below-the-knee amputation heals less successfully.

102. The proper method of suctioning a tracheostomy tube includes:
  1. Suctioning only while inserting the catheter.
  2. Suctioning only while withdrawing the catheter.
  3. Suctioning during both insertion and withdrawal of the catheter.
  4. Suctioning on insertion only if secretions are copious.

103. In assessing a woman in labor following the administration of spinal anesthesia, the nurse should realize that if she can wiggle her toes:
  1. The effect of the spinal anesthesia has dissipated.
  2. She may still become hypotensive.

3. This behavior is essentially meaningless.

4. She is prone to hypertension.

104. To help a preschooler cope most effectively with repeated painful injections of EDTA, the nurse should:

1. Teach the mother the importance of bringing favorite toys.

2. Encourage the child to spend most of the day in the playroom, engaged in free play.

3. Offer the opportunity for therapeutic play.

4. Allow play with other preschool children as much as the child wants.

105. Which arm position will best facilitate venous return on the operative side of a patient who has had a modified mastectomy, and reduce the occurrence of lymphedema?

1. Semi-Fowler's position with the elbow flexed and the arm across the chest.

2. Low Fowler's position with the arm elevated so that the hand and elbow are slightly higher than the shoulder.

3. High Fowler's position with the elbow flexed and the right hand positioned next to the head.

4. Adduction of the shoulder, extension of the elbow, and flexion of the wrist.

106. The most important aspect of treatment for a client who is a substance abuser is:

1. Teaching the client about the hazards of taking drugs.

2. Informing the client that using drugs is illegal.

3. Encouraging the client to want to change behavior.

4. Assisting the client to develop alternative coping mechanisms.

107. Two hours after a child returns to the unit following cardiac catheterization, the dressing is soaked with bright-red blood. The nurse first reinforces the dressing. What should the nurse do next?

1. Check vital signs.

2. Increase the flow rate of the IV.

3. Place the child in reverse Trendelenburg position.

4. Notify the cardiologist.

108. New parents express concern about when they can resume intercourse. After validating the information with the physician, the nurse would inform the couple that:

1. Generally it is a good idea to wait until after the sixth-week postpartum checkup.

2. If there are no unforeseen problems, 3 weeks is usually the recommended waiting time.

3. The couple may have sex as soon as they arrive home from the hospital, as long as the mother feels up to it.

4. The couple should wait until the mother ceases to breastfeed.

109. A patient is awaiting the insertion of a permanent pacemaker because of complete heart block. The nurse knows that isoproterenol hydrochloride (Isuprel) is used for this patient because of which effect?

1. Beta-mimetic.

2. Cardiac glycoside.

3. Anticholinergic.

4. Beta-blocker.

110. A pregnant woman is hospitalized for preeclampsia. She and her husband express anxiety about having limited insurance, which may not cover this hospitalization. The *most* appropriate nursing intervention would be to:

1. Refer the couple to social services for possible assistance.

2. Initiate a family-counseling referral.

3. Provide supportive counseling.

4. Assess the couple's needs through discussion.

111. A patient has had an above-the-knee amputation on the left side. While being repositioned onto the abdomen, the patient cannot turn because the "left foot is causing too much pain." The first response by the nurse should be:

1. To insist that the patient lie on the abdomen.

2. To ignore the comment and state that the nurse will return later.

3. To discuss the principle of phantom pain after amputation.

4. To offer some form of pain control.

112. During a predischarge teaching session for a patient who has had a permanent pacemaker inserted, the patient's wife states, "Don't worry, I'll be sure that he obeys the doctor's orders to the letter." The nurse's best response would be:

1. "I can see that with your help, he should do just fine."

2. "Are you worried?"

3. "I'm not worried. You both have a lot of common sense."

4. "This has been a difficult period for both of you. Can you foresee any problems with these instructions?"

113. In planning initial care for an adolescent client who is a substance abuser, the nurse should:

1. Be very direct with the client.

2. Allow the client to make all the decisions about his or her care.

3. Help the client to feel very secure to prevent anxiety.

4. Encourage the client to begin to depend on others.

114. Upon return from the OR at 11:30 A.M., a patient has 425 mL left in an IV bag of 5% dextrose and ½ NS. The postop MD orders include "IV to infuse at 320 mL every 8 hours." When should the nurse anticipate having to change the IV bag?

1. 3:00 P.M.

2. 6:00 P.M.

3. 9:00 P.M.

4. 12:00 midnight.

115. The nurse's assessment of a patient in pulmonary edema would reveal:

1. Rapid respiration, frequent cough, flushed face.

2. Persistent cough, rapid respiration, hemoptysis.

3. Dyspnea, hacking cough, purulent sputum.

4. Air hunger, orthopnea, elevated temperature.

116. Before entering a patient's room, the nurse should wash her or his hands for a minimum of:

1. 10 seconds.

2. 30 seconds.

3. 45 seconds.

4. 60 seconds.

117. The nurse in the recovery room is monitoring the patient's vital signs every 15 minutes. Which change should be reported immediately to the surgeon?

1. Dry, cool skin.

2. A systolic blood pressure that drops 20 mm Hg or more.

3. A diastolic pressure below 70.

4. A pulse rate that increases and decreases with respirations.

118. The preoperative medications ordered by the anesthesiologist are morphine sulfate, 15 mg, and atropine SO₄, 0.4 mg, subcutaneously. The nurse can expect to give these drugs:

1. Right before the patient leaves for surgery.

2. 45–60 minutes before anesthetic induction.

3. 20–30 minutes before anesthetic induction.

4. 10–15 minutes before anesthetic induction.

119. The nurse knows that a person who is on a bland diet may *lack* which essential nutrient?

1. Vitamin C.

2. Carbohydrates.

3. Protein.

4. Vitamin A.

120. When assessing a client who has been abusing amphetamines, the nurse would expect to see which symptom?

1. Bradycardia.

2. Increased irritability.

3. Hypotension.

4. Constipation.

121. Which action is *least* likely to be within the role and legal responsibilities of the nurse who is assisting with an amniocentesis?

1. Informing the woman about the risks involved in amniocentesis.

2. Explaining/reinforcing how the procedure will be done.

3. Monitoring the fetal heart rate.

4. Observing the woman for signs of bleeding or contractions after the procedure is completed.

122. When noticing that a patient's IV site appears red and swollen, the nurse should:

1. Apply warm soaks.

2. Decrease the flow rate.

3. Elevate the IV site.

4. Remove the IV.

123. Two weeks after a cast is applied, a foul odor is detected at the lower end of the cast. A window is made in the cast over the infected area and an antibiotic is prescribed. After 3 days on antibiotic therapy, which

effect would be most indicative of a therapeutic response?

1. White blood cell count is 7900/mm³.

2. Temperature is 99.4°F.

3. No complaints of pain.

4. Appetite is fairly good.

124. On completion of a nursing assessment, the nurse concludes that the patient is showing signs of increased intracranial pressure. Data to support this conclusion would include:

1. Decreased blood pressure, tachycardia, tachypnea.

2. Increase in level of consciousness.

3. Dilation of the pupil on the side opposite the hematoma.

4. Bradycardia, increased pulse pressure, and Biot's breathing.

125. Ten days after the birth of their infant, a new father is concerned about the mother's mood. He states that she is tearful and apathetic and does not eat much. What would be the nurse's most appropriate response?

1. "Many women experience some degree of depression after the birth of a baby."

2. "I will suggest a psychiatric referral to assist her in coping with this crisis."

3. "I will notify the physician of your concern and ask the physician to prescribe an antidepressant for her."

4. "You need to be patient since these symptoms will dissipate."

126. A patient with diabetes is NPO before surgery. An appropriate nursing measure on the day of surgery is:

1. To withhold the daily insulin dose.

2. To administer the daily insulin dose.

3. To administer the insulin and request that the patient drink a glass of juice.

4. To request specific orders regarding insulin administration.

127. A patient with hallucinatory behavior constantly asks the nurse to bring french fries and a piece of apple pie. The nurse should realize that this patient is probably:

1. Starving.

2. Hallucinating.

3. Disoriented.

4. Playing a game.

128. In caring for a patient with a double-lumen tracheostomy tube, the inner cannula should be removed and cleansed with hydrogen peroxide and normal saline:

1. Only as necessary.

2. Every 2–4 hours.

3. Once a day.

4. Never—do not remove the inner cannula for any reason.

129. Assessment of a woman in labor reveals the following: 4 cm dilated cervix, intact membranes, mild to moderate contractions every 4–6 minutes, alert affect. The

nurse determines that this woman is in which stage of labor?
1. First.
2. Second.
3. Third.
4. Fourth.

130. The best antimicrobial agent for the nurse to use in hand washing is:
    1. Soap and water.
    2. Isopropyl alcohol.
    3. Hexachlorophene (PhisoHex).
    4. Chlorhexidine gluconate (CHG) (Hibiclens).

131. The nurse knows that the proper technique for two-person CPR includes:
    1. Two full breaths followed by five compressions.
    2. A brief pause between rescue breathing and compressions.
    3. Rescuers changing positions every 5 minutes to prevent fatigue.
    4. A slower rate than is used in one-person CPR.

132. A patient is taking nitroglycerin to control angina. Patient teaching regarding administration of nitroglycerin includes the importance of notifying the physician if repeated doses do not relieve chest pain. Additional information would include:
    1. Notifying the physician if headaches occur.
    2. Storing the medication in the refrigerator.
    3. Taking nitroglycerin prophylactically before exercise.
    4. Ingesting the tablets with liquid.

133. The mother of a recently deceased infant insists on seeing the infant's body before leaving the hospital. The most therapeutic nursing action includes:
    1. Arranging for her to see the infant's body.
    2. Discussing this with the family's priest.
    3. Informing the father that seeing the infant's body would be detrimental to the mother's health.
    4. Telling the parents that hospital policy forbids her seeing the infant's body.

134. A woman is to have a cesarean birth. Her partner asks the nurse whether he will see any "gore" or blood during the operation. The most realistic response would be:
    1. "I'm not sure."
    2. "It depends on the technique the physician uses."
    3. "Probably not, because a drape keeps the operation from view by both of you, if you sit by her head."
    4. "Yes, blood and tissue will be all over the table."

135. If a patient's antihypertensive drug therapy is effective, the nurse would expect:
    1. A greater decrease in systolic than diastolic pressure.
    2. A greater decrease in diastolic than systolic pressure.
    3. An approximately equal decrease in both systolic and diastolic pressures.
    4. Little change in blood pressure initially, but pulse will slow.

136. When teaching a 3-year-old about a procedure, the nurse should realize that the *most* important factor influencing the child's ability to learn is:
    1. Chronological age.
    2. Developmental level.
    3. Present state of anxiety.
    4. Previous experience with illness and hospitalization.

137. What will the nurse encourage a patient who has had a modified right mastectomy to do as appropriate *initial* therapy 24 hours after surgery?
    1. Self-feeding and hair combing.
    2. Passive/active flexion and extension of the elbow and pronation and supination of the wrist.
    3. Abduction and external rotation of the right shoulder.
    4. Early ambulation and active extension and flexion of the elbow.

138. When teaching a young mother about a decrease in her milk production, the nurse should:
    1. Recommend weaning the baby onto formula.
    2. Assess the mother's feelings about breastfeeding.
    3. Refer the mother to La Leche League.
    4. Suggest supplemental feedings of glucose water.

139. Besides enhancing pacemaker automaticity and facilitating AV conduction during heart block, what other effect of isoproterenol (Isuprel) would the nurse look for?
    1. Increased peripheral vascular resistance.
    2. Decreased automaticity of Purkinje fibers.
    3. Decreased bronchoconstriction.
    4. Decreased oral secretion.

140. A pregnant woman at 29 weeks of gestation is concerned about her weight gain of 15 pounds during this pregnancy. The nurse will most likely determine that this woman is primarily concerned about:
    1. The baby's nutrition status.
    2. Her own body image.
    3. Her need to diet.
    4. Her need to gain more weight.

141. A patient who has had a myocardial infarction states, "I can hardly get my breath." Vital signs are BP 100/70, apical pulse 126, respirations 26. Pulmonary crackles and wheezes are heard halfway up the chest. The first nursing action is to:
    1. Administer morphine sulfate to allay the patient's apprehension.
    2. Assist the patient to a sitting position and lower the legs.
    3. Remove excess pulmonary secretions with suction.
    4. Administer oxygen at 10 liters, per mask instead of nasal catheter.

142. When a woman is in labor, which action requested by the nurse could cause a problem to the woman?
    1. Empty her bladder.
    2. Lie on her back to facilitate adequate ventilation.
    3. Not bear down until she enters the second stage.
    4. Breathe slowly and evenly.

143. A husband blames his wife for their son's problems with substance abuse, saying, "I always knew you were too easy on him. You see what giving him his way has done!" In understanding the father's response, the nurse should realize that this behavior indicates a nursing diagnosis of defensive coping as evidenced by:
    1. Guilt.
    2. Sublimation.
    3. Projection.
    4. Displacement.

144. The doctor orders Burow's solution soaks for a toddler with eczema. In order to gain the toddler's cooperation with this treatment, the nurse should tell the toddler:
    1. "Let's do this real fast and then you can see mommy and daddy."
    2. "You don't want to have to stay here forever, do you? Let's make you all better now!"
    3. "This medicine will help you get better so you can go home. Help me pour some on your arms."
    4. "This is magic medicine that will make all your boo-boos go away. Don't you want to chase away those boo-boos?"

145. When teaching parents how to provide CPR for their infant, it is important to stress:
    1. Applying systematic pressure to the chest with the heel of the hand.
    2. Compressing the chest at a rate of 100 compressions per minute.
    3. Placing the resuscitator's mouth over the infant's mouth to ensure an adequate seal.
    4. Blowing forcefully into the infant's air passages to fully inflate the lungs.

146. When planning to teach a client about the side effects of amphetamines, the nurse should emphasize that:
    1. Withdrawal from these drugs usually causes death.
    2. The body develops a tolerance to these drugs.
    3. An overdose of these drugs induces sleepiness.
    4. Physiological dependence may develop.

147. While preparing a patient's preoperative medication, the nurse notes that the atropine SO_4 on hand is in a strength of 0.6 mg/mL. The prescribed dosage is 0.4 mg. The correct amount of atropine to administer is:
    1. 1.5 mL.
    2. 1 mL.
    3. 10 minims.
    4. 8 minims.

148. If a pregnant woman remains essentially healthy, the nurse's health teaching about safeguards to maintain throughout pregnancy should be for her to:
    1. Stop working by week 32 of gestation.
    2. Avoid intercourse.
    3. Avoid alcohol and smoking.
    4. Eat a minimum of three full meals each day.

149. Given a diagnosis of pulmonary edema, the nurse knows that a patient's dyspnea is the result of:
    1. Increased lung compliance due to mechanical congestion.
    2. Decreased CO_2 retention.
    3. Decreased venous return.
    4. Fluid shift from systemic circulation to lungs.

150. The nurse realizes that the discharge of green amniotic fluid may indicate:
    1. Rh or ABO incompatibility.
    2. Fetal distress occurred approximately 36 hours ago.
    3. Recent or current hypoxia.
    4. Abruptio placentae has occurred.

151. The rationale for using humidified oxygen with tracheal tubes is that:
    1. It is a traditional procedure.
    2. It is a means of providing fluid intake.
    3. It decreases insensible water loss.
    4. The natural humidifying pathway has been bypassed.

152. Parents of a 6-month-old infant bring the baby in for a physical examination; all immunizations are up-to-date. This infant should receive three of the following immunizations at this time; which immunization should not be given?
    1. Hepatitis B.
    2. Diphtheria, tetanus, and pertussis (DTP).
    3. *H. influenzae* type b.
    4. Measles, mumps, rubella.

153. An IV rate is to be regulated to keep vein open (KVO). The nurse knows that the longest possible time that a single 1000 mL bottle or bag can infuse safely is:
    1. 24 hours.
    2. 5 hours.
    3. 18 hours.
    4. 12 hours.

154. The nurse should know that the best position to check an adolescent for scoliosis is:
    1. Standing up straight.
    2. Lying flat on the stomach.
    3. Standing and bending 90 degrees at the waist.
    4. Sitting in a straight-back chair.

155. A unit of blood is ordered for a patient when the BP drops to 90/60. What is the most important safeguard before administering blood?
    1. Refrigerate unit of blood until immediately before giving.
    2. Agitate the blood so it is well mixed.
    3. Carefully check labeled blood against patient's wristband.
    4. Infuse the blood through a blood warmer.

156. Potassium chloride is to be added to an infant's intravenous fluids. Before adding this electrolyte, the nurse should determine that:
    1. The infant has voided recently.
    2. Moro reflex is present.
    3. Respiratory rate is between 25 and 40.
    4. Mucous membranes are moist.

157. A young woman describes experiencing a heavy vaginal discharge and severe itching for the past 3 days. She is diagnosed as having *Trichomonas vaginalis* infection. Health teaching for this woman should include dosage, administration, and signs and symptoms of side effects of which medication as treatment for this condition?
    1. Tetracycline.
    2. Erythromycin.
    3. Nystatin.
    4. Metronidazole.

158. Immediately on returning to the recovery room, a patient's above-the-knee amputation stump should initially be:
    1. Elevated on a pillow to reduce occurrence of edema and hemorrhage.
    2. Placed in Buck's traction to prevent skin and muscle retraction.
    3. Firmly bandaged to a padded board to prevent contractures.
    4. Wrapped in an Ace bandage to reduce edema formation.

159. When a postop patient is admitted following an appendectomy, the *first* action the nurse should take is to:
    1. Attach nasogastric tube to suction.
    2. Calculate the IV flow rate and adjust the drip.
    3. Monitor vital signs.
    4. Check patient's ID band.

160. The nurse planning to administer a unit of blood to a child should know that after it is removed from the refrigerator, the blood should be transfused within:
    1. Six hours.
    2. Two hours.
    3. Four hours.
    4. One hour.

161. In observing women in the latent phase of the first stage of labor, the nurse would expect to see which behavior?
    1. Tendency to hyperventilate.
    2. Euphoria, excitement, and talkativeness.
    3. Fairly quiet and introverted behavior.
    4. Irritability and crying.

162. To which postoperative complication is a patient who has had a modified mastectomy predisposed because of the nature of her surgery?
    1. Peripheral thrombophlebitis.
    2. Wound dehiscence.
    3. Atelectasis.
    4. Paralytic ileus.

163. In teaching a couple about preparation for childbirth, the nurse should *first*:
    1. Evaluate the couple's knowledge base of childbirth techniques.
    2. Assess the couple's level of readiness to learn.
    3. Consult a childbirth nurse practitioner regarding what to tell the couple.
    4. Refer the couple to a Lamaze childbirth class.

164. Following surgery for a ruptured appendix, the nurse should place the patient in a semi-Fowler's position primarily to:
    1. Fully aerate the lungs.
    2. Promote drainage and prevent subdiaphragmatic abscesses.
    3. Splint the wound.
    4. Facilitate movement and reduce complications from immobility.

165. The nurse assessing a person who has a history of substance abuse would expect to find which characteristic?
    1. A very assertive individual.
    2. A very dependent individual.
    3. A very mature individual.
    4. A very aggressive individual.

166. The earliest signs of whole blood transfusion reaction a nurse would monitor for are:
    1. Headache and elevated temperature.
    2. Hypertension and flushing.
    3. Urticaria and wheezing.
    4. Oliguria and jaundice.

167. The nurse caring for a patient recovering from GI bleeding should:
    1. Plan care so the patient can receive at least 8 hours of uninterrupted sleep each night.
    2. Monitor vital signs every 2 hours.
    3. Make sure that the patient takes food and medications at prescribed intervals.
    4. Provide milk every 2–3 hours.

168. To monitor a patient's fluid volumes more closely, a CVP line has been inserted via the right subclavian vein. The nurse needs to know that CVP assesses the pressure in:
    1. The left atrium.
    2. The right atrium.
    3. The left ventricle.
    4. The right ventricle.

169. A patient is diagnosed as being mildly hypertensive. In assessing this patient's BP, the nurse most likely finds that the resting diastolic pressure is:
    1. Between 110 and 120 mm Hg.
    2. Between 90 and 100 mm Hg.
    3. Between 120 and 140 mm Hg.
    4. Between 100 and 115 mm Hg.

170. A patient has had a permanent pacemaker inserted, with the pacing catheter introduced into the right external jugular vein and positioned in the right ventricle. Which nursing care activity is the nurse's first priority in the *early* postimplantation period?
    1. Restricting activity to prevent pacing catheter displacement.
    2. Monitoring the ECG continually, noting rhythm, rate, appearance, and amplitude of pacing spike.
    3. Implementing passive range-of-motion exercise to the right arm to prevent "frozen shoulder."
    4. Maintaining sterile dressings over the operative site to prevent infection.

171. A client takes secobarbital (Seconal) whenever feeling "too stressed," such as whenever there is an exam or whenever the client feels too pressured, which happens at least four or five times a week. The nurse should be aware that large doses of secobarbital can cause:
    1. Tachycardia.
    2. Hypertension.
    3. Assaultive behavior.
    4. Increased respirations.

172. The nurse knows that angina pectoris, which occurs after eating, may be due to:
    1. Incomplete digestion of fats due to a decrease in pancreatic enzyme, thereby increasing reflux.
    2. Local blood flow regulators that shunt blood to gut during digestion, thereby decreasing coronary artery perfusion pressures.
    3. Abdominal distention from swallowing air during eating, thereby decreasing diaphragmatic excursion and arterial PO_2.
    4. Decreased heart rate and blood pressure, resulting in increased myocardial oxygen consumption.

173. A toddler is diagnosed as having iron deficiency anemia. In addition to teaching the parents to give this toddler Fer-In-Sol (ferrous sulfate) between meals, the nurse should also instruct them to give this medication with:
    1. Orange juice.
    2. Milk.
    3. Apple juice.
    4. Prune juice.

174. The nurse knows that the desired effects of morphine SO_4 and atropine SO_4 have been achieved preoperatively when:
    1. Pain is relieved and anxiety is reduced.
    2. Secretions are decreased and sensitivity to stimuli is reduced.
    3. Sleep occurs and oral secretions are reduced.
    4. Sensitivity to pain is reduced and muscular relaxation occurs.

175. A woman in labor has a history of undiagnosed vaginal bleeding. Which procedure may be *contraindicated* on her arrival in the labor room?
    1. Initiating intravenous therapy.
    2. Taking her blood pressure.
    3. Examining her vaginal canal.
    4. Monitoring FHR.

176. The mother of a child with eczema asks the nurse if she can bathe the child in the bathtub at home. The best response by the nurse would be:
    1. "It would probably be a good idea to check with your doctor first."
    2. "Perhaps in a week to 10 days you can begin tub baths; until then, a sponge bath will be adequate."
    3. "No, baths are not generally permitted for children with eczema."
    4. "Yes, frequent baths will help dry the lesions."

177. Crepitus in the neck and upper chest of a patient who has a new tracheostomy in place is caused by:
    1. Air from a displaced tracheal tube.
    2. An inadequately inflated tracheostomy cuff.
    3. An overinflated tracheostomy cuff.
    4. Edema from the trauma of surgery.

178. An expectant couple is concerned about what effect preeclampsia may have on the fetus. Which indicator or test of fetal well-being should the nurse teach the couple to expect most commonly during the rest of the prenatal period?
    1. Nonstress test.
    2. Amniocentesis.
    3. L/S ratio.
    4. Fetal blood gases.

179. The nursing aide caring for a child in Bryant's traction reports that the child's buttocks are resting on the mattress. The nurse would be most correct in telling the aide that:
    1. This is where the buttocks should be.
    2. The buttocks should be slightly off the mattress.
    3. This is the responsibility of the nurse.
    4. The child will need special skin care to avoid pressure areas or breakdown.

180. Which nursing intervention for a patient with a Hemovac is *inappropriate*?
    1. Observing and recording the amount and color of the drainage.
    2. Maintaining suction by emptying and recompressing the apparatus regularly.
    3. Increasing suction by attaching the Hemovac to wall suction as the drainage increases.
    4. Preventing traction on the drainage tubes by repositioning the Hemovac each time the patient is repositioned.

181. An adolescent boy was admitted for substance abuse and hallucinations. This client's mother asks the nurse to talk with her son's father when he arrives at the hospital. She says that she is afraid of what the father might say to the boy. The most appropriate nursing intervention would be to:
    1. Inform the mother that she and the father can work through this problem themselves.
    2. Refer the mother to the hospital social worker.
    3. Agree to talk with the mother and the father together.
    4. Suggest that the father and son work things out.

182. Following an amputation, a nursing measure to help reduce the size of the stump once the surgical wound is healed is:
    1. Elevation of the stump on a pillow when reclining.
    2. Pushing the stump against a hard surface.
    3. Wrapping moist, warm soaks on the thigh.
    4. Applying an elastic bandage.

183. The nurse would interpret a patient's central venous pressure (CVP) as normal if the pressure were:
    1. 4–10 cm H_2O.
    2. 20–30 mm Hg.

3. 10–20 cm H₂O.

4. 7–14 mm Hg.

184. The nurse working with a family that is using an apnea monitor should know that the monitor's most problematic side effect is:

1. Sounding the alarm whenever the infant moves around in the crib.

2. Overprotectiveness by the parents.

3. Developmental lag in the infant.

4. Unreliability of the monitor.

185. During an adolescent's hospitalization for treatment of substance abuse, the nurse must be able to handle a variety of behavior problems. In implementing care for this client, which action would be the *least* appropriate?

1. Allowing the client to select some of the food he or she wants to eat.

2. Restricting activity level.

3. Encouraging friends to visit.

4. Closely monitoring behavior.

186. The nurse knows that after administration of nitroglycerin, a patient's angina will be relieved because the drug:

1. Constricts cardiac chambers to reduce workload.

2. Stimulates the heart rate to increase blood supply to the myocardium.

3. Increases myocardial contractility.

4. Decreases workload of the heart through lowering the systemic blood pressure.

187. A patient is hospitalized with a BP of 170/100, difficulty breathing, dizziness, and weakness. The nurse establishing this patient's care should consider:

1. Ensuring that a different nurse takes care of the patient each day to prevent hospital fatigue.

2. Planning care to allow for periods of activity.

3. Identifying any misconceptions the patient may have regarding hypertension.

4. Instructing the patient to report only major symptoms to the physician.

188. In planning for discharge, the nurse should inform a patient who has had a right modified mastectomy of actions that may increase lymphedema. Which activity is *most likely* to increase symptoms?

1. Wearing gloves for household tasks or gardening.

2. Carrying heavy groceries in her right arm.

3. Wearing dresses with elasticized sleeves.

4. Driving to and from work.

189. A woman is in preterm labor and is bleeding. She requests a sip of water after being in labor for 2 hours in the hospital. The most appropriate nursing action would be:

1. Checking the physician's orders.

2. Giving her a small sip of water.

3. Offering her ice chips.

4. Telling her she cannot have fluids at this time.

190. A mother states that the pediatrician told her that her son has numerous allergies, including milk allergies. The nurse should offer him which formula?

1. Lofenalac.

2. Lonalac.

3. Similac with iron.

4. Isomil.

191. What would receive the *least* emphasis in the nurse's predischarge education plan for a patient who has had a permanent pacemaker inserted?

1. Rationale for pacemaker implantation.

2. Pacemaker function and signs indicating malfunction.

3. Therapeutic program, including medication, diet, activity schedule, and safety precautions.

4. Necessity for periodic follow-up visits to physician.

192. The nurse needs to know that SIDS usually occurs:

1. Within 2–4 weeks after birth.

2. Between 2 and 4 months after birth.

3. More than 6 months after birth.

4. Between 6 and 9 months after birth.

193. A patient's vital signs are BP 124/84, apical pulse 100 and regular, respirations 24. Given that this patient's normal BP is 144/96 and average pulse is 80, the nurse concludes that the present vital signs are related to:

1. Increased vagal stimulation of SA node.

2. Arrhythmias.

3. Cardiogenic shock.

4. Sympathetic nervous system response.

194. The nurse must recognize the side effects of morphine and atropine administration given preoperatively, which include:

1. Bradycardia, anorexia, and decreased urine output.

2. Hypertension, nausea, vomiting, tachycardia.

3. Hypotension, cotton mouth, nausea, and vomiting.

4. Dryness, cotton mouth, constricted pupils, and bradycardia.

195. In planning discharge care for a patient after treatment for hypertension, the nurse should emphasize:

1. Medication scheduling and side effects.

2. Need to change jobs.

3. Importance of smoking less.

4. Sexual activity restrictions.

196. The MD orders an IV of D₅W at 40 mL/hr. A 500 mL bag, with a pediatric microdrip chamber, is hung at 11:00 A.M. At 3:15 P.M., the nurse notes that the bag has 100 mL left. What should be the nurse's initial action?

1. Readjust the flow rate to 40 microdrops per minute.

2. Hang a new 500 mL bag of fluid.

3. Maintain the flow rate at 20 microdrops per minute until the IV is back on schedule.

4. Notify the physician.

197. The nurse knows that the *primary* advantage of Hemovac wound suction is that it:

1. Exerts high, even suction.

2. Allows easy mobility because it is lightweight.

3. Speeds wound healing by removing excess fluids.

4. Reduces the occurrence of postoperative infection.

198. The nurse would expect to find drug abuse *least* prevalent in:
1. An upper socioeconomic family.
2. An elderly individual.
3. A lower socioeconomic family.
4. An adolescent.

199. A toddler has been in the hospital 1 week and refuses to talk with anyone, including the family. The toddler sits in the corner of the crib crying and rocking back and forth. The most important nursing intervention at this time should be to:
1. Establish a one-to-one relationship with the toddler to develop trust.
2. Assign different staff to work with the toddler each day to promote socialization.
3. Ignore the behavior because it probably indicates normal regression.
4. Refer the toddler to the pediatric clinical nurse specialist for further evaluation.

200. Among the elderly, what is the most common postoperative complication following amputation?
1. Hemorrhage and shock.
2. Pulmonary embolus.
3. Disseminated intravascular clotting.
4. Thrombophlebitis.

ANSWERS/RATIONALE

1. (2) Hypertension is considerably more severe in men than women and tends to occur more frequently at an earlier age. **Answer 1** is incorrect because currently it is estimated that 20 to 25 million Americans (about 10% of the population) have hypertension. The low percentage is due largely to non-detection related to the slow onset and lack of specific symptoms in its early stages. **Answer 3** is incorrect because the prevalence in *every* age group is higher for American blacks than for whites. Likewise, the severity of hypertension in black men is three times that in white men and the severity in black women is almost six times that experienced by white women. Mortality rates for the American black population with hypertension are twice those of the white hypertensive population. **Answer 4** is incorrect because in many individuals hypertension goes undetected and untreated.

> **Test-taking tip**—Use a process of elimination.

AN, 6, PhI, Physiological Adaptation

2. (2) The date of the woman's last period is the most relevant question to ask in performing the initial assessment, because it will assist the nurse in making a preliminary determination of possible pregnancy. **Answer 1** is incorrect: whether the woman is presently taking oral contraceptives may be relevant, but it would be more pertinent to assess what *general* type of birth control the couple may be using and if they have been using it effectively. **Answers 3** and **4** are incorrect: whether she has been pregnant before and how much weight she has gained are both relevant to performing the assessment, but *not* essential to determining *whether* she is pregnant at the present time.

> **Test-taking tip**—Choose the answer that meets the condition of the stem: to find out *if* she is pregnant *now*. Review presumptive, probable, and positive signs of pregnancy.

AS, 5, HPM, Prevention and Early Detection

3. (2) Adequate oxygenation is foremost in importance. **Answer 1** is incorrect because the primary intervention should be to ensure a patent airway, *followed* by observation for signs and symptoms of shock. **Answer 3** is incorrect: liquids would be contraindicated because of the child's burns and possible shock. **Answer 4** is incorrect because a medical order would be needed to initiate intravenous therapy.

> **Test-taking tip**—Patent airway is always the priority of care.

IMP, 1, PhI, Physiological Adaptation

4. (3) Patients who abuse drugs react in various ways, depending on the amount and type of drug taken, the combination of drugs, and individual factors such as overall general health and age. However, seizures are common shortly after the ingestion of drugs such as narcotics and stimulants. Seizures may also accompany the withdrawal from drugs. **Answer 1** is incorrect because the patient is not in touch with reality. **Answer 2** is incorrect because maintaining a quiet environment is of secondary importance to taking precautions against seizures. **Answer 4** is incorrect because taking vital signs is of secondary importance to taking precautions against seizures. However, vital signs should be taken as soon as possible, to establish a baseline, and retaken at least every 1–2 hours thereafter until the patient is stable.

> **Test-taking tip**—*Primary* concern is seizure prevention.

PL, 2, SECE, Management of Care

5. (1) Because the patient has experienced some gastric bleeding, he or she should be observed closely for symptoms of shock. **Answer 2** is incorrect because paging the physician is secondary to the close monitoring of the patient's vital signs for symptoms of shock. **Answer 3** is incorrect because completing the appropriate assessment tool may be done when the patient is under less stress. **Answer 4** is incorrect because CPR is not indicated at this time—the patient is not experiencing cardiac or respiratory failure.

> **Test-taking tip**—Think priority and the first step in assessment—observation.

AS, 6, PhI, Physiological Adaptation

6. (2) The one factor that has been *highly* correlated to smoking cigarettes and marijuana is low birth weight. **Answers 1, 3, and 4** are incorrect because retardation, deformation, and malnourishment do *not* have a *high* correlation to smoking cigarettes and marijuana.

> **Test-taking tip**—Think *low* birth weight = *high* risk (i.e., high correlation). Choose the *least* serious consequence as the *highest* probability for causing the condition. Review teratogenic and high-risk substances women may use during pregnancy. Know the most common effects of these substances on the fetus/newborn.

EV, 5, HPM, Prevention and Early Detection

7. (1) Having established, by stimulating the patient, that he or she is unconscious rather than asleep, the nurse should immediately call for help. This may be done by dialing the operator from the patient's phone and giving the hospital code for cardiac arrest and the patient's room number to the operator, or if a phone is not available, by pulling the emergency call button. Noting the time is important baseline information for cardiac arrest procedure. **Answer 2** is incorrect because clearing the airway *follows* an unsuccessful attempt to ventilate. **Answer 3** is incorrect because checking the pulse *follows* after the airway has been established and ventilation has begun. **Answer 4** is incorrect because initial ventilation includes two full breaths.

> **Test-taking tip**—Remember the sequence for CPR—"help," then ABC.

IMP, 6, PhI, Physiological Adaptation

8. (1) If the IV infuses at the prescribed rate of 75 mL per hour from 7:00 P.M. to 7:00 A.M., or 12 hours, 75 mL × 12 hours = 900 mL infused. If a 1000 mL bag were hung and 900 mL infused, 1000 − 900 = 100 mL *left* in the bag. **Answers 2** and **3** are incorrect calculations. **Answer 4** is incorrect because there *is* enough information to determine this.

> **Test-taking tip**—Looks more difficult than it is. Just multiply and subtract.

EV, 6, PhI, Pharmacological and Parenteral Therapies

9. (1) The inherent rate of ventricular excitable tissue is between 20 and 40 and does not increase significantly with exertion in complete heart block. **Answers 2** and **3** are incorrect because this phenomenon results in decreased cardiac output despite increased diastolic filling time, coronary artery blood flow, and stroke volume with each ventricular contraction. **Answer 4** is incorrect because the decreased cardiac output results in stimulation of circulatory reflexes to increase venous return, which produces peripheral vasoconstriction, the cause of the patient's pallor and diaphoresis.

> **Test-taking tip**—Look for a similar idea in answer.

AN, 6, PhI, Physiological Adaptation

Key to codes following rationales *Nursing process:* **AS**, Assessment; **AN**, Analysis; **PL**, Plan; **IMP**, Implementation; **EV**, Evaluation. *Category of human function:* **1**, Protective; **2**, Sensory-perceptual; **3**, Comfort, Rest, Activity, and Mobility; **4**, Nutrition; **5**, Growth and Development; **6**, Fluid-Gas Transport; **7**, Psychosocial-Cultural; **8**, Elimination. **Client need: SECE**, Safe, Effective Care Environment; **PhI**, Physiological Integrity; **PsI**, Psychosocial Integrity; **HPM**, Health Promotion/Maintenance. See appendices for full explanation.

10. (3) Depending on the hospital, this is a physician's decision, especially in cases where the fetus, as well as the mother, may be in danger. **Answer 1** is incorrect because time may not permit a physician *referral* to occur. **Answer 2** is incorrect because although some hospitals and/or physicians require childbirth classes as a prerequisite to attending the birth, others do not require it. **Answer 4** is incorrect because it is an inappropriate nursing action without a physician's approval.

> **Test-taking tip**—This is the *MD's* decision, but the nurse's role is to act as an advocate by going to the MD.

IMP, 7, SECE, Management of Care

11. (3) The apnea monitor will sound an alarm during any periods of apnea to warn the parents or caretakers. **Answer 1** is incorrect. Although the alarm may startle the infant and stimulate breathing, it should not be relied on for this function. **Answer 2** is incorrect because the monitor screen displays the infant's respirations (and pulse, with some monitors) but not temperature. **Answer 4** is incorrect because the monitor will not maintain the infant's respirations.

> **Test-taking tip**—Review the function of an apnea monitor and narrow the choice to an option that has "breathing" and "alarm" (what a *monitor* does).

IMP, 2, PhI, Reduction of Risk Potential

12. (4) To repeat the breathing exercises until the patient is light-headed is inappropriate. It indicates hyperventilation, which may lead to tetany due to loss of volatile hydrogen ions. Patients *should,* however, be able to supply a rationale for deep breathing and coughing techniques (**Answer 1**), as well as demonstrate them correctly (**Answer 2**). **Answer 3** is also a desirable outcome.

> **Test-taking tip**—*Least* desired outcome will be low priority.

EV, 6, PhI, Physiological Adaptation

13. (1) The patient's pH is within normal range (pH 7.35–7.45). Therefore, even though the serum bicarbonate level is reduced, indicating metabolic acidosis, the lungs have been able to excrete enough CO_2 to keep the total pH within normal range. **Answer 2** is incorrect because P_{CO_2} in hyperventilation is reduced (less than 40 mm Hg), but serum bicarbonate levels are usually normal. **Answer 3** is incorrect because a pH *below* 7.35 would represent uncompensated metabolic acidosis. **Answer 4** is incorrect because in alveolar hypoventilation the P_{CO_2} is elevated and the condition of respiratory acidosis exists.

> **Test-taking tip**—Know *normals* and what "compensated" looks like.

EV, 6, PhI, Physiological Adaptation

14. (1) Lead poisoning primarily affects the CNS, causing increased intracranial pressure. This results in irritability and changes in level of consciousness, as well as seizure disorders, hyperactivity, and learning disabilities. **Answer 2** is incorrect because lead poisoning may affect the GI tract and cause constipation, *not* diarrhea. **Answer 3** is incorrect because lead poisoning may also cause anemia and tachycardia, *not* bradycardia. **Answer 4** is incorrect because lead poisoning does not cause bleeding tendencies.

> **Test-taking tip**—Think neurological signs and symptoms.

AS, 1, HPM, Prevention and Early Detection of Disease

15. (4) Although reducing environmental stimuli and activity is necessary for a woman with mild preeclampsia, she will most probably have bathroom privileges. **Answer 1** is incorrect because her vital signs and fetal heart rate and rhythm *should* be assessed at least once per shift during the time she is awake. **Answer 2** is incorrect because her daily weight *is* an indicator of her response to treatment and loss of edema. **Answer 3** is incorrect because deep-tendon reflexes do assist in assessing the degree of CNS hyperirritability.

> **Test-taking tip**—When a question asks for *least* likely, choose the response that is not necessary to do. Recall a plan of care for woman with mild preeclampsia vs. severe preeclampsia.

IMP, 6, PhI, Basic Care and Comfort

16. (2) The purpose of a tracheostomy is to provide more controlled ventilation and to ease removal of respiratory secretions. When long-term therapy is indicated, it reduces or prevents respiratory fatigue. A tracheostomy is done when intubation is necessary for longer than 3–5 days, when the patient is unable to handle respiratory secretions, or if there is upper-airway obstruction. **Answer 1** is incorrect because although anxiety will be decreased when ventilation is improved, this is not the primary purpose for a tracheostomy. **Answer 3** is incorrect because desired effects of improving ventilation include improved cerebral oxygenation. **Answer 4** is incorrect because a side effect of tracheostomy is increased risk of pulmonary infection, which is not true in the case of endotracheal intubation, though both may cause injury to mucous membranes.

> **Test-taking tip**—Look for the broadest choice—improve ventilation.

PL, 6, PhI, Physiological Adaptation

17. (4) Acknowledging her presence and discomfort is most important to provide emotional support. **Answer 1** is incorrect: privacy is important if she requests it; however, assuming that she wants to be isolated may cause feelings of rejection and loneliness. **Answer 2** is incorrect because an assessment of her overall level of functioning and coping abilities must be performed *before* any medication is prescribed. It is also the doctor's decision to give medication. **Answer 3** is incorrect: such a decision must be discussed with her.

> **Test-taking tip**—Most *appropriate* action is to provide emotional support.

IMP, 7, PsI, Psychosocial Adaptation

18. (3) Tight pressure dressing, discomfort, and fear of tearing the incision tend to limit chest expansion and the patient's willingness to cough. The nurse can assist the patient in this procedure by helping her sit upright and by supporting (with her hand) both the anterior and the posterior chest wall at the incisional site. Frequent turning will also facilitate mobilization of secretions and the prevention of atelectasis. **Answer 1** is incorrect because the dressing is on the chest wall and will not interfere with body alignment. **Answer 2** is incorrect because arm exercises initially will be isometric and can be done with the dressing in place. **Answer 4** is incorrect because vital signs should be checked on the *inoperative* arm.

> **Test-taking tip**—Visualize the patient (chest constricted).

EV, 6, PhI, Reduction of Risk Potential

19. (1) A local hypersensitivity reaction is angioedema, redness and swelling. **Answer 2** is incorrect because cardiovascular collapse is a systemic reaction. **Answer 3** is incorrect because nausea with vomiting and diarrhea represents a systemic reaction. **Answer 4** is incorrect because asthma-like symptoms also represent a systemic reaction.

> **Test-taking tip**—Key word is *local*. Three choices involve major systems.

AS, 1, PhI, Physiological Adaptation

20. (1) According to Nägele's rule (LMP - 3 months + 7 days), the calculations would be: 7/10 − 3 months = 4/10 + 7 days = 4/17. Nägele's rule assumes that the woman has a 28-day cycle and that pregnancy occurred on the fourteenth day. If the woman's cycle is longer or shorter than 28 days, appropriate adjustments must be made. Only about 4–5% of women give birth on the EDB plus or minus 7 days. **Answers 2, 3,** and **4** are incorrect calculations.

Test-taking tip—Use Nägele's rule. A simple method is to count +9 months from the LMP, + 7 days.

AN, 5, HPM, Growth and Development

21. **(3)** If the IV infusion was at the prescribed rate of 35 mL/hr for 4.5 hours, from 7:00 A.M. to 11:30 A.M., 35 mL × 4.5 hours = 157.5 mL absorbed. If 500 mL was hung at 7:00 A.M., and approximately 160 mL was infused, 500 − 160 = 340 mL left in the bag at 11:30 A.M. **Answers 1** and **2** are incorrect calculations. **Answer 4** is incorrect.

Test-taking tip—Use basic math, not a formula.

EV, 6, PhI, Pharmacological and Parenteral Therapies

22. **(3)** The patient may perceive this as avoidance, but it is more important to redirect back to the patient, especially in light of the manipulative behaviors of drug abusers and adolescents. **Answers 1** and **4** are incorrect because they provide information about the nurse's personal life that is irrelevant to the maintenance of a therapeutic relationship. **Answer 2** is incorrect because it plays into the patient's manipulation.

Test-taking tip—Review therapeutic communication. This is a technique to redirect focus back to the patient. **Answers 1** and **4** focus on the nurse.

IMP, 7, PsI, Coping and Adaptation

23. **(4)** Amniotic fluid is alkaline, which makes litmus paper turn blue. **Answer 1** is incorrect because the fluid is usually milky or opaque with small white flecks (vernix caseosa), *not* bloody. Bloody amniotic fluid may indicate abruptio placentae. **Answer 2** is incorrect because *no* offensive odor is usually apparent. **Answer 3** is incorrect because most amniotic fluid has a *thin* consistency, not thick.

Test-taking tip—Think amniotic = alkaline (blue litmus).

EV, 6, HPM, Growth and Development

24. **(3)** Although some complete or partial amputations may result from trauma (**Answer 1**), the majority are necessitated by arteriosclerosis obliterans. **Answer 2** is incorrect because long-standing complications of diabetes mellitus are peripheral vascular insufficiency and infections, which in turn may increase the likelihood of amputation. **Answer 4** is incorrect because bone tumors, particularly of the knee, necessitate amputation less often than arteriosclerosis obliterans.

Test-taking tip—Think broad and most encompassing.

AN, 3, PhI, Physiological Adaptation

25. **(1)** Initially, the nurse must obtain more information about the patient's pain before giving medication. **Answer 2** is incorrect because if the pain were due to compression of the leg by a cast that is too tight, medicating the patient could result in serious neurovascular complications. **Answers 3** and **4** are incorrect because offering reassurance or distraction is not appropriate at this time, or a sufficient nursing intervention.

Test-taking tip—Assessment is always the first step of the nursing process.

IMP, 3, PhI, Physiological Adaptation

26. **(3)** Diazepam is a CNS depressant, and in children and elderly adults, it may depress the respiratory center. Thus, when the patient returns to the unit, the nurse should first evaluate respirations. **Answers 1, 2,** and **4** are incorrect. After determining that the patient is breathing adequately, the nurse can then evaluate the temperature, pulse, and blood pressure.

Test-taking tip—Patent airway and respirations are always the priority of care.

EV, 1, PhI, Pharmacological and Parenteral Therapies

27. **(3)** Many times the physiological response to stress may be a decrease in milk production. This may rectify itself over time, provided the anxiety is controlled. However, as long as the system is under prolonged, intense stress, the milk supply will probably remain diminished. **Answers 1** and **4** are incorrect because the nurse does *not* have physiological evidence to substantiate the probability of a virus or of occluded lactation ducts. **Answer 2** is incorrect because the surviving infant is probably *too young* to react physiologically to the twin's death. However, it is possible that the infant is experiencing some emotional trauma in response both to the increase in familial tension and to not hearing or seeing the other twin.

Test-taking tip—Think funeral = increased stress. Note the similarity between the stem ("producing . . . milk") and **Answer 3** ("milk producing"). Review factors that might alter normal lactation.

IMP, 5, PsI, Coping and Adaptation

28. **(3)** Pyloric stenosis is not a congenital anatomical defect, but the precise etiology is unknown. It develops gradually during the *first few weeks* of life. **Answer 1** is incorrect because pyloric stenosis is not present *at* birth. **Answer 2** is incorrect because pyloric stenosis is not acquired due to a formula allergy. **Answer 4** is incorrect because the presence of pyloric stenosis is well known before surgery.

Test-taking tip—Know the facts about causation in order to answer correctly.

IMP, 4, HPM, Prevention and Early Detection of Disease

29. **(1)** Morphine sulfate acts on subcortical brain levels not only to inhibit perception of pain and to decrease apprehension and anxiety by inducing euphoria, but also to decrease sympathetic nervous system stimulation, thereby reducing peripheral arterial resistance and increasing venous capacitance. A side effect of this last action is hypotension. **Answer 2** is incorrect because morphine reduces arterial resistance. **Answer 3** is incorrect because a second side effect of morphine is respiratory *depression*. **Answer 4** is incorrect because it describes actions directly opposite to the effects of morphine.

Test-taking tip—Know expected effect of morphine on blood vessels.

PL, 6, PhI, Pharmacological and Parenteral Therapies

30. **(4)** In this case the nurse's calm, assured manner would be most therapeutic. It would serve to decrease the couple's anxiety and to facilitate an effective admission, labor, and birth. **Answer 1** is incorrect because the couple's anxiety level would probably interfere with effective learning at this time. However, reinforcing any previously learned material and answering questions may be used. **Answer 2** is incorrect because although the woman is in active labor, she is *not ready* to give birth at this time. **Answer 3** is incorrect because assessing the couple's level of preparation would be done *in conjunction* with answering questions. It would be more important to assess their level of *readiness rather* than preparation at this time.

Test-taking tip—When two answers are correct, select the one that encompasses them both (in this case, by answering whatever questions they have, the nurse will be able to assess their level of preparation).

IMP, 5, PsI, Coping and Adaptation

31. **(2)** In selecting the correct needle to administer an IM injection to a preschool child, the nurse should always look at the child and use judgment in evaluating muscle mass and amount of subcutaneous fat. In this case, in the absence of further data, the nurse would be most correct in selecting a needle gauge and length appropriate for the "average" preschool child. A medium-gauge needle (21 G) that is 1 inch long would be most appropriate. **Answer 1** is incorrect because a ⅝ inch needle would be too short. A 25 G needle would be too thin to use on most preschool children. **Answer 3** is incorrect because an 18 G needle would be too large (wide) to use on most preschool children and would be better suited for a school-age child or an adolescent. **Answer 4** is incorrect because a 1½ inch needle would be too long. An 18 G needle would also be too large (wide) to use on

most preschool children and would be better suited for a school-age child or an adolescent.

> **Test-taking tip**—Select the midpoint: not too long, not too short; not too narrow, not too wide.

IMP, 1, PhI, Pharmacological and Parenteral Therapies

32. **(1)** Before beginning any teaching plan, the nurse must assess the patient's current understanding of the procedure, as well as his or her interest and ability to comprehend different facets of it. The physician has generally given the patient an outline of the facts as to why the procedure is necessary. **Answer 2** is incorrect because the patient's husband, wife, or significant others may be invited to join the teaching session *if* the clinical situation allows; otherwise they should be informed separately. **Answer 3** is incorrect because several intervening variables, such as anxiety and decreased cerebral perfusion, may be affecting the patient's ability to absorb information. Therefore, it is frequently necessary not only to reinforce information given by the physician but also to reexplain the procedure. **Answer 4** is incorrect because *after* explanations of the procedure, the operative permit is signed, thereby ensuring *informed* consent.

> **Test-taking tip**—Think priority. What should be done before teaching?

IMP, 7, PhI, Reduction of Risk Potential

33. **(3)** When the patient knows what to expect or who will do the care on return from the operating room, anxiety decreases. **Answer 1** is incorrect because it would be difficult for the patient to relax in high Fowler's position, and at this time there is no documented evidence of respiratory distress. **Answer 2** is incorrect because the patient may be drowsy but may not be asleep. Assuring the patient that he or she will be asleep gives false information. **Answer 4** is incorrect because the patient should void *before* medication is given, not after.

> **Test-taking tip**—Look for safety and security.

IMP, 1, PhI, Reduction of Risk Potential

34. **(1)** When cardiac catheterization is performed, a cutdown must be performed on a major artery in either an arm or a leg; thus, essential nursing care following this procedure involves checking the pulse in the affected extremity to be sure there is adequate circulation. **Answer 2** is incorrect because following cardiac catheterization, during which the patient does not receive anesthesia, deep breathing is unnecessary and coughing is contraindicated, as it may cause hemorrhage at the cutdown site. **Answer 3** is incorrect because there is no need to sedate the patient following this procedure, although bed rest for several hours is usually recommended. **Answer 4** is incorrect because in general, cardiac catheterization should have little or no effect on urine output; therefore, there would be no specific need to monitor urine output.

> **Test-taking tip**—When there is more than one correct answer, determine which is *most* important to the patient immediately.

IMP, 1, PhI, Reduction of Risk Potential

35. **(1)** After opening the airway by head tilt and chin lift, the nurse must look, listen, and feel for any movement of air. Often opening the airway may be all that is needed. Giving two breaths (**Answer 2**) is done after establishing breathlessness, followed by checking the pulse (**Answer 3**). Finger sweeps (**Answer 4**) are only done if ventilation is unsuccessful and back blows have been done.

> **Test-taking tip**—Remember the ABCs of CPR.

IMP, 1, PhI, Physiological Adaptation

36. **(2)** The nurse should quickly turn the patient onto the left side, lowering the head of the bed to minimize the chance of air bubbles entering the cerebral circulation, and notify the physician. **Answer 1** is incorrect because, alone, Trendelen-

burg is insufficient; the air must be trapped in the right ventricle (left-side position). **Answer 3** is incorrect because turning the patient to the right side, head up, would facilitate movement of the air embolism through the circulation and potentially to the brain. **Answer 4** is incorrect because supine in high Fowler's position would facilitate movement of the air embolism through the circulation and potentially to the brain.

> **Test-taking tip**—Visualize where the air is in the heart and keep it there.

IMP, 6, PhI, Physiological Adaptation

37. **(1)** The woman is more apt to become irritable, uncooperative, and discouraged during the transitional phase. **Answers 2 and 3** are incorrect because excitement and euphoria are associated with the latent phase, *not* the transitional phase. **Answer 4** is incorrect because seriousness is associated with the active phase, *not* the transitional phase.

> **Test-taking tip**—The key element is *when* (i.e., timing). Match the stage (active labor, latent phase, *transitional* phase) with the corresponding expected emotional reaction.

EV, 5, PsI, Coping and Adaptation

38. **(4)** Although the nurse suspects that this behavior may occur, there is no valid concern unless the couple's behavior becomes inappropriate. The nurse needs to realize that kissing is a normal part of adolescence. **Answer 1** is incorrect because some privacy may be provided; however, periodic supervision is warranted because the patient is an adolescent. However, the patient still needs companionship. **Answer 2** is incorrect because he needs to feel trusted in order to develop into an independent and mature person. **Answer 2** also serves only to highlight mistrust, and the couple may already feel that intimacy is inappropriate in this setting. **Answer 3** is incorrect because privacy is needed, *but* with some supervision to promote responsible behavior.

> **Test-taking tip**—Choose "allow" rather than "do not allow" and "prohibit."

IMP, 7, PsI, Coping and Adaptation

39. **(1)** Fresh fish with scales would be permitted on a mildly restricted (2 g) to an extremely restricted (200 mg) sodium diet. Only shellfish are restricted. **Answers 2, 3,** and **4** are incorrect because foods to be avoided on a sodium-restricted diet include ethnic foods, particularly Chinese, which is usually prepared with soy sauce; commercially prepared soups, such as canned tomato soup; and hot dogs, which are a commercially prepared meat.

> **Test-taking tip**—Look for similarities in answers. Only one choice is fresh cooked.

EV, 4, PhI, Basic Care and Comfort

40. **(1)** During exercise there is a general increase in vasomotor tone, which increases venous return. To meet the increased metabolic needs of the body, the heart normally increases its rate and stroke volume. In this patient's case, left ventricular hypertrophy has compromised the heart's ability to increase its efficiency during exercise. Therefore, even though the heart rate is increased, the stroke volume does not increase sufficiently, so the increased venous return tends to back up into the pulmonary vasculature. This results in the perception of increased work of breathing, or shortness of breath. **Answer 2** is incorrect because venous return is increased with exercise. **Answer 3** is incorrect because asynergistic cardiac contractions occur when a portion of the heart is noncontractile, as with myocardial infarction with ventricular aneurysm. **Answer 4** is not correct because obesity and sedentary lifestyle are contributing factors to physiological phenomena underlying the symptoms.

> **Test-taking tip**—Visualize blood flow through the heart and lungs. Breathing problems will occur if . . .

AN, 6, PhI, Physiological Adaptation

41. (3) The best approach in administering an injection to a preschooler is to give a short, simple explanation immediately before giving the injection, being truthful that it will hurt. This helps maintain the child's sense of trust in the nurse. **Answer 1** is incorrect because the nurse should not rely on the mother to give an appropriate explanation. **Answer 2** is incorrect because the nurse should not give the injection without telling the child anything. **Answer 4** is incorrect because the nurse should not attempt to bribe the child.

> **Test-taking tip**—Use the process of elimination to omit "mother" (the question asks for a *nursing* action) and "must" (too mandatory). Then focus on "tell" vs. "not tell."

IMP, 5, PsI, Coping and Adaptation

42. (3) Skin preps are designed primarily to reduce the occurrence of postoperative infections by reducing the number of microorganisms on the skin and by removing any hair that may tend to harbor these organisms. **Answer 1** is incorrect because cleaning excess oils and hairs is a *secondary* objective of a skin prep. **Answer 2** is incorrect because skin preps do *not* sterilize the skin or kill all the microorganisms. **Answer 4** is incorrect because providing a clear field is a *secondary* objective of a skin prep.

> **Test-taking tip**—Look for the broadest and most important choice.

PL, 1, PhI, Reduction of Risk Potential

43. (1) It is of paramount importance to prevent the patient from hurting himself or herself or others. **Answer 2** is incorrect; the nurse cannot establish a trusting relationship at this time because the patient is unable to communicate effectively. **Answer 3** is incorrect because the patient cannot be oriented to time, place, and person until he or she is able to communicate. **Answer 4** is incorrect because to isolate the patient is only one aspect of maintaining a safe environment, which will prevent the patient from harming others, as well as protect the patient from overstimulation.

> **Test-taking tip**—"Safety" is a most appropriate intervention.

PL, 2, PsI, Psychosocial Adaptation

44. (3) Patients with permanent pacemakers are cautioned to avoid all sources of high electronic output because they may cause pacemaker malfunction. Other sources of high electronic output include older, noninsulated microwave ovens, running car engines, and dental drills. **Answers 1** and **4** are incorrect because activities such as swimming and golf can be resumed usually after 5 weeks. **Answer 2** is incorrect because creative hobbies such as fashioning lamps are indicated as long as precautions are taken to avoid electrical shocks.

> **Test-taking tip**—Look for a restricted or potentially "risky" activity.

IMP, 6, PhI, Reduction of Risk Potential

45. (1) The patient is kept NPO until shock and bleeding are controlled. Often a nasogastric tube is inserted to drain off blood and to provide a route for antacid therapy. **Answer 2** is incorrect because a liquid diet is started after shock and bleeding have been controlled. **Answer 3** is incorrect because a soft, bland diet is started after a liquid diet has begun. **Answer 4** is incorrect because milk is not given; it increases gastric acid production.

> **Test-taking tip**—This is a priority question—what is safest for the patient at this time?

IMP, 4, PhI, Basic Care and Comfort

46. (2) The "formula" for determining parity is *TPAL: T* is the number of *t*erm pregnancies (38 + weeks); *P* is the number of *p*reterm pregnancies (20–37 weeks); *A* is the number of *a*bortions (pregnancies that do not reach viability, 20–22 weeks of gestation); *L* is the number of *l*iving children. This woman's first pregnancy ended in abortion and she has no living children. Her parity is T = 0, P = 0, A = 1, L = 0; or 0-0-1-0. **Answers 1, 3,** and **4** are not correct according to this formula.

> **Test-taking tip**—Use the TPAL system: term, preterm, abortions, living children.

AN, 5, HPM, Growth and Development

47. (2) One-person or two-person CPR for adults is done at a minimum rate of 80 compressions per minute (up to a rate of 100). Sixty compressions per minute (**Answer 1**) is no longer considered adequate in CPR. **Answers 3** and **4** are both within the range of acceptable rates; however, the question asks for the *minimum* rate.

> **Test-taking tip**—Asks for minimum rate (know 80).

IMP, 6, PhI, Physiological Adaptation

48. (4) Following an appendectomy, the nurses' notes in the patient's chart should include the dressing changes, input and output, and return of bowel sounds. **Answer 1** is incorrect because dumping syndrome is not a common complication following an appendectomy. **Answer 2** is incorrect: mouth care and dressing changes should be noted but are not as critical as charting input and output and bowel sounds. **Answer 3** is incorrect: following a ruptured appendectomy, a patient will be NPO initially and then gradually advanced; a low-residue diet is not routine.

> **Test-taking tip**—Potentially life-threatening situation— think priority nursing assessment.

IMP, 8, PhI, Reduction of Risk Potential

49. (3) Lidocaine is the treatment of choice in this situation. Ventricular tachycardia is a serious arrhythmia. It must be treated at once because (a) it may compromise cardiac output and (b) it is considered a precursor of ventricular fibrillation. **Answer 1** is incorrect because standing coronary care unit orders generally cover the administration of lidocaine in this situation, so it is not necessary to notify the physician to obtain a verbal order. **Answer 2** is incorrect because O_2 flow rate is increased only if clinical signs indicate the patient is in distress, which is unlikely with a short burst of ventricular tachycardia. **Answer 4** is incorrect because research data indicate that morphine sulfate may stabilize the threshold for ventricular fibrillation, but it is not the drug of choice in this situation.

> **Test-taking tip**—Life-threatening situation requires *direct* (drug) action.

IMP, 6, PhI, Physiological Adaptation

50. (2) SIDS occurs most frequently in low-birth-weight, preterm infants, and in the lower, not middle (**Answer 3**), socioeconomic groups. **Answer 1** is incorrect because SIDS occurs most frequently in blacks and Native Americans, not Hispanics. **Answer 4** is incorrect because SIDS has a lower incidence in breastfed infants.

> **Test-taking tip**—Review risk factors; when in doubt, choose an objective risk factor.

AS, 5, HPM, Prevention and Early Detection of Disease

51. (2) Elevation of 20–30 degrees is the optimum position to reduce intracranial pressure, aid venous drainage from the brain, and facilitate respiration. **Answer 1** is incorrect because flat on the back may increase the chance of aspiration. A lateral or semiprone position may be indicated in the early postoperative period if there are no signs of cerebral edema. **Answers 3** and **4** are incorrect because they may increase the amount of hip flexion and can contribute to an increase in intracranial pressure.

> **Test-taking tip**—Picture the patient position. *Optimum* is key to head *and* limb positioning.

PL, 2, PhI, Reduction of Risk Potential

52. (1) Providing reassurance that it is normal for most people to fear the unknown may bolster the husband's confidence. If more time were available, the nurse would try to explore his fears and provide emotional support. **Answer 2** is inap-

propriate because it provides *false reassurance,* which may merely increase his anxiety. **Answer 3** is incorrect because it may stimulate feelings of *guilt.* **Answer 4** is incorrect because it may not necessarily be true and may provide *false reassurance.*

> **Test-taking tip**—Eliminate the clichés and false reassurances, and select the option that acknowledges feelings.

IMP, 7, PsI, Coping and Adaptation

53. **(3)** The choice of anesthesia depends on the surgeon's choice and the patient's condition. **Answer 1** is incorrect because IV regional blocks may not provide adequate blockage of impulses for this procedure, and the patient would be awake. **Answer 2** is incorrect: though a spinal anesthetic may be used, the sawing of the bone can be very distressing to the patient, so usually a general anesthetic is preferred. **Answer 4** is incorrect because muscle relaxants are administered in conjunction with general anesthesia.

> **Test-taking tip**—Look for an *ideal* choice.

PL, 1, PhI, Pharmacological and Parenteral Therapies

54. **(1)** The cast should be fully exposed to the air to help it dry properly. **Answer 2** is incorrect because the patient should be turned every 2 hours to help the cast to dry, not remain in one position. **Answer 3** is incorrect because the cast should be elevated and placed on pillows rather than a bedboard. **Answer 4** is incorrect because the cast should be handled with the palms of the hands to avoid pressure and making indentations with the fingers.

> **Test-taking tip**—Consider patient *comfort* and *proper* technique.

PL, 3, PhI, Reduction of Risk Potential

55. **(4)** Weighing the patient and instituting intake and output records are admission procedures; therefore, they are the least important. **Answer 1** is incorrect: providing sedation to relieve anxiety and promote relaxation *is* a greater priority than weighing the patient and instituting records. **Answer 2** is incorrect: instituting arm and leg range-of-motion exercises *is* a greater priority than weighing and instituting records. **Answer 3** is incorrect: establishing an intravenous line *is* a greater priority than weighing the patient and instituting records.

> **Test-taking tip**—Look for *lowest priority* at the *time.*

PL, 6, PhI, Reduction of Risk Potential

56. **(3)** Pressure dressings are never removed (**Answer 1**), but if saturated, they should be reinforced with sterile dressings. The possibility of hemorrhage is ever-present, and signs of increased bleeding should be immediately reported to the surgeon. This is not a normal occurrence. Vital signs and Hemovac drainage and function should also be assessed. **Answer 2** is incorrect: Hemovacs may be irrigated, but generally they are not milked. **Answer 4** is incorrect because this is not a normal occurrence.

> **Test-taking tip**—Gather data to interpret finding. Assess!

IMP, 6, PhI, Reduction of Risk Potential

57. **(2)** Providing and maintaining a patent airway and administering oxygen immediately are essential to establish regular respirations. **Answer 1** is incorrect because CPR *may not be necessary* if respirations are adequately established. **Answer 3** is incorrect because reassuring the parents *is not appropriate* now. No one can accurately predict the outcome at this point. **Answer 4** is incorrect because checking the mother's chart for type of drug, amount, and time given is more appropriately the job of a second staff member in attendance. The neonate may be a candidate for naloxone HCl (Narcan).

> **Test-taking tip**—Think ABCs—patent *airway.*

IMP, 6, PhI, Physiological Adaptation

58. **(3)** Presuctioning and postsuctioning ventilation with 100% oxygen is important in reducing hypoxemia, which occurs when the flow of gases in the airway is obstructed by the suctioning catheter. **Answer 1** is incorrect because it

describes the nursing action while suctioning the patient with an *endotracheal* tube rather than a tracheal tube. **Answer 2** is incorrect because it is a proper nursing action before suctioning the patient with an endotracheal tube, *not* a tracheal tube. **Answer 4** is incorrect; although it is a correct nursing procedure before suctioning any patient, it does not *prevent* hypoxemia.

> **Test-taking tip**—Look for key words in the stem. Prevent hypoxemia → give O_2.

IMP, 6, PhI, Physiological Adaptation

59. **(2)** This response allows the couple to become informed without infringing on the physician's role. The physician can then decide either to inform the couple of the procedure to be used or to have the anesthesiologist inform them. **Answer 1** is incorrect because time is limited and the physician may decide to inform the couple himself or herself. **Answers 3** and **4** are incorrect because it is not the nurse's role to discuss anesthesia of choice.

> **Test-taking tip**—Choose the appropriate nursing role rather than the MD's role when it deals with explaining emergency procedures.

IMP, 7, SECE, Management of Care

60. **(4)** In addition to the shock of the immediate crisis, the mother probably has never accepted the fact that her son was extensively involved with drugs. **Answer 1** is incorrect because it will take time to develop as she takes in the implications of the situation. **Answer 2** is incorrect because this is *part* of the shock process. **Answer 3** is incorrect *because* acceptance is unrealistic at this time.

> **Test-taking tip**—When two or more options may be correct, choose the broad, more inclusive option (shock instead of denial).

AS, 7, PsI, Coping and Adaptation

61. **(1)** In pyloric stenosis, the pyloric sphincter at the distal end of the stomach is thickened, or stenotic. This sphincter blocks the flow of formula into the small intestine, causing vomiting; it also blocks the flow of bile back into the stomach. Thus, the infant with pyloric stenosis characteristically vomits only stomach contents, not bile (**Answer 2**), blood (**Answer 3**), or feces (**Answer 4**).

> **Test-taking tip**—The correct choice is the one that is different ("only"). All of the other choices contain another element (that does not relate to correct anatomy and pathophysiology).

AS, 4, HPM, Prevention and Early Detection of Disease

62. **(1)** The primary nursing action would be to maintain a patent airway to ensure oxygen for the woman and fetus. **Answer 2** is incorrect because although observing bowel and bladder functioning may also be important for a thorough assessment of the convulsion, it is a lower priority than providing a patent airway or ensuring safety. **Answer 3** is incorrect: CPR may be needed if the woman progresses into cardiac arrest; however, in implementing CPR, maintaining a patent airway is again the foremost priority. **Answer 4** is incorrect: providing a safe environment is an important *second* priority.

> **Test-taking tip**—When the question asks for the *primary* action, choose the action that the nurse would do *first* and that is *most critical.* Remember the ABCs—*Airway* first.

PL, 2, PhI, Reduction of Risk Potential

63. **(2)** Although ECG changes can be used to identify the site, extent of changes, and acuteness of an infarct, the extent of the injury is usually approximated by the peak levels of serial enzymes (CPK, ALT [SGOT], LDH). Of these enzymes, CPK-MB or CPK2 gives the most specific information about the amount of myocardial necrosis. **Answer 1** is incorrect because sinus tachycardia may result from a number of factors, including emotional responses and heart failure. **Answer 3** is incorrect because the duration of chest pain is

dependent not only on the extent of tissue ischemia but also on other factors, such as affective responses and muscle spasm. **Answer 4** is incorrect because primary ventricular fibrillation does not indicate the extent of infarct; fibrillation occurs due to metabolic changes in the ischemic area.

Test-taking tip—Look for a pattern. Three choices could be ongoing. Correct answer: single point in time (early).

AS, 6, PhI, Physiological Adaptation

64. **(2)** EDTA and BAL work by binding to the heavy metal lead and promoting its excretion via the kidneys. Renal toxicity may occur as a result. The nurse should force fluids and monitor kidney function carefully. The other choices are incorrect because calcium disodium edetate (EDTA) and dimercaprol (BAL) do not adversely affect the neurological system (**Answer 1**), the cardiovascular system (**Answer 3**), or the hematological system (**Answer 4**).

Test-taking tip—Determine where the drug is excreted; omit neurological, cardiovascular, and hematological systems.

EV, 8, PhI, Pharmacological and Parenteral Therapies

65. **(2)** Modified radical mastectomy consists of removal of the breast and all or selected lymph nodes with preservation of the pectoralis major muscle. The other choices are incorrect because they are examples of a simple mastectomy (**Answer 1**), classic radical mastectomy (**Answer 3**), and supraradical mastectomy (**Answer 4**).

Test-taking tip—The key word is *modified,* something less than radical.

AS, 3, PhI, Physiological Adaptation

66. **(4)** Being direct with the adolescent about this issue is extremely important because the incident violates hospital policy, the law, treatment, and parents' rules. The patient should be directly confronted and the incident discussed with the patient and the medical staff. The health team will decide whether it is in the patient's best interest to inform the parents and/or the police. **Answer 1** is incorrect because avoidance will merely perpetuate the situation. **Answers 2** and **3** are incorrect because whether to inform the police or the parents is a health team decision.

Test-taking tip—Two options are opposite actions (ignore vs. confront); eliminate "ignore" because it is a situation where rules are being violated. Eliminate "parent" (**3**) because the focus should be on the *patient.*

IMP, 7, PsI, Psychosocial Adaptation

67. **(4)** The day following surgery, the patient who has had an above-the-knee (AK) amputation is turned onto his or her abdomen for a short period. Thereafter, he or she is turned to the prone position at least three times daily. While in this position, the patient should practice push-up exercises that strengthen arm and shoulder muscles, thereby facilitating both transfer procedures and preparation for crutch walking. **Answer 1** is incorrect; sandbags or blanket rolls are used after this surgery to *prevent* outward rotation of the stump. **Answer 2** is incorrect because hyperextension of the thigh and stump is encouraged for patients with *below-the-knee* amputations only. Patients with AK amputations may perform this exercise only on medical orders, because it tends to put undue stress on the suture line. **Answer 3** is incorrect because the patient is taught at a later time to lift the buttocks and stump off the bed while in a supine position, an exercise that develops abdominal muscles necessary for stabilizing the pelvis when the patient stoops or bends.

Test-taking tip—There is a pattern in three choices (stump); only one strengthens the arms.

IMP, 3, PhI, Reduction of Risk Potential

68. **(3)** The purpose of restraints for this child is to keep the toddler from scratching the affected areas. Mitten restraints would prevent scratching, while allowing the most movement permissible. **Answer 1** is incorrect because clove-hitch restraints would needlessly restrict the toddler's movements. **Answer 2** is incorrect: elbow restraints are generally inappropriate for children with eczema, because the inner aspect of the arm is usually affected. **Answer 4** is incorrect because a Posey jacket would not prevent the child from scratching the affected areas.

Test-taking tip—Choose the *least* restrictive restraint.

IMP, 1, SECE, Safety and Infection Control

69. **(2)** Contractions may affect the pulse, BP, and respiratory rate. If possible, take vital signs between contractions. **Answer 1** is incorrect because immediately before a contraction the mother is usually very excited and apprehensive. **Answer 3** is incorrect because after a contraction she may feel more comfortable, but her vital signs may be altered due to the contraction itself. **Answer 4** is incorrect because if the nurse waits for the mother to feel totally comfortable, the nurse may never be able to assess the maternal vital signs.

Test-taking tip—Choose the midpoint: *not* before, *not* after, but *between.*

PL, 5, HPM, Prevention and Early Detection

70. **(1)** The definitive diagnosis of intussusception is based on a barium enema, which clearly demonstrates the telescoping of the bowel wall, which blocks the flow of the barium. **Answer 2** is incorrect because although a secondary effect may be a nonsurgical reduction of the telescoping (which may occur due to hydrostatic pressure), this is uncertain and is not the main reason the procedure is performed. **Answers 3** and **4** are incorrect because a barium enema is not administered to ease the passage of stool or provide symptomatic relief.

Test-taking tip—Barium enema is a diagnostic procedure; therefore, the answer involves "diagnosis."

IMP, 8, PhI, Reduction of Risk Potential

71. **(3)** These are common symptoms of pregnancy. Eighty percent of pregnant women experience breast tingling sensation during the first few weeks of gestation. **Answer 1** is incorrect because quickening usually is not perceived until the *sixteenth to eighteenth* week of gestation. **Answer 2** is incorrect because lightening usually occurs about *2 weeks before* labor in the nullipara, and with the onset of labor in subsequent pregnancies. **Answer 4** is incorrect because nausea and vomiting are not necessarily experienced by *all* women.

Test-taking tip—Choose the nursing prenatal assessment that matches with the first trimester of pregnancy and the expected finding and outcome. The key is *when,* i.e., correct *timing.*

AS, 5, HPM, Growth and Development

72. **(2)** Before any operative procedure can proceed, however minor, a voluntary, informed consent must be given. **Answer 1** is incorrect: the nurse's *third* step is to check the time and the type of preoperative medication. **Answer 3** is incorrect because before the nurse initiates preoperative care, charts should be checked *first* for operative consent and *second* for laboratory results, noting any abnormalities. **Answer 4** is incorrect: the nurse must verify an informed consent in the chart *before* checking to be sure the patient has been placed on the NPO list. Once done, it is followed up by checking for the sign on the patient's bed when the nurse goes to help the patient prepare.

Test-taking tip—This is priority question: first check for evidence of consent.

IMP, 7, SECE, Management of Care

73. **(2)** Hypotension is even more severe when there has been bleeding. **Answer 1** is incorrect because one of the advantages of spinal anesthesia is that it causes *very little* fetal depression. **Answer 3** is incorrect because if administered properly, *very little* anesthesia should cross the placenta. **Answer 4** is incorrect because it is *irrelevant* unless the mother has an adverse reaction to the anesthesia.

Test-taking tip—First, decide if the effect is primarily on the mother or the fetus. Then eliminate the two options related to the fetus. Recall that spinal anesthesia affects BP, rather than respirations.

AN, 6, PhI, Pharmacological and Parenteral Therapies

74. (3) There are no definite answers, because there are many possible causes of drug abuse. Many times not even the abuser can say why he or she began using drugs. **Answer 1** is incorrect because although peer pressure may be a contributing factor, the nurse lacks validation. **Answer 2** is incorrect because inappropriate limits is an invalidated assumption that would need to be explored further. **Answer 4** is incorrect because although feelings of isolation and of being unloved may be contributing factors, the nurse again lacks validation.

Test-taking tip—There is insufficient information in the stem to choose three of the options. Focus on the most general answer, based on lack of definitive data in the stem.

IMP, 7, PsI, Psychosocial Adaptation

75. (1) If the IV infuses at the proper rate, 110 mL per hour, from 2:30 A.M. to 6:00 A.M., 110 mL × 3.5 hours = 385 mL infused. **Answers 2, 3,** and **4** are incorrect calculations.

Test-taking tip—Basic math, not a formula.

EV, 6, PhI, Pharmacological and Parenteral Therapies

76. (1) If the alarm sounds, the parents should always respond immediately. **Answer 2** is incorrect because they should first check the infant's breathing and, if the infant is not breathing, they must start CPR immediately to prevent brain damage. However, if the infant is breathing normally when the alarm sounds, something technical is responsible for the alarm, and it would be inappropriate to begin CPR. **Answer 3** is incorrect because having to remain with the infant at all times would defeat the alarm's purpose. The adult can leave the room if the infant is being monitored correctly. **Answer 4** is incorrect because in terms of follow-up care, the physician and/or emergency department should be contacted, but only after the apnea has been successfully resolved; it is *not* appropriate to call the emergency department *while* the infant is apneic.

Test-taking tip—*Assess* first; check the infant in response to the monitor alarm.

IMP, 2, PhI, Physiological Adaptation

77. (2) Anesthesia is divided into four stages. Most surgical procedures are carried out in stage III, during which time the patient is unconscious and reflexes are depressed. As the patient eliminates the anesthetic agent, she or he goes into stage II, which is the stage of delirium or excitement. Respirations are exaggerated and irregular, and muscle tone is increased. To prevent injury during this stage, nursing measures are designed to reduce stimulation by maintaining a quiet, well-regulated environment. **Answer 1** is incorrect because continued stimulation will only increase restlessness. **Answer 3** is incorrect because pain medication may delay elimination of the anesthetic secondary to decreased respiratory excursion. **Answer 4** is incorrect because although nailbeds should always be checked for signs of hypoxia, cyanosis only occurs with severe respiratory *depression*.

Test-taking tip—Always think patient safety first.

IMP, 3, PhI, Reduction of Risk Potential

78. (1) An early indication of cardiac decompensation is tachycardia. Therefore, the patient's vital signs, mentation, and pulmonary status should be assessed to rule out this complication of myocardial infarction. Other causes of tachycardia are hypovolemia, anxiety, and pain. Assessment of pain and emotional status can be determined during cognitive assessment. **Answers 2, 3,** and **4** are incorrect because actions such as encouraging verbalization of feelings, administering oxygen, and decreasing the rate of intravenous infusion will be determined by the nurse's assessment of vital signs.

Test-taking tip—Choose the first step of the nursing process: *assess*.

IMP, 6, PhI, Physiological Adaptation

79. (3) Signs and symptoms of a hemolytic reaction usually include chills, shaking, fever, red (or black) urine, headache, and flank pain. **Answer 1** is incorrect because urticaria is not a common sign in a hemolytic reaction, although it is common with an allergic reaction. **Answers 2** and **4** are incorrect because neither polyuria nor hypothermia is a common sign in a hemolytic reaction.

Test-taking tip—Recognize possible complications (kidney with hemolysis).

AS, 6, PhI, Pharmacological and Parenteral Therapies

80. (2) Both atropine and isoproterenol (Isuprel) are kept available in the preoperative period as drugs of choice should the ventricular rate decrease further. Isoproterenol enhances pacemaker automaticity and facilitates AV conduction in heart block. Atropine acts to enhance AV conduction by inhibiting parasympathetic nervous system innervation of the AV node. **Answer 1** is incorrect because lidocaine is an antiarrhythmic used to depress myocardial automaticity. Therefore, this drug would not be indicated should the patient's ventricular rate decrease in the preinsertion period. **Answer 3** is incorrect because digoxin enhances vagal stimulation of the AV node, decreasing conduction through the node, and therefore would not be indicated should the patient's ventricular rate decrease in the preinsertion period. **Answer 4** is incorrect because propranolol is a beta-blocker that depresses cardiac contractility and heart rate. This drug would not be indicated should the patient's ventricular rate decrease in the preinsertion period.

Test-taking tip—Note pattern in drug effects: three slow or depress cardiac function.

PL, 6, PhI, Pharmacological and Parenteral Therapies

81. (3) Bryant's traction is a form of skin traction used in infants and toddlers with fractured femurs; when applied correctly, adhesive material should be taped to the skin of both legs. **Answers 1** and **2** are incorrect because skeletal traction in the form of a Kirschner wire or Steinmann pin is not used in Bryant's traction. **Answer 4** is incorrect because adhesive material should be taped to the skin of both legs, not one leg.

Test-taking tip—Choose the option that is different: three options have *one* leg; one option involves *both* legs. Bryant's traction is always applied bilaterally.

AS, 3, PhI, Basic Care and Comfort

82. (2) Positive pregnancy test results are considered among the *probable* signs of pregnancy (with the exception of the bioassay test for the beta subunit of HCG, which is accurate). **Answers 1, 3,** and **4** are incorrect because hearing fetal heart sounds, feeling fetal movements, and seeing the fetus are all *positive* signs of pregnancy, not probable signs.

Test-taking tip—The positive pregnancy test is a *probable* sign. Compare presumptive, probable, and positive signs of pregnancy.

IMP, 5, HPM, Growth and Development

83. (1) Bland feedings should be given in small amounts on a frequent basis to neutralize the hydrochloric acid and to prevent overload. **Answer 2** is incorrect because clear liquids may not control the amount of acid in the stomach, would be monotonous, and may lack all the necessary nutrients. **Answer 3** is incorrect because a regular diet may overload the system. **Answer 4** is incorrect: NPO would promote the production of free acid in the stomach and increase the symptoms.

Test-taking tip—Consider time element (*first* diet).

PL, 4, PhI, Basic Care and Comfort

84. (4) This response does not contradict the patient's perceptions, is honest, and shows empathy. **Answer 1** is incorrect

because it "humors" the patient and is dishonest and non-therapeutic. **Answer 2** is incorrect because it makes fun of the patient. **Answer 3** is incorrect because it avoids the situation and makes the patient feel that the nurse does not care.

> **Test-taking tip**—Choose the answer that provides reality orientation and acknowledges feelings.

IMP, 2, PsI, Psychosocial Adaptation

85. **(3)** Dentures, hairpins, and combs must be removed. Nail polish must be removed so cyanosis can be easily monitored by observing nailbeds. **Answer 1** is incorrect because the wedding band is taped securely to the finger, not removed. **Answer 2** is incorrect because in the short time available before surgery, although the patient should be allowed to voice concerns and should be given any needed support, time will not permit an extensive exploration of the basis of the patient's concerns. **Answer 4** is incorrect because the patient should void before receiving medication, not afterward.

> **Test-taking tip**—Think patient safety first.

IMP, 1, PhI, Reduction of Risk Potential

86. **(1)** Hypertensive patients should be cautioned to make position changes slowly to prevent intermittent postural hypotension. **Answer 2** is incorrect because alcohol may *contribute* to hypotension, *not* prevent it. **Answer 3** is incorrect because cold causes *vasoconstriction*, not vasodilation associated with hypotension. **Answer 4** is incorrect because exercise increases, *not* decreases, vasodilation.

> **Test-taking tip**—Correct choice is a common activity.

IMP, 6, PhI, Pharmacological and Parenteral Therapies

87. **(3)** Atropine is a cholinergic blocker (parasympatholytic) used preoperatively to diminish secretions and to block cardiac vagal reflexes. Normal side effects include dry mouth; hot, dry, flushed skin; and tachycardia or palpitations. Thus, the patient can be safely told that these are normal, expected effects of atropine; in fact, this probably should have been included in the preop instructions, before the patient even received the medication. **Answer 1** is incorrect because it would be unnecessary to administer the atropine antidote, which is physostigmine salicylate. **Answer 2** is incorrect because it would be inappropriate to bathe the patient at this time. **Answer 4** is incorrect because it would be unnecessary to page the surgeon.

> **Test-taking tip**—Know both the expected and untoward effects. Three options imply that there is a problem; one does not. Choose the option that is different in this case.

EV, 1, PhI, Pharmacological and Parenteral Therapies

88. **(3)** Breast size is not as important as the amount of glandular tissue, because it is not the adipose tissue but the secreting tissues of the mammary glands that produce the milk. **Answers 1** and **2** are incorrect responses because adequate diet and rest *are* essential to promoting lactation. **Answer 4** is incorrect because she may ovulate and could become pregnant while lactating.

> **Test-taking tip**—When a question asks for the "need for further teaching," choose the *incorrect* answer; in this case eliminate the one that is a myth.

EV, 4, HPM, Growth and Development

89. **(2)** Having the legs elevated (20 degrees) in a straight line, and the trunk horizontal, improves venous return to the heart and prevents abdominal viscera from impinging on the diaphragm. **Answer 1** is incorrect because oxygen administration may have a palliative effect but does not affect venous return. **Answer 3** is incorrect because the Trendelenburg position, after initially increasing blood flow to the brain, initiates a reflex mechanism that causes cerebral vasoconstriction. **Answer 4** is incorrect: wrapping the patient in blankets will cause dilation of the peripheral vasculature, which will further decrease venous return.

> **Test-taking tip**—Visualize impact of choice on improving blood flow to *heart*.

IMP, 6, PhI, Physiological Adaptation

90. **(1)** To prevent exacerbating the eczema, it is generally recommended that the child wear pure, natural cotton clothing only. **Answers 2, 3,** and **4** are incorrect because linen, wool, and polyester blends are more likely to cause worsening of the eczema.

> **Test-taking tip**—Because of the allergic nature of eczema, any food or clothing should be hypoallergenic.

IMP, 1, PhI, Basic Care and Comfort

91. **(3)** Enemas are not administered when there is vaginal bleeding or preterm labor or when the fetus is in an abnormal presentation or position. **Answer 1** is incorrect for the same reason. **Answer 2** is incorrect: soapsuds enemas are contraindicated because they are potentially dangerous due to their physiological incompatibility with the lower gastrointestinal tract. **Answer 4** is incorrect: though the fetal position must be assessed before administering an enema, enemas are not administered in these circumstances.

> **Test-taking tip**—The decision to make in choosing the best answer here is whether or not enemas are OK in this case. Because they are *not*, choose the option in which the enema is *not* given (i.e., "Refuse . . .").

IMP, 1, PhI, Reduction of Risk Potential

92. **(3)** Broken ribs may occur *even with proper CPR technique,* particularly when performed on the elderly. The nurse should check that the hands are positioned properly, then continue CPR even if the cracking continues. Broken ribs will heal, whereas stopping compressions (**Answer 1**) will likely result in the patient's death. Compressing less than the standard of 1.5 to 2 inches (**Answer 2**) will be ineffective on an adult. Individual strength (**Answer 4**) is irrelevant; proper hand position and depth are essential for anyone doing CPR.

> **Test-taking tip**—First step in the nursing process—*assess* technique.

EV, 1, PhI, Physiological Adaptation

93. **(2)** This response is open ended and will elicit the most information. **Answer 1** is incorrect because it merely provides false reassurance and *trivializes* her feelings. **Answer 3** is incorrect: although it may be a therapeutic response, it is a short-term intervention unless the nurse consistently sits with the woman for a while every day. If possible, the same nurse should be assigned to her each day. **Answer 4** is an inappropriate nursing intervention because the nurse *can* work in conjunction with the physician to provide psychological support.

> **Test-taking tip**—*Eliminate* the response that minimizes the patient's concern (**1**); the response that is OK but it does not focus on the patient's feelings (**3**); and the response that "passes the buck" to the MD (**4**).

IMP, 7, PsI, Coping and Adaptation

94. **(4)** Periodic checks on pacemaker function are essential and may be accomplished by pulse taking, frequent ECGs, or telephone transmission of ECG. Generally, rate changes greater than ±15 beats should be reported to the physician; so should symptoms such as syncope, dizziness, hiccoughs (diaphragmatic stimulation), dyspnea, chest pain, and fluid retention. **Answer 1** is incorrect because it is incomplete. The patient must also report rate changes and symptoms. **Answer 2** is incorrect because drainage and discoloration refer to indicators of infection. **Answer 3** is incorrect: although estimating battery life indicates that the patient understands the battery pack has a limited life expectancy, the answer is incomplete.

> **Test-taking tip**—There are two correct responses; choose the one that is more complete.

EV, 6, PhI, Reduction of Risk Potential

95. **(1)** This is the most appropriate and honest response. However, it is essential to answer the question clearly, without stimulating unnecessary fear. **Answer 2** is incorrect because there is *no way to guarantee* the birth of a healthy infant. Furthermore, the woman smoked early in her pregnancy, the period of organogenesis when the conceptus is most susceptible to teratogenic effects. **Answer 3** is incorrect: there is *no way to absolutely validate* this. **Answer 4** is incorrect because there are no definitive *data* to support such a claim.

Test-taking tip—Look at the verbs and choose **Answer 1** as the least definitive in this case: "*could* affect" (1), "*is assured*" (2), "*is due to*" (3), "*is considered*" (4).

IMP, 1, HPM, Prevention and Early Detection

96. **(4)** In the three-point gait, both crutches and the affected "bad" leg and foot are moved together, with the unaffected "good" leg and foot following. **Answers 1 and 2** are incorrect because the crutches are both moved simultaneously, not independently. **Answer 3** is incorrect because the patient should not bear any weight on the fractured leg when using the three-point gait.

Test-taking tip—Visualize each answer. Which one avoids weight bearing?

IMP, 3, PhI, Basic Care and Comfort

97. **(1)** The airway tube should remain in place and the patient's head should be turned to the side to prevent obstruction of the airway by the tongue and to allow secretions to drain from the mouth. **Answer 2** is incorrect because the head is not turned to the side. **Answers 3 and 4** are incorrect because the airway tube should never be removed until the patient is alert enough to begin attempting to eject it. Leaving the airway tube in after this point may cause vomiting due to stimulation of the gag reflex.

Test-taking tip—Think patient safety as a priority.

IMP, 6, PhI, Reduction of Risk Potential

98. **(3)** Attempting to control the situation and do as the patient pleases is most likely the patient's primary goal, in light of the history of drug abuse. Bending the rules for a severe violation of hospital policy, the treatment, and the law is not justified. For **Answer 1** to be correct, the nurse would need further evidence of the patient's desire to change, such as overt, consistent changes in the patient's pattern of behavior and open verbalization of feelings. **Answers 2 and 4** are incorrect because they are aspects of manipulation.

Test-taking tip—Review the concept of manipulation.

AN, 7, PsI, Coping and Adaptation

99. **(4)** Tachycardia decreases diastole, which decreases ventricular filling time and stroke volume. A significant decrease in stroke volume will result in a concomitant fall in cardiac output and tissue perfusion. Decreased cerebral perfusion and cellular hypoxia will result in signs of increased restlessness, anxiety, apprehension, and irritability. **Answer 1** is incorrect because to prime the pump, venous return is *enhanced* by the activation of circulatory reflexes, not depressed. **Answer 2** is incorrect because tachycardia is the result of *increased* sympathetic nervous system stimulation of the heart and may result in the patient's awareness of his or her heartbeat, thus increasing anxiety. **Answer 3** is incorrect because decreased cardiac output and tissue perfusion only occur at very high rates or when myocardial contractility is compromised, as with myocardial infarction.

Test-taking tip—Recognize expected outcome from physiological response.

EV, 6, PhI, Physiological Adaptation

100. **(2)** Down syndrome is due to chromosomal aberration and, although trisomy 21 is more common in infants of older women, another form, mosaicism, occurs in pregnancies of women of all ages. **Answer 1** is incorrect because an extra chromosome *is* implicated in the development of Down syndrome. **Answer 3** is incorrect because amniocentesis at or after 16 weeks of gestation *can* successfully identify the presence of this abnormality. **Answer 4** is incorrect because varying degrees of mental retardation *do* accompany Down syndrome.

Test-taking tip—When the question asks when further teaching is necessary, choose the *incorrect* answer. Understand the chromosomal abnormalities associated with Down syndrome and incidence of occurrence.

EV, 5, HPM, Prevention and Early Detection

101. **(1)** Above-the-knee amputations are often necessary because of the extent of the disease. The most critical factor in determining the level of the amputation is the adequacy of the arterial blood supply. **Answer 2** is incorrect because it describes the advantages associated with a below-the-knee amputation. **Answer 3** is incorrect because an above-the-knee amputation requires *more* energy for rehabilitation and walking. **Answer 4** is incorrect because a below-the-knee amputation not only heals faster than does an above-the-knee amputation, but it is less painful postsurgically, less psychologically disturbing, and less prone to contractures.

Test-taking tip—See a pattern? Three choices deal with a postoperative concern. The correct choice explains the initial decision.

IMP, 6, PhI, Physiological Adaptation

102. **(2)** Suction is applied only after the catheter is in place and ready for withdrawal. Applying suction intermittently and rotating the suction catheter assist in reducing the negative pressure effects of suctioning. Suctioning should be limited to periods of 10–15 seconds. **Answers 1, 3, and 4** are incorrect because of the negative effects these actions would have on patient aeration.

Test-taking tip—Proper and safe technique: three choices include during "insertion."

IMP, 6, PhI, Physiological Adaptation

103. **(2)** Wiggling the toes indicates that the motor block caused by the spinal is wearing off. However, the autonomic block is still present, and the woman may experience hypotension (not hypertension). **Answer 1** is incorrect because the autonomic block is *still* present even though the effects of the anesthesia are wearing off. **Answer 3** is incorrect because wiggling the toes indicates that the motor block caused by the spinal is wearing off and is therefore *not meaningless*. **Answer 4** is incorrect because the woman may experience *hypo*tension.

Test-taking tip—In this question, focus on two contradictory options: *hypo*tensive vs. *hyper*tension. Remember: a spinal causes decreased BP.

EV, 2, PhI, Pharmacological and Parenteral Therapies

104. **(3)** The most effective intervention to help preschoolers cope with painful experiences during hospitalization is to offer the opportunity for therapeutic play with puppets or dolls and medical equipment. This type of play experience allows the child to "act out" frustrations and anger in a safe, controlled manner, enabling the child to work through feelings about a difficult experience. **Answers 1, 2, and 4** are incorrect because playing with toys, engaging in free play, and playing with other children are not as effective as offering an opportunity for therapeutic play.

Test-taking tip—*Therapeutic* release of feelings (pain) is accomplished best via *therapeutic* (medical) play.

IMP, 5, PsI, Coping and Adaptation

105. **(2)** Low Fowler's to semi-Fowler's position with the arm elevated on pillows so that the wrist and elbow are slightly higher than the shoulder best facilitates venous return, reducing the occurrence of edema. Some physicians may order that the patient be positioned so that the hand is raised above the head. **Answers 1, 3, and 4** are incorrect because venous return is not enhanced, or muscle contractures may possibly develop.

Test-taking tip—Visualize the position of the arm.

IMP, 6, PhI, Physiological Adaptation

106. **(3)** The treatment of drug abuse is only effective if the client is motivated to make changes in style and pattern of living. Although the hazards of drugs (**Answer 1**), the fact that using drugs is illegal (**Answer 2**), and developing alternative coping mechanisms (**Answer 4**) are all significant components to be incorporated in health teaching, the client must first be motivated to learn.

> **Test-taking tip**—Key phrase is "most important aspect of treatment"; in this question, "motivation" precedes other choices.

PL, 7, PsI, Psychosocial Adaptation

107. **(1)** After marking the original dressing (to indicate the extent of the bleeding) and reinforcing the dressing (to prevent infection), the nurse should check the vital signs to determine if the bleeding episode has had any effect on the child's physiological status. **Answer 2** is incorrect because in general the nurse should never change the flow rate of the IV without a physician's order. **Answers 3** and **4** are incorrect because *after* checking vital signs, depending on the status of the bleeding and the vital signs, the nurse might change the patient's position and notify the cardiologist.

> **Test-taking tip**—Look at the verbs; select a verb that assesses ("*check*" before "increase," "place," or "notify"). Assessment is the first step of the nursing process.

IMP, 6, PhI, Physiological Adaptation

108. **(2)** All physicians and institutions have their own guidelines. However, 3 weeks is generally appropriate if the lochia has decreased and becomes fairly clear in color, and if there are no other problems. **Answer 1** is incorrect because 6 weeks is *longer* than is usually necessary. **Answer 3** is incorrect because when they arrive home is *too soon*. **Answer 4** is incorrect because waiting until breastfeeding ceases is *longer* than is usually necessary.

> **Test-taking tip**—The key factor is best timing—*when*: not too soon ("as soon as . . . arrive home"); not too long (6 weeks, or when she stops breast feeding).

IMP, 5, HPM, Growth and Development

109. **(1)** Isoproterenol is categorized as a beta-mimetic, in that its action simulates beta-adrenergic discharge. Actions include increased strength of cardiac contraction, increased heart rate, and decreased venous pooling, which increases venous return. An additional effect of isoproterenol is increased myocardial consumption resulting from increased rate and contractility. Isoproterenol is not a cardiac glycoside (**Answer 2**) like *digoxin,* an anticholinergic (**Answer 3**) like *atropine,* or a beta-blocker (**Answer 4**) like *propanolol.*

> **Test-taking tip**—Recognize expected drug effects.

AS, 6, PhI, Pharmacological and Parenteral Therapies

110. **(4)** An effective assessment of the couple's needs is obtained through discussing the couple's own perceptions of those needs. **Answers 1** and **2** are incorrect: although referral to social services or family counseling may be an appropriate action once a thorough assessment is complete, it should *never precede* discussion with the couple. **Answer 3** is incorrect: although supportive counseling may be an appropriate action once a thorough assessment is complete, it also should *never precede* discussion with the couple.

> **Test-taking tip**—Choose "assess" *before* "refer" or "provide." Review the nurse's role as patient advocate and guidelines for proper referral.

IMP, 7, SECE, Management of Care

111. **(3)** Phantom limb pain or sensation is an unpleasant complication that sometimes follows amputation. This phenomenon is not completely understood but is believed to result from afferent nerve fibers (sensory) severed during surgery. The pain in the limb may be identical to that perceived by the patient before surgery. The patient needs to be aware of the nature of this discomfort. Sometimes the sensation will disappear if the patient looks at the stump and recalls that the limb has been amputated. In cases where discomfort persists, alcohol may be injected into the nerve endings for temporary relief, the nerve endings may be removed, or on rare occasions reamputation may be required. **Answers 1** and **2** are incorrect because they negate the patient's perceptions of discomfort and avoid the issue. **Answer 4** is incorrect: an explanation of the phenomenon and other palliative measures should *precede* the administration of a narcotic.

> **Test-taking tip**—*First* response: address the patient's comment.

IMP, 2, PhI, Basic Care and Comfort

112. **(4)** Conflicts concerning discharge instructions following myocardial infarction and pacemaker insertion are common. When the nurse prepares a patient for discharge, it is important to recognize that both patient and spouse may have several fears they have not verbalized. Allow time for and encourage verbalization of feelings. Likewise, be sure that discharge instructions are feasible for the individual's lifestyle; if they are not, work out a plan of modification with the patient, family, and physician. Referral to a community health nurse or local cardiac rehabilitation support group may also facilitate the rehabilitation. **Answers 1, 2,** and **3** are incorrect because they cut off the patient's and spouse's range of response and may therefore preclude obtaining pertinent data.

> **Test-taking tip**—Look for the broadest response.

IMP, 7, PsI, Coping and Adaptation

113. **(1)** Straightforward, direct communication is needed to keep the client from manipulating his or her care. The nurse needs to be honest and to set firm limits. **Answer 2** is incorrect because an adolescent drug abuser tends to be very manipulative; however, allowing the client to *assist* in the decision-making process is essential. **Answer 3** is incorrect because too much security will foster dependence. The client needs to identify and begin to cope with the anxiety, although anxiety generally cannot be eliminated entirely. **Answer 4** is incorrect because drug abusers are already characteristically very dependent individuals.

> **Test-taking tip**—Concept of manipulation is operative here, requiring direct communication.

PL, 7, PsI, Psychosocial Adaptation

114. **(3)** Per MD order, the IV should infuse at 320 mL every 8 hours, or 40 mL per hour. Thus, if there is 425 mL left in the IV and it runs at 40 mL per hour, the present bag should last 10 hours, or from 11:30 A.M. to 9:30 P.M. The nurse should plan to change the bag at 9:00 P.M., before it runs out completely. **Answers 1** and **2** are incorrect because changing it earlier would waste IV fluid, which is costly. **Answer 4** is incorrect because changing it later would mean the IV would run out completely, which may result in an embolism or a clogged IV line.

> **Test-taking tip**—Basic math, no formula required.

IMP, 6, PhI, Pharmacological and Parenteral Therapies

115. **(2)** As the capillary pressure in the lungs increases from cardiac decompensation, fluid pours from the circulatory system, across the capillary membrane into the alveoli, bronchi, and bronchioles. Typical manifestations include a respiratory rate as high as 60–70 breaths per minute and a persistent cough with expectoration of large amounts of frothy, blood-tinged sputum (hemoptysis). **Answer 1** is incorrect because the patient's face will be pale, not flushed. **Answer 3** is incorrect because the cough is productive, not hacking, and purulent sputum would be seen with an infection such as pneumonia. **Answer 4** is partially correct, except the patient in pulmonary edema will show signs of shock and be cold, most likely with a subnormal temperature.

> **Test-taking tip**—Use a process of elimination. Visualize lungs filling with fluid.

AS, 6, PhI, Physiological Adaptation

116. **(1)** To be sure a typical antimicrobial will have the desired effect, it must be in contact with the skin for a minimum of 10 seconds. **Answers 2, 3,** and **4** are incorrect because durations longer than 10 seconds are not necessary.

   Test-taking tip—The minimum duration of time for proper hand washing is approximately equal to the amount of time it takes to whistle one stanza of the tune "Yankee Doodle Dandy" (about 10 seconds)!
   IMP, 1, SECE, Safety and Infection Control

117. **(2)** A drop in the systolic blood pressure of 20 mm Hg or more below the preoperative blood pressure is indicative of impending shock. Shock may be due to hemorrhage, vasodilation caused by anesthesia, insufficient fluid replacement, or abnormal clotting. **Answer 1** is incorrect because skin may be dry and cool in the immediate postoperative period because of normal temperature-regulating mechanisms, that is, vasoconstriction due to skin exposure in the operating room. **Answer 3** is incorrect because a diastolic reading below 70 mm Hg is significant only if it is abnormal for the patient and is accompanied by a drop in systolic or a narrowing pulse pressure. **Answer 4** is incorrect because pulse rates normally increase and decrease with respirations to some extent because changes in intrathoracic pressures affect venous return. This phenomenon, however, is more evident in children.

   Test-taking tip—Recognize changes from normal—most life threatening.
   EV, 6, PhI, Reduction of Risk Potential

118. **(2)** To reduce anxiety and ensure ease of induction, a preoperative medication should be administered 45–60 minutes before anesthesia. Side rails should be raised after administration of medication, because the patient will begin to feel drowsy and light-headed. **Answers 1, 3,** and **4** are incorrect because giving medication less than 45–60 minutes before induction of anesthesia would not allow sufficient time for the medication to reach its peak effect.

   Test-taking tip—Correct answer is broadest and most optimal for desired outcome.
   PL, 1, PhI, Pharmacological and Parenteral Therapies

119. **(1)** The patient should be given diluted orange juice to ensure an adequate supply of ascorbic acid (vitamin C). **Answers 2, 3,** and **4** are incorrect because carbohydrates, protein, and vitamin A can be easily obtained by ensuring a variety of foods in the bland diet.

   Test-taking tip—Choose the option that would potentially increase acid (ascorbic *acid*).
   EV, 4, PhI, Basic Care and Comfort

120. **(2)** Although in moderation these drugs produce feelings of well-being and alertness, an overdose of amphetamines causes an increase in tension and irritability. **Answers 1** and **3** are incorrect because an increase in the heart rate and blood flow is exhibited (these drugs stimulate the release of norepinephrine). **Answer 4** is incorrect because diarrhea, not constipation, is a common side effect.

   Test-taking tip—Review signs and symptoms of amphetamine abuse.
   EV, 7, PhI, Physiological Adaptation

121. **(1)** Obtaining consent and informing the woman about the risks involved are legally the *physician's* role. The nurse's role is to reinforce the physician's teaching and to confirm that the information has been given to the woman. **Answer 2** is an incorrect response because it *is* an appropriate nursing action to reinforce the physician's teaching and to confirm that the information has been given to the woman. **Answers 3** and **4** are incorrect because monitoring the fetal heart rate and observing for bleeding *are* both appropriate nursing actions.

   Test-taking tip—When asked to choose the *least* likely, choose an *incorrect* answer. Review the nurse's legal responsibilities regarding informed consent for procedures.

PL, 7, SECE, Management of Care

122. **(4)** If it appears that the patient's IV has infiltrated (site is red and swollen), the only acceptable action by the nurse would be to remove the IV line. **Answer 1** is incorrect: *after* removing the IV line, the nurse might apply warm soaks if the area appeared reddened. **Answer 2** is incorrect because the nurse should not increase or decrease the flow rate without a physician's order. **Answer 3** is incorrect because elevating the site would further slow the flow rate, although IV fluids would continue to drip into tissue and might cause damage to the surrounding area.

   Test-taking tip—Priority: *immediate action*. Safety is the priority of care; only one action *stops* the procedure.
   IMP, 1, PhI, Pharmacological and Parenteral Therapies

123. **(1)** The most objective measure of the effectiveness of an antibiotic is a return of the white blood cell count to normal. **Answer 2** is incorrect because a low-grade temperature may indicate a lingering infection. **Answers 3** and **4** are incorrect because no pain and a good appetite are both good clinical indicators, but not as objective or as clearly measurable as the white blood cell count.

   Test-taking tip—Key term is "*most* indicative" of a therapeutic response (*no infection*).
   EV, 1, PhI, Pharmacological and Parenteral Therapies

124. **(4)** The classic vital sign changes in increased intracranial pressure are known as Cushing's reflex. The pressure on the vasomotor center in the brain produces a slowing of the heart rate (bradycardia), an increase in the pulse pressure in an attempt to increase cerebral perfusion pressure, and an irregular breathing pattern (e.g., Biot's or ataxic, Cheyne-Stokes, apneustic). **Answer 1** is incorrect because the vital sign changes indicate shock and are the opposite of increased intracranial pressure. **Answer 2** is incorrect because the level of consciousness, rather than increasing, will decrease, which may be indicated by an unconscious patient becoming nonresponsive to painful stimuli. **Answer 3** is incorrect because pupil dilation will occur when there is compression of cranial nerve III (oculomotor) on the same side as the injury or hematoma, not the opposite side.

   Test-taking tip—Recognize expected outcome; changes are opposite of shock.
   EV, 2, PhI, Physiological Adaptation

125. **(1)** Many women experience some slight to moderate depression. Sleep deprivation and an inadequate support system may contribute to the "blues." **Answer 2** is incorrect: if the behaviors become severe (i.e., persistent over a long period of time and increasingly exaggerated), *then* professional help should be initiated. **Answer 3** is incorrect because a physician's referral may not be necessary and it is not the nurse's job to ask the physician to prescribe antidepressants; medication may not even be needed. **Answer 4** is incorrect because the new father should be informed that patience, understanding, and *help with housework and care of the infant* are needed, and may help decrease some of the mother's anxiety.

   Test-taking tip—The key concept being tested is using a support system. Address the father's concern directly with correct health teaching rather than jump to make a referral (**Answers 2** and **3**).
   IMP, 7, PsI, Coping and Adaptation

126. **(4)** All insulin-dependent diabetics are to receive daily insulin. However, the physician should write specific orders for insulin coverage on the day of surgery. The reason for this is that both the physical and the psychological stresses of surgery tend to increase serum-glucose levels via glycogenolysis, and the patient's usual insulin may be insufficient. **Answer 1** is incorrect because all insulin-dependent diabetics are to receive daily insulin. **Answer 2** is incorrect because the physical and psychological stresses of surgery tend to increase serum-glucose levels via glycogenolysis, and the

patient's usual insulin may be insufficient. Frequently, a rainbow coverage of regular insulin is ordered to supplement or temporarily replace daily doses of NPH or other longer-acting insulins. **Answer 3** is incorrect because the patient is not given fluids before surgery, particularly if a general anesthetic is to be administered.

Test-taking tip—Correct choice is the broadest.
IMP, 4, PhI, Pharmacological Therapy

127. **(3)** The patient is disoriented to time, place, and person and needs constant monitoring and comprehensive support. **Answer 1** is incorrect: although the patient may be physiologically hungry, this is difficult to validate because the patient is confused. **Answer 2** is incorrect because although the patient may be hallucinating, the information given here merely implies that the patient is disoriented. **Answer 4** is incorrect because the patient does not appear to be in touch with reality.

Test-taking tip—Hallucinatory behavior and disorientation go together.
AN, 2, PsI, Psychosocial Adaptation

128. **(2)** During the early postinsertion period, the inner cannula is removed using aseptic technique every 2–4 hours for cleansing. If secretions are copious or very viscous, more frequent cleansing may be necessary. If the patient is receiving oxygen therapy or is on mechanical ventilation, these treatments are continued through the outer cannula. **Answer 1** is incorrect because routine cleansing is done, even when it appears unnecessary. **Answer 3** is incorrect because once a day is not frequent enough. **Answer 4** is incorrect because the cannula *must* be removed for cleansing.

Test-taking tip—Look for the "ideal" frequency of cleansing and secretion management.
PL, 1, PhI, Reduction of Risk Potential

129. **(1)** The first stage is the stage of the cervix. The woman's cervix is dilated only 4 cm, with contractions occurring every 4–6 minutes, and she is alert. **Answer 2** is incorrect because the second stage is the stage from a 10 cm dilated cervix to full birth of the baby. **Answer 3** is incorrect because the third stage is the stage of the placenta. **Answer 4** is incorrect because the fourth stage is the period of recovery, usually the first 2 hours after birth.

Test-taking tip—These are *early* changes; therefore, select the *earliest* phase.
AN, 5, HPM, Growth and Development

130. **(4)** CHG is a highly effective antimicrobial ingredient, especially when it is used consistently over time. **Answer 1** is incorrect because soap and water, although recommended for most general patient care, is not an antimicrobial. **Answer 2** is incorrect because alcohol will degerm skin rapidly but, because of its drying effect on the skin, it is not recommended for repeated washing. **Answer 3** is incorrect because hexachlorophene acts primarily on gram-positive bacteria and has also been associated with neurotoxicity; it is no longer recommended.

Test-taking tip—Use process of elimination (and the longest answer!).
IMP, 1, SECE, Safety and Infection Control

131. **(2)** The person doing compressions should allow for a full breath to be given before starting the compressions. Without the pause, the patient will not receive sufficient ventilation. The ratio is *one* full breath to five compressions, not two breaths (**Answer 1**). The persons doing CPR may change positions *as needed*; the protocol does *not* specify the time (**Answer 3**). The compression rate for two-person CPR is the *same* as the rate for one-person CPR: 80–100 compressions per minute, not slower (**Answer 4**).

Test-taking tip—Know the "recipe" for effective CPR.
IMP, 1, PhI, Physiological Adaptation

132. **(3)** Patients must be taught to place a nitroglycerin tablet under the tongue before exercising, eating a large meal, emo-

tionally stressful events, and sexual activity. **Answer 1** is incorrect because headaches following drug use are to be expected, but lessen over time. The physician does not need to be notified unless repeated dosages (3–5 tablets) do not relieve the pain. **Answer 2** is incorrect because the medication should be stored in a dark bottle in a dry location. Refrigeration is not appropriate. **Answer 4** is incorrect because the tablet is placed under the tongue and allowed to dissolve completely, and the saliva is retained briefly before swallowing. Swallowing whole with liquid will negate the drug's effectiveness.

Test-taking tip—Only one answer deals with *when* the drug should be taken.
PL, 1, PhI, Pharmacological and Parenteral Therapies

133. **(1)** This is a health team decision that needs to be supported by the hospital administration in order to assist the family in working through the grieving process. **Answer 2** is incorrect because it may be a violation of the family's privacy. The priest's input may be considered, if the family requests it. **Answer 3** is incorrect because it is an inappropriate assumption that would need further validation. **Answer 4** is incorrect because it should not be standard policy in any hospital today. It is essential for many families to see the deceased in order to work through their grief.

Test-taking tip—The concept here is *grief.* The best answer allows the *mother* (who is the focus of the question) to grieve. Eliminate **Answers 3** and **4** because these options do *not* allow the mother to grieve. Eliminate **Answer 2** (the priest) because it moves the focus away from the mother.
IMP, 7, PsI, Coping and Adaptation

134. **(3)** In most cesareans a drape is used and one can see very little "gore" or blood. **Answer 1** is incorrect because the nurse *needs to find* out what the procedure usually involves. **Answer 2** is incorrect because in almost all hospitals a drape of some type is used. **Answer 4** is incorrect because it is *not true.*

Test-taking tip—When the question asks for the most *realistic response,* identify and eliminate the ones that are not realistic first. In this case, the longest answer is the most complete, accurate, and realistic. You can also sound out the options and eliminate **Answers 1** and **4** because they are "turn-offs." **Answer 2** leaves the partner "hanging" without a helpful response.
IMP, 7, PsI, Coping and Adaptation

135. **(3)** Both systolic and diastolic pressures should decrease as a result of the pharmacological interventions. **Answer 1** is incorrect because vasodilation and decreases in fluid volume decrease peripheral resistance, thereby lowering the diastolic pressure. **Answer 2** is incorrect for the same reason, but a concomitant drop in systolic pressure also occurs because the left ventricle is delivering its stroke volume at considerably less resistance. **Answer 4** is incorrect because the goal of antihypertensive drug therapy is to lower pressure, not slow pulse.

Test-taking tip—Recognize the *expected* outcome—initially a concurrent *increase*—with treatment a concurrent *decrease.*
EV, 6, PhI, Pharmacological and Parenteral Therapies

136. **(3)** Anxiety is a significant factor; if it is too high, anxiety would negatively affect the child's ability to learn. Although the child's chronological age (**Answer 1**), developmental level (**Answer 2**), and previous experiences (**Answer 4**) are important for the nurse to assess in relation to the teaching style or techniques to be used, they are all *less* important in terms of the child's ability to learn.

Test-taking tip—The question asks about influence on *ability* to learn, i.e., *what* affects learning, *not when.* (i.e., age-related *time frame.* Choose the *present* over *previous* influences).
AN, 5, PsI, Coping and Adaptation

137. (2) The earliest exercises initiated are passive range of motion of the elbow, wrist, and hand; these exercises are begun on the first postoperative day. As the patient is able, she is encouraged to put those joints through active range of motion. These exercises assist in maintaining function and in reducing lymphedema. Progression to other exercises, such as hair combing and wall reaching, is dependent on wound healing, grafts, presence of drainage tubes, and the patient's tolerance. **Answers 1, 3,** and **4** are incorrect responses; they are implemented after a modified mastectomy, but are not appropriate *initial* therapy.

> **Test-taking tip**—When all are correct answers, consider the time period and patient limitations early postop.

PL, 3, PhI, Reduction of Risk Potential

138. (2) Any recommendation must be based on an assessment of the mother. This will ensure that her needs are met at an appropriate level and may prevent unnecessary stress and feelings of guilt at a later time. **Answer 1** is incorrect. It may be appropriate if she thinks she would rather wean or if the combination of breastfeeding and supplemental feeding proves inadequate for the infant or mother. **Answer 3** is incorrect. It may be appropriate *if* the mother has experienced a similar situation; however, this referral should be initiated only *after* assessing and validating the need and appropriateness with the patient and with the La Leche League. **Answer 4** is incorrect. It may be appropriate *after* assessing the mother's feelings about breastfeeding; however, the supplemental feedings will need to be validated with a physician, and they will probably consist of some type of formula rather than glucose water.

> **Test-taking tip**—"Assess" *before* "recommend," "refer," or "suggest." The last two options are OK, but a matter of *timing* (i.e., OK *after*).

PL, 4, PsI, Coping and Adaptation

139. (3) Actions of isoproterenol include relaxation (dilation) of smooth muscles in the bronchi, skeletal muscle vasculature, and alimentary tract, and thus decreased bronchoconstriction. **Answer 1** is incorrect: increased peripheral vascular resistance is the action of norepinephrine (Levophed) or metariminol (Aramine). **Answer 2** is incorrect: decreased automaticity of Purkinje fibers is the action of digoxin. **Answer 4** is incorrect: decreased oral secretion is the anticholinergic effect of a drug such as atropine.

> **Test-taking tip**—Know the expected effects of cardiac drugs on the heart and lungs.

EV, 6, PhI, Pharmacological and Parenteral Therapies

140. (2) Throughout pregnancy, especially after the second trimester, most women express anxiety over their change in body image. The nurse must be aware of the need to provide positive reinforcement and encouragement in order to facilitate and maintain the woman's self-esteem. **Answer 1** is incorrect because during this stage of pregnancy the mother is very *self*-focused. **Answer 3** is incorrect because most women realize that dieting during pregnancy is contraindicated unless prescribed by a physician. **Answer 4** is of no concern to the pregnant woman because she is gaining plenty of weight.

> **Test-taking tip**—Choose the psychosocial answer. Choose the answer that is *different* from the others (not nutrition, diet, or weight).

AN, 7, HPM, Growth and Development

141. (2) While summoning the physician, the nurse should ensure that the patient's head is elevated. A sitting position bent slightly forward is best (a bedside table with pillows can be used for the patient to rest on), because it allows for the greatest lung expansion and gravity aids in shifting fluids toward the base of the lungs. Lowering the legs tends to decrease venous return by pooling blood in the periphery. **Answer 1** is incorrect because morphine SO$_4$ may be given

only per physician order. **Answer 3** is incorrect because suctioning at this time is not indicated. **Answer 4** is incorrect: supplemental oxygen *may* be given while awaiting medical orders, but *initial* nursing actions should be directed toward decreasing venous return and improving ventilation.

> **Test-taking tip**—First priority: make the patient comfortable or safe.

IMP, 6, PhI, Physiological Adaptation

142. (2) The woman in labor is instructed to lie on her *side* to promote relaxation, to prevent supine hypotension, and to facilitate anterior rotation of the fetal head. Therefore, to tell the woman to lie on her back would cause a problem to the woman. **Answer 1** *is* an appropriate action. A full bladder may impede progress or result in trauma to the bladder. **Answer 3** *is* an appropriate action. Bearing down before the second stage is fruitless and serves only to expend energy and possibly damage the cervical opening. **Answer 4** *is* an appropriate action. Slow, even breathing promotes adequate ventilation for the maternal and fetal systems and lessens anxiety.

> **Test-taking tip**—In positioning a patient, decide what you are trying to *prevent* or *promote*. The question is asking the position that is contraindicated. Review venal caval syndrome and prevention by position changes.

EV, 1, PhI, Reduction of Risk Potential

143. (4) He is essentially blaming the situation on his son's mother because he is unable to cope effectively with his own feelings at this time. **Answer 1** is incorrect because it is usually not a coping mechanism because it does not help a person cope with anxiety or other feelings. **Answer 2** is incorrect because sublimation involves rechanneling a destructive or instinctual impulse that is socially unacceptable into an acceptable outlet, such as channeling anger into sports. **Answer 3** is incorrect because it involves denying one's own thought or emotion and seeing that thought or emotion in others.

> **Test-taking tip**—Eliminate "guilt," because it is *not* a coping mechanism. Next, by definition, select the correct term.

AN, 7, PsI, Coping and Adaptation

144. (3) To best gain the cooperation of a toddler, the nurse should help her or him focus on how the treatment will help the toddler go home; the nurse should also use distraction. **Answers 1, 2,** and **4** are incorrect because the nurse should never bribe, threaten, or lie to the child.

> **Test-taking tip**—Choose the one option that is *not* manipulative, frightening, or fantasy.

IMP, 5, PsI, Psychosocial Adaptation

145. (2) The rate for cardiac compressions for infants is 100 per minute. **Answer 1** is incorrect because pressure should be evenly applied with the fingers over the middle third of the sternum, not with the heel of the hand. **Answer 3** is incorrect because to form a seal, the resuscitator should place his or her mouth over the mouth and nose of the infant. **Answer 4** is incorrect because once the seal over the airway is made, the rescuer need only use gentle, not forceful puffs of air to inflate lungs.

> **Test-taking tip**—Visualize the procedure; omit incorrect steps; choose the one option that is different (option with a number—100/minute).

IMP, 6, PhI, Physiological Adaptation

146. (2) There is no physiological dependence, but the person has to increase the dose to receive the same effect because the body develops a tolerance. **Answer 1** is incorrect because withdrawal usually leads to severe exhaustion. **Answer 3** is incorrect because overdoses induce hyperactivity within the system. **Answer 4** is incorrect because psychological, not physiological, dependence develops from increased tolerance.

> **Test-taking tip**—Know side effects of amphetamines.

IMP, 7, PhI, Pharmacological Therapy

147. **(3)** Correct medication administration is extremely important. When the medication order is of a different strength from the supplies at hand, using the following formula will be helpful in determining the correct dose:

$$\frac{\text{Desired}}{\text{Available}} \times \frac{\text{Quantity}}{\text{on hand}} = \frac{0.4}{0.6} \times \frac{15 \text{ minims}}{1}$$

$$= \frac{2}{3} \times \frac{15}{1}$$

$$= \frac{30}{3}$$

$$= 10 \text{ minims}$$

Answers 1, 2, and 4 are inaccurate calculations.

Test-taking tip—Know the correct *ratio* formula.

IMP, 1, PhI, Pharmacological and Parenteral Therapies

148. **(3)** Alcohol and smoking are thought to present dangers to the fetus. **Answer 1** is incorrect: many women *do* work until they are about to give birth. **Answer 2** is incorrect because intercourse *is* permissible in the absence of vaginal bleeding. **Answer 4** is incorrect because *caloric requirements* for growth must be maintained.

Test-taking tip—Select the option that deals with risk factors.

IMP, 5, HPM, Prevention and Early Detection of Disease

149. **(4)** The patient's dyspnea is due to a shift of fluid from systemic circulation to lungs. With left ventricular failure, blood backs up in the pulmonary vasculature, causing increased pulmonary pressure and exudation of fluids into the interstitial space, alveoli, and bronchioles—that is, pulmonary edema. **Answer 1** is incorrect because the mechanical congestion of the lungs decreases expandability (compliance) and increases the work of breathing; that is, the patient becomes aware of his or her efforts at breathing (dyspnea). **Answer 2** is incorrect because pulmonary edema also decreases the amount of pulmonary membrane available for the diffusion of gases, thereby decreasing arterial oxygen and increasing the likelihood of CO_2 retention. **Answer 3** is incorrect because venous return is increased, not decreased.

Test-taking tip—Look for similar words in the stem and answer (e.g., "pulmonary" and "lung"; "edema" and "fluid").

AN, 6, PhI, Physiological Adaptation

150. **(3)** Green fluid is usually seen when the fetus is or has *recently* been in distress and hypoxic. **Answer 1** is incorrect because Rh or ABO incompatibility may result in a *yellow* fluid. **Answer 2** is incorrect because fetal distress that occurred *36 hours* ago also may result in a *yellow* fluid. **Answer 4** is incorrect because abruptio placentae usually results in a *port wine–colored* fluid.

Test-taking tip—The key word is *green*. Recall normal appearance of amniotic fluid. Recall what alteration in color (e.g., green, yellow, or port wine) is matched with what problem. Also *time* element is important: in fetal distress, green is *now* and yellow was *before* (36 hours ago).

AN, 6, PhI, Reduction of Risk Potential

151. **(4)** The natural pathway of humidification, the upper respiratory tract, has been bypassed. Therefore, to prevent drying out of the mucous membranes of the bronchi, as well as crusting of secretions, humidification by nebulization is provided. **Answer 1** is incorrect: although supplying humidification during oxygen therapy has become standard, it is not a rationale for its use. **Answers 2** and **3** are incorrect because they are not specific to this question, though probably true to some extent.

Test-taking tip—Identify the key concept—humidification.

AN, 6, PhI, Physiological Adaptation

152. **(4)** Measles, mumps, and rubella are first given at 12–15 months, and repeated at either 4–6 years or 11–12 years. Hepatitis B (**Answer 1**), DTP (**Answer 2**), and *H. influenzae* type b (**Answer 3**) *should* all be given at 6 months.

Test-taking tip—Knowing immunization schedule is the only way to select this answer. Note that the question asks which is *not* given.

IMP, 1, HPM, Prevention and Early Detection of Disease

153. **(1)** The likelihood of product contamination after opening the bottle or bag increases over time, but the bottle or bag can hang safely for a maximum of 24 hours. Bottles or bags used for intermittent IV medications should be timed and dated, and not left hanging at the bedside for over 24 hours. The use of the heparin lock has decreased the need for KVO IVs, and medications are administered with 50 mL or 100 mL single-use solution bags. **Answers 2, 3,** and **4** are incorrect because the times are all too soon and would unnecessarily increase the cost of hospitalization.

Test-taking tip—The best answer includes all the other choices.

EV, 6, PhI, Pharmacological and Parenteral Therapies

154. **(3)** To effectively screen for the S-shaped lateral curvature of scoliosis, the nurse should ask the adolescent to stand and bend over at the waist 90 degrees. The nurse should look for unevenness of the shoulders or hips, or any curves or humps, which require further follow-up and evaluation. **Answers 1, 2,** and **4** are incorrect because no other position is recommended.

Test-taking tip—Select the position that is not like the others; three describe a straight or flat position, only one involves bending.

AS, 3, HPM, Prevention and Early Detection of Disease

155. **(3)** Some of the most serious reactions occurring with blood transfusions are the result of human error. To reduce human error, it is essential for two nurses to verify that the patient's name and hospital number on the blood bag correspond exactly to that on the wristband. **Answers 1, 2,** and **4** are incorrect because although they are proper safeguards, they are not the *first* priority.

Test-taking tip—Only one choice deals with direct patient safety.

IMP, 6, PhI, Pharmacological and Parenteral Therapies

156. **(1)** Before adding potassium chloride to any IV line, the nurse must check that the patient's kidneys are functioning to avoid potassium overload and hyperkalemia. **Answers 2, 3,** and **4** are incorrect because it is not necessary to check reflexes, respiratory rate, or mucous membranes before adding potassium to the IV line.

Test-taking tip—Remember, "no pee = no potassium."

AN, 8, PhI, Pharmacological and Parenteral Therapies

157. **(4)** Metronidazole (Flagyl) is the drug of choice in treating *Trichomonas* vaginitis. **Answers 1** and **2** are incorrect because tetracycline and erythromycin are ineffective against *Trichomonas* infection and are more commonly used in treating *bacterial* disease. **Answer 3** is incorrect because nystatin has little effect on *Trichomonas vaginalis,* but is the drug of choice for *Candida* infection.

Test-taking tip—Choose the pharmacological agent commonly used for STDs and vaginal infections, rather than bacterial diseases (**1** and **2**).

IMP, 1, PhI, Pharmacological and Parenteral Therapies

158. **(1)** To reduce bleeding and edema, the stump is elevated for the first 24 hours; after 24 hours, however, hip flexion contracture may occur with prolonged elevation. **Answer 2** is incorrect because this procedure is not used for amputations. **Answer 3** is incorrect because this procedure is used with a below-the-knee amputation, to prevent contractures in the knee joint. **Answer 4** is incorrect: this is a standard

postoperative procedure *initiated by the surgeon in the operating room* to facilitate shrinkage of the stump and to prevent edema.

> **Test-taking tip**—Look for independent nursing actions—positioning.

IMP, 3, PhI, Reduction of Risk Potential

159. (4) When a nurse is admitting a new patient to the unit, the first action the nurse should take is to correctly identify the patient. If the patient is fully awake and alert, the nurse can ask the patient for his or her name; if the patient is a newly postop patient, still under the influence of anesthesia and medication, the nurse should first check the ID band. After identifying the patient, the nurse could *then* proceed to monitor vital signs (**Answer 3**), check the IV (**Answer 2**), and attach the Salem sump tube to suction (**Answer 1**).

> **Test-taking tip**—Focus on the patient, then the procedures with priority questions. Order of priority starts with a KIS (keep it simple) option (i.e., identify the *patient*).

IMP, 1, PhI, Reduction of Risk Potential

160. (3) Refrigerating blood assists in delaying the growth of bacteria. The blood must be administered within 4 hours, not 6 hours (**Answer 1**), but not so rapidly that the patient experiences overload (**Answers 2, 4**).

> **Test-taking tip**—Eliminate the "extremes" first (too short, too long time periods).

IMP, 6, PhI, Pharmacological and Parenteral Therapies

161. (2) Euphoria, excitement, and talkativeness are all seen *initially,* when the woman is fairly energetic and anxious to have labor begin. **Answer 1** is incorrect because a tendency to hyperventilate usually occurs during the *midactive* phase. Introverted behavior (**Answer 3**) and irritability or crying (**Answer 4**) usually occur in the *transitional* or deceleration period of the active phase of the first stage.

> **Test-taking tip**—The key is a *time* element. *First* stage, *first* euphoria. Review phases and stages of labor and a woman's expected responses.

EV, 5, PsI, Coping and Adaptation

162. (3) Splinting of the incision and tight pressure dressings tend to reduce lung expansion and ventilation. As a result, mucus can block off small bronchioles, causing atelectasis or collapse of distal alveoli. **Answer 1** is incorrect because peripheral thrombophlebitis is always a threat if the patient's legs are not exercised. In most patients, early ambulation prevents its occurrence. **Answer 2** is incorrect because wound dehiscence is more likely to occur with abdominal surgeries. **Answer 4** is incorrect because paralytic ileus is more likely to occur with abdominal surgeries, though it may occur as the result of the effects of anesthesia on autonomic nervous system function, or hypokalemia.

> **Test-taking tip**—Visualize the patient and location of surgery.

AN, 6, PhI, Reduction of Risk Potential

163. (1) In evaluating the couple's present knowledge base of childbirth and childbirth techniques, the nurse will be able to set up a more efficient and effective program of learning for the couple. The couple may have already investigated resources and may need more validation than primary health teaching. **Answer 2** is incorrect; a *secondary* goal would be to meet the couple at their level of readiness to ensure optimal learning. **Answer 3** is incorrect: *if* unsure of the information, the nurse may consult with or refer to a specialist in the area. **Answer 4** may be inappropriate if the couple desires an alternative method.

> **Test-taking tip**—First, evaluate *what* they know; then assess readiness to *learn*.

AS, 5, HPM, Growth and Development

164. (2) Following surgery for a ruptured appendix, the patient should be placed in a semi-Fowler's position to promote drainage and to prevent possible complications, such as

diaphragmatic abscess. **Answer 1** is incorrect: this position will help aerate the patient's lungs by allowing for maximum expansion, but it is not the *primary* reason for this position. **Answer 3** is incorrect because this position will *not* help splint the incision. **Answer 4** is incorrect because this position will *not* help facilitate movement or necessarily reduce complications.

> **Test-taking tip**—Visualize the position and how it would affect the operative site.

PL, 1, PhI, Reduction of Risk Potential

165. (2) Drug abusers tend to be excessively dependent and passive, become easily frustrated, and cannot cope with anxiety. **Answers 1, 3,** and **4** are incorrect because assertive, mature, or aggressive individuals are generally able to externalize their feelings and fears or to cope effectively with stress.

> **Test-taking tip**—Choose the option that is different (*dependent* vs. outgoing).

AS, 7, PsI, Coping and Adaptation

166. (1) The earliest indications of blood transfusion reactions are headache, chills, and elevation of temperature. The skin may also become pale and cool, and hypotension may develop quickly. Respirations generally increase in rate and depth. Should symptoms occur, stop transfusion, notify physician, and send a stat urine specimen to the lab for analysis. **Answer 2** is incorrect: hypertension and flushing are not indicators of a transfusion reaction. **Answer 3** is incorrect: wheezing and urticaria may occur, but are *not the earliest* indications of blood transfusion reaction. **Answer 4** is incorrect because oliguria and jaundice are *late* signs of transfusion reaction, *secondary* to *hemolysis* of red blood cells.

> **Test-taking tip**—Think timing. Stem asks for *earliest* signs.

EV, 6, PhI, Pharmacological and Parenteral Therapies

167. (3) Food and drug therapy will prevent the accumulation of hydrochloric acid or will neutralize and buffer the acid that does accumulate. **Answer 1** is incorrect because 8 hours would be too long without food/medication. **Answer 2** is incorrect because monitoring vital signs every 2 hours is not indicated unless bleeding or shock continues, and if those symptoms are present, vital signs should be taken more frequently. **Answer 4** is incorrect: milk is not a food of choice because it increases gastric acid production.

> **Test-taking tip**—Key word: *recovering*. Action should promote healing.

PL, 4, PhI, Basic Care and Comfort

168. (2) Central venous pressure (CVP) is a reflection of pressures in the right atrium and systemic veins. Although CVP is the least sensitive indicator of left ventricular end-diastolic pressures (increased with decreased ventricular compliance due to myocardial infarction and left ventricular failure), the CVP line is a safer one than a pulmonary artery (PA) line. In addition, it can be used to estimate blood volumes, obtain venous blood samples, and administer fluids. **Answer 1** is incorrect because a PA line reflects left atrial pressure. **Answer 3** is incorrect because a PA line indirectly reflects left ventricular pressure. **Answer 4** is incorrect because right ventricular pressure is *not* measured by a CVP line.

> **Test-taking tip**—Visualize the chambers of the heart. The CVP catheter tip "sits" at the entrance.

AS, 6, PhI, Physiological Adaptation

169. (2) The patient with mild hypertension usually has a diastolic pressure of between 90 and 100 mm Hg. **Answer 1** is incorrect because diastolic pressures of 110–120 mm Hg are considered moderately hypertensive. **Answer 3** is incorrect because diastolic pressures of 120–140 mm Hg are considered severely hypertensive. **Answer 4** is incorrect because diastolic pressures of 100–115 cross over two levels of hypertension; persons with these diastolic pressures would probably be considered to have mild to moderate hypertension.

Test-taking tip—Know normal values: "mild" would be something just at or above 90 mm Hg.
AS, 6, PhI, Physiological Adaptation

170. **(1)** Each of these activities (restricting activity, monitoring ECG, implementing passive range of motion, maintaining sterile dressings) is a priority in the early postinsertion period. However, because a transvenous approach was used with this patient, it is essential that activities be restricted for the first few days to reduce the risk of catheter dislodgement. To monitor for this complication, periodic comparisons of the patient's current rhythm strip should be made with the tracing taken at the time of insertion. Changes in either the pacemaker artifact or pacemaker-initiated QRS indicate a change in position. Although this may not always be significant, it becomes so if the pacemaker fails to capture, causing a decrease in heart rate and cardiac output. **Answers 2, 3, and 4** are incorrect because *restricting activity* is the nurse's *first priority*.

Test-taking tip—When all answers are correct, look for the most important at that point.
PL, 6, PhI, Reduction of Risk Potential

171. **(3)** With large dosages of secobarbital there may be an increase in anger or a deep sleep, depending on the individual's reaction. Secobarbital, a barbiturate, causes a depression of the CNS, so its effects usually include bradycardia (*not* tachycardia, **Answer 1**), hypotension (*not* hypertension, **Answer 2**), and depressed respiration (*not* increased respirations, **Answer 4**).

Test-taking tip—Look at the pattern of responses and choose the one that is different (in this case, the psychosocial answer).
EV, 7, PhI, Pharmacological Therapies

172. **(2)** Blood flow to the intestines is increased following ingestion of meals, to facilitate digestion and absorption. As a result of this circulatory shift, other organs receive less volume. This blood shift is partially responsible for feelings of sleepiness and lethargy following large meals. If a patient has a large atheromatous plaque in one of the coronary arteries, the decreased pressure and flow of blood may result in transient ischemia. **Answer 1** is incorrect because decreased pancreatic enzyme secretion results in diarrhea and steatorrhea (large amounts of fats in the stools). **Answer 3** is incorrect: swallowing air during eating can produce an uncomfortable feeling of fullness that can be relieved by eructation (belching), but should not decrease arterial oxygenation. **Answer 4** is incorrect because a decrease in heart rate and blood pressure will decrease rather than increase myocardial oxygen consumption.

Test-taking tip—Read the choices and look for clues: the correct answer mentions "digestion" and "coronary" perfusion.
AN, 6, PhI, Physiological Adaptation

173. **(1)** Liquid iron preparations such as Fer-In-Sol should be given with a citrus juice to enhance the absorption of the iron. **Answer 2** is incorrect because it may actually block the absorption of iron. **Answer 3** is incorrect because apple juice will not enhance the absorption of iron. **Answer 4** is incorrect because prune juice will not enhance the absorption of iron (however, iron does cause constipation, and prune juice may be given to treat or prevent this side effect).

Test-taking tip—Concept: *absorption is needed.* The best source of vitamin C is needed to accomplish this.
IMP, 4, PhI, Pharmacological and Parenteral Therapies

174. **(2)** The desired effect of morphine in this situation is to reduce sensitivity to stimuli in order to allay apprehension and, in some cases, to induce drowsiness. Atropine acts to dry oral and bronchial secretions, reducing the hazards of aspirations during anesthetic induction. **Answer 1** is incorrect because although morphine effectively relieves pain, pain relief is usually not an objective in administering a preoperative medication. **Answer 3** is incorrect because drowsiness, not sleep, may result. **Answer 4** is incorrect because morphine is not a muscle relaxant.

Test-taking tip—Know the desired and expected outcomes.
EV, 3, PhI, Pharmacological and Parenteral Therapies

175. **(3)** Examining her vaginal canal is contraindicated initially because of her preadmission history of bleeding. **Answer 1** is incorrect: initiating IV therapy *is* imperative to have a line available for any ordered medications or fluids. **Answers 2 and 4** are incorrect because taking her blood pressure and monitoring FHR *are* essential to establish baseline data and to monitor the mother's and infant's status.

Test-taking tip—The problem may be placenta previa or other bleeding abnormalities in pregnancy. Choose the answer that covers what the nurse would *not* do when the question asks for a procedure that is contraindicated. The problem is *vaginal* bleeding, so select the option that relates to the *vaginal* canal.
AN, 1, PhI, Reduction of Risk Potential

176. **(4)** Frequent baths will help lesions crust over, dry, and heal; thus bathing more frequently than usual is recommended. Baths will also reduce the bacterial count, thus reducing the risk of infection. However, no soap should be used, because it will cause excessive drying and cracking of both the affected areas and the healthy skin. **Answer 1** is incorrect because it is inappropriate for the nurse to tell the mother to check with the doctor first. The nurse can and should handle this question, because teaching is part of the *nurse's responsibility*. **Answer 2** is incorrect because it would be incorrect for the nurse to advise the mother that *sponge* baths are recommended for 10 days. **Answer 3** is incorrect because it would be incorrect for the nurse to advise the mother that baths are not permitted.

Test-taking tip—When in doubt, focus on two options that are opposites ("no" vs. "yes"). Eliminate "doctor" and "perhaps" options.
IMP, 1, PhI, Basic Care and Comfort

177. **(1)** Crepitus in the neck or upper chest is a sign that the tracheal tube is no longer in place and is delivering oxygen into the interstitial or mediastinal space. This condition may severely impair ventilation of the lungs. **Answer 2** is incorrect because an inadequately inflated cuff creates an air leak around the tracheal tube. **Answer 3** is incorrect because an overinflated cuff can cause necrosis of the trachea. **Answer 4** is incorrect because edema is characterized by fluid, not air, in the tissues.

Test-taking tip—Use a process of elimination. With 2 choices, make a mental picture: would air or fluid make a noise?
AN, 6, PhI, Physiological Adaptation

178. **(1)** The procedure most commonly used in assessing fetal well-being is the nonstress test, which provides valuable data without inducing hazard to mother or fetus. **Answer 2** is incorrect because amniocentesis is used *selectively*, that is, in cases where the information gained is vital to fetal *survival*. **Answer 3** is incorrect because the lecithin-sphingomyelin (L/S) ratio is an indicator of fetal *lung* maturity; it would require amniocentesis. **Answer 4** is incorrect because determination of fetal blood gases is *not a common* procedure and is most often done on scalp blood when the mother is in labor.

Test-taking tip—The key words are "most common." **Answers 2 and 3** involve the same procedure, amniocentesis, which can be hazardous and is not commonly used; neither is determination of fetal blood gases (**4**).
IMP, 5, PhI, Reduction of Risk Potential

179. **(2)** In Bryant's traction, the hips and buttocks should be raised slightly (1 inch) above the mattress, not resting on the

mattress (**Answer 1**), for the traction to be effective. **Answer 3** is incorrect because although the nurse is ultimately responsible, the aide should be commended for having brought this concern to the nurse's attention. **Answer 4** is incorrect: although it is true that this child will need special skin care due to prolonged immobility, the nurse should first take measures to correct the problem with the traction.

Test-taking tip—Remember that weights and pulleys must hang free and clear for traction to be most effective.

IMP, 3, PhI, Basic Care and Comfort

180. **(3)** The Hemovac is a portable suction system that provides low negative pressure (30–45 mm Hg) to gently remove excess fluid and debris from the wound. It does not require attachment to any other suction system. **Answers 1, 2,** and **4** are incorrect because they *are* standard and appropriate nursing measures.

Test-taking tip—Look for an *incorrect* nursing action.

IMP, 6, PhI, Reduction of Risk Potential

181. **(3)** By agreeing to talk with both parents, the nurse can provide emotional support and further assess and validate the family's needs. **Answer 1** is incorrect because it lacks empathy and makes the mother feel rejected. **Answer 2** is incorrect: it may be an appropriate action *after* doing further assessment. **Answer 4** is incorrect because this suggestion should be made only if, after further assessment and discussion with the physician and social worker, the health team thinks it is appropriate. However, at this time it is inappropriate.

Test-taking tip—Providing *support* and maintaining a *family* focus is the best answer.

IMP, 7, PsI, Psychosocial Adaptation

182. **(4)** After the stump has healed, an elastic bandage is applied to it to produce shrinkage and a conical shape. It is a compression dressing, with maximal compression at the distal end of the stump and minimal compression at the proximal end. The stump is wrapped with a clean bandage each day and rewrapped four times each day to maintain compression. **Answer 1** is incorrect: elevation of the stump *after* the first 24 hours is always contraindicated because of the risk of flexion contracture in the hip. **Answer 2** is incorrect: pushing the stump against a hard surface will facilitate toughening the skin for weight bearing once the prosthesis is applied, but it does not facilitate either reduction in size or shaping of the stump. **Answer 3** is incorrect: warm, moist soaks may be applied to reduce phantom pain discomfort, but they are *not applicable* to this situation.

Test-taking tip—Visualize the effect of each action on stump *size*.

IMP, 3, PhI, Basic Care and Comfort

183. **(1)** Central venous pressures of 4–10 cm H_2O are normal. Some clinicians consider up to 15 cm H_2O to be normal, but pressures over 15 cm H_2O (**Answer 3**) clearly indicate hypervolemia or heart failure. **Answers 2** and **4** are incorrect because CVP is measured by water, not mercury.

Test-taking tip—Know normal ranges to interpret changes.

EV, 6, PhI, Physiological Adaptation

184. **(2)** Many parents become "slaves" to the monitor and become overprotective to the infant. **Answer 1** is incorrect because faulty alarms should only occur if the electrodes are not properly placed. **Answer 3** is incorrect: the monitor should have very little effect on the infant's developmental level, provided it is used appropriately and the infant is environmentally stimulated. **Answer 4** is incorrect because most apnea monitors are reliable if properly used.

Test-taking tip—Picture what probably happens when the alarm sounds. The parents get alarmed and tend to "hover." Note the use of the words *problematic side effect* in this question.

EV, 2, PsI, Coping and Adaptation

185. **(3)** Encouraging friends to visit is inappropriate because they may bring drugs or encourage the client to act out by leaving the hospital or taking drugs. Visitation should not be completely curtailed but should be closely monitored. **Answer 1** allows the client to feel that he or she has some control over care, which is especially important during adolescence. **Answer 2** helps the client regain strength and decreases stimuli in the immediate environment. **Answer 4** allows the nurse to monitor care more closely.

Test-taking tip—Key phrase: "*least* appropriate."

IMP, 7, PsI, Psychosocial Adaptation

186. **(4)** Nitroglycerin causes vasodilation and a decrease in systemic blood pressure, which subsequently decreases the amount of work the heart must perform. **Answer 1** is incorrect because constriction of the cardiac chambers would increase cardiac resistance and workload. **Answer 2** is incorrect because nitroglycerin does not increase heart rate. That effect would be seen with isoproterenol (Isuprel) or atropine. **Answer 3** is incorrect because to increase myocardial contractility, digoxin would be given.

Test-taking tip—Look for an effect of vasodilation (e.g., decreased pressure).

AN, 6, PhI, Pharmacological and Parenteral Therapies

187. **(3)** Understanding the condition will increase the patient's compliance with the treatment regimen. **Answer 1** is incorrect because it is important to provide consistency in assigning nurses to care for the person with hypertension, to minimize stress and provide constant and consistent reinforcement of care and health teaching. **Answer 2** is incorrect: the nurse should plan care to reduce the number of situations that create or increase physical stress. **Answer 4** is incorrect because the patient must report minor symptoms as well as major ones.

Test-taking tip—Do not pass the buck to the MD. Think immediate *need*.

PL, 7, PsI, Coping and Adaptation

188. **(2)** Carrying anything heavy, such as groceries or even a purse, on the affected side may increase the occurrence of lymphedema. **Answer 1** is incorrect because wearing gloves for household tasks or gardening is encouraged to prevent lymphedema or possible infection *if* the skin is broken. **Answer 3** is incorrect because elasticized sleeves *may* be worn if they are *not* tight. However, any constricting garment or jewelry should be avoided. **Answer 4** is incorrect because driving, particularly if the affected arm is kept high on the steering wheel, should *not* increase lymphedema.

Test-taking tip—Do not read any additional facts into the choices. The stem does not say *tight*.

IMP, 3, PhI, Reduction of Risk Potential

189. **(1)** Fluid orders vary among hospitals, physicians, and childbirth methods. Because the woman is in preterm labor and is bleeding, the orders will probably maintain her NPO with an IV. **Answers 2** and **3** are incorrect because giving her a small sip of water or ice chips may be contraindicated at this time. **Answer 4** is incorrect because the physician may allow sips of water or ice chips.

Test-taking tip—Look at the verbs: "check" with the MD, "give," "offer," "tell . . . cannot have." Two options *give* the water; one option *withholds* it. The best answer is to *check* with the MD because this is a complicated labor.

IMP, 6, PhI, Reduction of Risk Potential

190. **(4)** Infants or children with milk allergies should be offered a lactose-free formula such as Isomil. **Answers 1, 2,** and **3** are incorrect because these formulas are lactose based and are contraindicated for infants or children with milk allergies.

Test-taking tip—Know which formulas are lactose free: Isomil, Prosobee, and Nutramigen.

IMP, 4, PhI, Basic Care and Comfort

191. (1) The rationale for pacemaker implantation is presented in the preinsertion period and is reinforced in the postinsertion period and therefore receives the least emphasis in the predischarge plan. **Answers 2, 3, and 4** are incorrect: they *are* essential components of a predischarge teaching plan, because the patient must focus on management of the pacemaker, and they all receive great emphasis.

> **Test-taking tip**—Look for a pattern. The *least* emphasis would be on a preinsertion education topic.

PL, 6, PhI, Reduction of Risk Potential

192. (2) SIDS usually occurs within the first year of life. The peak time appears to be between 2 and 4 months after birth. **Answer 1** is incorrect because SIDS rarely occurs before 4 weeks after birth. **Answers 3 and 4** are incorrect because SIDS is comparatively unusual after 6 months of age; 95% of all cases occur by 6 months of age.

> **Test-taking tip**—Answers 3 and 4 are virtually the same; therefore, neither choice is the correct answer.

AS, 5, HPM, Prevention and Early Detection of Disease

193. (4) Baroreceptors in the carotid sinus and aortic arch constantly monitor and respond to variations in blood pressure. Decreased cardiac output results in a drop in blood pressure. These receptors transmit afferent signals to the cardiovascular center in the medulla. Activation of these centers results in increased vasoconstriction, heart rate, and force of cardiac contraction via adrenergic efferents in the sympathetic nervous system. **Answer 1** is incorrect because vagal stimulation of the SA node decreases heart rate. **Answer 2** is incorrect because arrhythmias generally produce an irregularity in heart rhythm. **Answer 3** is incorrect because these vital signs do not indicate shock at this time.

> **Test-taking tip**—Know the differences between sympathetic and parasympathetic responses.

AN, 6, PhI, Physiological Adaptation

194. (3) Morphine sulfate acts not only to reduce pain and anxiety by blocking the activity of the reticular substance in the brainstem, but also to relax vascular smooth muscle, thereby decreasing blood pressure. Nausea and vomiting are common adverse side effects of this medication. Atropine is an anticholinergic whose drying effects tend to cause the patient to complain that the mouth feels like cotton. **Answers 1 and 4** are incorrect because atropine also blocks vagal effects on the heart, increasing pulse rate, not decreasing it. **Answer 2** is incorrect because blood pressure is decreased, not increased.

> **Test-taking tip**—Look for side effects that relate to the drug action: vasodilation (morphine) and decreased secretions (atropine)

EV, 1, PhI, Pharmacological and Parenteral Therapies

195. (1) Teaching regarding medications is essential if the patient is going to recognize side effects. The patient must be told that medications must continue even though he or she "feels" fine. **Answer 2** is incorrect because changing jobs is unrealistic in most cases. The patient should be taught stress-reduction or relaxation techniques to better handle work-related stress. **Answer 3** is incorrect because the patient should quit smoking, not just lessen the amount. **Answer 4** is incorrect because there are generally no limitations on sexual activities merely due to hypertension; unless restrictions are warranted because of an individual's specific condition, this is considered irrelevant when teaching the average hypertensive patient.

> **Test-taking tip**—Look for a pattern: only one choice emphasizes *treatment*.

PL, 6, PhI, Reduction of Risk Potential

196. (1) If the IV infused at the correct rate of 40 mL/hr from 11:00 A.M. to 3:15 P.M., the patient should have received 170 mL of IV fluid; because the patient has received twice the prescribed amount, the nurse should *first* correct the

rate, *then* notify the physician (**Answer 4**). (The nurse should also check at this time to see if the IV line is being affected by the position of the limb.) If, after contacting the physician, a new rate is ordered, only then would the nurse adjust the rate to a level lower than originally prescribed (**Answer 3**). **Answer 2** is incorrect because there is no reason to hang a new bag at this time.

> **Test-taking tip**—First, decide whether this is OK or *not* OK. Next, choose a corrective action *before* calling the MD. Look for a choice that *first* addresses the patient's safety.

IMP, 6, PhI, Pharmacological and Parenteral Therapies

197. (3) The primary advantage of Hemovac suction is that it removes excess fluid and debris from the wound site that could retard tissue granulation and healing. If serum is allowed to accumulate under the skin, the pressure can cause sloughing of tissue flaps. **Answer 1** is incorrect because the Hemovac exerts low, even pressure. **Answer 2** is incorrect because the Hemovac is also lightweight (which is an advantage in postoperative ambulation), but this is *not* its *primary* advantage. **Answer 4** is incorrect because the removal of excess sera reduces the likelihood of postoperative infection but is a *secondary* advantage.

> **Test-taking tip**—With more than one plausible choice, think of the purpose of the device.

PL, 1, PhI, Reduction of Risk Potential

198. (2) Although drug abuse may be found at every age level, the elderly seem least likely to abuse substances. This is probably due to generational differences in cultural norms and morals. (It was thought that one was "weak" or "sick" to rely on drugs to escape problems.) However, many times the elderly use alcohol as an escape mechanism. **Answers 1 and 3** are incorrect because drug abuse is found among all socioeconomic classes. **Answer 4** is incorrect because many adolescents use drugs to escape reality, cope with stress, identify with their peers, etc. The reasons for abuse vary from individual to individual, depending on their particular needs.

> **Test-taking tip**—Note key phrase: "*least* prevalent."

AN, 7, PsI, Coping and Adaptation

199. (1) The toddler is probably experiencing severe separation anxiety and is exhibiting symptoms of despair. A consistent one-to-one relationship will develop trust in the nurse; in addition, rooming-in by the mother should be encouraged. **Answer 2** is incorrect because assigning different staff would increase anxiety stemming from feelings of uncertainty and lack of trust. **Answer 3** is incorrect because ignoring the behavior may worsen the age-related separation anxiety. **Answer 4** is incorrect: referral to the pediatric clinical nurse specialist may not be necessary at this time, as long as appropriate interventions are implemented.

> **Test-taking tip**—Choose one (consistent) staff nurse over *different* staff.

IMP, 5, PsI, Coping and Adaptation

200. (2) The most common complication occurring in the postoperative period is pulmonary embolus. This is a particularly significant problem in elderly patients with a history of vascular insufficiency. Therefore, an antiembolism stocking is applied to the unaffected limb, and early physiotherapy and ambulation with a walker are encouraged. **Answer 1** is incorrect because hemorrhage and shock are always potential problems after *any* surgery. To assess for this problem in *this* case, any bright-red drainage on the stump dressing should be outlined so that the rate of bleeding can be determined. **Answer 3** is incorrect because disseminated intravascular clotting is a problem associated with *prolonged shock*. **Answer 4** is incorrect because thrombophlebitis tends to occur with *long bed rest* and can be prevented.

> **Test-taking tip**—Think timing (postoperative) and age-specific problems.

EV, 6, PhI, Physiological Adaptation

This chart gives a quick overview of what is normal and the conditions that result in high or low values.

Test	Normal Values	Possible Significance	
		Increases	Decreases
Hematology			
Aspartate aminotransferase (AST)—formerly called serum glutamic oxaloacetic transaminase (SGOT)	*Men:* 10–40 U/L *Women:* 9–25 U/L	Myocardial infarction, cardiac surgery, hepatitis, cirrhosis, trauma, severe burns, progressive muscular dystrophy, infectious mononucleosis, acute renal failure	Uremia, chronic dialysis, ketoacidosis
Bleeding time—indication of hemostatic efficiency	1–9 min	Hemorrhagic purpura, acute leukemia, aplastic anemia, DIC, oral anticoagulant therapy	
Hematocrit—volume of packed red blood cells/100 mL of blood	*Men:* 45% (40–50%) *Women:* 40% (38–47%)	Dehydration, polycythemia, congenital heart disease	Anemia, hemorrhage, leukemia, dietary deficiencies
Hemoglobin—oxygen-combining protein	*Men:* 13.5–18 g/dL *Women:* 12–16 g/dL	Same as for Hematocrit	Same as for Hematocrit
Activated partial thromboplastin time (aPTT)—tests coagulation mechanism; stage I deficiencies	*aPTT:* 25–41	Deficiency of factors VIII, IX, X, XI, XII; anticoagulant therapy	Extensive cancer, DIC
Platelets—thrombocytes	150,000–400,000/mm³	Polycythemia vera, postsplenectomy, anemia	Leukemia, aplastic anemia, cirrhosis, multiple myeloma, chemotherapy
Prothrombin time—tests extrinsic clotting; stages II and III	10–13 sec	Anticoagulant therapy, DIC, hepatic disease, malabsorption	Digitalis therapy, diuretic reaction, vitamin K therapy
Red blood cell count—number of circulating erythrocytes in 1 μL of whole blood	*Men:* 4.5–6.2 million/μL *Women:* 4.2–5.4 million/μL	Polycythemia vera, anoxia, dehydration	Leukemia, hemorrhage, anemias, Hodgkin's
Sedimentation rate—speed at which red blood cells settle in uncoagulated blood	*Men:* 0–15 mm/hr *Women:* 0–20 mm/hr	Acute bacterial infection, cancer, infectious disease, numerous inflammatory states	Polycythemia vera, sickle cell anemia
White blood cell count—number of leukocytes in 1 μL	4.5–11 × 10³/μL	Leukemia, bacterial infection, severe sepsis	Viral infection, overwhelming bacterial infection, lupus erythematosus, antineoplastic chemotherapy, bone marrow depression

Test	Normal Values	Possible Significance	
		Increases	**Decreases**
White blood cell differential—enumeration of individual leukocyte distribution			
Neutrophils	56% mean cell count 1800–7800/µL	Bacterial infection, tumor, inflammation, stress, drug reaction, trauma, metabolic disorders	Acute viral infection, anorexia nervosa, radiation therapy, drug induced, alcoholic ingestion
Eosinophils	2.7% cell count 0–450/µL	Allergic disorder, parasitic infestation, eosinophilic leukemia	Acute or chronic stress; excess ACTH, cortisone, or epinephrine; endocrine disorder
Basophils	25–100/µL, or 0–1% cell count 0–200/µL	Myeloproliferative disease, leukemia	Anaphylactic reaction, hyperthyroidism, radiation therapy, infections, ovulation, pregnancy, aging
Lymphocytes	20–40% cell count 1000–4800/µL	Chronic lymphocytic leukemia, infectious mononucleosis, chronic bacterial infection, viral infection	Leukemia, systemic lupus erythematosus, immune deficiency disorders
Blood Chemistry			
Alkaline phosphatase (ALP)	32–92 U/L	Hyperparathyroidism, Paget's disease, cancer with bone metastasis, obstructive jaundice, cirrhosis, hepatitis A, rickets	Malnutrition, scurvy, celiac disease, chronic nephritis, hypothyroidism, cystic fibrosis
Amylase	80–180 IU/L	Acute pancreatitis, mumps, duodenal ulcer, pancreatic cancer, perforated bowel, renal failure	Advanced chronic pancreatitis, chronic alcoholism
Bilirubin, serum	*Direct:* 0.0–0.4 mg/dL *Indirect:* 0.2–0.8 mg/dL *Total:* 0.3–1.0 mg/dL	Massive hemolysis, low-grade hemolytic disease, cirrhosis, obstructive liver disease, hepatitis, biliary obstruction, neonatal (physiological) jaundice	
Calcium, serum	8.2–10.2 mg/dL	Hyperparathyroidism, multiple myeloma, bone metastasis, bone fracture, thiazide-diuretic reaction, milk-alkali syndrome	Hypoparathyroidism, renal failure, pregnancy, massive transfusion
Carbon dioxide	22–30 mEq/L	Emphysema, salicylate toxicity, vomiting	Starvation, diarrhea
Chloride, serum	98–107 mEq/L	Hyperventilation, diabetes insipidus, uremia	Heart failure, pyloric obstruction, hypoventilation, vomiting, chronic respiratory acidosis
Creatine, serum	*Men:* 0.7–1.3 mg/dL *Women:* 0.5–1.0 mg/dL	Chronic glomerulonephritis, nephritis, heart failure, muscle disease	Debilitation, long-term corticosteroid therapy
Creatine kinase (CK) (creatine phosphokinase [CPK])	*Men:* 17–148 IU/L *Women:* 10–79 IU/L	Acute myocardial infarction, acute stroke, convulsions, surgery, muscular dystrophy, hypokalemia	Addison's disease
Isoenzymes			
CPK-MM/CK-MM	100%	Muscular dystrophy, delirium tremens, surgery, hypokalemia, crush injuries, hypothyroidism	
CPK/MB/CK-MB	0.6% of total CPK	Acute myocardial infarction, cardiac defibrillation, myocarditis, cardiac ischemia	
CPK-BB/CK-BB	0%	Pulmonary infarction, brain surgery, stroke, pulmonary embolism, seizures, intestinal ischemia	
Fibrinogen, serum	0.2–0.4 g/100 dL or 200–400 mg/dL	Pneumonia, acute infection, nephrosis, rheumatoid arthritis	Cirrhosis, toxic liver necrosis, anemia, obstetric complications, DIC, advanced carcinoma

Test	Normal Values	Possible Significance	
		Increases	**Decreases**
Glucose (fasting)	60–110 mg/100 mL (serum)	Acute stress, Cushing's syndrome, hyperthyroidism, acute or chronic pancreatitis, diabetes mellitus, hyperglycemia	Addison's disease, liver disease, reactive hypoglycemia, pituitary hypofunction
Glycosylated hemoglobin (HbA$_{1c}$)	4.0–7.0%	Newly diagnosed or poorly controlled diabetes mellitus	Iron deficiency anemia, chronic blood loss
Iron-binding capacity (total)	218–385 g/dL	Lead poisoning, hepatic necrosis	
Lactic dehydrogenase (LDH)	60–120 U/mL (Wacker Scale) 150–450 U/mL (Wroblewski)	Myocardial infarction, pernicious anemia, chronic viral hepatitis, pneumonia, pulmonary emboli, stroke, renal tissue destruction, leukemia, non-Hodgkins lymphoma, shock, trauma	
LDH-1	17–27%		
LDH-2	27–37%		
LDH-3	18–25%		
LDH-4	3–8%		
LDH-5	6–16%		
Lipids			
Cholesterol (total serum)	<200 mg/dL	Hypercholesterolemia, hyperlipidemia, myocardial infarction, uncontrolled diabetes mellitus, high-cholesterol diet, hypothyroidism, atherosclerosis, stress, glomerulonephritis (nephrotic stage), familial biliary obstruction	Malnutrition, cholesterol-lowering medication, anemia, liver disease, hyperthyroidism
Low-density lipoprotein (LDL)	<130 mg/dL		
High-density lipoprotein (HDL)	35–75 mg/dL		
Triglycerides	40–150 mg/100 mL		
Phosphorus, inorganic serum	3.0–4.5 mg/dL	Chronic glomerular disease, hypoparathyroidism, milk-alkali syndrome, sarcoidosis	Hyperparathyroidism, rickets, osteomalacia, renal tubular necrosis, malabsorption syndrome, vitamin D deficiency
Potassium, serum	3.5–5.0 mEq/L	Diabetic ketosis, renal failure, Addison's disease, excessive intake	Thiazide diuretics, Cushing's syndrome, cirrhosis with ascites, hyperaldosteronism, steroid therapy, malignant hypertension, poor dietary habits, chronic diarrhea, diaphoresis, renal tubular necrosis, malabsorption syndrome, vomiting
Protein, serum (albumin/globulin)	*Total:* 6.4–8.3 g/dL *Albumin:* 3.5–5.0 g/dL *Globulin:* 2.8–4.4 g/dL	Dehydration, multiple myeloma	Chronic liver disease, myeloproliferative disease, burns
Serum glutamic oxaloacetic transaminase (SGOT)—*see AST*	—	—	—
Sodium, serum	136–145 mEq/L	Increased intake, either orally or IV; Cushing's syndrome, excessive sweating, diabetes insipidus	Addison's disease, sodium-losing nephropathy, vomiting, diarrhea, fistulas, tube drainage, burns, renal insufficiency with acidosis, starvation with acidosis, paracentesis, thoracentesis, ascites, heart failure, SIADH
T$_3$ uptake	24–34%	Hyperthyroidism, thyroxine-binding globulin (TBG) deficiency	Hypothyroidism, pregnancy, TBG excess
Thyroxine	5–12 μg/dL	Hyperthyroidism, pregnancy	Hypothyroidism, renal failure
Urea nitrogen, serum (BUN)	5–20 mg/dL	Acute or chronic renal failure, heart failure, obstructive uropathy, dehydration	Cirrhosis, malnutrition

Test	Normal Values	Possible Significance	
		Increases	**Decreases**
Uric acid, serum	*Men:* 4.5–8 mg/dL *Women:* 2.5–6.2 mg/dL	Gout, chronic renal failure, starvation, diuretic therapy	
Blood Gases			
Bicarbonate (HCO_3)	21–28 mEq/L	Metabolic alkalosis	Metabolic acidosis
Carbon dioxide pressure (PCO_2), whole blood, arterial	35–45 mm Hg	Primary respiratory acidosis, loss of H^+ through nasogastric suctioning or vomiting	Primary respiratory alkalosis
Oxygen pressure (PO_2), whole blood, arterial	80–100 mm Hg	Oxygen administration in the absence of severe lung disease	Chronic obstructive lung disease, severe pneumonia, pulmonary embolism, pulmonary edema, respiratory muscle disease
pH, serum	7.35–7.45	Metabolic alkalosis–alkali ingestion, respiratory alkalosis–hyperventilation	Metabolic acidosis–ketoacidosis, shock, respiratory acidosis–alveolar hypoventilation
Immunodiagnostic Studies Carcinoembryonic antigen	<2.5 ng/mL	*Cancer* of: colon, lung, metastatic breast, pancreas, stomach, prostate, ovary, bladder, limbs; also neuroblastoma, leukemias, osteogenic carcinoma; *noncancer* conditions such as: hepatic cirrhosis, uremia, pancreatitis, colorectal, polyposis, peptic ulcer disease, ulcerative colitis, regional enteritis	
Urinalysis			
pH	4.5–7.8	Metabolic alkalosis	Metabolic acidosis
Specific gravity	1.003–1.029	Dehydration, pituitary tumor, hypotension	Distal renal tubular disease, polycystic kidney disease, diabetes insipidus, overhydration
Glucose	Negative	Diabetes mellitus	
Protein	Negative	Nephrosis, glomerulonephritis, lupus erythematosus	
Casts	0–0.4 hyaline casts per LPF	Nephrosis, glomerulonephritis, lupus erythematosus, infection	
Red blood cells	Negative	Renal calculi, hemorrhagic cystitis, tumors of the kidney	
White blood cells	Negative	Inflammation of the kidneys, ureters, or bladder	
Color	Normal yellow, clear	*Abnormal:* red to reddish brown—hematuria; *brown to brownish* gray—bilirubinuria or urobilinuria; *tea colored*—possible obstructive jaundice	*Almost colorless:* chronic kidney disease, diabetes insipidus, diabetes mellitus
Sodium	40–220 mEq/L/24 hr	Salt-wasting renal disease, SIADH, dehydration	Heart failure, primary aldosteronism
Chloride	110–250 mEq/24 hr	Chronic obstructive lung disease, dehydration, salicylate toxicity	Gastric suction, heart failure, emphysema
Potassium	25–125 mEq/L/24 hr	Diuretic therapy	Renal failure
Creatinine clearance	90–139 mL/min		Renal disease
Hydroxycorticosteroids	2–10 mg/24 hr	Cushing's disease	Addison's disease
17-Ketosteroids	*Men:* 4.5–12 mg/24 hr *Women:* 2.5–10 mg/24 hr	Hirsutism, adrenal hyperplasia	Thyrotoxicosis, Addison's disease
Catecholamines (VMA)	*Epinephrine:* <20 µg/24 hr *Norepinephrine:* <100 µg/24 hr	Pheochromocytoma, severe anxiety, numerous medications	
Urine Test			
Schilling test	Excretion of 8–40% or more of test dose should appear in urine		Gastrointestinal malabsorption, pernicious anemia

D. PHYSIOLOGICAL INTEGRITY

See also **Appendix H,** Eight Detailed Areas of Human Functions Definitions/Descriptions—*Sensory-Perceptual; Comfort, Rest, Activity, and Mobility; Nutrition; Fluid-Gas Transport; Elimination.*

The nurse meets the physiological integrity needs of clients with potentially life-threatening or chronically recurring physiological conditions, and of clients at risk for the development of complications or untoward effects of treatments or management modalities, by providing and directing nursing care that promotes achievement of the following client needs:

7. **Basic care and comfort**—providing comfort and assistance in the performance of activities of daily living, including those that have been modified because of health deviations; providing assistance to clients and families or significant others to promote client self-care; supporting families or significant others in order to enhance the overall management of client care, including self-care–related teaching provided in any care delivery environment.

8. **Pharmacological and parenteral therapies**—managing and providing care related to the administration of medications and parenteral therapies.

9. **Reduction of risk potential**—reducing the likelihood that clients will develop complications or health problems related to existing conditions, treatments, or procedures. Also included are those activities that involve monitoring changes in status and preparing or caring for clients undergoing diagnostic procedures and invasive therapies.

10. **Physiological adaptation**—managing and providing care to clients with acute, chronic, or life-threatening physical health conditions.

Knowledge, Skills, and Abilities

To meet client needs for physiological integrity, the nurse should possess knowledge, skills, and abilities that include but are not limited to the following areas:

7. *Basic care and comfort*
   - Assistive Devices
   - Elimination
   - Mobility/Effects of Immobility
   - Nonpharmacological Comfort Interventions
   - Nutritional Therapies and Oral Hydration
   - Personal Hygiene
   - Rest and Sleep; Activities of Daily Living

8. *Pharmacological and parenteral therapies*
   - Administration of Blood and Blood Products
   - Central Venous Access Devices
   - Chemotherapy
   - Expected Effects
   - Intravenous Therapy
   - Medication Administration
   - Parenteral Fluids
   - Pharmacological Actions
   - Pharmacological Agents
   - Side Effects
   - Total Parenteral Nutrition
   - Untoward Effects

9. *Reduction of risk potential*
   - Alterations in Body Systems
   - Diagnostic Tests
   - Lab Values
   - Pathophysiology
   - Potential Complications of Diagnostic Tests, Procedures, Surgery, and Health Alterations
   - Skin and Wound Care
   - Therapeutic Procedures
   - Use of Special Equipment

10. *Physiological Adaptation*
    - Alterations in Body Systems
    - Fluid and Electrolyte Imbalances
    - Hemodynamics
    - Infectious Diseases
    - Medical Emergencies
    - Normal Body Function and Structure
    - Pathophysiology
    - Radiation Therapy
    - Respiratory Care
    - Unexpected Response to Therapies

The practice questions in this book (end-of-unit questions, **Pre Test, Practice Test,** and **Final Test**) are coded as to the client need being tested; the codes are found following the answer/rationale for each question. *Key to client need codes:*

SECE	Safe, Effective Care Environment
HPM	Health Promotion and Maintenance
PsI	Psychosocial Integrity
PhI	Physiological Integrity

For an index to *questions* relating to each general client need, see **Appendix D.**

For page references for specific *topics (content, theory) to review* relating to each client need, see **Appendix C.**

Index: Content Related to Four General Client Needs and 10 Subcategories (with Detailed Knowledge, Skills, and Abilities)

The following outline of content (nursing knowledge, skills, and abilities) is organized in terms of **four categories of client need:** *Safe, Effective Care Environment* (SECE), *Health Promotion/Maintenance* (HPM), *Psychosocial Integrity* (PsI), and *Physiological Integrity* (PhI). Included in the outline of topics are **10** numbered **subcategories** and corresponding task statements. These items are derived from study of nursing tasks and are *used in the development of the NCLEX-RN test plan.*

Students who have taken and evaluated their performance on the **Pre Test, Practice Test,** or **Final Test** in this book will find this outline a useful guide for a concentrated review of specific problem topics. **Repeat NCLEX-RN test takers** will also find this outline to be a useful guide for review of their areas of weakness. Refer to the pages listed in the right column for review of content in a particular topic.

Integrated Concepts and Processes

The following concepts and processes are basic to nursing practice. They are integrated throughout the four major categories of *client needs*:

For an index to *questions* relating to each client need, see **Appendixes D** and **E.**

Index: Questions Related to Four General Client Needs

Use this index to locate *practice questions* throughout the book in each of the four general categories of *client needs* that are tested on NCLEX-RN.

FOUR CATEGORIES OF CLIENT NEEDS

Unit	Safe, Effective Care Environment (SECE)	Health Promotion and Maintenance (HPM)	Psychosocial Integrity (PsI)	Physiological Integrity (PhI)
	Question No.	Question No.	Question No.	Question No.
Unit 1: Orientation and Pre Test (Q/A: 1–200)	12, 37, 58, 70, 128, 135, 139, 180	1, 19, 47, 49, 52, 57, 62, 63, 65, 69, 76, 90, 107, 111, 115, 149, 170, 189, 194	8, 11, 21, 24, 31, 33, 46, 48, 50, 51, 77, 83, 85, 86, 91, 95, 99, 102, 104, 106, 117, 122, 129, 132, 140, 142, 151, 152, 157, 174, 179, 184, 187, 199	2, 3, 4, 5, 6, 7, 9, 10, 13, 14, 15, 16, 17, 18, 20, 22, 23, 25, 26, 27, 28, 29, 30, 32, 34, 35, 36, 38, 39, 40, 41, 42, 43, 44, 45, 53, 54, 55, 56, 59, 60, 61, 64, 66, 67, 68, 71, 72, 73, 74, 75, 78, 79, 80, 81, 82, 84, 87, 88, 89, 92, 93, 94, 96, 97, 98, 100, 101, 103, 105, 108, 109, 110, 112, 113, 114, 116, 118, 119, 120, 121, 123, 124, 125, 126, 127, 130, 131, 133, 134, 136, 137, 138, 141, 143, 144, 145, 146, 147, 148, 150, 153, 154, 155, 156, 158, 159, 160, 161, 162, 163, 164, 165, 166, 167, 168, 169, 171, 172, 173, 175, 176, 177, 178, 181, 182, 183, 185, 186, 188, 190, 191, 192, 193, 195, 196, 197, 198, 200
Unit 3: Management of Care, Ethical and Legal Aspects in Nursing (Q/A: 1–55)	1, 2, 3, 4, 5, 6, 8, 9, 10, 11, 12, 13, 14, 15, 16, 17, 18, 19, 20, 21, 22, 23, 24, 25, 26, 27, 28, 29, 30, 31, 32, 33, 34, 35, 36, 37, 38, 39, 40, 41, 42, 43, 44, 45, 46, 47, 48, 49, 50, 51, 52, 53, 54, 55			7

FOUR CATEGORIES OF CLIENT NEEDS

Unit	Safe, Effective Care Environment (SECE) Question No.	Health Promotion and Maintenance (HPM) Question No.	Psychosocial Integrity (PsI) Question No.	Physiological Integrity (PhI) Question No.
Unit 4: Nursing Care of the Childbearing Family (Q/A: 1–109)	91, 92, 99	1, 2, 4, 5, 6, 7, 11, 15, 20, 21, 25, 26, 29, 32, 33, 34, 35, 38, 43, 44, 45, 47, 50, 51, 56, 59, 60, 61, 62, 66, 68, 69, 70, 71, 73, 74, 77, 78, 81, 82, 84, 86, 90, 97, 100, 101, 102, 103, 104, 105, 109	36, 48, 52, 53, 54, 55, 65, 98	3, 8, 9, 10, 12, 13, 14, 16, 17, 18, 19, 22, 23, 24, 27, 28, 30, 31, 37, 39, 40, 41, 42, 46, 49, 57, 58, 63, 64, 67, 72, 75, 76, 79, 80, 83, 85, 87, 88, 89, 93, 94, 95, 96, 106, 107, 108
Unit 5: Nursing Care of Children and Families (Q/A: 1–145)	1, 7, 9, 14, 32, 36, 58, 61, 62, 75, 87, 110, 111, 116, 117, 120, 122, 123, 124, 126, 129, 131, 132, 133, 134, 135, 136, 142, 143, 144, 145	5, 8, 10, 11, 22, 24, 30, 42, 43, 57, 59, 60, 63, 68, 72, 76, 77, 80, 81, 83, 88, 89, 90, 93, 100, 104, 105, 106, 107, 113, 114, 115, 119	3, 18, 19, 26, 28, 29, 34, 37, 46, 74, 84, 92, 95, 99, 118, 130	2, 4, 6, 12, 13, 15, 16, 17, 20, 21, 23, 25, 27, 31, 33, 35, 38, 39, 40, 41, 44, 45, 47, 48, 49, 50, 51, 52, 53, 54, 55, 56, 64, 65, 66, 67, 69, 70, 71, 73, 78, 79, 82, 85, 86, 91, 94, 96, 97, 98, 101, 102, 103, 108, 109, 112, 121, 125, 127, 128, 137, 138, 139, 140, 141
Unit 6: Nursing Care of Behavioral and Emotional Problems Throughout the Life Span (Q/A: 1–159)	11, 24, 59, 96, 101, 102, 118, 133, 145, 153, 154, 155, 157	12, 20, 22, 53, 80, 91, 112, 116, 132	2, 3, 4, 6, 7, 8, 9, 13, 14, 15, 16, 17, 18, 19, 21, 23, 25, 27, 28, 29, 30, 31, 32, 33, 34, 35, 36, 37, 38, 39, 40, 41, 42, 43, 44, 45, 46, 47, 48, 49, 50, 51, 52, 54, 55, 56, 58, 60, 61, 62, 63, 64, 65, 66, 67, 68, 69, 70, 71, 72, 73, 74, 75, 76, 77, 78, 79, 81, 82, 83, 84, 85, 86, 87, 88, 89, 90, 92, 94, 95, 97, 98, 100, 103, 104, 105, 106, 107, 109, 110, 111, 113, 114, 115, 117, 119, 120, 121, 122, 123, 124, 125, 126, 127, 128, 129, 130, 131, 135, 136, 137, 138, 139, 140, 141, 142, 143, 146, 147, 148, 149, 150, 152, 156, 158, 159	1, 5, 10, 26, 57, 93, 99, 108, 134, 144, 151
Unit 7: Nursing Care of the Acutely Ill and the Chronically Ill Adult (Q/A: 1–132)	1, 100, 106, 114, 125	51, 99, 126	3, 9, 42, 48, 52, 53, 73, 76, 86, 129	2, 4, 5, 6, 7, 8, 10, 11, 12, 13, 14, 15, 16, 17, 18, 19, 20, 21, 22, 23, 24, 25, 26, 27, 28, 29, 30, 31, 32, 33, 34, 35, 36, 37, 38, 39, 40, 41, 43, 44, 45, 46, 47, 49, 50, 54, 55, 56, 57, 58, 59, 60, 61, 62, 63, 64, 65, 66, 67, 68, 69, 70, 71, 72, 74, 75, 77, 78, 79, 80, 81, 82, 83, 84, 85, 87, 88, 89, 90, 91, 92, 93, 94, 95, 96, 97, 98, 101, 102, 103, 104, 105, 107, 108, 109, 110, 111, 112, 113, 115, 116, 117, 118, 119, 120, 121, 122, 123, 124, 127, 128, 130, 131, 132
Unit 9: Review of Nutrition 🍽 (Q/A: 1–9)				1, 2, 3, 4, 5, 6, 7, 8, 9

FOUR CATEGORIES OF CLIENT NEEDS

Unit	Safe, Effective Care Environment (SECE) Question No.	Health Promotion and Maintenance (HPM) Question No.	Psychosocial Integrity (PsI) Question No.	Physiological Integrity (PhI) Question No.
Unit 10: Review of Pharmacology (Q/A: 1–64)		29, 51	54	1, 2, 3, 4, 5, 6, 7, 8, 9, 10, 11, 12, 13, 14, 15, 16, 17, 18, 19, 20, 21, 22, 23, 24, 25, 26, 27, 28, 30, 31, 32, 33, 34, 35, 36, 37, 38, 39, 40, 41, 42, 43, 44, 45, 46, 47, 48, 49, 50, 52, 53, 55, 56, 57, 58, 59, 60, 61, 62, 63, 64
Unit 11: Common Diagnostic Procedures, Intravenous and Oxygen Therapy, Isolation Precautions, and Hands-on Nursing Care (Q/A: 1–13)	10			1, 2, 3, 4, 5, 6, 7, 8, 9, 11, 12, 13
Unit 12: Practice Test (Q/A: 1–100)	10, 27, 35, 58	1, 11, 13, 16, 18, 26, 29, 31, 36, 41, 45, 47, 53, 60, 62, 74, 81, 83, 85, 90, 95, 97	6, 14, 17, 19, 20, 22, 24, 34, 37, 42, 43, 44, 52, 54, 55, 59, 64, 68, 70, 72, 75, 79, 84, 89, 91, 96, 99	2, 3, 4, 5, 7, 8, 9, 12, 15, 21, 23, 25, 28, 30, 32, 33, 38, 39, 40, 46, 48, 49, 50, 51, 56, 57, 61, 63, 65, 66, 67, 69, 71, 73, 76, 77, 78, 80, 82, 86, 87, 88, 92, 93, 94, 98, 100
Unit 13: Final Test (Q/A: 1–200)	4, 10, 59, 68, 72, 110, 116, 121, 130	2, 6, 14, 20, 23, 28, 46, 50, 61, 69, 71, 82, 88, 95, 100, 108, 129, 140, 148, 152, 154, 163, 192	17, 22, 27, 30, 37, 38, 41, 43, 52, 60, 66, 74, 84, 93, 98, 104, 106, 112, 113, 125, 127, 133, 134, 136, 138, 143, 144, 161, 165, 181, 184, 185, 187, 198, 199	1, 3, 5, 7, 8, 9, 11, 12, 13, 15, 16, 18, 19, 21, 24, 25, 26, 29, 31, 32, 33, 34, 35, 36, 39, 40, 42, 44, 45, 47, 48, 49, 51, 53, 54, 55, 56, 57, 58, 62, 63, 64, 65, 67, 70, 73, 75, 76, 77, 78, 79, 80, 81, 83, 85, 86, 87, 89, 90, 91, 92, 94, 96, 97, 99, 101, 102, 103, 105, 107, 109, 111, 114, 115, 117, 118, 119, 120, 122, 123, 124, 126, 128, 131, 132, 135, 137, 139, 141, 142, 145, 146, 147, 149, 150, 151, 153, 155, 156, 157, 158, 159, 160, 162, 164, 166, 167, 168, 169, 170, 171, 172, 173, 174, 175, 176, 177, 178, 179, 180, 182, 183, 186, 188, 189, 190, 191, 193, 194, 195, 196, 197, 200

For an index to *topics* (i.e., content, theory) relating to each client need, see **Appendix C.**

APPENDIX **E**

Index: Questions Related to 10 Subcategories Under Four General Client Needs

Use this index to locate *practice questions* throughout the book in each of the 10 subcategories of *client needs* that are tested on NCLEX-RN.

CLIENT NEEDS: 10 SUBCATEGORIES

Unit	1. Management of Care Question No.	2. Safety and Infection Control Question No.	3. Growth and Development Question No.	4. Prevention and Early Detection of Disease Question No.	5. Coping and Adaptation Question No.	6. Psychosocial Adaptation Question No.	7. Basic Care and Comfort Question No.	8. Pharmacological and Parenteral Therapies Question No.	9. Reduction of Risk Potential Question No.	10. Physiological Adaptation Question No.
Unit 1: Orientation and Pre Test (Q/A: 1–200)	12, 37, 58, 135	70, 128, 139, 180	49, 57, 63, 65, 76, 115, 149, 189, 194	1, 19, 47, 52, 62, 69, 90, 107, 111, 170	8, 21, 24, 31, 33, 46, 48, 50, 51, 77, 83, 86, 91, 95, 99, 102, 104, 116, 117, 122, 129, 132, 140, 142, 151, 152, 157, 174, 179, 184, 187	11, 66, 85, 106, 199	41, 44, 101, 133, 143, 145, 154, 166, 197	14, 78, 82, 94, 100, 118, 123, 126, 131, 144, 147, 167, 168, 191	7, 10, 17, 18, 22, 25, 28, 35, 40, 42, 43, 45, 53, 55, 59, 60, 61, 64, 67, 68, 73, 81, 87, 89, 93, 96, 97, 103, 108, 109, 110, 113, 120, 124, 127, 130, 134, 136, 137, 138, 141, 146, 148, 150, 153, 156, 159, 162, 163, 164, 165, 172, 175, 176, 182, 188, 190, 193, 198	2, 3, 4, 5, 6, 9, 13, 15, 16, 20, 23, 26, 27, 29, 30, 32, 34, 36, 38, 39, 54, 56, 71, 72, 74, 75, 79, 80, 84, 88, 92, 98, 105, 112, 114, 119, 121, 125, 155, 158, 160, 161, 169, 171, 173, 177, 178, 181, 183, 185, 186, 192, 195, 196, 200
Unit 3: Management of Care, Ethical and Legal Aspects of Nursing; Cultural Diversity (Q/A: 1–55)	3, 4, 5, 6, 8, 9, 11, 12, 13, 14, 15, 16, 17, 18, 20, 21, 22, 23, 24, 26, 27, 28, 29, 30, 31, 32, 33, 34, 35, 38, 40, 42, 44, 46, 47, 48, 49, 50, 52, 53, 54, 55	1, 2, 10, 19, 25, 36, 37, 39, 41, 43, 45, 51						7		

For an index to *topics* relating to each client need, see **Appendix C**.

CLIENT NEEDS: 10 SUBCATEGORIES

Unit	1. Management of Care — Question No.	2. Safety and Infection Control — Question No.	3. Growth and Development — Question No.	4. Prevention and Early Detection of Disease — Question No.	5. Coping and Adaptation — Question No.	6. Psychosocial Adaptation — Question No.	7. Basic Care and Comfort — Question No.	8. Pharmacological and Parenteral Therapies — Question No.	9. Reduction of Risk Potential — Questio...	10. — Questio...
Unit 4: Nursing Care of the Childbearing Family (Q/A: 1–109)	92	91, 99	1, 2, 6, 7, 11, 15, 20, 21, 25, 26, 29, 33, 43, 44, 47, 50, 51, 56, 59, 60, 61, 62, 69, 70, 71, 73, 77, 78, 84, 86, 90, 97, 100, 101, 102, 103, 104, 105, 109	4, 5, 32, 34, 35, 38, 45, 66, 68, 74, 81, 82	36, 48, 52, 53, 54, 55, 65	98	10, 14, 17, 19, 27, 57, 58, 63, 64, 80, 89, 106, 107	88, 94	8, 12, 23, 24, 30, 31, 39, 40, 41, 42, 46, 49, 72, 75, 76, 79, 83, 87, 93, 95, 108	3, 9, 13, 16, 18, 22, 28, 37, 67, 85, 96
Unit 5: Nursing Care of Children and Families (Q/A: 1–145)	36, 120, 123, 124, 126, 129, 131, 132, 133, 134, 135, 136, 144, 145	1, 7, 14, 32, 58, 61, 62, 75, 87, 110, 111, 116, 117, 122, 142	8, 11, 22, 24, 42, 59, 60, 63, 72, 76, 77, 80, 90, 114, 115, 119	5, 10, 30, 43, 57, 68, 81, 83, 88, 89, 93, 100, 104, 105, 106, 107, 113	3, 18, 19, 26, 28, 29, 34, 37, 46, 74, 84, 92, 95, 99, 118	130	2, 6, 25, 44, 51, 55, 79, 102, 103, 128	15, 17, 27, 35, 38, 50, 53, 65, 69, 70, 82, 98, 101, 108, 109, 112, 125, 138, 139, 140, 141	16, 33, 41, 47, 48, 52, 54, 64, 66, 67, 85, 86, 91, 94, 96, 97, 121, 127, 137, 143	4, 9, 12, 13, 20, 21, 23, 31, 39, 40, 45, 49, 56, 71, 73, 78
Unit 6: Nursing Care of Behavioral and Emotional Problems Throughout the Life Span (Q/A: 1–159)	24, 96, 101, 133, 153, 154, 157	11, 59, 118, 145, 155	12, 20, 22, 53, 80, 91, 112, 116, 132		2, 4, 8, 9, 13, 15, 16, 17, 18, 19, 23, 25, 27, 28, 31, 37, 38, 39, 40, 41, 43, 44, 46, 47, 48, 50, 52, 55, 56, 58, 60, 62, 63, 69, 70, 71, 72, 78, 82, 83, 87, 88, 90, 92, 94, 95, 98, 100, 103, 104, 106, 107, 109, 110, 111, 113, 114, 120, 122, 123, 125, 126, 127, 128, 129, 130, 136, 137, 139, 140, 142, 149, 152, 158, 159	3, 6, 7, 14, 21, 29, 30, 32, 33, 34, 35, 36, 42, 45, 49, 51, 54, 61, 64, 65, 66, 67, 68, 73, 74, 75, 76, 77, 79, 81, 84, 85, 86, 89, 97, 105, 115, 117, 119, 121, 124, 131, 135, 138, 141, 143, 146, 147, 150, 156	5, 57, 93, 134	144, 151	26, 99	1, 10, 102, 108

Appendices

CLIENT NEEDS: 10 SUBCATEGORIES

Unit	1. Management of Care	2. Safety and Infection Control	3. Growth and Development	4. Prevention and Early Detection of Disease	5. Coping and Adaptation	6. Psychosocial Adaptation	7. Basic Care and Comfort	8. Pharmacological and Parenteral Therapies	9. Reduction of Risk Potential	10. Physiological Adaptation
	Question No.	Question No.	Question No.	Question No.	Question No.	Question No.	Question No.	Question No.	Question No.	Question No.
Unit 12: Practice Test (Q/A: 1–100)	10, 35, 58	27	1, 11, 16, 26, 29, 31, 41, 45, 47, 53, 62, 74, 83, 90, 97	13, 18, 36, 60, 81, 85, 95	14, 19, 22, 37, 43, 44, 54, 55, 59, 68, 70, 72, 75, 84, 89, 91	6, 17, 20, 24, 34, 42, 52, 64, 79, 96, 99	28, 40, 56, 57, 63, 65, 66, 77, 82, 92, 100	25, 32, 39, 48, 73, 87	2, 3, 4, 5, 8, 9, 23, 33, 46, 78, 88, 93	7, 12, 15, 21, 30, 38, 49, 50, 51, 61, 67, 69, 71, 76, 80, 86, 94, 98
Unit 13: Final Test (Q/A: 1–200)	4, 10, 59, 72, 110, 121	68, 116, 130	20, 23, 46, 71, 82, 88, 108, 129, 140, 163	2, 6, 14, 28, 50, 61, 69, 95, 99, 148, 152, 154, 192	22, 27, 30, 37, 38, 41, 52, 60, 93, 98, 104, 112, 125, 133, 134, 136, 138, 143, 161, 165, 184, 187, 198, 199	17, 43, 66, 74, 84, 106, 113, 127, 144, 181, 185	15, 39, 45, 81, 83, 90, 96, 111, 119, 167, 176, 179, 182, 190	8, 21, 26, 29, 31, 53, 64, 73, 75, 79, 80, 86, 87, 103, 109, 114, 118, 122, 123, 126, 132, 135, 139, 146, 147, 153, 155, 156, 157, 160, 166, 171, 173, 174, 186, 194, 196	11, 18, 32, 33, 34, 42, 44, 48, 51, 54, 55, 56, 62, 67, 70, 77, 85, 91, 94, 97, 117, 128, 137, 142, 150, 158, 159, 162, 164, 170, 175, 178, 180, 188, 189, 191, 195, 197	1, 3, 5, 7, 9, 12, 13, 16, 19, 24, 25, 35, 36, 40, 47, 49, 57, 58, 63, 65, 76, 78, 89, 92, 99, 101, 102, 105, 107, 115, 120, 124, 131, 141, 145, 149, 151, 168, 169, 172, 177, 183, 193, 200

For an index to *topics* (i.e., content, theory) relating to each of the 10 subcategories above, see **Appendix C.**

NCLEX-RN Test Plan:
◆ Nursing Process
Definitions/Descriptions

The phases of the nursing process include:

I. Assessment: establishing a database.
  A. *Gather objective and subjective information relative to the client:*
    ▪ Collect information from the client, significant others, and health care team members; current and prior health records; and other pertinent resources.
    ▪ Use assessment skills appropriate to client's condition.
    ▪ Recognize *symptoms* and significant findings.
    ▪ Determine client's ability to assume care of daily health needs.
    ▪ Determine health team member's ability to provide care.
    ▪ Assess environment of client.
    ▪ Identify own or staff reactions to client, significant others, and health care team members.
  B. *Confirm data:*
    ▪ Verify observation or perception by obtaining additional information.
    ▪ Question prescriptions and decisions by other health care team members when indicated.
    ▪ Observe condition of client directly when indicated.
    ▪ Validate that an appropriate client assessment has been made.
  C. *Communicate information gained in assessment:*
    ▪ Document assessment findings thoroughly and accurately.

Source: Adapted from National Council of State Boards of Nursing: NCLEX-RN Test Plan. National Council of State Boards, Chicago, 1994.

    ▪ Report assessment findings to relevant members of the health care team.

II. Analysis: identifying actual or potential health care needs and problems based on assessment.
  A. *Interpret data:*
    ▪ Validate data.
    ▪ Organize related data.
    ▪ Determine *need for additional* data.
    ▪ Determine client's unique needs or problems.
  B. *Formulate client's nursing diagnoses:*
    ▪ Determine significant relationship between data and client needs or problems.
    ▪ Use *standard taxonomy* for formulating nursing diagnoses.
  C. *Communicate results of analysis:*
    ▪ *Document client's nursing diagnoses.*
    ▪ Report results of analysis to relevant members of the health care team.

III. Planning: setting goals for meeting client's needs and designing strategies to achieve these goals.
  A. *Prioritize nursing diagnoses:*
    ▪ Involve client, significant others, and health care team members when establishing nursing diagnoses.
    ▪ Establish priorities among nursing diagnoses.
    ▪ Anticipate needs and problems on the basis of established priorities.
  B. *Determine goals of care:*
    ▪ Involve client, significant others, and health care team members in setting goals.
    ▪ Establish *priorities among goals.*
    ▪ Anticipate needs or problems on the basis of established priorities.

C. *Formulate outcome criteria for goals of care:*
  - Involve client, significant others, and health care team members in formulating outcome criteria for goals of care.
  - Establish *priorities* among *outcome criteria* for goals of care.
  - Anticipate needs or problems on the basis of established priorities.

D. *Develop plan of care and modify as necessary:*
  - Involve the client, significant others, and health care team members in designing strategies.
  - Individualize the plan of care based on such information as *age, gender, culture, ethnicity, and religion.*
  - Plan for client's safety, comfort, and maintenance of optimal functioning.
  - Select nursing interventions for delivery of client's care.
  - Select *appropriate teaching* approaches.

E. *Collaborate with other health care team members when planning delivery of client's care:*
  - Identify health or social resources available to the client and significant others.
  - Select appropriate health care team members when planning assignments.
  - Coordinate care provided by health care team members.

F. *Communicate plan of care:*
  - Document plan of care thoroughly and accurately.
  - Report plan of care to relevant members of the health care team.
  - Review plan of care with client.

IV. **Implementation: initiating and completing actions necessary to accomplish the defined goals.**

A. *Organize and manage client's care:*
  - Implement a plan of care.
  - Arrange for a client care conference.

B. *Counsel and teach client, significant others, and health care team members:*
  - Assist client, significant others, and health care team members to recognize and manage stress.
  - Facilitate client relationships with significant others and health care team members.
  - *Teach* correct principles, procedures, and techniques for maintenance and promotion of health.
  - Provide client with health status information.
  - Refer client, significant others, and health care team members to appropriate *resources.*

C. *Provide care to achieve established goals of care:*
  - Use safe and appropriate techniques when administering client care.
  - Use precautionary and *preventive* interventions in providing care to client.
  - *Prepare client for surgery,* delivery, or other procedures.
  - Institute *interventions* to compensate for *adverse* responses.
  - Initiate *lifesaving interventions* for emergency situations.

  - Provide an environment conducive to attainment of goals of care.
  - Adjust care in accord with client's expressed or implied needs, problems, and preferences.
  - Stimulate and motivate client to achieve self-care and independence.
  - Encourage client to follow a treatment regimen.
  - Assist client to maintain optimal functioning.

D. *Supervise and coordinate the delivery of client's care provided by nursing personnel:*
  - Delegate nursing interventions to appropriate nursing personnel.
  - Monitor and follow up on delegated interventions.
  - Manage health care team members' reactions to factors influencing therapeutic relationships with clients.

E. *Communicate nursing interventions:*
  - Record actual client responses, nursing interventions, and other information relevant to implementation of care.
  - Provide complete, accurate reports on assigned client(s) to relevant members of the health care team.

V. **Evaluation: determining the extent to which goals have been achieved and interventions have been successful.**

A. *Compare actual outcomes with expected outcomes of care:*
  - Evaluate responses (expected and unexpected) in order to determine the degree of success of nursing interventions.
  - Determine impact of therapeutic interventions on the client and significant others.
  - Determine need for modifying the plan of care.
  - Identify factors that may interfere with the client's ability to implement the plan of care.

B. *Evaluate the client's ability to implement self-care:*
  - Verify that tests *or measurements are performed correctly* by the client and other caregivers.
  - Ascertain client's and others' understanding of information given.

C. *Evaluate health care team members' ability to implement client care:*
  - Determine impact of teaching on health care team members.
  - Identify factors that might alter health care team members' response to teaching.

D. *Communicate evaluation findings:*
  - Document client's response to therapy, care, and teaching.
  - Report client's response to therapy, care, and teaching to relevant members of the health care team.
  - Report and document others' responses to teaching.
  - Document other caregivers' responses to teaching.

The practice questions in this book (end-of-unit questions, **Pre Test, Practice Test,** and **Final Test**) are coded as to the phase of the nursing process being tested; the codes are found following the answer/rationale for each question. *Key to nursing process codes:*

- ◆ AS   Assessment
- ◆ AN   Analysis
- ◆ PL   Planning
- ◆ IMP   Implementation
- ◆ EV   Evaluation

For an index to questions relating to each phase of the nursing process, see **Appendix G.**

Index: Questions Related
·to Nursing Process

Use this index to locate *practice questions* throughout the book in each of the
five phases of the *nursing process.*

FIVE PHASES OF THE NURSING PROCESS AND THEIR CODES

Unit	Assessment (AS) Question No.	Analysis (AN) Question No.	Plan (PL) Question No.	Implementation (IMP) Question No.	Evaluation (EV) Question No.
Unit 1: Orientation and Pre Test (Q/A: 1–200)	1, 10, 27, 32, 43, 51, 53, 73, 76, 92, 99, 111, 112, 113, 114, 126, 161, 162, 167, 176, 177, 183, 185, 190, 195, 198	2, 3, 5, 6, 9, 13, 15, 16, 18, 20, 26, 28, 30, 36, 38, 46, 48, 49, 50, 57, 59, 62, 65, 71, 72, 74, 80, 82, 84, 102, 104, 105, 107, 109, 115, 117, 118, 121, 125, 129, 130, 138, 141, 144, 150, 151, 155, 159, 160, 164, 166, 169, 178, 182, 184, 186, 196, 200	8, 11, 12, 17, 21, 22, 41, 61, 67, 79, 81, 85, 87, 89, 95, 103, 106, 110, 116, 127, 134, 135, 143, 148, 152, 156, 157, 165, 173, 187, 188	4, 7, 19, 23, 24, 25, 29, 31, 33, 34, 35, 37, 40, 42, 44, 45, 52, 54, 56, 58, 60, 64, 66, 68, 70, 75, 77, 78, 83, 86, 88, 96, 98, 100, 101, 108, 119, 120, 122, 123, 124, 128, 131, 132, 133, 136, 137, 139, 145, 146, 147, 153, 154, 158, 163, 168, 170, 172, 174, 175, 179, 180, 181, 189, 191, 193, 197, 199	14, 39, 47, 55, 63, 69, 90, 91, 93, 94, 97, 140, 142, 149, 171, 192, 194
Unit 3: Management of Care, Ethical and Legal Aspects of Nursing (Q/A: 1–55)	41	15, 16, 18, 22, 23, 24, 25, 38, 40, 51	5, 42, 43, 48, 50, 53	1, 2, 3, 4, 7, 11, 12, 17, 19, 36, 37, 39, 44, 45, 46, 47, 49, 54, 55	6, 8, 9, 10, 13, 14, 20, 21, 27, 33, 52
Unit 4: Nursing Care of the Childbearing Family (Q/A: 1–109)	2, 3, 5, 15, 25, 30, 33, 39, 44, 48, 49, 55, 61, 62, 65, 70, 71, 77, 82, 84, 86, 87, 89, 95, 97, 105, 108	7, 9, 11, 13, 16, 18, 20, 21, 22, 24, 26, 28, 29, 37, 41, 43, 45, 50, 51, 52, 60, 67, 73, 74, 75, 76, 79, 85, 90, 91, 92, 93, 96, 101, 102, 103, 104, 106, 107	54, 88, 98, 99, 109	1, 4, 6, 8, 10, 12, 14, 17, 19, 23, 27, 31, 32, 34, 35, 36, 38, 40, 46, 47, 53, 56, 57, 58, 59, 63, 64, 66, 68, 69, 72, 78, 83, 94, 100	42, 80, 81
Unit 5: Nursing Care of Children and Families (Q/A: 1–145)	12, 27, 40, 90, 93, 104, 119	6, 7, 14, 16, 17, 19, 21, 22, 23, 35, 47, 48, 52, 56, 58, 60, 62, 75, 76, 77, 78, 80, 89, 100, 103, 105, 109, 112, 116, 117, 118, 121, 127, 130, 133, 138, 139, 144	25, 28, 49, 61, 65, 71, 108, 134	1, 2, 3, 5, 8, 11, 13, 15, 18, 20, 24, 26, 29, 31, 32, 33, 36, 39, 41, 42, 44, 45, 46, 51, 53, 54, 55, 59, 63, 66, 69, 70, 72, 74, 79, 81, 82, 83, 84, 85, 86, 87, 88, 91, 92, 94, 95, 96, 97, 99, 101, 102, 106, 107, 110, 111, 113, 115, 120, 124, 128, 129, 131, 135, 136, 137, 141, 145	4, 9, 10, 30, 34, 37, 38, 43, 50, 57, 64, 67, 68, 73, 98, 114, 122, 123, 125, 126, 132, 140, 142, 143
Unit 6: Nursing Care of Behavioral and Emotional Problems Throughout the Life Span (Q/A: 1–159)	4, 15, 39, 45, 52, 71, 102, 108, 128, 136, 143	8, 9, 12, 20, 25, 27, 36, 37, 38, 40, 41, 43, 44, 46, 47, 53, 55, 56, 57, 60, 62, 63, 65, 69, 70, 72, 76, 78, 80, 83, 99, 103, 104, 106, 107, 110, 111, 112, 113, 114, 123, 125, 127, 129, 130, 132, 137, 147, 148, 149, 152, 153, 154, 156	1, 10, 17, 21, 26, 29, 32, 33, 34, 49, 59, 64, 67, 73, 74, 75, 81, 89, 91, 92, 98, 105, 115, 117, 118, 124, 138, 140, 141, 157, 158	2, 3, 5, 6, 7, 11, 13, 14, 16, 19, 22, 23, 24, 28, 30, 31, 35, 42, 50, 51, 54, 58, 61, 66, 68, 77, 79, 84, 85, 86, 87, 88, 90, 94, 96, 97, 100, 101, 119, 120, 121, 122, 126, 133, 134, 135, 139, 142, 145, 146, 150, 151, 155, 159	18, 48, 82, 93, 95, 109, 116, 131, 144
Unit 7: Nursing Care of the Acutely Ill and the Chronically Ill Adult (Q/A: 1–132)	4, 13, 35, 41, 53, 72, 77, 78, 79, 84, 90, 98, 99, 107, 109, 113, 119, 127	5, 8, 9, 10, 11, 15, 17, 19, 23, 29, 30, 32, 37, 39, 45, 56, 58, 65, 71, 74, 80, 82, 85, 86, 93, 95, 100, 101, 102, 104, 105, 110, 112, 116, 128, 132	2, 3, 6, 12, 20, 21, 27, 40, 44, 62, 108, 114, 118	1, 7, 14, 18, 24, 25, 26, 28, 36, 38, 42, 43, 46, 48, 49, 52, 54, 55, 57, 59, 60, 63, 69, 70, 73, 75, 81, 89, 92, 97, 103, 106, 115, 120, 121, 123, 124, 125, 126, 129, 130, 131	16, 22, 31, 33, 34, 47, 50, 51, 61, 64, 66, 67, 68, 76, 83, 87, 88, 91, 94, 96, 111, 117, 122

FIVE PHASES OF THE NURSING PROCESS AND THEIR CODES

Unit	Assessment (AS) Question No.	Analysis (AN) Question No.	Plan (PL) Question No.	Implementation (IMP) Question No.	Evaluation (EV) Question No.
Unit 9: Review of Nutrition (Q/A: 1–9)	8		2, 4, 5, 7, 9	1, 3, 6	
Unit 10: Review of Pharmacology (Q/A: 1–64)	1, 11, 20, 29	14, 19, 23, 35, 36, 37, 41, 44, 47, 50, 59, 60	2, 4, 9, 13, 27, 31, 33, 39, 40, 45, 49, 56	3, 6, 8, 12, 16, 21, 22, 24, 25, 26, 30, 32, 38, 46, 48, 51, 52, 53, 54, 55, 57, 58, 61, 62, 63, 64	5, 7, 10, 15, 17, 18, 28, 34, 42, 43
Unit 11: Common Diagnostic Procedures, Intravenous and Oxygen Therapy, Isolation Precautions, and Hands-on Nursing Care (Q/A: 1–13)	9	1, 6	2, 3, 8, 12	4, 5, 10, 11	7, 13
Unit 12: Practice Test (Q/A: 1–100)	8, 13, 14, 33, 36, 37, 51, 59, 79, 80, 98	10, 16, 19, 21, 22, 24, 26, 31, 41, 53, 60, 67, 69, 70, 72, 74, 75, 76, 93, 94	6, 11, 20, 29, 45, 46, 52, 54, 57, 82, 83, 86, 92, 99	2, 3, 4, 5, 7, 17, 23, 25, 28, 30, 32, 34, 35, 38, 39, 40, 43, 44, 47, 49, 55, 56, 61, 62, 64, 65, 66, 68, 71, 73, 77, 78, 81, 84, 85, 88, 89, 91, 95, 96, 97, 100	1, 9, 12, 15, 18, 27, 42, 48, 50, 58, 63, 87, 90
Unit 13: Final Test (Q/A: 1–200)	2, 5, 14, 19, 50, 60, 61, 63, 65, 71, 79, 81, 109, 115, 154, 163, 165, 168, 169, 192	1, 9, 20, 24, 40, 46, 73, 98, 127, 129, 136, 140, 143, 149, 150, 151, 156, 162, 172, 175, 177, 186, 193, 198	4, 16, 29, 42, 43, 51, 53, 54, 55, 62, 69, 80, 83, 106, 113, 118, 121, 128, 132, 137, 138, 164, 167, 170, 187, 191, 195, 197	3, 7, 10, 11, 15, 17, 22, 25, 27, 28, 30, 31, 32, 33, 34, 35, 36, 38, 41, 44, 45, 47, 48, 49, 52, 56, 57, 58, 59, 66, 67, 68, 70, 72, 74, 76, 77, 78, 82, 84, 85, 86, 89, 90, 91, 93, 95, 96, 97, 101, 102, 104, 105, 107, 108, 110, 111, 112, 114, 116, 122, 125, 126, 130, 131, 133, 134, 141, 144, 145, 146, 147, 148, 152, 155, 157, 158, 159, 160, 173, 176, 178, 179, 180, 181, 182, 185, 188, 189, 190, 196, 199	6, 8, 12, 13, 18, 21, 23, 26, 37, 39, 64, 75, 87, 88, 92, 94, 99, 100, 103, 117, 119, 120, 123, 124, 135, 139, 142, 153, 161, 166, 171, 174, 183, 184, 194, 200

Eight Detailed Areas of Human Functions Definitions/Descriptions

The following detailed eight detailed areas are incorporated under specific client needs (see Appendix B: **A** 1, 2; **B** 3, 4; **C** 5, 6; **D** 7, 8, 9, 10). These functions are *detailed* areas of eight selected topics included under the 10 client need subcategories (i.e., they provide a **further breakdown of the most important concepts to master** related to client needs).

1. **Protective Functions** (A2—Safety and Infection Control; B4—Prevention and Early Detection of Disease)

   Client's ability to maintain defenses and prevent physical and chemical *trauma, injury, infection,* and threats to health status. Examples: *communicable* diseases (including sexually transmitted diseases), *immunity, physical trauma* and *abuse,* asepsis, *safety hazards, poisoning,* skin disorders, and preoperative care and postoperative complications.

2. **Sensory-Perceptual Functions** (C5—Coping and Adaptation)

   Client's ability to perceive, interpret, and respond to sensory and cognitive stimuli. Examples: *auditory, visual,* and verbal impairments, sensory *deprivation,* sensory *overload, aphasia, brain tumors, laryngectomy, dementia, body image, reality orientation,* learning disabilities, and *seizure* disorders.

3. **Comfort, Rest, Activity, and Mobility Functions** (D7—Basic Care and Comfort)

   Client's ability to maintain mobility, desirable level of activity, and adequate sleep, rest, and comfort. Examples: joint impairment, body alignment, *pain, sleep* disturbances, *activities of daily living, neuromuscular* impairment, *musculoskeletal* impairment, and *endocrine* disorders that affect activity.

4. **Nutrition** (D7—Basic Care and Comfort)

   Client's ability to maintain the intake and processing of essential nutrients. Examples: *normal* nutrition, diet in *pregnancy* and *lactation, obesity,* conditions such as *diabetes, gastric* disorders, and *metabolic* disorders that affect primarily the nutritional status.

5. **Growth and Development** (B3—Growth and Development Throughout the Life Span)

   Client's ability to maintain maturational processes throughout the life span. Examples: *childbearing, child rearing,* conditions that interfere with the maturation process, maturational crises, changes in *aging, psychosocial development,* sterility, and conditions of the *reproductive system.*

6. **Fluid-Gas Transport Functions** (D10—Physiological Adaptation)

   Client's ability to maintain fluid-gas transport. Examples: *fluid volume deficit and overload, cardiopulmonary* diseases, *acid-base balance,* cardiopulmonary resuscitation, *anemias, hemorrhagic* disorders, leukemias, and *infectious pulmonary* diseases.

7. **Psychosocial-Cultural Functions** (C5—Coping and Adaptation; C6—Psychosocial Adaptation)

   Client's ability to function in intrapersonal, interpersonal, intergroup, and sociocultural relationships. Examples: *grieving, death and dying, psychopathology, self-concept,* therapeutic *communication, group* dynamics, *ethical-legal* aspects, *community resources, spiritual* needs, situational *crises,* and *substance abuse.*

8. **Elimination Functions** (D10—Physiological Adaptation)

   Client's ability to maintain functions related to relieving the body of waste products. Examples: conditions of the *gastrointestinal* system, such as vomiting, diarrhea, constipation, ulcers, neoplasms, colostomy, and hernia; conditions of the *urinary* system, such as kidney stones, transplants, renal failure, and prostatic hyperplasia.

The practice questions in this book (end-of-unit questions, **Pre Test, Practice Test,** and **Final Test**) are coded as to the category of human function being tested; the codes are found following the answer/rationale for each question. *Key to category of human function codes:*

1	Protective
2	Sensory-Perceptual
3	Comfort, Rest, Activity, and Mobility
4	Nutrition
5	Growth and Development
6	Fluid-Gas Transport
7	Psychosocial-Cultural
8	Elimination

For an index to *questions* relating to each human function, see **Appendix J.**

For page references of specific *topics to review* relating to each human function, see **Appendix I.**

Index: Content Related to Eight Detailed Areas of Human Functions

These eight detailed areas of human functions/concepts provide detailed examples of *content* areas incorporated under the 10 subcategories of the four general areas of client needs on which the NCLEX-RN test plan is based.

How to use this index: If, for example, after you take the tests in this book, you notice that you are mostly missing questions under VI (6) *Fluid-Gas Transport Functions,* this means that you have identified your *specific* problem area under the general client need of **Physiological Integrity,** subcategory 10, *Physiological Adaptation.* In other words, **Appendix I** will lead you to the pages in this book that cover the specific problem area that you identified for extra focus in your exam prep.

To summarize, this is a diagram of how these various categories relate to each other:

First, there are the:

| 4 general **Client Needs** |

This breaks down into:

| 10 subcategories of Client Needs |

Finally, these are detailed areas to master:

| 8 detailed areas (concepts of human function) under the 10 subcategories |

For an index to *questions* relating to each category of human function, see **Appendix J.**

Appendices

Index: Questions Related to Eight Detailed Areas of Human Functions

This index lists *practice questions* for you to use in reviewing the eight detailed areas of *human functions* (which are detailed examples of what is covered by the four broad client needs and 10 subcategories.)

EIGHT CATEGORIES OF HUMAN FUNCTIONS

Unit	Protective Functions (1) Question No.	Sensory-Perceptual Functions (2) Question No.	Comfort, Rest, Activity, and Mobility Functions (3) Question No.	Nutrition (4) Question No.	Growth and Development (5) Question No.	Fluid-Gas Transport Functions (6) Question No.	Psychosocial-Cultural Functions (7) Question No.	Elimination Functions (8) Question No.
Unit 1: Orientation and Pre Test (Q/A: 1–200)	19, 23, 25, 37, 42, 43, 52, 53, 54, 60, 69, 70, 74, 75, 87, 90, 97, 110, 120, 125, 126, 128, 134, 135, 139, 156, 167, 170, 186, 191	21, 38, 72, 111, 124, 147, 148, 163, 180	7, 17, 18, 22, 26, 41, 45, 68, 89, 96, 99, 101, 108, 136, 138, 160, 190, 197	3, 6, 15, 20, 27, 30, 34, 36, 44, 56, 59, 82, 100, 103, 118, 141, 143, 145, 162, 166, 168, 175, 193	14, 47, 48, 49, 57, 58, 62, 63, 76, 98, 107, 115, 116, 149, 151, 189, 194, 196, 198	2, 10, 12, 13, 28, 29, 31, 32, 35, 64, 71, 72, 73, 78, 79, 80, 84, 86, 88, 92, 93, 94, 105, 109, 113, 114, 119, 121, 123, 127, 130, 131, 133, 137, 146, 150, 153, 159, 161, 164, 165, 171, 172, 176, 181, 182, 183, 185, 188, 192, 195, 200	8, 11, 24, 33, 46, 50, 51, 65, 66, 83, 85, 91, 95, 102, 104, 106, 117, 122, 129, 132, 140, 142, 152, 157, 174, 179, 184, 187, 199	1, 4, 5, 9, 16, 39, 40, 55, 61, 67, 81, 112, 144, 154, 155, 158, 169, 173, 177, 178
Unit 3: Management of Care, Ethical and Legal Aspects of Nursing (Q/A: 1–55)	1, 2, 4, 7, 19, 21, 22, 25, 51		54	53			3, 5, 6, 8, 9, 10, 11, 12, 13, 14, 15, 16, 17, 18, 20, 23, 24, 26, 27, 28, 29, 30, 31, 32, 33, 34, 35, 36, 37, 38, 39, 40, 41, 42, 43, 44, 45, 46, 47, 48, 49, 50, 52, 55	
Unit 4: Nursing Care of the Childbearing Family (Q/A: 1–109)	5, 24, 41, 56, 67, 92, 94, 108	12, 40, 49, 95	14, 26, 27, 62, 64, 68, 73, 80	10, 11, 17, 18, 29, 42, 58, 63, 106, 107	1, 2, 3, 6, 7, 15, 19, 20, 21, 25, 32, 33, 34, 36, 43, 44, 45, 47, 48, 50, 51, 52, 57, 59, 60, 61, 66, 69, 70, 71, 74, 77, 78, 84, 86, 88, 90, 97, 100, 101, 102, 103, 105	4, 8, 9, 13, 16, 23, 28, 30, 31, 37, 38, 39, 46, 72, 75, 76, 79, 81, 82, 83, 85, 87, 91, 93, 96, 99, 104	53, 54, 55, 65, 98, 109	22, 35, 89
Unit 5: Nursing Care of Children and Families (Q/A: 1–145)	2, 5, 10, 14, 15, 16, 17, 32, 33, 35, 37, 41, 48, 53, 58, 61, 62, 71, 72, 79, 82, 88, 89, 95, 110, 112, 116, 117, 120, 122, 124, 126, 134, 135, 136, 140, 145	52, 93, 105, 143, 144	1, 7, 74, 91, 100, 106, 133, 138, 139	20, 25, 44, 56, 70, 73, 94, 113, 125, 128, 137	8, 11, 17, 24, 26, 42, 50, 59, 63, 76, 77, 80, 90, 99, 114, 115, 118, 119, 132	4, 6, 9, 12, 13, 21, 22, 27, 30, 31, 38, 39, 40, 43, 45, 49, 51, 54, 55, 57, 65, 66, 67, 69, 77, 78, 81, 83, 85, 86, 87, 96, 97, 101, 104, 107, 108, 109, 111, 121, 127, 129, 141	3, 18, 19, 29, 34, 46, 60, 84, 130, 131	23, 28, 36, 47, 64, 68, 75, 92, 98, 102, 103, 123, 142

Appendices

Unit								
Unit 6: Nursing Care of Behavioral and Emotional Problems Throughout the Life Span (Q/A: 1–159)	11, 30, 118, 141, 145, 153, 154, 155, 156	2, 4, 6, 9, 14, 21, 26, 33, 35, 39, 49, 57, 67, 87, 123	100, 108, 119, 121, 151	5, 148	12, 20, 25, 44, 86, 112, 136	1, 59	3, 7, 8, 10, 13, 15, 16, 17, 18, 19, 22, 23, 24, 27, 28, 29, 31, 32, 34, 36, 37, 38, 40, 41, 42, 43, 45, 46, 47, 48, 50, 51, 52, 53, 54, 55, 56, 58, 60, 61, 62, 63, 64, 65, 66, 68, 69, 70, 71, 72, 73, 74, 75, 76, 77, 78, 79, 80, 81, 82, 83, 84, 85, 88, 89, 90, 91, 92, 93, 94, 95, 96, 97, 98, 99, 101, 102, 103, 104, 105, 106, 107, 109, 110, 111, 113, 114, 115, 116, 117, 120, 122, 124, 125, 126, 127, 128, 129, 130, 131, 132, 133, 134, 135, 137, 138, 139, 140, 142, 143, 144, 146, 147, 149, 150, 152, 157, 158, 159	
Unit 7: Nursing Care of the Acutely Ill and the Chronically Ill Adult (Q/A: 1–132)	8, 21, 22, 28, 46, 81, 88, 105, 125, 126	2, 11, 26, 31, 36, 51, 56, 59, 60, 61, 65, 67, 77, 98, 99, 109, 110, 129, 132	6, 16, 18, 24, 27, 30, 45, 49, 50, 55, 62, 63, 69, 70, 74, 75, 78, 79, 80, 82, 83, 84, 90, 93, 100, 102, 111, 120, 130, 131	1, 7, 10, 12, 19, 25, 29, 39, 44, 68, 72, 73, 96, 97, 124	101	4, 15, 17, 20, 23, 32, 33, 35, 37, 38, 40, 41, 47, 58, 64, 66, 85, 87, 91, 92, 94, 95, 103, 104, 107, 108, 112, 113, 114, 115, 117, 118, 119, 121, 123, 127, 128	3, 9, 42, 48, 52, 53, 76, 86	5, 13, 14, 34, 43, 54, 57, 71, 89, 106, 116, 122
Unit 9: Review of Nutrition (Q/A: 1–9)				1, 2, 3, 4, 5, 6, 7, 8, 9				
Unit 10: Review of Pharmacology (Q/A: 1–64)	22, 24, 30, 31, 32, 37, 38, 39, 40, 44, 45, 46, 51, 52, 53, 55	10, 21, 26	1, 3, 14, 17, 56	9, 13, 16, 23, 27, 57, 62	29, 33, 34, 35, 36, 54	4, 5, 6, 11, 12, 25, 41, 42, 47, 48, 49, 50, 58, 59, 60, 61, 64	43	2, 7, 8, 15, 18, 19, 20, 28, 63

EIGHT CATEGORIES OF HUMAN FUNCTIONS

Unit	Protective Functions (1) Question No.	Sensory-Perceptual Functions (2) Question No.	Comfort, Rest, Activity, and Mobility Functions (3) Question No.	Nutrition (4) Question No.	Growth and Development (5) Question No.	Fluid-Gas Transport Functions (6) Question No.	Psychosocial-Cultural Functions (7) Question No.	Elimination Functions (8) Question No.
Unit 11: Common Diagnostic Procedures, Intravenous and Oxygen Therapy, Isolation Precautions, and Hands-on Nursing Care (Q/A: 1–13)				5, 6, 7, 8, 12		2, 3, 4, 13		1, 9, 10, 11
Unit 12: Practice Test (Q/A: 1–100)	2, 8, 13, 27, 51, 60, 69, 73, 82, 85, 95	23, 43, 56	12, 30, 32, 35, 40, 63, 65, 66, 81, 88, 100	18, 25, 77	1, 10, 11, 16, 29, 31, 33, 36, 41, 44, 45, 47, 53, 62, 84, 89, 93	3, 5, 7, 21, 26, 28, 38, 49, 50, 61, 67, 71, 76, 80, 94, 98	6, 14, 17, 19, 20, 22, 24, 34, 37, 39, 42, 52, 54, 55, 59, 64, 68, 70, 72, 74, 75, 78, 79, 83, 87, 90, 91, 96, 97, 99	4, 9, 15, 46, 48, 57, 58, 86, 92
Unit 13: Final Test (Q/A: 1–200)	3, 14, 19, 26, 31, 33, 34, 35, 42, 53, 68, 85, 87, 90, 91, 92, 95, 116, 118, 122, 123, 128, 130, 131, 132, 142, 147, 152, 157, 159, 164, 175, 176, 194, 197	4, 11, 43, 51, 62, 76, 84, 103, 111, 124, 127, 184	24, 25, 54, 65, 67, 77, 81, 96, 137, 154, 158, 174, 179, 182, 188	28, 39, 45, 61, 83, 88, 119, 126, 138, 167, 173, 190	2, 6, 20, 27, 30, 37, 41, 46, 50, 69, 71, 82, 100, 104, 108, 129, 136, 144, 148, 161, 163, 178, 192, 199	1, 5, 6, 8, 9, 12, 13, 15, 16, 18, 21, 23, 29, 36, 40, 44, 47, 49, 55, 56, 57, 58, 63, 73, 75, 78, 79, 80, 86, 89, 94, 97, 99, 101, 102, 105, 107, 109, 114, 115, 117, 135, 139, 141, 145, 149, 150, 151, 153, 155, 160, 162, 166, 168, 169, 170, 172, 177, 180, 183, 186, 189, 191, 193, 195, 196, 200	10, 17, 22, 32, 38, 52, 59, 60, 66, 72, 74, 93, 98, 106, 110, 112, 113, 120, 121, 125, 133, 134, 140, 143, 146, 165, 171, 181, 185, 187, 198	48, 64, 70, 156

For an index to *content* (theory) related to each of the above, see **Appendix I.**

Reduction of Risk Potential: Index to Diagnostic Procedures/Tests

This is an important area to review because it is a **subcategory** of the **NCLEX-RN** Test Plan that is often tested. Refer also to **Unit 11.** These tests below are listed in chronological order by unit.

Common Acronyms and Abbreviations

This list provides a review of what you need to know about acronyms and abbreviations used in charting, verbal directives, and study guides.

a	Before (*ante*)
Ab	Antibody/Abortion
Abd	Abdomen/Abdominal
ABG	Arterial blood gas
ac	Before meals (*ante cibum*)
ACTH	Adrenocorticotropic hormone
ADH	Antidiuretic hormone
ad lib	As much as desired (*ad libitum*)
ADLs	Activities of daily living
AFB	Acid-fast bacillus
Afib	Atrial fibrillation
Aflutter	Atrial flutter
AFP	Alpha-fetoprotein
AG	Antigen
AGA	Average for gestational age
AGE	Acute gastroenteritis
AIDS	Acquired immunodeficiency syndrome
AK (or AKA)	Above-the-knee (amputation)
ALL	Acute lymphocytic (lymphoblastic) leukemia
AMA	Against medical advice
AML	Acute myelogenous leukemia
ANP	Adult Nurse Practitioner
A&O × 3	Alert, oriented to person, place, time
AP	Anteroposterior/Alkaline phosphatase
aPPT	Activated partial thromboplastin time
APSGN	Acute poststreptococcal glomerulonephritis
ARC	AIDS-related complex
ARDS	Adult respiratory distress syndrome
ARF	Acute renal failure
AROM	Artificial rupture of membranes
ASA	Acetylsalicylic acid (aspirin)
ASAP	As soon as possible
ASD	Atrial septal defect
AV	Atrioventricular/Arteriovenous/Aortic valve
AVB	Atrioventricular block
AVM	Arteriovenous malformation

BBT	Basal body temperature
bid	Twice daily (*bis in die*)
BK (or BKA)	Below-the-knee (amputation)
BM	Bowel movement/Bone marrow
BMI	Body mass index
BOM	Bilateral otitis media
BMR	Basal metabolic rate
BMT	Bone marrow transplant
BP	Blood pressure
BPD	Bronchopulmonary dysplasia
BPH	Benign prostatic hyperplasia
bpm	Beats per minute
BPP	Biophysical profile
BRP	Bathroom privileges
BSE	Breast self-examination
BUN	Blood urea nitrogen
$\bar{c}$	With (*cum*)
CA	Carcinoma/Cancer
CABG	Coronary artery bypass graft operation (×1, 2, 3, 4 = number of grafts)
CAD	Coronary artery disease
CBC	Complete blood count
CC	Chief complaint
cc	Cubic centimeter
CCU	Cardiac (intensive) care unit
CF	Cystic fibrosis
CHD	Congenital heart disease
CHF	Congestive heart failure
CMV	Cytomegalovirus
CNS	Central nervous system/Coagulase-negative *Staphylococcus*
C/O	Complains of
COPD	Chronic obstructive pulmonary disease
CPD	Cephalopelvic disproportion
CPK	Creatine phosphokinase (now creatine kinase [CK])
CPR	Cardiopulmonary resuscitation
CRF	Chronic renal failure/Cardiac risk factors
CRP	C-reactive protein
CSF	Cerebrospinal fluid
CST	Contraction stress test
CT	Computerized tomography

CVA	Cerebrovascular accident/Costovertebral angle
CVP	Central venous pressure
Δ	Change (Greek letter delta)
D/C	Discharge/Discontinue
D&C	Dilation and curettage
DDH	Developmental dysplasia of the hip
D&E	Dilation and evacuation
DI	Diabetes insipidus
DIC	Disseminated intravascular coagulation
Dig	Digitalis
DKA	Diabetic ketoacidosis
DM	Diabetes mellitus
DMD	Duchenne muscular dystrophy
DNR	Do not resuscitate
DOA	Dead on arrival
DOB	Date of birth
DOE	Dyspnea on exertion
DPT	Diphtheria, pertussis, and tetanus
DRG	Diagnosis-related group
DTs	Delirium tremens
DTR	Deep-tendon reflex
DVT	Deep vein thrombosis
D5W/D₅W	5% dextrose in water
Dx	Diagnosis
ECG	Electrocardiogram (purist's version)
Echo	Echocardiogram
ECMO	Extracorporeal membrane oxygenation
ECT	Electroconvulsive therapy
ED	Emergency department (commonly called *emergency room*)
EDB	Estimated date of birth
EEG	Electroencephalogram
EFM	Electronic fetal monitoring
EKG	Electrocardiogram (common version)
EMG	Electromyogram
EMT	Emergency medical technician
ENT	Ear, nose, and throat
ER	Emergency room
ESR	Erythrocyte sedimentation rate
ETOH	Alcohol (ethanol)
FAS	Fetal alcohol syndrome
FBS	Fasting blood sugar
FEV₁	Forced expiratory volume in 1 second
FHR	Fetal heart rate
FNP	Family nurse practitioner
FRC	Functional residual capacity
FSH	Follicle stimulating hormone
FTT	Failure to thrive
FUO	Fever of unknown origin
FVC	Forced vital capacity
Fx	Fracture
g	Gram
G	Gravida
GABS	Group A beta-hemolytic streptococcus
GB	Gallbladder

GBS	Group B streptococcus
GBS	Guillain-Barré syndrome
GC	Gonococcus/Gonorrhea
GER	Gastroesophageal reflux
GI	Gastrointestinal
gr	Grain
GTT	Glucose tolerance test
gtt(s)	Drop(s) (*guttae*)
GU	Genitourinary
GYN	Gynecological
HAV	Hepatitis A virus
HBGM	Home blood glucose monitoring
HBV	Hepatitis B virus
HCG	Human chorionic gonadotropin
Hct	Hematocrit
HDL	High-density lipoprotein
HEENT	Head, eyes, ears, nose, throat
Hgb	Hemoglobin
HgbA₁c	Glycosylated hemoglobin
HIB	*Haemophilus influenzae* type B
HIV	Human immunodeficiency virus
HMO	Health maintenance organization
HOB	Head of bed
HPL	Human placental lactogen
HPS	Hypertrophic pyloric stenosis
HPV	Human papilloma virus
HR	Heart rate
HRT	Hormone replacement therapy
hs	Bedtime (*hora somni*)
HSP	Henoch-Schönlein purpura
HSV	Herpes simplex virus
HTN	Hypertension
Hx	History
ICP	Intracranial pressure
ICU	Intensive care unit
I&D	Incision and drainage
IDDM	Insulin-dependent diabetes mellitus
Ig	Immunoglobulin
IM	Intramuscular
INH	Isoniazid
I&O	Intake and output
IPPB	Intermittent positive-pressure breathing
IUD	Intrauterine device
IV	Intravenous
IVC	Inferior vena cava
IVP	Intravenous pyelogram/Intravenous push
IVH	Intraventricular hemorrhage
JCAHO	Joint Commission on Accreditation of Healthcare Organizations
JRA	Juvenile rheumatoid arthritis
KUB	Kidneys, ureters, bladder (flat/upright abdominal x-ray)
LGA	Large for gestational age
LLL	Left lower (lung) lobe
LLQ	Left lower quadrant
LMP	Last menstrual period

LOC	Loss of consciousness; level of consciousness
LPN	Licensed practical nurse
LTB	Laryngotracheobronchitis
LTE	Life-threatening event
LUL	Left upper (lung) lobe
LUQ	Left upper quadrant
MAP	Mean arterial pressure
MCL	Midclavicular line
MDI	Metered-dose inhaler
Med	Medication
MI	Myocardial infarction
mL	Milliliter
MMR	Measles, mumps, rubella
MOM	Milk of magnesia
Mono	Mononucleosis
MR	Mitral regurgitation/Mental retardation
MRI	Magnetic resonance imaging
MS	Mental status/Mitral stenosis/Multiple sclerosis/Morphine sulfate
NA	Not applicable
NEC	Necrotizing enterocolitis
NG	Nasogastric
NICU	Neonatal intensive care unit
NIDDM	Non–insulin-dependent diabetes mellitus
NL	Normal
NOC	Night (nocturnal)
NPH	Neutral-protamine-Hagedorn (intermediate-acting insulin)
NPO	Nothing by mouth (nil per os)
NS	Normal saline
NSAID	Nonsteroidal anti-inflammatory drug
NSR	Normal sinus rhythm
NST	Nonstress test
NTG	Nitroglycerin
N/V	Nausea, vomiting
NVD	Nausea, vomiting, diarrhea
O$_2$	Oxygen
OB	Obstetrics
OD	Right eye (oculus dexter); Overdose
OFTT	Organic failure to thrive
OOB	Out of bed; out of breath
O&P	Ova and parasites
OR	Operating room
OS	Left eye (oculus sinister)
OT	Occupational therapy
OU	Both eyes (oculo utro)
P	Para/Pulse
p	Post (after)
PA	Posteroanterior/Physician's assistant/Pulmonary artery
PAC	Premature atrial contraction
PAF	Paroxysmal atrial fibrillation
PAo$_2$	Alveolar oxygen pressure
Pao$_2$	Arterial partial pressure of oxygen
PAS	Para-aminosalicylic acid
PAT	Paroxysmal atrial tachycardia
pc	After meals (post cibum)

PCA	Patient-controlled analgesia (pump); Patient care assistant
PCP	Pneumocystis carinii pneumonia/Phencyclidine
PDA	Patent ductus arteriosus
PE	Pulmonary embolus
PEEP	Positive end-expiratory pressure
PERRL(A)	Pupils equally round and reactive to light (and accommodation)
PICU	Pediatric intensive care unit
PID	Pelvic inflammatory disease
PIH	Pregnancy-induced hypertension
PKU	Phenylketonuria
PMI	Point of maximum impulse
PMS	Premenstrual syndrome
PND	Paroxysmal nocturnal dyspnea
PNP	Pediatric nurse practitioner
PO	By mouth (per os)
PPD	Purified protein derivative (TB skin test)
PPHN	Persistent pulmonary hypertension of the newborn
PPO	Preferred provider organization
prn	When necessary (pro re nata)
PSA	Prostate-specific antigen
Pt	Patient
PT	Prothrombin time/Physical therapy
PTA	Prior to admission
PTCA	Percutaneous transluminal coronary angioplasty
PTL	Preterm labor
PTSD	Posttraumatic stress disorder
PTT	Partial thromboplastin time
PUD	Peptic ulcer disease
PVC	Premature ventricular contraction
q	Each, every (quaque)
qd	Each day (quaque die)
qhs	Every night before sleep (quaque hora somni)
qid	Four times a day (quarter in die)
qod	Every other day
R	Respirations
RA	Rheumatoid arthritis/Right atrium
RAD	Reactive airway
RBC	Red blood cell
RDA	Recommended dietary allowances
RDS	Respiratory distress syndrome
RHD	Rheumatic heart disease
RLL	Right lower (lung) lobe
RLQ	Right lower quadrant
RML	Right middle (lung) lobe
R/O	Rule out
ROM	Range of motion/Rupture of membranes
ROP	Retinopathy of prematurity
ROS	Review of systems
RSV	Respiratory syncytial virus
RUL	Right upper (lung) lobe
RUQ	Right upper quadrant
Rx	Prescription/Therapy/Treatment

s	Without (*sine*)	TID	Three times a day (*ter in die*)
S₁	First heart sound	TKO	To keep open
S₂	Second heart sound	TLC	Total lung capacity/Tender loving care
S₃	Third heart sound	TORCH	Toxoplasmosis, other (hepatitis B, syphilis), rubella, cytomegalovirus, herpes simplex 2
S₄	Fourth heart sound		
SAB	Spontaneous abortion		
SBE	Subacute bacterial endocarditis	TPN	Total parenteral nutrition
SC	Subcutaneously	TPR	Temperature, pulse, respirations
SCA	Sickle cell anemia	TSH	Thyroid-stimulating hormone
SGA	Small for gestational age	TSS	Toxic shock syndrome
SIADH	Syndrome of inappropriate antidiuretic hormone	TURP	Transurethral resection of prostate
		TV	Total volume/Tidal volume
SICU	Surgical intensive care unit	Tx	Treatment
SIDS	Sudden infant death syndrome		
SL	Sublingually	UA	Urinalysis
SLE	Systemic lupus erythematosus	UAP	Unlicensed assistive personnel
SOB	Short(ness) of breath	UGI	Upper gastrointestinal
SQ	Subcutaneously	UQ	Upper quadrant
SR	Sinus rhythm	URI	Upper respiratory infection
SROM	Spontaneous rupture of membranes	UTI	Urinary tract infection
S/S	Signs, symptoms	UV	Ultraviolet
Stat	Immediately (*statim*)		
STD	Sexually transmitted disease	VBAC	Vaginal birth after cesarean
SVG	Spontaneous vaginal delivery	VC	Vital capacity
Sx	Symptoms	VF, Vfib	Ventricular fibrillation
		VS	Vital signs
T	Temperature	VSD	Ventricular septal defect
TAB	Therapeutic abortion	VZV	Varicella-zoster virus
TAR	Total all routes (intake)		
T&A	Tonsillectomy and adenoidectomy	WHO	World Health Organization
TB	Tuberculosis	WIC	Women, infants, and children
TEF	Tracheoesophageal fistula	WBC	White blood cell; White blood (cell) count
TENS	Transcutaneous electrical nerve stimulation	WNL	Within normal limits
TIA	Transient ischemic attack	w/o	Without

Many clinical signs have been named for the physicians who first described them, or the phenomena they resemble. Following is a list of *33 of the most common clinical signs* for use as a quick reference as you review.

Babinski reflex   Dorsiflexion of the big toe after stimulation of the lateral sole; associated with *corticospinal tract lesions.*

Barlow test   *Developmental hip dysplasia* is present if femoral head moves in and out of the back of the acetabulum while exerting pressure from the front.

Blumberg's sign   Transient pain in the abdomen after approximated fingers pressed gently into abdominal wall are suddenly withdrawn—rebound tenderness; associated with *peritoneal inflammation.*

Braxton-Hicks contractions   Irregular painless uterine contractions.

Brudzinski's sign   Flexion of the hip and knee induced by flexion of the neck; associated with *meningeal irritation.*

Brushfield's spots   Speckling of iris associated with *Down syndrome.*

Chadwick's sign   Cyanosis of vaginal and cervical mucosa; associated with *pregnancy.*

Cheyne-Stokes respiration   Rhythmic cycles of deep and shallow respiration, often with apneic periods; associated with *central nervous system respiratory center dysfunction.*

Chvostek's sign   Facial muscle spasm induced by tapping on the facial nerve branches; associated with *hypocalcemia.*

Coppernail's sign   Ecchymoses on the perineum, scrotum, or labia; associated with *fracture of the pelvis.*

Cullen's sign   Bluish discoloration of the umbilicus; associated with *acute pancreatitis* or *hemoperitoneum,* especially *rupture of fallopian tube* in ectopic pregnancy.

Doll's-eyes sign   Dissociation between the movements of the head and eyes: as the head is raised the eyes are lowered, and as the head is lowered the eyes are raised; associated with *global-diffuse disorders of the cerebrum.*

Fluid wave   Transmission across the abdomen of a wave induced by snapping the abdomen; associated with *ascites.*

Goldstein's sign   Wide distance between the great toe and the adjoining toe; associated with *cretinism* and *trisomy 21.*

Harlequin sign   In the newborn infant, reddening of the lower half of the laterally recumbent body and blanching of the upper half, due to a *temporary vasomotor disturbance.*

Hegar's sign   Softening of the fundus of the uterus; associated with the *first trimester of pregnancy.*

Homans' sign   Pain behind the knee, induced by dorsiflexion of the foot; associated with peripheral vascular disease, especially *venous thrombosis* in the calf.

Kehr's sign   Severe pain in the left upper quadrant, radiating to the top of the shoulder; associated with *splenic rupture.*

Kernig's sign   Inability to extend leg when sitting or lying with the thigh flexed on the abdomen; associated with *meningeal irritation.*

Knie's sign   Unequal dilation of the pupils; associated with *Graves' disease.*

Kussmaul's respiration   Paroxysmal air hunger; associated with acidosis, especially *diabetic ketoacidosis.*

Lasègue's sign   Straight leg raising with hip flexed and knee extended will elicit sciatic pain associated with *herniated lumbar disk.*

McBurney's sign   Tenderness at McBurney's point (located two-thirds of the distance from the umbilicus to the anterior-superior iliac spine); associated with *appendicitis.*

Murphy's sign Pain on taking a deep breath when pressure is applied over location of the gallbladder; a sign of *gallbladder disease*.

Ortolani's maneuver Manual procedure performed to rule out the possibility of congenital hip dysplasia. A "click" sound sometimes is heard if *hip dysplasia* is present; on assessment, head of femur can be felt (or heard as a click) as it slips forward in the acetabulum and slips back when pressure is released and legs are returned to their original position.

Osler's sign Small painful erythematous swellings in the skin of the hands and feet; associated with bacterial endocarditis.

Psoas sign Pain induced by hyperextension of the right thigh while lying on the left side; associated with *appendicitis*.

Setting-sun sign Downward deviation of the eyes so that each iris appears to "set" beneath the lower lid, with white sclera exposed between it and the upper lid; associated with *increased intracranial pressure* or irritation of the *brainstem;* also seen in *hydrocephalus*.

Simian crease Transverse palmar or plantar crease; associated with *Down syndrome.*

Tinel's sign Tingling sensation felt from light percussion on the radial side of the palmaris longus tendon; associated with *carpal tunnel syndrome.*

Trendelenburg sign When child bears weight on affected hip, pelvis tilts downward on the unaffected side instead of upward, as it should; associated with *developmental hip dysplasia.*

Trousseau's sign Carpopedal spasm develops when BP cuff is inflated above systolic pressure for 3 minutes; associated with *hypocalcemia.*

Williamson's sign Markedly diminished blood pressure in the leg as compared with that in the arm on the same side; associated with *pneumothorax* and *pleural effusions.*

Acid-base—*"RAMS"* (*Respiratory Alternate, Metabolic Same*)

	Respiratory (alternate)		Metabolic (same)	
Acidosis	$\downarrow$pH	$\uparrow$Pco$_2$	$\downarrow$pH	$\downarrow$HCO$_3$
Alkalosis	$\uparrow$pH	$\downarrow$Pco$_2$	$\uparrow$pH	$\uparrow$HCO$_3$

Alcohol withdrawal: clinical features—*"HITS"*[a]

Hallucinations (visual, tactile)

Increased vital signs and insomnia

Tremens → delirium tremens (potentially lethal)

Shakes/Sweats/Seizures/Stomach pains (nausea, vomiting)

Angina: precipitating factors—*"three E's"*

Eating

Emotion

Exertion (Exercise)

Anorexia nervosa: clinical features—*"ANOREXIC"*[a]

Adolescent women/Amenorrhea

NGT alimentation (most severe cases)

Obsession with losing weight/becoming fat though underweight

Refusal to eat ($\geq$5% die)

Electrolyte abnormalities (e.g., $\downarrow$ K$^+$, cardiac arrhythmia)

$\uparrow$eXercise

Intelligence often above average/Induced vomiting

Cathartic use (and diuretic abuse)

Appendicitis: assessment—*"PAINS"*

Pain (RLQ)

Anorexia

Increased temperature, WBC (15,000–20,000)

Nausea

Signs (McBurney's, Psoas)

Arterial occlusion: symptoms—*"six P's"*

Pain

Pale

Pulseless

Paresthesia

Poikilothermic

Paralysis

Blood glucose (*rhyme*)

Symptom	Implication
Cold and **clammy** ...	give hard **candy**.
Hot and **dry** ...	glucose is **high**.

Blood vessels in umbilical cord—*"AVA"*

Artery

Vein

Artery

[a]From Rogers, PT: The Medical Student's Guide to Top Board Scores. Little, Brown, Boston, 1996.

Cancer: focus of patient care—"CANCER"

Chemotherapy

Assess body image disturbance (related to alopecia)

Nutritional needs when N/V present

Comfort from pain

Effective response to Tx? (Evaluate)

Rest (for patient and family)

Car seats for children

Use if under:

6 years old, or

60 pounds

Cholecystitis: risk factors—"five F's"

Female

Fat

Forty

Fertile

Fair

Cleft lip: nursing care plan (postoperative)—"CLEFT LIP"

Crying, minimize

Logan bow

Elbow restraints

Feed with Breck feeder

Tent, croup

Liquid (sterile water), rinse after feeding

Impaired feeding (no sucking)

Position—*never* on abdomen

Cognitive disorders: assessment of difficulties—"JOCAM"

Judgment

Orientation

Confabulation

Affect

Memory

Coma: causes—"A-E-I-O-U TIPS"[b]

Alcohol, acidosis (hyperglycemic coma)

Epilepsy (also electrolyte abnormality, endocrine problem)

Insulin (hypoglycemic shock)

Overdose (or poisoning)

Uremia and other renal problems

Trauma; temperature abnormalities (hypothermia, heat stroke)

Infection (e.g., meningitis)

Psychogenic ("hysterical coma")

Stroke or space-occupying lesions in the cranium

Cushing's syndrome: symptoms—"three S's"

Sugar (hyperglycemia)

Salt (hypernatremia)

Sex (excess androgens)

Diabetes: signs and symptoms—"three P's," "three poly's"

Polydipsia (very thirsty)

Polyphagia (very hungry)

Polyuria (urinary frequency)

Diarrhea: diet—"BRAT"

Banana

Rice (cereal)

Applesauce

Toast/Tea

Diet: low cholesterol—*avoid the three C's:*

Cake

Cookies

Cream (dairy, e.g., milk, ice cream)

Dystocia: etiology—"three P's"

Power

Passageway

Passenger

---

[b]Adapted from Caroline, NL: Emergency Care in the Streets, ed 5. Little, Brown, Boston, 1995.

Dystocia: general aspects (maternal)—*"three P's"*

Psych

Placenta

Position

Eardrops: administering—*UP/DOWN*

pull ear | **A D U L T S** | **P**

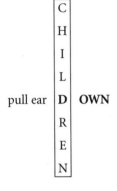

pull ear | **C H I L D R E N** | **OWN**

Episiotomy assessment—*"REEDA"*

Redness

Edema

Ecchymosis

Discharge

Approximation of skin

Eye medications

My**d**riatic = **d**ilated pupils

Mio**t**ic = **t**iny (constricted) pupils

Complication of severe preeclampsia—*"HELLP"* syndrome

Hemolysis

Elevated **L**iver enzymes

Low **P**latelet count

Hypertension: complications—*"four C's"*

CHF (congestive heart failure)

CVA (cardiovascular accident)

CAD (coronary artery disease)

CRF (chronic renal failure)

Hypertension: nursing care plan—*"I TIRED"*

Intake and output (urine)

Take blood pressure

Ischemia attack, transient (watch for TIAs)

Respiration, pulse

Electrolytes

Daily weight

Hypoglycemia: signs and symptoms—*"DIRE"*

Diaphoresis

Increased pulse

Restless

Extra hungry

Infections during pregnancy—*"TORCH"*

Toxoplasmosis

Other (hepatitis B, syphilis)

Rubella

Cytomegalovirus

Herpes simplex virus

IUD: potential problems with use—*"PAINS"*ᶜ

Period (menstrual: late, spotting, bleeding)

Abdominal pain, dyspareunia

Infection (abnormal vaginal discharge)

Not feeling well, fever or chills

String missing

Manipulation: nursing plan—promote the *"three C's"*:

Cooperation

Compromise

Collaboration

Medication administration—*"five rights"*

RIGHT medication

RIGHT dosage

RIGHT route

RIGHT time

RIGHT patient

ᶜFrom Hatcher, RA, et al: Contraceptive Technology. ed 16. Irving, New York, 1994.

Mental retardation: nursing care plan—*"three R's"*

Regularity (provide routine and structure)

Reward (positive reinforcement)

Redundancy (repeat)

Newborn assessment components: *"APGAR"*

Appearance

Pulse

Grimace

Activity

Respiratory effort

Obstetric (maternity) history: *"GTPAL"*

Gravida

Term

Preterm

Abortions (SAB, TAB)

Living children

Oral contraceptives: signs of potential problems—*"ACHES"*

Abdominal pain (possible liver or gallbladder problem)

Chest pain or shortness of breath (possible pulmonary embolus)

Headache (possible hypertension, brain attack)

Eye problems (possible hypertension or vascular accident)

Severe leg pain (possible thromboembolic process)

Pain: assessment—*"PQRST"*

What	Provokes the pain?
What is the	Quality of the pain?
Does the pain	Radiate?
What is the	Severity of the pain?
What is the	Timing of the pain?

Pain: management—*"ABCs"*

Ask about the pain

Believe when patients say they have pain

Choices—let patients know their choices

Deliver what you can, when you said you would

Empower/Enable patients' control over pain

Postoperative complications: order—*"four W's"*

Wind (pulmonary)

Wound

Water (urinary tract infection)

Walk (thrombophlebitis)

Preterm infant: anticipated problems—*"TRIES"*

Temperature regulation (poor)

Resistance to infections (poor)

Immature liver

Elimination problems (necrotizing enterocolitis [NEC])

Sensory-perceptual functions (retinopathy of prematurity [ROP])

Psychotropic medications: common antidepressives (tricyclics)—*"VENT"*

Vivactil

Elavil

Norpramin

Tofranil

Schizophrenia: primary symptoms—*"four A's"*

Associative looseness

Affect

Ambivalence

Autism

Sprain: nursing care plan—*"ICE"*

Immobilize (and rest)

Cool (with ice)

Elevate

Stool assessment—*"ACCT"*

Amount

Color

Consistency

Timing

Tracheoesophageal fistula: assessment—*"three C's"*

Coughing

Choking

Cyanosis

Traction: nursing care plan—*"TRACTION"*

Trapeze bar overhead to raise and lower upper body

Requires free-hanging weights; body alignment

Analgesia for pain, prn

Circulation (check color and pulse)

Temperature (check extremity)

Infection prevention

Output (monitor)

Nutrition (alteration related to immobility)

Transient ischemic attacks: assessment—*"three T's"*

Temporary unilateral visual impairment

Transient paralysis (one-sided)

Tinnitus → vertigo

Trauma care: complications—*"TRAUMA"*

Thromboembolism/Tissue perfusion, altered

Respiration, altered

Anxiety related to pain and prognosis

Urinary elimination, altered

Mobility impaired

Alterations in sensory-perceptual functions and skin integrity (infections)

Wernicke-Korsakoff syndrome (alcohol-associated neurological disorder)—*"COAT RACK"*[d]

Wernicke's encephalopathy (acute phase): clinical features:

Confusion

Ophthalmoplegia

Ataxia

Thiamine is an important aspect of Tx

Korsakoff's psychosis (chronic phase): characteristic findings:

Retrograde amnesia (↓recall of some old memories)

Anterograde amnesia (↓ability to form new memories)

Confabulation

Korsakoff's psychosis

[d]From Rogers, PT: The Medical Student's Guide to Top Board Scores. Little, Brown, Boston, 1996.

APPENDIX O

Directory of State Boards of Nursing

Alabama

Alabama Board of Nursing
PO Box 303900
Montgomery, AL 36130-3900

Alaska

Alaska Board of Nursing
Department of Commerce and
    Economic Development
Division of Occupational Licensing
3601 C Street, Suite 722
Anchorage, AK 99503

American Samoa

American Samoa Health Service
Regulatory Board
LBJ Tropical Medical Center
Pago Pago, AS 96799

Arizona

Arizona State Board of Nursing
1651 E Morten Avenue, Suite 150
Phoenix, AZ 85020

Arkansas

Arkansas State Board of Nursing
University Tower Building, Suite 800
1123 S University
Little Rock, AR 72204

California

California Board of Registered
    Nursing
PO Box 944210
Sacramento, CA 94244-2100

Colorado

Colorado Board of Nursing
1560 Broadway, Suite 670
Denver, CO 80202

Connecticut

Examinations and Licensure Division
    of Medical Quality Assurance
Connecticut State Department of
    Public Health
PO Box 340308
Mail Stop 12 APP
Hartford, CT 06134-0308

Delaware

Delaware Board of Nursing
Margaret O'Neill Building
PO Box 1401
Dover, DE 19903

District of Columbia

District of Columbia Board of Nurs-
    ing
825 North Capital Ave., NE
Washington, DC 20002

Florida

Florida Department of Professional
    Regulation
1940 N Monroe Street
Tallahassee, FL 32399-0750

Georgia

Georgia Board of Nursing
166 Pryor Street, SW
Atlanta, GA 30303

Guam

Guam Board of Nurse Examiners
PO Box 2816
Agana, GU 96910

Hawaii

Hawaii Board of Nursing
PO Box 3469
Honolulu, HI 96801

Idaho

Idaho Board of Nursing
PO Box 83720
Boise, ID 83720-0061

Illinois

Illinois Department of Professional
    Regulation
320 W Washington Street, 3rd Floor
Springfield, IL 62786

Indiana

Indiana State Board of Nursing
Health Professions Bureau
402 W Washington Street
Room 41
Indianapolis, IN 46204

Iowa

Iowa Board of Nursing
State Capitol Complex
1223 E Court Avenue
Des Moines, IA 50319

Kansas

Kansas State Board of Nursing
Landon State Office Building
900 SW Jackson, Suite 551-S
Topeka, KS 66612-1230

Kentucky

Kentucky Board of Nursing
312 Wittington Parkway, Suite 300
Louisville, KY 40222-5172

Louisiana

Louisiana State Board of Nursing
3510 North Causeway Boulevard,
   Suite 501
Metairie, LA 70002

Maine

Maine State Board of Nursing
State House Station 158
Augusta, ME 04333-0158

Maryland

Maryland Board of Nursing
4140 Patterson Avenue
Baltimore, MD 21215-2299

Massachusetts

Massachusetts Board of Registration
   in Nursing
239 Causeway St., Suite 400
Boston, MA 02114-2130

Michigan

Office of Testing Services
Michigan Department of Commerce
PO Box 30018
Lansing, MI 48909

Minnesota

Minnesota Board of Nursing
2829 University Avenue, SE 500
Minneapolis, MN 55114-3253

Mississippi

Mississippi Board of Nursing
1935 Lakeland Dr., Ste. B
Jackson, MS 39216-5014

Missouri

Missouri State Board of Nursing
PO Box 656
Jefferson City, MO 65102

Montana

Montana State Board of Nursing
111 N Jackson
PO Box 200513
Helena, MT 59620-0513

Nebraska

Bureau of Examining Boards
Nebraska Department of Health
PO Box 95007
Lincoln, NE 68509

Nevada

Nevada State Board of Nursing
PO Box 46886
Las Vegas, NV 89114

New Hampshire

New Hampshire Board of Nursing
78 Regional Drive, Building B
PO Box 3898
Concord, NH 03302-3898

New Jersey

New Jersey Board of Nursing
PO Box 45010
Newark, NJ 07101

New Mexico

New Mexico Board of Nursing
4206 Louisiana Boulevard, NE
Suite A
Albuquerque, NM 87109

New York

Division of Professional Licensing
   Services
State Education Department
Cultural Education Center
Albany, NY 12230

North Carolina

North Carolina Board of Nursing
PO Box 2129
Raleigh, NC 27602

North Dakota

North Dakota Board of Nursing
919 S 7th Street, Suite 504
Bismarck, ND 58504-5881

Northern Mariana Islands

Commonwealth Board of Nurse
   Examiners
Public Health Center
PO Box 1458
Saipan, MP 96950

Ohio

Ohio Board of Nursing
77 S High Street, 17th Floor
Columbus, OH 43266-0316

Oklahoma

Oklahoma Board of Nursing
2915 N Classen Boulevard, Suite 524
Oklahoma City, OK 73106

Oregon

Oregon State Board of Nursing
Suite 465
800 NE Oregon Street, Box 25
Portland, OR 97232

Pennsylvania

Pennsylvania State Board of Nursing
PO Box 2649
Harrisburg, PA 17105-2649

Puerto Rico

Commonwealth of Puerto Rico
Board of Nurse Examiners
Call Box 10200
Santurce, PR 00908

Rhode Island

Rhode Island Board of Nurse
   Registration and Nursing Education
Cannon Health Building
Three Capitol Hill, Room 104
Providence, RI 02908-5097

South Carolina

South Carolina State Board of Nursing
220 Executive Center Drive, Suite 220
Columbia, SC 29210

South Dakota

South Dakota Board of Nursing
4300 S Louise Avenue, Ste. C1
Sioux Falls, SD 57106-3124

Tennessee

State of Tennessee Board of Health
425 5th Ave., North
Cordell Hull Bldg.
Nashville, TN 37247

Texas

Texas Board of Nurse Examiners
333 Guadalupe, 3-460
Austin, TX 78701

Utah

Utah State Board of Nursing
Division of Occupational and
    Professional Licensing
PO Box 45805
Salt Lake City, UT 84145-0805

Vermont

Vermont State Board of Nursing
109 State Street
Montpelier, VT 05609-1106

Virgin Islands

Virgin Islands Board of Nurse
    Licensure
PO Box 4247, Veterans Drive Station
St Thomas, US VI 00803

Virginia

Virginia Board of Nursing
6606 W Broad Street, 4th Floor
Richmond, VA 23230-1717

Washington

Washington State Nursing Care
    Quality Assurance Commission
Department of Health
PO Box 47864
Olympia, WA 98504-7864

West Virginia

West Virginia Board of Examiners for
    Registered Professional Nurses
101 Dee Drive
Charleston, WV 25311-1620

Wisconsin

Wisconsin Department of Regulation
    and Licensing
1400 E Washington Avenue
PO Box 8935
Madison, WI 53708-8935

Wyoming

Wyoming State Board of Nursing
2020 Corey Ave.
Cheyenne, WY 82001-3617

Index

A "*t*" following a page number indicates a table.